OBSTETRICS

A Text-Book for the Use of Students and Practitioners

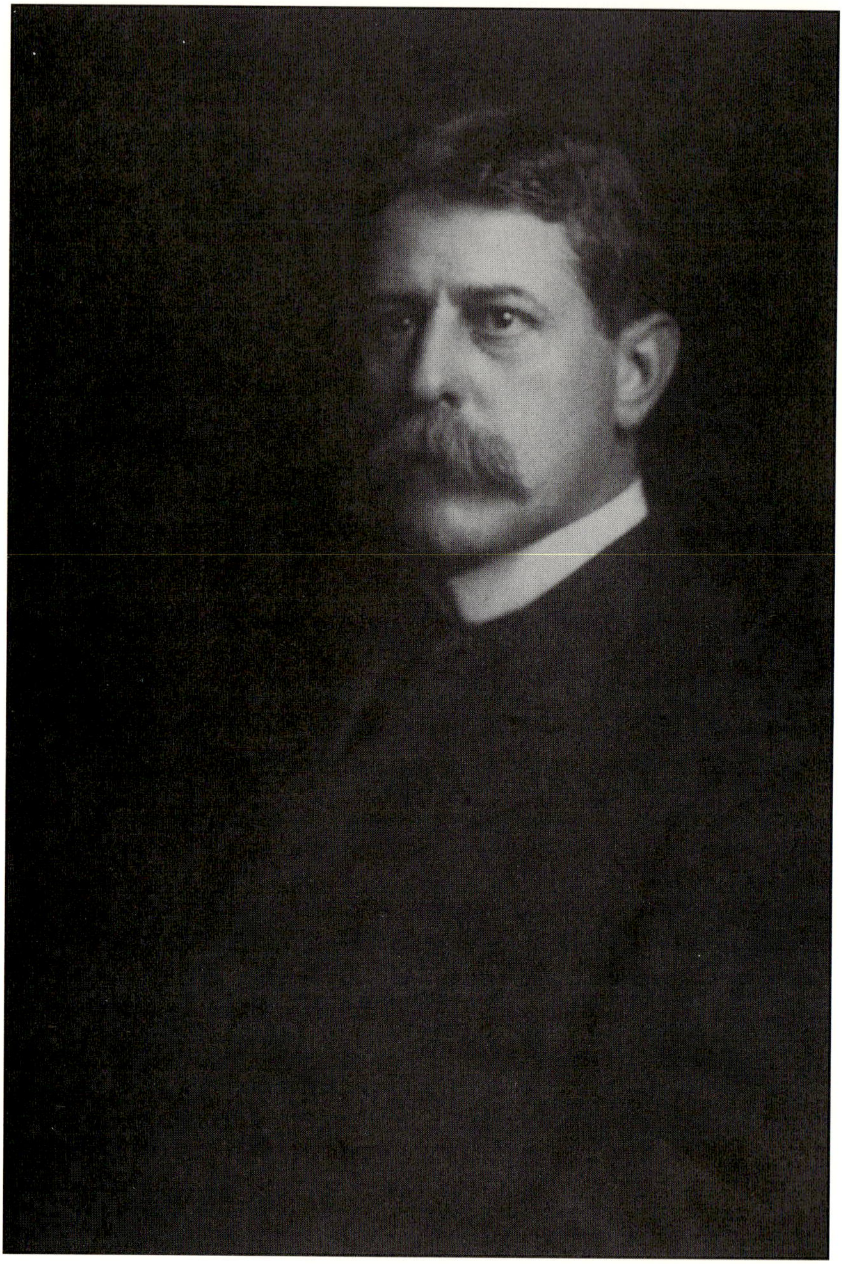

Photograph courtesy of the Alan Mason Chesney Medical Archives of The Johns Hopkins Medical Institutions

J. Whitridge Williams
(1866-1931)

OBSTETRICS

A Text-Book for the Use of Students and Practitioners

By

J. WHITRIDGE WILLIAMS

With an Introduction by

STEVEN L. CLARK, MD
PROFESSOR, DEPARTMENT OF OBSTETRICS AND GYNECOLOGY
UNIVERSITY OF UTAH SCHOOL OF MEDICINE
DIRECTOR,
INTERMOUNTAIN HEALTH CARE PERINATAL CENTERS
LATTER DAY SAINTS HOSPITAL
SALT LAKE CITY, UTAH

GARY D.V. HANKINS, MD
PROFESSOR AND VICE CHAIRMAN,
DEPARTMENT OF OBSTETRICS AND GYNECOLOGY
CHIEF, MATERNAL–FETAL MEDICINE
UNIVERSITY OF TEXAS
MEDICAL BRANCH AT GALVESTON
GALVESTON, TEXAS

APPLETON & LANGE
Stamford, Connecticut

97 98 99 00 01 / 10 9 8 7 6 5 4 3 2 1

Prentice Hall International (UK) Limited, *London*
Prentice Hall of Australia Pty. Limited, *Sydney*
Prentice Hall Canada, Inc., *Toronto*
Prentice Hall Hispanoamericana, S.A., *Mexico*
Prentice Hall of India Private Limited, *New Delhi*
Prentice Hall of Japan, Inc., *Tokyo*
Simon & Schuster Asia Pte. Ltd., *Singapore*
Editora Prentice Hall do Brasil Ltda., *Rio de Janeiro*
Prentice Hall, *Upper Saddle River, New Jersey*

Williams, J. Whitridge (John Whitridge), 1866--1931
Obstetrics : a text-book for the use of students and practitioners / by J. Whitridge Williams. ---Facsimile ed. / introduction by Steven L. Clark, Gary D.V. Hankins.
p. cm.
Originally published: New York : D. Appleton and Co., 1903.
Includes bibliographical references and index.
ISBN 0-8385-7199-9 (alk. paper)
1. Obstetrics. I. Title.
[DNLM: 1. Obstetrics. 2. Pregnancy--physiology. 3. Pregnancy Complications. WQ 100 W7280 1903F]
RG524.W7 1997
618.2--dc20
DNLM/DLC 96-28900
for Library of Congress CIP

ISBN 0-8385-7199-9

Designer: Mary Skudlarek

PRINTED IN THE UNITED STATES OF AMERICA

Collector's Edition

This Edition of *Obstetrics: A Text-Book for Students and Practitioners* is limited to two thousand five hundred numbered copies, of which this is

No. 81

INTRODUCTION

Throughout our professional lifetimes, and we suspect those of most readers as well, *Williams Obstetrics* has been the standard against which all other textbooks of obstetric practice are judged. Even today, with the recent proliferation of fine works dealing with clinical obstetrics, *Williams* remains dominant; while some may justifiably differ in their approaches to specific obstetric dilemmas, few, if any, would criticize an obstetrician who follows this text to the letter. There is still no phrase that will silence criticism at a weekly morbidity and mortality conference like "that's what they recommend in *Williams.*" End of conversation. Action justified.

It is thus with a sense of awe and a good deal of trepidation that we undertake to comment upon the first edition of this classic text. The reader of this edition will be fascinated by the account of the way things were in the beginning, and better appreciate the historical continuity which, even today, gives this text unique strength. We found ourselves both proud of the contributions our specialty has made to the care of women and their unborn infants in the past century and at the same time discouraged by our lack of progress in a number of fundamental areas. We sense that the reader will share our emotions.

Obstetrics: A Text-Book for the Use of Students and Practitioners, first published in 1903, represents the very beginning of the scientific approach to clinical obstetrics. While a rare study is cited as evidence for a specific practice pattern, a more common treatment of clinical controversy involves statements such as "it is my practice (for delivery) to render the patient completely unconscious" (using chloroform or cocaine), backed up, where necessary by affirmations that authorities such as "Eppinger, Nagel, Gebhard, Pretti and Waldeyer" agree with a certain course of action. Unfortunately this tendency to emphasize anecdotal experience over outcome-based research has not yet disappeared from obstetric writings.

For the student of medical history, this first edition of *Williams Obstetrics* is a special delight, for it is obvious that, even in his day, J. Whitridge Williams was also a student of past obstetrical practices and practitioners. We share his amusement with a quote from the 17th century writer Viardel, who explained the invariable diammniotic nature of unlike sex twins as the doing of Providence which "took this means of guarding their morals in-utero." It is further fascinating to read Williams' extensive history of forceps, as well as his then current recommendations for the contents of an "obstetrical valise."

Thinking of practicing backwoods medicine? This first edition details everything you need for a home birth, from the correct number of basins (five: four for the use of the physician and one for the patient) to the proper amount of oxalic and boric acid. Following delivery, Dr. Williams recommended that the puerperal woman not be allowed to sit up until the tenth day, or occasionally a day or so earlier. He cited a new idea recently proposed before the German Gynecologic Congress in 1899 that the patient be allowed to get up on the third or fourth day (the speaker obviously worked for an early HMO), but noted that "no one who spoke upon the subject endorsed these views."

Readers of this first edition will also become familiar with unfamiliar terms (Naegle's obliquity) and long-lost conditions (lactational insanity) which will enrich their historical perspective, and, more importantly, give them new tools with which to torment residents on rounds.

In Dr. Williams' era, basic science was synonymous with anatomic, as opposed to physiologic, description; almost 15 percent of the text is devoted to normal and abnormal anatomy of the bony pelvis. The histologic and embryologic descriptions of the female reproductive tract are virtually identical to those provided in the 20th edition of *Williams.* On the other hand, in what for the modern reader is an almost poignant passage, Dr. Williams struggles for several pages with the problem of relating menstruation to ovulation with no knowledge of the existence of reproductive hormones, and concludes that "the entire process is under some central control, and that both are dependent upon some general and as yet unknown cause." We feel similarly sympathetic to his concern regarding the mystique of "multiparous women who have repeatedly given birth to very large dead children." How many of our most profound mysteries will, in the next 100 years, be explainable by a simple but as yet undiscovered hormone, microorganism, or DNA sequence?

Despite this understandable lack of data, Dr. Williams was as undaunted as many of us today by the prospect of making definitive statements on a wide variety of subjects. Some of his conclusions were scientifically incorrect; "it now appears fairly certain that the kidneys normally play little, if any part in the production of the liquor amnii" or "conception usually occurs either soon after the last appearance of the menses, or shortly before the first period which is missed. In rare instances it takes place in the middle of the intermenstrual period. These views have been confirmed . . . ."

At other times, this early scientist made some distinctly bad calls; when describing the preferred treatment for placenta previa (the forcible dilation of the cervix, followed by internal version and breech extraction), he concluded "as the results obtained by the methods of treatment outlined above are quite satisfactory so far as the mother is concerned, it seems doubtful whether Caesarean section will come into very general use."

On the other hand, some of Dr. Williams' observations were amazingly prescient; the modern obstetrician would do well to heed his five rules of asepsis, designed to avoid puerperal infection, as well as his observation that he sees "no advantage in the procedure (of routine episiotomy)." Further, his list of bacteriologic causes of puerperal infection is little different than that provided by present-day data. Tired obstetricians can also sympathize with his stern admonition that except for emergencies, in managing the laboring woman, the obstetrician "should direct the nurse not to send for him if the labor commences at night, between 11 PM and 7 AM."

As you read the text, we encourage you to ask yourself, "what would it be like to practice under these conditions?" Principles of antisepsis were rudimentary—the use of gloves for pelvic examination appears not to have been universally accepted. Imagine an obstetric world without effective birth control, ultrasound, antibiotics, or blood transfusions. Dr. Williams' world had no pregnancy tests, in fact had virtually no laboratory tests at all. Consider the practice of obstetrics when cesarean section was an operation of last resort with a mortality of 10 percent (deemed by Dr. Williams to represent "excellent results.") In an era where most newborn intensive-care units consistently produce intact neonatal survival beyond 26 weeks gestation, can we comprehend practice in a time when "premature children weighing less than 1500 grammes have practically no chance of life?"

Given these limitations, we can perhaps understand some of the treatments proposed by Dr. Williams. For preeclampsia, recommended treatment included a diet of milk only, chloroform, diuresis, Epsom salts, enemas, and in recalcitrant cases, phlebotomy, performed to remove as much of the poison as possible. For postpartum endometritis (puerperal sepsis), curettage, and "a douche of several liters of boiled water" were the treatments of choice. We may marvel at the resilience of young women that with this treatment alone, Dr. Williams lost only 2 of 52 patients with bacteriologically confirmed streptococcal endometritis! Nevertheless, he reports that "in 1873, 20% of all women dying in Chicago between the ages of 20–50 succumbed to puerperal sepsis." For postpartum hemorrhagic shock, treatment included strychnine, hypodermic whisky, and enemas of black coffee and salt solution.

It is clear from a reading of this first edition that three basic paradigms pervaded the thinking of the 19th century obstetrician, and were the foundation of much of the clinical practice of that time. (1) An overriding and almost all-consuming fear of puerperal infection—this theme recurs throughout the text.

(2) An understandable reluctance to perform cesarean section except as a last ditch effort to avoid **maternal** (but virtually never **fetal)** mortality. (3) A clear distinction between "term" and "premature" infants, with neonatal mortality rising exponentially prior to full term.

Several fascinating examples illustrate this thinking. Dr. Williams' fear of cesarean section and its resultant complications was so great that in cases of persistent mentum posterior or transverse lie after failed version, "decapitation becomes the procedure of choice, even if the child is alive." Further, in those rare cases when cesarean section is to be performed, "when there is any possibility of infection, complete or at least supravaginal hysterectomy should be done." To achieve a maternal mortality of 10 percent, most cesarean sections appear to have been performed following a pre-labor diagnosis of pelvic contraction, the operation being "contraindicated when the patient has been subjected to repeated vaginal examinations during labor . . . even though no signs of infection are apparent at the time."

No description of turn-of-the-century obstetrics would be complete without a discussion of a procedure which for the modern obstetrician, is nothing short of horrifying: **accouchement forcé.** This procedure involved placing two fingers in the cervix at dilatation of about 3 cm or greater, and forcible manual dilatation, followed by either forceps delivery, or internal version and extraction. There is a nice diagram of the procedure on page 348. If the cervix was insufficiently dilated to permit the introduction of two fingers, a Reynolds cervical dilator was available. "In this way," Dr. Williams assures the reader "complete dilatation can be readily and harmlessly accomplished in a surprisingly short space of time, often within eight or ten minutes." This was the treatment of choice for placenta previa, eclampsia, and a variety of other conditions where expeditious termination of the pregnancy was required. Despite his assurances regarding the safety of this procedure, he also observed that 21 percent of cases of uterine rupture followed vaginal operative procedures of various types.

If this is our origin as a specialty, we may next ask, "How far have we come?" A careful reading of *Obstetrics: A Text-Book for the Use of Students and Practitioners* suggests the following to be the most important advances of the past century, probably in this order:

1. A refinement of the principles of asepsis and aseptic technique.
2. The availability of safely administered regional and general anesthesia.
3. The introduction of effective antibiotics for the treatment of postpartum endometritis.
4. The development of safe blood-banking techniques.
5. The clinical synthesis of the above developments which allowed the performance of safe cesarean section.
6. Earlier recognition and effective intrapartum management of preeclampsia, and the resultant reduction in eclampsia, a condition occurring in Dr. Williams' day in 1/60 to 1/500 labors, with a mortality of 20–25 percent.
7. The invention and widespread availability of real-time sonography.
8. The transition from anecdotal to evidence-based practice.

The modern reader also will wonder at statements such as (in describing sterilization at the time of cesarean section) "If the patient is intelligent, the decision should be left to her or her family; whereas with the ignorant it is incumbent upon the physician to do what he thinks is best under the circumstances," and, concerning the application of forceps, "It is usually not advisable to consult the patient upon the subject, as she is not in a condition to make an intelligent decision." Clearly, Dr. Williams' idea of informed consent differed from ours today.

Yet while we, as a specialty, have come far, we have even further to go. Dr. Williams observed "From time immemorial inquiring minds have sought an explanation for the fact that labour usually ensues about two hundred and eighty days after the appearance of the last menstrual period, but thus far no satisfactory universal cause has been discovered." It is discouraging to realize that we have little better explanation for the onset of labor today, and that we are no closer to effective preterm birth prevention than was Dr. Williams. We are little better at preventing preeclampsia than he was, do not know the cause of most stillbirths, and can do very little for the woman with recurrent pregnancy loss. Dr. Williams' recommended cocktail for threatened abortion (codeine sulphate, extract of hyoscyamine, and viburni prunifolii with a dash of oil of theobromine) is as effective as anything either of these writers can come up with today. The prevalence of cerebral palsy remains unchanged, and we are little better than was Dr. Williams in relieving the misery of hyperemesis gravidarum.

The speciality of obstetrics is sometimes belittled due to the observation that most of our patients would do just as well without us. While this observation is correct, the understanding of the historical context of modern obstetrics provided by this first edition brings sharply into focus the converse: those patients who do need our help need it badly, and the difference we make in these cases is profound. The first edition reminds us of an oft-forgotten fact, that the natural consequences of obstructed labor, placenta previa and abruption, and many cases of malpresentation is death of the fetus and mother. How many other specialists can truthfully claim that their intervention directly saves the lives of 10 percent of their patients, and saves two lives at that, with a combined future life expectancy of over 100 years? Think of that the next time you perform a cesarean section or arrest a dilatation at 2:00 AM—it will ease the fatigue.

Although we can take pride in the dramatic advances that characterize obstetrics in the past 100 years, an objective analysis reveals a darker side as well. Most of the dramatic advances in obstetric practice since the publication of the first edition have been made by non-obstetric specialists and then adapted into our specialty. In terms of clinical medicine, we have taken more from our colleagues in other specialties than we have given back. It is possible that the field of perinatal genetics will offer us, as a specialty, the greatest opportunity to make important, original contributions to medicine.

Further, an entire generation of the best minds in our specialty wasted a great deal of time and money in the study of subtle changes in the fetal heart rate during labor, findings of immense intellectual interest which have proven to have little, if any, clinical values in the prevention of childhood neurologic impairment. This was the era of well-funded government research, now gone forever, when pediatricians were developing a cure for childhood leukemia and infectious disease specialists eliminated smallpox from the earth. Let us hope that similar mistakes can be avoided in the future by a more diligent pursuit of the scientific practice of obstetrics and insistence upon outcome-based research as a foundation for clinical practice.

Perhaps most importantly, a study of the first edition suggests to these reviewers the need for a critical reanalysis of the paradigms that have heretofore governed obstetric practice. Too often, cesarean section is seen as a failure, something to avoid at all costs, when in reality, a scheduled cesarean section with epidural anesthesia today carries a lower maternal mortality risk than unselected vaginal delivery. Too often we fight "prematurity" with therapies that place mother and fetus at risk, at gestational ages where intact neonatal survival is today identical to full term. And we still fall prey to the tendency demonstrated so well in this first edition, to rely in our practice upon anecdotal experience, rather than evidence-based science.

We encourage all practitioners of obstetrics to read this first edition; truly a study of our origins lights the path for our future.

STEVEN L. CLARK, MD
GARY D.V. HANKINS, MD

A Note from the Publisher

This facsimile reproduces in its entirety *Obstetrics: A Text-Book for the Use of Students and Practitioners*, the first edition of the text now known as *Williams Obstetrics.* The eight color plates have been faithfully reproduced and tipped in so that their position matches that of the 1903 edition.

Six editions of this text were written by J. Whitridge Williams:

Obstetrics: A Text-Book for the Use of Students and Practitioners. With Eight Coloured Plates and Six Hundred and Thirty Illustrations in the Text. New York and London. D. Appleton and Company, 1903.

Obstetrics: A Text-Book for the Use of Students and Practitioners. Second Enlarged and Revised Edition. With Sixteen Plates and Six Hundred and Sixty-Six Illustrations in the Text. New York and London. D. Appleton and Company, 1908.

Obstetrics: A Text-Book for the Use of Students and Practitioners. Third Enlarged and Revised Edition. With Sixteen Plates and Six Hundred and Sixty-Eight Illustrations in the Text. New York and London. D. Appleton and Company, 1912.

Obstetrics: A Text-Book for the Use of Students and Practitioners. Fourth Enlarged and Revised Edition. With Seventeen Plates and Six Hundred and Eighty-Five Illustrations in the Text. New York and London. D. Appleton and Company, 1917.

Obstetrics: A Text-Book for the Use of Students and Practitioners. Fifth Enlarged and Revised Edition. With Seventeen Plates and Six Hundred and Ninety Illustrations in the Text. New York and London. D. Appleton and Company, 1923.

Obstetrics: A Textbook for the Use of Students and Practitioners. Sixth Enlarged and Revised Edition. With Seventeen Plates and Seven Hundred and Thirty Illustrations in the Text. New York and London. D. Appleton-Century Company Incorporated, 1930.

OBSTETRICS

A Text-Book for the Use of Students and Practitioners

PLATE I.

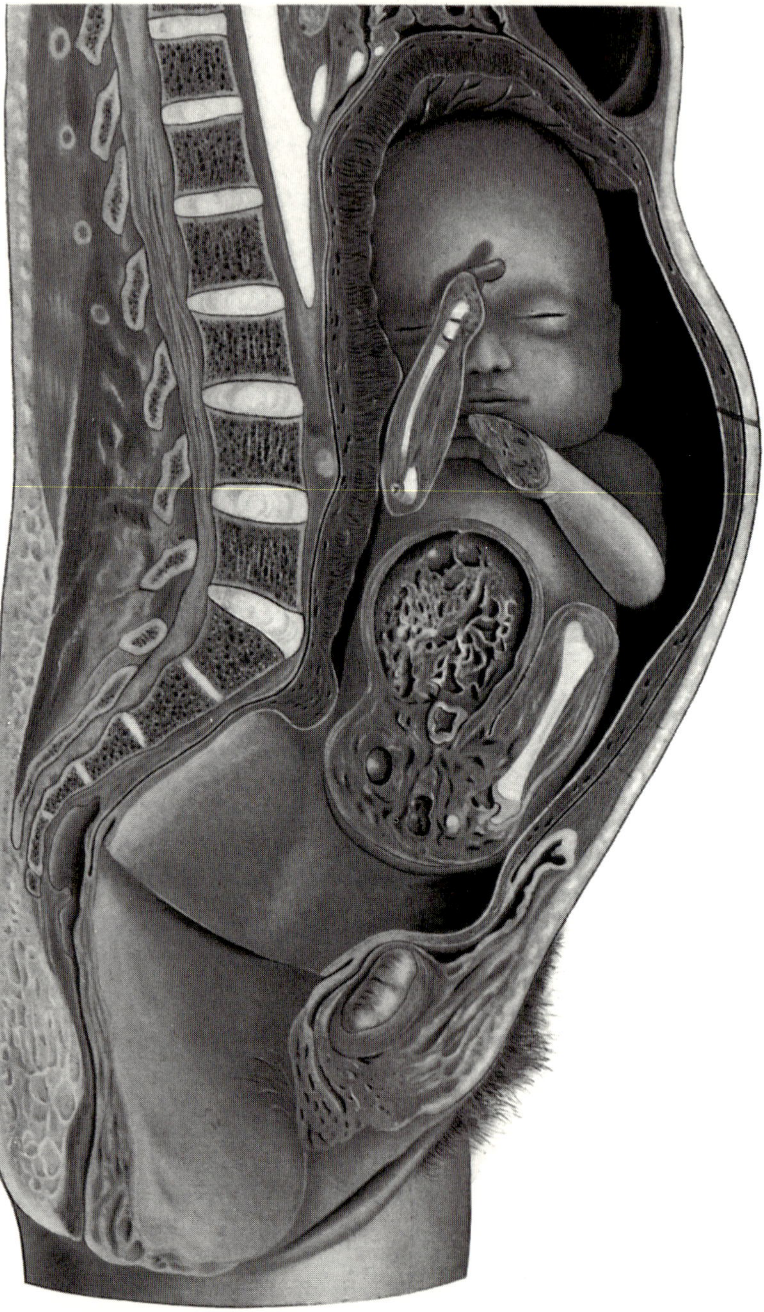

VERTICAL MESIAL SECTION THROUGH BODY OF WOMAN DYING IN LABOUR, WITH UNRUPTURED MEMBRANES PROTRUDING FROM VULVA.

OBSTETRICS

A TEXT-BOOK FOR THE USE OF STUDENTS AND PRACTITIONERS

BY

J. WHITRIDGE WILLIAMS

PROFESSOR OF OBSTETRICS, JOHNS HOPKINS UNIVERSITY; OBSTETRICIAN-IN-CHIEF TO THE JOHNS HOPKINS HOSPITAL; GYNÆCOLOGIST TO THE UNION PROTESTANT INFIRMARY, BALTIMORE, MD.

WITH EIGHT COLOURED PLATES AND
SIX HUNDRED AND THIRTY ILLUSTRATIONS IN THE TEXT

NEW YORK AND LONDON
D. APPLETON AND COMPANY
1903

Published February, 1903

Printed at The Appleton Press

TO

WILLIAM H. WELCH,

PROFESSOR OF PATHOLOGY,
JOHNS HOPKINS UNIVERSITY,

AND

WILLIAM T. COUNCILMAN,

PROFESSOR OF PATHOLOGY,
HARVARD UNIVERSITY,

AS A SLIGHT EXPRESSION OF
RESPECT AND AFFECTION.

PREFACE

In the following pages I have attempted to set forth, as briefly as seemed to be consistent with thoroughness, the scientific basis for and the practical application of the obstetrical art.

Especial attention has been devoted to the normal and pathological anatomy of the generative tract, in the hope that the book may prove serviceable as a laboratory guide for students. At the same time I have endeavoured to present the more practical aspects of obstetrics in such a manner as to be of direct service to the obstetrician at the bedside.

No pains have been spared in illustrating the work, although mere artistic effect has necessarily often been sacrificed to accuracy and practical teaching qualities. With the exception of those relating to pure embryology, all illustrations representing microscopical sections have been drawn from my own specimens under my direct personal supervision, and are accurate reproductions of the originals. The drawings and diagrams illustrating labour and its mechanism for the most part represent the woman on her back, thus affording a closer correspondence with the actual conditions encountered in practice. The representations of the various operative procedures have been redrawn from photographs taken from life.

Although no attempt has been made to present a complete bibliography, I have endeavoured to give at the end of each chapter such references to the early history as well as to the most recent advances in each subject, as to enable the student to refer readily to the most important original sources. In order to insure accuracy, the individual articles have been consulted in every case.

In conclusion, I desire to express my appreciation of the excellent work of Miss Katherine M. Montague and Mr. F. S. Lockwood in the preparation of the illustrations, and to thank my various assistants and my stenographer for most valuable aid. I am under very many obligations to my friend, Dr. Frank R. Smith, for the revision of the text and for many suggestions which have added materially to its clearness.

Baltimore.

CONTENTS

SECTION I

ANATOMY

SECTION II

PHYSIOLOGY AND DEVELOPMENT OF OVUM

SECTION III

PHYSIOLOGY OF PREGNANCY

SECTION IV

PHYSIOLOGY OF LABOUR

SECTION V

OBSTETRIC SURGERY

SECTION VI

PATHOLOGY OF PREGNANCY

SECTION VII

PATHOLOGY OF LABOUR

SECTION VIII

PATHOLOGY OF THE PUERPERIUM

LIST OF PLATES

LIST OF TEXT ILLUSTRATIONS

SECTION I.—ANATOMY

Section II.—Physiology and Development of Ovum

Section III.—Physiology of Pregnancy

Section IV.—Physiology of Labour

Section V.—Obstetric Surgery

Section VI.—Pathology of Pregnancy

Section VII.—Pathology of Labour

Section VIII.—Pathology of the Puerperium

OBSTETRICS

ANATOMY

CHAPTER I

THE PELVIS

Historical.—As the mechanism of labour is essentially a process of accommodation between the fœtus and the passage through which it must pass, it is apparent that obstetrics lacked a scientific foundation until the anatomy of the bony pelvis and of the soft parts connected with it was clearly understood.

We are indebted to Andreas Vesalius (1543) for the first accurate description of the pelvis. Prior to the publication of his observations it had generally been believed that the birth of the child could not be effected until the pelvic cavity had become increased in size by the separation and gaping of the pelvic bones. Vesalius demonstrated the fallacy of this conception, and showed that the pelvis, for practical purposes, should be considered as an unyielding bony ring. His work was still further elaborated by his successor at the University of Padua, Realdus Columbus, who also demonstrated that each innominate bone was originally composed of three separate portions: the ilium, ischium, and pubis, which fused together just before the age of puberty. Julius Cæsar Arantius, Professor of Anatomy in Bologna (1559), also made important contributions to the subject, and was the first to recognise the existence of contracted pelves.

That the teachings of these three great anatomists did not exert so great an influence as might have been expected, was largely due to the fact that no less an authority than Ambroise Paré still continued to adhere to the doctrine of the separation of the pubic bones during labour, and promulgated it in his obstetrical writings.

Among obstetricians, Heinrich Deventer was the first to make a thorough study of the anatomy of the pelvis. In his New Light for Midwives (1701) he dwelt upon it in detail, and also described the main varieties of contracted pelves. At that time, he felt called upon to apologize for taking up what was apparently so useless a consideration.

Smellie was the first English authority to devote particular attention to the subject. In his work on midwifery, published in 1752, he gave a most accurate description of the pelvis and its various measurements, and also introduced the method of determining the antero-posterior diameter which we still employ. A few years previously (1735), Johann Huwé had gone over somewhat the same ground, but his work had not received anything like the consideration which was accorded to Smellie's investigations.

Almost simultaneously with Smellie, Levret, the great French obstetrician, published the results of his observations, and was one of the first to promulgate the conception of the axis and the planes of the pelvis. The value of his work, however, was considerably impaired by many inaccuracies. Among the Germans, Stein the younger was apparently the first to give a thoroughly accurate description of the pelvis, and since his time correct ideas upon the subject have gradually become popularized. Practically, therefore, an attempt to follow the further development of our knowledge concerning the pelvis would resolve itself into writing a history of obstetrics. To do this would go far beyond the scope of the present work; and let it here suffice to say that among the more modern authors Naegele, Luschka, Michealis, and Litzmann in Germany, and Hodge in this country, deserve particular mention.

General Considerations.—In both sexes the pelvis forms the bony ring through which the body weight is transmitted to the lower extremities, but

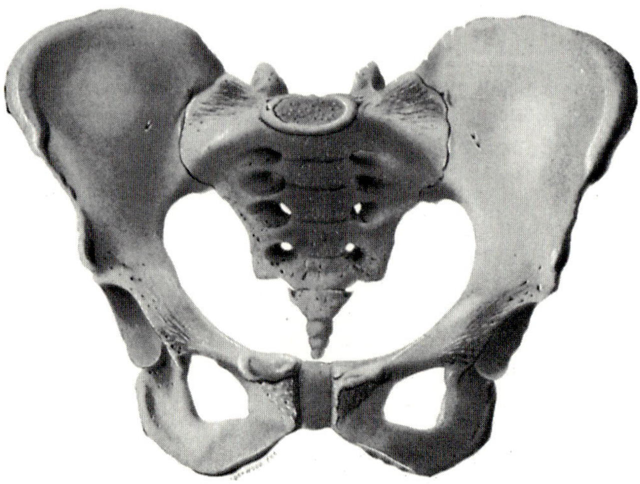

FIG. 1.—NORMAL FEMALE PELVIS. × ⅓.

in the female it assumes a peculiar form which adapts it to the purposes of childbearing.

It is composed of four bones: the sacrum, the coccyx, and two innominate bones, the last two being united at the sacro-iliac synchondroses and the symphysis pubis by strong articulations. The purely anatomical characteristics of the pelvis are dealt with at length in the standard works on anatomy, and more especially in the recent text-book of Joessel and Waldeyer, so that we shall limit our considerations to the peculiarities of the female pelvis, which are of importance in childbearing.

The Pelvis from an Obstetrical Point of View.—The linea terminalis forms the boundary between the false and the true pelvis, the former lying above and the latter below it. The *false pelvis* is bounded posteriorly by the lumbar vertebræ and laterally by the iliac fossæ, while in front the boundary is formed by the lower portion of the anterior abdominal wall. It possesses no particular obstetrical significance, but serves to support the intestines in the non-pregnant woman, and the enlarged uterus in the pregnant condition. It varies considerably in size in different individuals, according to the flare of the iliac bones; but ordinarily in dried specimens the distances between the anterior superior spines of the ilium and between the most widely distant portions of the iliac crests measure 23 and 26 centimetres respectively.

The *true pelvis* lies beneath the linea terminalis, and is the portion concerned in childbearing. It is bounded above by the promontory and alæ of the sacrum, the linea terminalis, and the upper margins of the pubic bones, and below by the pelvic outlet. Its cavity, roughly speaking, may be compared to an obliquely truncated cylinder with its greatest height posteriorly, since its anterior wall at the symphysis pubis measures 4½ to 5 centimetres, and its posterior wall 10 centimetres. With the woman in the upright position, in its upper portion the pelvic canal is directed downward and backward, while in its lower course it curves and becomes directed downward and forward.

The walls of the true pelvis are partly bony and partly ligamentous. Its posterior boundary is furnished by the anterior surface of the sacrum, its lateral limits are formed posteriorly by the sacro-sciatic notches and ligaments, and anteriorly by the inner surface of the ischial bones; while in front it is bounded by the obturator foramina, the pubic bones, and the ascending rami of the ischial bones.

The only part of the lateral wall of the pelvis which is entirely bony is made up of part of the ischium, the inner surface of which, with the woman in the upright position, forms an inclined plane which is directed from above downward and inward, and from behind forward. Considerable importance was attached to these surfaces by Hodge, who designated them as the inclined planes of the pelvis, and considered that they exercised a good deal of influence in causing internal rotation of the head during labour. This view, however, has since been abandoned. If the planes of the ischial bones were extended downward they would meet somewhere about the region of the knee. Extending from the middle of the posterior margin of each ischium are the ischial spines, which are of no little obstetrical importance, inasmuch as a line drawn between them represents the shortest diameter of the pelvic cavity. Moreover, since they can be readily felt on vaginal examination, they can be made to serve as valuable landmarks in determining the extent to which the presenting part has descended into the pelvis.

The sacrum forms the posterior wall of the pelvic cavity. Its upper anterior portion, corresponding to the body of the first sacral vertebra, and designated as the promontory, can be felt on vaginal examination, and offers a landmark which serves as the basis of internal pelvimetry. Normally, the sacrum presents a marked vertical and a less pronounced lateral concavity, which, in abnormal pelves, may undergo variations. A straight line drawn from the promontory to the tip of the sacrum usually measures 10 centimetres, whereas if the concavity be followed the distance averages 12 centimetres. The sacrum was formerly regarded as the "keystone" of the pelvic arch, but Matthews Duncan showed that this conception was erroneous, and that it represents an inverted keystone, inasmuch as it is wider along its anterior than along its posterior surface, so that it would tend to slip downward and forward into the pelvic cavity under the influence of the body weight were it not held in position by the strong posterior ilio-sacral ligaments (Fig. 2).

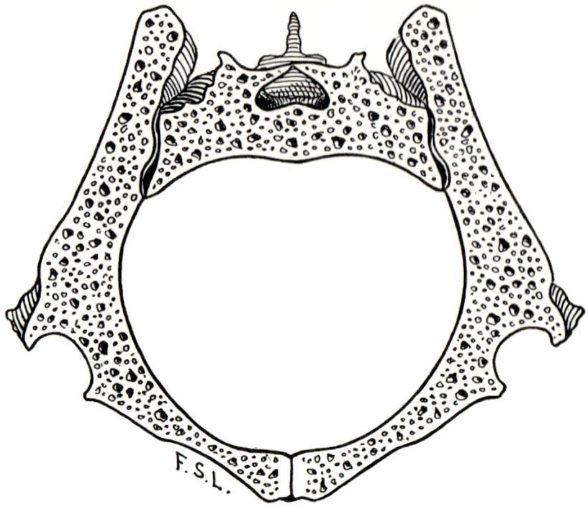

Fig. 2.—Drawing showing that the Sacrum is not the Keystone of the Arch.
Modified from Duncan. × ⅓.

In the female the pubic arch presents a characteristic appearance. The descending rami of the pubis unite at an angle of 90 to 100 degrees, and form a rounded opening through which the head can readily pass. Its margins are more delicate than in the male, and are considerably everted.

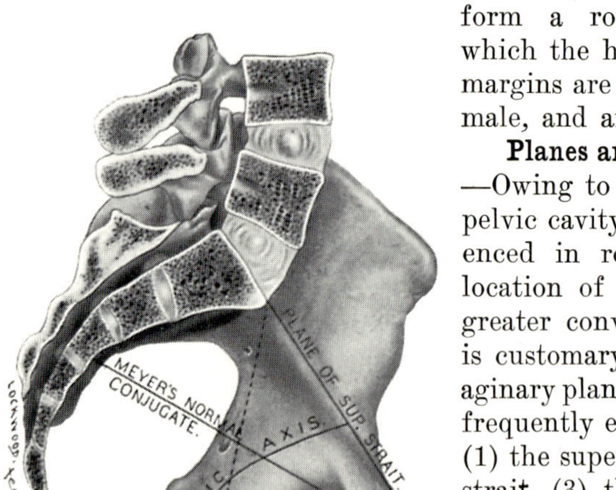

Fig. 3.—Sagittal Section through Normal Pelvis. × ⅓.

Planes and Diameters of the Pelvis.—Owing to the peculiar shape of the pelvic cavity and the difficulty experienced in rendering clear the exact location of a body occupying it, for greater convenience in description it is customary to construct certain imaginary planes through it. Those most frequently employed are designated as (1) the superior strait, (2) the inferior strait, (3) the plane of greatest, and (4) the plane of least, pelvic dimensions (Figs. 3 and 5).

The superior strait represents the upper boundary of the cavity, and is frequently spoken of as the pelvic inlet. It is somewhat oval in shape, with a depression on its posterior border corresponding to the promontory of the sacrum, and is occasionally described as blunt heart-shaped. It is bounded posteriorly by the promontory and alæ of the sacrum; laterally by the linea terminalis; anteriorly by the horizontal rami of the pubic bones and the symphysis pubis. Strictly speaking, it is not a mathematical plane, since its lateral margins, as represented by the linea terminalis, are at a lower level than its central portion between the promontory and symphysis pubis.

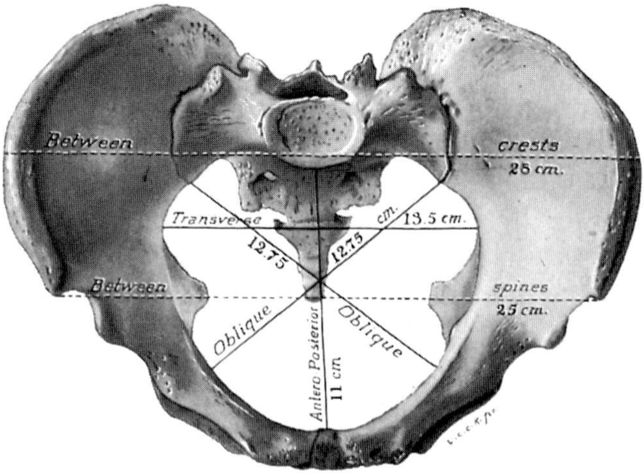

FIG. 4.—NORMAL FEMALE PELVIS SHOWING DIAMETERS OF THE SUPERIOR STRAIT. × ⅓.

Four diameters are usually described as traversing the superior strait: the antero-posterior, the transverse, and two oblique diameters. The antero-posterior diameter extends from the middle of the promontory of the sacrum to the upper margin of the symphysis pubis, and is designated as the *conjugata vera* or *true conjugate*. This term was first employed by Roederer, who likened the superior strait to an ellipse, whose shorter diameter ran antero-posteriorly. Normally, the conjugata vera measures 11 centimetres, but it may become markedly shortened in abnormal pelves. From a practical point of view it is the most important diameter, inasmuch as it is the point of departure for all attempts to estimate the size of the pelvis in actual practice. The transverse diameter is constructed at right angles to the conjugata vera, and represents the greatest distance between the linea terminalis on either side; it usually intersects the conjugata vera at a point a short distance in front of the promontory. Normally it measures 13.5 centimetres. Each of the oblique diameters extends from one of the sacro-iliac synchondroses to the ilio-pectineal eminence on the opposite side of the pelvis. They measure 12.75 centimetres, and are designated as right and left respectively, according as the starting-point is the right or left sacro-iliac synchondrosis. Instead of employing the terms right and left, the Germans usually speak of the first and second oblique diameters. The sacro-cotyloid diameters are sometimes described; they extend from the middle of the promontory of the sacrum to the ilio-pectineal eminence on either side, and measure from 8.75 to 9 centimetres.

Normally these two diameters are of equal length, but in certain forms of contracted pelves they may present marked variations.

The antero-posterior diameter of the superior strait is frequently described as the *anatomical conjugate* or the *conjugata vera.* This does not represent the shortest distance between the promontory of the sacrum and symphysis pubis, which is along a line drawn from the former to a point on the inner surface of the symphysis a few millimetres below its upper margin. The latter is the shortest diameter through which the head must pass in descending into the superior strait, and was designated by Michealis as the *obstetrical conjugate.* It is a few millimetres shorter than the anatomical or true conjugate, but for practical purposes the distinction is rarely made, and the obstetrician simply speaks of the conjugata vera.

Unfortunately, in the living woman, the conjugata vera cannot be measured directly with the examining finger, and various more or less complicated instruments have been devised for its determination, only a few of

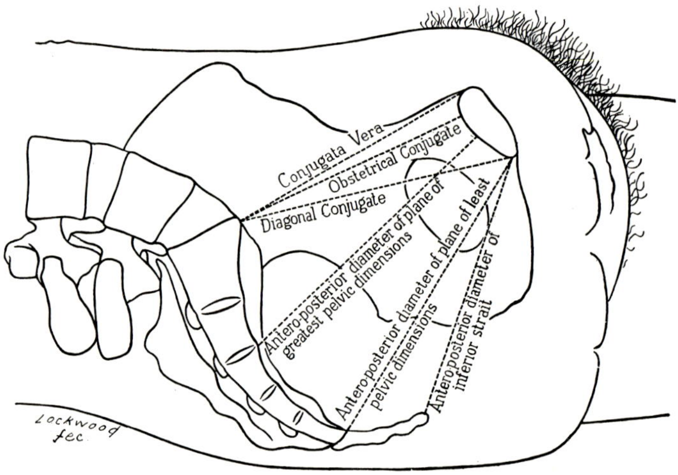

Fig. 5.—Diagram showing Pelvic Planes. × ⅓.

which give satisfactory results. For clinical purposes, therefore, we are content to estimate its length indirectly, by measuring the distance from the lower margin of the symphysis to the promontory of the sacrum, and subtracting from the result 1.5 to 2 centimetres, according to the height and inclination of the symphysis pubis. This diameter is the *conjugata diagonalis* or *oblique conjugate,* the importance of which was first emphasized by Smellie.

The outlet of the pelvis is designated the inferior strait. It is not a plane in a mathematical sense, but consists of two triangular planes whose bases would meet on a line drawn between the two ischial tuberosities. It is bounded posteriorly by the tip of the coccyx, laterally by the greater sacro-sciatic ligaments and the ischial tuberosities, and anteriorly by the lower margin of the pubic arch (Fig. 6). For the pelvic outlet two diameters are described: the antero-posterior and the transverse. The former extends from the lower margin of the symphysis pubis to the tip of the coccyx, and the latter between the inner margins of the ischial

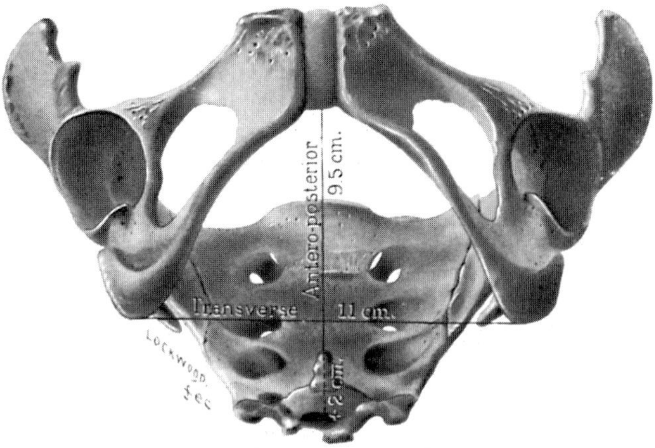

FIG. 6.—PELVIC OUTLET. × ⅓.

tuberosities. With the coccyx in its normal position, the antero-posterior diameter measures 9.5 centimetres, which is increased to 11.5 centimetres during labour by the backward displacement of the tip of the coccyx. The transverse diameter measures 11 centimetres.

The plane of greatest pelvic dimensions was first described by Levret, and, as its name implies, represents the roomiest portion of the pelvic cavity. It extends from the middle of the posterior surface of the sym-

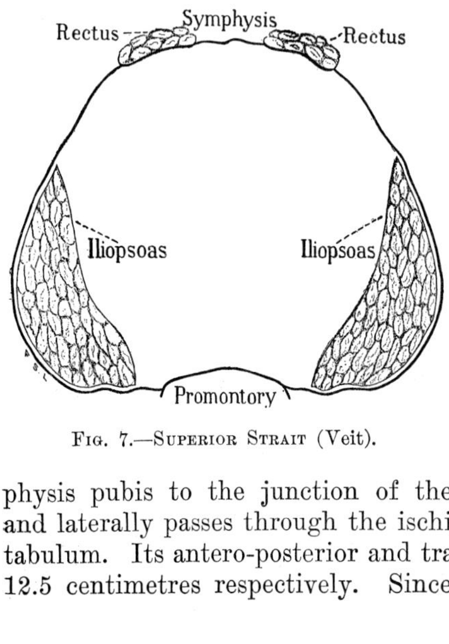

FIG. 7.—SUPERIOR STRAIT (Veit).

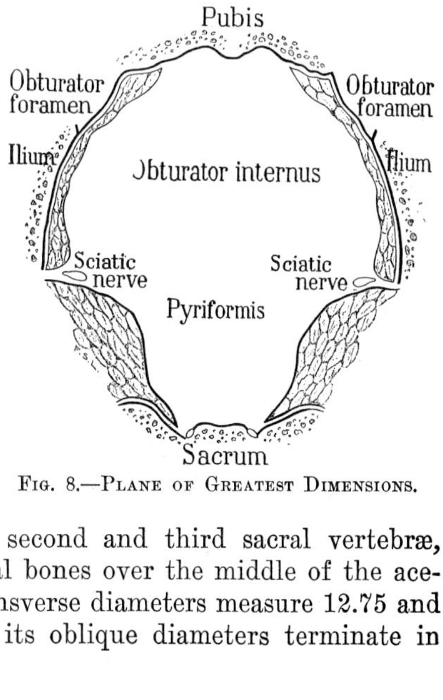

FIG. 8.—PLANE OF GREATEST DIMENSIONS.

physis pubis to the junction of the second and third sacral vertebræ, and laterally passes through the ischial bones over the middle of the acetabulum. Its antero-posterior and transverse diameters measure 12.75 and 12.5 centimetres respectively. Since its oblique diameters terminate in the obturator foramina and the sacro-sciatic notches, they are subject to marked variations in length.

The plane of least pelvic dimensions extends through the lower margin of the symphysis pubis, the tip of the sacrum, and the ischial spines. Its antero-posterior diameter measures 11.5 and its transverse diameter 10.5 centimetres, the latter being the shortest diameter in the normal pelvic cavity.

Hodge designated as the *second parallel*, another plane which passes through the lower margin of the symphysis pubis parallel to the plane of the superior strait. Very closely related to it is that described by Veit as the main plane of the pelvis, which extends from the lower margin of the symphysis pubis to the junction of the first and second sacral vertebræ. According to Veit this, from an obstetrical stand-point, is the largest plane of the pelvis, inasmuch as it is not encroached upon by the pelvic

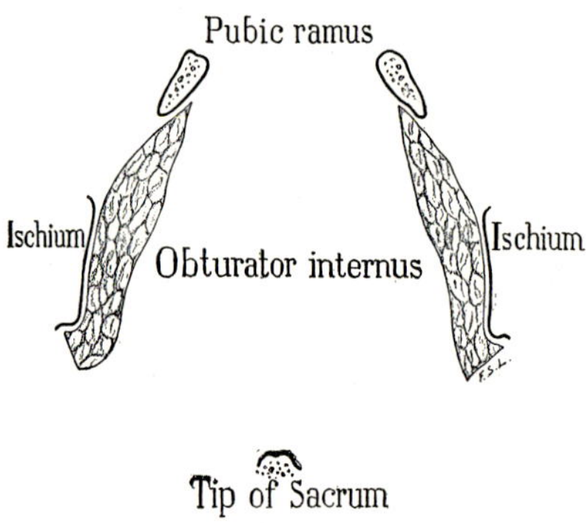

Fig. 9.—Plane of Least Dimensions (Veit).

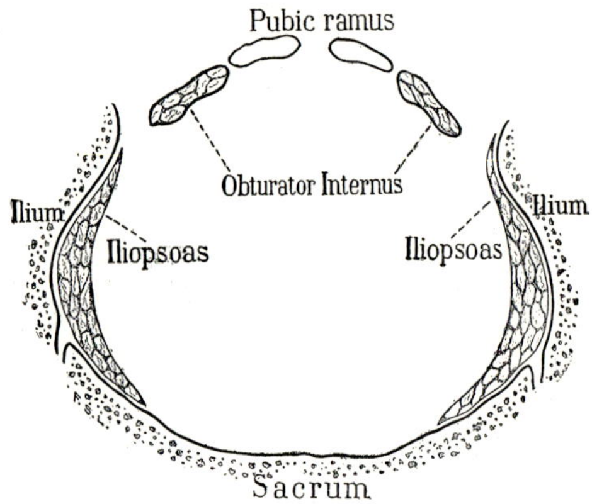

Fig. 10.—Veit's Main Plane.

soft parts, but passes above the obturator and pyriformis and below the ilio-psoas muscles.

Most pelves present slight individual variations in size, and perfectly normal and symmetrical examples are rarely seen. The measurements which we have given are those of Schroeder, and are the averages obtained from the accurate mensuration of 50 normal pelves.

Pelvic Inclination.—The normal position of the pelvis, with the woman in the erect posture, can be reproduced by holding the specimen in such a way that the incisions of the acetabula look directly downward. According to Meyer, the pelvis is in its normal position when the anterior superior spines of the ilium and the pubic spines are in the same vertical plane. Under these conditions the promontory of the sacrum is 9.5 to 10 centimetres higher than the upper margin of the symphysis pubis.

By the term *pelvic inclination* we understand the angle which the plane of the superior strait forms with the horizon (see Fig. 3). This conception was first introduced by J. J. Müller and Roederer, and the early statements concerning it were very conflicting. According to Meyer, the centre of gravity of the body passes along an imaginary vertical plane just posterior to the acetabula, so that under the influence of the body weight the pelvis would tend to rotate backward were it not held in position by the strong ilio-femoral ligaments. It is therefore apparent that the pelvic inclination must vary according to the degree of tension of these structures; it will be diminished when they are relaxed, and *vice versa*. It is least marked when the legs are slightly rotated inward and spread a little apart, and markedly increased when the knees are pressed tightly together, or when the legs are widely spread apart or rotated strongly either inward or outward. With the woman in the upright position the pelvic inclination is usually estimated at 45 to 50 degrees, but may vary from 40 to 100 degrees according to the degree of tension exerted by the ilio-femoral ligaments. In certain diseased conditions it may be obliterated, and the plane of the superior strait may become parallel to the horizon.

The first accurate work upon this subject was done by Naegele, who measured the distance from the floor to the lower margin of the symphysis pubis and the tip of the sacrum respectively, and in this way estimated the inclination which the inferior strait formed with the horizon. He then placed a normal pelvis in a similar position and estimated the inclination of its superior strait, which was usually about 60 degrees.

In view of the marked variations to which the pelvic inclination is subject, Meyer introduced a new conception concerning it, and stated that it was considerably influenced by the extent to which the sacrum rotated about its transverse axis. As this passes through the centre of the body of the third sacral vertebra, it is apparent that this portion of the sacrum retains approximately the same position, no matter to what extent its upper or lower portions may be displaced. Meyer, therefore, constructed a diameter extending from the upper margin of the symphysis to the middle of the third sacral vertebra, and designated it the *normal conjugate*. Its inclination he estimated at 30 degrees, and stated that it remained practically constant in all positions of the body.

Except when markedly abnormal, the pelvic inclination possesses no practical obstetrical significance, and is of value only in the study of atypical pelves and anthropology. Several complicated instruments have been invented for determining it, but Prochownick has suggested that it may be approximately estimated by drawing a line from the spine of the last lumbar vertebra to the upper margin of the symphysis, and estimating the angle which this forms with the horizon.

Since the lower margin of the symphysis occupies a lower level than the tip of the sacrum, the plane of the inferior strait is also inclined to the horizon, forming an acute angle, which is usually estimated at 10 degrees. Much more important, however, is the angle which is formed between the posterior surface of the symphysis pubis and the conjugata vera; this is usually estimated at 90 to 100 degrees, but varies considerably according to the shape, height, and inclination of the symphysis pubis. It must always be taken into consideration in estimating the length of the conjugata vera from that of the conjugata diagonalis, since it is evident that the amount to be subtracted from the latter will vary with the size of the angle between the symphysis and the conjugata vera.

The Pelvic Axis.—Deventer introduced the conception of a pelvic axis, which he obtained by erecting perpendiculars at the centres of innumerable planes, extending from the symphysis to the sacrum (see Fig. 3). At the end of pregnancy the axis of the superior strait, if extended directly upward, would pass through the abdominal wall at about the region of the umbilicus, while the axis of the inferior strait would impinge upon the promontory of the sacrum. The direction of the pelvic axis, therefore, would follow a curved line, which was formerly believed to represent the course which the child pursued in its passage through the pelvis. The work of Naegele, Hegar, Pinard, and others, however, has shown that this is not the case, so that at present this axis possesses only an historical interest.

The Pelvic Joints.—Anteriorly the pelvic bones are held together by the symphysis pubis, which consists of a mass of fibro-cartilage, and by the superior and inferior pubic ligaments, the latter being frequently designated as the ligamentum arcuatum pubis. Luschka demonstrated the presence of a synovial cavity in the fibro-cartilage, and therefore classed the symphysis among the true joints (Fig. 11). Joessel, on the other hand, denies its existence, and states that the fluid in the interior of the symphysis is simply a product of degeneration. Whether it be a true joint or not, in any case the symphysis admits of a certain amount of motility, which becomes particularly marked during pregnancy. This fact was demonstrated by Budin, who showed that if the finger were inserted into the vagina of a pregnant woman, and she were made to walk, one could distinctly feel the ends of the pubic bones move up and down with each step.

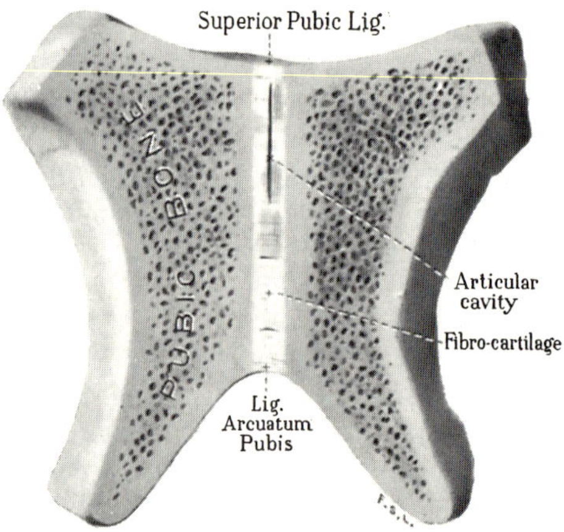

Fig. 11.—Frontal Section Symphysis Pubis (Spalteholz). × 1.

The articulations between the sacrum and innominate bones were formerly described as synchondroses, but Luschka conclusively demonstrated the presence of a synovial cavity within them, and therefore classed them among the true joints (Fig. 12). These articulations possess a certain amount of motility which plays a not unimportant part in practical obstetrics.

Walcher, in 1889, stated that the diagonal conjugate varied about 1 centimetre in length, according as it was measured with the woman in the usual obstetrical position, or with her buttocks resting on the edge of the table and her legs hanging down without any support, which has since been known as the Walcher or hanging position. His observations have been confirmed by nearly all who have repeated his work, among whom may be mentioned Klein, Wehle and Leopold and Küttner. The subject was chosen as one of the main themes for discussion at the International Gynæcological and Obstetrical Congress held at Amsterdam in 1899. The speakers, almost without exception, admitted the general correctness of Walcher's statements, differing only as to the extent of the changes, while Bar was the only one to deny their occurrence.

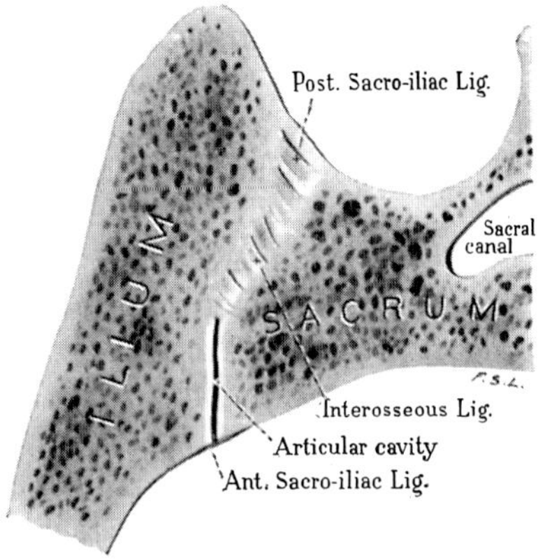

Fig. 12.—Sacro-iliac Synchondrosis (Spalteholz). × 1.

This slight amount of motility is utilized in dealing with contracted pelves; and not infrequently the increase in the size of the conjugata vera, brought about by Walcher's position, has proved sufficient to permit the engagement of the presenting part, which otherwise could not occur. The effect of Walcher's position upon the size of the pelvic cavity has recently been studied very carefully by Küttner, who showed in three cases that the conjugata vera was respectively 1.4, 0.9, and 1 centimetre longer when measured in the hanging than in the lithotomy position. Fig. 13 gives a graphic illustration of the changes in shape in one of these pelves.

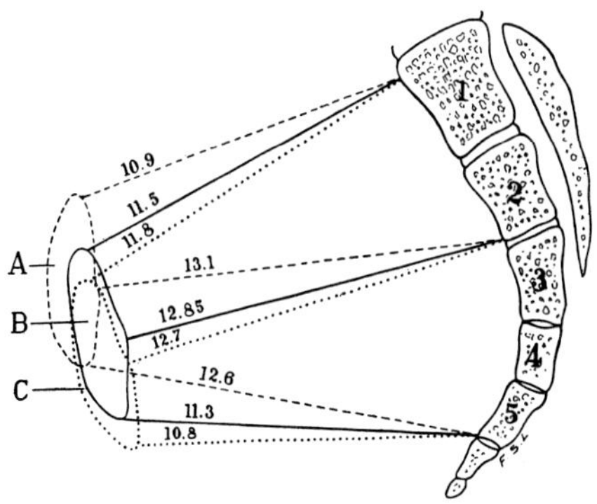

Fig. 13.—Diagram showing Variation of Antero-posterior Diameter of Pelvis in Various Positions (Küttner). × ⅛.

A, lithotomy; *B*, horizontal; *C*, Walcher's position.

Methods of Comparing Pelves.—Inasmuch as the normal pelvis usually presents slight individual variations in its form and dimensions, and as contracted pelves differ markedly from one another in shape, several devices have been employed to enable us to readily compare their points of difference. The decimal method, suggested by Litzmann, is very satisfactory for most purposes. In it the various diameters are expressed in terms of the conjugata vera, which is reckoned as 100 (see table on the following page).

Breisky introduced a graphic method for comparing pelves and constructed three diagrams, representing a vertical mesial section of the pelvis, the plane of the superior strait, and a frontal view of the pelvis. The first is constructed upon Meyer's normal conjugate, the second upon the distance between the sacro-iliac synchondroses, and the third upon the transverse diameter of the pelvic outlet.

Comparison of Various Diameters of Normal Pelvis by Litzmann's Decimal Method.	Diameters.		
	Antero-posterior.	Transverse.	Oblique.
Superior strait	100	122.7	113
Plane of greatest pelvic dimension	115	113.6	
Plane of least pelvic dimension	105.5	95.5	
Inferior strait	105.5	100	

Individual Variations in the Pelvis.—With the exception of the skull, no portion of the skeleton presents greater individual variations than the pelvis. This is due partly to the fact that it is developed from a considerable number of bones, and partly to the varying mechanical and developmental influences to which it is subjected during the early years of life.

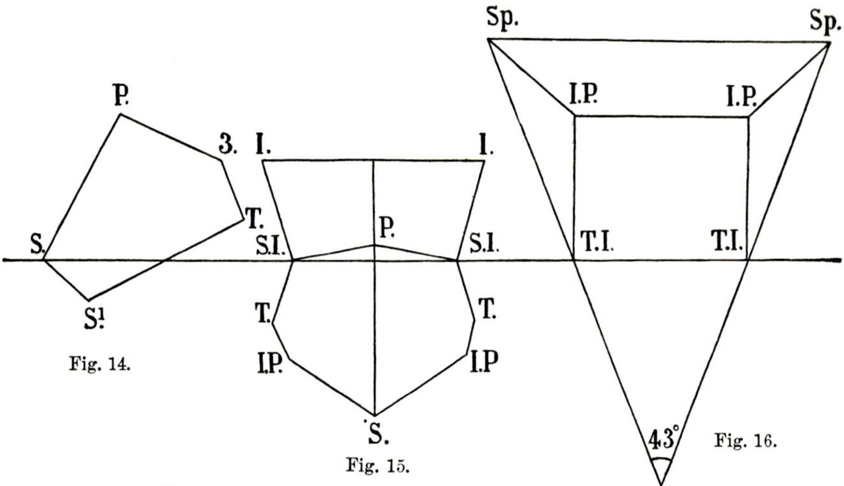

Fig. 14. Fig. 15. Fig. 16.

Figs. 14–16.—Breisky's Diagrams for Comparing Pelves.

I., inclination of iliac bones; *I.P.*, ilio-pectineal eminence; *P.*, promontory of sacrum; *S.*, upper margin of symphysis; *S.*[1], lower margin of symphysis; *S.I.*, sacro-iliac synchondrosis; *Sp.*, iliac spines; *T.*, transverse diameter, superior strait; *T.I.*, tuber ischii; *3*, bend in body of third sacral vertebra.

Indeed, we may say that no two pelves are exactly alike, and that perfectly normal pelves are rarely seen; so that an accurate conception of the form and dimensions of what may be termed the normal type can be obtained only from averages based upon the examination of numerous approximately normal pelves.

Owing to the greater employment of the right half of the body, the corresponding side of the pelvis is more developed than the left. Individual variations may be observed in the form, consistence, and general character of the pelvic bones, in the angles which the iliac fossæ form with the walls of the pelvic basin, in the shape of the sacrum, and particularly in that of the cavity itself. In view, therefore, of the varying thickness of the pelvic bones, and especially of the degree of flaring of the ilia, accurate conclusions cannot be based upon external pelvimetry.

Sexual Differences in the Adult Pelvis.—The pelvis presents marked sexual differences. Speaking generally, we may say that in the male the pelvis is heavier, higher, less graceful than in the female, and presents a

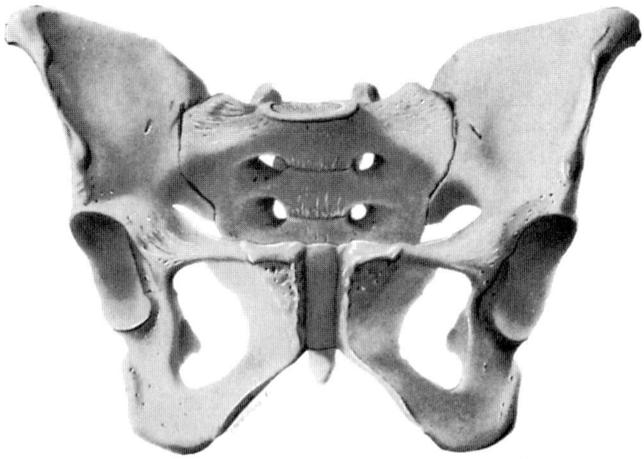

Fig. 17.—Front View Female Pelvis. × ⅓.

more conical appearance. In the male the muscular attachments are much more strongly marked, and the iliac bones are less flared than in the female. The pubic arch is more angular in shape, and presents an aperture of 70 to 75 degrees, as compared to 90 to 100 degrees in the female.

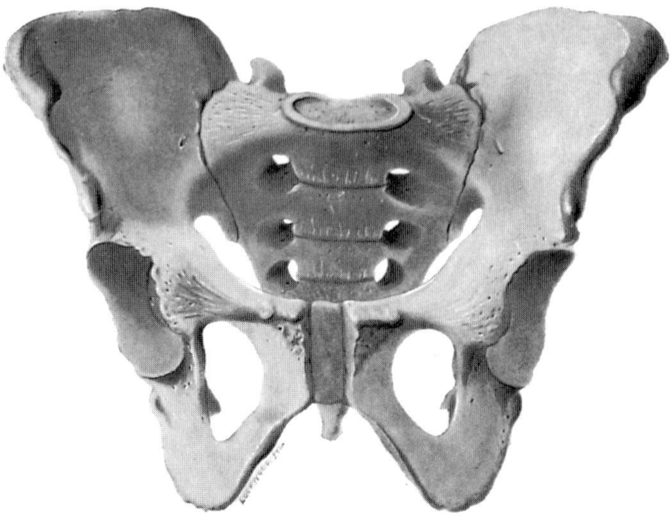

Fig. 18.—Front View Male Pelvis. × ⅓.

This difference is so marked that one usually speaks of the pubic angle in the male and the pubic arch in the female. In the male pelvis the superior strait is smaller and more triangular in outline, while the pelvic cavity is deeper and more conical in shape. These differences are readily noted in Figs. 17, 18, and 19, and may be especially emphasized by a comparison of the various measurements in the two sexes.

Broadly speaking, the external measurements are practically alike in both sexes, though the distance between the anterior superior spines of

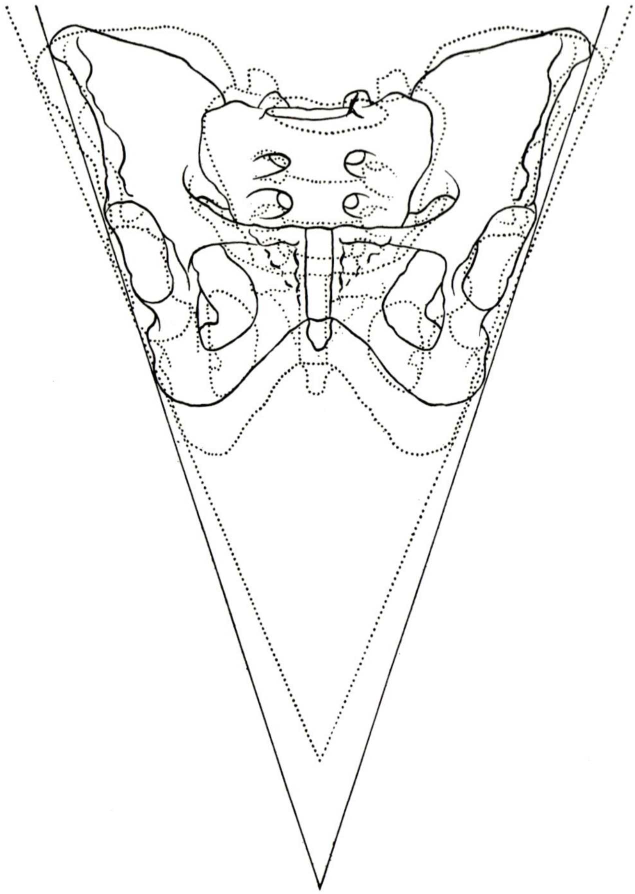

FIG. 19.—DIAGRAM SHOWING DIFFERENCE IN SHAPE OF MALE [....] AND FEMALE [——] PELVIS.

the ilium is somewhat less in the male; while all the diameters of the pelvic cavity are shorter, as is shown by the following table:

COMPARISON OF MALE AND FEMALE PELVIS.	DIAMETERS.		
	Antero-posterior.	Transverse.	Oblique.
Superior strait:			
Male	10.5	12.5	12 cm.
Female	11	13.5	12.75 cm.
Inferior strait:			
Male	9.5	8 cm.	
Female	11.5	11 cm.	

It is therefore apparent that the outlet of the male pelvis is contracted to such a degree as to render it impossible for a living child to pass through it, particularly in being forced out under the pubic angle. Occasionally the female pelvis may approach the male type, and under such circumstances may offer insuperable obstacles to the birth of the child, and necessitate radical operative procedures to effect delivery.

Numerous not very satisfactory attempts have been made to explain the cause of the differences between the male and female pelvis. According to Fehling and most subsequent investigators, sexual differences make their appearance as early as the fourth or fifth month of intra-uterine life, so that the sex can be ascertained long before term by examination of the pelvis. Arthur Thompson has recently made the same statement, and my own investigations have led me to similar conclusions. On the other hand, Schroeder and other authorities attribute the characteristic shape of the female pelvis to the presence of the internal genitalia, and state that the pelves of female eunuchs, as well as those of individuals in whom the uterus is congenitally absent, conform to the male type. While the correctness of such statements cannot be doubted, it nevertheless seems probable that the greater part of the sexual differences must be due to inherent developmental and hereditary factors.

Racial Differences.—Considerable variations may be observed in the form of the pelvis in various races, and especially upon comparing those obtained from aboriginal and civilized peoples. But in spite of the researches of Weber, Stein, Verneau, Topinard, Turner, and others, our knowledge upon the subject is still fragmentary. Stein distinguished four groups of pelves:

1. Blunt heart-shaped.
2. Elliptical, with the greatest diameter transverse.
3. Round.
4. Elliptical, with the greatest diameter antero-posterior.

Topinard attempted to classify pelves according to their "general index"—that is, the relation between their height and width, as represented by the distance between the iliac crests. His careful measurements showed that the pelvis becomes increasingly lower and broader the more civilized the race from which it is obtained.

Turner based his classification upon the relation between the transverse and antero-posterior diameters of the superior strait, and divided pelves into three great groups: dolichopellic, in which the conjugata vera is greater than the transverse diameter; mesatipellic, in which the conjugata vera and transverse diameters are of equal length; and platypellic, in which the conjugata vera is shorter than the transverse diameter. He stated that the first variety had not been observed in women, though it is not infrequent in men. The mesatipellic variety is observed in the women of the lower races, notably among the Bushmen, Hottentots, and the lower classes of negroes; while the platypellic forms are found in all the higher races. But even among civilized whites considerable racial differences are not infrequently noted, and it is generally stated that the pelves of the English and Holstein women are broader than those of other nationalities; while the

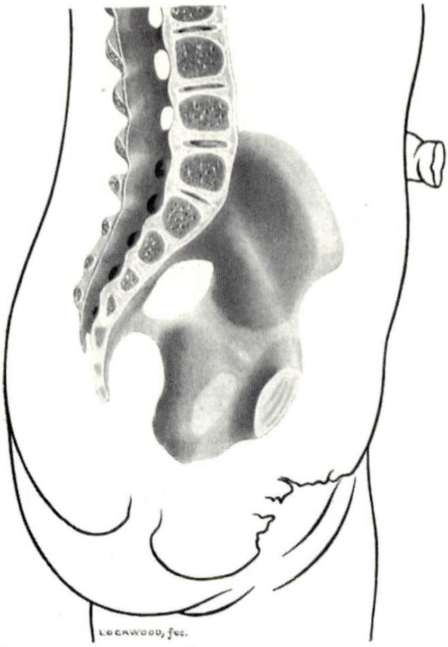

FIG. 20.—SAGITTAL SECTION SHOWING RELATIVE PROPORTION OF BONE AND CARTILAGE IN THE PELVIS OF A NEWLY BORN CHILD. × 1.

Jewesses living in the vicinity of Dorpat have extremely small pelves.

While the study of the racial differences in the pelvis presents a marked anthropological interest, it is, as yet, of little practical obstetrical value, as no extended studies have been made concerning the form and size of the heads of children which are born through them. My own experience in Baltimore has shown that contracted pelves occur several times more frequently among black than white women (21 per cent to 7 per cent), while operative delivery is more frequently required among the latter. This is probably due to the fact that the heads of negro children are somewhat smaller and more compressible, and thus compensate for the smaller size of the pelvis.

Pelvis of the New-born Child.—The pelvis of the child at birth is partly bony and partly cartilaginous. The innominate bone does not exist as such, its place being taken by the ilium, ischium, and pubis, which are united by a large Y-shaped cartilage, the three bones meeting in the acetabulum. The iliac crests and the acetabula, as well as the greater part of the ischiopubic rami, are entirely cartilaginous in structure. Figs. 20 and 21 clearly show the extent to which the infantile pelvis is ossified.

The cartilaginous portions of the pelvis gradually give place to bone, but complete union in the neighbourhood of the acetabulum does not occur until about the age of puberty, and occasionally even at a later period. Indeed, we may say that the innominate bones do not become completely ossified and fully developed until between the twentieth and twenty-fifth years.

Each innominate bone is developed from 12 centres of ossification.

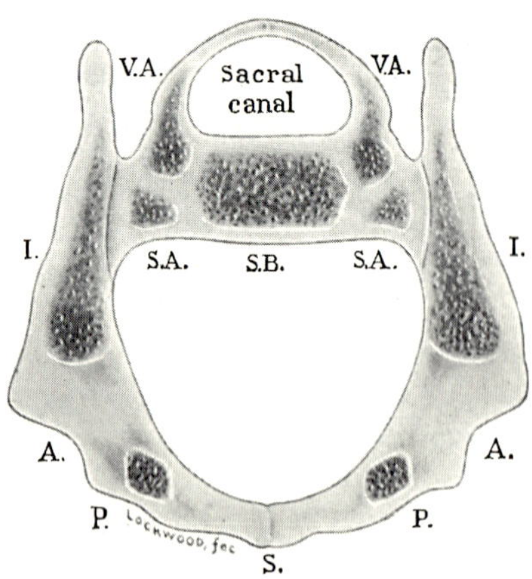

FIG. 21.—SECTION THROUGH INFANTILE PELVIS PARALLEL TO SUPERIOR STRAIT, SHOWING RELATIVE PROPORTIONS OF BONE AND CARTILAGE. × 1.

A., acetabulum; *I.*, ilium; *P.*, pubic bone; *S.*, symphysis pubis; *S.A.*, ala of sacrum; *S.B.*, body of sacrum; *V.A.*, vertebral arch.

Three of these are primary and give rise to the ilium, ischium, and pubis. They make their appearance by the end of the first half of pregnancy. The remaining 9 centres—the so-called epiphyseal centres—are secondary, and do not develop until a considerably later period, some of them not until after the age of puberty.

The sacrum at birth is likewise partly bony and partly cartilaginous. It is made up of 21 distinct bones, each of which is derived from a single centre of ossification. The 21 centres are arranged as follows: 1 for each vertebral body (5); 3 for the alæ on either side (6); and 2 for the arches of each vertebra (10). To these must be added the various epiphyseal centres which appear later. The cartilage gradually becomes ossified, and the various component parts of the sacrum fuse together. The alæ are the first portions to become united, after which the vertebral bodies gradually become welded together, the fusion extending from below upward. According to Litzmann, the bodies of the sacral vertebræ are not entirely united until the seventh year, and complete ossification of the sacrum is not effected until the twenty-fifth year. Fig. 22 represents the disarticulated pelvis of a child three years old, and clearly shows the extent to which ossification has progressed at that age.

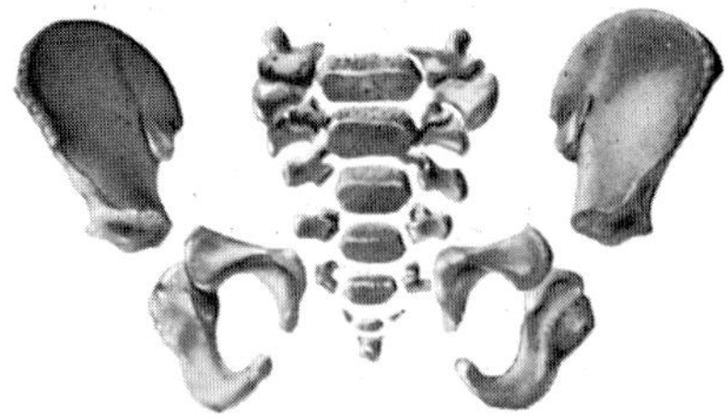

FIG. 22.—DISARTICULATED PELVIS OF THREE-YEAR-OLD GIRL. × ⅓.

The pelvis of the new-born child differs from that of the adult not only in being made up of a large number of bones which are united by cartilage, but more particularly in its characteristic shape. This is clearly seen upon comparing Figs. 24 and 25, which represent vertical mesial sections through the pelvis of a new-born child and an adult woman. In the former the vertebral column is almost vertical, and its lumbar curvature practically absent. The promontory is very slightly marked, and is situated at a much higher level than in the adult. The sacrum is almost straight from above downward, but presents a more marked lateral concavity than in the adult. Its alæ are only slightly developed, and as a consequence the pelvis is relatively narrower. The iliac fossæ are almost vertical, and the horizontal rami of the pubis are far shorter than in the adult. The pubic arch is much more angular, while the pelvic inclination is decidedly greater. The superior strait is narrower and more angular in shape, the relation between the conjugata vera and the transverse diameter being 100 to 105, instead of 100 to 122.5, as in the normal adult pelvis. The cavity of the pelvis is relatively much smaller, and is distinctly funnel-shaped. The antero-posterior and transverse diameters of the pelvic outlet, when expressed in terms of the con-

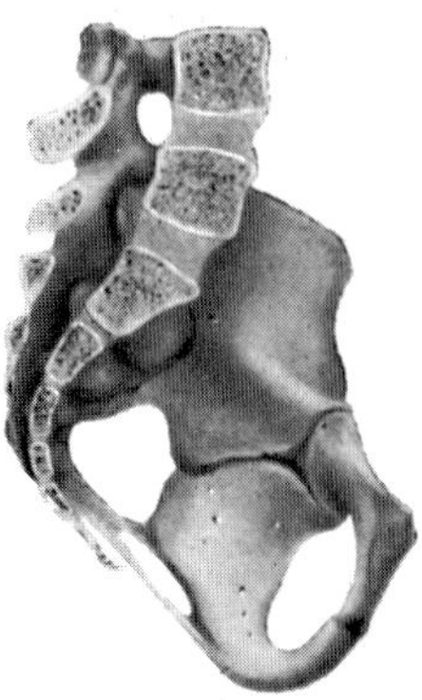

FIG. 23.—SAGITTAL SECTION THROUGH PELVIS OF FIVE-YEAR-OLD GIRL. × ⅓.

jugata vera, are respectively 93 and 73, instead of 104.5 and 100 as in the adult.

As we have already indicated, sexual differences make their appearance at a very early period. Fehling showed that they could be detected as early as the fourth month, when he found that the first sacral vertebra was wedge-shaped in the female, instead of cuboidal as in the male. His results have since been confirmed by a number of observers, among whom Balandin, Jürgens, and Arthur Thompson may be mentioned; my own work also corroborates their statements.

The pelvis of the female fœtus or new-born child presents the following characteristics as compared with that of the male: The pelvic canal

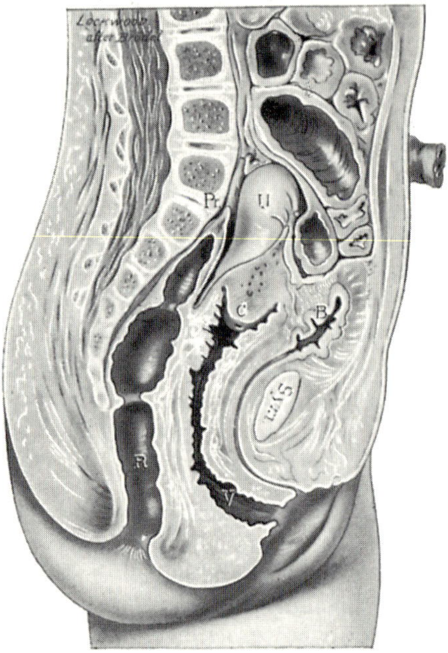

FIG. 24.—SAGITTAL SECTION THROUGH BODY OF NEWLY BORN CHILD.

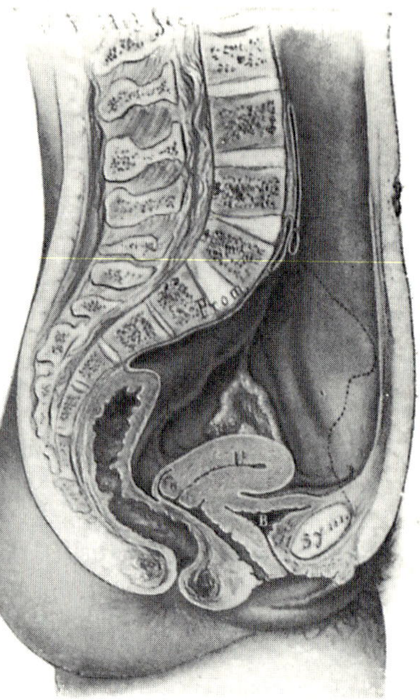

FIG. 25.—SAGITTAL SECTION THROUGH ADULT WOMAN (KELLY), REDUCED TO THE SAME SIZE AS FIG. 24 FOR COMPARISON.

is less funnel-shaped, the pubic arch is wider, the sacro-sciatic notches are larger, and the lumbar region of the spinal column is more markedly curved.

Transformation of Fœtal into Adult Pelvis.—The mechanism by which the pelvis of the fœtus is converted into the adult form is of interest, not only from a scientific but also from a practical point of view, as it affords important information concerning the mode of production of certain varieties of deformed pelves.

The earliest investigations upon this subject were made by De Fremery and Denman, who were followed by Litzmann, Duncan, Fehling, Schroeder, Veit, Von Meyer, and others. At present it is generally believed that in the evolution of the form of the pelvis two sets of factors—

developmental and inherent tendencies, and mechanical influences—are concerned. That the process is not entirely the result of the action of mechanical forces is manifested by the existence of sexual and racial differences in the adult pelvis, but especially by the presence of the former in the fœtal pelvis, long before it has been subjected to the usual mechanical influences. Moreover, the mechanical influences which come into play after birth are identical in both sexes, but despite this fact the sexual differences become still more accentuated as puberty is approached.

The part played by developmental and hereditary influences was clearly demonstrated by Litzmann, who showed that the female sacrum was characterized by a marked increase in width as compared with that of the male. At birth, in both sexes, the body of the first sacral vertebra is twice as broad as the alæ (100 to 50), but in the adult the relation becomes 100 to 76 in the female, and 100 to 56 in the male, indicating a much more rapid growth of the alæ in the former.

The effect exerted by mechanical influences has been particularly studied by Duncan, Meyer, Veit, and Schroeder, while Kehrer has insisted upon the part played by muscular action. According to Schroeder, three mechanical forces take part in bringing about the final shape of the pelvis—namely, the body weight, the upward and inward pressure exerted by the heads of the femora, and the cohesive force exerted at the symphysis pubis.

So long as the child remains constantly in the recumbent position these forces are in abeyance, but as soon as it sits up or walks, the body weight is transmitted through the vertebral column to the sacrum, and, as the centre of gravity is anterior to its promontory, the force transmitted is resolved into two components, one of which is directed downward and the other forward. Accordingly, the two together tend to force the promontory of the sacrum downward and forward, a process which can only be accomplished by the sacrum rotating slightly about its transverse axis so that its tips would become directed upward and backward. The displacement of the latter, however, is limited, as it is resisted by the strong sacro-sciatic ligaments which permit of only slight extension, with the result that the partly cartilaginous sacrum becomes bent upon itself just in front of its axis—i. e., about the middle of its third vertebra—so that its anterior surface becomes markedly concave from above downward, instead of flat as it was previously. At the same time the body weight forces the bodies of the sacral vertebra forward, so that they project slightly beyond the alæ and thus tend to diminish the lateral cavity of the sacrum.

As the anterior surface of the sacrum is wider than its posterior, the bone tends to sink down into the pelvic cavity under the influence of the body weight, and would prolapse completely into it were it not held in place by the strong posterior ilio-sacral ligaments which suspend it, so to speak, from the posterior superior spines of the ilium. As the sacrum is pushed downward into the pelvic cavity it exerts marked tension upon the ilio-sacral ligaments, which in turn drag the posterior superior spines inward towards the middle line, and consequently tend to rotate the anterior portions of the innominate bones outward. Excessive outward rotation is prevented, however, by the cohesive force exerted at the symphysis, but particularly by the upward and inward pressure exerted by the heads of the femora. Practically, then, the iliac bone becomes converted into a two-armed lever, with the articular surface of the sacrum as a fulcrum; as a consequence it bends at its point of least resistance, which is just anterior to the articulation, and thus gives the pelvis a greater transverse and a lesser antero-posterior diameter (Figs. 26, 27). At the same time it must be remembered that a considerable part of the transverse widening

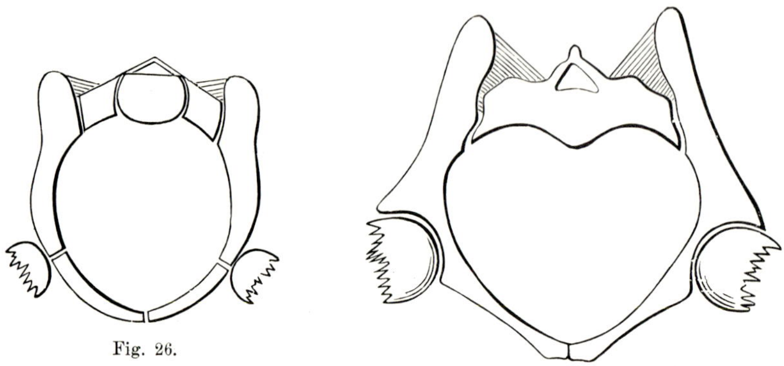

Fig. 26.

Fig. 27.

Figs. 26, 27.—Diagrammatic Representations of Sections through the Infantile and Adult Pelves (Schroeder).

is more apparent than real, and is due to the relative shortening of the conjugata vera by the downward and forward displacement of the promontory of the sacrum.

It is apparent that the forces just mentioned must act in identically the same manner in the two sexes, so that while they may serve to explain many points in the transformation of the fœtal into the adult pelvis, they fail to give a satisfactory explanation of its sexual differences, and we are therefore compelled to agree with Fehling, Freund, Joessel, and Breus and Kolisko that the latter must owe their origin to certain congenital tendencies concerning whose nature we are as yet absolutely ignorant.

The effect of the mechanical factors is particularly emphasized in certain abnormal types, more especially in the production of certain varieties of contracted pelves, and has been exhaustively studied by Von Meyer and Schroeder. In rare instances, as in a case recorded by Gurlt, none of the mechanical forces came into play, and we then have an opportunity of studying the development of the pelvis in their absence. In Gurlt's case of a thirty-one-year-old hydrocephalic woman, who had been bedridden since infancy and had never sat or walked, the autopsy showed that the pelvis had retained its fœtal characteristics.

The cohesive force exerted at the symphysis pubis cannot act by itself, as it is manifested only when the force exerted by the body weight causes a tendency towards gaping of the pubic bones. Likewise the effect of the upward and inward force exerted by the femora cannot be observed by itself, as this force comes into play only when it has to react against that resulting from the body weight. Thus far the action of the body weight alone has never been observed, though theoretically it might be noted in an individual presenting a split pelvis (congenital lack of union at the symphysis pubis) who had never walked. Its action, however, has been studied experimentally by Freund, who suspended a cadaver by the iliac crests after cutting through the symphysis, and found that the innominate bones gaped widely.

The effect of the combined action of the body weight and the force exerted by the femora has been studied by Litzmann in cases of congenital absence of the symphysis pubis. In such pelves there is a marked transverse widening of the posterior portion, while the force exerted by the femora causes the anterior portions of the innominate bones to become almost parallel.

The action of the body weight and the cohesive force exerted at the symphysis, without the upward and inward pressure exerted by the femora, can be studied in individuals whose lower extremities are absent, and occasionally in cases of congenital dislocation of the hips. Holst has described a case in which the lower extremities were congenitally absent, the pelvis being characterized by a marked increase in width and a marked decrease in its antero-posterior diameter. Owing to the excessive pressure exerted upon the tubera ischii in the absence of the counteracting force exerted by the femora, the innominate bones were rotated in such a manner as to turn their crests inward and the tubera ischii outward, thus producing a marked transverse widening of the inferior strait. More or less similar changes may be observed in the cases of congenital dislocation of the hip, in which the patients have never walked.

The effect of the various mechanical influences is particularly emphasized when they are exerted upon pelves whose bones are softened by disease, as in rhachitis and osteomalacia. But the consideration of the changes so produced will be deferred until the study of the deformed pelves is taken up.

LITERATURE

Arantius. Anatomicae observationes. Cap. XXXIX, Venetiis, 1857.

Balandin. Klinische Vorträge, Heft 1, St. Petersburg, 1883.

Bar. Influence de la position de la femme sur la forme, l'inclinaison et les dimensions du bassin. L'Obstétrique, iv, 529–542, 1899.

Breisky. Zeitschrift der Gesell. der Aerzte, Wien, i, 21, 1865.

Breus and Kolisko. Die pathologische Beckenformen, Bd. I, Theil I, Leipzig u. Wien, 1899.

Columbus. De re anatomica, Libri XV, Venetiis, 1559.

De Fremery. De mutationibus figuræ pelvis. D. I., Lugd. Batav., 1793.

Denman. An Introduction to the Practice of Midwifery. London, 1787–1795.

Deventer. Neues Hebammenlicht, etc. III. Aufl., Jena, 1728.

Duncan. Researches in Obstetrics. Edinburgh, 1868.
(On the Os Sacrum, 55–82.)
(On the Development of the Female Pelvis, 95–113.)

Fehling. Die Form des Beckens beim Fötus und Neugeborenen. Archiv f. Gyn., x, 1–80, 1876.

FREUND. Ueber das sogenannte kyphotische Becken, etc. Gynäkologische Klinik, i, 1-113, 1885.

GURLT. Ueber einige Missgestaltungen des weiblichen Beckens. Berlin, 1854.

HEGAR. Zur Geburtsmechanik. (Die Beckenaxe.) Archiv f. Gyn., i, 193-223, 1870.

HODGE. The Principles and Practice of Obstetrics. Philadelphia, 1860.

HOLST. Beschreibung des Beckens u. der Geburtstheile eines 40 Jahre alten weiblichen Amelus. Holst's Beiträge, Heft 2, 145-148, 1869.

HUWÉ. Onderwys der vrouwen, etc. Haarlem, 1735.

JOESSEL and WALDEYER. Lehrbuch der topographisch-chirurgischen Anatomie. Bonn, 1899. II. Theil, Das Becken.

JÜRGENS. Beiträge zur normalen und path. Anatomie des menschlichen Beckens. Virchow's Festschrift, Berlin, 1891.

KEHRER. Beiträge zur vergl. u. exper. Geburtshülfe, Heft 3, 1869; und Heft 5, 1875.

KLEIN. Zur Mechanik des Ileosacralgelenkes. Zeitschr. f. Geb. u. Gyn., xxi, 74-118, 1891.

KÜTTNER. Experimentell-anat. Untersuchungen über die Veränderlichkeit des Beckenraumes Gebärender. Hegar's Beiträge, i, 210-229, 1898.

LEVRET. L'art des accouchements. Paris, 1751.

LITZMANN. Die Formen des Beckens. Berlin, 1861.
Das gespaltene Becken. Archiv f. Gyn., iv, 266-284, 1872.
Die Geburt bei engem Becken. Leipzig, 1884.

LUSCHKA. Die Anatomie des menschlichen Beckens. Tübingen, 1864.

MEYER. Statik und Mechanik des menschlichen Knochengerüstes. Leipzig, 1873.

MICHEALIS. Das enge Becken. Leipzig, 1851.

MÜLLER, J. J. Diss. sist. casum rarissimum uteri in partu rupti. Basileae, 1745.

NAEGELE. Das weibliche Becken, etc. Carlsruhe, 1825.

PROCHOWNICK. Ueber Beckenneigung. Archiv f. Gyn., xix, 1-95, 1882.

ROEDERER. De axi pelvis. Goettingae, 1751.
Elementa artis obstetriciae. Goettingae, 1766.

SCHROEDER. Lehrbuch der Geburtshülfe. XIII. Aufl., 1899.

SMELLIE. A Treatise on the Theory and Practice of Midwifery. London, 1752.

STEIN, D. J. Lehre der Geburtshülfe. Elberfeld, 1825.

THOMPSON. The Sexual Differences of the Fœtal Pelvis. Journal of Anat. and Physiol., xxxiii, 359-381, 1899.

TOPINARD. Des proportions générales du bassin chez l'homme, etc. Bull. de la Soc. d'Anthropologie, 504-521, 1875.

TURNER. The Index of the Pelvic Brim as a Basis of Classification. Journal of Anat. and Physiol., xx, 1886.

VEIT. Die Entstehung der Form des Beckens. Zeitschr. f. Geb. u. Gyn., ix, 347-372, 1883.

VEIT, J. Die Anatomie des Beckens. Stuttgart, 1887.

VERNEAU. Le bassin dans les sexes et dans les races. Paris, 1875.

VESALIUS. De humani corporis fabrica libri septem. Basilae, 1543.

WALCHER. Die Conjugata eines engen Beckens ist keine konstante Grösse, etc. Centralbl. f. Gyn., 1889, 892, 893.

WEBER. Die Lehre von Ur- und Racenformen des Schädels und Beckens des Menschen. Düsseldorf, 1830.

WEHLE. Die Walcher'sche Hängelage und ihre praktische Verwerthung bei geburtshülflichen Operationen. Archiv f. Gyn., xlv, 323-336, 1894.

WILLIAMS. The Frequency of Contracted Pelves, etc. Obstetrics, i, Nos. 5, 6, 1899.

CHAPTER II

THE FEMALE ORGANS OF GENERATION

For convenience in description and on account of their differences in function, the female organs of generation are divided into two groups—the external and the internal—the vagina being usually classed with the former. The external organs, together with the vagina, serve more especially for copulation, while the internal organs are directly concerned with the development and birth of the fœtus.

THE EXTERNAL GENERATIVE ORGANS

The term pudendum is occasionally applied to the external organs of generation, although the more common designation is the *vulva.* This includes everything which is visible externally from the lower margin of the pubis to the perinæum—namely, the Mons Veneris, the labia majora and minora, the clitoris, vestibule, hymen, urethral opening, and various glandular and vascular structures.

Mons Veneris.—The Mons Veneris is the name given to the fatty cushion which rests upon the anterior surface of the symphysis pubis. After puberty the skin over it is covered by a thicker or thinner growth of crinkly hair, which is sometimes described as the "*escutcheon.*" Generally speaking, the distribution of the pubic hairs differs considerably in the two sexes. In the female they occupy a triangular area whose base corresponds to the upper margin of the symphysis, while a few hairs extend down over the outer surface of the labia majora. In the male, on the other hand, the escutcheon is not so circumscribed, as the hairs composing it extend triangularly upward towards the umbilicus and downward over the inner surface of the thighs. These differences were described in detail by Ploss, and at one time it was believed that they might be of value in determining the sex in doubtful cases. But Schultze showed that such variations were not absolutely characteristic, and my own experience has convinced me that the female escutcheon not infrequently approaches the male type.

Vulva.—In the restricted sense, the term vulva (from the Latin *valva,* or folding-door), or rima pudendi, is applied only to the structures lying beneath the Mons Veneris. Its position varies according to the inclination of the pelvis, but it usually runs horizontally when the woman is in the erect position. It presents marked individual variations in appearance, but its most noteworthy differences are dependent upon the age of the person and whether or not she has borne children.

Labia Majora.—On either side of the vulva extends a rounded mass of tissue, the labium majus. The labia majora vary markedly in appearance, according to the amount of fat beneath them. They are less prominent after childbearing, and in old age usually assume a shrivelled appearance. Ordinarily they measure 7 to 8 centimetres in length, 2 to 3 centimetres in width, and 1 to 1.5 centimetres in thickness. They are somewhat lozenge-shaped, and become narrower at their lower extremities. In children and virginal adults they usually lie in close apposition and completely conceal the underlying parts, whereas in multiparous women they often gape widely. Until recently it was usually stated that they were connected above and below by the anterior and posterior commissures of the vulva, but Luschka has shown that they are directly continuous with the Mons Veneris above, and fade away into the perinæum posteriorly.

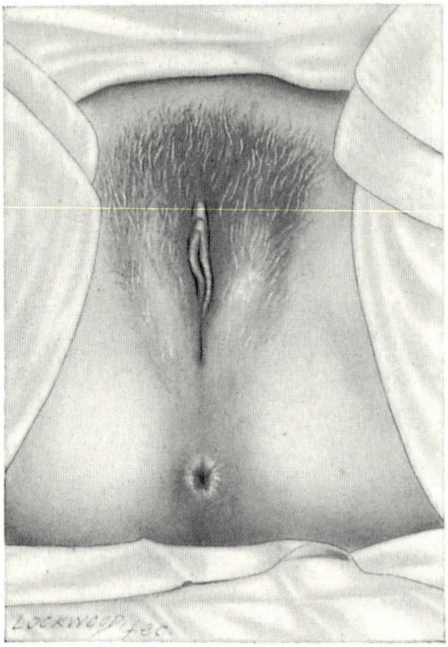

Fig. 28.—External Genitalia of Multiparous Woman, Labia in Contact.

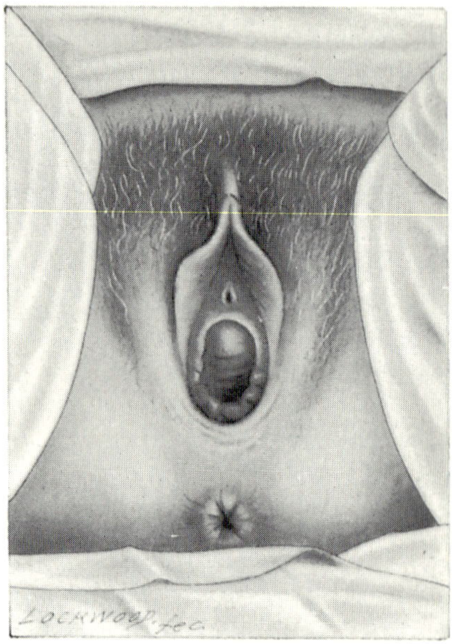

Fig. 29.—External Genitalia of Multiparous Woman, Labia spread Apart.

Each labium majus presents two surfaces, an outer and an inner. The outer surface corresponds in structure to the adjacent skin, and after the age of puberty is more or less thickly covered with hair. In women who have never borne children the inner surface is moist and resembles a mucous membrane in appearance; whereas in multiparæ it becomes more skin-like, but is not covered with hair. It is richly supplied with sebaceous glands. Beneath the skin there is a layer of dense connective tissue, which is rich in elastic fibres and adipose tissue, but does not contain muscular elements. Beneath this layer, which corresponds to the tunica dartos of the scrotum, is a tolerably dense mass of fat, to which the labium owes the greater part of its size. This fatty tissue is supplied with an abundant plexus of veins, which may rupture as the result of external violence or injury sustained during labour, and give rise to an extravasation of blood or hæmatoma.

The labia majora are analogous to the scrotum in the male, and at their upper ends receive the termination of the round ligaments. Exceptionally one or both of the inguinal canals, which in the female are designated as the canals of Nuck, may remain patent, so that in rare instances there results a hernial sac which usually contains intestine, but occasionally the tube or ovary, and possibly even the uterus.

Labia Minora.—On spreading apart the labia majora two triangular structures are seen, which meet together at the uppermost portion of the vulva and more or less resemble a cockscomb in appearance. These are the labia minora or *nymphæ*, so called because they were supposed to direct the course of the urine. They vary markedly in size and shape, and in nulliparous women are usually hidden by the labia majora. In multiparæ, on the other hand, they project beyond them.

The labia minora consist of thin folds of tissue, which when protected present a moist, reddish appearance, similar to that of a mucous membrane. They are, however, covered by stratified epithelium, into which project numerous papillæ. They have no hairs upon them, but contain many sebaceous follicles and occasionally a few sweat glands. Their interior portions are made up of connective tissue, in which are many vessels and a few non-striated muscular fibres, so that they are classed among the erectile structures. They are extremely sensitive, and are abundantly supplied with the several varieties of terminal nerve-endings, as has been shown by the work of Krause, Carrard, and Webster.

The labia minora converge anteriorly, each dividing towards its upper extremity into two lamellæ. Of these the two lower fuse together and form the *frenulum clitoridis*, while the upper ones make the *præputium*. Posteriorly they either pass almost imperceptibly into the labia majora, or approach the middle line as low ridges, which fuse together and form the *frenulum labiorum* or *fourchette* (Luschka, Cullingworth, and Nagel).

According to Nagel, the labia minora are homologous with the skin upon the under surface of the penis. Not infrequently they become considerably hypertrophied, either from unknown causes or as a result of masturbation. Among the Hottentots they assume immense proportions, and project from the vulva in the form of an apron some centimetres long. Among certain uncivilized races, voluminous labia minora are considered to enhance the beauty of their possessors, and artificial means are employed to bring about an increase in their size. According to Ploss, the Nubians and many other races practise *infibulation* as part of their religious ceremonial. In this operation, which is performed just before the age of puberty, the edges of the labia are freshened with a knife, and then sutured together in such a manner as to leave an opening only large enough to permit the escape of the menstrual flow. Under such circumstances a second operation is necessary before marriage can be consummated.

Clitoris.—The clitoris is situated at the most anterior portion of the vulva, and projects through the branched extremities of the labia minora which form its prepuce and frenulum. It is the analogue of the penis in the male, from which it differs in not possessing a corpus spongiosum, and in not being perforated by the urethra. It consists of a glans, a corpus, and two crura. The crura are long, narrow structures which arise from the inferior surface of each ischiopubic ramus and fuse together in the middle line, just below the pubic arch, to form the body of the clitoris. The clitoris is usually a very rudimentary organ and rarely exceeds 2 centimetres in length, even when in a state of erection. It is sharply bent on itself, owing to traction exerted upon it by the labia minora, whose anterior extremities, as has already been said, furnish the prepuce and frenulum. As a result, its free end looks downward and inward towards the vaginal opening. At the end of the body is the glans, which rarely exceeds a small pea in size. It is covered by squamous epithelium, is richly supplied with nerve-endings, and is extremely sensitive. The entire clitoris is very erectile, and its vessels are connected with the vestibular bulbs by means of the pars intermedia. Fig. 30 gives a good idea of the relations of the clitoris, its crura, and the vestibular bulbs. We are indebted to Kobelt for most of our knowledge concerning this organ, and since the appearance of his monograph, in 1844, the clitoris has been regarded as the chief seat of voluptuous sensation.

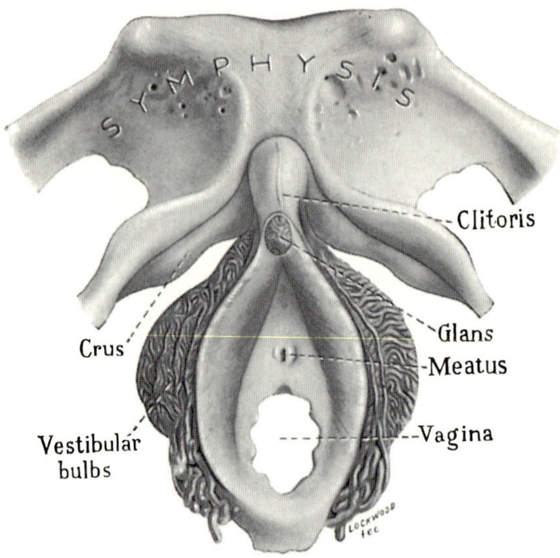

Fig. 30.—Preparation showing Clitoris and its Vascular Supply.

(Modified from Chrobak and Rosthorn.)

About the middle of the last century Baker Brown proposed its amputation as a panacea for nearly all the ills to which women are subject, and for a short time the operation of *clitoridectomy* enjoyed a marked vogue, but has since been completely abandoned. Among many of the aboriginal races the same operation had been performed from time immemorial as a religious rite, and was designated as "girl circumcision." Occasionally the clitoris may become considerably hypertrophied, so as to markedly resemble the penis, and not a few cases of so-called hermaphroditism are to be explained by this condition.

Vestibule.—The vestibule is the almond-shaped area which is inclosed between the labia minora and extends from the clitoris to the fourchette. It is the remnant of the uro-genital sinus of the embryo, and is perforated by four openings—the urethra, the vaginal opening, and the ducts of Bartholin's glands. Considerable uncertainty exists as to its boundaries, for the reason that the French anatomists usually describe it as a triangular area, bounded above by the labia minora and below by the vaginal opening. The posterior portion of the vestibule, between the fourchette and the vaginal opening, is called the *fossa navicularis*. It is rarely observed except in nulliparous women, as it usually becomes obliterated after childbirth.

Vestibular Glands.—In connection with the vestibule, certain glandular structures—the *glandulæ vestibulares majores* and *minores*—are usually described. The former are designated as *Bartholin's glands*, or the glands of Duverney, who first described them in the cow. They are two small structures varying from a pea to a small bean in size, and are situated beneath the vestibule, opposite the lateral margins of the vaginal opening. They lie under the constrictor muscle of the vagina, and in a few instances are found to be partially covered by the vestibular bulbs. They are compound racemose glands; their ducts, from 1.5 to 2 centimetres long, open upon the sides of the vestibule just outside the lateral margin of the vaginal orifice. In calibre they are usually small, and the lumen will admit only a bristle. Under the influence of sexual excitement the glands secrete a small amount of yellowish material. The ducts not infrequently harbour gonococci, which may gain access to the gland and cause it to suppurate, so that the entire labium becomes markedly distended by a collection of pus.

The glandulæ vestibulares minores are a number of small mucous glands which open upon the upper portion of the vestibule. Their orifices are occasionally several millimetres in diameter, and in such cases they are designated as lacunæ.

Urethral Opening.—The mouth of the urethra, or *urinary meatus*, is situated in the middle line of the vestibule, 1 to 1.5 centimetre below the pubic arch and a short distance above the vaginal opening. It usually presents a puckered appearance, and its orifice appears as a vertical slit, which on distention is 4 or 5 millimetres in diameter. The *para-urethral ducts* open upon the vestibule on either side of the urethra, and occasionally upon its posterior wall, just inside its mouth. They are of small calibre, $\frac{1}{2}$ millimetre in diameter, of varying length, and in this country are generally known as Skene's ducts. They were, however, described by Malpighi in the last century. Considerable discussion has arisen as to their origin, and certain observers, notably Kocks, believe that they represent the lower extremities of the Wolffian ducts. Most authorities, however, do not share this view, and believe that they are simply exaggerated lacunæ.

Vestibular Bulbs.—Lying beneath the mucous membrane of the vestibule, on either side, are the vestibular bulbs. These are almond-shaped, erectile bodies, 3 to 4 centimetres long, 1 to 2 centimetres wide, and 0.5 to 1 centimetre thick. They lie in close apposition to the ischio-pubic rami, and are partially covered by the ischio-cavernosus and constrictor vaginæ muscles. Their lower ends usually terminate about the middle of the vaginal opening, while their anterior extremities extend upward towards the clitoris, where they are united by the pars intermedia through which the blood from them reaches that organ. They were first described by Kobelt, and their vascular connections have been exhaustively studied by Gussenbauer.

Embryologically they correspond to the corpus spongiosum of the penis. During parturition they are usually pushed up beneath the pubic arch, but as their posterior ends partially encircle the vagina, they are liable to be injured to a greater or less extent, and their rupture may give rise to a hæmatoma of the vulva or to profuse external hæmorrhage if the tissues covering them are torn through.

Vaginal Opening and Hymen.—The vaginal opening occupies the lower portion of the vestibule and varies markedly in size and shape in different individuals. In virgins it is entirely hidden from view by the overlapping labia minora, and, when exposed by folding them back, appears almost completely closed by a membranous structure known as the hymen.

The hymen presents marked differences in shape and consistence. In the new-born child it is a redundant structure which projects considerably beyond the surrounding parts, while in adult virgins it is a membrane of varying thickness which closes the vaginal opening more or less completely, and presents an aperture which varies in size from a pin's point to a calibre which will readily admit the tip of one or even two fingers. The hymeneal opening is usually crescentic or circular in shape—*hymen semilunaris* or *annularis*. In rare instances it may assume other forms, which have been studied more particularly by Dohrn and Budin; the most important varieties being the cribriform, septate, and denticulate or fimbriated hymen. In very rare instances the membrane may be imperforate and lead to the retention of the menstrual discharges. Dohrn devoted particular attention to the fimbriated variety, and stated that it might be mistaken by an inexperienced observer for a ruptured hymen, so that this type possesses some little medico-legal interest.

According to the embryological researches of Nagel, the hymen represents the lowest portion of the vagina, which in early embryos is composed of a solid mass of epithelial cells. After proliferating rapidly for a time the most centrally situated cells begin to degenerate and a lumen is produced, except at the lower extremity of the mass, where the cells persist and give rise to the hymen. The hymen, therefore, is a fold of tissue presenting a structure similar to that of the vagina—namely, a connective-tissue core which is covered on either side by a layer of stratified epithelium, in which are numerous papillæ containing vessels and nerve-endings.

The hymen may vary markedly in consistence in different individuals. According to Dohrn, many types are observed—from a delicate structure resembling a spider's web to a fleshy, ligamentous, or even cartilaginous membrane, which in rare instances has even been described as "bony."

PLATE II.

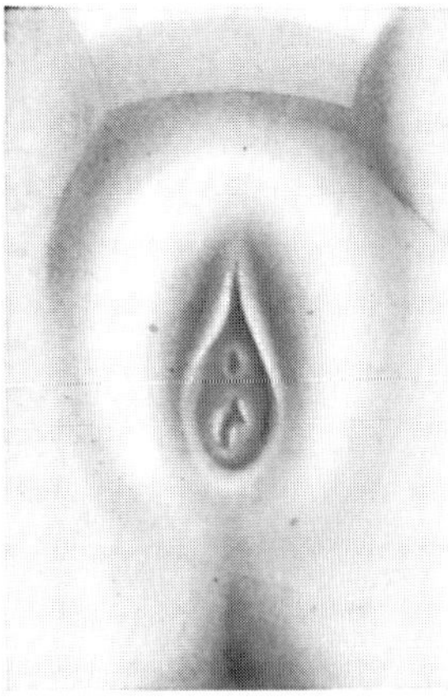

Infantile.

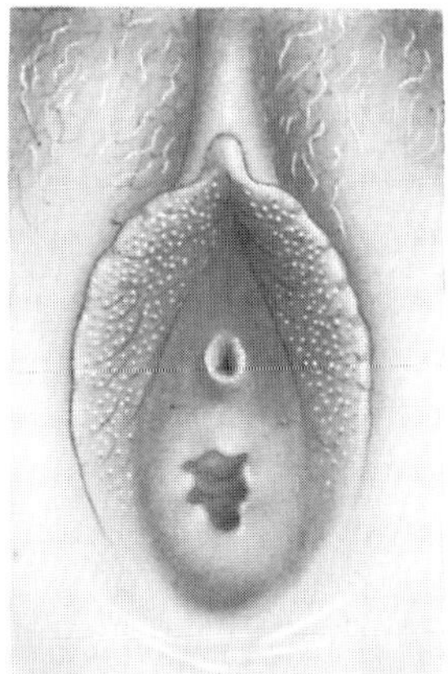

Annular.

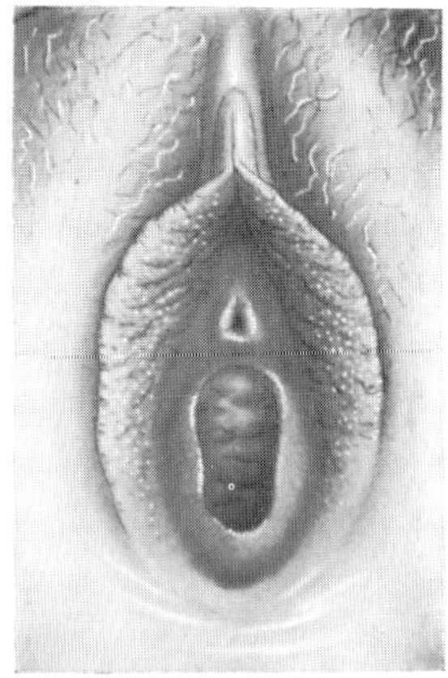

Semilunar.

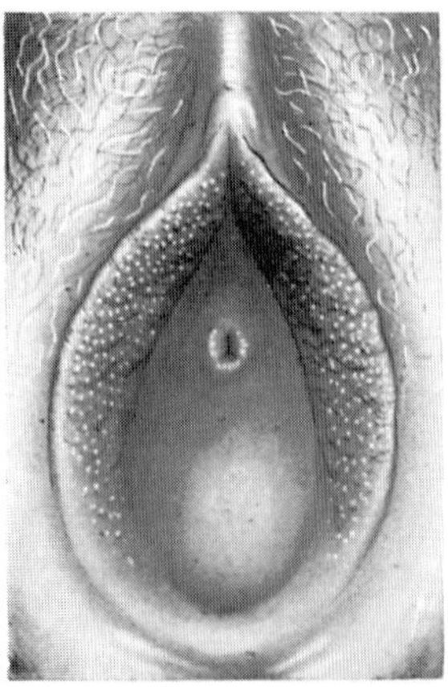

Imperforate.

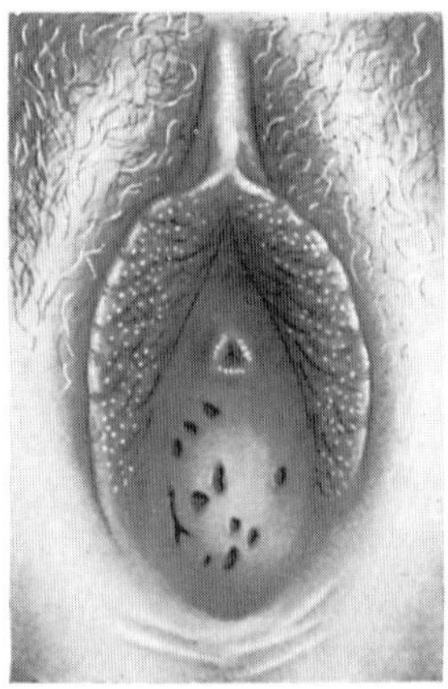

Cribriform.

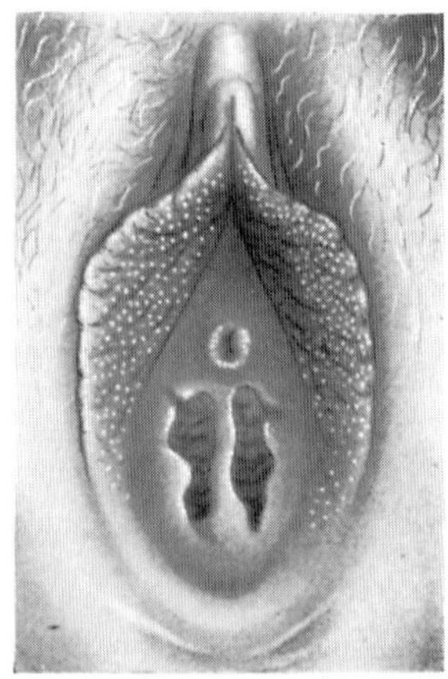

Septate.

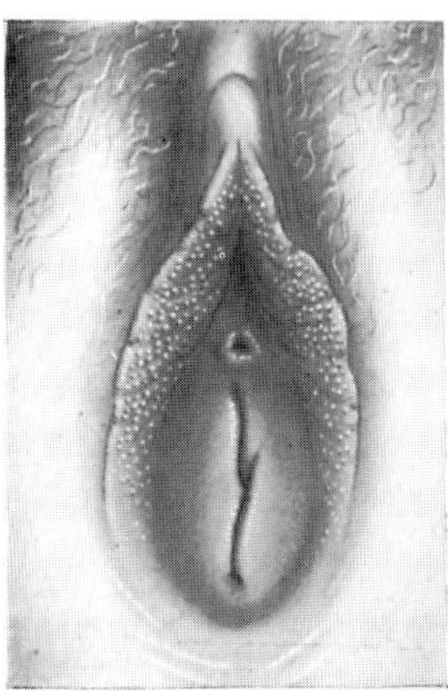

Vertical.

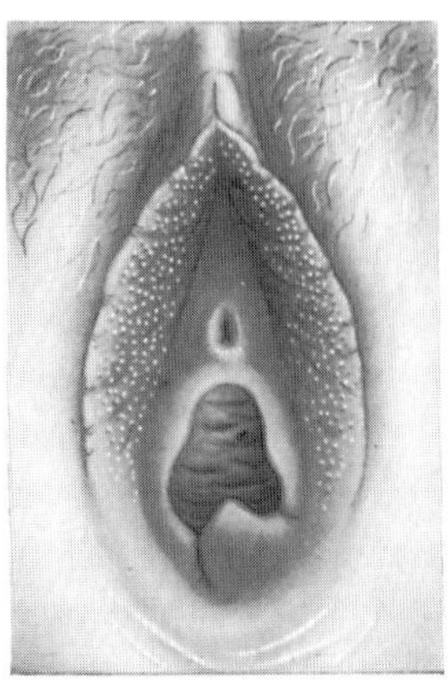

Normal injury at coitus.

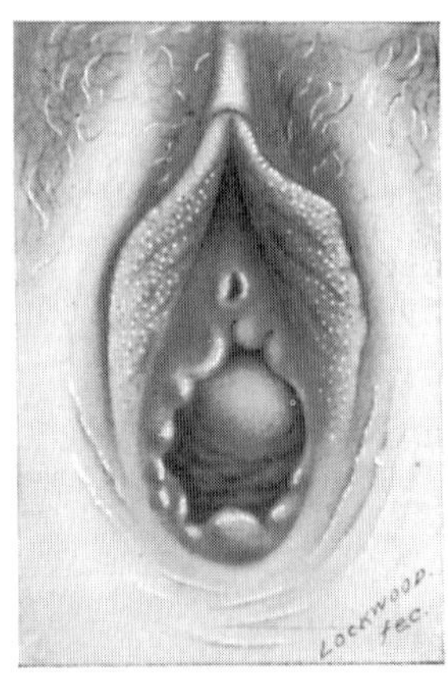

Carunculæ myrtiformes.

SHOWING SEVERAL VARIETIES OF HYMEN.

In the matter of elasticity again, wide variations are met with, some hymens being so delicate that they rupture upon the slightest touch, while others, though capable of considerable distention, still remain unbroken, and later may even regain their original appearance.

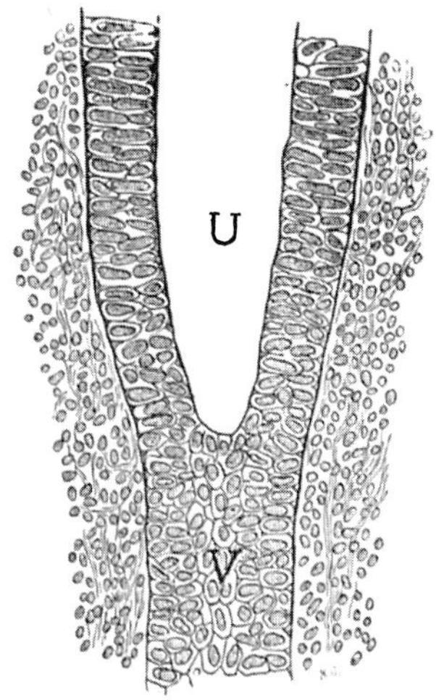

Fig. 31.—Longitudinal Section showing Transition from the Cylindrical Epithelium of the Uterus to the Cuboidal Epithelium of the Vagina.

From a 10-centimetre embryo (Nagel). *U.*, uterus; *V.*, vagina.

As a general rule the hymen ruptures at the first coitus, tearing at several points, usually in its posterior portion. The edges of the tears soon cicatrize, and the hymen becomes permanently divided into two or three portions, which are separated by narrow slits extending down to its base. (Plate II.) The extent to which rupture occurs varies with the structure of the hymen and the degree to which it is distended, being most marked when it is delicately formed.

Although it is generally believed by the laity that its rupture is associated with hæmorrhage, this is by no means always the case, though in rare instances such a profuse loss of blood may occur as to lead to profound anæmia and even death. This idea is probably based upon the biblical statement that loss of virginity is always associated with loss of blood. Nor is it unreasonable to suppose that considerable bleeding usually occured among the Hebrews of the biblical period, inasmuch as the girls married very young, and not infrequently before the age of puberty, so that marked disproportion must often have existed between the size of the male and female organs. On the other hand, it must be remembered that where Western civilization prevails full sexual development has usually been attained before marriage.

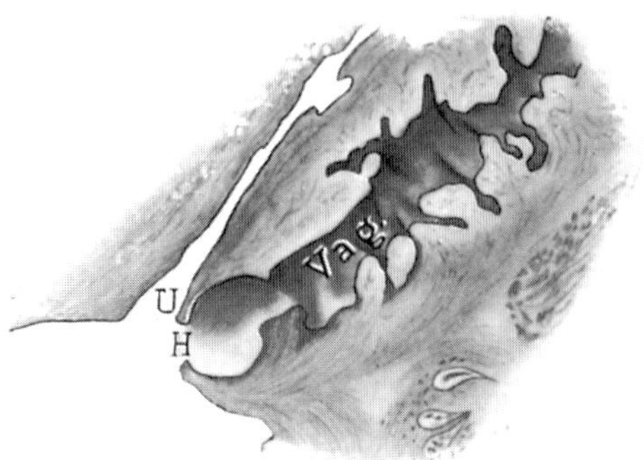

Fig. 32.—Sagittal Section through the Lower Portion of the Vagina of a 14-Centimetre Embryo (Nagel).

U., urethra; *H.*, hymen; *Vag.*, vagina.

In rare instances the membrane may be very resistant and surgical interference be required before coitus can be accomplished. Obertaufer, in 1802, reported a case in which the hymen was so tough that it creaked under the knife. Occasionally, instead of giving way in the middle, it may be torn loose from its base in the attempt at coitus, while in other cases the penis may dilate the urethral canal instead of entering the vagina. Neugebauer has lately collected an interesting series of injuries occurring during coitus, many of which were due to the presence of a very resistant hymen.

The changes in the hymen following coitus are often of medico-legal interest, as the physician is occasionally called upon to testify as to the virginity of an individual. Unfortunately, however, it is not always possible to arrive at a decisive conclusion as to this point. In occasional instances the hymen may be destroyed in early childhood, either as the result of masturbation or as a consequence of attempting to get rid of seat-worms. Among certain Eastern races, again, it is ruptured in early childhood for purposes of cleanliness. On the other hand, the hymen may not be torn, despite repeated coitus; whereas, in other instances, the denticulate or fimbriated type may be mistaken for a hymen which has been ruptured. Haberda, the Professor of Legal Medicine in Vienna, lately stated that he was able to make a positive diagnosis of loss of virginity in only about 50 per cent of the medico-legal cases which he had examined in the last five years. He believes that in many instances it is impossible to determine whether coitus has taken place or not, unless the individual is seen immediately after the attempt, before the torn surfaces have had an opportunity to unite. Achenbach, in a recent dissertation, collected 25 instances of pregnancy occurring in women with unruptured hymens; while Kanony has collected 43 similar reports from the literature. Some years ago I saw a case in which conception had occurred through an elastic hymen which presented only a pin-point opening.

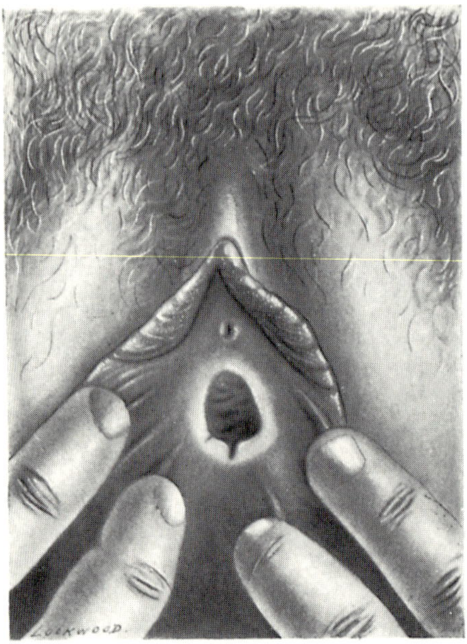

Fig. 33.—Almost Unruptured Hymen after Childbirth (Budin).

The changes produced by childbirth are much more marked than those following coitus, and, as a rule, are readily recognised. As the result of the distention incident to the birth of the child, the hymen undergoes pressure necrosis in various places, and after the puerperium the remnants are represented by a number of cicatrized nodules of varying size—the *carunculæ myrtiformes* (Plate II). Their significance was first emphasized by Schroeder. Practically speaking, they are infallible signs of previous childbearing, as they can be produced only by marked distention and long-continued pressure. In rare instances the injuries resulting from childbirth are extremely slight, and very exceptionally are entirely lacking. Such cases have been reported by Hyerneaux, Tolberg, Hyrtl, and Budin. Fig. 33 shows the external organs of one of Budin's patients who had given birth to a full-term child.

LITERATURE

ACHENBACH. 25 Fälle von Schwangerschaft und Geburt bei undurchbohrtem Hymen. D. I., Marburg, 1890.

BUDIN. Recherches sur l'hymen et l'orifice vaginale. Le Progrès Médical, août, 1879.

Description d'un cas dans lequel l'accouchement n'a déterminé, chez une primipare, que de légères fissures de l'orifice hyménal. Femmes en couches et Nouveau-nés, Paris, 1897, 1–4.

CARRARD. Beitrag zur Anatomie und Pathologie der kleinen Labien. Zeitschr. f. Geb. u. Gyn., x, 62–93, 1884.

CULLINGWORTH. A Note on the Anatomy of the Hymen and on that of the Posterior Commissure of the Vulva. Journal of Anat. and Physiol., xxvii, April, 1893.

DOHRN. Die Bildungsfehler des Hymens. Zeitschr. f. Geb. u. Gyn., xi, 1–19, 1885.

GUSSENBAUER. Ueber das Gefässsystem der aüsseren weiblichen Genitalien. Sitzungsbericht der k. k. Akad. der Wissenschaften, Wien, lx, 1869.

HABERDA. Ueber den anat. Beweis der erfolgten Defloration. Monatsschr. f. Geb. u. Gyn., xi, 69–88, 1900.

KANONY. De la fréquence des cas de persistance de l'hymen et de leur importance en médicine légale. Thèse de Montpellier, 1899.

KOBELT. Die männliche und weibliche Wollustorgane. Freiburg, 1844.

KOCKS. Ueber die Gärtner'schen Gänge beim Weibe. Archiv f. Gyn., xx, 487–492, 1882.

KRAUSE. Die Nervenendigung innerhalb der terminalen Körperchen. Archiv f. mikr. Anatomie, xix, 1881.

NAGEL. Die weiblichen Geschlechtsorgane, Bardeleben's Handbuch der Anatomie, 1896.

Ueber die Entwickelung des Uterus und der Vagina beim Menschen. Archiv f. mikr. Anat., Bd. XXXVII.

NEUGEBAUER. Ein Beitrag zur Lehre von den Verletzungen der weiblichen Sexualorgane sub coitu. Mit Kasuistik von 157 Beobachtungen. Monatsschr. f. Geb. u. Gyn., ix, 221, 1899.

PLOSS. Das Weib in der Natur und Völkerkunde. IV. Aufl., Bd. I, Leipzig, 1895.

SCHROEDER. The Condition of the Hymen and its Remains after Cohabitation, Childbearing, etc. Trans. Edinburgh Obst. Soc., 1878.

SCHULTZE. Zur forensischen Diagnose des Geschlechts. Jen. Zeitschr. f. Medizin und Naturwissensch., iv, 1868.

SKENE. The Anatomy and Pathology of Two Important Glands of the Female Urethra. Amer. Jour. of Obst., xiii, 265–270, 1880.

WEBSTER. The Nerve-Endings in the Labia Minora and Clitoris. Edinburgh Med. Journal, 1891.

THE VAGINA

The vagina is a musculo-membranous tube which extends from the vulva to the uterus, and is interposed between the bladder and the rectum. It serves three important functions: it represents the excretory duct of the uterus, through which its secretion and the menstrual flow escape; it is the female organ of copulation; and, finally, it forms part of the birth canal at labour. Its course runs almost entirely within the pelvic floor, and it is therefore practically outside of the pelvic cavity. The vaginal canal presents a somewhat S-shaped curvature. The common statement that its course corresponds in direction to that of the pelvic axis is incorrect, since its lower third is parallel to the plane of the superior strait, while its upper portion presents a concavity corresponding to the curve of the rectum.

Anteriorly, the vagina is in contact with the bladder and urethra, from which it is separated by the vesico-vaginal septum. Posteriorly, between its lower portion and the rectum, we have the perinæum and recto-vaginal septum; in its median portion it lies in close apposition with the rectum, while its upper portion is separated from it by Douglas's *cul-de-sac*. In view of these relations, Schauta, for the purposes of description, has divided its anterior wall into two parts—urethral and vesical—and its posterior wall into three—perineal, rectal, and peritoneal respectively. The urethral portion of the vagina is firmly united to the urethra and vesico-vaginal septum, from which it can be separated only with some difficulty; whereas the vesical portion is loosely attached to the bladder and can be readily detached from it.

The anterior and posterior walls of the vagina lie in contact, a slight space intervening between their lateral margins. When not distended the canal presents an H-shaped appearance on transverse section, as was first pointed out by Henle. The vagina is capable of marked distention, as is manifested at childbirth or when one attempts to pack it with gauze. The vagina and uterus meet at an acute angle, with its opening looking forward. The upper end of the vagina ends as a blind vault into which the lower portion of the cervix uteri projects. The vaginal vault, or, as it is usually designated, the *fornix*, for convenience of description, is subdivided into the anterior, posterior, and two lateral fornices. As the vagina is attached higher up upon the posterior than upon the anterior wall of the cervix, the posterior fornix is considerably deeper than the anterior.

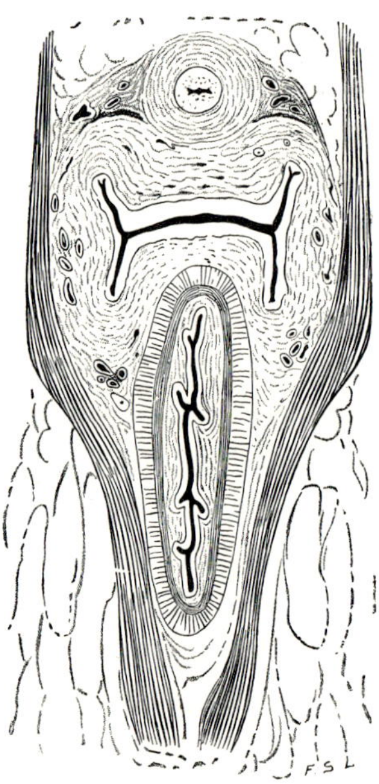

FIG. 34.—H-SHAPED LUMEN OF VAGINA (Henle).

The vagina presents considerable individual variations in length. Since it is united to the uterus at an acute angle, its anterior is always shorter than its posterior wall—6 to 8 or 7 to 10 centimetres respectively. The vagina is relatively longer in the new-born child than in the adult, and according to Luschka forms about $\frac{1}{9}$ of the body length in the former as compared with $\frac{1}{15}$ in the latter (Figs. 24 and 25).

Projecting from the middle line of both the anterior and posterior walls is a prominent longitudinal ridge—the anterior and posterior vaginal columns, the latter not infrequently being divided into two parts by a longitudinal furrow. In women who have not borne children, numerous transverse ridges or *rugæ* extend outward from and almost at right angles to the vaginal columns, gradually fading away as they approach the lateral walls. They give to the surface a corrugated appearance, which is more marked in the early years of life, and gradually becomes obliterated after repeated childbirth, so that in old multiparæ the vaginal walls are often perfectly smooth.

The vaginal wall itself is composed of three layers—the mucous, the muscular, and the connective-tissue layers. The mucosa is covered by numerous layers of stratified epithelium, and closely resembles the skin in structure; but, as its surface is not exposed to the air, the horny layer is absent. The lowest layer of epithelium is distinctly columnar in ap-

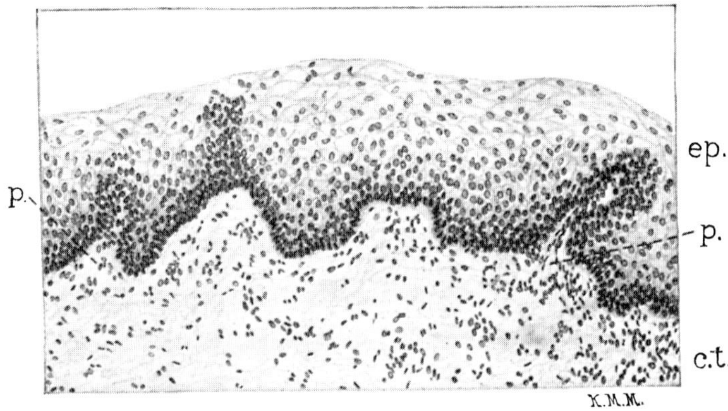

FIG. 35.—VAGINAL MUCOSA. × 90.
ep., epithelium ; *p.*, papilla ; *c.t.*, connective tissue.

pearance, while the cells immediately above it are polygonal in shape, and gradually become more and more flattened as the free surface is approached. Beneath the epithelium is the submucosa, a thin layer of connective tissue, which is tolerably rich in blood-vessels. Offshoots from it extend up into the epithelium and form papillæ, just as in the skin, and scattered here and there through the submucosa are small lymphoid nodules. The mucosa is very loosely attached to the underlying connective tissue, as is manifested by the ease with which it can be peeled off at operations.

According to Eppinger, Nagel, Gebhard, Pretti, and Waldeyer, the vaginal mucosa is absolutely devoid of glands, nor has the writer, in any of the large number of specimens examined, ever encountered them. Hennig and Preuschen, on the other hand, affirm that they are not infrequently present, but the statements of these writers have not been confirmed. It is true that in rare instances Veit and Davidsohn found a few, but the latter considered that they merely represented aberrant cervical glands.

The muscular layer is not very sharply marked, and is usually described as being composed of two layers of non-striated muscle—an outer, longitudinal, and an inner, circular layer. At the lower extremity of the vagina, Luschka described a thin band of voluntary muscle, the constrictor or *sphincter vaginæ*. This can always be found in perineal dissections, but for practical purposes the levator ani muscle is the real closer of the vagina.

Outside of the muscular layer is a layer of connective tissue which serves to connect the vagina with the surrounding parts. It is quite rich in elastic fibres, and contains an abundant venous plexus.

In the non-pregnant condition the vagina is kept moist by a small amount of secretion from the uterus; but in pregnancy a well-marked vaginal secretion is present, which, according to Döderlein and most subsequent observers, normally consists of a dry, thick, white, curdlike material composed of cast-off epithelium and many bacteria, and presents a markedly acid reaction. A great deal of work has been done upon the bacterial flora of the vaginal secretion in pregnancy, and all observers agree that bacillary forms predominate, though cocci are not infrequently seen. The consensus of opinion is that the ordinary pyogenic organisms are never present in the vaginal secretion of healthy pregnant women (Krönig and Williams). The subject will be considered in detail in the chapter on Puerperal Infection.

The vagina possesses an abundant vascular supply, its upper third being supplied by the cervico-vaginal branches of the uterine arteries, its middle third by the inferior vesical arteries, and its lower third by the median hæmorrhoidal and internal pudic arteries. Immediately surrounding the vagina is an abundant venous plexus, the vessels from which follow the course of the arteries and eventually empty into the hypogastric veins.

The distribution of lymphatics has been very accurately studied by Poirier, who found that the lymphatics from the lower third of the vagina empty into the inguinal lymph glands, those from its middle third into the hypogastric, and those from its lower third into the iliac glands.

The vagina is formed by the fusion of the terminal ends of the Müllerian ducts, which, according to Nagel, reach the uro-genital sinus in embryos 2.5 to 3 centimetres long. As has already been said, when considering the development of the hymen, the vagina is originally solid, and is made up of a mass of polygonal epithelial cells, its lumen resulting from their degeneration, which commences at about the third month of gestation. (See Fig. 31.)

LITERATURE

Davidsohn. Zur Kenntniss der Scheidendrüsen, etc. Archiv f. Gyn., lxi, 418–433, 1900.

Döderlein. Das Scheidensekret. Leipzig, 1892.

Eppinger. Zeitschr. f. Heilkunde, Bd. III.

Gebhard. Path. Anatomie der weiblichen Sexualorgane. Leipzig, 1899, 494.

Henle. Eingeweidelehre des Menschen. Braunschweig, 1873.

Krönig und Menge. Bakteriologie des weiblichen Genitalkanales. Leipzig, 1897.

Luschka. Die Anatomie des menschlichen Beckens. Tübingen, 1861.

Nagel. Die weiblichen Geschlechtsorgane. (Bardeleben's Handbuch der Anatomie.) Jena, 1896.

Poirier. Lymphatiques des organes génitaux de la femme. Paris, 1890.

Pretti. Beitrag zur histologischen Veränderungen der Scheide. Zeitschr. f. Geb. u. Gyn., xxxviii, 250–269, 1898.

Von Preuschen. Virchow's Archiv, lxx.

Schauta. Lehrbuch der gesammten Gynäkologie. Leipzig u. Wien, 1896, 51.

Veit. Cysten der Scheide. Handbuch der Gyn., i, 341, 1897.

WALDEYER und JOESSEL. Lehrbuch der topographisch-chirurg. Anatomie, II. Theil, 819. Bonn, 1899.

WILLIAMS, J. WHITRIDGE. The Bacteria of the Vagina and their Practical Significance. Amer. Jour. of Obst., xxxviii, 449–483, 1898.

INTERNAL GENERATIVE ORGANS

The Non-pregnant Uterus.—The uterus is a muscular structure, partially covered by peritonæum, and presents a small cavity lined by mucous membrane. It is the organ of menstruation, and during pregnancy serves for the reception, retention, and nutrition of the ovum, which it expels at the time of labour by its contractions.

The uterus is situated in the pelvic cavity between the bladder and rectum, its inferior extremity projecting into the vagina. Almost its entire posterior wall is covered by peritonæum, the lower portion of which

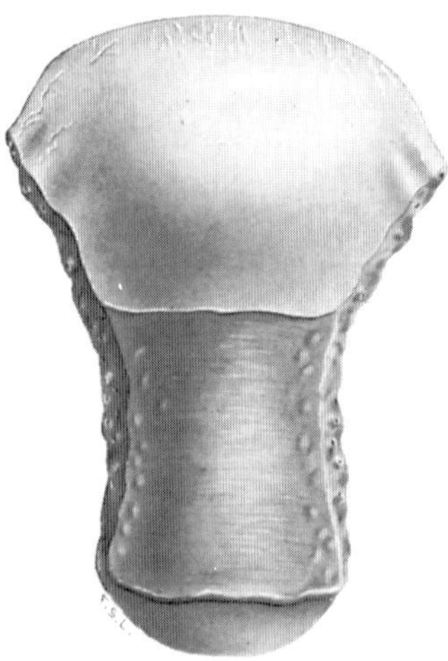

FIG. 36.—ANTERIOR ASPECT OF UTERUS. × 1.

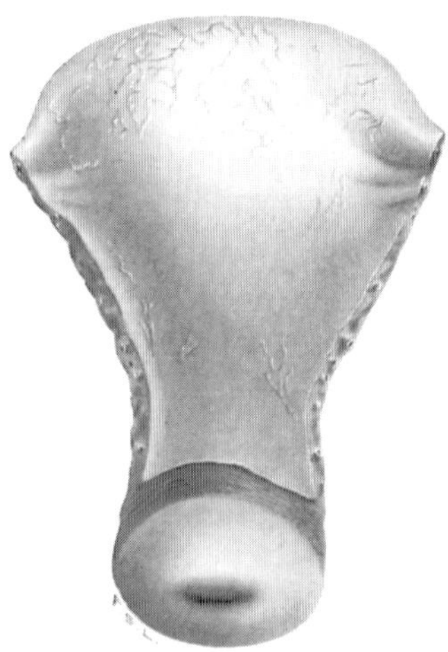

FIG. 37.—POSTERIOR ASPECT OF UTERUS. × 1.

forms the anterior boundary of Douglas's *cul-de-sac*; while only the upper portion of the anterior wall is so covered, its lower portion being united to the posterior wall of the bladder by a tolerably thick layer of connective tissue.

Roughly speaking, the uterus resembles a flattened pear in appearance, and consists of two unequal parts: an upper triangular portion—the *corpus*—and a lower, cylindrical, or fusiform portion—the *cervix*. The anterior surface of the corpus is almost flat, while its posterior surface is markedly convex. In view of the fact that the former, which looks downward and forward, rests upon the bladder, while the latter is in contact with the intestines, His has suggested that the surfaces be described as vesical and intestinal, instead of anterior and posterior respectively. The Fallopian tubes come off from the *cornua* of the uterus—i. e., at the junction of the superior and lateral margins on either side—the convex upper margin between their points of insertion being known as the *fundus uteri*.

The lateral margins extend from the insertion of the Fallopian tubes on either side to the pelvic floor. They are not covered by peritonæum, but receive the attachments of the broad ligaments.

The uterus presents marked variations in size and shape, according to the age of the individual, and whether or not she has borne children. The infantile organ varies from 2.5 to 3 centimetres in length; that of adult virgins measures from 5.5 to 8, 3.5 to 4, and 2 to 2.5 centimetres in its greatest vertical, transverse, and antero-posterior diameters respectively, as compared with 9 to 9.5, 5.5 to 6, and 3 to 3.5 centimetres in multiparous women. Virginal and parous uteri also differ considerably in weight, the former ranging from 40 to 50, and the latter from 60 to 70 grammes. The relation between the length of the corpus and that of the cervix likewise varies widely. In the young child the former is only half as long as the cervix; in young virgins the two are of equal length, or the corpus may be slightly longer. In multiparous women, on the other hand, the relation is reversed, and the cervix represents only a little more than $\frac{1}{3}$ of the total length of the organ.

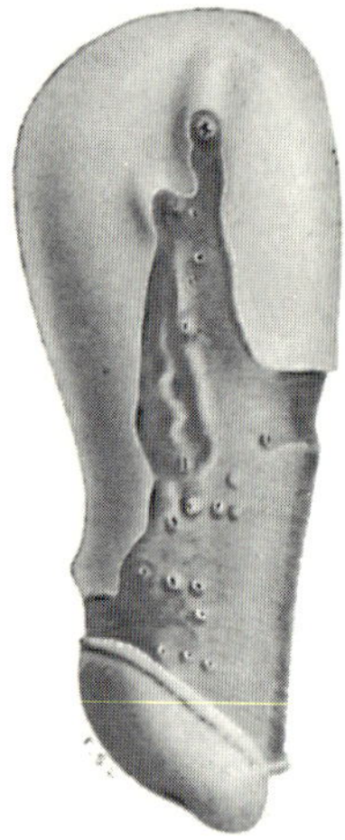

FIG. 38.—LATERAL ASPECT OF UTERUS, SHOWING SUPRAVAGINAL AND INFRAVAGINAL PORTIONS OF CERVIX AND ARRANGEMENT OF PERITONEAL COVERING. ×1.

On sagittal section it is seen that the great bulk of the uterus is made up of muscular tissue, and that the anterior and posterior walls of its body lie almost in contact, the cavity between them appearing as a mere slit, while that of the cervix is fusiform in shape with a small opening above and below—the internal and the external os.

On frontal section the cavity of the body of the uterus presents a triangular appearance, while that of the cervix retains its fusiform shape. After childbearing, the triangular appearance becomes less marked, and its margins become concave instead of convex, as in the vaginal condition.

Cervix Uteri.—The cervix is the portion of the uterus which lies below the internal os. Anteriorly its upper boundary is indicated by the point at which the peritonæum is reflected from the uterus on to the bladder.

It is divided, by the attachment of the vagina, into two parts: the supravaginal and infravaginal portions of the cervix. The former is covered on its posterior surface by peritonæum, while its lateral and anterior surfaces are in contact with connective tissue of the broad ligaments and bladder.

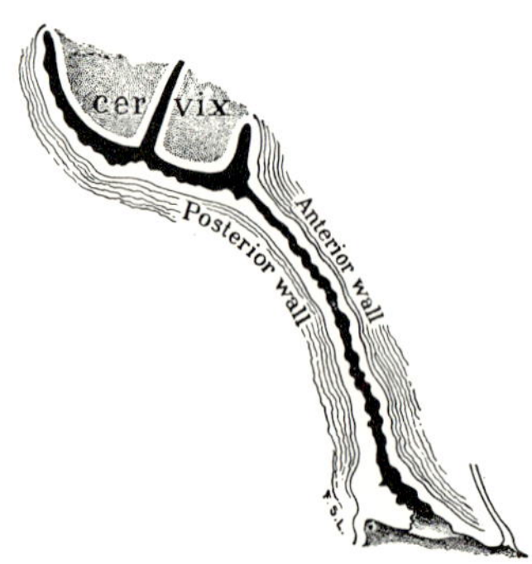

FIG. 39.—SHOWING JUNCTION OF VAGINA AND CERVIX (Skene).

The infravaginal portion of the cervix, which is usually designated as the *portio vaginalis*, projects into the vaginal fornix, and at its tip presents a small transverse opening, the *external os,* bounded in front and behind by the so-called anterior and posterior lips of the cervix. Owing to the fact that the posterior fornix is deeper than the anterior, the posterior lip appears longer than the anterior.

The external os may vary greatly in appearance. In the virgin it is a small, oval opening resembling a tench's mouth, whence the name, *os tincæ.* On vaginal examination it gives a sensation similar to that obtained on feeling the cartilage at the end of one's nose. After childbirth the orifice becomes converted into a transverse slit, and when the cervix has been markedly torn during labour, it may present an irregular nodular or stellate appearance. These changes are very characteristic, and enable one to assert with tolerable accuracy whether a woman has borne children or not (Figs. 43 and 44).

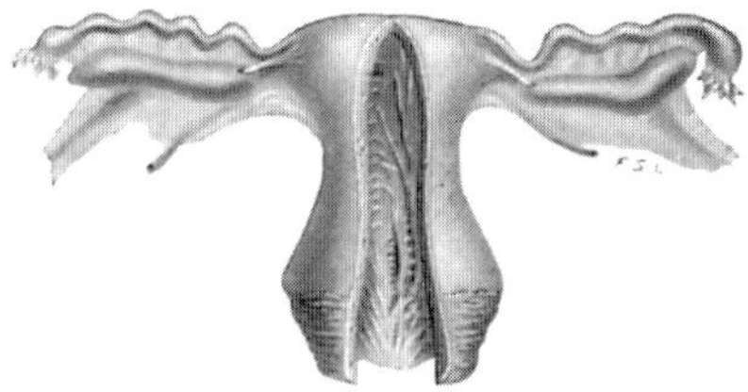

FIG. 40.—UTERUS AND APPENDAGES OF YOUNG CHILD. $\times \frac{2}{3}$.

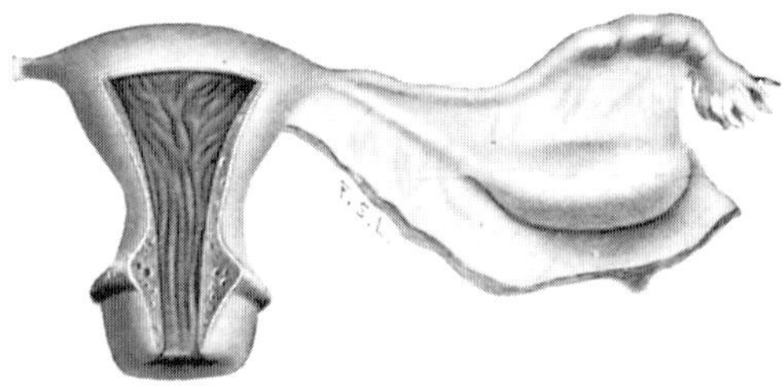

FIG. 41.—UTERUS AND APPENDAGES OF FOURTEEN-YEAR-OLD GIRL. $\times \frac{2}{3}$.

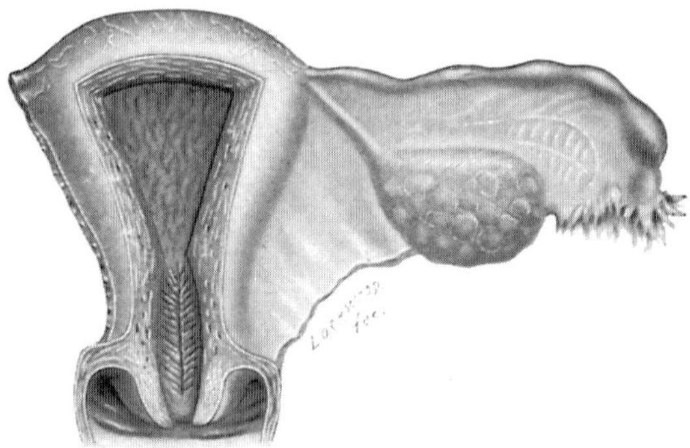

FIG. 42.—UTERUS AND APPENDAGES OF TWENTY-YEAR-OLD MULTIPARA. $\times \frac{2}{3}$.

The cervix is composed of connective tissue in which are many nonstriated muscle fibres and a certain amount of elastic tissue, a large part of its distensibility being due to the presence of the latter. The cervical canal, as has already been said, is fusiform in shape, and presents a longitudinal ridge upon its anterior and posterior surfaces, from which numerous others run off transversely, giving the membrane a corrugated appearance—the *arbor vitæ uterina* or *plicæ palmatæ.*

In the adult the arbor vitæ is limited to the cervical canal; but in childhood it extends throughout the entire cavity of the uterus, from which it begins to disappear as puberty is approached. In time, after repeated childbirths, it gradually becomes obliterated, even in the cervical canal, whose walls become almost smooth (see Figs. 40 to 42).

The mucosa of the cervical canal, embryologically speaking, is a direct continuation of the lining of the uterine cavity, but has become differentiated from it and possesses a characteristic appearance, so that sections through the canal present a honeycomb-like structure (Fig. 45). The mucosa is composed of a single layer of very high and narrow columnar epithelium, which rests upon a thin basement membrane. The oval nuclei are situated near the base of the columnar cells, the upper portions of which present a clear, more or less transparent appearance due to the presence of mucus. It is usually stated that these cells are abundantly supplied with cilia.

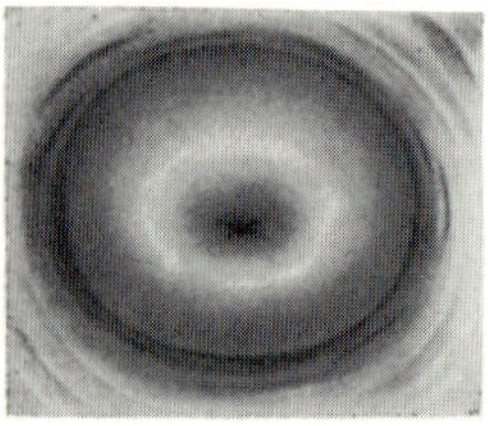

Fig. 43.—Virginal External Os.

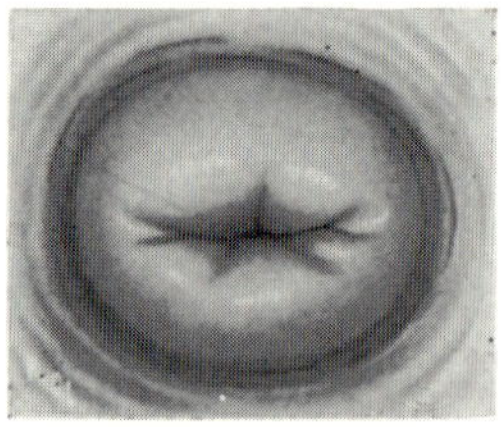

Fig. 44.—Parous External Os.

The cervical glands extend down from the surface of the mucosa into the stroma. They are of the branching, racemose variety, and are merely reduplications of the surface epithelium, being lined by epithelium of the same character. Friedländer was the first to demonstrate that it was made up of true "beaker" or mucous cells, which furnish the thick, tenacious secretion of the cervical canal. There is no submucosa in the cervix, the mucosa resting directly upon the underlying tissue.

The mucosa of the vaginal portion of the cervix is directly continuous with that of the vagina, and, like it, consists of many layers of stratified epithelium. Normally, there are no glands beneath it, but occasionally those from the cervical canal may extend down almost to its surface, and if their ducts are occluded, may become converted into retention cysts, which shimmer through it and appear as rounded protuberances the size of small peas. These are the so-called Nabothian follicles or *ovula Nabothi*.

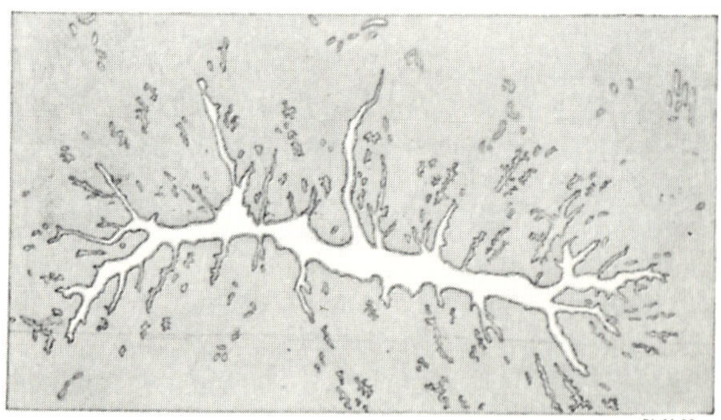

Fig. 45.—Cross-section through Cervical Canal. × 6.

Normally, the stratified epithelium of the vaginal portion and the cylindrical epithelium of the cervical canal meet at the external os. This, however, is the case only in early life, as in older persons the stratified epithelium gradually extends up the cervical canal until its lower third, and occasionally its lower half, is covered by it (Friedländer). This change is more especially marked in multiparous women, in whom the lips of the cervix are not infrequently markedly everted; and occasionally in cases of this character, almost the entire cervical canal may be lined by stratified epithelium.

In rare instances the junction of the two varieties of epithelium may be upon the vaginal portion, outside the external os. This condition was first described by Fischel, who designated it as *congenital ectropion,* and stated that he had observed it in 10 out of 28 uteri of young persons which he had examined. Still more rarely, the entire vaginal portion may be covered by cylindrical epithelium, which may even extend down over the vaginal walls. This anomaly was first described by Ruge in a case of imperforate hymen, associated with *hæmato-kolpos,* in which the entire vagina and the inner surface of the hymen were covered by a single layer of columnar, ciliated epithelium.

Corpus Uteri.—The wall of the uterine body is made up of three layers: serous, muscular, and mucous. The serous layer is formed by the peritonæum covering the uterus, to which it is firmly adherent except at the margins, where it is deflected to the broad ligaments.

Endometrium.—The innermost or mucous layer, which serves as a lining for the uterine cavity, is commonly known as the endometrium. It is a thin, pinkish, velvety membrane, which on close examination is seen to be perforated by large numbers of minute openings—the mouths of the uterine glands. On account of the constant changes to which it is subject during the sexual life of woman, the endometrium varies markedly in thickness, and may measure anywhere from 0.5 to 2 or 3 millimetres without being necessarily abnormal. It consists of a surface epithelium, glands, and interglandular tissue, in which are found numerous blood-vessels and lymphatic spaces.

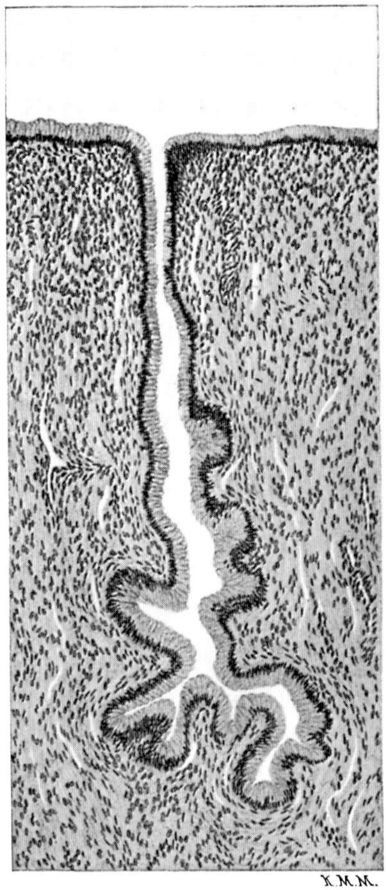

FIG. 46.—CERVICAL GLAND. × 90.

As the endometrium does not possess a submucosa, it is attached directly to the underlying muscular layer in such a manner that its outer boundary presents irregularities in outline corresponding with the interstices between the muscle bundles. This arrangement is of considerable importance in connection with the operation of curettage; for, as Düvelius and Werth have shown, it is from the portions included between the muscle bundles that the endometrium is regenerated after the procedure.

The surface epithelium of the uterine mucosa is composed of a single layer of high columnar ciliated cells, which are closely packed together. The oval nuclei are situated in the lower portions of the cells, but not so near their bases as in the cervix. Beneath the epithelium is a thin basement membrane with narrow, spindle-shaped nuclei.

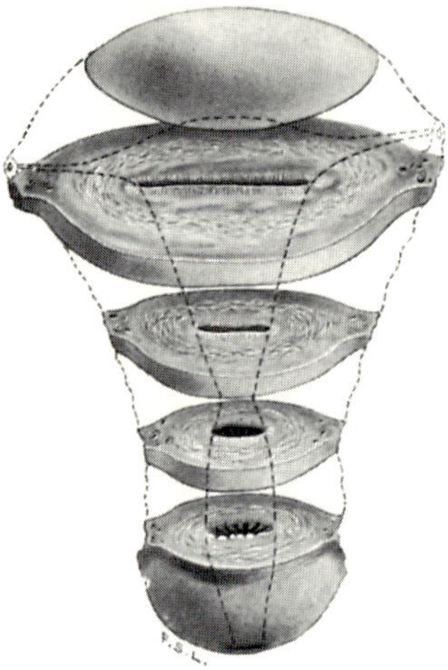

Fig. 47.—Reconstruction of Uterus, showing Shape of Uterine Cavity and Cervical Canal. × 1.

The existence of *cilia* was first demonstrated by Nylander in the sow, but they have since been found in nearly all animals. Although Wyder stated that they were not present in the new-born child, the recent researches of Meyer show that they are demonstrable at variable periods, being sometimes present at birth, but sometimes not appearing until much later. They persist throughout the entire period of sexual activity, and, according to Parviainen, disappear eight or ten years after the menopause.

Up to 1893, it was generally taught that the current produced by them was directed from below upward—namely, from the cervix towards the fundus; but Hofmeier conclusively demonstrated that it is in the opposite direction, and his researches have since been confirmed

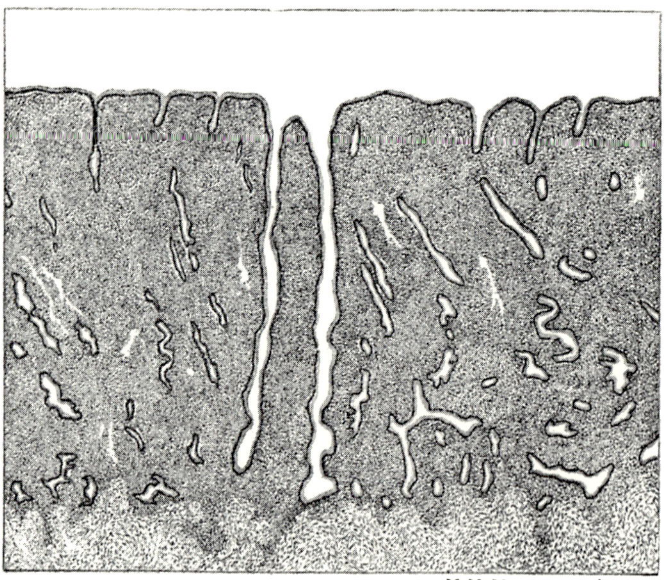

K. M. Montague, fec.

Fig. 48.—Normal Endometrium. × 16.

by Mandl. It may therefore be considered as a definitely established fact that the ciliary current in both the tubes and the uterus is in the same direction, and extends downward from the fimbriated end of the tubes to the external os.

In very exceptional instances, the uterine cavity may be lined by stratified epithelium, as in the cases reported by Zeller and F. Friedländer.

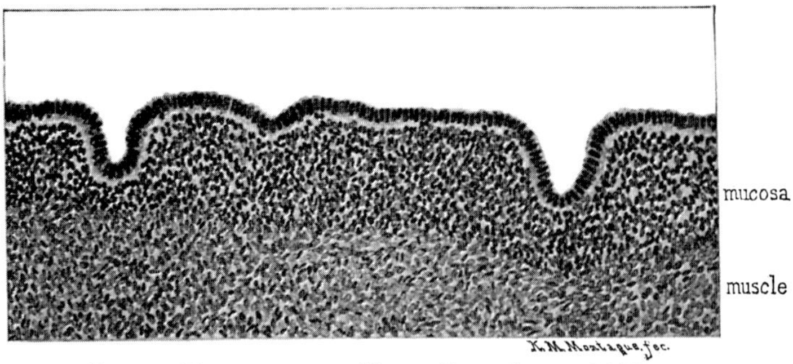

FIG. 49.—ENDOMETRIUM OF NEWLY BORN CHILD. × 150.

Such a condition readily explains the possible occurrence of flat-celled carcinoma of the body of the uterus.

Projecting down from the surface of the endometrium are large numbers of small tubular glands—the *uterine glands.* These must be regarded as mere invaginations of the surface epithelium and resemble the fingers of a glove, though occasionally they branch slightly at their deeper ex-

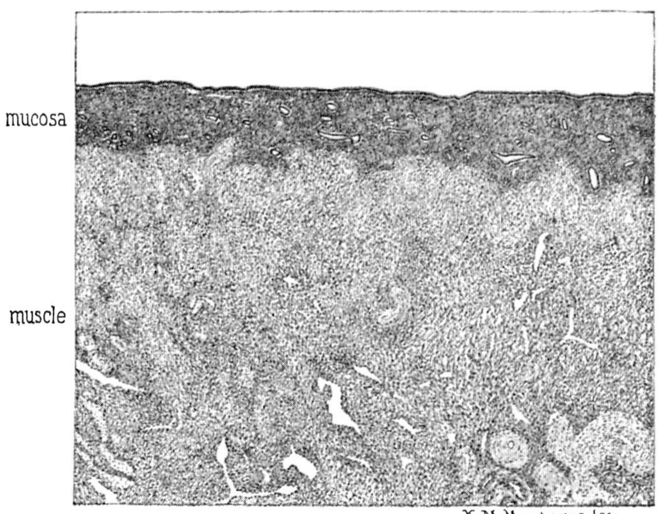

FIG. 50.—SENILE ENDOMETRIUM. × 17.

tremities. They extend through the entire thickness of the endometrium to the muscular layer, which they occasionally penetrate for a short distance. They present the same histological structure as the surface epithelium, and are lined by a single layer of high, columnar, ciliated epithelium, which rests upon a thin basement membrane. They secrete small quantities of a thin, alkaline secretion, which serves to keep the uterine cavity moist.

In studying microscopic sections, it must be remembered that the glands are not always cut vertically, and that their appearance will vary according to the direction of the section. Thus, they not infrequently appear as round or oval openings, and when hypertrophied may present a corkscrew-like appearance.

In the child the uterine glands are mere shallow depressions, which, according to Kundrat and Engelman, do not appear until the third year; but the researches of Meyer, which are confirmed by my own studies, show that they are not infrequently present at birth. At the menopause the en-

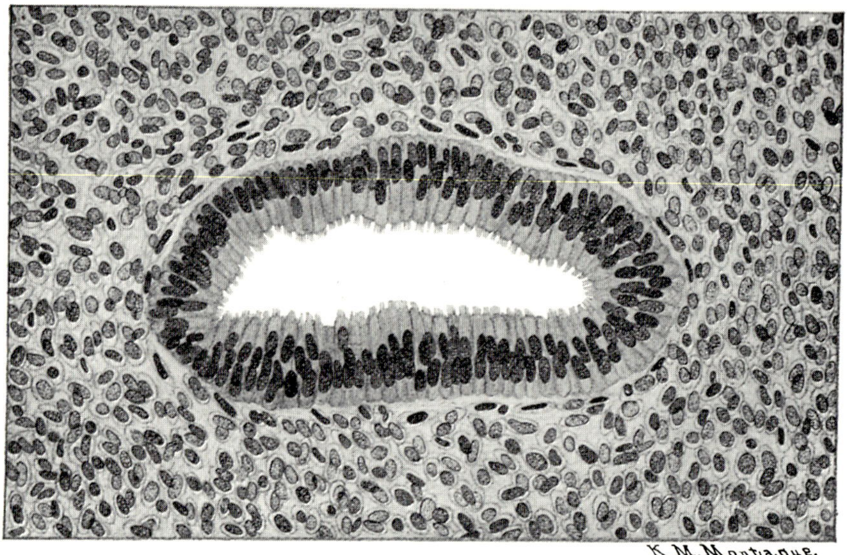

FIG. 51.—UTERINE GLAND AND STROMA. × 420.

tire endometrium undergoes atrophic changes; its epithelium becomes flatter, its glands gradually disappear, and its interglandular tissue takes on a more fibrous appearance (see Fig. 50).

The portion of the endometrium lying between the surface epithelium and the underlying muscle, which is not occupied by glands, is filled by an *interglandular tissue* or stroma of an embryonic type. Under the microscope (Figs. 48 and 51) it is seen to be made up of closely packed oval and spindle-shaped nuclei, around which there is very little protoplasm. When the tissues are spread apart by œdema, it is readily seen that the cells present a stellate appearance, with branching protoplasmic processes which anastomose one with another. These cells are more closely packed around the glands and blood-vessels than elsewhere. Occasionally larger or smaller collections of round cells may be seen between them, though it is uncertain whether or not these are to be regarded as *lymphoid nodules.*

The exact nature of the interglandular tissue has given rise to a great deal of discussion, concerning which the authorities are not yet fully agreed. Minot looks upon it as nothing but embryonic tissue, while Nagel sees in it a resemblance to lymphoid tissue, and Arthur W. Johnstone holds that it is of an adenoid type. On the other hand, Leopold, Championnière, Poirier, and others consider that it represents a lymphatic surface. According to Leopold, the " uterine mucosa should be considered as a spread-out lymph-gland (Lymphdrüsenfläche), which does not contain true lymph vessels, but consists of spaces lined by endometrium." There is a certain amount of evidence in support of all of these views, but I am inclined to agree with Minot in considering it as merely an embryonic type of connective tissue.

When preparations from the endometrium are treated by appropriate methods, an abundant reticulum can be demonstrated throughout its entire extent, which forms the scaffolding upon which it is constructed.

The endometrium contains many blood-vessels. The arteries pursue a spiral course and break up into a capillary network just beneath the surface epithelium, from which the blood is returned by a few comparatively large vessels.

Musculature of the Uterus — Myometrium. — The major part of the uterus is made up of bundles of non-striated muscle, which are united by a greater or lesser amount of connective tissue, in which are found many elastic fibres (Pick). On section the uterine wall presents a thick, felt-like structure, in which definite layers cannot be distinguished.

A great deal of work has been done upon the arrangement of the musculature both of the pregnant and non-pregnant uterus. Tarnier and Ribemont-Dessaignes were unable to make out definite layers of muscle bundles in the non-pregnant organ, while Bayer, Kreitzer, Veit, and others distinguished several, but did not agree as to their arrangement. All admit, however, that the greater part of the uterine wall is made up of a mass of muscle which is perforated in all directions by blood-vessels, and in which it is impossible to make out any definite arrangement of the bundles—*stratum vasculare.*

Roesger studied the question from a developmental point of view, and demonstrated that the muscle fibres are developed along the course of the blood-vessels, but failed to distinguish any definite arrangement. Similar studies by Werth and Grusdew go to show that the musculature of the fœtal and infantile uterus presents a very simple arrangement, which becomes much more complicated as puberty is approached. During gestation, on the other hand, the uterus undergoes marked hypertrophy, when it becomes possible to distinguish certain distinct layers which will be considered in the chapter on the changes incident to pregnancy.

Ligaments of the Uterus.—Extending from either half of the uterus are three ligamentous structures—the broad, round, and utero-sacral ligaments (ligamenta lata, teretia, and utero-sacralia).

The broad ligaments, or *ligamenta lata,* are two wing-like structures which extend from the lateral margins of the uterus to the pelvic walls, and serve to divide the pelvic cavity into an anterior and a posterior compartment. Each broad ligament consists of a fold of peritonæum inclosing various structures within it, and presents four margins for examination—a superior, lateral, inferior, and median. The superior margin, for its inner two thirds, is occupied by the Fallopian tube, while its outer third, extending from the fimbriated end of the tube to the pelvic wall, is known as the *infundibulo-pelvic ligament*—the suspensory ligament of the ovary (Henle)—and serves to transmit the ovarian vessels. The portion of the broad ligament beneath the Fallopian tube is called the *mesosalpinx,* and consists of two layers of peritonæum which are united by a small amount of loose connective tissue, in which is embedded the *parovarium* or organ of Rosenmüller (see Fig. 41).

At its lateral margin, the peritoneal covering of the broad ligament is reflected upon the side of the pelvis. The inferior margin, which is quite thick, is continuous with the connective tissue of the pelvic floor. Through it pass the uterine vessels. Its lower portion—the cardinal ligament of Kocks or the *ligamentum transversale colli* of Mackenrodt—is composed of dense connective tissue which is firmly united to the supravaginal portion of the cervix. The median margin is connected with the lateral margin of the uterus, and incloses the uterine vessels; through it certain muscular and connective tissue bands extend from the uterus into the broad ligament.

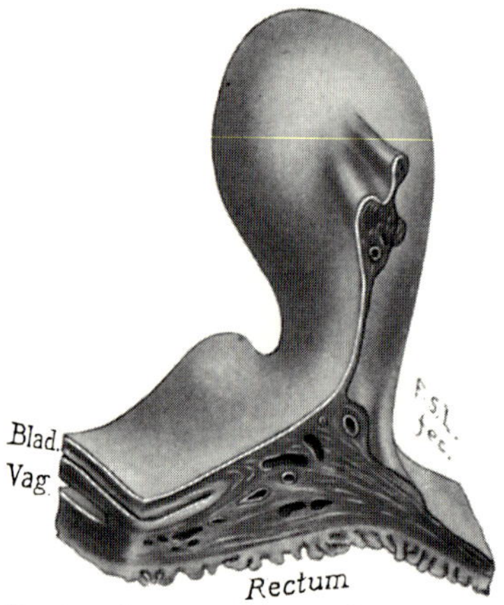

Fig. 52.—Section through Uterine End of Broad Ligament. $\times \frac{2}{3}$.

A vertical section through the uterine end of the broad ligament is triangular in shape, with the apex directed upward, while its base is broad and contains the uterine vessels; it is widely connected with the connective tissue covering the pelvic floor and lying behind the bladder, which is designated as the *parametrium.* A vertical section through the middle portion of the broad ligament shows that its upper part is made up mainly of three branches in which the tube, ovary, and round ligament are situated, while its lower portion is not so thick as in the previous section.

The *round ligament,* or *ligamentum teres,* extends from the anterior and lateral portions of the uterus, just below the insertion of the tubes. It lies in a fold of the broad ligament and runs in an upward and outward direction to the inguinal canal, through which it passes, to terminate finally in the upper portion of the labium majus. The round ligament varies from 3 to 5 millimetres in diameter; it is composed of connective tissue and a certain amount of non-striated muscle, which is directly continuous with that of the uterine wall. In the non-pregnant condition it appears as a lax cord, but in pregnancy it undergoes considerable hypertrophy and seems to act as a stay for the uterus. It can be palpated during pregnancy, and by its varying position aids us in diagnosing the location of the placenta.

The *utero-sacral ligaments—retractores uteri* (Luschka)—are two structures which extend from the upper portion of the cervix, encircle the rectum, and are inserted into the fascia covering the second and third sacral vertebræ. They are likewise composed of connective tissue and muscle, and are covered by peritonæum. They form the lateral boundaries of Douglas's *cul-de-sac,* and are believed to play a part in retaining the uterus in its normal position by exerting traction upon the cervix.

Position of the Uterus.—After many years of discussion, anatomists and gynæcologists have agreed that the normal position of the uterus, whether pregnant or not, is one of slight anteflexion. With the woman standing upright, the uterus occupies an almost horizontal position and is somewhat bent upon its vesical surface, the fundus resting upon the posterior surface of the bladder, while the cervix is directed backward towards the sacrum (see Fig. 25). The position of the organ varies markedly according to the degree of distention of the bladder and rectum, but when these are empty the uterus always tends to resume its normal position.

The causes which bring about its anteflexed position have not as yet been definitely determined. Normally, as long as it is *in situ,* the organ is anteflexed, but when removed from the body it immediately straightens out. Schauta would attribute the anteflexion to the action exerted by the vessels when filled with blood, but his explanation does not appear altogether satisfactory. According to Nagel and most embryologists, the anteflexion exists from the earliest stages of development, and is to be accounted for by the fact that the entire body is developed along a curved line. The pressure of the intestines upon the uterus is also believed to play a part, as the light corpus is readily movable; while the comparatively large cervix is held in a fixed position by the small pelvis.

The uterine ligaments were formerly supposed to play an important part in maintaining the uterus in its characteristic position. We have already indicated the functions of the round and utero-sacral ligaments. The upper portion of the broad ligament appears to have no influence upon the position of the uterus, since Mackenrodt has demonstrated that it can be cut through without causing any change in position, which only occurs when its deeper portion—the ligamentum transversale colli—is divided.

Blood-vessels of the Uterus.—The vascular supply of the uterus is derived from two sources: principally from the uterine, and to a lesser extent from the ovarian arteries. The uterine artery is the main branch of the hypogastric, which, after descending for a short distance, enters the base of the broad ligament, crosses the ureter, and makes its way to the side of the uterus. Just before reaching the supravaginal portion of the cervix, it divides into a larger and a smaller branch, the latter—the cervico-vaginal artery—supplying the lower portion of the cervix and the upper portion of the vagina. The main branch turns abruptly upward and extends as a very convoluted vessel along the margin of the uterus, giving off a branch of considerable size to the upper portion of the cervix, and numerous smaller ones, which penetrate the body of the uterus. Just before reaching the tube it divides into three terminal branches—the fundal, tubal, and ovarian—the last of which anastomoses with the terminal branch of the ovarian artery; the second, making its way through the mesosalpinx, supplies the tube, and the fundal branch is distributed to the upper portion of the uterus.

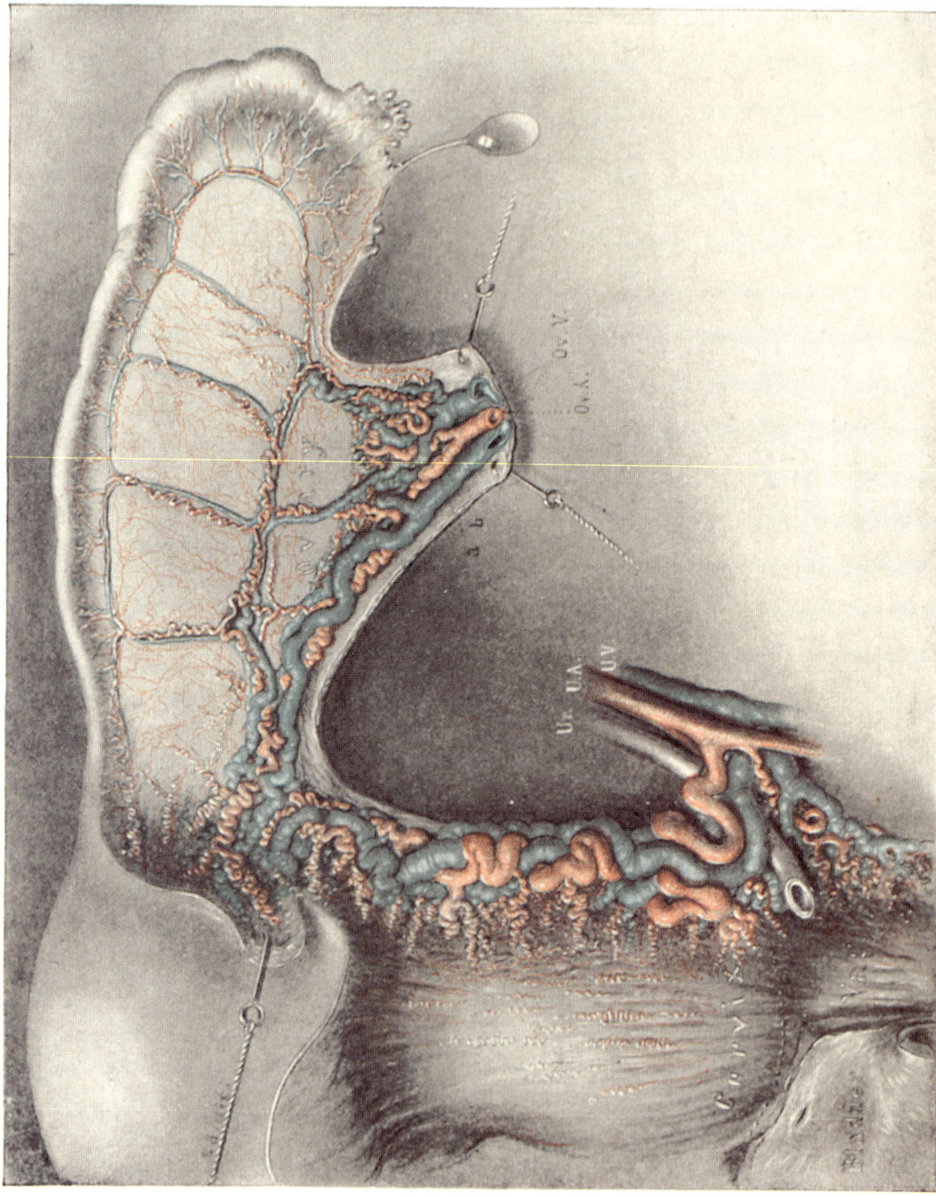

Fig. 53.—Blood Supply of Uterus (Kelly).

The ovarian or internal spermatic artery is a branch of the aorta and enters the broad ligament through the infundibulo-pelvic ligament. On reaching the hilum of the ovary it breaks up into a number of small branches which enter the organ, while its main stem traverses the entire length of the broad ligament and makes its way to the upper portion of the margin of the uterus, where it anastomoses with the ovarian branch of the uterine artery.

It is generally stated that there is very little communication between the vessels on the two sides of the uterus, but the recent experiments of Clark have positively demonstrated that such is not the case. This ob-

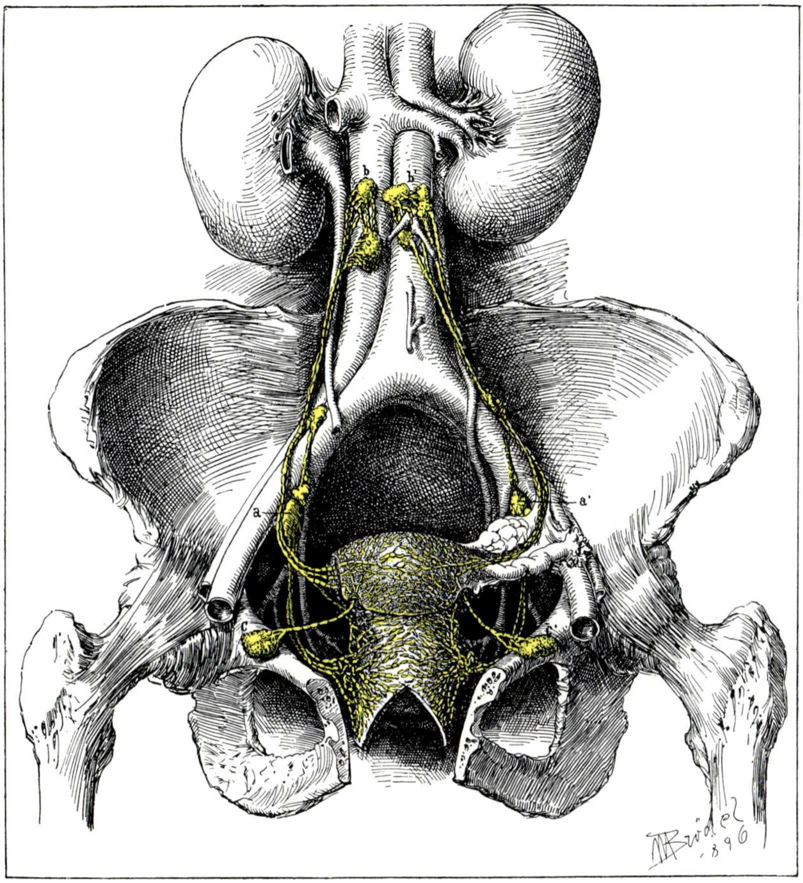

FIG. 54.—LYMPHATICS OF UTERUS (Kelly).

server found that when the uterine artery on one side was injected, the fluid escaped from the opposite uterine artery before it began to flow from the veins, thus indicating the presence of numerous arterial anastomoses in the substance of the uterus.

The veins from the uterus form an abundant plexus around each uterine artery, and unite to form the uterine vein on either side, which then empties into the hypogastric vein, which makes its way into the internal iliac. The blood from the ovary and upper part of the broad ligament is collected by a number of veins, which form a large plexus within the broad ligament—the *pampiniform plexus*—the vessels from which terminate in the ovarian vein. The right ovarian vein empties into the vena cava, while the left empties into the renal vein.

Lymphatics.—The careful work of Leopold, Poirier, Bruhns, and others has given us a fairly definite idea of the lymphatic system of the uterus.

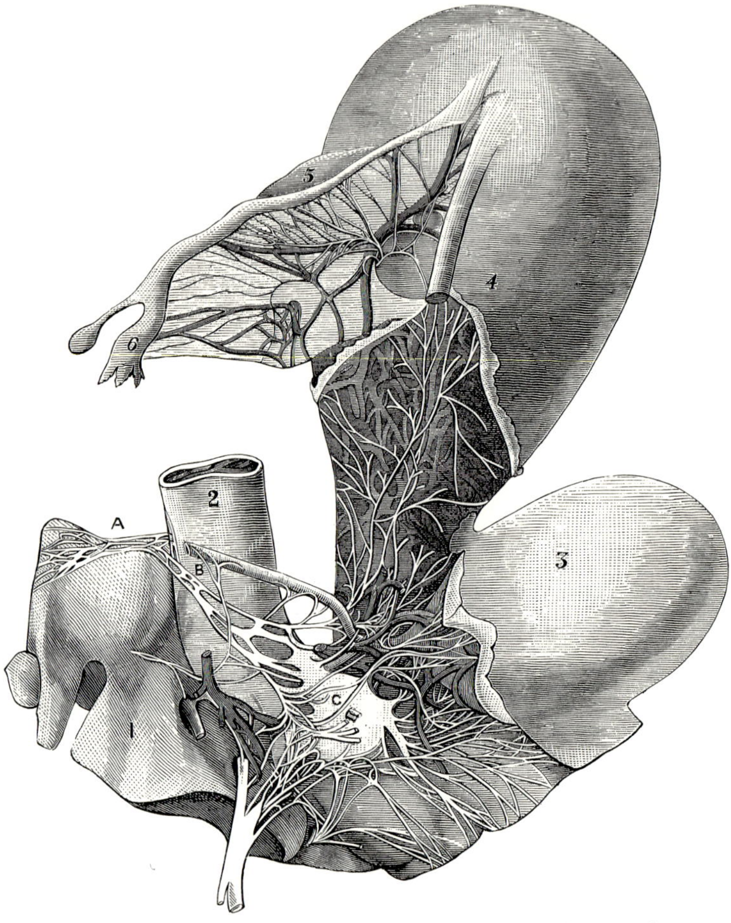

Fig. 55.—Nervous Ganglia of Pregnant Uterus (Frankenhäuser). *A*, plexus uterinus magnus; *B*, plexus hypogastricus; *C*, cervical ganglion.

The endometrium is abundantly supplied with lymph spaces, but possesses no true lymphatic vessels. Immediately beneath it in the muscularis a few lymphatics may be found, which become better defined as the peritonæum is approached, and form an abundant lymphatic plexus just beneath it, which is especially marked on the posterior or intestinal wall of the uterus.

The lymphatics from the various portions of the uterus are connected with several sets of glands—those of the cervix terminating in the hypogastric glands, which are situated in the spaces between the external iliac and hypogastric arteries. The lymphatics from the body of the uterus are distributed to two groups of glands, one set of vessels making their way to the hypogastric glands, while another set, after joining certain lymphatics from the ovarian region, terminate in the lumbar glands, which are situated in front of the aorta at about the level of the lower portion of the kidneys (see Fig. 54).

Innervation.—The nerve supply of the uterus is derived partly from the cerebro-spinal, but principally from the sympathetic nervous system. The cerebro-spinal system is represented by a few fibres from the third and fourth sacral nerves, and Herlizka has lately demonstrated the presence of medullated nerve-fibres in the uterine wall, which showed free endings between the muscle bundles.

The greater portion of the nerve supply, however, is derived from the sympathetic system, and has been studied particularly by Lee, Frankenhaüser, and Rein. According to these authors, large nerve-trunks from the inter-iliac plexus pass down on either side of the rectum, and following the course of the utero-sacral ligaments, terminate in the large *cervical ganglion*. This structure was first discovered by Lee; it lies to the side of and behind the cervix, and from it numerous fibres make their way to the uterus, as is readily seen in Fig. 55.

Herff and Gawronsky have recently described ganglionic cells in the muscularis, and the latter has been able to follow isolated nerve-fibres into the epithelial cells of the endometrium.

Development of the Uterus.—It is universally admitted by embryologists that both the tubes and the uterus are derived from the Müllerian ducts. According to His, the first signs of their development can be noted in embryos having a body length of from 7 to 7.5 millimetres, when a thickening may be noticed in the cœlomic epithelium on the outer margin of each Wolffian body. These gradually become converted into two epithelial ducts, which converge and eventually meet together in the middle line, terminating in the uro-genital sinus.

The Müllerian ducts reach the uro-genital sinus in embryos having a body length of 2.5 to 3.5 centimetres. Their upper ends form the Fallopian tubes, while their lower portions fuse together to form the uterus and vagina. The fusion of the Müllerian ducts is usually completed at about the third month, though the point at which the process is to occur is indicated at a much earlier period by the position of the round ligaments.

LITERATURE

Bayer. Zur physiol. und path. Morphologie der Gebärmutter. Freund's Gynäkologische Klinik, 1885, 369–662.

Bruhns. Ueber die Lymphgefässe der weiblichen Genitalien. Archiv f. Anat. u. Physiol., Anat. Abtheil, 1898, 57.

Championniere. Les lymphatiques utérines. Paris, 1875.

Clark. The Causes and Significance of Uterine Hæmorrhage in Cases of Myoma Uteri. Johns Hopkins Hospital Bulletin, 1899, 11–20.

DÜVELIUS. Zur Kenntniss der Uterusschleimhaut. Zeitschr. f. Geb. u. Gyn., x, 175–187, 1884.

ENGELMAN. The Mucous Membrane of the Uterus. Amer. Jour. Obst., viii, 30–86, 1875.

FISCHEL. Beiträge zur Morphologie der Portio vaginalis uteri. Archiv f. Gyn., xvi, 192–202, 1880.

FRANKENHÄUSER. Die Nerven der Gebärmutter. Jena, 1867.

FRIEDLÄNDER, C. Phys. anat. Untersuchungen über den Uterus. Leipzig, 1870.

FRIEDLÄNDER, F. Abnorme Epithelbildung im kindlichen Uterus. Zeitschr. f. Geb. u. Gyn., xxxviii, 8–16, 1898.

GAWRONSKY. Ueber Verbreitung und Endigung der Nerven in den weiblichen Genitalien. Archiv f. Gyn., xlvii, 271–283, 1894.

HERFF. Ueber das anat. Verhalten der Nerven in dem Uterus, etc. Münch. med. Wochenschr., Nr. 4, 1892.

HERLIZKA. Quoted by Joessel-Waldeyer, Das Becken. Bonn, 1899, 764.

HIS. Die anatomische Nomenclatur. Leipzig, 1895.

HOFMEIER. Zur Kenntniss der normalen Uterusschleimhaut. Centralbl. f. Gyn., 764–766, 1893.

JOHNSTONE. The Menstrual Organ. Brit. Gyn. Jour., November, 1886.

The Function and Patholog of the Reticular Tissue. Amer. Gyn. and Obst. Jour., ix, 166–187, 1896.

KOCKS. Die normale und path. Lage des Uterus, etc. Bonn, 1880.

KREITZER. Anatomische Untersuchungen über die Muskulatur der nicht schwangeren Gebärmutter. Petersburger med. Zeitschrift, 1871, 113.

LEE. The Anatomy of the Nerves of the Uterus. Philosophical Transactions, 1841, 1842, 1846.

LEOPOLD. Die Lymphgefässe des normalen, nicht schwangeren, Uterus. Archiv f. Gyn., vi, 1–55, 1874.

Studien über die Uterusschleimhaut. Berlin, 1878.

LUSCHKA. Die Anatomie des Beckens. Karlsruhe, 1873.

MACKENRODT. Ueber die Ursachen der normalen und path. Lagen des Uterus. Archiv f. Gyn., xlviii, 393-421, 1895.

MANDL. Ueber die Richtung der Flimmerbewegung im menschlichen Uterus. Centralbl. f. Gyn., 1898, 322–328.

MEYER. Ueber die fötale Uterusschleimhaut. Zeitschr. f. Geb. u. Gyn., xxxviii, 234–249, 1898.

MINOT. Human Embryology, 3, 1892.

NAGEL. Die weiblichen Geschlechtsorgane (Bardeleben's Handbuch der Anatomie), Jena, 1896, 87-90.

PARVIAINEN. Zur Kenntniss der senilen Veränderungen der Gebärmutter. Berlin, 1897.

PICK. Ueber das elastische Gewebe in der normalen und path. veränderten Gebärmutter. Volkmann's Sammlung klin. Vorträge, N. F., Nr. 283, 1900.

POIRIER. Lymphatiques des organes génitaux de la femme. Paris, 1890.

REIN. Notes sur le plexus nerveux fondamental de l'utérus. Comptes rendus de la Soc. de Biologie, 1882, 161.

RIBEMONT-DESSAIGNES. Précis d'obstétrique, 30. Paris, 1894.

ROESGER. Zur fötalen Entwickelung des menschlichen Uterus. Festschrift zum 50-jährigen Jubiläum der Gesellsch. f. Geb. u. Gyn. in Berlin, 9–52, 1894.

RUGE. Zur Erosionsfrage. Zeitschr. f. Geb. u. Gyn., vii, 231–233, 1882.

SCHAUTA. Lehrbuch der gesammten Gynäkologie, Wien, 1896, 5–14.

TARNIER. Traité de l'art des accouchements. T. I., 106, Paris, 1888.

VEIT. Uterusmuskulatur. Müller's Handbuch der Geburtshülfe, i, 122–129, 1888.

WERTH. Untersuchungen über die Regeneration der Schleimhaut nach Ausschabung der Uteruskörperhöhle. Archiv f. Gyn., xlix, 369, 370, 1895.

Werth und Grusdew. Untersuchungen über die Entwickelung und Morphologie der menschlichen Uterusmuskulatur. Archiv f. Gyn., lv, 325–413, 1898.

Wyder. Beiträge zur normalen u. path. Histologie der menschlichen Uterusschleimhaut. Archiv f. Gyn., xiii, 1–56, 1878.

Zeller. Plattenepithel im Uterus. Zeitschr. f. Geb. u. Gyn., xi, 56–88, 1885.

THE FALLOPIAN TUBES

The Fallopian or uterine tubes are more or less convoluted muscular canals which extend from the uterine cornua to the ovaries. They are covered by peritonæum and possess a lumen lined by mucous membrane. They represent the excretory ducts of the ovaries, as it is through them that the ova gain access to the uterine cavity. They are more or less cylindrical in shape, and vary from 8 to 14 centimetres in length.

For convenience in description, each tube may be divided into several parts—the uterine portion, isthmus, ampulla, and infundibulum. The uterine portion is included within the muscular wall of the uterus, and extends from the cornu to the upper angle of the uterine cavity. Its lumen is so small that it will admit only the finest probe. The *isthmus* is the narrow portion of the tube immediately adjoining the uterus, and gradually passes into the wider lateral portion or *ampulla*. The *infundibulum*, or fimbriated extremity, is the funnel-shaped opening of the lateral end of the tube, the margins of which present a dentate appearance (see Figs. 39 to 41).

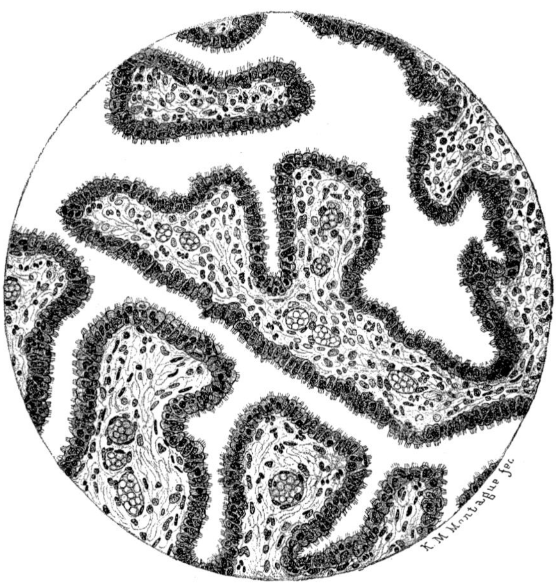

Fig. 56.—Tubal Mucosa. × 280.

The tube varies considerably in thickness, the narrowest portion of the isthmus measuring from 2 to 3 millimetres, and the widest portion of the ampulla from 5 to 7 or 8 millimetres in diameter.

With the exception of its uterine portion, the tube, throughout its entire length, is included within the upper margin of the broad ligament; it is completely surrounded by peritonæum except at its lower portion, corresponding to the mesosalpinx. The fimbriated extremity opens freely into the abdominal cavity, and one of its fimbriæ—the *fimbria ovarica*—which is considerably longer than the others, forms a shallow gutter which extends almost or quite to the ovary.

Generally speaking, the musculature of the tube is arranged in two layers—an inner, circular, and an outer, longitudinal layer. In its uterine

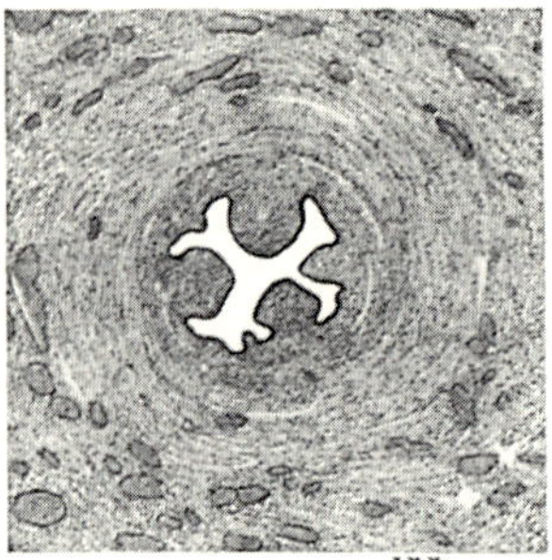

Fig. 57.

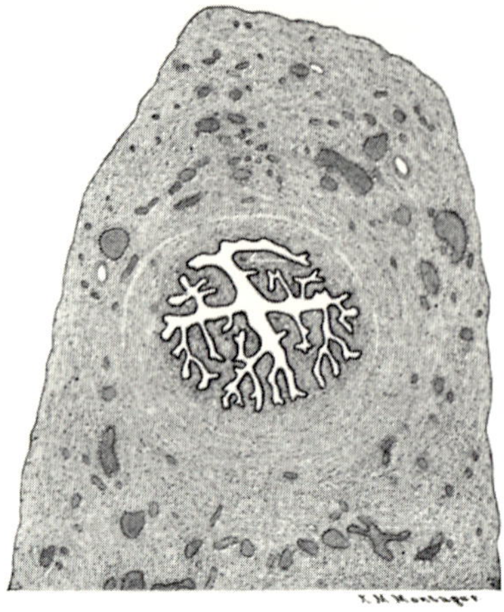

Fig. 58.

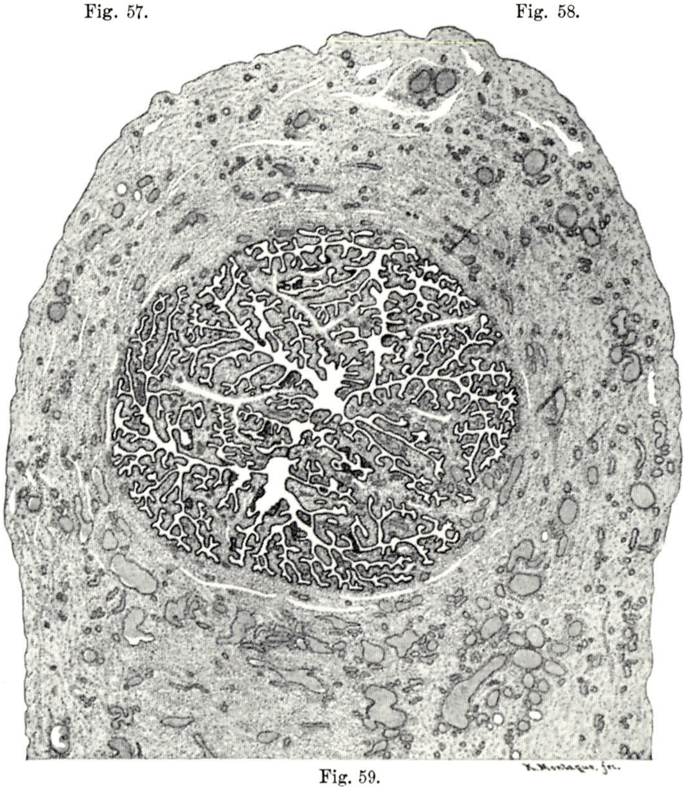

Fig. 59.

Figs. 57–59.—Sections through Uterine, Isthmic, and Ampullar Portions of Tube. × 15.

portion a third layer, lying between the circular layer and the mucosa, and composed of longitudinal fibres, may be distinguished. In the lateral portion of the tube the two primary layers become less marked, and in the neighbourhood of the fimbriated extremity are replaced by an interlacing network of muscle fibres. The writer was the first to call attention to the presence of the inner longitudinal layer in the uterine portion of the tube, and his observations have been confirmed by Ballantyne, Mandl, and Grusdew.

The lumen of the tube is lined with a mucous membrane whose epithelium is composed of a single layer of high, columnar, ciliated cells, which rest upon a thin basement membrane (Fig. 56). There is no submucosa, the epithelium being separated from the underlying muscle by a layer of connective tissue of varying thickness.

The mucosa is arranged in folds which become more complicated as the fimbriated end is approached. The appearance of the lumen varies according to the portion of the tube examined. In the uterine portion four elevations are seen, which together make a figure resembling a Maltese cross. In the isthmic portion of the tube a more complicated appearance

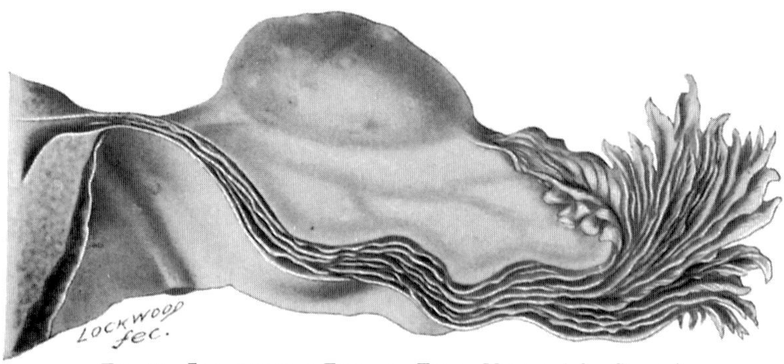

Fig. 60.—Longitudinal Folds of Tubal Mucosa (after Sappey).

can be noted; while in the ampulla the lumen is almost completely occupied by the arborescent mucosa, which upon careful examination is seen to be made up of four very complicated tree-like folds.

Fig. 60 represents a longitudinal section through the tube, and gives a good idea of the increasing complexity of its folds.

The statements of Hennig and Bland-Sutton that the tube possesses glands have since been found to be erroneous, inasmuch as the structures, which they considered as such, are merely depressions between folds of the mucosa. The absence of glands was conclusively demonstrated by Frommel, who showed that the glandular appearance disappeared when the tube was markedly distended, and that the greater part of its lumen became perfectly smooth, with four arborescent folds of mucosa arising from its sides. It is interesting to note that Nature not infrequently performs a similar experiment in cases of hydrosalpinx.

The current produced by the cilia of the tube is directed towards the uterus, as was conclusively demonstrated by the experiments of Pinner, Jani, and Lode, who showed that foreign bodies injected into the abdominal cavity of animals made their way into the tubes and were gradually carried down into the uterus and thence into the vagina.

The tubes are richly supplied with blood-vessels and lymphatics, and the latter not infrequently become so dilated as to fill up almost entirely certain folds of the mucosa.

Occasionally, as Richard first pointed out, the tube may possess a second fimbriated extremity, which is known as an accessory ostium (Fig. 61). Again, not infrequently small tube-like structures, with miniature fimbriated extremities, are found projecting from the exterior of the tube. As a rule, these are mere *culs-de-sac*, but occasionally one is met with possessing a lumen which communicates with that of the main tube. Henrotin and Herzog have lately reported a case of extra-uterine pregnancy in which the fertilized ovum had been arrested in such a structure.

Similar formations are frequently observed upon the anterior surface of the mesosalpinx, but have no connection with the tube. They have been studied more particularly by Kossmann, who designated them as

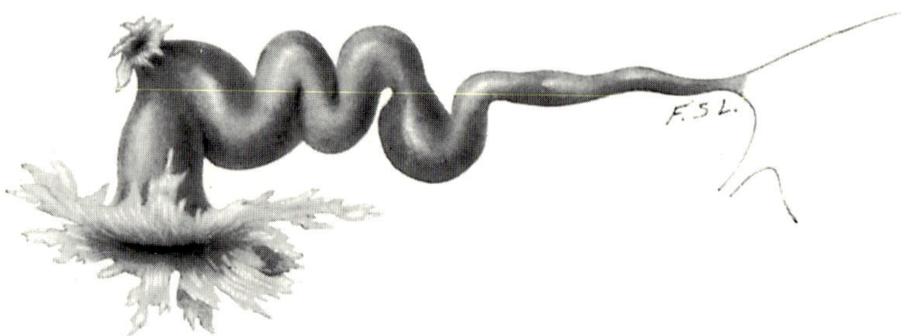

Fig. 61.—Tube with Accessory Ostium.

accessory tubes. They are probably derived from aberrant portions of the cœlomic epithelium.

In very exceptional instances there may be two tubes on one side, as in the cases reported by Pick and Both.

Diverticula may occasionally extend from the lumen of the tube for a variable distance into its muscular wall, and reach almost to its peritoneal covering. Such structures were first described by Landau and Rheinstein and myself. The suggestion that they might play a part in the production of tubal pregnancy would seem plausible, inasmuch as a fertilized ovum, which might chance to make its way into such a diverticulum, would be arrested at its tip and there develop, if suitable conditions existed. Similar structures have also been described by Henrotin and Goebel.

In rare instances the main canal of the tube may branch, and two or even three lumina may be seen in sections. After extending for a certain distance, more or less parallel to the main lumen, they usually rejoin it. It should always be borne in mind that such appearances are usually due to the fact that two or more twists or bends of the tube have been included in one section; although in several instances, by the use of the serial method, I have been able to demonstrate that more than one lumen really existed.

In the new-born child the tubes are markedly convoluted, and present a corkscrew-like appearance, as shown in Fig. 39. This gradually disappears with age, but occasionally the fœtal condition persists and may play a not unimportant part in the production of sterility and tubal disease, as was first pointed out by Freund and Schober.

LITERATURE

Ballantyne and Williams. The Histology and Pathology of the Fallopian Tubes. British Medical Journal, January 17 and 24, 1891.

Both. Rechtsseitige Tubarschwangerschaft, etc. Monatsschr. f. Geb. u. Gyn., ix, 782–794, 1899.

Frommel. Beiträge zur Histologie der Eileiter. Verh. der deutschen Gesell. f. Gyn., 1886, 95.

Freund. Ueber die Indicationen zur operativen Behandlung der erkrankten Tuben. Volkmann's Sammlung klin. Vorträge, Nr. 323, 1888.

Goebel. Beitrag zur Anatomie und Aetiologie der Graviditas tubaria, etc. Archiv f. Gyn., lv, 658–713, 1898.

Grusdew. Zur Histologie der Fallopia'schen Tuben. Centralbl. f. Gyn., 1897, 257.

Hennig. Ueber die Blindgänge der Eileiter. Archiv f. Gyn., xiii, 156, 1878.

Henrotin et Herzog. Anomalies du canal de Müller, comme cause des grossesses ectopiques. Revue de Gyn., 633–649, 1898.

Jani. Ueber das Vorkommen von Tuberkelbacillen im gesunden Genitalapparat bei Lungenschwindsucht, etc. Virchow's Archiv, ciii, 522.

Kossmann. Ueber accessorische Tuben und Tubenostien. Zeitschr. f. Geb. u. Gyn., xxix, 253–268, 1894.

Landau und Rheinstein. Beiträge zur path. Anatomie der Tuben. Archiv f. Gyn., xxxix, 273–290, 1891.

Lode. Exp. Beiträge zur Lehre von der Wanderung des Eies vom Ovarium zur Tube, Archiv f. Gyn., xlv, 295–324, 1894.

Mandl. Ueber den feineren Bau der Eileiter, etc. Monatsschr. f. Geb. u. Gyn., v. Ergänzungs Heft, 130–140, 1897.

Pick. Ein neuer Typus des voluminösen paroophoralen Adenomyoms. Archiv f. Gyn., liv, 117–206, 1897.

Pinner. Ueber den Eintritt des Eies aus dem Ovarium in die Tube, etc. Archiv f. Anat. u. Phys., Physiol. Abth., 1880, 241.

Richard. Pavillons multipliés. Gaz. Méd. de Paris, No. 26, 1851.

Schober. Ueber Erkrankungen gewundener Tuben. D. I., Strassburg, 1889.

Sutton. Glands of the Fallopian Tube and their Function. Trans. London Obst. Soc., xxx, 207–213, 1888.

Williams. Contributions to the Normal and Pathological Histology of the Fallopian Tubes. Amer. Jour. Med. Sciences, October, 1891.

THE OVARIES

General Anatomy.—The ovaries are two flattened, more or less almond-shaped organs, whose chief function is the development and extrusion of ova. They vary considerably in size, and during the childbearing period measure from 2.5 to 5 centimetres in length, 1.5 to 3 centimetres in breadth, and 0.6 to 1.5 centimetres in thickness (see Fig. 41). After the menopause they diminish markedly in size, and in old women are often scarcely larger than peas.

Normally, the ovaries are situated in the upper part of the pelvic cavity, one surface of each ovary resting in a slight depression in the upper portion of the inner surface of the obturator muscle—the *fossa ovarica* of Waldeyer. With the woman standing, the long axes of the ovaries occupy an almost vertical position, which become horizontal when she is on her back. Their situation, however, is subject to marked variations, and it is rare to find both ovaries at exactly the same level.

Each ovary presents for examination two surfaces, two margins, and two poles. The surface which is in contact with the ovarian fossa is called the lateral, and the one directed towards the uterus is known as the median surface. The margin which is attached to the mesovarium is more or less straight, and is designated as the *hilum*, while the free margin is markedly convex and is directed backward and inward towards the rectum. The extremities of the ovary are termed the upper and lower, or tubal and uterine poles respectively.

The ovary is attached to the broad ligament by the *mesovarium*, which forms the posterior leaf of that structure. The *ovarian ligament* extends from the lateral and posterior portion of the uterus, just beneath the tubal insertion, to the uterine or lower pole of the ovary. It is usually several centimetres long and 3 to 4 millimetres in diameter. It is covered by peritonæum, and is made up of muscle and connective-tissue fibres, which are continuous with those of the uterus. The *infundibulo-pelvic* or *suspensory ligament* of the ovary extends from its upper or tubal pole to the pelvic wall. It represents the portion of the upper margin of the broad ligament which is not occupied by the tube, and through it the ovarian vessels gain access to the broad ligament.

For the most part the ovary projects freely into the abdominal cavity, and is not covered by peritonæum except near its hilum, where a narrow band may be observed which is continuous with the peritonæum covering the mesosalpinx. It follows, therefore, that over its lower portion only can be noted the glistening appearance characteristic of peritonæum, while the greater part of its surface is of a dull white colour and looks moist. This distinction was discovered by Farre, but its importance was first emphasized by Waldeyer (Fig. 66), who showed that the ovary above the peritoneal line was covered by cuboidal epithelium.

In many of the lower animals the ovary does not project freely into the abdominal cavity, but is more or less completely inclosed in a peritoneal sac, into which opens the fimbriated end of the tube. In the cow, dog, and cat there is more or less free communication between it and the peritoneal cavity.

The exterior of the ovary varies in appearance according to the age of the individual. In young women the organ presents a smooth, dull white surface, through which glisten a number of small, clear vesicles—the Graafian follicles. As the woman grows older it takes on a more corrugated appearance, which in the aged may become so marked as to be suggestive of the convolutions of the brain.

The general structure of the ovary can best be studied in cross-sections, when the organ is seen to be made up of two portions: the cortex and medulla, or zona parenchymatosa and zona vasculosa. The *cortex* or outer layer varies in thickness according to the age of the individual, becoming thinner with advancing years. In this layer the ova and Graafian follicles are situated. It is composed of spindle-shaped connective-tissue cells, through which are scattered primordial and Graafian follicles in various stages of development, which become less numerous as the woman grows older. The most external portion of the cortex presents a dull whitish appearance, and is designated as the *albuginea*; on its surface is a single layer of cuboidal epithelium—the ovarian epithelium of Waldeyer.

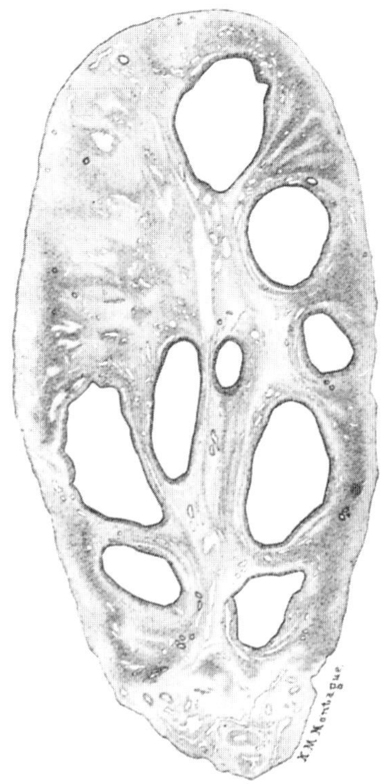

FIG. 62.—CROSS-SECTION ADULT OVARY, SHOWING GRAAFIAN FOLLICLES. × 4.

The *medulla* or central portion of the ovary is composed of loose connective tissue, which is continuous with that of the mesovarium. It contains large numbers of blood-vessels, both arteries and veins; and, according to His, Köllicker, and Rouget, a considerable number of non-striated muscle-fibres, whose presence caused the last-named observer to class it among the erectile tissues. The arrangement of the blood-vessels has lately been studied exhaustively by Clark, to whose admirable monograph we would refer those interested in the subject.

In the neighbourhood of the hilum, epithelial structures are occasionally observed which consist of short tubes or ducts lined by a single layer of columnar, ciliated epithelium. These are the *medullary cords* (Markstränge) of Köllicker, and represent portions of the Wolffian body which have become included within the ovary.

The nerves of the ovary are derived in great part from the sympathetic plexus which accompanies the ovarian artery, while a few are derived from the plexus surrounding the ovarian branch of the uterine artery. Their finer anatomy, after they enter the ovary, has lately been studied by numerous investigators, among whom may be mentioned Von Herff, Gawronsky, Mandl, Winterhalter, and Vallet. The consensus of these researches shows that the ovary is very richly supplied with non-medullated nerve-fibres, which for the most part accompany the blood-vessels, and are merely vascular nerves; whereas a few form wreaths around the follicles and give off many minute branches, which have been traced up to, but not through, the membrana granulosa.

Elizabeth Winterhalter has described a collection of ganglionic cells in the medulla of the ovary which she designates as the ovarian ganglion.

She believes that these cells play an important part in the production of menstruation, although the majority of investigators do not share her views.

Accessory Ovaries.—Waldeyer, in 1870, directed attention to the occasional presence of accessory bodies which are sometimes found on the broad ligament in the neighbourhood of the main ovary. These structures are usually small, although in rare instances they may attain a considerable size. Occasionally they result from faulty development, but more frequently are to be attributed to inflammatory changes occurring during fœtal life, as a consequence of which small portions of the ovary have been cut off from the body of the organ. The subject has lately been considered in detail by Engström and Thumin, the latter stating that Keppler and Falk have described cases in which there was found a typical third ovary connected with the uterus by a separate tube.

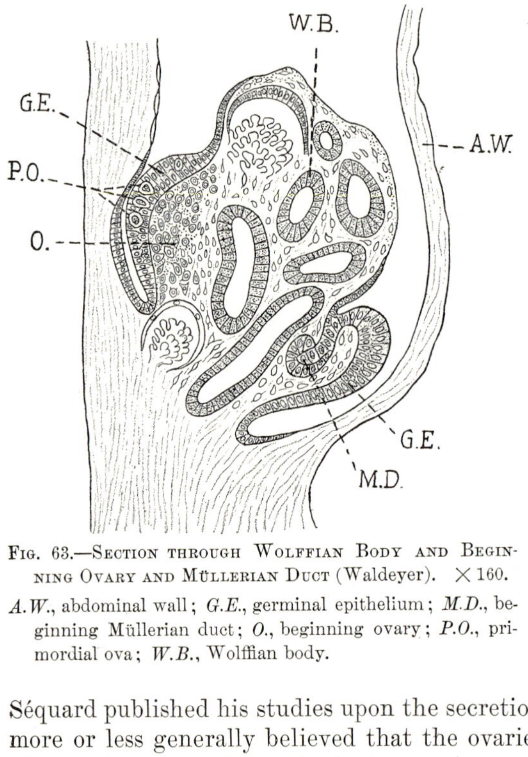

Fig. 63.—Section through Wolffian Body and Beginning Ovary and Müllerian Duct (Waldeyer). × 160.
A.W., abdominal wall; *G.E.*, germinal epithelium; *M.D.*, beginning Müllerian duct; *O.*, beginning ovary; *P.O.*, primordial ova; *W.B.*, Wolffian body.

Transplantation of Ovaries.—Experimental studies undertaken recently by Grigorieff, Morris, Knauer, and others have shown that the ovaries of animals and women may be excised from their original position and transplanted to other portions of the body, and that in their new situation they can establish vascular connections and continue their functional activity. In several cases pregnancy has followed the operation in animals.

Internal Secretion.—From the time that Brown-Séquard published his studies upon the secretion of the testicles, it has been more or less generally believed that the ovaries likewise elaborate a somewhat analogous product, which plays an important part in the female economy. Indeed, Knauer's recent work renders it probable that this secretion is directly concerned in maintaining the integrity of the other generative organs; inasmuch as he has shown that atrophy of the uterus and vagina rapidly follows the removal of the ovaries, whereas this does not occur when the ovaries are removed from their normal position and transplanted to other portions of the body. Knauer therefore concludes that in such cases the absence of atrophy must be attributed to the action of the internal secretion of the transplanted ovaries, since all nerve connections were severed at the time of operation. Upon this same idea is based the therapeutic application of ovarian extracts. A full *résumé* of the literature dealing with this subject is to be found in the thesis of Bestion de Camboulas (1898).

Development of the Ovary.—An accurate idea of the structure of the ovary can be gained only through the study of its development. To Waldeyer we are indebted for most of our knowledge concerning the subject, though important preliminary work has been done by Valentin and Pflüger.

In 1870, Waldeyer published his monograph upon the Ovary and Ovum (Eierstock und Ei), which was based in great part upon the embryology of the chicken. He found that by the fourth day of development the cœlomic epithelium covering the inner surface of the Wolffian body is differentiated from the surrounding tissue, its cells becoming larger and more cuboidal in shape, and some of them assuming a considerable size. Within a short time the epithelium proliferates to such an extent as to form a distinct elevation, which indicates the situation of the future ovary (Fig. 63). This epithelium Waldeyer designated as *germinal epithelium*, and the large, clear cells found within it as *primordial ova*. As the proliferation continues, a mass of cells is formed consisting of large primordial ova and smaller germinal epithelial cells. At the same time, bands of connective tissue and blood-vessels grow upward from the Wolffian body and divide the epithelial mass into numerous smaller portions, the so-called egg-balls or egg-nests.

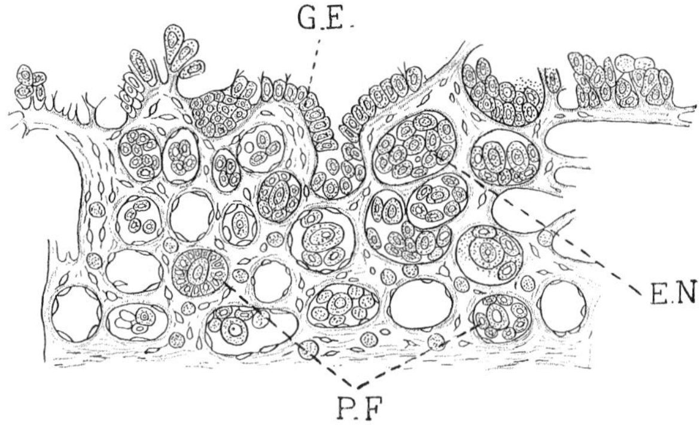

Fig. 64.—Vertical Section through Ovary of Eight-months' Fœtus (Waldeyer).

E.N., egg-nests; *G.E.*, germinal epithelium; *P.F.*, primordial follicle.

Each egg-nest at this stage of development consists of a mass of primordial ova, which are indiscriminately mixed with smaller epithelial cells, while the surface or germinal epithelium continues to proliferate. Continued growth of the connective tissue gradually subdivides the egg-nests into smaller and smaller masses, until eventually isolated primordial ova are found which are surrounded by a single layer of more or less flattened epithelium. These represent the *primordial follicles* (Fig. 64).

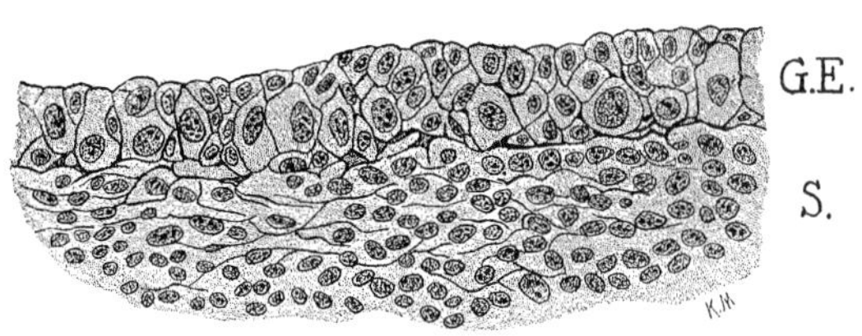

Fig. 65.—Section through the Ovary of a Pig Embryo (Nagel).

G.E., germinal epithelium; *S.*, stroma of Wolffian body.

Practically the same process has been observed in human beings by all embryologists. For full information concerning it the student is referred to the works of Nagel, Wendeler, and Clark.

The ovary, therefore, in its earliest stages, consists of two layers, a single layer of germinal epithelium covering an underlying connective tissue (Fig. 65). In human beings the formation of primordial ova ceases

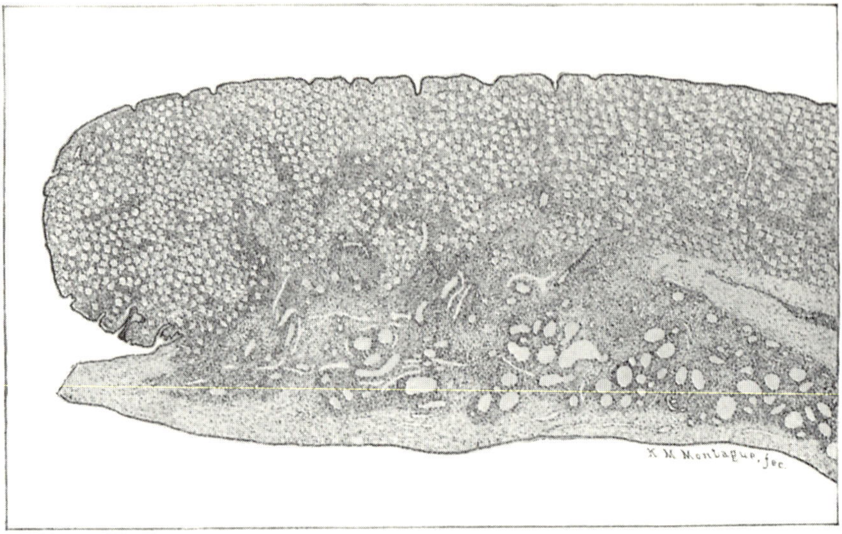

FIG. 66.—OVARY OF NEW-BORN GIRL. ×22.

at birth, but in some of the lower animals, especially in the bat, the process may continue throughout life.

At birth the greater part of the ovary consists of the cortex, which is made up of closely packed primordial follicles, which are separated from one another by very thin bands of connective tissue, although occasionally small groups of follicles may be in direct contact. At this period the surface of the ovary is covered by a single layer of cuboidal epithelium which shows no signs of proliferation (Figs. 66 and 67).

All authorities agree that the primordial ova are derived from the germinal epithelium, but there is still considerable discussion as to the origin of the epithelium surrounding them. According to Waldeyer and the majority of other observers, the *follicular epithelium* is derived from the cells of the germinal epithelium, which have not been converted into primordial ova. Köllicker, on the other hand, believed that it originated from the epithelium of the Wolffian bodies, and that the medullary cords in the adult ovary represented portions of the Wolffian body which were not utilized in this way. Foulis, in 1878, stated that the so-called follicular epithelium was derived from the connective tissue of the ovary, and the recent studies of Wendeler and Clark tend to confirm this view. Clark bases his conclusions upon his observation that the cells surrounding the primordial follicles are spindle-shaped and differ but little in appearance from the adjacent stroma cells; and more especially upon the fact that in the earlier stages of the ovary many of the primordial ova are not surrounded by epithelium at all, but are in direct contact with the surrounding connective tissue.

Waldeyer's view, however, has obtained almost universal acceptance; nor would it seem advisable that Foulis's theory should be adopted until more convincing evidence has been adduced in support of it, as its acceptance would necessitate the recasting of all our ideas concerning the pathology of the ovary.

In rare instances the surface epithelium of the ovary may be ciliated, and now and again, as has been pointed out by Von Velits and myself, the follicular epithelium may likewise be found to possess cilia. These observations, in spite of their rarity, speak strongly against the connective-tissue origin of the follicular cells.

Microscopic Structure of Ovary.—From the first stages of its development until after the menopause the ovary is undergoing constant change. According to Waldeyer, each ovary at birth contains at least 100,000 primordial ova, the majority of which disappear before the age of puberty; so that at that time only 30,000 to 40,000 remain. The changes concerned in their disappearance will be considered more fully when we consider the corpus luteum.

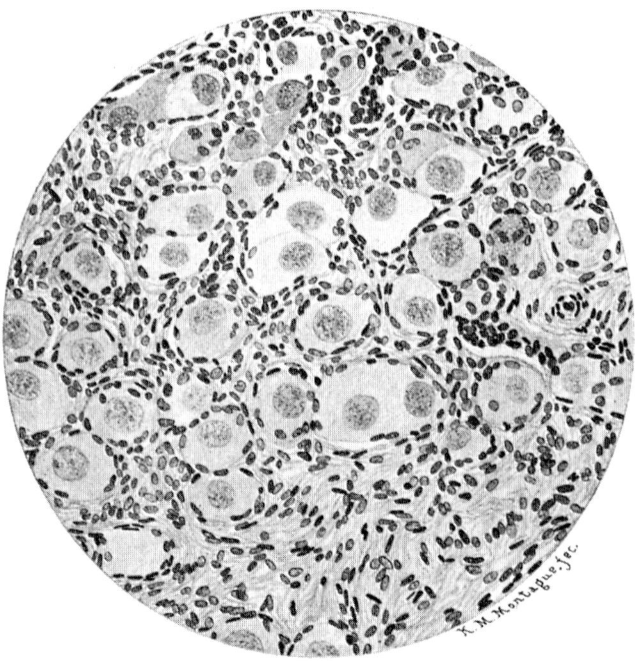

Fig. 67.—Ovary at Birth, showing Primordial Follicles. × 300.

Before taking up the consideration of the evolution of the mature follicle, it may be well to mention certain historical points in connection with it. The Graafian follicle was first described in 1672 by De Graaf, a physician of Delft, who not only observed the vesicles, but demonstrated the presence of ova in the tubes of rabbits. The human ovum was first recognised by Von Baer in 1827, its nucleus or germinal vesicle by Purkyne in 1830, and its nucleolus or germinal spot a few years later by Wagner.

In the young child the greater portion of the ovary is composed of the cortex, which is filled with large numbers of closely packed primordial follicles, those nearest the central portion of the ovary showing the most advanced stages of development. As was mentioned above, the majority are destroyed before the time of puberty.

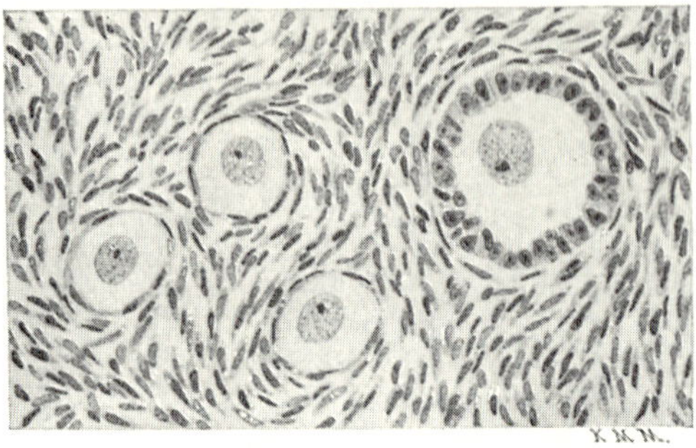

Fig. 68.—Ovary of Young Woman, showing Primordial Follicles on Left Side and Follicle just beginning to develop on Right. × 210.

In young women the cortex contains large numbers of primordial follicles separated by thicker or thinner bands of connective tissue, which is made up of cells with spindle-shaped or oval nuclei. Each primordial follicle consists of an ovum and its surrounding epithelium. The ovum is a single cell, more or less round in shape, with a clear protoplasm and a tolerably large nucleus occupying its central portion. The nucleus presents a marked network, and at one point a well-defined nucleolus and numerous accessory nucleoli, which are formed at the intersections of the nuclear thread-work.

According to Nagel, the ovum remains constant in size from birth until the transformation of the primordial into the typical Graafian follicle, no matter at what period of life this change may occur. The ova measure from 48 to 69 microns, and their nuclei from 29 to 32 microns in diameter. The primordial ovum is sur-

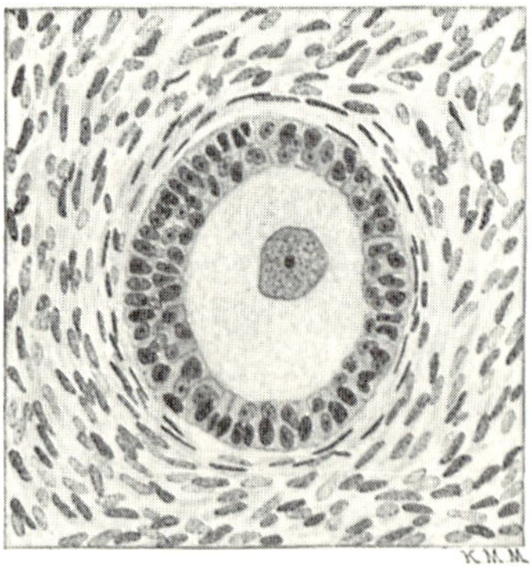

Fig. 69.—Developing Follicle. × 210.

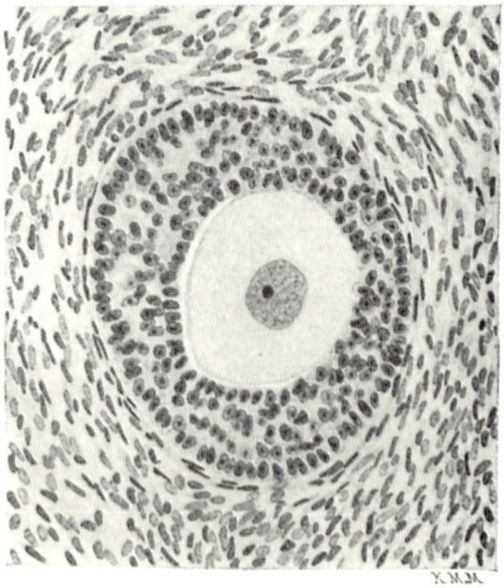

Fig. 70.—Developing Follicle. × 210.

rounded by a single layer of small, spindle-shaped, epithelial cells, which are somewhat sharply differentiated from the still smaller spindle-shaped cells of the surrounding stroma (Fig. 68).

Occasionally a primordial ovum may contain two nuclei or germinal vesicles, as has been shown by Nagel, Klein, von Franqué, and others. Again, occasionally two and sometimes three distinct ova may be found in a single primordial follicle, and it is from such structures that multiple pregnancies not infrequently develop.

When, under the influence of factors with which we are as yet unacquainted, the primordial follicle begins to develop, we notice in the first

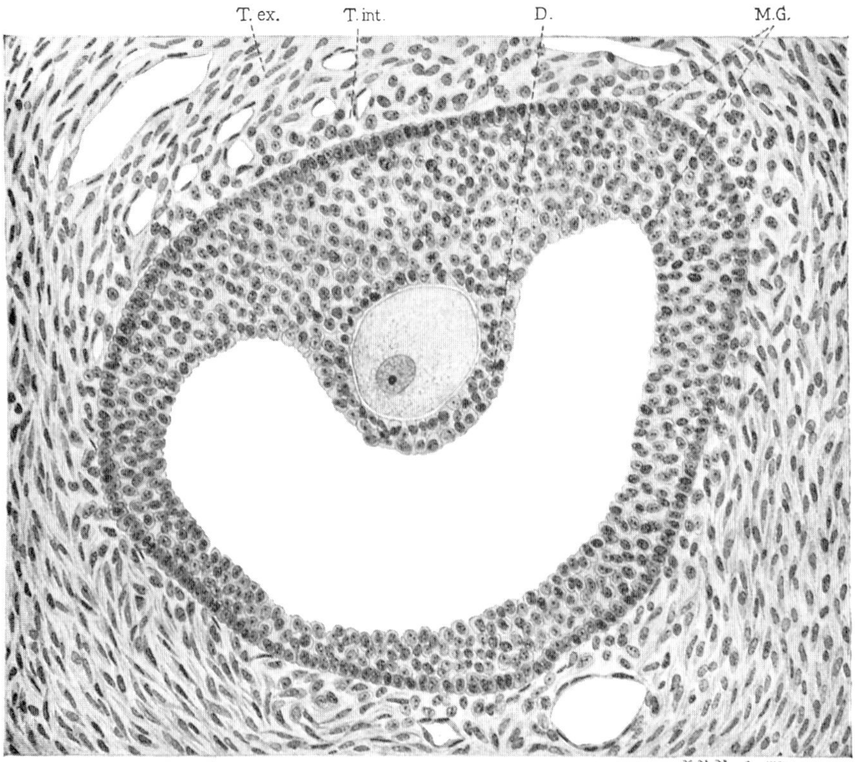

FIG. 71.—NEARLY MATURE FOLLICLE. ×210.
D., discus proligerus; *M.G.*, membrana granulosa; *T.ex.*, tunica externa; *T.int.*, tunica interna.

place that its epithelium becomes converted into a single layer of cuboidal cells (Fig. 68). Nuclear figures soon make their appearance, and the cells begin to proliferate rapidly, so that in a very short time the ovum becomes surrounded by a number of layers of epithelial cells. Certain of these cells undergo degeneration, and vacuolated areas are not infrequently observed between them. This process continues until a considerable portion of the follicle is filled with fluid, which is formed partly by the degeneration of the follicular cells and partly by transudation from surrounding vessels.

Coincident with the development of the fluid, the so-called *liquor folliculi*, the ovum becomes pushed to one side of the follicle, where it is surrounded by a mass of cells—the *discus proligerus* or *cumulus oophorus*—while the rest of the epithelium is arranged in a number of layers around the interior of the follicle, and is known as the *membrana granulosa* (Fig. 71).

While these changes are taking place, the ovum itself becomes larger, yolk granules or deutoplasm are deposited in its protoplasm, and a thin, transparent structure—the *vitelline membrane*—appears about its periphery. At the same time, the stroma immediately surrounding the growing follicle becomes vascular, and its cells show marked evidences of proliferation. The membrana granulosa is separated from the stroma by a thin basement membrane consisting of a single layer of flattened, spindle-shaped, connective-tissue cells. Just between the basement membrane and the outermost layer of the membrana granulosa there not infrequently appears a thin, transparent layer, which was first described by Grohe and Slavjansky. This, no less than the vitelline membrane, is a species of exudate from the granulosa cells.

Mature Graafian Follicle.—From birth until the cessation of sexual life, Graafian follicles are constantly being developed. Before the age of puberty they are found only in the deeper portions of the cortex, and do not reach the surface of the ovary; later, however, they develop in the superficial portions of the cortex and make their way to the surface, where they appear as transparent vesicles, varying from 2 or 3 to 10 or 15 millimetres in diameter. As the follicle approaches the surface of the ovary its walls become thinner and more abundantly supplied with vessels, except in its most prominent projecting portion, which appears almost bloodless and is designated as the *stigma*, the spot where rupture is to occur.

The mature Graafian follicle consists of a connective-tissue covering—the theca folliculi; an epithelial lining—the membrana granulosa; the ovum, and the liquor folliculi. The *theca folliculi* is readily divided into two layers: an outer, the tunica externa, and an inner, the tunica interna. The tunica externa consists of the ordinary ovarian stroma, which is arranged concentrically about the follicle, while the connective-tissue cells of the tunica interna have undergone marked changes.

Almost as soon as the primordial follicle shows signs of development, nuclear figures appear in the stroma immediately surrounding it, and a considerable multiplication of cells occurs. These become considerably larger than the surrounding connective-tissue cells, and as the follicle increases in size assume a granular appearance, which is due to the presence of a yellowish pigment. These cells are designated as *lutein cells* and, as will be seen later, play an important part in the formation of the corpus luteum. In most hardened specimens the colouring matter has been dissolved out, and the cells appear not unlike those of the suprarenal capsules (see *T.I.*, Fig. 72). At the same time there is a marked increase in the vascularity of the theca, and numerous lymphatic spaces make their appearance.

The epithelial lining of the follicle, or *membrana granulosa*, consists of a number of layers of small polygonal or cuboidal cells, with round, darkly staining nuclei, which are arranged in fewer layers the larger the follicle.

At one point the membrana granulosa is much thicker than elsewhere, and forms a more or less pyramidal mound in which the ovum is included. This is the *discus proligerus* or *oophorus*, and is usually situated at the portion of the follicle farthest removed from the surface of the ovary (see Fig. 71). The follicle is filled with a clear, albuminous fluid, the liquor folliculi, which is partly the product of the degenerated follicular epithelium and partly a transudate from surrounding vessels. As the follicle approaches

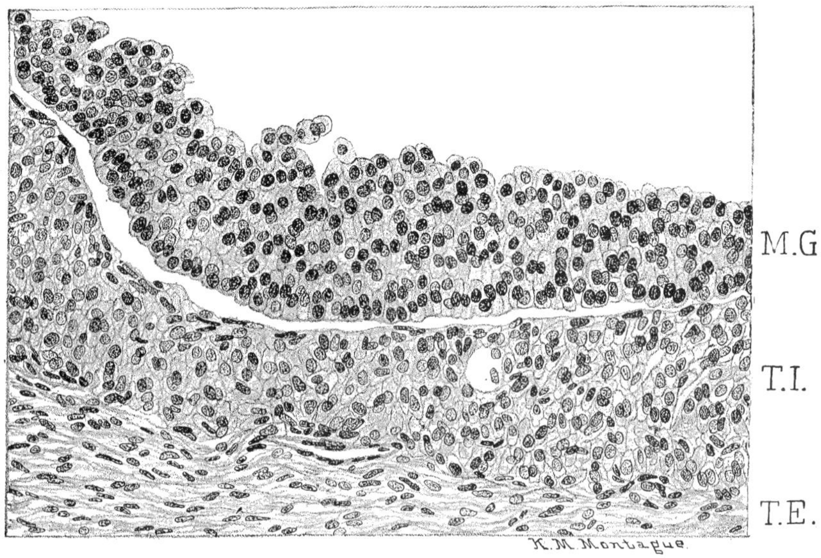

FIG. 72.—SECTION THROUGH WALL OF MATURE FOLLICLE (highly magnified).

M.G., membrana granulosa; *T.I.*, tunica interna; *T.E.*, tunica externa.

its highest development, marked alterations appear in the follicular epithelium, which by appropriate methods can be demonstrated as due to fatty degenerative changes.

The ovum becomes much larger as it approaches maturity, and, according to Nagel, measures from 150 to 250 microns ($\frac{1}{5}$ millimetre) in diameter, as compared with 48 to 69 microns in its primordial condition.

If the *mature ovum* be examined in the liquor folliculi or in normal salt solution, the following structures, according to Nagel, may be distinguished in and about it: (*a*) a corona radiata; (*b*) a zona pellucida; (*c*) a perivitelline space; (*d*) a small, clear zone of protoplasm; (*e*) a broad, finely granulated zone of protoplasm; (*f*) a central, deutoplasmic zone; and (*g*) the germinal vesicle with its germinal spot.

The *corona radiata* consists of a number of layers of follicular epithelium which adhere to the ovum, and was so designated by Bischoff, by whom it was first described. Inside of the corona radiata comes a transparent zone—the *zona pellucida*—which is a product of the granulosa cells, and does not belong to the ovum itself. Separating the ovum from the zona pellucida is a clear, narrow space, the *perivitelline space*, within which the ovum is freely movable, so that no matter what position it may assume its germinal vesicle will always point upward. Inside of the perivitelline space is the ovum proper, which differs markedly from the primordial ovum, not only by its increased size, but more especially by the presence of a yolk or deutoplasm which fills the greater part of its interior. The *deutoplasm* occupies the central portion of the ovum, and is made up of large numbers of irregularly shaped, highly refractive granules. As it develops it pushes the germinal vesicle to one side, so that the latter always assumes an eccentric position in the ovum.

Outside of the deutoplasm comes a narrow zone of finely granular protoplasm, which owes its peculiar appearance to the presence of very small yolk-granules; external to this, again, is a still narrower zone of clear protoplasm.

The *germinal vesicle* presents a distinct nuclear network, the intersections of which appear as very darkly staining points. The nucleolus or *germinal spot* is much larger than in the primordial ovum, and according to Auerbach presents typical amœboid movements.

A follicle presenting the above characteristics is generally described as mature, but is not capable of fertilization and further development until its nucleus has undergone certain changes which are manifested by the formation and casting off of the polar bodies.

Graafian follicles, as we have already pointed out, develop throughout childhood, and occasionally attain a considerable size; but they rarely rupture at this time on account of their position in the depths of the ovary and the intervention of a thick layer of cortex between them and the surface. In adults, on the other hand, the developing follicle makes its way to the surface, and when it has attained its highest development ruptures and extrudes its ovum into the peritoneal cavity or the tube, where it may be fertilized.

Formerly it was believed that *rupture of the follicle* was brought about by the increased tension resulting from the rapid formation of the liquor folliculi, which, according to Nagel, was markedly accentuated by the pressure exerted by the lutein cells developing about its periphery. Clark, however, has lately shown that rupture of the follicle is a complex process, and is due primarily to circulatory changes. As the period of ovulation approaches, the ovary becomes engorged with blood, and the intra-ovarian tension being markedly increased, the growing ovum is forced to the surface; at the same time the circulation in the most distended portion of the wall of the follicle is interfered with, whence results necrosis at the point designated as the stigma, which eventually gives way.

Corpus Luteum.—The corpus luteum is a structure which is formed at the site of a ruptured follicle. Its function would appear to be the preservation of the cortical circulation of the ovary, by preventing an excessive formation of scar tissue.

When the mature follicle ruptures, the ovum, liquor folliculi, and a considerable portion of the degenerated membrana granulosa make their escape, and the walls of the empty follicle collapse. In a short time, however, its cavity becomes filled with blood, which is derived partly from the vessels at the point of rupture, but principally from those of the tunica interna of the theca.

The corpus luteum, therefore, in its earliest stages is simply a ruptured follicle filled with blood, outside of which is a narrow yellow ring formed by the lutein cells of the theca, which, however, proliferate rapidly and invade the blood-filled follicle, forming a festooned layer about its central blood-clot (Fig. 73). This layer is yellowish in colour, whence the term "corpus luteum." As the structure becomes older, the yellow

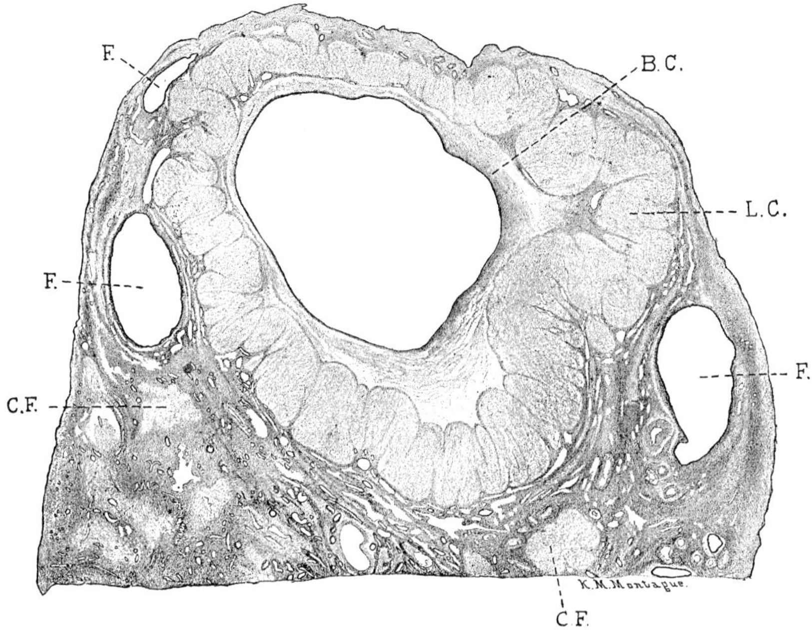

Fig. 73.—Portion of Ovary, showing a Corpus Luteum of Pregnancy, with Cystic Centre. × 4.

B.C., blood-clot; *C.F.*, corpus fibrosum; *F.*, Graafian follicles; *L.C.*, lutein cells.

ring becomes thicker and thicker, until at last it almost entirely fills the interior of the follicle, the central blood-clot remaining being now quite small.

At its greatest development the corpus luteum is always larger than the original follicle, and not infrequently occupies a considerable portion of the ovary, sometimes as much as one-third of the entire organ.

Microscopic sections through a well-developed example show that its centre is occupied by a compressed blood-clot, immediately outside of which is a thin layer of newly formed connective tissue. The greater part of the structure, however, is occupied by the festooned yellow ring, which is made up of large polygonal epithelioid cells, with small, round, somewhat faintly staining nuclei. These are the *lutein cells*, whose protoplasm has taken on a granular appearance due to the presence of a peculiar yellow pigment which is soluble in chloroform, alcohol, and ether. The layer of lutein cells is traversed by numerous radiate, tolerably thick, connective-tissue partitions, to which it owes its festooned appearance. They are richly supplied with blood-vessels and lymphatics (Fig. 74).

As the cavity of the follicle is encroached upon by the growing lutein cells, the blood-clot becomes more and more compressed, and vascular loops extend into it and soon cause its organization. At the same time, the blood pigment is removed by leucocytes, which can be found in the surrounding tissue with their bodies filled with particles of it. Occasionally hæmorrhage does not take place into the ruptured follicle, and a corpus

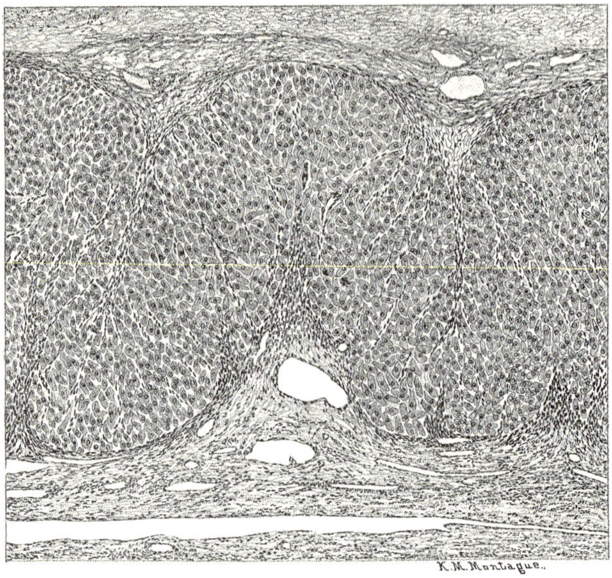

Fig. 74.—Section through Yellow Layer of Corpus Luteum, showing Lutein Cells.

luteum is formed without a central blood-clot. This is the exception in human beings, but the rule in many of the lower animals, as in the rabbit and mouse.

After the cavity of the follicle has become obliterated by the ingrowth of the lutein cells and connective tissue, degenerative changes soon make their appearance in the former, some of which undergo hyalin and others fatty degeneration. In young women, in whom the circulation is active, the degenerated lutein cells are rapidly absorbed, so that in a short time the corpus luteum becomes replaced by newly formed connective tissue which corresponds closely in appearance to the surrounding ovarian stroma. But in more advanced life, when the ovarian circulation has become impaired, absorption goes on less rapidly; and not infrequently the degeneration extends to the intervening connective tissue and blood-vessels until the entire structure is converted into an almost homogeneous mass of hyalin in which only a few connective-tissue cells and degenerated blood-vessels can be seen (Fig. 75). These structures—the so-called *corpora fibrosa* or *albicantia*—present on fresh section a dull white appearance, somewhat suggestive of old scar tissue. They are, however, gradually invaded by the surrounding stroma, and become broken up into smaller and smaller hyalin masses, which are eventually absorbed, the site of the original fol-

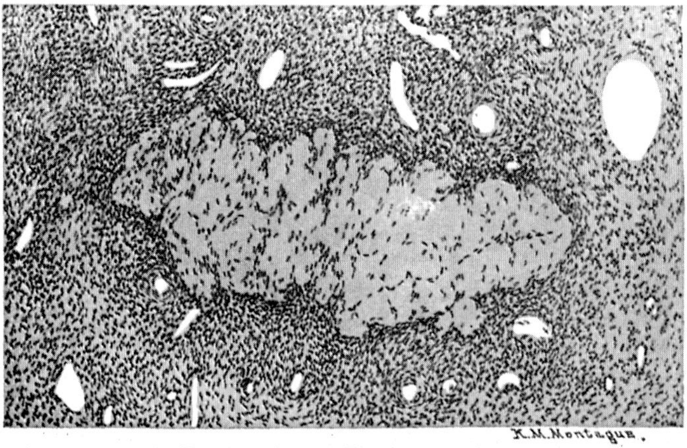

FIG. 75.—CORPUS FIBROSUM. × 75.

licle being indicated only by an area of slightly thickened connective tissue. When the circulation is very defective, absorption takes place much more slowly, so that it is not uncommon to find the ovaries of women near the menopause almost filled by corpora fibrosa of varying size. Not infrequently the small hyalin bodies resulting from the breaking up of these structures assume peculiar and bizarre forms, and very often present a curved and twisted appearance suggestive of a degenerated artery (Fig. 76). Similar structures are sometimes left after the obliteration of non-ruptured follicles.

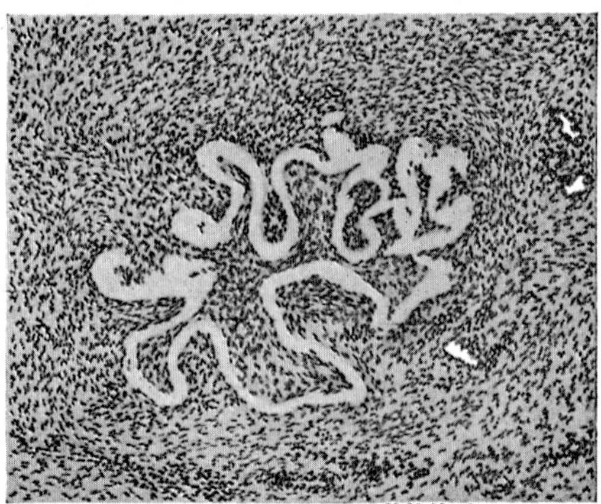

FIG. 76.—LATER STAGE OF CORPUS FIBROSUM. × 75.

Practically all authorities are agreed as to the life-history of the corpus luteum, and the only point which still remains unsettled deals with the *origin of the lutein cells.* The earlier observers considered that the changes were analogous to the organization of a blood-clot which was followed by the formation of cicatricial tissue, but at present this view possesses only an historical interest.

The majority of investigators believe that the lutein cells are of connective-tissue origin and represent the cells of the theca interna. This view was first advanced by von Baer, and has been confirmed by the work of Köllicker, His, Beigel, Benckiser, Nagel, Clark, and many others. A few authors, on the other hand, following the example of Bischoff, consider that they originate from epithelial cells and are derived from those of the membrana granulosa. This explanation has been advocated more particularly by Sobotta, and has lately received additional support from the work of Kreis. Full details of the discussion are contained in the recent papers of Clark and Doering. I shall content myself with giving the evidence in favour of the former view.

The connective-tissue origin of the lutein cells is based upon two facts: first, the cells of the tunica interna of the theca begin to undergo marked changes as soon as the follicle commences to develop; and secondly, the membrana granulosa presents extensive degenerative changes, and is usually cast off in great part at the time of rupture.

In the early stages of follicular development, the cells of the theca interna become larger and assume an epithelioid appearance. Nuclear figures soon appear and rapid proliferation ensues. At the same time their protoplasm becomes more granular, and pigment is deposited within them, so that they closely resemble the lutein cells. That they first appear in the theca would argue against their derivation from the membrana granulosa, but even more so the fact that they are separated from it by a definite barrier of unchanged connective tissue, the upper layer of which forms the basement membrane of the follicle (see Figs. 72 to 74).

The mature follicle, then, is surrounded by actively proliferating lutein cells, while its membrana granulosa shows signs of fatty degeneration. In many instances, before rupture, a narrow yellow ring may be found surrounding the periphery of the follicle, from which it is separated by a thin layer of connective tissue. As soon as the follicle ruptures the lutein cells proliferate more rapidly, and with the vessels included between them, speedily invade the follicular cavity.

Observations based upon the study of several hundred human corpora lutea have convinced me that the connective-tissue origin of the lutein cells is established beyond all reasonable doubt. Strong support in favour of this view is also to be obtained from the changes which are observed in follicles which develop in the deeper portions of the ovary, and degenerate without rupture. This process has been studied by a number of observers, notably Slavjansky, Schottländer, Clark, and others, and is usually designated as *follicular atresia.* Under such circumstances, precisely the same changes are observed as in the formation of the corpus luteum, except that hæmorrhage is absent and that the process is less marked. In many instances the entire membrana granulosa is separated from the walls of the follicle and lies free in its cavity, presenting marked signs of fatty degeneration, while the cells of the theca are actively proliferating and are being converted into lutein-like cells.

The function of the corpora lutea is to bring about the obliteration of the spaces left by the ruptured follicles without the formation of cicatricial tissue; for if they healed by the latter process it is evident that in a very short time the entire ovary would be converted into a mass consisting of nothing but scar tissue, the very nature of which would effectually prevent further ovulation. It has been estimated by Clark that if each follicle healed in this manner, and if ovulation could continue under such conditions, a fibroma would eventually be produced 5,000 times as large as the original ovary.

It is usual to distinguish between *true* and *false* corpora lutea—namely, those following impregnation and menstruation respectively. This distinction is based entirely upon their relative size, and not upon any inherent anatomical difference, as they both present exactly the same structure, the larger size of the so-called true corpus luteum being simply due to the increased vascular supply incident to pregnancy.

Not infrequently the corpus luteum of pregnancy contains in its centre a small cyst filled with clear fluid, the walls of which are composed of connective tissue, outside of which are the typical lutein cells. Such cysts are due to the liquefaction of the central blood-clot (see Fig. 73).

In rare instances the corpus luteum, instead of disappearing in the manner just described, may be the starting-point of cystic formations, to which attention was first directed by Rokitansky, and with which every gynæcologist is now familiar.

The corpus luteum was first described by De Graaf as a conglomerate glandular body, and was considered by him and all earlier authorities as positive evidence of previous childbearing. Moreover, it was generally believed that the number of children which a woman had borne could readily be estimated by counting the number of corpora lutea in her ovaries. This view was held for many years, and was so firmly established, even at the end of the eighteenth century, that such eminent authorities as Abernethy, Sir Astley Cooper, and Denman, had no hesitancy in swearing in a medico-legal case that a woman had been pregnant because a corpus luteum was found in one ovary. Even after the more frequent performance of autopsies, and the closer attention directed to the condition of the ovaries had led to the abandonment of this view, it was for a time believed that the presence of corpora lutea indicated that the individual had indulged in sexual relations, or had at least been under marked sexual excitement. Finally, as a result of the work of Bischoff, Raciborski, Négrier, and Pouchet (1840–'47), it was definitely established that the corpus luteum was not necessarily a sign of pregnancy, but occurred after each menstrual period in virginal as well as married women. For fuller information on this point the works of Montgomery and Dalton may be consulted.

LITERATURE

Auerbach. Quoted by Nagel.

Von Baer. De ovi mammalium et hominis genesi. Leipzig, 1827.

Beigel. Zur Naturgeschichte des Corpus luteum. Archiv f. Gyn., xiii, 109–122, 1878.

Benckiser. Zur Entwickelungsgeschichte des Corpus luteum. Archiv f. Gyn., xxiii, 350–367, 1884.

Bestion de Camboulas. Le suc ovarian. Paris, 1898.

Bischoff. Entwickelungsgeschichte der Säugethiere und des Menschen, 1842.

Beweis der von der Begattung unabhängigen periodischen Reifung und Loslösung der Eier als der ersten Bedingung ihrer Fortpflanzung, etc. Giessen, 1844.

CLARK. The Origin, Growth, and Fate of the Corpus Luteum. Johns Hopkins Hospital Reports, vii, 181–220, 1898.

The Origin, Development and Regeneration of the Blood-vessels of the Ovary. Contributions to the Science of Medicine, by pupils of William H. Welch, 1900, 593–676.

CORNIL. Note sur l'histologie des corps jaunes de la femme. Annales de Gyn. et d'Obst., lii, 373–381, 1899.

DALTON. On the Corpus Luteum of Menstruation and Pregnancy. Philadelphia, 1851.

DOERING. Beitrag zur Streitfrage über die Bildung des Corpus luteum. D. I., Königsberg, 1898.

ENGSTRÖM. Ueberzählige Ovarien. Mittheil. der gyn. Klinik des Prof. Engström, i, 55, 1897.

FARRE. Uterus and its Appendages. Todd's Cyclopædia of Anatomy and Physiology, Parts XLIX and L, 1858.

FOULIS. The Development of the Ova, etc., with Special Reference to the Origin and Development of the Follicular Epithelial Cells. Jour. of Anat. and Physiol., xiii.

VON FRANQUÉ. Beschreibung einiger seltenen Eierstockspräparate. Zeitschr. f. Geb. u. Gyn., xxxix, 326–346, 1898.

GAWRONSKY. See Anatomy of Uterus.

DE GRAAF, REGNERUS. De mulierum organis generationi inservientibus tractatus novus, etc. Lugd., 1672.

GRIGORIEFF. Schwangerschaft bei der Transplantation der Eierstöcke. Centralbl. f. Gyn., 1897, 663.

GROHE. Ueber den Bau und das Wachstum des menschlichen Eierstockes, etc. Virchow's Archiv, xxvi, 1863.

VON HERFF. Ueber den feineren Verlauf der Nerven im Eierstocke des Menschens. Zeitschr. f. Geb. u. Gyn., xxiv, 289–308, 1892.

HIS. Beobachtungen über den Bau des Säugethiere-Eierstockes. Archiv f. mikros. Anat., i, 1865.

KLEIN. Ueber mehreiige Graaf'sche Follikel beim Menschen. Münchener med. Abhandlungen, IV. Reihe, Heft 4, 1893.

KNAUER. Die Ovarientransplantation. Archiv f. Gyn., lx, 322–376, 1900.

KÖLLICKER. Entwickelungsgeschichte des Menschen und der höheren Thiere. II. Aufl., Leipzig, 1879.

KREIS. Die Entwickelung und Rückbildung des Corpus luteum spurium beim Menschen. Archiv f. Gyn., lviii, 411–427, 1899.

MANDL. Ueber Anordnung und Endigungsweise der Nerven im Ovarium. Arch. f. Gyn., xlviii, 276–292, 1895.

MONTGOMERY. An Exposition of the Signs and Symptoms of Pregnancy. 2d ed., London, 1863, 419–489.

MORRIS. The Ovarian Graft. New York Medical Journal, October, 1895.

NAGEL. Das menschliche Ei. Arch. f. mikros. Anat., xxxi.

Die weiblichen Geschlechtsorgane. Jena, 1896.

NÉGRIER. Recherches anatomiques et physiologiques sur les ovaries dans l'espèce humaine. Paris, 1840.

PFLÜGER. Ueber die Eierstöcke der Säugethiere und des Menschen. Leipzig, 1867.

POUCHET. Théorie positive de l'ovulation spontanée et de la fécondation, etc. Paris, 1847.

PURKYNE. Symbolae ad ovi avium historiam ante incubationem. Lipsiae, 1830.

RACIBORSKI. De la puberté et de l'âge critique chez la femme, et de la ponte périodique chez les mammifères. Paris, 1844.

ROKITANSKY. Ueber Abnormitäten des Corpus luteum. Allg. Wiener med. Zeitung, iv, Nr. 34, 35, 1859.

ROUGET. Recherches sur les organes érectiles de la femme, etc. Jour. de la Physiol., i, 1858.

SCHOTTLÄNDER. Ueber den Graaf'schen Follikel, etc. Archiv f. mikros. Anat., xxxi, 219–294.

SLAVJANSKY. Zur normalen u. path. Histologie der Graaf'schen Bläschen des Menschen. Virchow's Archiv, li, 1870.

SOBOTTA. Ueber die Bildung des Corpus luteum bei der Maus. Archiv f. mikros. Anat., xlvii, 1897.

THUMIN. Ueberzählige Eierstöcke. Archiv f. Gyn., lvi, 342–354, 1898.

VALENTIN. Handbuch der Entwickelungsgeschichte des Menschen. Berlin, 1835.

VALLET. Nerfs d'ovaire, etc. Thèse de Paris, 1900.

VON VELITS. Beiträge zur Histologie u. Genese der Flimmerpapillärkystomen des Eierstocks. Zeitschr. f. Geb. u. Gyn., xvii, 232–278, 1889.

WALDEYER. Eierstock und Ei. Leipzig, 1870.

Beiträge zur Kenntniss der Lage der weiblichen Beckenorgane. Bonn, 1892.

WALDEYER und JOESSEL. Lehrbuch der topographisch-chirurg. Anatomie, Theil II, 790–804, 1899.

WENDELER. Entwickelungsgeschichte und Physiologie der Eierstöcke. Martin's Die Krankheiten des Eierstocks u. Nebeneierstocks, Leipzig, 1899, 16–105.

WILLIAMS, J. WHITRIDGE. Papillomatous Tumours of the Ovary. Johns Hopkins Hospital Reports, iii, 1–84, 1892.

WINTERHALTER. Ein sympathisches Ganglion im menschlichen Ovarium. Archiv f. Gyn., li, 49–55, 1896.

PHYSIOLOGY AND DEVELOPMENT OF THE OVUM

CHAPTER III

MENSTRUATION AND OVULATION—MIGRATION OF THE OVUM AND PLACE OF MEETING OF OVA AND SPERMATOZOA

Menstruation.—By menstruation we understand a process characterized by a discharge of blood from the genitalia, which recurs at regular intervals, except during pregnancy and lactation, from the time of puberty until the menopause. Ordinarily it comes on every four weeks and lasts from three to five days, though there are marked individual variations as to its frequency and duration.

The age at which the menses are established varies in different countries, being earlier in warm and later in cold climates. In the temperate zone, the first menstruation does not usually occur before the fourteenth or fifteenth year. Not a few instances of a much earlier appearance of the function, however, are to be found in the literature, and are usually associated with precocious sexual development. One of the most notable cases of this character is that of Anna Mummenthaler, who, according to Haller, menstruated regularly from her second year; and gave birth to a full-term child at the age of nine.

Not infrequently a bloody vaginal discharge is observed in new-born infants, which ceases after a few days, no further discharge being noted until puberty. To describe these as instances of precocious menstruation, however, would be incorrect.

In this country the menopause usually occurs about the forty-fifth year. In rare instances, however, the menstrual flow may cease as early as the twenty-eighth or thirtieth year, while not very infrequently it continues until well into the fifties, and occasionally until even a later period. Thus, Kennedy reports the case of a woman who gave birth to her twenty-second child when she was sixty-three years old, after which she still continued to menstruate. For various interesting historical and ethnological points concerning menstruation, the reader is referred to the works of Ploss and Ottokar Alt.

The menstrual flow is derived from the uterine mucosa, and consists of blood mixed with mucus, which, under ordinary circumstances, will not coagulate.

Anatomical Changes in Menstruation.—The statements concerning the extent of the changes occurring in the endometrium during menstruation are very contradictory. Sir John Williams believes that the entire mucosa

PLATE III.

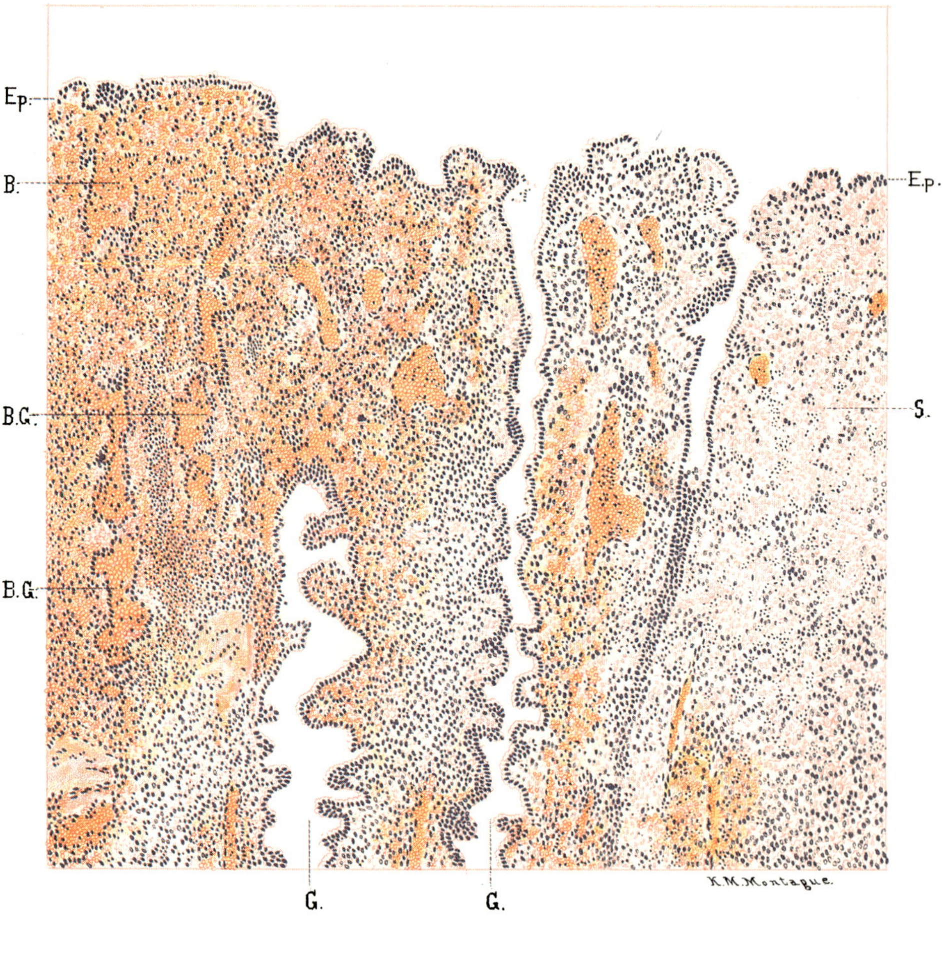

SECTION THROUGH ENDOMETRIUM ON THIRD DAY OF MENSTRUATION.

× 52.

B, blood; *B. G.*, gland filled with blood; ***Ep.***, surface epithelium; *G.*, hypertrophied glands; ***S.***, stroma.

is cast off at each menstrual period, while Moericke and numerous other observers state that there is little or no destruction of tissue. Between these extremes, we find a number of authors stating that a greater or lesser portion undergoes disintegration. Generally speaking, the older authorities held that the entire mucosa, or at least a considerable part of it, was cast off. Their adoption of this view is probably explained by the fact that their conclusions were drawn from the study of uteri in which post-mortem changes had taken place, since De Sinéty was the only observer among those whose work was based upon autopsy specimens, who stated that there was but little destruction of tissue.

In 1882 Moericke expressed the opinion that menstruation was accompanied by little or no destruction of tissue, basing his statements upon the examination of 45 specimens of the menstruating endometrium which he obtained by curettage. His views were soon confirmed by other observers, among whom may be mentioned De Sinéty, Löhlein, Westphalen, Strassmann, Gebhard, and Findley. Meerdevoort and Mandl consider that the extent to which the tissue is destroyed varies within wide limits, the loss being almost imperceptible in some individuals and quite marked in others; while Kahlden and Christ believe that the destruction is always considerable.

My own experience, based upon the examination of several uteri removed during the menstrual period and numerous specimens obtained by curettage, is such that I have no hesitation in adopting the views of Moericke and his supporters.

Plate III, which represents a section through the endometrium of a uterus removed on the third day of menstruation, shows very distinctly that but little destruction of tissue has occurred. The entire mucosa is markedly thickened, and its superficial portion is infiltrated with blood. The surface epithelium is intact, but in places it has been separated from the underlying tissue by small collections of blood—the so-called subepithelial hæmatomata of Gebhard. The uterine glands are markedly hypertrophied, as is shown by their twisted and corkscrew-like course; this hypertrophy is associated with a considerable increase in the interglandular tissue, the cells of which, however, do not appear to have undergone changes in shape. There is marked engorgement of the blood-vessels, and just beneath the surface epithelium may be seen capillaries which are distended almost to the point of bursting, while considerable quantities of blood have escaped from the vessels and lie free in the tissues. From these and similar observations, then, it would seem evident that menstruation is not attended by any great loss of tissue, but consists essentially in marked hypertrophy of the mucosa, engorgement of its superficial vessels and the consequent escape of blood, partly following rupture, but in great measure by diapedesis.

After the menstrual flow has ceased, a certain amount of degeneration takes place in the superficial layers of the mucosa, which, however, is soon repaired, nuclear figures appearing in the cells of the epithelium and interglandular tissue, which begin to multiply and replace the degenerated cells, so that regeneration is rapidly effected.

As menstruation occurs every twenty-eight days, it is apparent that the endometrium is subjected to an almost continuous change, the process being described by Leopold and others as the *menstrual cycle.* This covers a period of sixteen days, five of which are needed for the preliminary swelling, four for the menses proper, and seven for the period of regeneration, so that the endometrium remains quiescent only about twelve days in each month. For further particulars concerning the anatomical details observed in menstruation, the exhaustive article of Gebhard should be consulted.

Relation between Menstruation and Ovulation.—By ovulation we understand the rupture of a mature Graafian follicle and the extrusion of the ovum. The relation between menstruation and ovulation has given rise to a great deal of controversy, and while many interesting facts have been added to our information, it must be conceded that the subject is still far from being satisfactorily understood.

The fact that young girls do not usually conceive until after the appearance of the menses, and the extreme rarity of impregnation after their cessation, rendered it natural for the earlier observers to suppose that conception could not occur without menstruation, and that the menstrual flow represented the female semen. This view, however, was soon abandoned, and the discharge was regarded as a process of purification.

It was not until the doctrine of periodical ovulation had been established by the work of Gendrin, Négrier, Bischoff, Pouchet and others, that definite ideas could be formulated concerning the relation between ovulation and menstruation. From that time on, however, it was generally believed that menstruation was brought about by the ripening of the Graafian follicles; that the two processes occurred almost, if not quite, simultaneously, and that menstruation should be considered as analogous with the heat or rut of animals.

This doctrine culminated in 1865 with the appearance of Pflüger's article upon the significance and cause of menstruation, in which he stated that the flow resulted from a reflex stimulation, which owed its origin to the pressure exerted by the growing follicle upon the nerves of the ovary. This theory obtained almost immediate acceptance, and for years was the predominant belief; upon it was based our method of calculating the expected date of confinement, the rule being to date the beginning of pregnancy from the last menstrual period.

Pflüger's theory, however, was somewhat shaken by the work of Leopold, Prochownick, and De Sinéty, whose careful studies of the condition of ovaries removed at operation proved conclusively that the two processes were not necessarily synchronous, but might occur quite independently of one another, and accordingly ovulation could not be considered the unvarying cause of menstruation. Clinical experience also lent further probability to this view, since it has shown that ovulation and subsequent pregnancy might take place without menstruation, as was demonstrated by the instances of conception occurring before the first menstrual period and after the menopause, as well as during lactation, when the menstrual flow is usually absent. Moreover, a few cases were recorded in which pregnancies had occurred in such rapid succession that menstruation did not occur for years. Ahlfeld has reported the case of a woman who gave birth to numerous children, but did not menstruate until her thirty-second year; and one of Leviot's patients did not menstruate for fourteen years, and yet during that time became pregnant no less than four times.

Sigismund, Löwenhardt, Löwenthal, and Aveling next advocated the theory that ovulation preceded menstruation, and that the latter was due to the failure of conception. Aveling designated the process as nidation and denidation, and considered that a *menstrual decidua* was formed each month for the reception of the fertilized ovum, and that if conception did not occur it degenerated and was cast off with the menstrual flow. The gist of these theories was tersely expressed by Powers in the dictum, "Women menstruate because they do not conceive." This view was also adopted by His and most embryologists as true, for a certain number of cases at least. They found on examining ova which were nominally of the same age, as estimated from the last menstrual period, that some presented a stage of development several weeks in advance of the others; they held, therefore, that this difference could be explained only by supposing that the former resulted from conception soon after the last menstrual period, and the latter from conception just before the first period missed. This view is also confirmed by the reproductive history of the orthodox Jewesses, who are noted for their fertility. According to their laws women are considered unclean during the entire menstrual period and the seven days following it, so that in them conception probably occurred just before the first missed menstrual period.

In 1894, Leopold and Mironoff made an extended study of the condition of ovaries removed at operation from 42 women whose menstrual history had been carefully noted. In 30 cases they found that menstruation and ovulation were synchronous; in 11 menstruation occurred without any trace of ovulation; while in 1 case ovulation occurred in the middle of the intermenstrual period.

Strassmann, in a recent study, has more or less rehabilitated the original Pflüger theory, by showing that rut can be produced by injecting gelatine into the ovaries of animals. His views have received a certain sort of confirmation from the discovery by Elisabeth Winterhalter of a sympathetic ganglion in the ovary.

From the evidence before us, we must conclude that the two processes usually occur about the same time, but that one not infrequently antedates the other by a few days; while in exceptional cases they may occur quite independently.

Some years ago Stevenson advanced the so-called menstrual-wave theory, which has been accepted by Johnstone, Webster, Ott, and others. According to this idea, the metabolic processes in women present a distinct rhythm, and gradually increase in intensity up to the time of the menstrual flow, when they suddenly drop and reach their lowest point; after this they gradually rise again and attain their maximum intensity just before the next menstrual period, thus indicating that the entire process is under some central control, and that neither menstruation nor ovulation are directly dependent upon one another, but upon some general and as yet unknown cause.

The results following various operations upon the genital tract tend to show that menstruation is dependent upon the presence of the ovaries, but that ovulation may take place without the presence of the uterus; as it is generally admitted that the complete removal of both ovaries, which necessarily stops ovulation, is always associated with cessation of the menses. On the other hand, the total removal of the uterus, while associated with abolition of the menstrual flow, exerts no effect upon ovulation, as is manifested by the regular occurrence of the so-called menstrual molimina.

A number of observers have attempted to show that menstruation may occur independently of ovulation, basing their contention upon the occasional continuance of menstruation after the removal of the ovaries. This conclusion, however, is fallacious, as in such cases either the ovaries had not been completely removed, or an accessory ovary was present. The now well-established fact that a very small portion of ovary will suffice for ovulation has been demonstrated by the occurrence, in rare instances, of pregnancy after the removal of both ovaries by competent operators, two cases of which have lately been reported by Gordon.

Such observations conclusively demonstrate the fallacy of the view advanced by Tait, Johnstone, and Savage, that menstruation is regulated by the so-called menstrual nerve, and that its persistence after operation was due to the fact that this nerve had not been included within the ligature.

Ordinarily, the Fallopian tubes take no part in the menstrual function, and in none of my specimens were there any traces of a bloody fluid in them. Occasionally, however, the tubal mucosa may share in the process, as has been shown by the experience of Thompson, who recently reported a case in which a pyosalpinx had ruptured through the abdominal wall, leaving a fistulous opening which did not heal, and through which a slight amount of bloody fluid exuded at each menstrual period.

Migration of the Ovum.—The mechanism by which the ovum gains access to the tube after escaping from the ruptured follicle is a question of extreme interest, and one which has given rise to a great deal of discussion. The process is readily understood in those animals in which the ovaries are more or less completely inclosed in a peritoneal sac into which the tube opens; but in women, and in animals in which the ovary projects freely into the peritoneal cavity, the question presents greater difficulties and has not as yet received a thoroughly satisfactory solution.

As we have already shown, the fimbriated extremity of the tube lies in the neighbourhood of the ovary, but is not necessarily in direct contact with it, the only organic connection between the two structures being furnished by the *fimbria ovarica,* which is attached to the upper or tubal pole of the ovary.

Numerous theories have been advanced to explain the manner in which the ovary enters the tube. Rouget believed that the latter became engorged with blood at the menstrual period, and that as a result of its becoming erectile, the fimbriæ applied themselves to the portion of the ovary in which the ripe follicle was situated—so that after its rupture, the ovum was immediately taken up by the fimbriated extremity of the tube. This view, however, has been abandoned, as it is difficult to suppose that the tube could instinctively pick out the exact portion of the ovary to which it should apply itself. Kehrer believed that the ovum was ejected from the follicle at the time of rupture, with sufficient force to be thrown directly into the fimbriated end of the tube. This, the so-called ejaculation theory, for a time enjoyed considerable vogue, but has likewise been abandoned.

At present it is generally believed that the cilia upon the fimbriated end of the tube give rise to a current in the capillary layer of fluid which lies between the various pelvic organs, so that the ovum, on escaping from the follicle, is taken up by the current and wafted towards one or the other tube, whence it is carried to the uterus. The correctness of this view has been substantiated by the experimental work of Pinner, Jani, and Lode. The former injected cinnabar and the latter the ova of ascarides into the peritoneal cavity of animals, and found that they made their way to the pelvis, where they were taken up by the tubes, through which they were carried to the uterus, and eventually appeared in the vagina. This experimental evidence is re-enforced by the fact that in certain amphibians large tracts of the peritonæum become covered by the ciliated epithelium shortly before the time of ovulation. It is more than likely, however, that a considerable proportion of the ova which escape from the ruptured follicle fail to gain access to the tubes, but remain in the peritoneal cavity where they perish.

In 1844, Bischoff directed attention to the fact that not infrequently in animals possessing bicornuate uteri one finds that the corpora lutea are in one ovary, while the embryos are developed in the uterine horn on the opposite side. He supposed in such cases that the fertilized ova had come from the ovary in which the corpora lutea were found, and had made their way into the cornu of the opposite side instead of into the one corresponding to the ovary from which they came. This process he designated as *migration of the ovum.*

The possibility of such an occurrence in women was first carefully studied by Kussmaul, who stated that it might be brought about in two ways: either by the ovum making a circuit through the pelvic cavity and thus gaining access to the opposite tube, or passing down one tube, traversing the uterine cavity, and then making its way up the opposite tube. The former he designated as external, the latter as internal, migration of the ovum.

External migration of the ovum is not infrequently observed, whereas there is considerable discussion as to the possibility of the occurrence of internal migration. We are unable to ascertain how frequently external migration takes place in normal uterine pregnancies, though it is probably by no means rare. On the other hand, its occurrence has been repeatedly demonstrated in cases of bicornuate uteri, and those presenting a rudimentary horn; and not infrequently in normal uteri, when one tube is markedly diseased and the other more or less normal, as in cases of hydrosalpinx and inflammatory lesions of one tube associated with occlusion of its fim-

6

briated extremity. In such cases when the corpus luteum is found on the side of the diseased tube, it is inferred that the ovum gained access to the uterus through the normal or only slightly diseased tube of the opposite side. Moreover, the same event has not infrequently been observed in extra-uterine pregnancy.

External migration of the ovum has been produced experimentally in animals by Leopold, who excised one ovary and the opposite tube, and found in a number of such cases that the animals became pregnant after the operation. A very convincing case has been recorded by Kelly, who removed the diseased left ovary and right tube from a patient, leaving the normal right ovary and left tube behind. Fifteen months later the woman was delivered at term, and seventeen months after delivery the remaining tube was removed for a ruptured extra-uterine pregnancy.

I have examined specimens from 6 cases of extra-uterine pregnancy, which apparently offered incontrovertible evidence of external migration of the ovum, the corpus luteum being found in the ovary of one side and the pregnancy in the opposite tube. The same condition was beautifully exemplified in a specimen which Dr. H. C. Coe sent me for examination. In this case the right tube had twice been the seat of extra-uterine pregnancy. The first pregnancy, which dated from several years before, was situated in the isthmic portion of the tube, the fœtus having become converted into a lithopædion which completely blocked the lumen. External to this, and occupying the lateral portion of the tube, was a freshly ruptured four months' pregnancy. The right ovary was small, atrophic, and covered by adhesions, while the left contained the corpus luteum of pregnancy. It was apparent in this case that the ovum must have been fertilized, soon after leaving the left ovary, by a spermatozoon which had made its way up the left tube; after which it had been carried to the right tube and had passed down it until arrested by the lithopædion, when it underwent further development.

Satisfactory evidence has not yet been adduced in favour of the occurrence of *internal migration* of the ovum, and it is hardly possible that such proof can ever be brought in the future, though its theoretical possibility cannot be denied. Schaeffer and Veit have conclusively demonstrated that the specimens which were formerly relied upon to establish its occurrence are open to other and simpler explanations.

Place of Meeting of the Ovum and Spermatozoa.—During coitus the semen is deposited in the vagina, and the question arises, How do the spermatozoa contained in it make their way into the uterus, and when and where do they come in contact with the ovum?

The number of spermatozoa contained in a single ejaculation is marvellous, and has been estimated by Lode at 226,257,900. Various explanations of the method by which they gain access to the uterine cavity have been advanced, the most widely known being the aspiration theory of Litzmann, Wernich, and Beck, and the mucus-plug theory of Kristeller. The first-mentioned observers held that the external muscles of the uterus contract forcibly during coitus and compress the uterine cavity, into which the spermatozoa are aspirated when relaxation occurs. Kristeller believed that at the height of the orgasm the thick tenacious mucus, which is usually found in the cervix, is forced down for a short distance into the vagina, where it becomes covered with spermatozoa, after which it returns to its original position and carries them with it.

It cannot be denied that spermatozoa may gain access to the uterine cavity in either of these ways in a certain number of cases; but in the majority of instances it is probable that they may make their way thither by their own activity. That this view is correct is demonstrated by the instances of pregnancy following imperfect coitus, and those which have been observed in women with unruptured hymens. Furthermore, it has been shown by Henle that spermatozoa can move at quite a rapid rate, being able to travel a distance of 1 centimetre in three minutes.

It was formerly taught that *impregnation* normally occurred in the uterine cavity, and it was believed by Tait, Wyder, and other observers that conjugation was favoured by the direction of the currents produced by the cilia of the uterus and the tubes, the former being directed from below upward, and the latter from above downward, so that the two met in the upper part of the uterine cavity. Thus, the ciliary current would favour the entrance of spermatozoa into the uterus, while rendering impossible their entry into the tubes, except in diseased conditions. But in view of the observations of Hofmeier, Mandl, and others, which show that the ciliary current is directed from above downward, in the uterus as well as in the tubes, it is apparent that this theory must be abandoned, and it must be admitted that the spermatozoa have to make headway against the current from the time they enter the internal os.

It is probable that spermatozoa can nearly always be found in the tubes of married women, into which they make their way by their own motility. Living spermatozoa have been observed in the tubes of women by Birch-Hirschfeld and Dührssen, and it is a well-known fact that they retain their activity in the tubes of the bat for many months. Years ago Bischoff showed that they could be found on the surface of the ovaries of animals for a certain length of time after copulation, and the occurrence of ovarian pregnancy demonstrates that the same may occur in women.

From the evidence available, it appears to be tolerably satisfactorily demonstrated that in women who copulate at frequent intervals the tube must be regarded as a species of *receptaculum seminis*, in which spermatozoa are always present and waiting for the ovum, and that fertilization usually occurs in the tubes and only rarely in the uterus.

LITERATURE

AHLFELD. Lehrbuch der Geburtshülfe, II. Aufl., 2, 1898.

ALT. Ueber das Vorkommen und die Bedeutung der Menstruation bei der Völkern der Altenwelt. Monatsschr. f. Geburtskunde, vi, 161–179, 1855.

AVELING. Obst. Jour. of Great Britain and Ireland, July, 1874, 209.

BECK. How do the Spermatozoa enter the Uterus? American Jour. of Obst., viii, 353–391, 1875.

BISCHOFF. Die Entwickelung des Kaninchen-Eies, 1842.

See literature on the Anatomy of Ovaries.

BIRCH-HIRSCHFELD. Quoted by Zweifel, Lehrbuch der Geburtshülfe, II. Aufl., 20, 1889.
CHRIST. Das Verhalten der Uterusschleimhaut während der Menstruation. D. I., Giessen, 1892.
COE. Internal Migration of the Ovum. Trans. Amer. Gyn. Soc., xviii, 262–278, 1893.
DÜHRSSEN. Lebendige Spermatozoen in der Tube. Centralbl. f. Gyn., 593, 1893.
FINDLEY. Anatomy of the Menstruating Uterus. Amer. Jour. Obst., 1902, xlv, 509–512.
GEBHARD. Die Menstruation. Veit's Handbuch der Gyn., iii, 1–94, 1898.
GENDRIN. Traité philosophique de médecine pratique. Paris, 1839.
GORDON. Two Pregnancies following the Removal of Both Tubes and Ovaries. Trans. Amer. Gyn. Soc., xxi, 104–108, 1896.
HALLER. Quoted by Ahlfeld, Lehrbuch, II. Aufl., 1, 1898.
HENLE. Lehrbuch der Anatomie.
HIS. Anatomie menschlicher Embryonen, 1880.
HOFMEIER. See literature on Anatomy of Uterus.
JANI. See literature on Anatomy of Uterus.
JOHNSTONE. The Menstrual Organ. British Gyn. Jour., November, 1886.
The Pathological Aspect of Stevenson's Wave. Amer. Jour. Obst., xxxi, 662–668, 1895.
The Clinical Importance of the Menstrual Wave. Trans. Amer. Gyn. Soc., xxi, 57–65, 1896.
KAHLDEN. Ueber das Verhalten der Uterusschleimhaut während und nach der Menstruation. Hegar's Festschrift, Beiträge zur Geb. u. Gyn., Stuttgart, 1889.
KEHRER. Die Zusammenziehungen des weiblichen Genitalcanals. Beiträge zur vergleich. u. exp. Geburtskunde, Heft 1, 1864.
KELLY. Operative Gynecology, vol. ii, 189, 1898.
KENNEDY. Edinburgh Medical Journal, xxvii, 1085, 1882.
KRISTELLER. Berliner klin. Wochenschr., 1871, Nr. 27, 28.
KUSSMAUL. Von dem Mangel, der Verkümmerung und Verdoppelung der Gebärmutter und der Ueberwanderung des Eies. Würzburg, 1859.
LEOPOLD. Studien über die Uterusschleimhaut. Berlin, 1878.
Die Ueberwanderung des Eies. Arch. f. Gyn., xvi, 22–44, 1880.
Untersuchungen über Menstruation u. Ovulation. Arch. f. Gyn., xxi, 347–408, 1885.
LEOPOLD und MIRONOFF. Beitrag zur Lehre von der Menstruation u. Ovulation. Arch. f. Gyn., xlv, 506–538, 1894.
LÉVIOT. Ovulation sans menstruation pendant une période de 14 ans. Bull. de la Soc. d'Obst. et de Gyn., Paris, 1893, 202.
LITZMANN. Wagner's Handwörterbuch der Physiologie, iii, 53.
LODE. Wiener klin. Wochenschr., 1891, 907.
See literature on Anatomy of Uterus.
LÖHLEIN. Das Verhalten der Uterusschleimhaut während der Menstruation. Gynäkolog. Tagesfragen, Heft 2, Nr. 6.
LÖWENHARDT. Die Berechnung und die Dauer der Schwangerschaft. Arch. f. Gyn., iii, 356–391, 1872.
LÖWENTHAL. Eine neue Deutung des Menstruationprocess. Archiv f. Gyn., xxiv, 169–261, 1884.
MANDL. Beitrag zur Frage des Verhaltens der Uterusmucosa während der Menstruation. Arch. f. Gyn., lii, 557–578, 1896.
See literature on Anatomy of Uterus.
MEERDERVOORT. Quoted by Gebhard.
MOERICKE. Die Uterusschleimhaut in verschiedenen Altersperioden und zur Zeit der Menstruation. Zeitschr. f. Geb. u. Gyn., vii, 84–137, 1882.
NÉGRIER. See literature on Anatomy of Ovaries.
OTT. Gesetz der Periodicität der physiologischen Functionen im weiblichen Organismus. Verh. des X. internat. med. Congresses, Bd. III, Abt. viii, 33, Berlin, 1891.
PFLÜGER. Ueber die Bedeutung u. Ursache der Menstruation. Berlin, 1865.

PINNER. See literature on Anatomy of Uterus.

PLOSS. Das Weib in der Natur- und Völkerkunde, IV. Aufl., Bd. I, 266–334, 1895.

POUCHET. See literature on Anatomy of Ovaries.

PROCHOWNICK. Fall von Menstruatio praecox. Archiv f. Gyn., xvii, 330–381, 1881.

ROUGET. Recherches sur les organes érectiles de la femme. Jour. de la Physiologie, i, 320, 1858.

SAVAGE. The Female Pelvic Organs. 3d ed., New York, 1880.

SCHAEFFER. Ueber die innere Ueberwanderung des Eies. Zeitschr. f. Geb. u. Gyn., xvii, 13–42, 1889.

SIGISMUND. Ideen über das Wesen der Menstruation. Berliner klin. Wochenschr., 1871, 824, 825.

DE SINÉTY. Recherches sur la muqueuse utérine pendant la menstruation. Gazette méd. de Paris, No. 7, 1881.

STEVENSON. On the Menstrual Wave. Amer. Jour. Obst., xv, 287–294, 1882.

STRASSMANN. Beiträge zur Lehre von der Ovulation, Menstruation und Conception. Archiv f. Gyn., lii, 134–234, 1896.

TAIT. See literature on Anatomy of Uterus.

THOMPSON. Zur Frage der Tubenmenstruation. Centralbl. f. Gyn., 1898, 1227, 1228.

VEIT. Die Frage der inneren Ueberwanderung des Eies. Zeitschr. f. Geb. u. Gyn., xxiv, 327–355, 1892.

WEBSTER. The Biological Basis of Menstruation. Montreal Med. Journal, April, 1897.

WERNICH. Ueber die Erectionsfähigkeit des unteren Uterusabschnittes, etc. Beiträge zur Geb. u. Gyn., Berlin, 1872, 297–307.

WESTPHALEN. Zur Physiologie der Menstruation. Archiv f. Gyn., lii, 35–70, 1896.

WILLIAMS. The Normal Structures of the Uterine Mucosa, and its Periodical Changes. Obst. Journal of Great Britain and Ireland, 1875.

WINTERHALTER. See literature on Anatomy of Ovaries.

WYDER. See literature on Anatomy of Ovaries.

CHAPTER IV

MATURATION, FERTILIZATION, AND DEVELOPMENT OF THE OVUM

Formation of the Fœtal Membranes.—In the present work we shall not attempt to trace the development of the ovum through all its stages, but shall consider only those changes which are directly concerned in the formation of the fœtal membranes and the placenta. For detailed information concerning the general development of the embryo, the student is referred to the standard works upon embryology.

Maturation of Ovum.—The ovum, as it occurs in the mature Graafian follicle, is not adapted for fertilization and further development until it has undergone certain changes more especially noticeable in its nucleus, which may be regarded as signs of maturation. The process has not as yet been proved for human beings; but, as it has been observed in all the lower animals which have been studied, it is reasonable to suppose that it also occurs in man. The changes are supposed to begin just before the

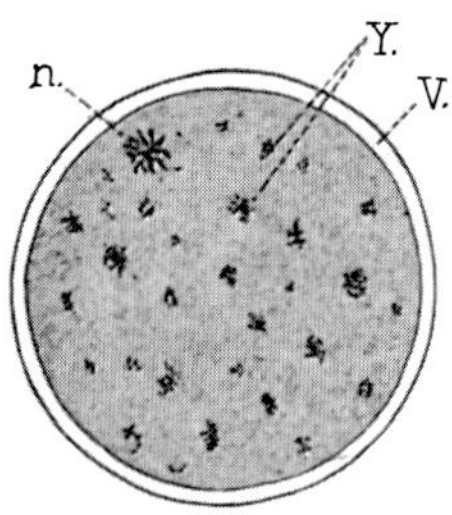

Fig. 77.

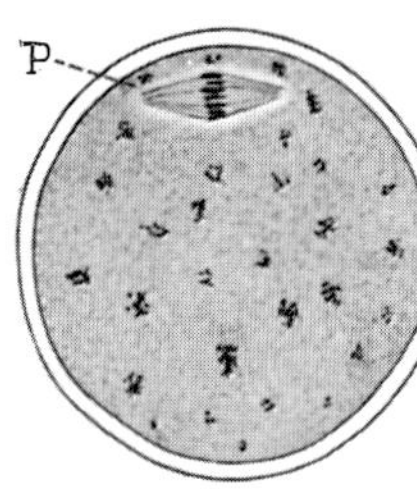

Fig. 78.

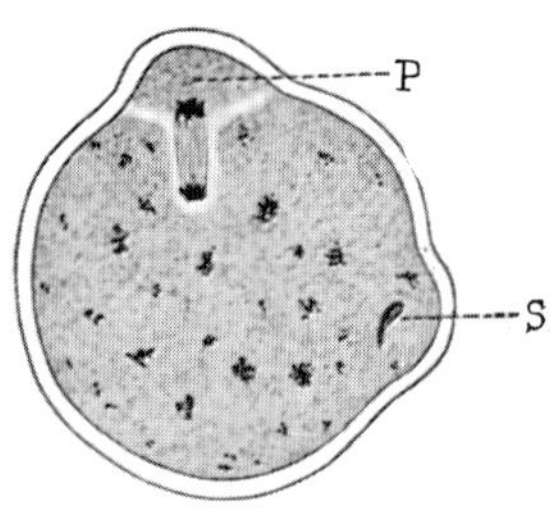

Fig. 79.

Figs. 77–79.—Formation of Polar Body (Sobotta). × 500.

n., nucleus ; *V.*, vitelline membrane ; *Y.*, yolk granules ; *P.*, polar spindle : *S.*, head of spermatozoon.

rupture of the follicle, and to be completed while the ovum is in the upper portion of the tube, though occasionally they may take place while it is still within the ovary. Sobotta has recently made an exhaustive study of the process in the mouse, and it is from his article that most of our statements are taken.

When the process of maturation is about to begin, the germinal vesicle approaches the surface of the ovum and appears to become smaller, while at the same time its membrane disappears. It gradually becomes less and less distinct, until finally its situation is indicated by a clear area surrounded by deutoplasm, which is traversed by many radiating lines. In a short time this area becomes transformed into a typical caryocinetic or mitotic figure (Fig. 77), which undergoes the usual changes and soon becomes spindle-shaped. The spindle, when it first appears, is situated tangentially to the surface of the ovum, but later turns and becomes per-

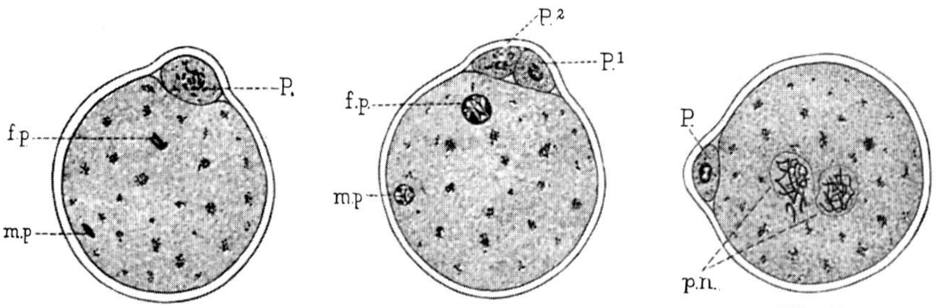

Fig. 80. Fig. 81. Fig. 82.

FIGS. 80–82.—FORMATION OF FEMALE PRONUCLEUS AND ITS FUSION WITH MALE PRONUCLEUS (Sobotta). × 500.

P., polar body; *P.*², second polar body; *f.p.* female and *m.p.* male pronucleus; *p.n.*, pronuclei about to fuse.

pendicular to it. The chromatin of the spindle then becomes rearranged and a typical dyaster is formed. Division rapidly ensues, and the new nucleus nearest the surface, with the portion of protoplasm surrounding it, is cut off from the rest of the ovum and comes to lie between it and the vitelline membrane. In this way is formed the first *polar body*.

Within a short time similar changes take place in the remaining portion of the nucleus of the ovum, and a second polar body is formed and cast off. The portion of the original nucleus, which remains within the ovum, is known as the *female pronucleus*.

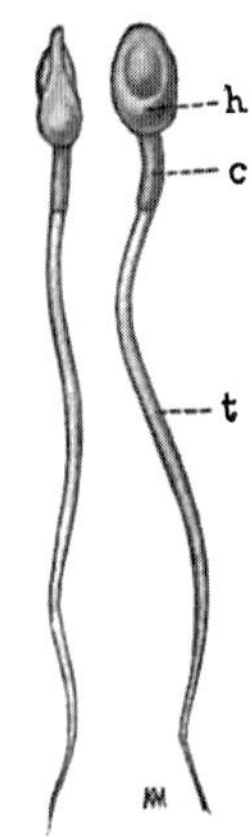

FIG. 83.—HUMAN SPERMATOZOA.

h., head; *c.*, intermediate portion; *t.*, tail.

The number of polar bodies which are cast off varies. In most animals two are usually found, but in the mouse, according to Sobotta, it is exceptional to find more than one. The polar bodies are the result of typical division of the ovum, and their whole history forces us to regard them as cells homologous with ova. Consequently, when two polar bodies are formed, the female pronucleus, and more especially the chromatin bodies, which are constant and can be counted, represent half of the original germ nucleus before the polar bodies were given off, and half of the number of nuclei characteristic of the given species. The ovum is a quarter of the primitive germ cell, which in maturing has been broken up by two divisions into two polar bodies and the ovum.

Various theories have been advanced by Minot, Weismann, Kollmann, and others in explanation of the process, but none of them are very satisfactory. In the present state of our knowledge it must be admitted that we are ignorant of its cause or significance, and must be content with the knowledge that its occurrence is a necessary preliminary to the fertilization and further development of the ovum.

Fertilization.—By fertilization we understand the union of a spermatozoon and the mature ovum. Each *spermatozoon* consists of three portions —the head, tail, and intermediate portion. The head is somewhat triangular in shape and flattened from side to side; it contains a certain amount of chromatin, which is derived from the mother cells of the testicle (Fig. 83). Each spermatozoon must be regarded as a distinct cell, and

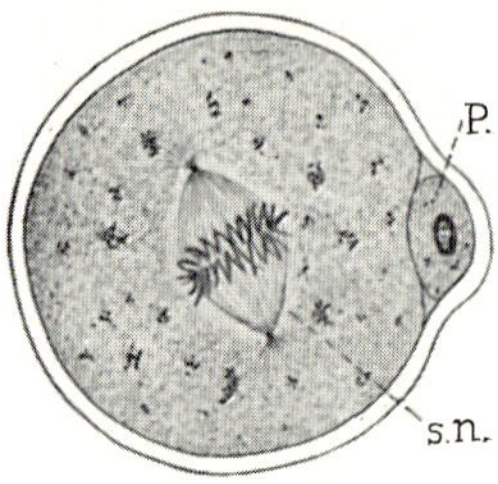

Fig. 84.

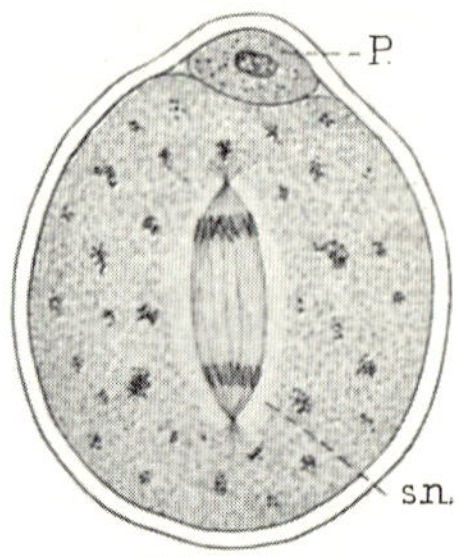

Fig. 85.

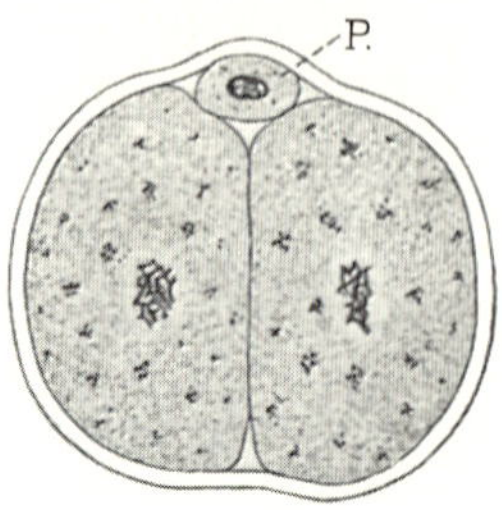

Fig. 86.

Figs. 84–86.—Changes in the Segmentation Nucleus (Sobotta). × 500.
P., polar body; *s.n.*, segmentation nucleus.

each germ, as compared with the ovum, represents a fourth part of the primitive germ cell, from which four sperms arise by two divisions. Its structure is one half of that characteristic of the nuclei of the species. Interpolated between the long tail and the head is a small cylindrical body, the intermediate portion, to which is attached the tail. The spermatozoa are endowed with marked motility, derived from the rapid vibration of their tails, and, according to Henle, can traverse a distance of 1 centimetre in three minutes.

As has already been pointed out, the spermatozoa and ovum usually come together in the lateral portion of the tube, which may be regarded as a species of receptaculum seminis, although in rare instances the meeting may take place on the surface of the ovary or even in the Graafian

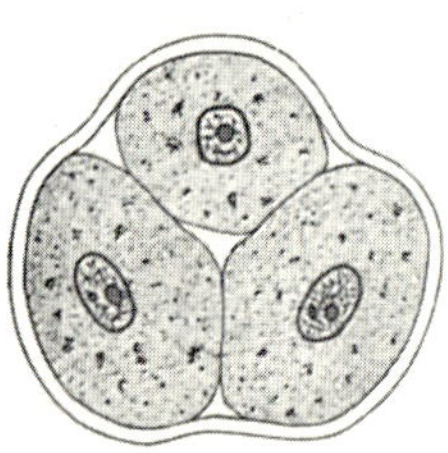
Fig. 87.

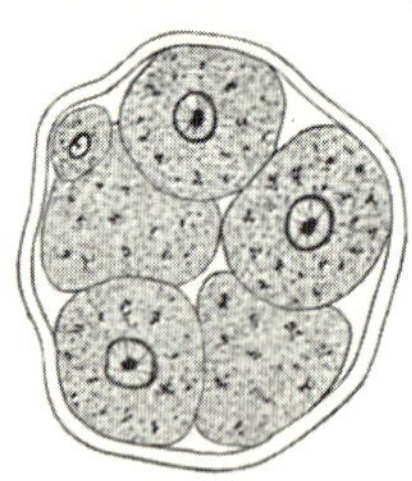
Fig. 88.

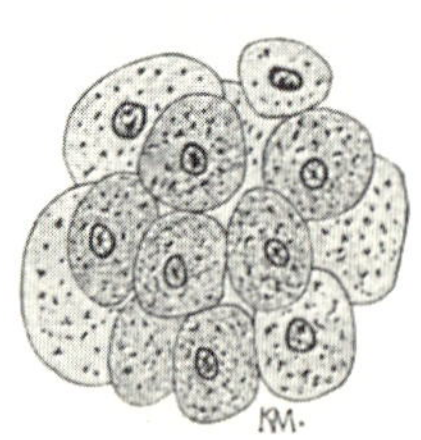

Fig. 89.

Figs. 87–89.—Formation of Mulberry Mass (Sobotta). × 500.

follicle, as is demonstrated by the occurrence of ovarian pregnancy. Moreover, Stratz has shown that in Sorex their union on the surface of the ovary is not of infrequent occurrence.

In the lower animals in which the process of fertilization has been studied, the ovum is found in the lateral end of the tube, surrounded by a considerable number of spermatozoa, as many as 60 having been counted about a single ovum. They rapidly penetrate the vitelline membrane, but it appears that only one of them makes its way into the ovum, and that after its entry the superficial portion of the latter becomes impervious to other spermatozoa.

After the head has entered the ovum the tail rapidly disappears, and in a short time nothing is left of the original spermatozoon but a small spindle-shaped mass, the *male pronucleus* (Fig. 79). This rapidly makes its way to the centre of the ovum, where it meets and fuses with the female pronucleus to form the segmentation nucleus (Figs. 81 and 82). It is therefore apparent that in the species studied half of the chromatin of the segmentation nucleus is derived from the original nucleus of the ovum, and half from the head of the spermatozoon.

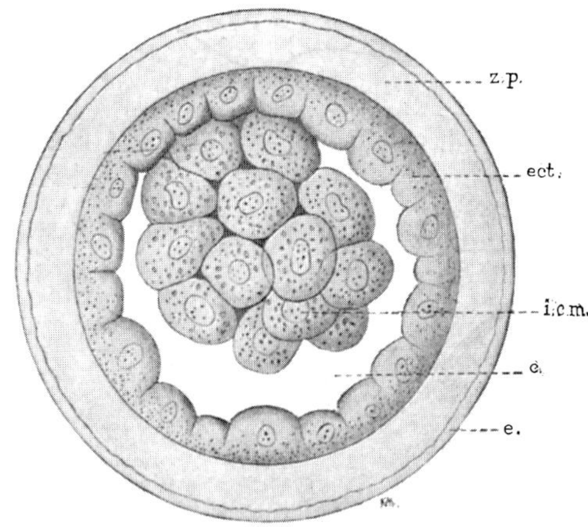

FIG. 90.—BLASTODERMIC VESICLE OF RABBIT (v. Beneden).

c., cavity of vesicle; *ect.*, primitive ectoderm; *i.c.m.*, internal cell mass; *z.p.*, zona pellucida; *e.*, albuminous envelope.

Development of the Ovum.—Soon after the appearance of the segmentation nucleus, caryocinetic changes take place within it and give rise to a typical nuclear spindle, which is soon converted into a dyaster, to be speedily followed by the division of the ovum into two cells (Figs. 85 and 86). Each of these in turn divides, giving rise to four cells, though Sobotta's investigations on the mouse show that one of the original cells segments earlier than the other, so that we next have three cells. This process of cell division or segmentation goes on until the original ovum becomes converted into a mass of cells, which is designated as the *morula* or *mulberry mass* (Fig. 89).

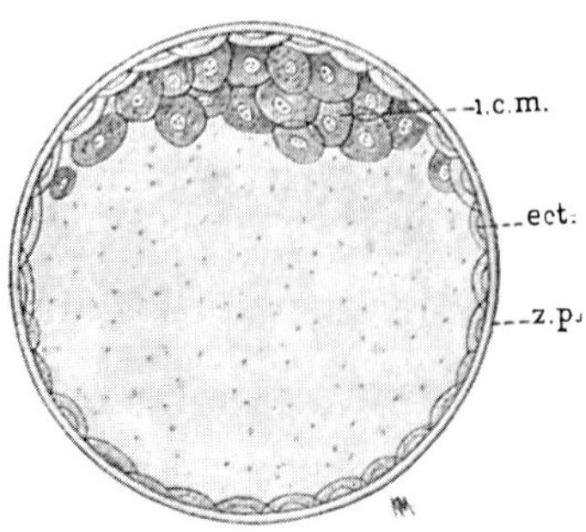

FIG. 91.—MAMMALIAN BLASTODERMIC VESICLE (v. Beneden).

ect., primitive ectoderm; *i.c.m.*, internal cell mass (embryonic area); *z.p.*, zona pellucida.

Fluid soon appears in the mulberry mass and forces the cells to the periphery, thus giving rise to a vesicular structure consisting of a single layer of cells which surround a cavity filled with fluid—the segmentation cavity. The entire structure at this time is known as the *blastodermic vesicle*, which in the rabbit and many other animals is still surrounded by the vitelline membrane (Fig. 90), whereas in the mouse the latter disappears before the formation of the mulberry mass.

In a short time a collection of cells can be noted at one point on the inner surface of the blastodermic vesicle. This is known as the *internal cell-mass*; while the single layer of cells forming the wall of the vesicle is frequently spoken of as the primitive chorion (Fig. 91). When viewed by transmitted light the internal cell-mass appears darker than the rest of the surface of the blastodermic vesicle, and hence is called the *macula embryonalis.* Sections made through it at this point show that it is composed of several layers of cells, those nearest the exterior being ectodermal, and those nearest the segmentation cavity entodermal.

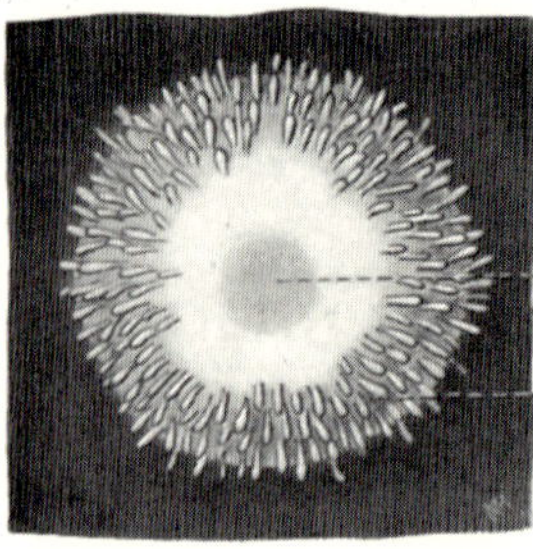

Fig. 92.—Human Ovum (Reichert). × 6.

e.a., embryonic area ; *v.*, villi.

This stage of development has not as yet been observed in the human ovum, but as it has been demonstrated in the ova of the various species of animals which have been available for study, there is no doubt that it occurs in all mammals. These changes are supposed to take place while the ovum is making its way through the tubes, which is believed to occupy a period of from five to seven days, since the only human ovum thus far found in transit through the Fallopian tube was discovered by Hyrtl in its uterine end five days after the cessation of the menstrual period. The earliest human ovum appearing in the uterine cavity was recently described by Peters, and, although he considers it to be only three days old, certainly presents a tolerably advanced stage of development.

As the cells composing the internal cell-mass proliferate, they give rise to a round or oval area at one point on the surface of the blastodermic

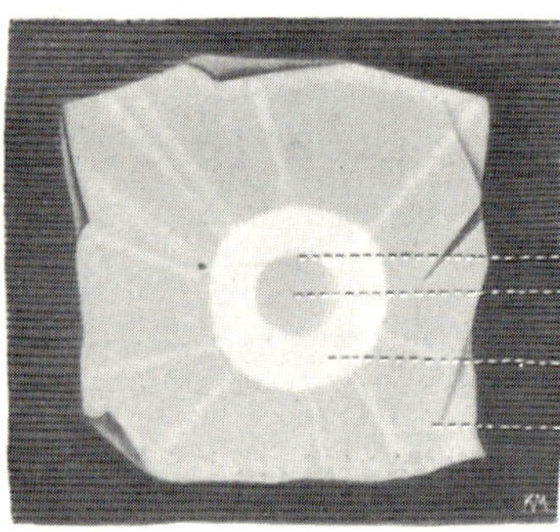

Fig. 93.

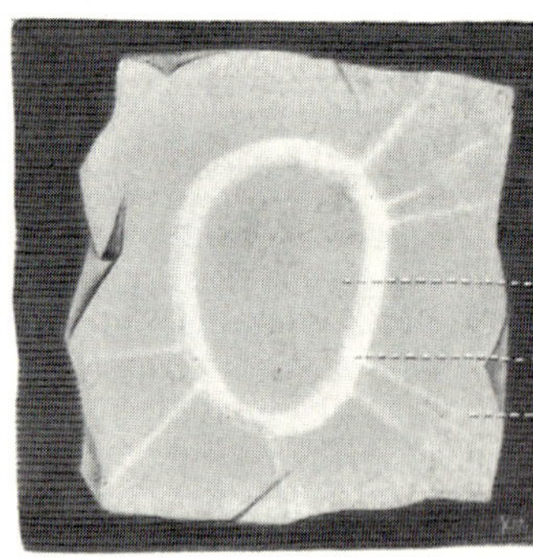

Fig. 94.

Figs. 93, 94.—Embryonic Area of Rabbit (Kollmann). × 30.

A.o., area opaca ; *A.p.*, area pellucida ; *B.v.*, wall of blastodermic vesicle ; *E.s.*, embryonic shield.

vesicle—the *embryonic area*—which at first consists of two layers of cells representing the ectoderm and entoderm respectively. One of the earliest human ova showing this condition was described by Reichert. It was oval in shape, about the size of a pea, and partially covered by villi (Fig. 92).

Specimens presenting this stage of development are readily obtained from the lower animals, especially rabbits. In them the embryonic area, when viewed by transmitted light, is first round, but later oval in shape, and presents a dark centre and a light periphery, which are designated respectively as the *area opaca* and the *area pellucida* (Figs. 93 and 94).

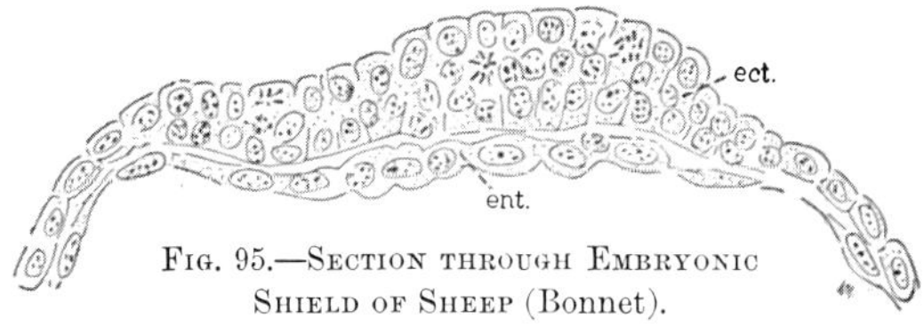

FIG. 95.—SECTION THROUGH EMBRYONIC SHIELD OF SHEEP (Bonnet).
ect., ectoderm ; *ent.*, entoderm.

The embryonic area soon becomes slightly elevated above the general surface of the blastodermic vesicle, and now forms what is known as the *embryonic shield*; its differentiation into the area opaca and the area pellucida is due to the varying number of cells composing it, inasmuch as they are arranged in several layers in the former, whereas in the latter only two can be made out. A few hours later a darker zone appears at one end of the embryonic shield and soon exceeds it in size (Fig. 96). This is the *mesodermic area*, which on section is seen to be made up of spindle-shaped and triangular cells. Fig. 97, representing a section through the embryonic area of a rabbit at this stage, shows distinctly that it is made up of three layers — ectoderm, mesoderm, and entoderm. The mesodermic area rapidly increases in size, and soon forms a complete layer inside the blastodermic vesicle just beneath the ectoderm.

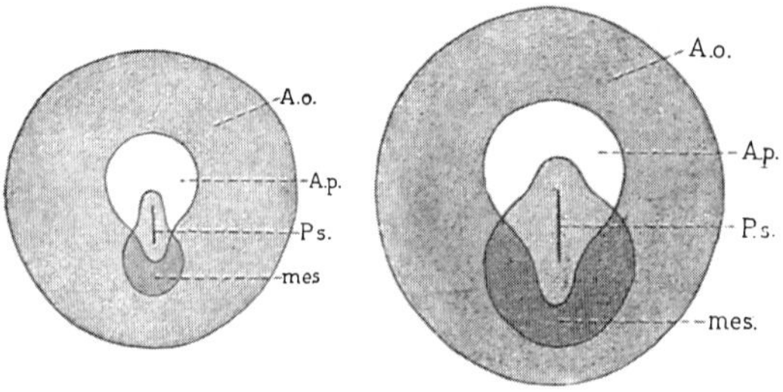

FIG. 96.—DIAGRAMS SHOWING EXTENSION OF MESODERM (Duval).
A.o., area opaca; *A.p.*, area pellucida; *mes.*, mesoderm; *P.s.*, primitive streak.

A little later there appears in the middle of the embryonic area a slight depression—the *primitive streak*—which is bounded on either side by a slight elevation—the *primitive folds*. Graf Spee has described a human ovum from the early part of the second week, which presented this stage of development. In it the embryonic area was 0.4 millimetre long, and the primitive streak extended throughout its entire length (Figs. 98 and 103). A little later a second depression—the *medullary groove*—appears in front of the primitive streak. It is bounded on either side by an elevated fold—the medullary ridges—which converge anteriorly to form the head-folds. The medullary groove is in the same line with the primitive streak,

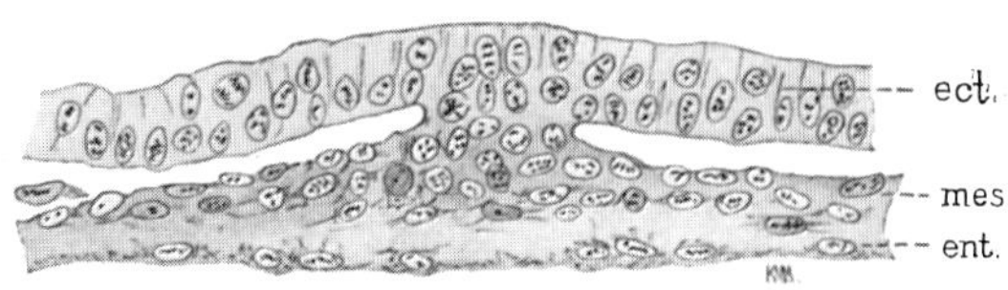

FIG. 97.—RABBIT'S OVUM, SHOWING THREE LAYERS (Rabl).
ect., ectoderm ; *ent.*, entoderm ; *mes.*, mesoderm.

but never unites with it; while the medullary folds diverge posteriorly and inclose the anterior end of the primitive streak. As the ovum becomes older the medullary groove and folds rapidly increase in size, while the primitive streak remains stationary, so that in a short time it occupies only a small portion of the embryonic area.

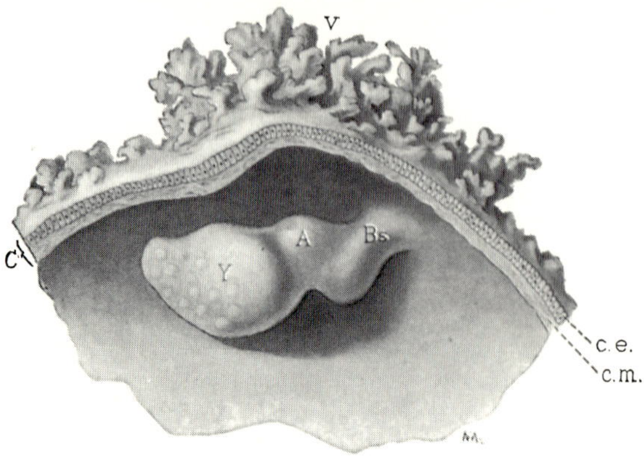

Fig. 98.—Spee's Human Ovum, Embryonic Area, 0.4 Millimetre Long. × 24.

A., amnion; *Bs.*, abdominal pedicle; *C.*, chorion; *c.e.*, chorionic epithelium; *c.m.*, chorionic mesoderm; *V.*, chorionic villi; *Y.*, yolk-sac.

Graf Spee has also described a human ovum belonging to a stage a little later than that represented in Fig. 98, in which the embryonic area was 2 millimetres long. The structures occupying it are clearly shown in Fig. 100. The medullary groove and primitive streak are not in the same plane, but the latter is bent almost at right angles to the former and occupies the inferior end of the embryonic area. Between the two is a small opening, the *neurenteric canal*, which serves to connect the ectoderm with the entoderm.

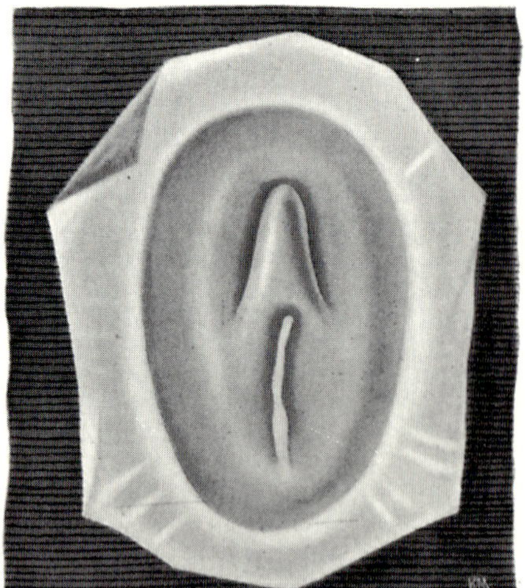

Fig. 99.—Embryonic Shield of Rabbit, showing Primitive Streak and Medullary Folds (Kollmann). × 28.

The medullary groove and folds result from the proliferation of the ectoderm, and from them the central nervous system is developed.

While these changes are taking place on the surface of the embryonic area, others of no less importance are going on in its depths, which result in the formation of the mesodermic structure. On either side of the medullary canal can be observed a slight thickening—the segmental layer (the Stammzone of the Germans), outside of which is a thinner layer—the parietal zone (Fig. 101). The segmental layer soon becomes divided up into a number of more or less cuboidal masses of tissue on either side of the medullary groove, which are variously designated as *protovertebræ*, primary segments, or mesoblastic somites; from these the musculature of the dorsal portion of the body is developed. The parietal zone is also made up of mesoderm, and soon becomes divided into two layers which inclose a cavity, the *cœlome*. The outer layer is covered by ectoderm, and is designated as the *somatopleure*, while the inner is lined by entoderm and is called the *splanchnopleure*. From a part of the former the anterior and lateral abdominal walls are developed, while in many of the lower animals its greater portion gives rise to the chorion and amnion.

Thus far we have considered the growing ovum as seen from without; but the study of the microscopical sections through it aid us still further in understanding its development. Fig. 95 represents a section through the embryonic area at an early period, and shows that the greater part of the blastodermic vesicle is composed of two layers of cells, the *ectoderm* and the *entoderm*. In the region of the embryonic area the ectoderm is arranged in several layers, whereas the entoderm consists of a single layer. Fig. 97 represents a section through the embryonic area of a rabbit at a little later stage, and shows three distinct layers —ectoderm, mesoderm, and entoderm. In Fig. 102 the embryonic area of a chicken is shown at a still later period of development; the medullary groove and notochord are well marked, and the mesoderm has become thickened to form the segmental layer.

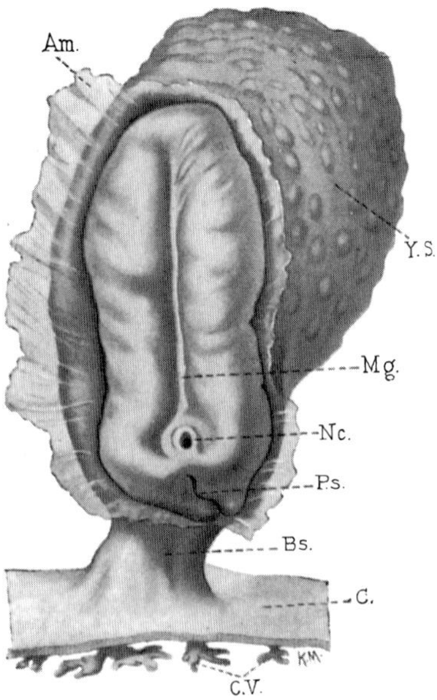

FIG. 100.—HUMAN EMBRYO 2 MILLIMETRES LONG (Graf Spee). × 30.

A., amnion; *C.*, chorion; *C.V.*, chorionic villi; *B.s.*, Bauchstiel; *M.g.*, medullary groove; *N.c.*, neurenteric canal; *P.s.*, primitive streak; *Y.s.*, yolk-sac.

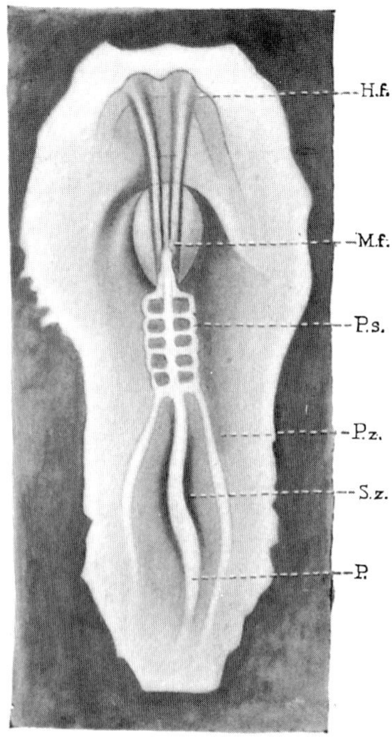

FIG. 101.—CHICKEN EMBRYO WITH FIVE SEGMENTS (Kollmann).

H.f., head fold; *M.f.*, medullary folds; *P.*, primitive streak; *P.s.*, primitive segments; *P.z.*, parietal zone; *S.z.*, segmental zone.

Fig. 103 shows a section through Graf Spee's youngest ovum, in which the three layers are clearly differentiated, and the dorsal portion of the

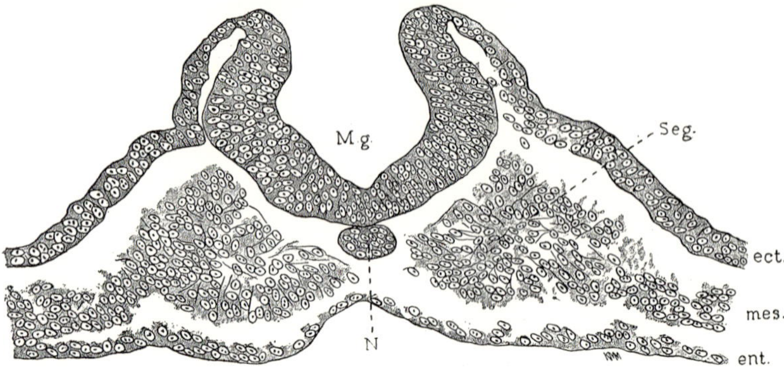

FIG. 102.—CROSS-SECTION THROUGH CHICKEN EMBRYO WITH SEVEN SEGMENTS (Minot). × 220. *ect.*, ectoderm; *ent.*, entoderm; *mes.*, mesoderm; *M.g.*, medullary groove; *N.*, notochord; *Seg.*, primitive segment.

embryo is covered by amnion. Fig. 104 shows a human ovum at a later period, with a well-defined medullary canal and a marked increase in the mesodermic structures.

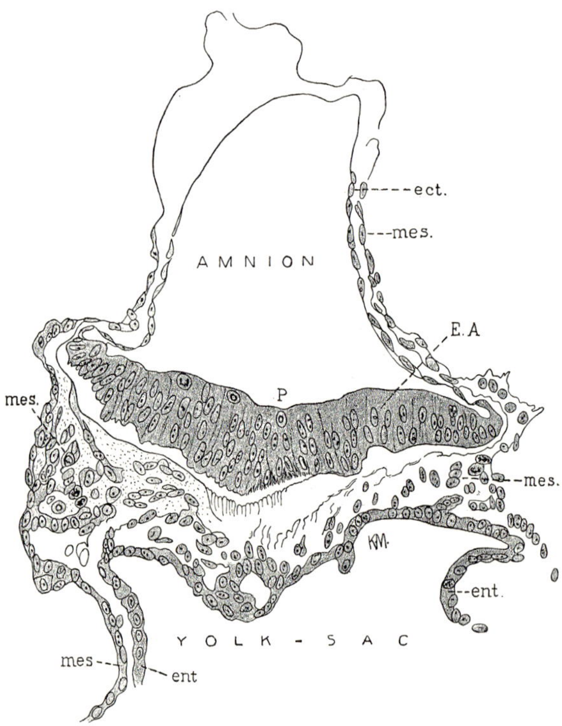

FIG. 103.—CROSS-SECTION THROUGH GRAF SPEE'S YOUNGEST OVUM. *E.A.*, embryonic area; *P.*, primitive streak; *ect.*, ectoderm; *ent.*, entoderm; *mes.*, mesoderm.

From the ectoderm are developed the central nervous system and the cutaneous structures; from the mesoderm are derived the muscular and circulatory portions of the body, the reproductive organs and the connective-tissue framework of the various other organs; while the entoderm gives rise to the digestive tract and the organs which are more or less intimately connected with it.

In the chicken and many mammals the *chorion* and *amnion* are not formed until the parietal layer of the mesoderm has become well developed and, together with the ectoderm, has been differentiated into the somatopleure and splanchnopleure; but in all of the very early human ova thus far described, the chorion and amnion are well developed, while the embryo itself is in a very rudimentary condition. This would appear to indicate that in man and certain mammals they are formed in a manner different from that usually described for the lower animals.

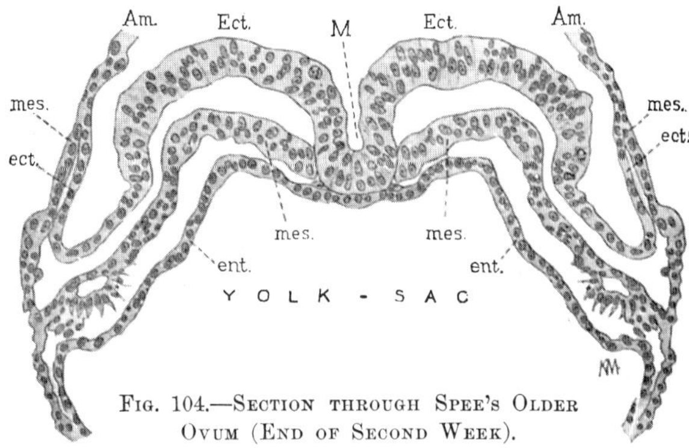

FIG. 104.—SECTION THROUGH SPEE'S OLDER OVUM (END OF SECOND WEEK).

Am., amnion; *ect.*, ectoderm; *mes.*, mesoderm; *ent.*, entoderm; *M.*, medullary groove.

Amnion and Chorion in the Chick.—We shall now briefly consider the formation of the chorion and amnion in the chicken and many of the mammals. While the changes which we have just described are taking place in the embryonic area, the entoderm and mesoderm extend around the interior of the blastodermic vesicle, so that in a short time its walls are made up of three layers, except in the region of the embryonic area, where quite a

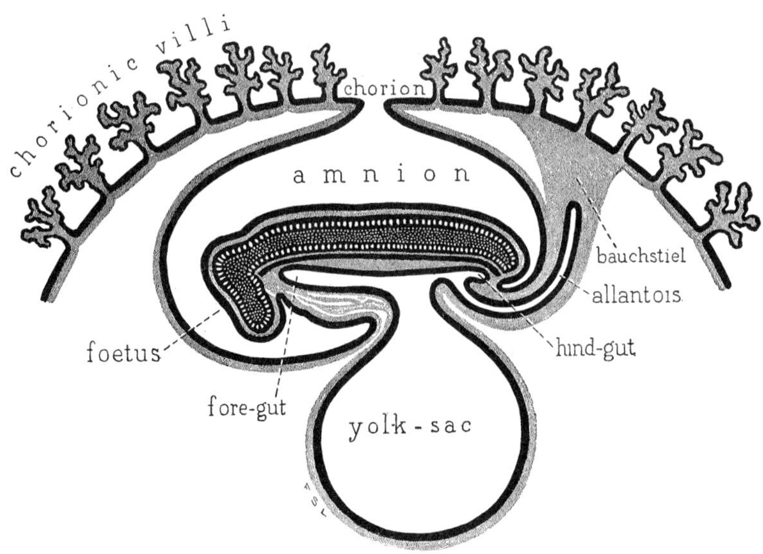

FIG. 105.—DIAGRAM SHOWING LONGITUDINAL SECTION THROUGH MAMMALIAN EMBRYO, SHOWING FORMATION OF AMNION.

number are present. At this period the cavity lined by entoderm occupies the greater part of the ovum and is designated as the *yolk-sac*.

After the segmental and parietal zones have been developed, and the latter has become differentiated into the *somatopleure* and *splanchnopleure,* the formation of the fœtal membranes begins, and part of the yolk-sac is taken up into the embryo to form the intestinal tract.

At either end of the embryonic area a fold of somatopleure makes its appearance and gradually arches over the cephalic and caudal extremities until the two portions meet together in the middle and thus form a double-layered sac which surrounds the embryo. The inner layer consists of ectoderm within and mesoderm without, and is designated as the amnion; the outer layer consists of mesoderm within and ectoderm without, and is known as the chorion; while the cavity between the two is called the extra-embryonic cœlome. According to Minot, therefore, "the chorion is all of the extra-embryonic portion of the somatopleure which does not enter into the formation of the amnion." While the outer por-

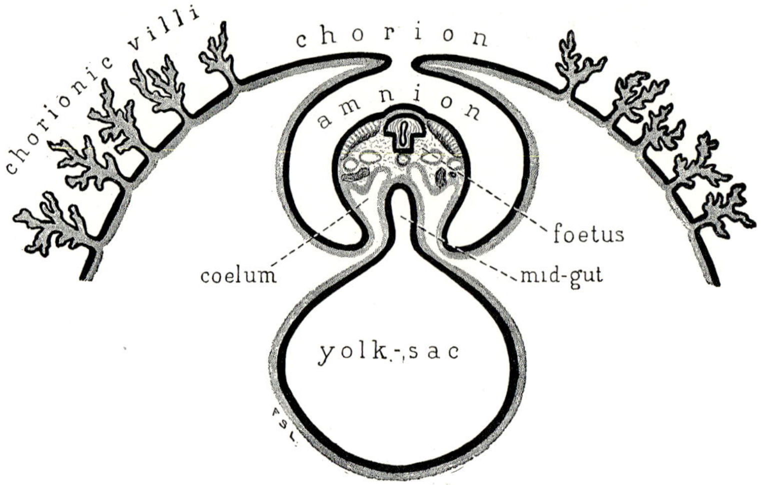

Fig. 106.—Diagram showing Transverse Section through Mammalian Embryo, showing Formation of Amnion.

tions of the somatopleure are taking part in the formation of the amnion and chorion, those nearer the embryo become folded inward and downward to form its abdominal walls.

Coincident with these changes the splanchnopleure becomes separated throughout the entire extent of the ovum, so that it completely surrounds the yolk-sac, which then becomes a definite organ lined within by entoderm and without by mesoderm, and separated from the chorion by the cœlome.

As the body walls become developed at the head and tail ends and sides of the embryo, the upper portion of the yolk-sac becomes included within its body, where it forms the primitive gut and becomes more or less separated from the rest of the yolk-sac by the infolding of the somatopleure which forms the abdominal walls. This condition of affairs is well illustrated in Figs. 105 and 106.

Almost as soon as the formation of the hindgut is begun, a small off-

PLATE IV.

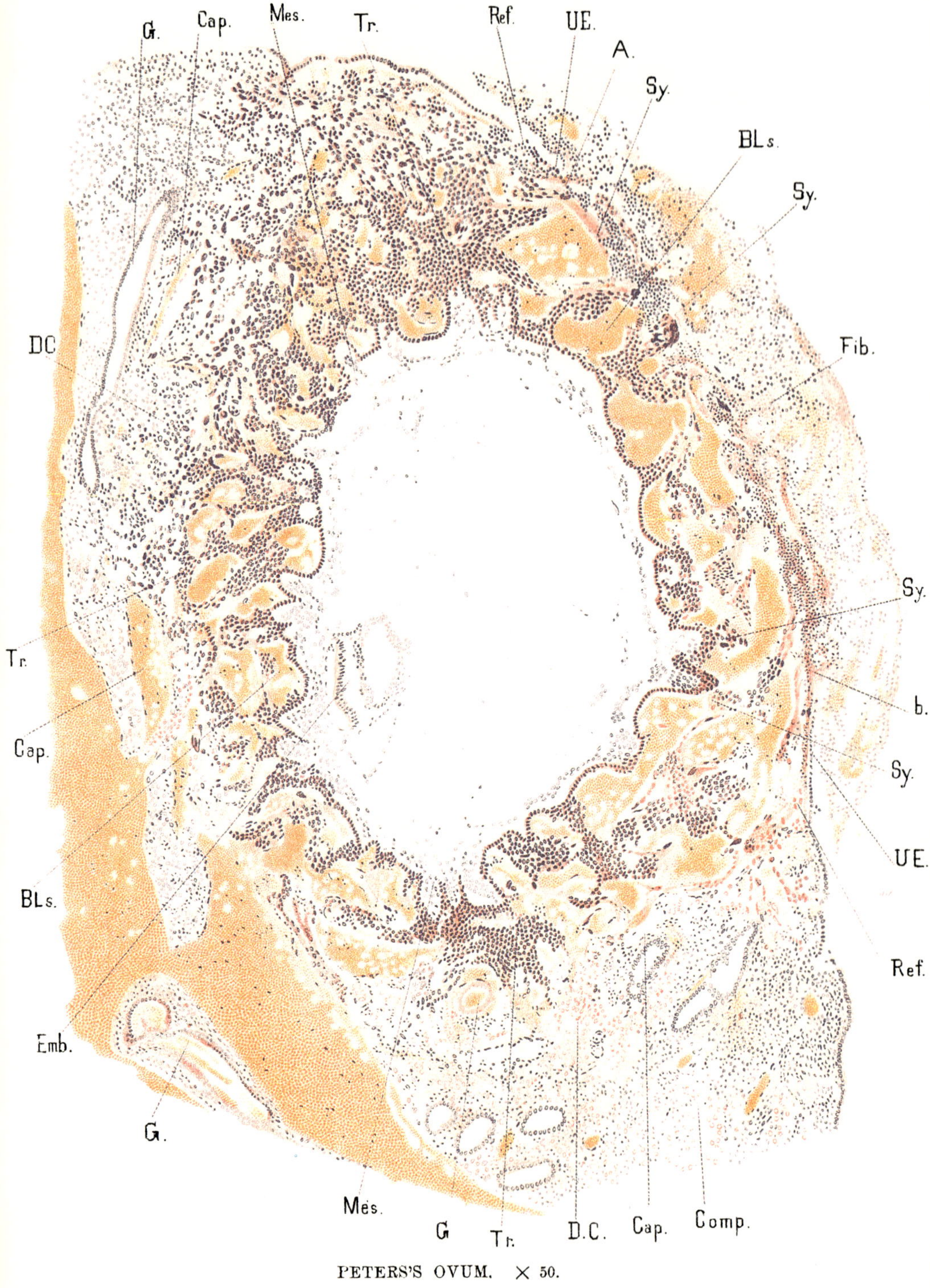

PETERS'S OVUM. × 50.

Bl.S., blood spaces; *Cap.*, capillary; *Comp.*, compact layer of decidua; *D. C.*, decidual cells; ***Emb.***, beginning embryo; ***Fib.***, mass of fibrin covering point of entry of ovum into decidua; ***Mes.***, connective-tissue layer of chorion; ***Ref.***, decidua reflexa; ***Syn.***, syncytium; ***Tr.***, trophoblast; ***U. E.***, uterine epithelium.

shoot extends from its caudal extremity, which is made up of entoderm internally and mesoderm externally. This is the *allantois*, which undergoes marked development in many animals, but in man remains in a rudimentary condition. In many animals it becomes converted into a vesicular structure which soon occupies a considerable portion of the extra-embryonic cœlome, until it reaches the inner surface of the chorion, to which it applies itself, and with which it soon becomes intimately connected. The umbilical vessels spread out over the allantois, through which they are ultimately distributed to the chorion and thus bring about intimate vascular connections between the vessels of the embryo and those of the mother.

When the allantoic vesicle is highly developed, as in the calf, it also serves another important function, as into it a large part of the urinary secretion of the embryo is passed.

Formation of Chorion and Amnion in Man.—The earliest human ova thus far described possess a well-developed chorion and amnion, while the embryo itself is in a far more rudimentary stage of development than is the case with most mammals at the time of the formation of the somatopleure and splanchnopleure. Accordingly, it appears reasonable to suppose that these structures are formed in man in a manner different from that which obtains for most of the lower animals.

Peters's specimen, which was found in the uterus of a woman who committed suicide three days after missing her menstrual period, is the *youngest human ovum* with which we are acquainted. It measured $1.6 \times 0.8 \times 0.9$ millimetre in its various diameters, and presented a well-developed chorion and a very small amnion. Plate IV represents a section through the portion of decidua in which it was embedded, and shows that the chorion is made up of two layers—a thin, inner layer of connective tissue which is poor in cells and forms the lining of the cœlomic cavity, and an outer layer composed of many layers of epithelial cells. These cells form a capsule of varying thickness about the periphery of the ovum, and are designated as the *trophoblast*, which in Peters's opinion represents the primitive ectoderm of the ovum. The majority of the cells are distinctly epithelial in appearance and possess well-marked roundish or cuboidal bodies and vesicular nuclei. Scattered between them are masses of protoplasm which show no sign of division into individual cells, and contain irregularly shaped, darkly staining nuclei. The trophoblast has invaded the surrounding decidual tissue and opened up numerous blood-vessels, so that many comparatively large blood spaces have been formed in it.

From the underlying connective tissue of the chorion, numerous small processes project into the trophoblast and represent the earliest stages in the formation of *chorionic villi*.

Merttens, Reichert, Leopold, and Spee have all described ova from the second week of pregnancy, none of which exceeded 4 millimetres in diameter. Each possessed a well-developed chorion with typical branching villi. The ova of Reichert and Spee were cast off as early abortions, while those of Merttens and Leopold were found in the uterus, the former being discovered accidentally in the scrapings obtained by curettage, and the latter in a uterus removed for carcinoma; both were completely surrounded by decidual tissue. Fig. 92 gives a representation of Reichert's ovum, which is lenticular in shape and surrounded at its equator by short villi. Fig. 109 represents a section through Leopold's ovum, and shows that it is surrounded by villi which are in contact with the decidua serotina and reflexa. In all of these ova the chorion consists of a membranous sac composed of mesoderm within and ectoderm without, from whose periphery numerous villi project which are covered by two layers of epithelium.

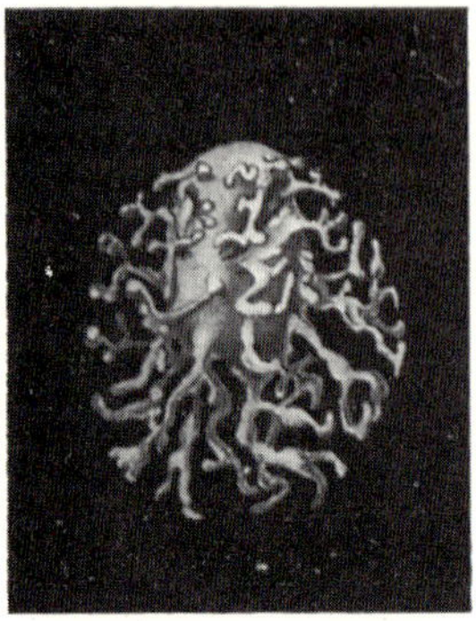

FIG. 107.—SEVEN- TO EIGHT-DAYS' HUMAN OVUM (Leopold).

From the study of these, which are the youngest ova at present at our disposal, it is apparent that definite information concerning the development and origin of the human chorion is still lacking, though it is probable that the earliest stages in its formation are completed while the ovum is still in the tube. Furthermore, it is highly probable that the changes which result in its formation are among the very first which the human ovum undergoes, and that the chorionic epithelium corresponds to the primary ectoderm of the blastodermic vesicle.

Kollmann believes that the ovum, by the time it reaches the uterus, is surrounded by a distinct chorion possessing short but definitely formed villi; while Ruge and Peters hold that the villi do not appear until after the implantation of the ovum upon the decidua. Further particulars concerning the structure of the chorion will be given later.

Nor have the earliest stages in the formation of the amnion been observed in the earliest human ova yet obtainable, inasmuch as in all of them a closed amniotic sac had already been formed which arched over the embryonic area. In Peters's ovum the amnion was represented by a closed, flattened sac, which was almost in contact with the embryonic area on the one side and with the connective-tissue layer of the chorion on the other (Fig. 110).

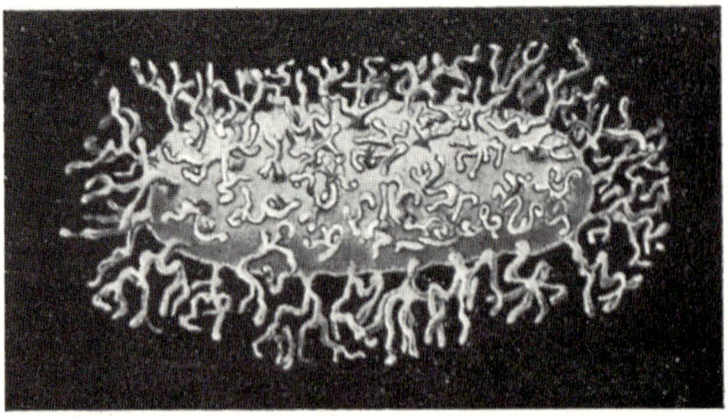

FIG. 108.—TWO-WEEKS' HUMAN OVUM (Leopold).

The ovum from the second week, described by Graf Spee, gives us important information concerning the amnion, and although it does not present the earliest stages in its formation, it enables us to theorize as to its origin. The entire ovum in this case measured 6 × 4.5 millimetres in diameter, and possessed a well-developed chorion, a portion of which is shown in Fig. 98. Projecting from one point of its interior is a small vesicular structure—the beginning embryo.

Fig. 111 represents a section through the same ovum, and shows clearly the relations of its various parts. The embryo is attached to the inner surface of the chorionic membrane by a mesodermic pedicle, which represents the earliest stage of the *abdominal pedicle* (the Bauchstiel of the Germans), which is the precursor of the umbilical cord. The greater portion of the embryo is occupied by the yolk-sac, from one end of which a small process, lined by entoderm, extends into the pedicle, which must be considered as a rudimentary allantois. Occupying one side of the pedicle is a small cavity lined by a single layer of epithelium, which corresponds

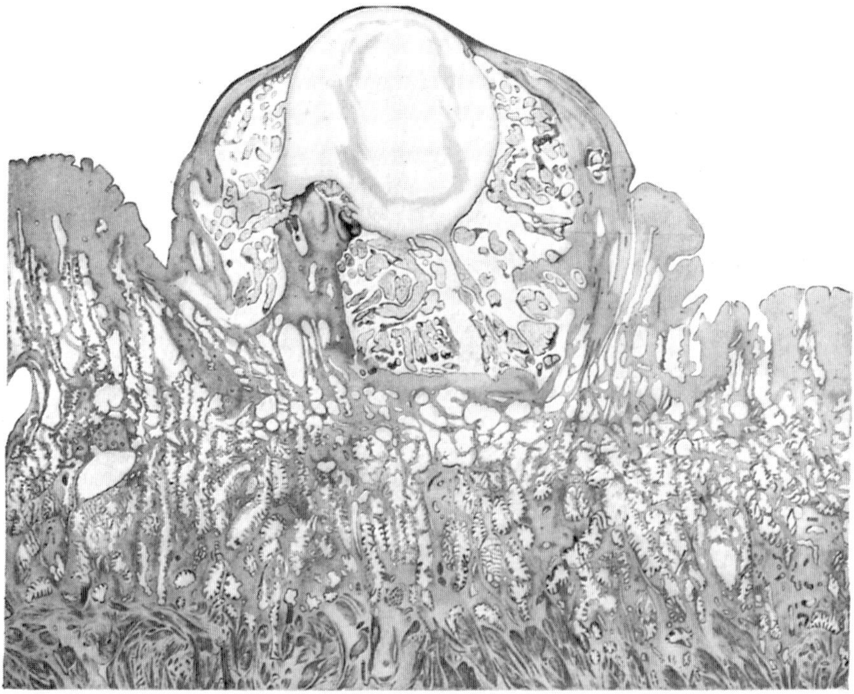

Fig. 109.—Microscopic Section, showing Seven-days' Ovum Embedded in Decidua and Surrounded by Decidua Reflexa (Leopold).

to the amnion. On one side of this, again, is a mass of cells arranged in several layers, which represents the embryonic area, in which there is a primitive streak 0.4 millimetre long. It is apparent from this specimen that the amnion could not have resulted from the formation and fusion of the two folds of somatopleure, as is usually stated, for the embryonic area is in a far too rudimentary state to admit of such an explanation.

Figs. 100 and 112 represent an older ovum which was also described by Graf Spee, and which he believed belonged to the third week of pregnancy. In it the relations are essentially the same, except that the outlines of the embryo are clearly indicated and all the parts are larger. The amnion appears as a flattened sac, which is closely applied over the dorsal surface of the embryonic area.

Graf Spee, in describing his youngest ovum, stated that it was possible that the amnion might be formed by an inversion of a portion of the wall of the original blastodermic vesicle, and the recent investigations

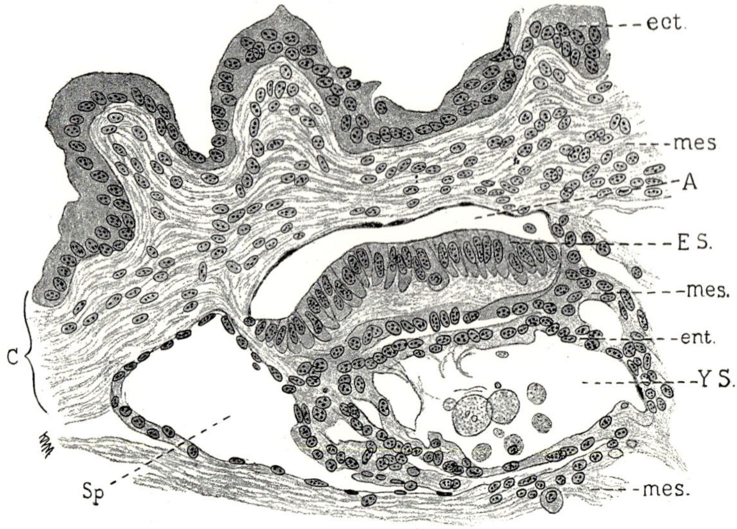

Fig. 110.—Portion of Peters's Ovum, Highly Magnified, showing Early Stage in Development of Embryo.

A., amnion ; *C.*, chorion ; *ect.*, ectoderm ; *ent.*, entoderm ; *mes.*, mesoderm ; *E.S.*, embryonic shield *Y.S.*, yolk-sac ; *Sp.*, portion of cœlum.

of Selenka upon the monkey tend to confirm this view. Fig. 113, representing a section through a very young monkey embryo, shows an earlier stage of development than Graf Spee's youngest ovum; here the amnion is represented by an inversion from the surface of the blastodermic vesicle. It is only necessary to suppose that the upper margins of the inverted

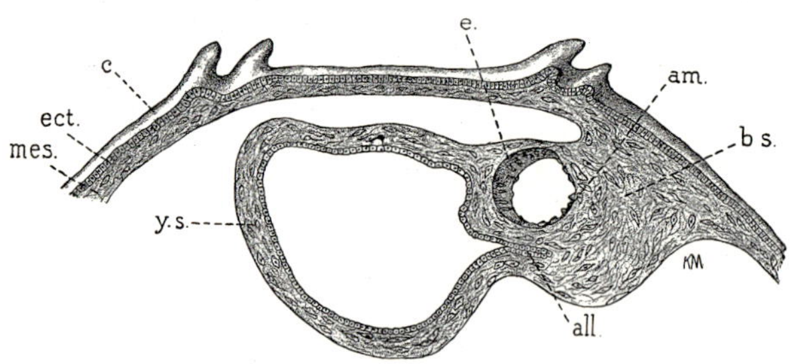

Fig. 111.—Section through Spee's Youngest Ovum, shown in Fig. 98. × 24.

c., chorionic membrane ; *ect.*, ectoderm ; *mes.*, mesoderm ; *am.*, amnion ; *e.*, beginning embryo ; *bs.*, abdominal pedicle ; *all.*, allantois ; *y.s.*, yolk-sac.

portion of the ectoderm had become adherent in order to produce a condition similar to that observed in Spee's ovum.

Structure of the Chorion.—In its very earliest stages, and while the ovum is still in the tube, the chorion probably consists of the single layer of ectodermal cells forming the wall of the blastodermic vesicle, which soon becomes lined by a mesodermic layer. In the uterus, however, as shown by the researches of Hubrecht, Heukelom, and Peters, the chorionic epithelium rapidly proliferates and forms the many-layered trophoblast. In its earliest stages the chorion is probably a smooth membranous sac without villi; but in a short time buds of connective tissue make their way into the trophoblast and give rise to rudimentary villi.

Fig. 114 represents a section through the chorion from a seventeen-days'-old pregnancy. In it can be distinguished two portions—the chorionic membrane and the villi projecting from it. The chorionic membrane consists of two layers—the inner of connective tissue, the outer

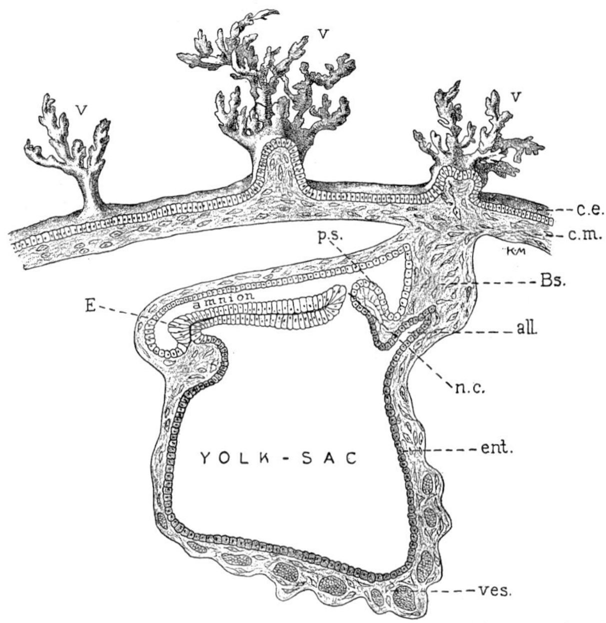

FIG. 112.—SECTION THROUGH HUMAN OVUM, SHOWN IN FIG. 100 (Spee).
all., allantois; *c.e.*, chorionic epithelium; *c.m.*, chorionic mesoderm; *Bs.*, abdominal pedicle; *E.*, beginning embryo; *ent.*, entoderm; *n.c.*, neurenteric canal; *p.s.*, primitive streak; *v.*, chorionic villi; *ves.*, vessels in wall of yolk-sac.

of epithelium. Its connective tissue is composed of spindle- and star-shaped cells embedded in a mucoid intercellular substance, and at this period does not contain blood-vessels. Its epithelium is arranged in two layers: an inner one adjoining the connective tissue, which is composed of sharply marked cuboidal or roundish cells with clear protoplasm and lightly staining vesicular nuclei, and an outer layer made up of coarsely granular protoplasm, which shows no signs of division into cells, and through which are scattered irregularly shaped, darkly staining nuclei.

Each villus arises from the chorionic membrane as a single stem, giving origin to numerous branches which result in a more or less arborescent form, the complexity of which increases with advancing age. The villi consist of a connective-tissue stroma and an epithelial covering, the former being continuous with and analogous in structure to the connective tissue of the chorionic membrane, while the epithelium is composed of the same two layers.

Projecting here and there from the surface of the villi are epithelial buds, usually consisting of a mass of protoplasm which is not divided into distinct cells, and which, when seen in cross or tangential section, resemble giant cells. These buds indicate proliferation of the outer layer of the chorionic epithelium, and represent the first stage in the development of new villous branches. Here and there in the spaces between the villi, larger and smaller masses of small, clear cells with vesicular nuclei are seen. They are usually described as *decidual islands,* and are supposed to represent sections through decidual septa, which project upward towards the chorionic membrane. It is more than probable, however, that they are really masses of trophoblast which have not been converted into villi.

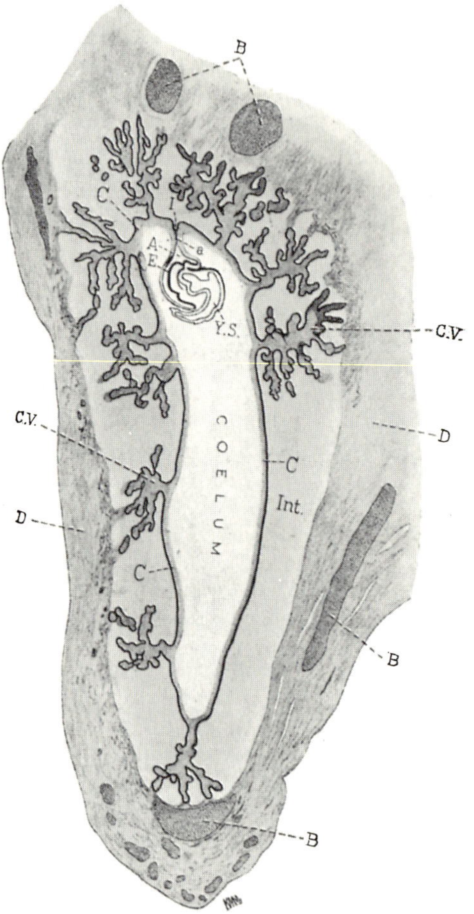

Fig. 113.—Section through Young Ovum of Hylobates, showing Formation of Amnion (Selenka). × 8.

A., amnion; *a.*, amniotic pedicle; *B.*, blood-vessel; *C.*, chorion; *C.V.*, chorionic villi; *D.*, decidua; *E.*, embryo; *I.*, point of inversion of blastodermic vesicle; *Int.*, Intervillous space; *Y.S.*, yolk-sac.

In early ova the embryo is connected with the connective-tissue layer of the chorion by a mesodermic pedicle, which was first described by His as the *abdominal pedicle* (Bauchstiel). In it can be observed a small process of entoderm which represents an extension of the hindgut, and which corresponds to the allantois of lower vertebrates. Through the abdominal pedicle the umbilical vessels of the embryo make their way to the interior of the chorion, which then becomes vascularized.

For our first definite information concerning the structure of the *fully developed human chorion* we are indebted to Langhans, who showed that it was made up of four layers: a gelatinous, a fibrillar, a vascular, and an epithelial layer. The gelatinous is the innermost layer and is composed of star- and spindle-shaped connective-tissue cells embedded in a mucoid intercellular substance. External to this the cells become more fusiform in shape and relatively abundant, so that the membrane assumes a more fibrillar appearance. Scattered through the portion just outside of this second layer are numerous vessels, both arteries and veins; while still more externally comes the epithelial covering, which is composed of the two layers already described in the seventeen-days'-old chorion.

Projecting from the outer surface of the chorionic membrane are numerous villi, which at first are pretty equally distributed over its periphery. As pregnancy advances, however, they become more abundant over the portion which is in contact with the decidua serotina, the site of the future

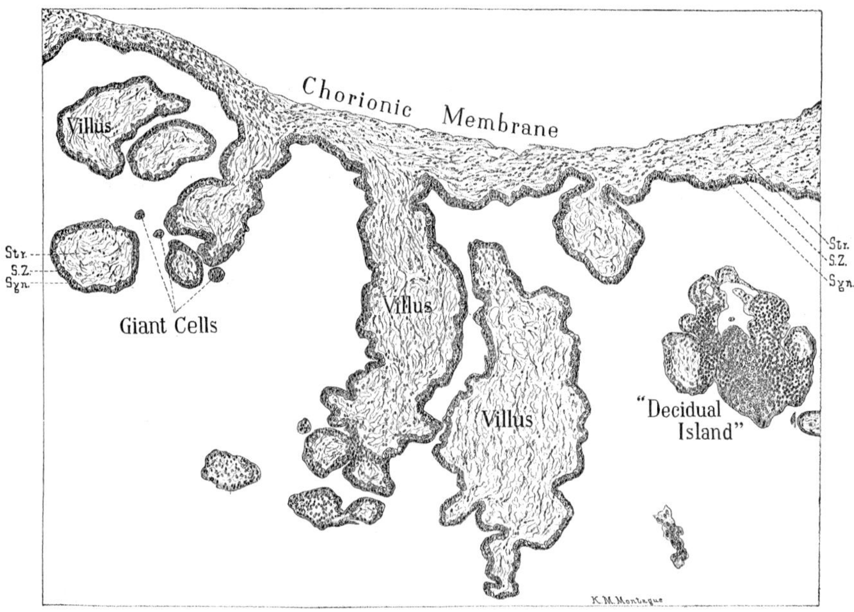

FIG. 114.—SECTION THROUGH CHORION OF TWO-WEEKS, HUMAN OVUM. × 50. *Str.*, stroma; *S.Z.*, Langhans's layer; *Syn.*, syncytium.

placenta. This portion of the chorion is designated as the *chorion frondosum,* while the remainder, which is in contact with the decidua reflexa, is termed the *chorion læve,* since the villi covering it eventually undergo complete degeneration.

A certain number of villi extend from the chorionic membrane to the underlying decidua, attaching the ovum to it, and hence are designated as *fastening villi.* The majority of the villi, however, spring from the chorionic membrane as arborescent structures, whose free endings do not reach the decidua, and which increase in complexity as pregnancy advances.

In early pregnancy the villi are short and plump and represent simply the main stems, which later give off numerous branches and assume an arborescent appearance. Thus, sections through a young chorion show only a few large villi, while those through an older one are filled with a multitude of smaller villi. This change in appearance is due to the increasing arborescence, and may be compared to what takes place in a clump of trees, which at an early period are represented by a number of almost isolated trunks, but later give off innumerable branches and twigs. These differences have been particularly emphasized by De Loos, who has shown that with a little practice one can roughly estimate the age of the chorion by its appearance on section.

The stroma of the chorionic villi is made up of connective tissue which varies in appearance according to the age of the chorion. In the earlier stages the cells are branching in shape, and are separated from one another by a large amount of mucoid intercellular substance; later on they become more spindle-shaped and more closely packed together, so that the stroma assumes a denser appearance (Figs. 115 and 117). After the first few weeks blood-vessels appear in the stroma, and in the later months of pregnancy the arteries present thick walls possessing the typical three layers. The arteries and veins extend to the tips of the villi, where they break up into

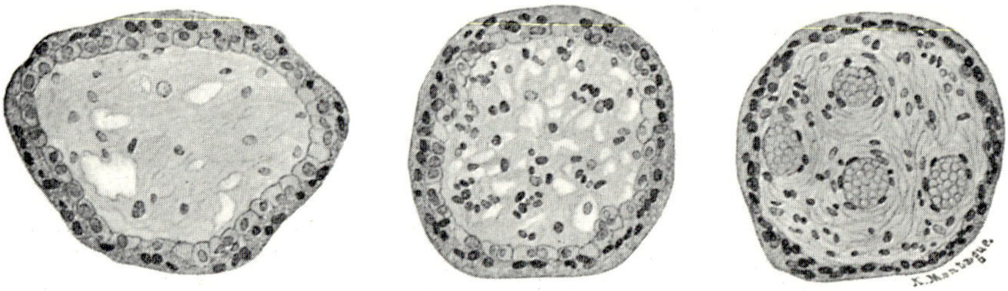

Fig. 115. Fig. 116. Fig. 117.

FIGS. 115–117.—CHORIONIC VILLI AT THIRD WEEK AND THIRD AND NINTH MONTHS. × 375.

capillaries, but there is no anastomosis between the vascular supply of the various villi any more than between the branches of different trees in a forest.

The *epithelium* covering the villi was mentioned by Dalrymple in 1842, but was first definitely described by Langhans many years later. The latter pointed out that it was made up of two layers similar to those which have been described in the seventeen-days'-old chorion. The inner layer was designated as the *cell-layer* (Zellschicht), and is now generally known as *Langhans's layer*; while the outer layer is usually known as the *syncytium*. The term "syncytium" was introduced in 1893–'94 by Kossmann and Merttens, although the characteristics of the tissue had been recognised years before by Kastschenko, who described it as *plasmodium*.

During the first half of pregnancy the two are readily distinguished, but in the second half Langhans's layer becomes more and more indistinct, so that at the end of pregnancy the majority of the villi are covered only by a single layer of syncytium. Figs. 115, 116, and 117 give a good idea of the successive changes in the stroma and epithelium of the villi at different ages.

The origin of the two layers of chorionic epithelium has given rise to a great deal of discussion, but it has been established by the work of

Langhans, Kastschenko, Minot, Webster, Heukelom, His, Ruge, and Peters that they are both of fœtal origin, and are derived from the ectoderm. Peters has demonstrated that they both come from the original trophoblastic covering of the ovum. He believes that this was originally made up of individual cells, which, however, became converted into syncytium where they came in contact with the maternal blood.

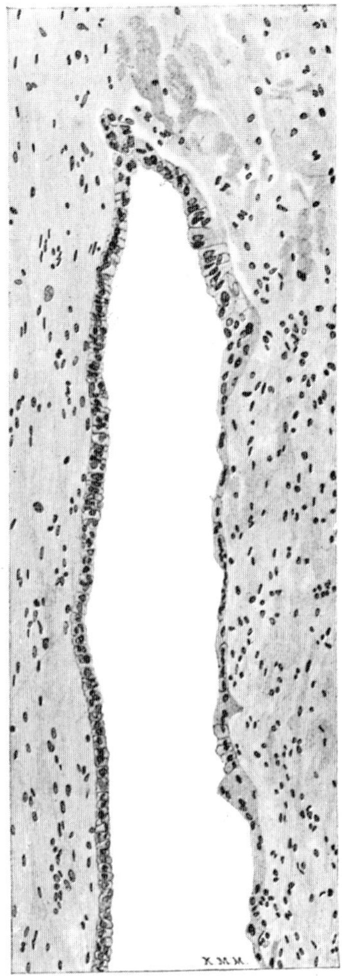

FIG. 118.—TUBAL MUCOSA, SHOWING CONVERSION OF EPITHELIUM INTO SYNCYTIUM.

Normal epithelium on left, syncytium on right side.

The fœtal origin of the two layers of chorionic epithelium has also been confirmed by the work of Hubrecht for the hedgehog, Duval for dogs, Fränkel for many species of animals, and Opitz for the guinea-pig, cat, and rabbit, and is at present the prevailing view.

In 1893, Kossmann advanced the theory that the syncytium was derived from the epithelium of the uterus, while Langhans's layer represented the original fœtal ectoderm. His work was apparently confirmed by Merttens a year later, who showed conclusively that a certain amount of uterine epithelium was converted into syncytium, and thought himself justified in concluding that it grew up over the villi, which up to that time were covered by only a single layer of Langhans's cells or fœtal ectoderm, and thus gave them their second or outer layer. The work of Kossmann and Merttens was very plausibly set forth and accompanied by numerous excellent illustrations, and their conclusions were soon adopted by many authorities, among whom we may mention Marchand and Kollmann. It would seem, however, that this view is untenable, inasmuch as the work of Hubrecht, Heukelom, and Peters has shown that the ovum is surrounded by the many-layered trophoblast before the formation of the villi begins, and that the syncytium represents only a modification of it. Moreover, it must be remembered that during pregnancy the greater part of the uterine epithelium gradually loses its cylindrical shape and becomes cuboidal or flattened, and eventually disappears.

On the other hand, it must be admitted that the small areas of uterine epithelium may occasionally assume a distinctly syncytial appearance, and not a few of my specimens confirm this view. This occurrence, however, must be regarded as the exception, and even when portions are so converted, satisfactory evidence has not been adduced to show that the tissue grows up over the villi and gives rise to their syncytial covering. The formation of syncytium is not necessarily characteristic of pregnancy, and may occur in other conditions, as Gebhard has shown that similar changes are occasionally observed in carcinoma of the non-pregnant uterus.

The theory of Kossmann and Merttens is only one of a large number which have been advanced in explanation of the origin of the chorionic epithelium. Those who are interested in the subject are referred to the article of Waldeyer, who in 1890 was able to arrange in ten groups the numerous theories which had been advanced up to that time.

Structure of the Amnion.—In the very early stages of pregnancy, as we have already shown, the amnion is a small sac which arches over the dorsal surface of the embryo, and later becomes larger and completely surrounds it. At first the amnion is minute and occupies only a small portion of the entire ovum; but as pregnancy advances it increases in size, until eventually it comes in contact with the interior of the chorion and obliterates the extra-embryonic portion of the cœlome. When the outer surface of the amnion has applied itself to the inner surface of the chorion, the two membranes become slightly adherent, but are never very intimately connected, for even at the end of pregnancy they can be readily separated from one another.

From its earliest stages the amnion consists of two layers: an outer layer of mesoderm and an inner layer, made up of flattened, almost spindle-shaped ectodermal cells. The mesodermic layer eventually becomes converted into mucoid-like tissue, which does not contain blood-vessels; while the ectodermal portion changes into a single layer of small cuboidal epithelial cells, which by their origin represent simply an extension of the body walls of the embryo.

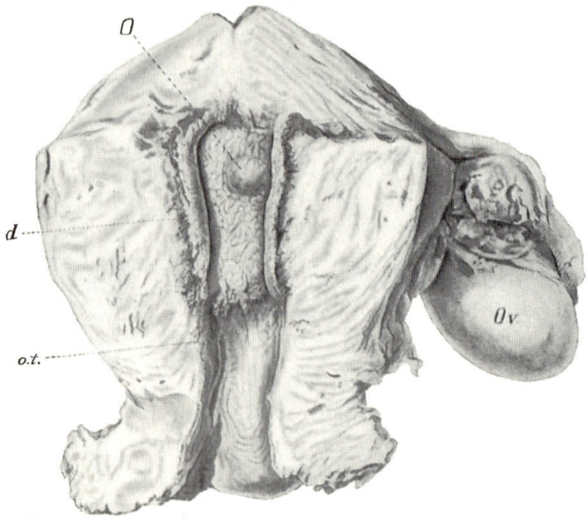

FIG. 119.—UTERUS LINED BY DECIDUA, CONTAINING SEVEN- TO EIGHT-DAYS' OVUM (Leopold). × 1.

Soon after its formation, a certain amount of clear fluid collects within the amniotic cavity —the amniotic fluid— which increases in quantity as pregnancy advances. The amount varies within wide limits, and according to Fehling averages about 600 cubic centimetres at the end of pregnancy, although it may be as much as 2,300 or as little as 265 cubic centimetres. Its specific gravity ranges from 1.002 to 1.028, and it contains a certain amount of albumin, urea, kreatin, and various salts. The origin and function of the amniotic fluid will be considered when we take up the physiology of the fœtus.

Thus far we have been describing the fœtal membranes. Before taking up the study of the placenta, it will be necessary to consider the changes which the uterine mucous membrane undergoes to prepare it for the reception of the ovum.

Decidua.—The decidua is the mucous membrane of the uterus which has undergone marked changes under the influence of pregnancy, to fit it for the implantation and nutrition of the ovum. It is so named from the fact that it is cast off after labour. The older writers usually distinguished between the decidua of menstruation and that of pregnancy, but the em-

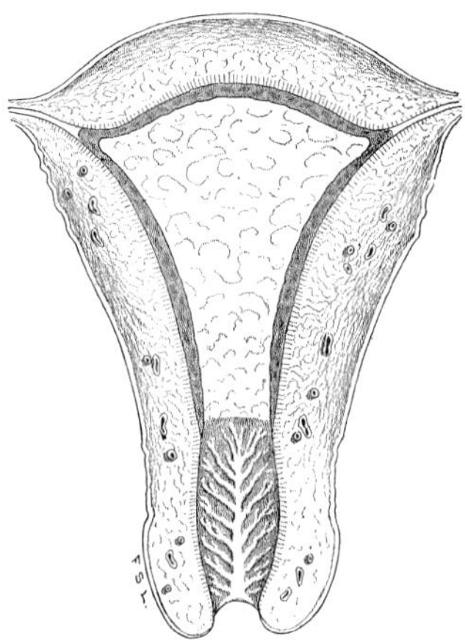

Fig. 120.

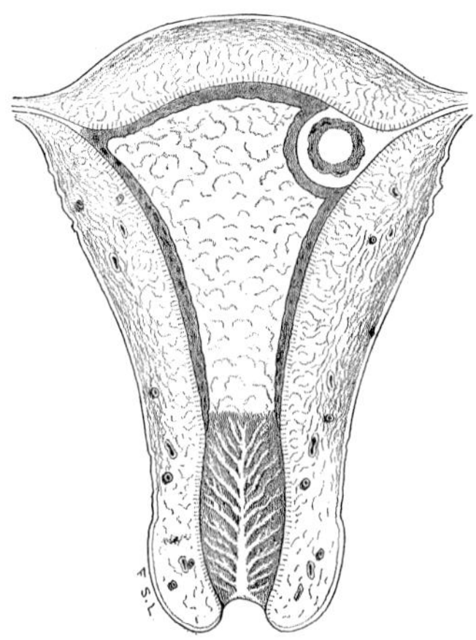

Fig. 121.

Figs. 120, 121.—Diagrams illustrating Hunterian Theory of Formation of Decidua Reflexa.

ployment of the former term is no longer justified, since it has been shown that there is no great loss of tissue at the menstrual period.

The conversion of the mucous membrane of the uterus into decidua occurs shortly after the fertilization of the ovum, though we are unable to state exactly when the process commences, inasmuch as a fairly well-marked decidua was present in all of the early pregnancies which have thus far been described, being well developed in the specimens described by Peters and Leopold, which belonged to a three- and a seven- or eight-days' pregnancy respectively.

Very shortly after conception, the smooth velvety endometrium becomes markedly thicker and its surface is indented by furrows of considerable depth, which give the entire membrane a mamelonated appearance. Under the magnifying-glass numerous small openings can be distinguished which are the mouths of the uterine glands. The decidual formation is limited to the body of the uterus, and does not extend below the internal os, though in rare instances, as in the cases reported by von Franqué and von Weiss, isolated decidual cells are found beneath the cervical epithelium.

For purposes of description the decidua is usually divided into several portions: that lining the greater part of the cavity of the uterus being designated as the *decidua vera*; that beneath the ovum as the *decidua serotina*; while the portion which surrounds the ovum and shuts it off from the rest of the uterine cavity is known as the *decidua reflexa*.

The terms *reflexa* and *serotina* date from the time of William Hunter, who gave excellent drawings of the decidual membrane in his atlas. Unfortunately, the author died just after its appearance and before the completion of the explanatory text, which was prepared by John Hunter and Matthew Baillie, who considered that the decidua represented a fibrinous exudate from the lining membrane of the uterus, which formed a complete cast of the uterine cavity and completely covered the tubal openings. They supposed, therefore, that when the ovum reached the uterine end of the tube its further passage was opposed by the decidua vera, which it was obliged to push before it as it entered the uterus, whence the term reflexa; and that after the reflexa had been pushed forward, a new exudate was developed behind the ovum, to which the term serotina was applied.

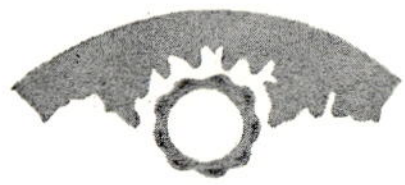

Fig. 122.

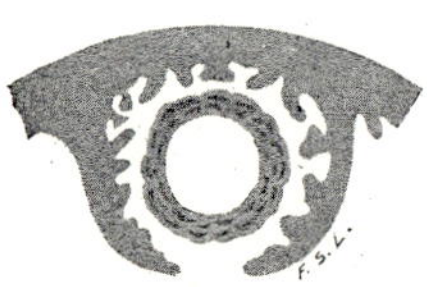

Fig. 123.

Figs. 122, 123.—Diagrams showing Formation of Decidua Reflexa (Coste).

This conception was universally accepted until 1846, when Weber in Germany, and Sharkey in England, demonstrated that the decidua was not an exudate, inasmuch as it contained glandular structures which they identified with the uterine glands. It having therefore become necessary to explain the formation of the reflexa in a different manner, it was assumed that the ovum, on reaching the uterus, found its entire cavity lined by decidua vera, to which it became attached at a point on the anterior or posterior wall somewhere in the neighbourhood of the fundus; and that immediately after its attachment the vera began to proliferate and to form a wall around the ovum, which gradually increased until it completely inclosed and surrounded it. Notwithstanding the new ideas concerning the formation of the decidua, the terms reflexa and serotina are still retained, though in the new anatomical nomenclature of His they are designated as the *decidua capsularis* and *basalis* respectively.

Decidua Vera.—The microscopic structure of the decidua vera was first studied by Hegar and Maier, but it was not until the work of Friedländer and Kundrat and Engelmann that its structure was definitely understood. Friedländer, in 1870, pointed out that the decidua vera was composed of two portions: a *compact* layer superimposed upon a *spongy* or *glandular* layer, the latter being nearer to the muscular wall of the uterus, and mainly forming the thickness of the membrane. Furthermore, he was of the opinion that the separation of the decidua at the time of labour took place at the junction between the two layers. He showed that the compact layer was made up of large round, oval, or polygonal cells, with large, lightly staining, vesicular nuclei—the *decidual cells*; while the spongy layer was composed of the dilated and hyperplastic uterine glands.

The decidua vera increases markedly in thickness during the first three or four months of pregnancy, so that at the end of that time it has attained a thickness of about 1 centimetre. Figs. 48 and 124 show very graphically the difference between the normal endometrium and decidua vera from a uterus four months pregnant. After the fourth month, owing to the marked increase in the size of the uterus, the vera gradually becomes thinner, so that at term it is rarely more than 2 millimetres thick.

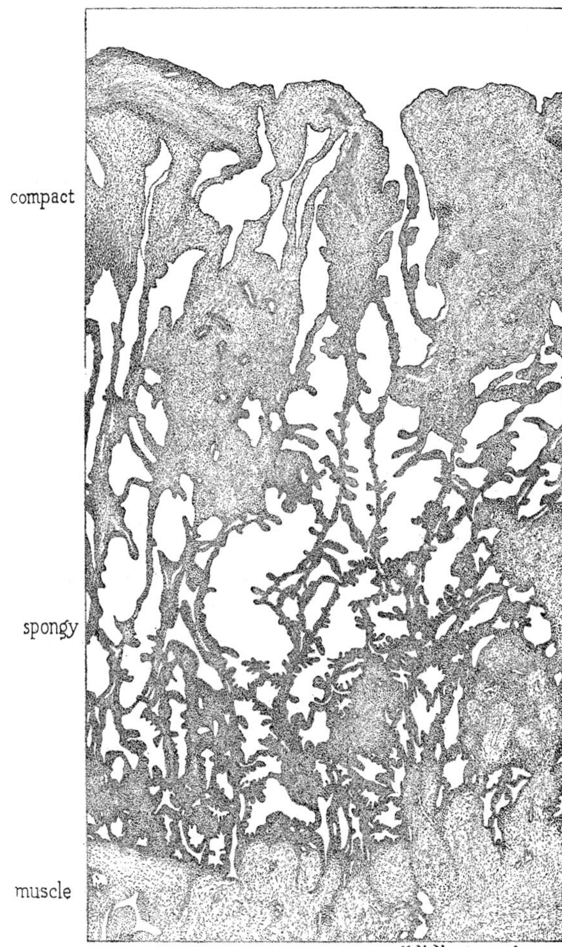

FIG. 124.—DECIDUA VERA, FOURTH MONTH. × 16.

Under the microscope the compact layer is seen to be made up of somewhat closely packed, large, round, oval, or polygonal cells, which are distinctly epithelioid in appearance, and possess round, vesicular nuclei, which stain but slightly with the ordinary reagents. When the tissue has been distended by hæmorrhage or œdema, it is seen that many of the decidual cells present a stellate appearance, and are provided with long protoplasmic outgrowths which anastomose with similar processes from neighbouring cells. In the early months of pregnancy the ducts of the uterine glands may be seen traversing the compact layer, but they soon disappear, so that in the later months all trace of them is lost.

The spongy layer is made up of the distended and hyperplastic glands of the endometrium, which are separated from one another by a minimal amount of stroma. In many instances the glandular hyperplasia is so marked that the spongy layer suggests an adenoma in appearance. At first the glands are lined by typical cylindrical uterine epithelium, which, however, gradually becomes more cuboidal in shape and undergoes fatty degeneration, and is cast off in great part into their lumina. A certain amount of epithelium, however, remains intact throughout pregnancy, and

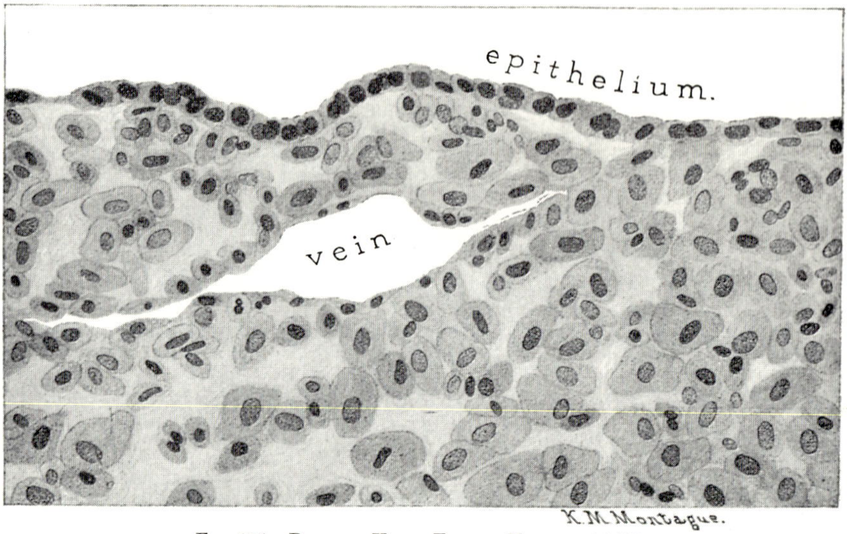

Fig. 125.—Decidua Vera, Fourth Month. × 420.

from it the endometrium is regenerated after labour. In many instances the stroma between the dilated glands has undergone but little change, and closely resembles that of the non-pregnant uterus.

Under the influence of pregnancy, the surface epithelium covering the decidua gradually loses its cylindrical shape and becomes cuboidal or flattened, sometimes even resembling endothelium. Klein first directed attention to this condition, and held that it was a characteristic microscopic evidence of pregnancy. All subsequent investigators have confirmed his observations.

Fig. 125 represents a section through the compact layer of the decidua vera at the fourth month, while Fig. 126 shows a gland with its surrounding stroma from a non-pregnant uterus, drawn under the same magnification. On comparing them, it is readily seen that the decidua differs from the non-pregnant endometrium by a marked increase in size of the stroma cells, and a marked decrease in size of the epithelial cells.

As a result of the work of Hegar and Maier, Leopold, Minot, and others, it is now generally admitted that the decidual cells are derived from the stroma cells of the endometrium, which have undergone marked increase in size but only slight increase in number. Ruge directed attention to the resemblance which they bear to sarcoma cells, and stated that "the decidual cell represents the physiological type of the sarcoma cell."

The connective-tissue origin of the decidual cell was established only after prolonged investigation, and has been further re-enforced by observations made in certain cases of early tubal pregnancy, in which decidual cells may be seen developing in the smaller folds of the tubal mucosa. Such specimens show clearly that they are derived from the ordinary connective-tissue cells and result from the hypertrophy of pre-existing units rather than from their proliferation. Furthermore, Schmorl, Kinoshita, Lindenthal, and others have described, in women dying soon after childbirth, small nodules, varying from structures just visible to the naked eye to bodies 1 to 2 millimetres in diameter, which are scattered over the peritonæum, covering the posterior surface of the uterus, Douglas's *cul-de-sac*, and the anterior surface of the rectum, and occasionally also over the ovaries. Schmorl considers that these structures are always found at full-term pregnancy, and has demonstrated that they are made up of decidual tissue. But, whereas they develop beneath the peritonæum, it is evident that they must be derived from connective-tissue cells.

Before the true nature of the decidual cells was definitely proved, various theories were advanced as to their origin: Hennig believing that they were derived from leucocytes, Frommel and Overlach from the uter-

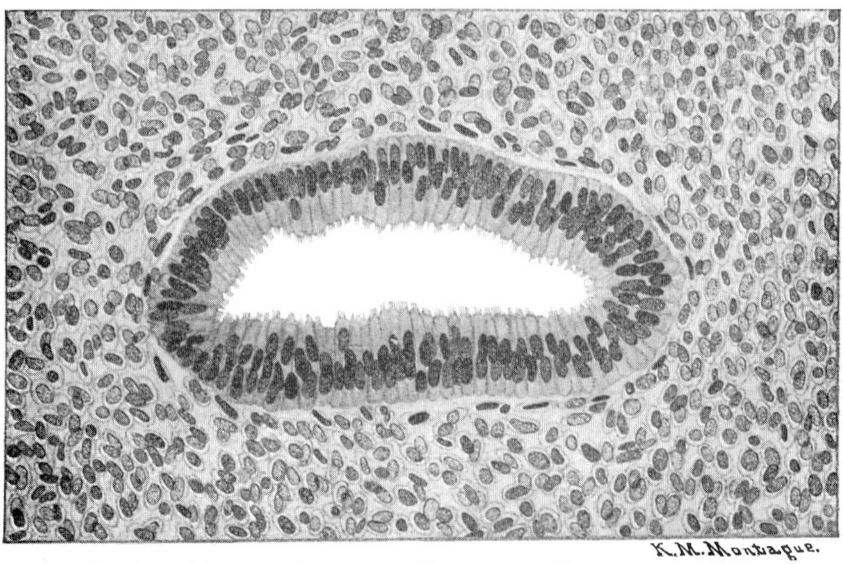

Fig. 126.—Gland and Stroma from Non-pregnant Endometrium. × 420.

ine epithelium, and Ercolani from the endothelium of the blood-vessels. At the present time, these views are of interest only from an historical stand-point.

Decidua Reflexa.—Except for the first few hours after its entry into the uterus, the ovum is shut off from the rest of the uterine cavity by the decidua reflexa, which forms a capsule of decidual tissue around it. Fig. 119 shows a seven-days' pregnancy in which the reflexa is quite apparent, and Fig. 127 a seventeen-days' pregnancy in which it is well developed.

During the early months of pregnancy the decidua reflexa does not entirely fill the uterine cavity, so that a space of varying size exists between it and the vera. This is well shown in Fig. 128, which represents a section through a six- to seven-weeks' pregnant uterus. At the fourth month of pregnancy, however, the growing ovum entirely fills the uterine

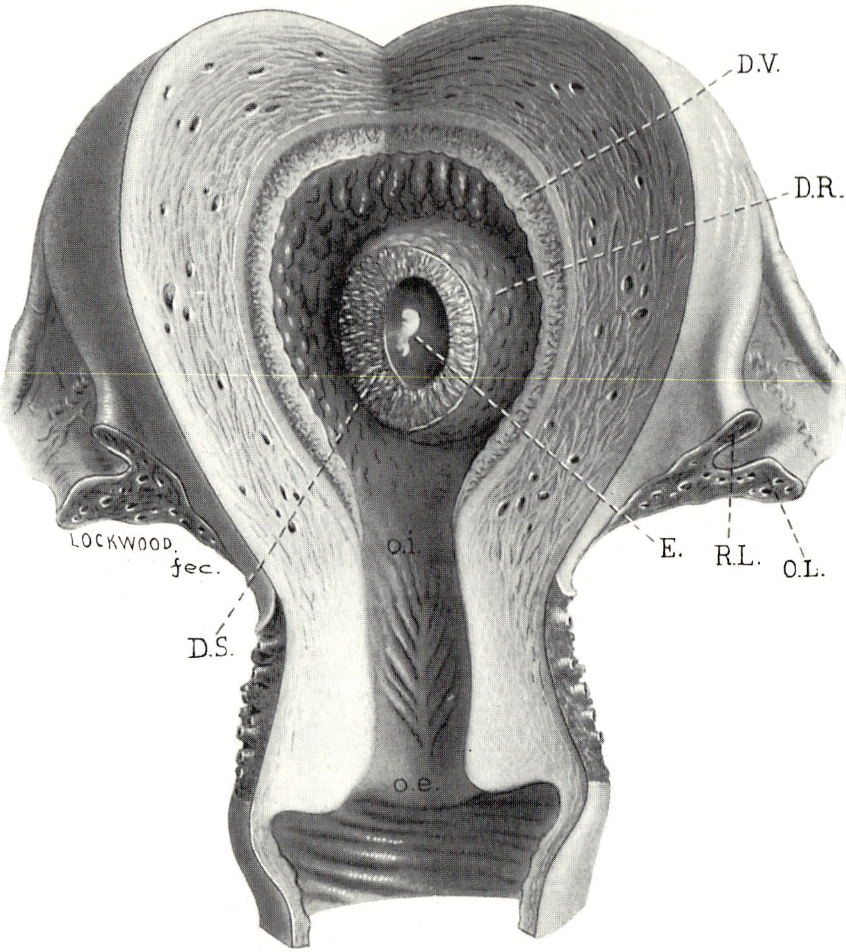

Fig. 127.—Seventeen-days' Pregnant Uterus. × 1. (Anatomical Museum Johns Hopkins University.) Embryo drawn relatively too large.

D.R., decidua reflexa; *D.S.*, decidua serotina; *D.V.*, decidua vera; *E.*, embryo; *O.L.*, ovarian ligament; *R.L.*, round ligament.

cavity, so that the reflexa and vera are brought into intimate contact, and the part of the uterine cavity which has remained unoccupied up to this time becomes obliterated. In a short time the two structures fuse together, when the reflexa gradually degenerates and disappears. This view was first advocated by Minot, and appears to be well founded, inasmuch as sections through the wall of the full-term uterus outside of the placental site show that the entire decidua is only 2 to 3 millimetres thick, and no trace of the decidua reflexa can be discovered. (See Fig. 133.)

The decidua reflexa usually attains its greatest thickness at about the second month. Sections through it at this time show that it is made up of decidual cells and is covered on its exterior by a single layer of flattened or cuboidal epithelial cells; while internally it is in contact with the fœtal villi, and at no time shows any trace of uterine epithelium. In its lowest portion, where it is connected with the vera, a few glands may be found, whose ducts, when they are present, are seen to open only upon the outer surface of the membrane.

Up to a few years ago it was universally believed that the reflexa originated from the proliferation of the vera, which grew up around and gradually inclosed the ovum. Selenka, however, pointed out that in monkeys and in certain other animals, the decidua reflexa was not formed in this way, but that the ovum penetrated the surface epithelium and burrowed down into the depths of the vera, almost immediately after its implantation, and thus came to be surrounded by the stroma cells. According to this view the reflexa would be merely the portion of the decidua vera which covers the ovum. Von Herff then stated, upon theoretical grounds, that possibly a more or less similar process takes place in human beings. He believed, however, that the ovum did not become implanted upon the free surface of the vera, but sank down into one of the depressions by which the latter is marked.

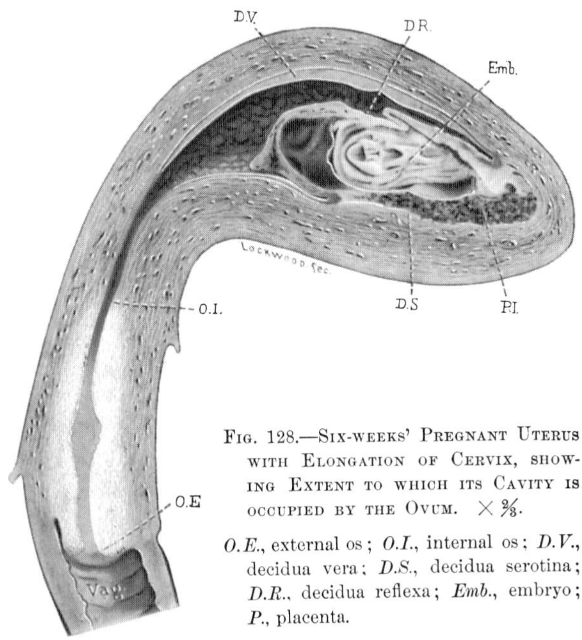

Fig. 128.—Six-weeks' Pregnant Uterus with Elongation of Cervix, showing Extent to which its Cavity is occupied by the Ovum. × ⅝.

O.E., external os; *O.I.*, internal os; *D.V.*, decidua vera; *D.S.*, decidua serotina; *D.R.*, decidua reflexa; *Emb.*, embryo; *P.*, placenta.

It was not, however, until Peters described a specimen representing, as he believed, a three-days' pregnancy, in which the ovum was embedded in the decidua vera, that anything like positive proof in support of Selenka's views was adduced for human beings. Plate IV, taken from a section through Peters's three-days' pregnant uterus, shows distinctly that the ovum has burrowed down beneath the surface of the decidua vera and is lying in the interglandular stroma. Such pictures clearly indicate that the reflexa is not formed by the proliferation of the decidua vera as is generally stated, but simply represents the portion of it which covers the ovum, and which undergoes passive enlargement as the latter increases in size. I have not had an opportunity of examining the pregnant uterus in its earliest stages, but in several very early cases of tubal pregnancy I have seen conditions which tend to confirm Peters's views.

Decidua Serotina.—The decidua serotina is the portion of the decidua which lies immediately beneath the ovum; from it the maternal portion of the placenta is developed. Broadly speaking, it presents the same gen-

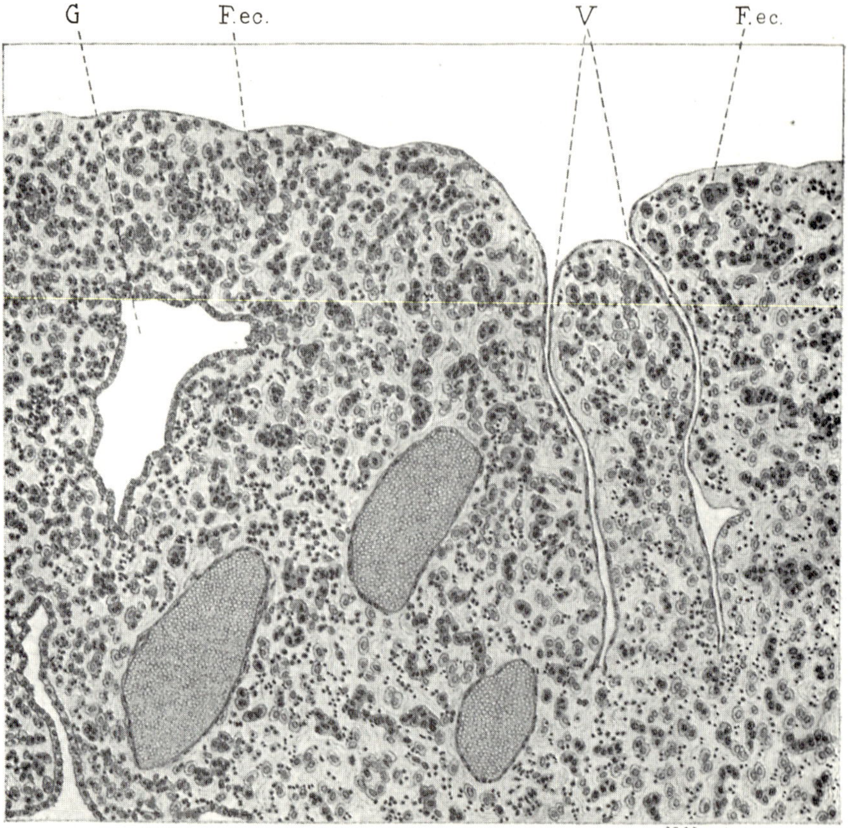

Fig. 129.—Decidua Serotina, showing Mixture of Fœtal and Maternal Cells. × 75. *G.*, gland; *V.*, vessel; *F.ec.*, fœtal ectoderm.

eral structure as the decidua vera, except that it has been invaded by fœtal tissue, so that its superficial portions are composed of decidual cells and fœtal ectoderm.

Friedländer and Leopold stated in their original monographs that giant cells appeared in the serotina about the middle of pregnancy. These, they thought, made their way into the vessels and gave rise to thrombosis. Their interpretation, however, is no longer accepted, and it is now generally believed that the majority of the so-called giant cells are not of decidual origin, but represent portions of fœtal ectoderm—the so-called syncytium—which have made their way down into the decidua. Fig. 129, representing a section through the decidua serotina in the last month of pregnancy, shows clearly that its superficial portions are composed of a mixture of both fœtal and maternal cells.

In the decidua serotina large numbers of blood-vessels are observed. The arteries pursue a spiral course, and usually penetrate the entire thickness of the membrane; while many of the veins become markedly dilated and form large sinuses. In Fig. 129 two small vessels may be seen which, after pursuing their course through the superficial layer of the serotina, open into the intervillous spaces of the placenta. The consideration of the vascular connections between the fœtus and the uterus, however, will be deferred until we take up the study of the placenta.

Development of the Placenta.—When the fertilized ovum reaches the uterus it finds the endometrium transformed into decidua in anticipation of its reception. At this time, as has already been pointed out, the exterior of the ovum is represented by the chorionic membrane, whose epithelium is arranged in many layers—the trophoblast. We are unable to state as yet whether it possesses villi or not, though if such are present, they must be in a very rudimentary condition.

The ovum, as a rule, becomes attached to the decidua vera covering the anterior or posterior wall of the uterus, somewhere in the neighbourhood of the fundus, and only exceptionally in the lower portion of the uterine cavity. It is very rarely implanted in the angles, since these present only a slight decidual reaction as compared with the anterior and posterior walls. At present we are absolutely ignorant concerning the factors which cause the arrest of the ovum at a given point.

There are two theories as to what occurs immediately after the implantation of the ovum upon the decidua vera. According to the one recently promulgated and advocated by Peters, the trophoblast soon destroys the surface epithelium of the decidua, so that the ovum almost immediately comes in contact with its stroma, into which it rapidly burrows (Plate IV). According to the older view, which has obtained universal acceptance until recently, and which has been considered in detail by Ruge and His, the ovum becomes attached at some point on the surface of the decidua vera, which immediately begins to proliferate around it and soon surrounds it as the decidua reflexa.

The evidence at our disposal renders it probable that Peters's explanation is correct, especially as the same process has been observed by Selenka in the monkey, by Opitz in the guinea-pig, and upon theoretical grounds was advocated by von Herff for human beings. Under these circumstances the reflexa would simply represent the portion of the decidua vera which covers the ovum, its further growth being passive and due to the force exerted by the growing ovum. This view has also been adopted by Leopold, Marchesi, and Bott, who consider that the seven-days'-old ovum described by the former was probably implanted in this manner.

My own observations tend to show that this is the course of events in tubal pregnancy, as in several instances I have found the ovum embedded in the wall of the tube and separated from its lumen by a thin layer of tissue. Several drawings illustrating this condition will be found in the chapter on Extra-uterine Pregnancy. At first I was inclined to regard such findings as evidence of the development of the ovum in a diverticulum from the lumen of the tube; but, after the appearance of Peters's monograph, more careful examination of my specimens led me to believe that my former conclusion was incorrect.

In a short time, no matter what the mode of implantation may have been, the ovum becomes completely surrounded by decidua, the portion separating it from the uterine cavity being known as the reflexa, and that immediately beneath it as the serotina. Almost immediately after the implantation of the ovum, its trophoblast begins to proliferate and invade the surrounding decidual tissue, as was shown by the work of Hubrecht, Heukelom, and Peters. As it does so, it breaks through the walls of maternal capillaries, from which the blood escapes and forms cavities, which are bounded partly by trophoblast and partly by decidua (Plate IV). As the process goes on, more vessels are opened up, so that in a short time the trophoblast presents a sieve-like appearance due to the presence of large numbers of blood spaces filled with maternal blood. As a result, the trophoblastic cells become compressed into irregularly shaped masses of varying size, some of which extend from the surface of the ovum to the surrounding decidua, and afford the epithelial basis from which the villi are developed.

The maternal blood spaces established in this manner represent the earliest stages in the formation of the *intervillous blood spaces* of the future placenta, and were abundantly present in the early ova examined by Peters and Leopold. Coincidently with their formation, the irregularly shaped masses of trophoblast are invaded by connective-tissue offshoots from the chorionic membrane, and are thus converted into *villi.* The cells surrounding them become arranged in two layers, the inner corresponding to Langhans's layer, the outer one being composed of syncytium.

As we have already indicated, a considerable number of the primary villi extend from the chorionic membrane to the surrounding decidua, while the majority project freely into the blood spaces. The former are designated as *fastening villi* (Haftzotten), and serve to attach the ovum to the decidua. Where they come in contact with the latter, the trophoblast at their tips, which is now designated as chorionic epithelium, undergoes marked proliferation, and like the roots of a tree invades the decidual tissue still further, until the two structures become firmly united. The proliferated trophoblast may be observed in placentæ in all stages of development, and is represented by what are usually known as the *cell nodes* or *cell columns.* Their formation was carefully studied by Heukelom in the early ovum which he described.

During the first few weeks of pregnancy, branching villi project from the entire periphery of the ovum, as is well seen in the figures taken from Leopold's work. They come in contact not only with the decidua serotina, but also with the reflexa; so that intervillous blood spaces surround the entire ovum, as is particularly well shown in the section through

PLATE V.

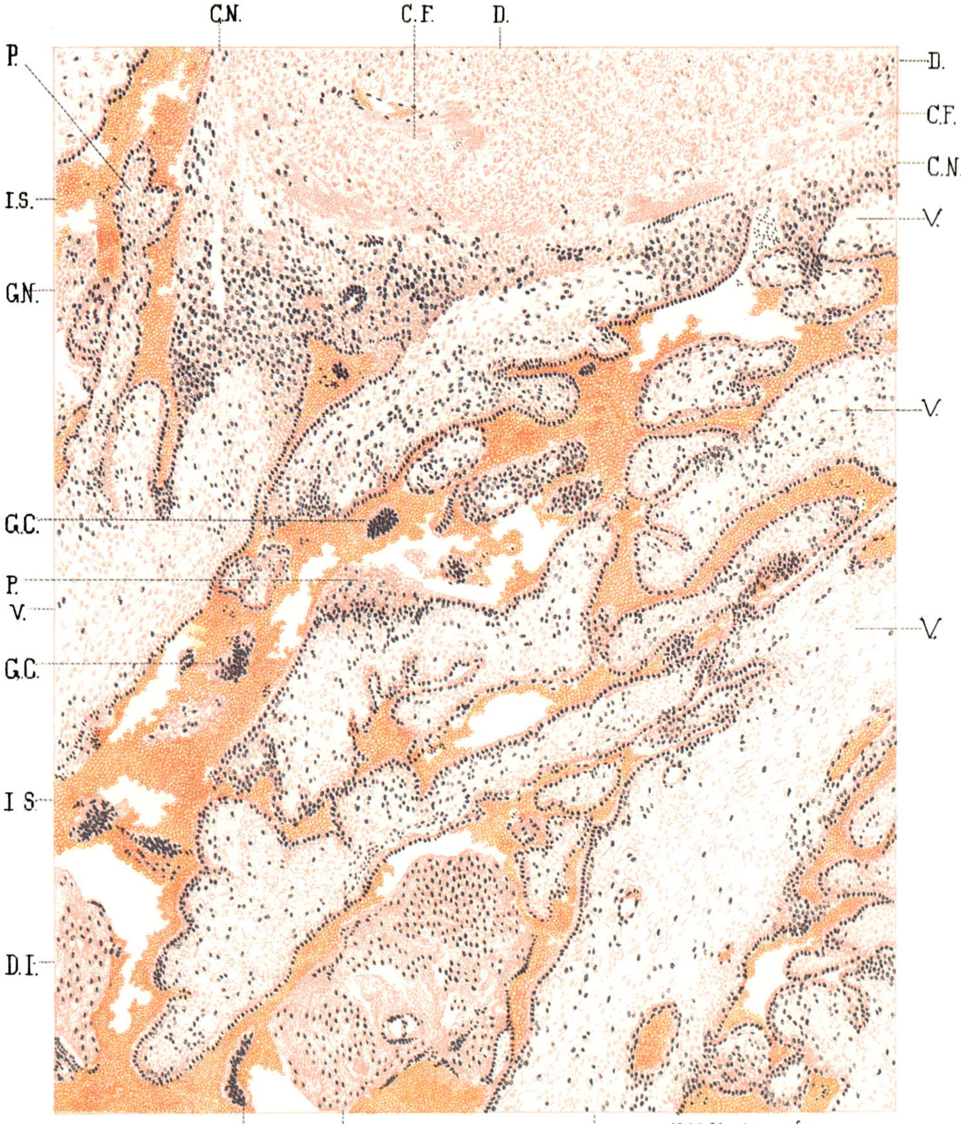

SECTION THROUGH FOUR MONTHS' PLACENTA, SHOWING JUNCTION OF CHORION AND DECIDUA. × 56.

C. F., canalized fibrin; *C. N.*, cell nodes; *D.*, decidua serotina; *D. I.*, decidual island; *G. C.*, giant cell; *I. S.*, intervillous space; *P.*, proliferating villous epithelium; *V.*, chorionic villi.

a seven-days' pregnancy (Fig. 109). During this period the chorionic villi are devoid of blood-vessels, and the ovum is nourished by osmosis from the maternal blood.

As pregnancy advances, the blood supply of the decidua serotina becomes more and more abundant, while that of the reflexa is diminished; as a consequence the villi in contact with the former are better nourished and begin to grow more luxuriantly than those upon the rest of the ovum, the process thus leading to the formation of the *chorion frondosum*. At the same time the villi covering the rest of the ovum develop less rapidly, so that this portion becomes known as the *chorion læve*. As the ovum increases in size, the intervillous spaces in the chorion læve become smaller and smaller, and by the time the decidua reflexa has come in contact with the vera, which happens at some time in the fourth month of pregnancy, they become obliterated, and the villi which project into them undergo almost complete degeneration. In sections through the fœtal membranes at term (Fig. 133), the chorion læve consists of several layers of epithelial cells, which represent the chorionic epithelium, and through which are scattered, here and there, round or oblong hyaline bodies, in which a few spindle-shaped nuclei can be distinguished. These are the remains of the earlier villi. At the same time degenerative changes take place in the epithelium of the chorion læve, which result in the formation of a fibrin-like material which will be considered in detail a little later.

On the other hand, the villi of the chorion frondosum increase in size and number, and become vascularized by branches of the umbilical vessels of the embryo; so that after the first few weeks the fœtal circulation extends to the tips of the smallest villi.

The *placenta* is formed by the union of the chorion frondosum and the decidua serotina, and therefore is composed of fœtal and maternal tissues. In the third or fourth month of pregnancy it constitutes a distinct structure, although its site is indicated at a much earlier period by the increased thickness of the chorion at that point.

We can probably best understand the structure of the placenta by studying sections through it at the fourth month of pregnancy, one of which is shown in Plate V. Here we see that the organ is made up in great part of chorionic villi, whose stroma presents a somewhat mucoid appearance, and contains spindle- and star-shaped connective-tissue cells, between which well-developed arteries, veins, and capillaries may be observed. At this stage the villous epithelium is arranged in two layers—Langhans's layer and the syncytium—and from the latter many buds protrude which, when seen in cross or tangential section, appear as giant cells lying free in the intervillous spaces.

In the upper part of the plate is the decidua serotina, with which some of the larger villi—the fastening villi—are connected. At their ends can be noted a marked proliferation of Langhans's layer, which invades the underlying decidua, giving rise to the *cell nodes* or *cell columns*, and corresponds to the trophoblastic formation of the early days of pregnancy. The cell nodes are apparently composed almost exclusively of Langhans's cells, as the syncytium does not follow them down into the depths of the decidua. The spaces between the villi and the decidua, and between the villi themselves, are designated as the *intervillous spaces.* These are filled with maternal blood and their walls are lined by syncytium. Scattered through them are isolated giant cells—the so-called placental giant cells—whose origin we have already considered. Here and there are seen a few large areas composed of cuboidal or polygonal cells with vesicular nuclei, which frequently present marked signs of degeneration. These are the so-called *decidual islands,* and are usually supposed to represent sections through decidual septa, which project upward from the surface of the decidua serotina towards the chorionic membrane. But, as has already been pointed out, it is more than probable that many of them are masses of trophoblast, into which the chorionic connective tissue has not grown, and which therefore have not developed into typical villi.

At the junction between the cell nodes and the decidual tissue, areas are noted which stain deeply with eosin, and which, on closer examination, are seen to be made up of fibrin, honeycombed in various directions by small spaces—the so-called *canalized fibrin*—which probably results from the degeneration of the deeper layers of the cell nodes. This is known as Nitabuch's fibrin layer, from the author who first called attention to its presence in the decidua. Its existence has been confirmed, and its characteristics have been studied by Langhans, Rohr, Tussenbroeck, Ulesko-Stroganowa, and others, and it is generally considered to mark the border line between the fœtal and maternal tissues.

Until comparatively recently the participation of fœtal tissue in the decidua serotina was not recognised, and when fœtal cells were found beneath the chorionic membrane they were considered as being of decidual origin. Accordingly, Winckler and other observers believed that decidual tissue extended from the margins of the decidua serotina over the whole of the outer surface of the chorionic membrane, so that the entire intervillous space was included between decidual or maternal tissue. Winckler designated the superficial portion of the decidua as the *basal,* and the portion covering the chorionic membrane as the *closing plate* of the decidua. We have already shown that the tissue in question is composed of fœtal ectoderm, and the conception of decidual plates should therefore be abandoned.

At one point (Plate V) a maternal vessel is seen which, after reaching the surface of the decidua, opens directly into the intervillous spaces. At present it is universally admitted that the blood in these spaces is exclusively maternal in origin.

The fœtal blood in the vessels of the chorionic villi at no time gains access to the maternal blood in the intervillous spaces, the two being separated from one another by the double layer of chorionic epithelium, a portion of the stroma of the villus and the vessel walls (Plate VI).

Structure of Placenta in Latter Half of Pregnancy and at Full Term.—Except in its increased size, the placenta in the second half of pregnancy differs but slightly from that of the fourth month. Microscopic sections at this period, however, show certain points of difference. These are well illustrated in Fig. 130, which represents a section through a seven-and-a-half-months' placenta and the adjacent uterine wall. Studying it from

PLATE VI.

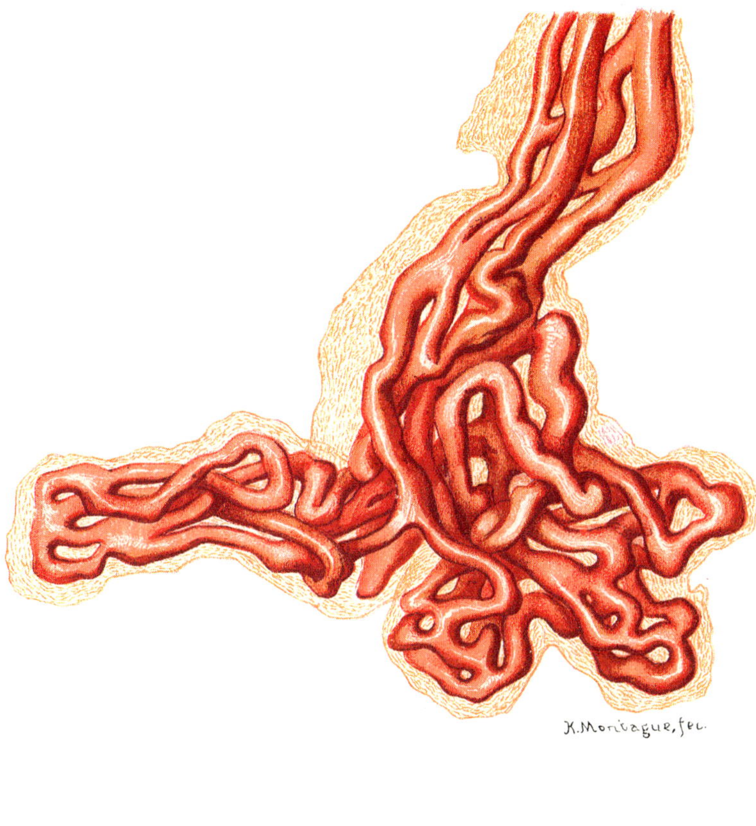

TERMINAL CHORIONIC VILLUS, WITH INJECTED VESSELS.

within outward, we see that it is composed of the following structures: amnion, chorionic membrane, villi, intervillous blood spaces, and decidua serotina.

The amnion covers the inner or fœtal surface of the placenta, and consists of a single layer of cuboidal epithelium, below which comes a layer of more or less fibrillar connective tissue, containing no blood-vessels. The chorionic membrane presents essentially the same structure as in the earlier months of pregnancy, differing only in the presence of a large amount of canalized fibrin immediately beneath its epithelium.

The great bulk of the placenta is made up of chorionic villi, which are much more abundant, but at the same time considerably smaller than at the fourth month. Their stroma, which is made up of spindle-shaped cells, is denser in appearance, is occupied in great part by blood-vessels, and differs markedly from the mucoid tissue of the earlier months. These changes have already been referred to, and are clearly shown in Figs. 116 and 117.

The epithelium covering the villi has also undergone marked change; Langhans's layer has almost completely disappeared and only a thin layer of syncytium remains,

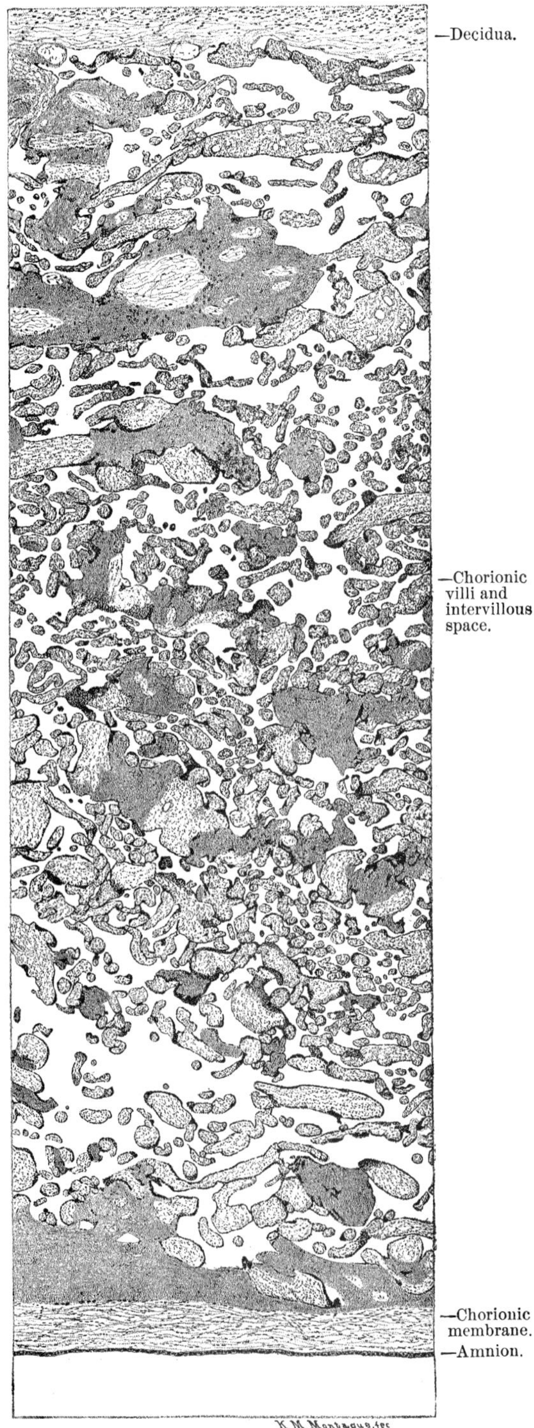

Fig. 130.

Fig. 130.—Section through Entire Thickness of Placenta at Eighth Month. × 33.

which gives rise to fewer buds than previously. In many villi immediately under the epithelium, and occupying the former position of Langhans's layer of cells, a thicker or thinner layer of canalized fibrin may be observed. This was described by Langhans, and is of constant occurrence in the latter half of pregnancy. It appears to indicate senile degeneration of the placenta. At the same time, many of the arteries show marked changes and present all stages of an obliterating endarteritis, to which, in great part, the formation of the tissue in question should be attributed.

The superficial portions of the decidua at this period are covered by canalized fibrin, which probably results from coagulation necrosis of the cell nodes and columns. In the deeper layers numerous giant cells are observed, which occasionally extend into the connective-tissue septa between the muscle fibres. They are of various shapes, and represent portions of syncytium which have wandered down into the decidua.

From the free surface of the decidua numerous elevations of varying shapes and sizes extend upward for a greater or less distance into the placenta. They are composed of cuboidal or polygonal cells, with round vesicular nuclei, and only rarely contain blood-vessels; in many places they have undergone degeneration and become converted into canalized fibrin. They are usually described as decidual septa, but in all probability are derived from fœtal ectoderm or trophoblast.

The entire space between the chorionic membrane and the free surface of the decidua serotina is designated as the *placental space*, into which the chorionic villi dip, thereby subdividing it into myriads of irregularly shaped cavities which communicate freely with one another—the intervillous spaces. They are lined by the syncytium covering the chorionic membrane and villi, except at those portions of the decidua serotina which have become converted into canalized fibrin, and which are only partially covered by it. The syncytium is thinner than in the earlier months of pregnancy, and under high powers of the microscope its protoplasm presents a vacuolated appearance, which, according to Marchand, is due to the glycogen normally contained in it having been dissolved out by the fluids used in hardening the placenta.

The intervillous spaces are at no time lined by endothelial cells, except for very short distances on the surface of the decidua serotina, over which the endothelium of maternal vessels may extend to a slight extent. It is probable, however, that a great part of this tissue in reality represents thinned-out syncytium. Hence, it would appear that the intervillous spaces are lined entirely by fœtal tissue, and that the maternal blood, which is circulating through them, lies outside of the body of the mother. The maternal blood gains access to the placental space by branches of the uterine arteries, which pursue a convoluted course through the decidua serotina and, after their walls have gradually become reduced to a single layer of endothelium, open upon the sides of the decidual septa. The blood escapes from the intervillous spaces through more or less funnel-shaped openings upon the surface of the decidua, which can be traced directly into the large venous sinuses in its depths. It is therefore apparent that there is a distinct circulation through the intercommunicating inter-

PLATE VII.

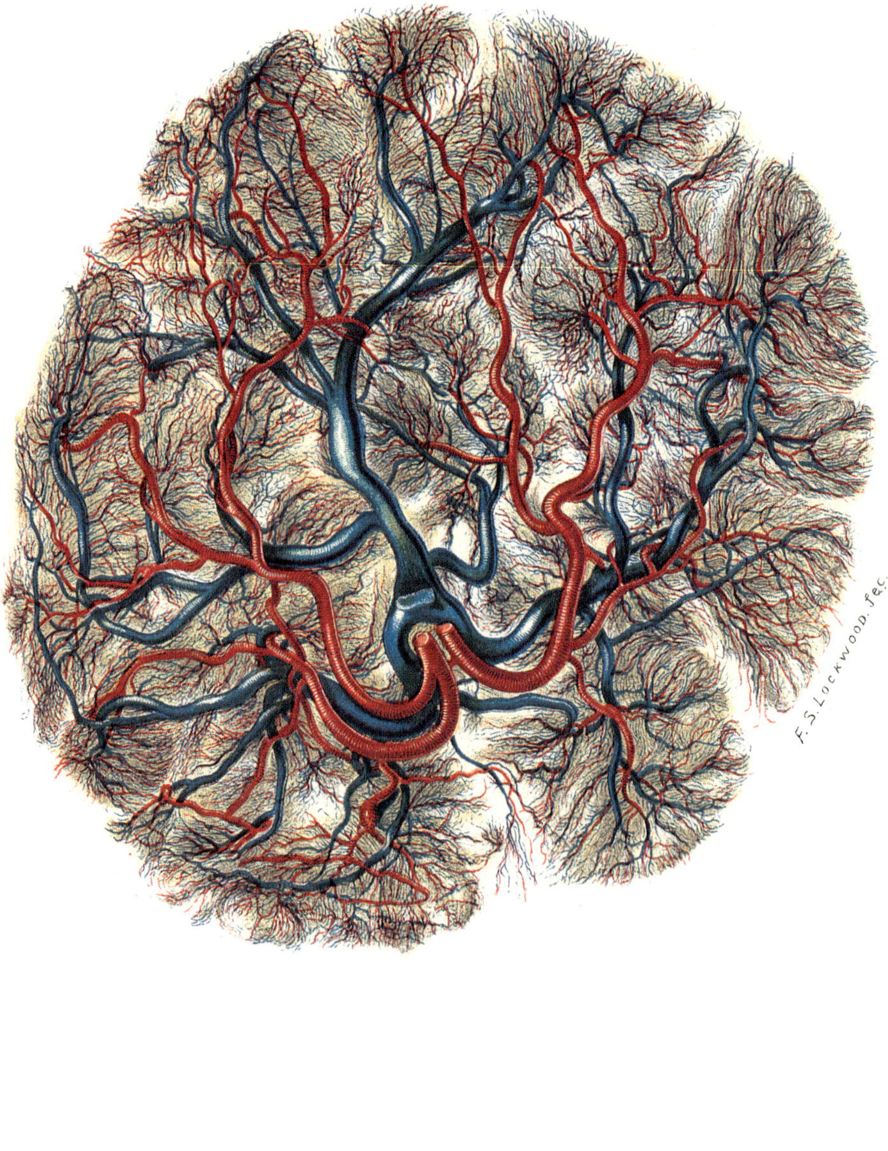

CORROSION PREPARATION OF MATURE PLACENTA, TO SHOW FŒTAL VESSELS. × ¾.

villous spaces, though it is necessarily more sluggish than elsewhere in the body.

The nature of the *intervillous spaces* and the question as to whether they contained maternal blood have given rise to a great deal of discussion. Vater, Noortwyk, and William and John Hunter, in the eighteenth century, expressed an affirmative opinion; and the last two investigators conclusively demonstrated it by injection experiments. Similar results were obtained by E. H. Weber in 1842. But this work was gradually lost sight of, and all sorts of theories were evolved concerning the nature and contents of the intervillous spaces. Braxton Hicks, Ercolani, and others believed that they did not contain blood, but some substance derived from the mucous membrane of the uterus which they designated as *uterine milk*.

Correct conceptions as to the nature of the placenta were finally established by the work of Farre, Turner, Waldeyer, Nitabuch, Rohr, Bumm, Leopold, and others, who showed conclusively that the intervillous spaces contained maternal blood, and that vessels from the mother could be traced into them. This was especially well demonstrated by Waldeyer, who, in five pregnant cadavers, was able to inject them from the maternal vessels. Furthermore, the recent work of Peters, Leopold, and others, has placed the question beyond all doubt.

In view of these facts, then, the placenta must be regarded as a collection of maternal blood, included between the chorionic membrane and the decidua serotina, into which the villi dip and by which they are surrounded. Some idea of the complexity of its vascular arrangement may be gained from Plate VII, which represents a corrosion preparation of the fœtal portion of a full-term placenta, which was injected through the umbilical arteries and veins with red and blue celloidin. (Also see Plate VI.)

Normally there is no communication between the fœtal blood contained in the chorionic villi and the maternal blood in the intervillous spaces, and it would appear that the transmission of substances from one to the other is accomplished partly by osmosis and partly by the direct cellular activity of the syncytium, the process being analogous to that which takes place in the tubules of the kidney and other organs. The effete materials from the fœtus are carried by the umbilical arteries to the capillaries of the terminal villi, whence they are transmitted to the maternal blood in the manner just described. At the same time the oxygen and the materials needed for the nutrition of the fœtus are taken up from the former and carried by the umbilical vein to the fœtus. Thus, in a general way we may say that the placenta represents the lungs, stomach, and excretory organs of the unborn child.

Placenta at Full Term.—The placenta, as it is cast off from the uterus after the birth of the child, is a flattened, roundish, or oval organ—15 to 18 centimetres in diameter, and 2 to 3 centimetres in height at its thickest part—from the margins of which the membranes extend. Ordinarily its weight is about $\frac{1}{6}$ of that of the fœtus, so that when the latter is normally developed the placenta weighs from 500 to 600 grammes.

It presents for examination two surfaces and a margin—the surface in contact with the decidua serotina being designated as the maternal or

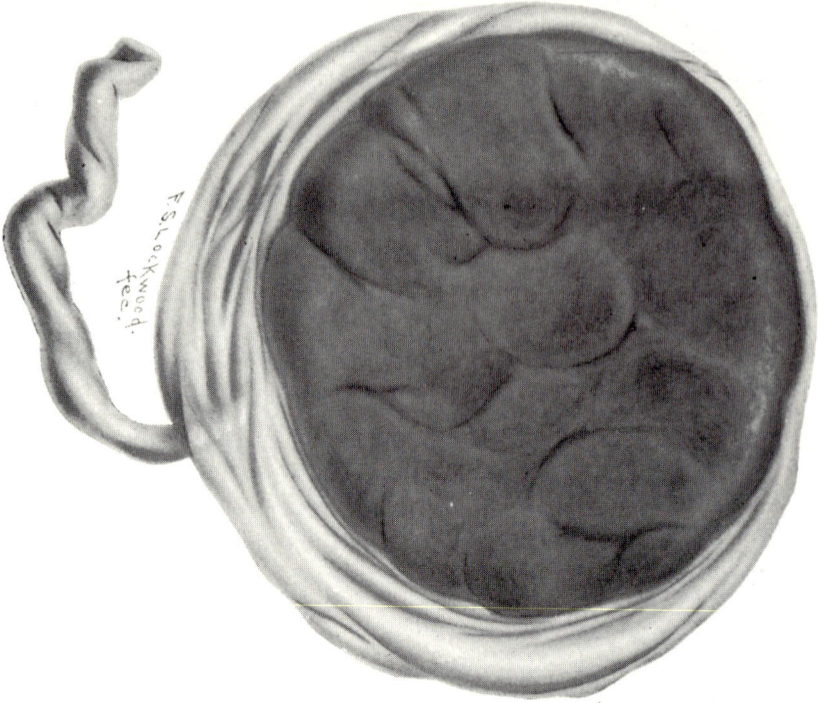

FIG. 131.—MATERNAL SURFACE OF MATURE PLACENTA, SHOWING COTYLEDONS; MEMBRANES TURNED BACK. × ⅔.

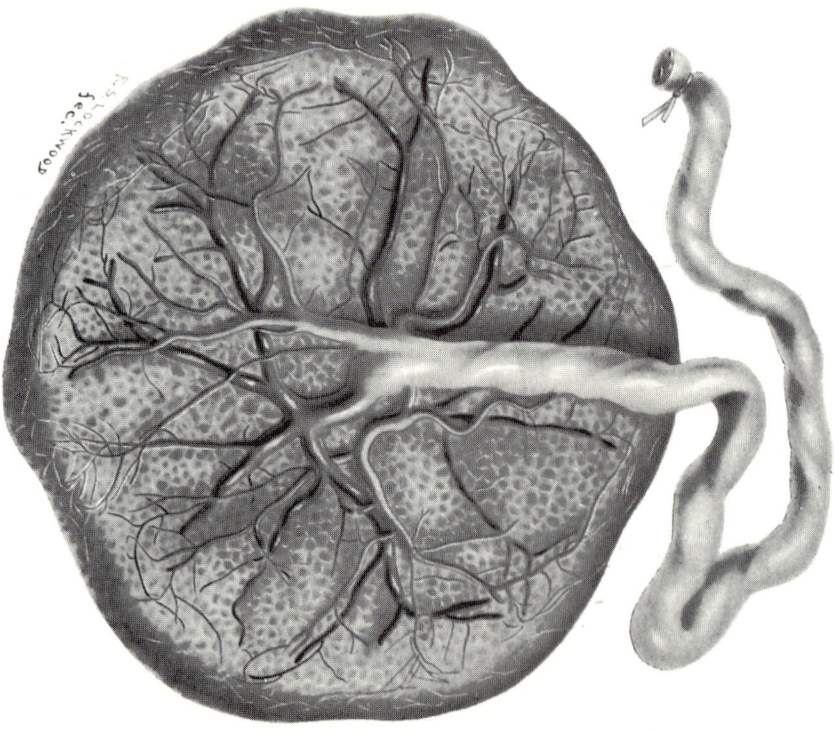

FIG. 132.—FŒTAL SURFACE OF MATURE PLACENTA. × ⅔.

outer, and that directed towards the cavity of the ovum as the fœtal or inner surface. The former is covered by a thin layer of decidua and presents a ragged, torn appearance, being divided by depressions of varying depth into a number of irregularly shaped areas, the so-called *cotyledons*, which vary considerably in number, as many as twenty being sometimes observed. On careful examination of the decidual surface, numerous vessels may be seen which have been torn through when the

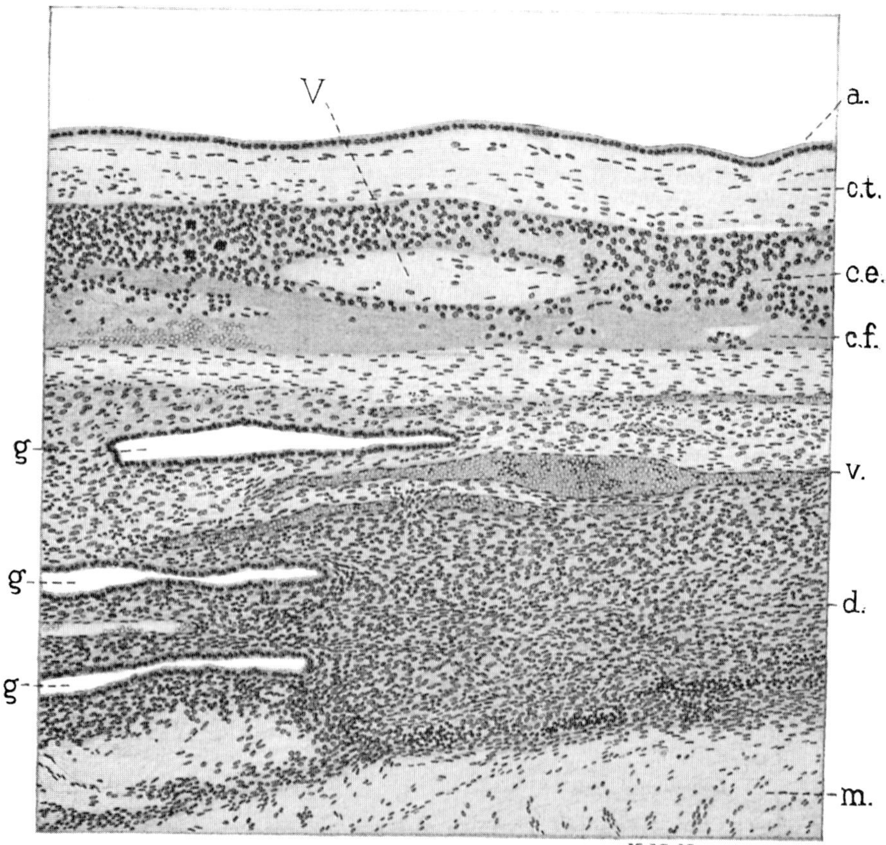

FIG. 133.—FŒTAL MEMBRANES AND UTERINE WALL. × 75.

a., amnion; *c.t.*, connective tissue of amnion and chorion; *c.e.*, chorionic epithelium; *c.f.*, canalized fibrin; *d.*, decidua; *g.*, gland; *m.*, muscularis; *v.*, vein; *V.*, atrophic villus.

placenta was separated. Thus, Klein was able to count 51 arteries and 53 veins in a single specimen.

The fœtal or inner surface presents a glistening appearance, owing to the fact that it is covered by amnion, which, however, is only slightly adherent. When the latter is removed, it leaves a coarsely granular surface, upon which the umbilical cord is usually inserted somewhat eccentrically, though it may be just at the centre of the organ and occasionally near its margin. The various modes of insertion will be considered when we take up the abnormalities of the placenta.

The vessels composing the umbilical cord spread out beneath the amnion and rapidly divide, but the main branches remain upon the fœtal surface of the placenta until its margin is reached. In many instances a large vein, which is usually known as the *circular sinus*, extends around a considerable portion of the periphery of the placenta, but only in very rare cases completely encircles the organ.

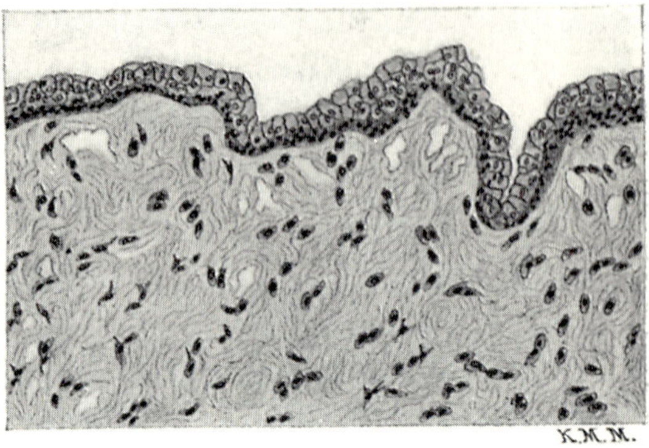

FIG. 134.—EPITHELIUM OF UMBILICAL CORD. × 110.

The *fœtal membranes* consist of the amnion, chorion, and a thin layer of decidua. The amnion, the innermost of the membranes, is a thin, transparent, glistening structure, which is rarely thicker than a sheet of writing paper. Its outer surface is closely applied to the chorion, from which, however, it can usually be separated without difficulty. The chorion is more opaque and thicker than the amnion, though it rarely exceeds 1 millimetre in thickness. It represents the chorion læve of the early months, and under the microscope is seen to possess a number of degenerated villi. Clinging to its outer surface are a few shreds of tissue—the portion of the decidua which is cast off after the birth of the child. Fig. 133 is taken from a section through the fœtal membranes and the uterine wall outside of the placental site, and gives a good idea of their composition.

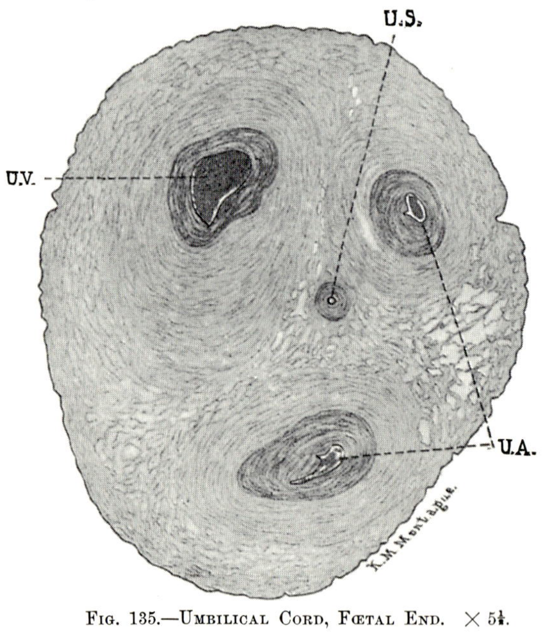

FIG. 135.—UMBILICAL CORD, FŒTAL END. × 5¼.
U.A., umbilical artery; *U.S.*, remnant of umbilical stalk; *U.V.*, umbilical vein.

Umbilical Cord.—The umbilical cord, or funis, extends from the navel of the child to the fœtal surface of the placenta. Its exterior presents a dull white, moist appearance, and through it shimmer the umbilical vessels—two arteries and a vein. It varies from 1 to 2.5 centimetres in diameter, and averages about 55 centimetres in length; though in extreme cases it may vary from 0.5 to 198 centimetres. The average length of 1,000 cords, which were measured at the Johns Hopkins Hospital, was 55 centimetres, the shortest being 12 and the longest 100 centimetres.

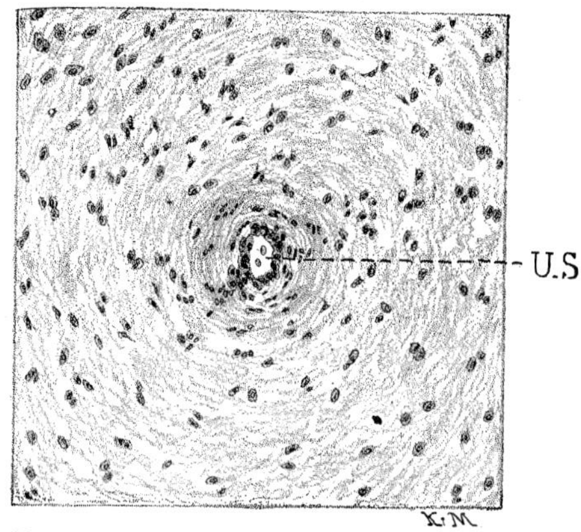

Fig. 136.—Section through Umbilical Cord, showing Stalk of Umbilical Vesicle. × 110.

The cord frequently presents a twisted appearance, the coiling usually being from left to right. As the vessels are usually longer than the cord, they are frequently folded upon themselves, thus giving rise to nodulations upon the surface which are designated as false knots.

The cord is covered by several layers of epithelium, which is a direct continuation of the skin covering the abdomen of the embryo; its interior is made up of a mucoid connective tissue—the so-called Whartonian jelly.

Microscopic sections through the fœtal and placental ends of the cord at term present a somewhat different appearance. In the former, besides the vessels, one usually sees two small, darkly staining areas, which under higher magnification appear as small ducts lined by cuboidal or flattened epithelial cells. One is the remnant of the allantois, and the other the duct or stalk of the umbilical vesicle; at the placental end only the latter is present.

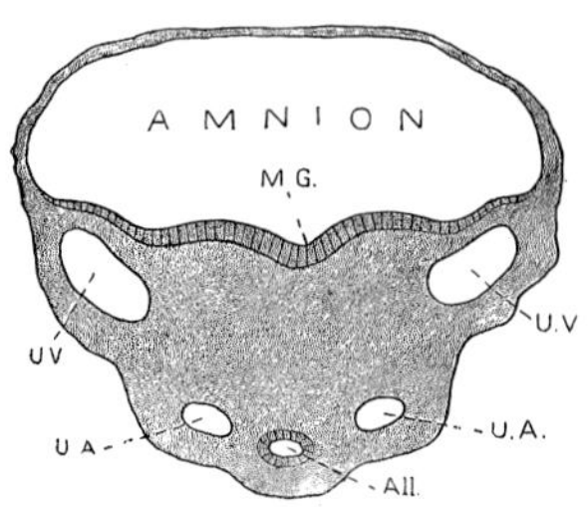

Fig. 137.—Section through Abdominal Pedicle of 2.25-Millimetre Embryo (His). × 50.

All., allantois; *M.G.*, medullary groove; *U.A.*, umbilical artery; *U.V.*, umbilical vein.

In most text-books, it is stated that the cord is derived from the allantois, and is covered by a sheath of amnion. The researches of His have definitely shown that such is not the case in man, but that the fœtus, in the earliest stages of pregnancy, is connected with the inner surface of the chorion by a tolerably thick mass of tissue, only a small portion of which is occupied by the allantois. This His designated as the abdominal pedicle (*Bauchstiel*), and showed that it represents merely an extension of the caudal end of the embryo.

Fig. 137 represents a section through the abdominal pedicle of one of the early embryos studied by His, and clearly shows its analogy with the embryonic area. The great bulk of the structure is made up of mesodermic tissue in which the umbilical vessels and the allantois are embedded; its dorsal surface is covered by a single layer of ectoderm, showing at its middle a slight depression which represents a continuation of the medullary groove, while arching over it is the amnion. In its further development the ectodermal portion extends downward and inward, eventually inclosing a small portion of the cœlome in a way similar to that in which the abdominal walls are formed in the embryo itself. In this cavity the stalk of the umbilical vesicle or yolk-sac is included. In the meantime the amnion is likewise extending around the entire structure, but is not in contact with it; and as the former becomes more and more distended by the amniotic fluid, it becomes farther and farther separated from the abdominal pedicle, or as we may now call it, the umbilical cord. Eventually the amnion is connected only with the portion of the cord which is attached to the fœtal surface of the placenta.

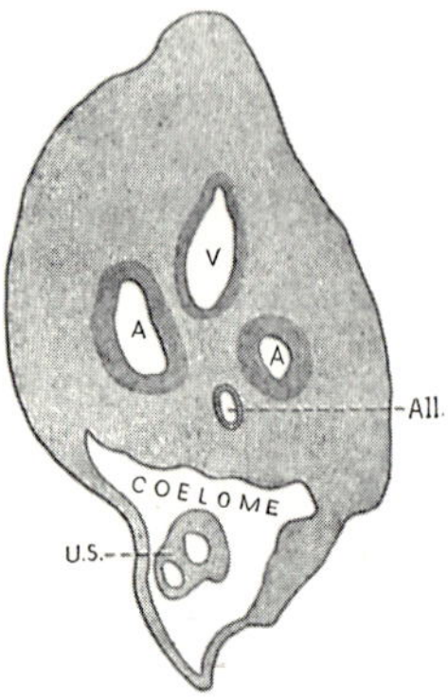

Fig. 138.—Section through Young Umbilical Cord (Minot).

A., artery; *All.*, allantois; *U.S.*, stalk of umbilical vesicle; *V.*, vein.

Fig. 139 represents a thirty-days' embryo described by His, and gives a very good idea of the manner in which the stalk of the umbilical vesicle becomes included within the cord.

Umbilical Vesicle.—The yolk-sac, or, as it becomes later, the umbilical vesicle, is a very prominent organ at the beginning of pregnancy, and is present in all the early ova which have been described. In its earliest stages it occupies all of the blastodermic vesicle which is not taken up by the embryonic area. But, as the embryo develops, it becomes relatively smaller, and, as we have already shown, is taken up in great part to form the intestinal canal, so that after the formation of the abdominal walls it protrudes from the umbilicus as a rounded sac with a distinct stalk. As pregnancy advances the sac becomes smaller and its stalk longer.

The structure persists throughout pregnancy, and can nearly always be found at full term, when it is represented by a small oval sac, 3 to 5 millimetres in diameter, which usually lies on the fœtal surface of the placenta, between the chorion and amnion, but occasionally in the membranes just beyond the placental margin. It is connected with the umbilical cord by a fine pedicle, which, as has been already shown, may be seen in sections through the cord at term. Schultze, in 1861, was able to

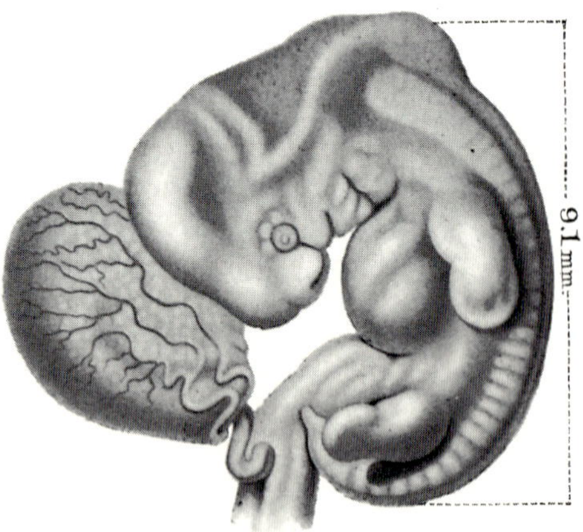

Fig. 139.—Stalk of Umbilical Vesicle being included in the Umbilical Cord (His).

demonstrate the umbilical vesicle in 146 out of 150 mature placentæ examined.

The intra-abdominal portion of the duct of the umbilical vesicle, which extends from the umbilicus to the intestine, usually atrophies and disappears, but occasionally it remains patent, forming what is known as *Meckel's diverticulum,* which may play an important pathological part in later life.

In animals whose ova possess a large amount of yolk, the umbilical vesicle is the main source of nutrition for the embryo; but in those of women its significance is not so clear, since the proportion of yolk is exceedingly small. It must, however, play an important part in the economy of the embryo, as it develops a considerable circulation, and, as Selenka has shown, forms numerous crypts from its entodermal lining. As yet, however, we are unacquainted with its functions.

LITERATURE

Bumm. Zur Kenntniss der Utero-placentar-gefässe. Archiv f. Gyn., xxxvii, 1–15, 1890.
Ueber die Entwickelung der mütterlichen Blutkreislaufes in der menschl. Placenta. Archiv f. Gyn., xliii, 181–195, 1893.

Dalrymple. Medico-chir. Transactions, xxv, 21, 1842 (quoted by Waldeyer).

Duval. Le placenta des carnassiers. Annales de Gyn. et d'Obst., xlv, 167–182, 1896.

Engelmann. The Mucous Membrane of the Uterus, etc. Amer. Jour. Obst., viii, 30–87, 1875.

Ercolani. Della struttura anat. della caduca uterina, etc. Bologna, 1874.
Quoted by Waldeyer, p. 5.

Farre. Uterus and its Appendages. Todd's Cyclopædia of Anat. and Physiol., Parts XLIX and L.

Fehling. Ueber die physiologische Bedeutung des Fruchtwassers. Archiv f. Gyn., xiv 221–244, 1879.

Fränkel, L. Vergleichende Untersuchungen des Uterus- und Chorion-epithels. Archiv f. Gyn., lv, 269–316, 1898.

von Franqué. Cervix und unteres Uterinsegment, Stuttgart, 1897.

Friedländer. Physiol. anat. Untersuchungen über den Uterus. Leipzig, 1870.

Frommel. Verh. d. deutschen Gesellschaft f. Gyn., i, 306, 1886.

Gebhard. Ueber das sogenannte Syncytioma malignum. Zeitschr. f. Geb. u. Gyn., xxxvii, 480–518, 1897.

Hegar. Beiträge zur Pathologie des Eies, etc. Monatsschr. f. Geburtskunde, xxi, Supplement Heft. 1–66, 1863.

Hennig. Die weissen Blutkörperchen und die Deciduazellen. Archiv f. Gyn., vi, 508, 509, 1874.

Herff. Beiträge zur Lehre von der Placenta und von den mütterlichen Eihüllen. Zeitschr. f. Geb. u. Gyn., xxxv, 268–297 and 325–372, 1896.

Heukelom. Ueber die menschliche Placentation. Arch. f. Anat. u. Physiol., Anat. Abth., 1898, 1–36.

Hicks. The Anatomy of the Human Placenta. Trans. London Obst. Soc., xiv, 149–189, 1873.

His. Bauchstiel und Nabelstrang, Anatomie menschlicher Embryonen, iii, 222–226, 1885.
Die Umschliessung der menschl. Frucht während der frühesten Zeiten der Schwangerschaft. Arch. f. Anat. u. Physiol., Anat. Abth., 1897, 399–430.

Hubrecht. The Placentation of Erinaceus Europaeus, with remarks on the Phylogeny of the Placenta. Quart. Jour. of Microscop. Science, xxx, 1889.

HUBRECHT. Die Rolle des embryonalen Trophoblasts bei der Placentation. Centralbl. f. Gyn., 1897, 1206.

HUNTER, JOHN. Observations on Certain Parts of the Animal Economy. London, 1778.

HUNTER, WM. Anatomy of the Human Gravid Uterus. London, 1774.

HYRTL. See Kollmann.

KASTCHENKO. Das menschliche Chorionepithel und dessen Rolle bei der Histogenese der Placenta. Arch. f. Anat. u. Physiol., Anat. Abth., 1885.

KINOSHITA. Ueber grosszellige decidua-ähnliche Wucherungen auf dem Peritoneum. Monatsschr. f. Geb. u. Gyn., viii, 500–509, 1898.

KLEIN. Entwickelung und Rückbildung der Decidua. Zeitschr. f. Geb. u. Gyn., xxii. 247–295, 1891.

KOLLMANN. Lehrbuch der Entwickelungsgeschichte des Menschen. Jena, 1898.

KOSSMANN. Zur Histologie der Chorionzotten des Menschen. Leuckhart's Festschrift, 1892.

Zur Histologie der Extrauterinschwangerschaft, nebst Bemerkungen über ein sehr junges mit der Decidua gelöstes Ei. Zeitschr. f. Geb. u. Gyn., xxvii, 266–286, 1893.

KUNDRAT u. ENGELMANN. Untersuchungen über die Uterusschleimhaut. Stricker's med. Jahrb., 1873.

LANGHANS. Untersuchungen über die menschliche Placenta. Arch. f. Anat. u. Entwickelungsgesch., Leipzig, 1877, 188–276.

Ueber die Zellschicht des menschlichen Chorions. Beiträge zur Anat. und Embryologie. (Henle's Festgabe), Bonn, 1882.

LEOPOLD. Studien über die Uterusschleimhaut, etc. Berlin, 1878.

Ueber den Bau der Placenta. Verh. d. deutschen Gesell. f. Gyn., iii, 257, 1890.

Uterus u. Kind. Leipzig, 1897.

LEOPOLD, MARCHESI, u. BOTT. Zur Entwickelung und der Bau der menschlichen Placenta. Arch. f. Gyn., lix, 516–544, 1899.

LINDENTHAL. Ueber Decidua ovarii. Monatsschr. f. G. u. G., xiii, 707–723, 1901.

DE LOOS. Das Wachstum der menschlichen Chorionzotten. D. I., Freiburg in B., 1897.

MARCHAND. Ueber die sogenannten "decidualen" Geschwülste. Monatsschr. f. Geb. u. Gyn., i, 419–513, 1895.

Beiträge zur Kenntniss der Placentarbildung. Marburg, 1898.

MERTTENS. Beiträge zur normalen u. path. Anatomie der menschlichen Placenta. Zeitschr. f. Geb. u. Gyn., xxx, 1–97, 1894.

MINOT. Uterus and Embryo. Jour. of Morphology, ii, No. 3, 1889.

Human Embryology. New York, 1892.

NITABUCH. Beiträge zur Kenntniss der menschlichen Placenta. D. I., Bern, 1887.

NOORTWYK. Quoted from Waldeyer.

OPITZ. Vergleich der Placentarbildung bei Meerschweinchen, etc., mit derjenigen beim Menschen. Zeitschr. f. Geb. u. Gyn., xli, 120–144 and 153–173, 1899.

OVERLACH. Die pseudomenst. Mucosa uteri. D. I., München, 1885.

PETERS. Ueber die Einbettung des menschlichen Eies. Wien, 1899.

REICHERT. Beschreibung einer frühzeitigen menschlichen Frucht. Abhandlungen d. königl. Akad. d. Wissenschaften, Berlin, 1873.

ROHR. Die Beziehungen der mütterlichen Gefässe zu den intervillösen Räumen der reifen Placenta, speciell zur Thrombose derselben ("weisser Infarct"). D. I., Bern, 1889.

RUGE. Ueber die menschliche Placenta. Zeitschr. f. Geb. u. Gyn., xxxix, 550–588, 1898.

SCHMORL. Ueber grosszellige (decidua-ähnliche) Wucherungen auf dem Peritoneum u. den Ovarien bei intrauteriner Schwangerschaft. Monatsschr. f. Geb. u. Gyn., v, 46, 1897.

SCHULTZE. Das Nabelbläschen ein constantes Gebilde in der Nachgeburt des ausgetragenen Kindes. Leipzig, 1861.

SELENKA. Studien über Entwickelungsgeschichte der Thiere, Heft 5, Wiesbaden, 1891. Menschen-Affen, 11, Wiesbaden, 1899.

SHARKEY. English translation of Müller's Handbuch der Physiologie, according to Schroeder's Lehrbuch, XIII. Aufl., 1899.

SOBOTTA. Die Befruchtung und Furchung des Eies der Maus. Archiv f. mikro. Anat., 1895, xlv, 15–93.

SPEE. Beobachtungen an einer menschl. Keimscheibe mit offener Medullarrinne, etc. Archiv f. Anat. u. Phys., Anat. Abth., 1899, 159–176.

Neue Beobachtungen über sehr frühe Entwickelungsstufen des menschlichen Eies Arch. f. Anat. u. Physiol., Anat. Abth., 1896, 1–30.

TURNER. Observations on the Structure of the Human Placenta. Jour. Anat. and Physiol., vii, 120, 1873; also xi, 1877.

TUSSENBROECK. Die Decidua uterina bei ektopischer Schwangerschaft, etc. Virchow's Archiv, cxxxiii, 207–236, 1893.

ULESKO-STROGANOWA. Beiträge zur Lehre vom mikros. Bau der Placenta. Monatsschr. f. Geb. u. Gyn., iii, 207, 1896.

VATER. Quoted from Waldeyer.

WALDEYER. Bemerkungen über den Bau der Menschen- und Affen-Placenta. Archiv f. mikros. Anat., xxxv, 1–52, 1890.

WEBER. Zusätze vom Bau und den Verrichtungen der Geschlechtsorgane. Abh. der kgl. sächsischen Akademie, 1846.

WEBSTER. The Changes in the Uterine Mucosa during Pregnancy and in the Attached Fœtal Structures. Amer. Gyn. and Obst. Journal, x, 168–264 and 535–662, 1897.

Human Placentation. Chicago, 1901.

VON WEISS. Zur Kasuistik der Placenta praevia centralis. Centralbl. f. Gyn., 641–649, 1897.

WINCKLER. Textur, Structur und Zellleben in den Adnexen des menschlichen Eies. Jena, 1870.

CHAPTER V

THE FŒTUS

The Fœtus in the Various Months of Pregnancy.—It is a matter of considerable importance that the physician be able to tell approximately the age of embryos and prematurely born children, and we shall therefore give a short description of the fœtus at its various periods of development.

The average duration of pregnancy, from the commencement of the last menstrual flow to the onset of labour, is two hundred and eighty days, or ten lunar months, though a considerable number of children are born shortly before or after the expiration of that period.

The following details concerning the development of the unborn child are taken in great part from His, who distinguished three periods in its evolution. Thus, during the first two weeks of pregnancy the product of conception is designated as the ovum; from the third to the fifth week—the period during which the various organs are developed and a definite form is assumed—it is known as the embryo; after the fifth week it becomes the fœtus.

First Two Weeks.—The earliest human ova with which we are acquainted were described by Peters, Leopold, Reichert, and Spee. These

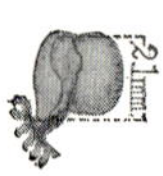

Fig. 140.

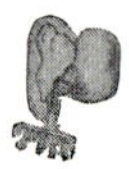

Fig. 141.

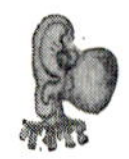

Fig. 142.

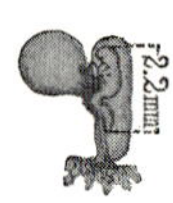

Fig. 143.

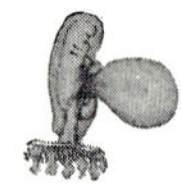

Fig. 144.

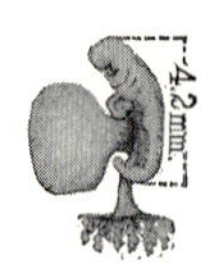

Fig. 145.

Figs. 140–145.—Early Embryos described by His.

were vesicular structures whose most prominent feature was the chorion, to one side of which was attached the future embryo, so small a body that its component parts could be distinguished only with the aid of the microscope. In each of these ova the embryonic area was covered by a well-developed amnion, and the great bulk of the structure consisted of the yolk-sac. Spee's ovum presented the earliest stages in the formation of the embryo itself—namely, the primitive streak. Figs. 140 to 145 represent early ova described by His.

Third Week.—The embryonal period begins with the third week, in the early part of which can be detected the beginning formation of the medullary groove and canal, soon to be followed by the appearance of the head-folds. At this stage of development the abdominal pedicle is seen coming off from the tail end of the embryo, and lying almost in the same axis with it. The embryo is concave on its dorsal surface, and is made up in great part of the yolk-sac.

A little later, the formation of the double heart may be noted; while in the latter part of the week the cerebral and optic vesicles appear, as well as the visceral arches and clefts. The yolk-sac becomes more and more constricted, and is connected with the ventral surface of the embryo by a broad pedicle. At the very end of the third week (about the twenty-first day) the limbs make their appearance as small buds upon the surface of the embryo.

Fourth Week.—This week is characterized by a great increase in the size of the embryo, which becomes markedly flexed upon its ventral sur-

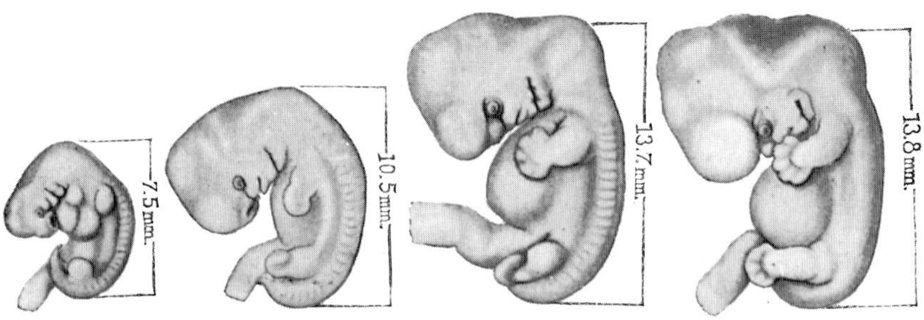

Fig. 146. Fig. 147. Fig. 148. Fig. 149.

FIGS. 146–149.—EMBRYOS FROM FOURTH AND FIFTH WEEKS (His). × 2.

face, so that its head and tail ends come almost in contact. The rudiments of the eyes, ears, and nose now make their appearance, and the umbilical vesicle becomes still more pedunculated. At the end of the first lunar month the embryo measures from 7.5 to 10 millimetres (0.3 to 0.4 inch) in length.

Second Month.—In the first half of the second month the human embryo does not differ essentially in appearance from that of other animals. It is still markedly bent on itself, and the visceral clefts and arches are the most prominent characteristics of its cephalic region, while the extremities are in a very rudimentary condition. In the latter part of the month, owing to the development of the brain, the head becomes considerably larger, and assumes a certain resemblance to that of a human being. At the same time the nose, mouth, and ears become less prominent and the extremities more developed, so that it can be seen that they are made up of three portions. The external genitalia also make their appearance in the latter part of this month, and at its end the fœtus has attained a length of 2.5 centimetres (1 inch).

Third Month.—At the end of this month the entire product of conception is about as large as a goose's egg, and the embryo measures from 7 to 9 centimetres in length. Centres of ossification have appeared in most of the bones; the fingers and toes become differentiated and are supplied with nails; the external genitalia are beginning to show definite signs of sex.

Fourth Month.—By the end of the fourth month the fœtus is from 10 to 17 centimetres long, and weighs about 120 grammes. An examination of the external genital organs will now definitely reveal the sex.

Fifth Month.—The fœtus varies from 18 to 27 centimetres in length, and weighs about 280 grammes. Its skin has become less transparent, a

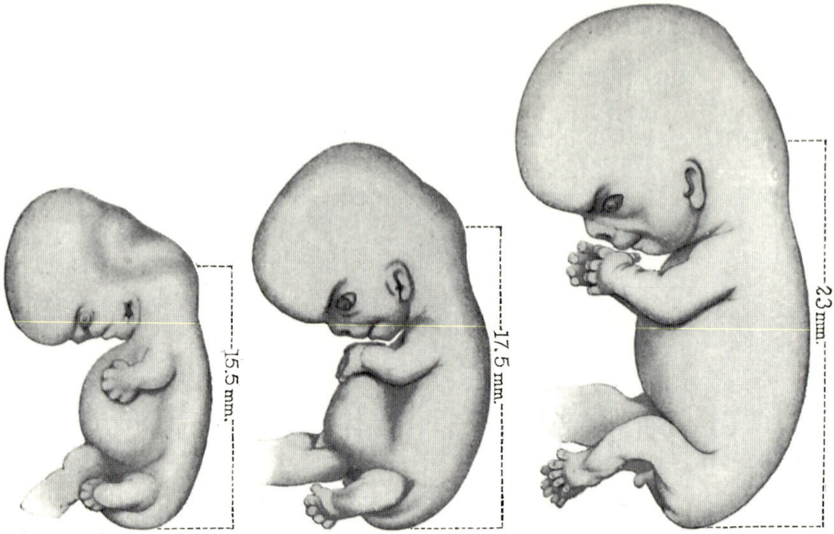

Fig. 150. Fig. 151. Fig. 152.

Figs. 150–152.—Embryos from Second Month (His). × 2.

downy covering is seen over its entire body, while a certain amount of typical hair has made its appearance on the head.

Sixth Month.—At the end of the sixth month the fœtus varies from 28 to 34 centimetres in length, and weighs about 634 grammes. The skin presents a markedly wrinkled appearance, and fat begins to be deposited beneath it; the head is still comparatively quite large. A fœtus born at this period will attempt to breathe and move its limbs, but always perishes within a short time.

Seventh Month.—The length during this month varies from 35 to 38 centimetres, and the fœtus attains a weight of over 1,200 grammes. The entire body is very thin, the skin is reddish and covered with vernix caseosa. The pupillary membrane has just disappeared from the eyes. A fœtus born at this period moves its limbs quite energetically and cries with a weak voice; but, as a rule, it cannot be raised, even with the most expert care, although an occasional successful case is found in the records.

It is generally believed among the laity that a child born at the end of the seventh month has a better chance of living than when it comes into the world four weeks later. This idea is a remnant of the old Hippocratic doctrine and is absolutely erroneous, as the more developed the child the greater are its chances for life.

Eighth Month.—At the end of the eighth month the fœtus has attained a length of 42.5 centimetres, and a weight of about 1,900 grammes. The surface of the skin is still red and wrinkled, and the child resembles an old man in appearance. Children born at this period may live if properly cared for, though their chances are not very promising.

Ninth Month.—At the end of the ninth month the fœtus is 46.75 centimetres long, and weighs about 2,500 grammes. Owing to the presence of considerable fat, the body has become more rotund and the face has lost its previous wrinkled appearance. Children born at this time have a very fair chance of life if properly cared for.

Tenth Month.—Full term is reached at the end of this month. The fœtus is now fully developed, and presents the appearances which we shall consider in detail when we describe the new-born child.

According to Ahlfeld, the average weight and length of the fœtus in the last four months of its development are as follows:

Week.	Weight.	Length.
27th....	1,142 grammes.	36.3 centimetres.
28th..............................	1,635 "	40.4 "
29th	1,576 "	39.6 "
30th..............................	1,868 "	42 "
31st..............................	1,872 "	43.7 "
32d	2,107 "	43.4 "
33d	2,084 "	43.88 "
34th..............................	2,424 "	46.07 "
35th..............................	2,753 "	47.03 "
36th..............................	2,806 "	48.3 "
37th..............................	2,878 "	48.3 "
38th..............................	3,016 "	49.9 "
39th..............................	3,321 "	50.6 "
40th..............................	3,168 "	50.5 "

These figures possess only an approximate value, and generally speaking the length affords a more accurate criterion of the age of a child than its weight. Haase has suggested a very simple method of determining the size of the embryo at its various periods of development. According to him, the length in centimetres may be roughly approximated during the first five months by squaring the number of the month to which the pregnancy has advanced; in the second half of pregnancy, by multiplying the month by 5, as is shown in the following table:

At the end of the first month	1 × 1,	1 centimetre.
" " " second month......................	2 × 2,	4 centimetres.
" " " third month....................	3 × 3,	9 "
" " " fourth month	4 × 4,	16 "
" " " fifth month	5 × 5,	25 "
" " " sixth month....................	6 × 5,	30 "
" " " seventh month	7 × 5,	35 "
" " " eighth month	8 × 5,	40 "
" " " ninth month	9 × 5,	45 "
" " " tenth month	10 × 5,	50 "

The Child at Full Term.—The average child at full term is 50 to 51 centimetres (20 to 21 inches) long, and weighs 3,250 grammes (7 pounds). The skin is smooth and polished in appearance, and shows no lanugo, except occasionally about the shoulders. Over the entire surface is spread a whitish, greasy material, the *vernix caseosa*, which is a mixture of epithelial cells, lanugo hairs, and the secretion of the sebaceous glands. The head is usually covered by darkish hairs 2 to 3 centimetres in length, and the cartilages of the nose and ears are well developed. The fingers and toes possess well-developed nails, which project beyond their tips. In male children the testicles are usually found within the scrotum; in girls the labia majora are well developed and are in contact with one another, and usually conceal the rest of the genitalia. The bones of the head are well ossified, and are in close contact at the various sutures. At autopsy a centre of ossification, 0.5 centimetre in diameter, is found in the lower epiphysis of the femur. This was first described by Blécard, in 1826, as a diagnostic sign of maturity. It is not infallible, however, as Hartmann has shown that it was absent in 12 out of 102 full-term children which he examined. No one of these conditions affords indisputable proof of the maturity of a child, but when the majority of them are present the evidence becomes fairly convincing.

Soon after its birth, and occasionally just after the head emerges from the vulva, and before the expulsion of the entire body, the child makes inspiratory movements and begins to cry loudly. It moves its extremities freely, and after a short time passes urine and meconium.

Negro babies at birth differ somewhat in appearance from white children, but not so markedly as one would expect. Their skin presents a dusky, bluish-red hue, but does not at all suggest the darker colour which it will assume in the course of a few weeks. Where there is a considerable admixture of white blood, the dusky hue may be entirely absent, and the only evidence of negro ancestry will be found in an increased pigmentation about the external genitalia.

Weight of the New-born.—The average infant at birth weighs about 3,250 grammes (7 pounds), boys being usually 100 grammes (3 ounces) heavier than girls. Marked variations are frequently observed, which are dependent upon the race and size of the parents, the number of children which the mother has borne, her mode of life, and her nutrition and general condition during the later months of pregnancy. In 500 full-term white children born at the Johns Hopkins Hospital, the average weight was 3,409 grammes (7 pounds 5 ounces), the smallest child weighing 2,180 grammes (4 pounds 11 ounces) and the largest 4,553 grammes (9 pounds 12 ounces).

It appears that coloured children weigh considerably less than white, a fact that, in large cities, at least, is indicative of the physical degeneration which characterizes the race. Five hundred full-term coloured children born at the Johns Hopkins Hospital averaged 3,023 grammes (6 pounds 8 ounces) in weight, a difference of 386 grammes (13 ounces) in favour of the white race.

Similar but less marked differences may be observed in the different countries and even in various portions of the same country. Thus Schroeder found that the children born in Bonn averaged 71 grammes ($2\frac{1}{2}$ ounces) less in weight than those observed by Hecker in Munich.

Perfectly healthy full-term children may vary from 2,300 to 5,000 grammes (5 to $10\frac{3}{4}$ pounds) in weight. They rarely exceed the latter figure, although it is not unusual to hear of children weighing 15, 16, and even 20 pounds at birth. The majority of these cases, however, must be regarded as apocryphal, and careful inquiry will usually show that the weight has been only roughly estimated by lifting the child in the hand, and not based upon accurate determination. Hecker in 1,096 cases found only 2 children that weighed over 5,000 grammes, and Winckel only 5 in 30,500 deliveries. According to Ludwig, out of 15,166 children born in Chrobak's clinic in Vienna, only 1 weighed 5,300 grammes ($11\frac{1}{8}$ pounds), and Varnier states that in seven years, at the Baudelocque Clinic in Paris, there were only 6 children that exceeded 5,000 grammes at birth, the largest weighing 6,150 grammes (13 pounds 3 ounces).

Out of nearly 3,000 children delivered under my supervision, the largest weighed 5,833 grammes, or 12 pounds 8 ounces; though several of my friends have met with babies which were considerably heavier. Dubois, in 1897, collected from the literature 28 cases in which the child weighed 5,600 grammes (12 pounds) or more at birth, and stated that the heaviest children on record were reported by Ortega, Rachel and Neumer and Beech, and weighed respectively 11,300 (24 pounds 3 ounces), 11,250 (24 pounds 2 ounces), and 10,750 grammes (23 pounds 12 ounces). Ortega's child was 70 centimetres (28 inches) long, and Beech's 76 centimetres (30 inches). Ludwig, a few years ago, reported a case in which he was obliged to perform Cæsarean section, after craniotomy and amputation of the extremities, in order to deliver a child weighing 7,700 grammes (16 pounds 8 ounces). But in spite of these exceptional cases, one should be extremely sceptical in accepting reports concerning phenomenally heavy children, unless one is convinced that the reporter is a truthful person and has weighed the child upon an accurate balance.

On the other hand, children are frequently met with under 3,250 grammes (7 pounds) in weight, and it is not unusual to see healthy full-term babies weighing from 2,333 to 2,800 grammes (5 to 6 pounds). Any weight below 5 pounds, in the case of an infant born at term, should always lead one to suspect some disease on the part of the mother or fœtus, as nephritis or syphilis.

Generally speaking, premature children weighing less than 1,500 grammes (3 pounds 3 ounces) have practically no chance of life, though exceptional cases have been reported in which such infants have done well. Piering, in a recent article, reports raising a premature child that weighed only 1,120 grammes at birth, and mentions cases under the charge of Ritter, Rodman, and D'Outrepont in which children weighing only 717, 719, and 750 grammes respectively were successfully reared.

The size of the fœtus increases with the age of the mother up to the twenty-eighth or thirtieth year, if pregnancies have not followed in too rapid succession; the children of succeeding pregnancies usually follow the same rule.

The size of the fœtus is also dependent, to a considerable extent, upon that of the parents, especially the father; and in many instances its head closely resembles that of the father in shape.

The social condition of the mother and the comforts by which she is surrounded also exert a marked influence upon the child's weight, heavier children being more common in the upper walks of life. Thus, on looking over the records of my private cases, which are almost exclusively among the well-to-do classes, I found that 133 healthy full-term children, which I had weighed upon the same pair of scales, averaged 3,795 grammes (8 pounds 2 ounces) in weight, as compared with 3,409 and 3,023 grammes for the white and coloured children in hospital practice—a difference of 386 and 772 grammes, respectively. The heaviest child weighed 5,833 grammes (12 pounds 8 ounces), and the lightest 2,536 grammes (5 pounds 8 ounces). Eleven weighed 4,666 grammes (10 pounds), and 15 weighed 3,266 grammes (7 pounds) or less, leaving 107 between the two limits.

Pinard and Bachimont, from a study of 4,445 cases observed in the Baudelocque Clinic, have lately arrived at more or less similar conclusions. They found that the children of women who had lived in the hospital for three months prior to confinement averaged 500 grammes (1 pound 2 ounces) heavier than those of patients who had entered the hospital just

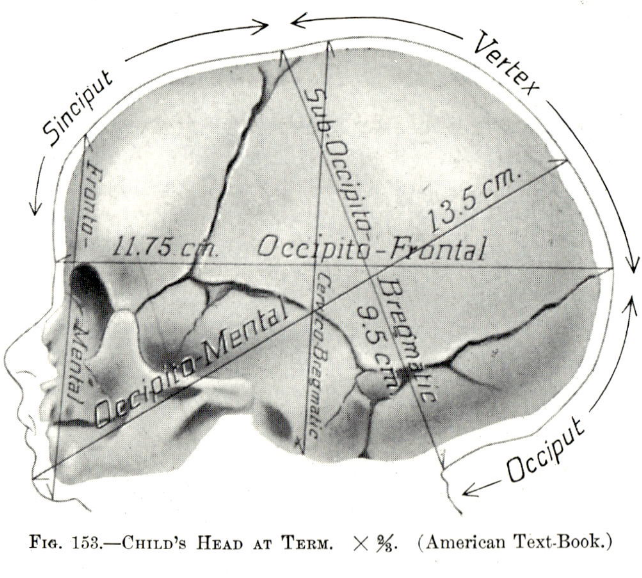

Fig. 153.—Child's Head at Term. × ⅜. (American Text-Book.)

before or during labour. They consider that this difference is due to the better nourishment of the former class of patients, and to the absence of hard work and the consequent tendency to premature labour. Fuchs, of Halle, obtained approximately the same results.

Provided the pelvis is normal, it is unusual for children weighing less than 5,000 grammes (10 pounds) to cause difficult labour simply from their size, since Varnier has shown that the diameters of the head do not increase in the same ratio as the weight of the child.

The Head of the Child.—From an obstetrical point of view the head of the child is its most important part, as the essential feature of labour is a process of adaptation between it and the various portions of the pelvis through which it passes. An accurate knowledge of its characteristics and size is therefore of capital importance.

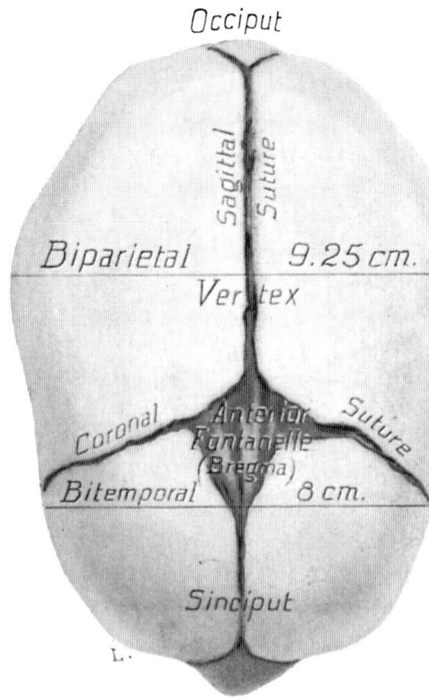

FIG. 154.—CHILD'S HEAD AT TERM. × ⅔. (American Text-Book.)

Only a comparatively small part of the head of the child at term is represented by the face, the rest being composed of the firm, hard skull, which is made up of two frontal, two parietal, two temporal bones, the upper portion of the occipital, and the wings of the sphenoid. These bony portions are not firmly united together, but are separated from one another by spaces filled with membrane—the *sutures*. Of these the most important are the *frontal*, between the two frontal bones; the *sagittal*, between the two parietal bones; the *coronal*, between the frontal and parietal bones; and the *lambdoid* suture, between the posterior margins of the parietal bones and the upper margin of the occipital bone. All of these sutures can be felt during labour; whereas the *temporal* suture, which is situated on either side between the inferior margin of the parietal and the upper margin of the temporal bones, is covered by soft parts and cannot be felt on the living child.

Where several sutures meet together an irregular space is formed, which is closed by a membrane and designated as a *fontanelle*. We usually distinguish four such structures: the greater and lesser, and the two temporal fontanelles. The *greater* or *anterior fontanelle* is a lozenge-shaped space situated at the junction of the sagittal and the coronal sutures. The *lesser* or *posterior fontanelle* is represented by a small triangular area at the intersection of the sagittal and lambdoid sutures. These are readily felt during labour, and their recognition gives important information concerning the position and presentation of the child. The *temporal* or *Gasserian fontanelles*, which are situated at the junction of the lambdoid and temporal sutures, cannot be felt on vaginal examination.

Arnold Lea has lately directed attention to the occasional presence of what he designates as the *sagittal fontanelle*, which is a lozenge-shaped space found in the sagittal suture at a point about half-way between the greater and lesser fontanelles. He considers that it results from faulty ossification of the parietal bones, and states that it occurs quite frequently—in 22 out of 500 fœtal skulls which he examined (4.4 per cent). I have met with a similar structure in only two instances, and in one it gave rise to a serious error in diagnosis. Since that time I have examined several hundred fœtal heads just after birth, but have not encountered other examples of the abnormality, so that it would seem probable that Lea's experience was very exceptional.

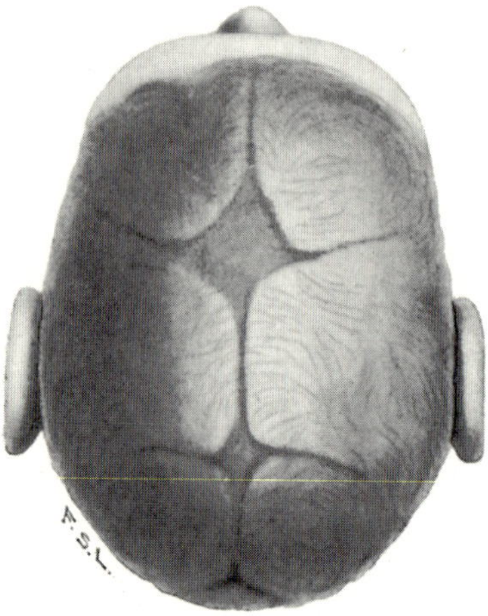

Fig. 155.—Head at Term, showing Small, Sagittal, and Large Fontanelles. × ½.

To aid us in forming definite ideas concerning the shape and size of the fœtal head, it is customary to measure certain *diameters* and *circumferences.* The diameters most frequently used are: (1) the fronto-occipital, which follows a line extending from the root of the nose to the most prominent portion of the occipital bone; (2) the biparietal, which represents the greatest transverse diameter of the head, and usually extends from one parietal boss to the other; (3) the bitemporal, which represents the greatest distance between the two temporal sutures; (4) the mento-occipital, from the chin to the most prominent portion of the occiput; and (5) the suboccipito-bregmatic, which follows a line drawn from the middle of the large fontanelle to the under surface of the occipital bone, just where it joins the neck. For convenience the various diameters are frequently designated by initials, which, with their several average measurements, are given in the following table:

Fronto-occipital, F. O.	11.75	centimetres.
Biparietal, B. P.	9.25	"
Bitemporal, B. T.	8	"
Mento-occipital, M. O.	13.5	"
Suboccipito-bregmatic, S. O. B.	9.5	"

The greatest *circumference of the head,* which corresponds to the plane of the fronto-occipital diameter, is 34.5 centimetres, while the least circumference, corresponding to the plane of the suboccipito-bregmatic diameter, is 32 centimetres. The figures just given are based upon the average measurements of a large number of heads just after birth, individual variations being frequently encountered. As a rule, boys have somewhat larger heads than girls, and the children of multiparæ than those of primiparæ.

A certain amount of motility exists at the sutures between the various bones composing the skull. This may vary within relatively wide limits in different individuals, so that heads which afford the same diameters on actual measurement not infrequently differ markedly in the obstacle which they offer to labour, as the bones of one may be soft, compressible, and readily displaced, while those of another are firmly and densely ossified and admitting of but little motility, the former being readily moulded to the genital canal, while the latter is incapable of reduction in size.

Physiology of the Fœtus.—Our knowledge concerning the physiology of the fœtus has been markedly enriched during recent years; nevertheless, when compared with that of the adult, it offers many points concerning which we are but slightly informed or profoundly ignorant.

Nutrition of the Fœtus.—Owing to the small amount of yolk contained in the human ovum, the growth of the fœtus is almost entirely dependent upon the amount of nutritive material which it obtains from its mother.

During the first few months of pregnancy, as Fehling first pointed out, the embryo consists almost entirely of water, and it is during this period that it grows most rapidly. In the later months of pregnancy, when more solids are being added, the increase in size becomes gradually slower. Fehling's conclusions were confirmed by Michel, who analyzed fœtuses at various periods of their development. Some of his results are shown in the following table:

	Water.	Albuminoids.	Salts.	Fats.
At 2½ months...	93.82 per cent.	4.39 per cent.	Trace.	Trace.
3d to 4th month	89.95 "	7.05 "	1.729 per cent.	.0379 per cent.
7th month	84.75 "	10.04 "	2.487 "	1.823 "
At term........	69.16 "	13.96 "	3.373 "	11.75 "

It is therefore apparent that, as the fœtus increases in age, it contains relatively less water and a markedly increased quantity of albuminoid materials, salts, and fats.

During the first few weeks after the implantation of the ovum upon the uterine mucosa its nutrition is entirely dependent upon osmosis. From the end of the first week it is surrounded by decidua, and between it and the chorion are developed the intervillous blood spaces which are filled with maternal blood. At this period the chorionic villi are devoid of vessels, and the only way in which nutritive material can be taken up from the maternal blood, by which these are surrounded, is by osmosis.

In the third week of pregnancy the omphalo-mesenteric vessels make their appearance upon the surface of the umbilical vesicle, and whatever nutritive materials the latter may contain are conveyed to the embryo by them. During the fourth week branches of the umbilical vessels appear in the chorionic villi, and from this time on the greater part of the nutrition of the fœtus is received from the maternal blood, which in the earlier weeks of pregnancy surrounds the entire ovum, but soon becomes limited to the placental site.

The Fœtal Circulation.—Owing to the fact that the materials needed for the nutrition of the fœtus are brought to it by the umbilical vein, the fœtal circulation differs materially from that of the adult (Plate VIII).

The blood is purified and laden with nutritive material in the placenta, and is then carried to the fœtus through the umbilical vein, which, after penetrating the abdominal wall, divides into two branches. Of these the smaller unites with the portal vein, the blood from which circulates through the liver and then gains access to the inferior vena cava through the hepatic vein. The other, the larger branch, which is designated as the ductus venosus, empties directly into the vena cava. The contents of the vena cava above the hepatic vein, therefore, consist of a mixture of arterial blood from the placenta and venous blood returning from the lower extremities of the fœtus. This is carried into the right auricle, and owing to the intervention of the Eustachian valve is directed through the foramen ovale into the left auricle, whence it passes into the left ventricle, which forces it into the aorta. The greater part of this blood makes its way into the vessels which supply the head and neck, while only a small portion of it passes by way of the arch of the aorta to nourish the lower portions of the body.

The blood which is returned from the head and upper extremities by way of the superior vena cava is poured into the right auricle, and crossing the current from the inferior vena cava passes into the right ventricle, whence it is forced into the pulmonary arteries. But so long as the lungs do not function, only a small portion of this blood gains access to them, the greater part of it passing through the ductus arteriosus to the arch of the aorta, and being then carried to the rest of the body of the embryo.

The blood which has gained access to the aorta directly from the left and also from the right ventricle, through the ductus arteriosus, is propelled down the aorta and given off to the various organs according to their needs; but the bulk of it enters the internal iliac and hypogastric arteries—the latter after passing the umbilicus being designated as the umbilical arteries—and through them gains access to the placenta.

From the foregoing description it is apparent that the blood circulating in the fœtus is at no time strictly arterial or strictly venous, but that the content of the inferior vena cava is far purer than that of the aorta.

The distinctive features of the fœtal circulation are connected with the ductus venosus and arteriosus, the foramen ovale, the hypogastric arteries, and the umbilical cord. After birth these structures undergo marked changes. As soon as the child is born and begins to breathe, the pulmonary circulation becomes established. As a result, a much greater quantity of blood is pumped by the right ventricle into the pulmonary arteries, while a lessened amount passes through the ductus arteriosus. Moreover, as soon as the circulation in the cord is abolished, the umbilical vein becomes functionless, and a diminished quantity of blood is returned to the right auricle by the inferior vena cava. This change leads to a diminution in the tension in the right auricle, while that in the left side of the heart is increased, bringing about the closure of the valve-like foramen ovale.

As the circulation through the umbilical arteries ceases almost immediately after the pulmonary circulation is established, the function of the hypogastric arteries is rendered useless, and their distal ends rapidly

PLATE VIII.

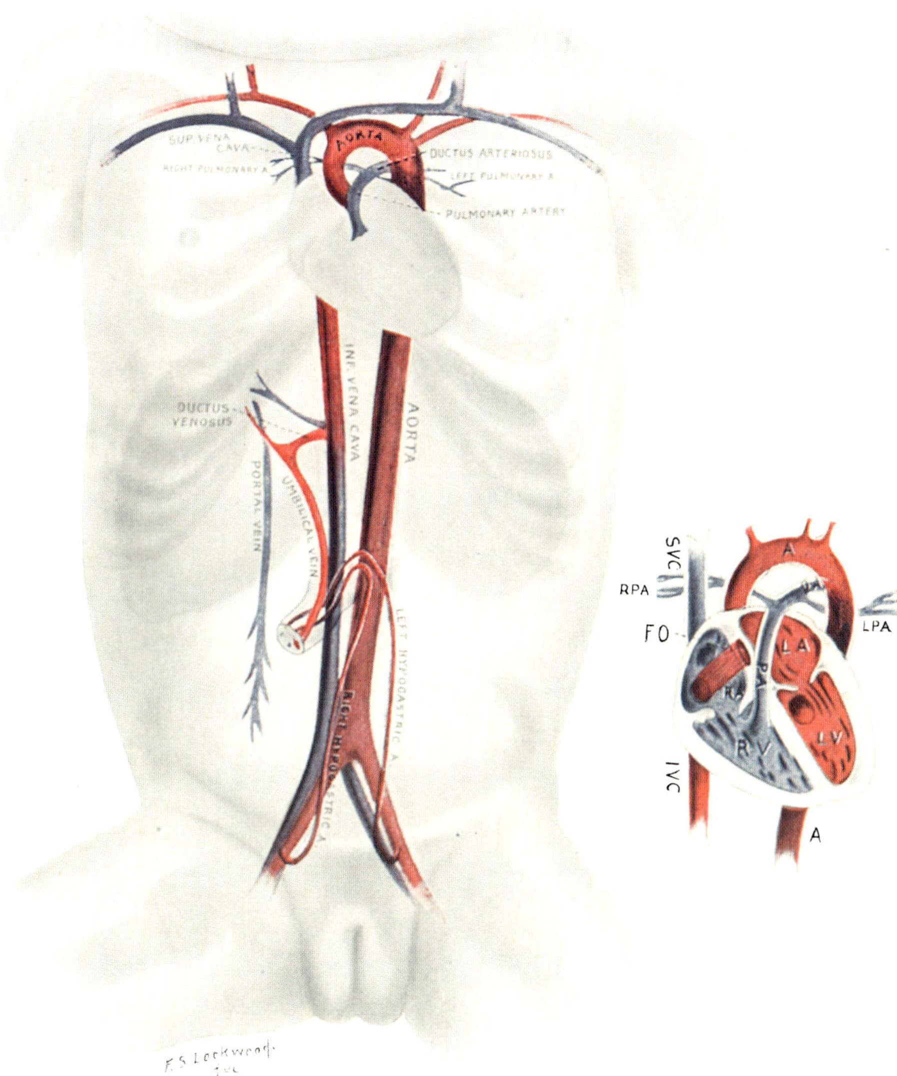

FŒTAL CIRCULATION.

undergo atrophy and obliteration, which is usually complete three or four days after birth. The ductus venosus and umbilical vein also become occluded during the first week, whereas the closure of the ductus arteriosus is more gradual, and frequently its opening does not become impervious until several weeks after birth. Permanent closure of the foramen ovale does not occur for some time, and not rarely months elapse before it is completed. Occasionally it remains more or less patent, and circulatory disturbances of greater or less gravity result from its persistence.

Transmission of Substances through the Placenta.—As was shown when considering the structure of the placenta, there is no direct communication between the vessels of the chorionic villi and the intervillous blood spaces. In the first half of pregnancy fœtal and maternal blood are separated from one another by the syncytium, Langhans's layer of cells, a thicker or thinner leaflet of the stroma of the villus, and the walls of the fœtal capillaries, while in the second half Langhans's layer gradually disappears.

The independence of the two circulations is readily demonstrated on examining the contents of the fœtal vessels and the intervillous spaces. In the former large numbers of nucleated red corpuscles are found, which are never present in the latter. In order that substances may pass from the mother to the fœtus, or in the reverse direction, it is necessary for them to traverse the layers of tissue which we have just mentioned. It would appear that gases and substances in solution pass by osmosis directly from the maternal blood to the vessels of the chorionic villi, and *vice versa*, but that formed substances must undergo certain changes in the chorionic epithelium before they can be transmitted.

The transmission of gaseous substances has been definitely demonstrated both by clinical observation and experimental work. Comparison of the blood in the umbilical vein and arteries, respectively, shows that the former is lighter in colour, indicating that it is richer in oxygen than the latter. This fact has also been demonstrated experimentally by Zweifel, who showed that the blood in the umbilical vein, when examined by means of the spectroscope, contained oxyhæmoglobin. Again, Cohnstein and Zuntz have demonstrated that the blood of the umbilical vein in the sheep is richer in oxygen and poorer in carbon dioxide than that contained in the umbilical arteries. Zweifel has also shown that chloroform administered to the mother is rapidly transmitted to the fœtus.

The increase in the size of the fœtus affords conclusive evidence that materials in solution must pass from the maternal to the fœtal circulation, and this has been demonstrated experimentally for a number of substances. The first work of this character we owe to Mayer, who in 1817 proved the passage of cyanide of potassium. Since then conclusive evidence of such transmission has been adduced for iodide and ferrocyanide of potassium, salicylic acid, corrosive sublimate, methylene blue, and many other substances.

Krönig and Füth in 1901 investigated the molecular concentration of the fœtal and maternal blood by determining their freezing points. They found that both fluids froze at the same temperature, a fact which indicates that they possess the same osmotic pressure, and that osmosis can occur equally readily in either direction.

The evidence concerning the passage of formed substances through the placenta is conflicting, but the general belief is that such does not occur, unless the material has first undergone marked changes under the influence of the chorionic epithelium, or the placenta presents lesions. The occurrence of intra-uterine small-pox was urged by John Hunter and many subsequent observers as proof in support of the affirmative view. Formerly it was not infrequent for mothers who suffered from small-pox during pregnancy to give birth to children bearing marks of the disease, and one of the most celebrated cases of this character was that of Mauriceau, the well-known obstetrician of the seventeenth century, who was born pock-marked. The significance of this occurrence, however, is by no means clear, inasmuch as we are not as yet acquainted with the *materies morbi* concerned.

It has been already pointed out that the nucleated red corpuscles of the fœtus do not gain access to the intervillous spaces, and Sänger has shown that maternal blood-cells do not enter the chorionic vessels, by demonstrating in a case of pernicious leucæmia that the leucocytes of the mother did not pass to the fœtus; and the same fact holds good in malaria, as there is no evidence that in the case of a pregnant woman suffering from this disease the specific parasites can pass from the maternal to the fœtal blood. A large amount of experimental work has been done with such substances as powdered cinnabar, India-ink, and sulphindigodate of sodium, the earlier investigators having reported positive, and the more recent investigators negative, results. It appears probable that the former were due to injuries sustained by the placenta during the manipulation.

The passage of bacteria from the mother to the fœtus has of late years been a fruitful field for experimentation, and it is now generally admitted that the transmission occurs only in exceptional instances. Lubarsch, in a recent article, has shown that the organisms of anthrax, pneumonia, typhoid fever, relapsing fever, and the various infections due to pyogenic organisms, may be transmitted now and again, but regards such an occurrence as exceptional.

This is particularly well shown in tuberculosis, and so far as the literature shows, out of the large number of tuberculous women who are delivered every year, only 18 have given birth to children or placentæ which gave evidence of the disease. Birch-Hirschfeld, Schmorl, and Lehmann have described tuberculosis of the fœtal portion of the placenta, and Sarwey recognised a case of congenital tuberculosis in a deformed fœtus. But in none of the placentæ from tuberculous women which I have examined have I been able to find the slightest trace of tuberculosis in the fœtal portion, even when the decidua was affected by the disease.

The same applies to typhoid fever, though it would appear that in this disease the transmission of organisms occurs more frequently than in tuberculosis. Speier, in 1897, found the specific bacilli in the organs of a fœtus whose mother was suffering with typhoid fever, and collected 11 similar cases from the literature. We have lately observed an instance of the same character at the Johns Hopkins Hospital, which has been reported by F. W. Lynch.

From the evidence before us it would appear that so long as the placenta is normal and the epithelium covering its villi intact, the transmission of disease germs does not occur, but that when lesions of the placenta are present it is quite possible. It remains to be decided, however, whether the lesions that were demonstrated had existed prior to the disease, or had resulted from toxines produced by the bacteria circulating in the intervillous spaces.

The transmission of materials from the fœtus to the mother has also been experimentally demonstrated for animals. Thus Savory and Gusserow showed, by injecting strychnine into embryos still within the uterus, that the mother died within a short time from strychnine poisoning. Similar results were also obtained by Preyer with hydrocyanic acid.

The Nature and Functions of the Amniotic Fluid.—In addition to the materials received from the placenta, it is generally believed that the fœtus obtains a great part of the fluid necessary for its development from that contained in the amniotic sac. Spiegelberg, Ahlfeld, Zweifel and others have demonstrated that considerable quantities of it are swallowed, inasmuch as they found lanugo hairs, epidermic cells, etc., in the stomach and intestines of the fœtus. Ahlfeld believes that the amniotic fluid is swallowed in such large quantities that even the small amount of albumin which it contains is of some benefit in the nutrition of the fœtus; but this point is very doubtful.

According to Hoppe-Seyler, the amniotic fluid is clear, alkaline in reaction, having a specific gravity of 1.006 to 1.008, and consisting of 98.48 per cent water, 0.19 per cent albuminoid material, 0.556 per cent soluble inorganic salts, 0.8 per cent extractives, and 0.024 per cent insoluble organic salts.

It is generally admitted that it represents in great part a transudation from the maternal vessels, but many authorities consider that a portion of it is derived from the urinary secretion of the fœtus. The solution of the question in the case of human beings presents very serious difficulties; though Döderlein has conclusively shown that in the calf the fœtal kidneys function during the latter part of pregnancy, as in this animal the urinary excretions are passed into the allantoic vesicle and do not mingle with the contents of the amnion. But in the human fœtus, which does not possess a vesicular allantois, it is evident that, if the kidneys secrete, the urine must be passed into the amniotic cavity, and this problem has not yet been definitely solved. The question has been answered in the affirmative by Schroeder, Nagel, and others, their conclusions being based in great part upon the formation of retention cysts in embryos which presented some abnormality in the lower portion of the urinary tract. Chemical analysis of the amniotic fluid, however, shows that it contains very small quantities of urea, and indicates that the fœtal urine, if secreted at all, differs markedly from that of extra-uterine life.

The experiments of Schaller, in 1899, have rendered it extremely doubtful whether the fœtal kidneys function at all. This observer availed himself of the well-known fact that the administration of phloridzin gives rise to a transient diabetes, which results from the action of the drug upon the renal epithelium, and not from changes produced in the blood. He showed that after the drug had been injected into the mother its presence could readily be demonstrated in the tissues of the fœtus, while the amniotic fluid rarely contained traces of sugar, which should have been present in large quantity had the fœtal kidneys functioned.

In addition to supplying water to the tissues, the amniotic fluid plays an important part by surrounding the fœtus with a medium of constant temperature, which serves to prevent loss of heat while at the same time affording a protection against sudden shocks from without. It also subserves an important function by preventing the formation of adhesions between the fœtus and the walls of the amniotic sac, which, when they occur, often give rise to serious deformities to be considered later.

Respiratory and Digestive Functions.—It would appear that the fœtus *in utero* requires a relatively small quantity of oxygen to support life, so there is but little tissue waste. Again, the fact that it is surrounded by amniotic fluid makes it necessary for the fœtus to produce but little warmth, as only a small amount of energy is expended during its restricted movements. Its need of oxygen, however, is demonstrated by the rapid occurrence of death, with symptoms of asphyxia, whenever the circulation of the umbilical cord is interfered with even for a short time.

It has been demonstrated that the fœtus actually produces warmth, as Wurster showed that its temperature exceeded that of the interior of the uterus by 0.5° C. or 0.9° F. Vicarelli has lately arrived at a similar conclusion, although he puts the excess at only 0.2° C. or 0.36° F.

Very little is known concerning the functions of the intestinal tract of the fœtus, though it has been demonstrated that the stomach contains pepsin and rennin after the fifth month, their presence indicating a certain amount of glandular activity. The large amount of blood which circulates through the liver would go to show that this organ serves some important purpose, and the formation of bile is conclusively demonstrated by the presence of biliary materials in the meconium.

While the fœtus remains in the uterus its movements are restricted within narrow limits, though such undoubtedly occur, being felt by the mother as " life " from the middle of pregnancy, and at a little later period by the physician when he places his hand upon the abdomen. Ahlfeld demonstrated, by the use of the sphygmograph, that the fœtus makes very rapid superficial movements—at the rate of sixty to the minute—which he considered represented an abortive type of respiration; but his conclusions have not been accepted by other observers.

Sex of the New-born Child.—Statistics show that more boys are born than girls, the proportion, according to the figures given by Rauber, being 106 to 100. Ahlfeld has pointed out that this ratio is still further increased in elderly primiparæ; for when the first child is born between the thirtieth and fortieth years, the proportion is 120–130 to 100, which increases to 130–140 to 100 between the fortieth and fiftieth years.

Various theories have been advanced from time to time in explanation of this fact, but none of them are altogether satisfactory. Those who are interested in the subject are referred to the monograph of Rauber for detailed information.

At present we are almost absolutely ignorant concerning the causation of sex, though certain observers are inclined to suppose that the determining factor must be sought for in the ovum. Probability is lent to this view by the fact that twins derived from the same ovum are always of the same sex; but when each is derived from a separate ovum, the sex may or may not be the same. We do not know, however, whether the determination of sex resides in the ovum before fertilization, or takes place soon after it, though it must occur at a very early period, since the researches of Clark and others have shown that embryos do not present an indifferent stage of sexual development, as was formerly believed; for examination of the internal generative organs enables one to differentiate the sex at a much earlier period than was formerly believed possible.

Several years ago Schenk startled the world by stating that sex could be determined at will, as it was entirely dependent upon the condition of nutrition of the mother, and could therefore be influenced by appropriate dietetic treatment. Further investigation, however, has shown that his conclusions were visionary.

LITERATURE

Ahlfeld. Bestimmungen der Grösse und des Alters der Frucht vor der Geburt. Archiv f. Gyn., ii, 353–372, 1871.

Die Geburten älterer Erstgeschwängerten. Archiv f. Gyn., iv, 510–520, 1872.

Ueber die Bedeutung des Fruchtwassers als Nahrungsmittel für die Frucht. Berichte u. Arbeiten, ii, 22, Leipzig, 1885.

Atem-bewegungen des Fötus. Lehrbuch der Geb., II. Aufl., 57, 1898.

Bachimont. De la puériculture intrautérine au cours de la grossesse gémellaire. Thèse de Paris, 1898.

Birch-Hirschfeld. Quoted by Lubarsch. See below.

Blécard. Quoted by Schroeder, Lehrbuch des Geburtshülfe, XIII. Aufl., 67, 1899.

Cohnstein und Zuntz. Untersuchungen über das Blut, den Kreislauf und die Athmung beim Säugethier-Fötus. Pflüger's Archiv, xxxiv, 173, 1884.

Döderlein. Vergleichende Untersuchungen über das Fruchtwasser, etc. Archiv f. Gyn., xxxvii, 141–174, 1890.

Dubois. Les gros enfants. Thèse de Paris, 1897.

Fehling. Beiträge zur Physiologie des placentären Stoffverkehrs. Archiv f. Gyn., xi, 523–557, 1877.

Fuchs. Die Abhängigkeit des Geburtsgewichtes des Neugeborenen vom Stand und Beschäftigung der Mutter. D. I., Halle, 1899.

Haase. Charité-Annalen, ii, 686.

Hartmann. Beiträge zur Osteologie der Neugeborenen. D. I., Tübingen, 1869.

Hecker. Klinik der Geburtskunde, 49, Leipzig, 1861.

His. Anatomie menschlichen Embryonen. Leipzig, 1880–1885.

Hoppe-Seyler. Physiologische Chemie, I. Theil, 609, 1877.

Krönig and Füth. Vergleichende Untersuchungen über den osmotischen Druck im mütterlichen und kindlichen Blute. Monatsschr. f. Geb. u. Gyn., xiii, 39–54, 1901.

Lea. The Sagittal Fontanelle in the Heads of Infants at Birth. Trans. London Obst. Soc., xl, 263–270, 1898.

LEHMANN. Ueber einen Fall von Tuberculose der Placenta. Deutsche med. Wochenschr., No. 9, 1893. Also Berliner klin. Wochenschr., 1894, 601.

LUBARSCH. Uebertragung von Infektionskrankheiten von Ascendenten auf Descendenten. Lubarsch-Ostertag, Ergebnisse der Allg. Path. u. Path. Anat., i, 427-455, 1896.

LUDWIG. Sectio caesarea bei übermässig entwickelter todtfauler Frucht. Centralbl. f. Gyn., 1896, 64, 65.

LYNCH. Placental Transmission, with Report of a Case during Typhoid Fever. Johns Hopkins Hospital Reports, 1902, x, 203–322.

MAYER. Quoted by Preyer. See below.

MICHEL. Sur la composition organique et minérale du fœtus et du nouveau-né. L'Obstétrique, v, 252–261, 1900.

NAGEL. Beitrag zur Lehre von der Herkunft des Fruchtwassers. Archiv f. Gyn., xxxv, 131–148, 1889.

PIERING. Ueber die Grenzen des Körpergewichtes Neugeborener. Monatsschr. f. Geb. u. Gyn., x, 303–311, 1899.

PINARD. Note pour servir à l'histoire de la puériculture pendant la grossesse. Annales de Gyn. et d'Obst., l, 81–89, 1898.

PREYER. Specielle Physiologie des Embryo. Leipzig, 1885.

RAUBER. Der Ueberschuss an Knabengeburten u. Seine biologische Bedeutung. Leipzig, 1900.

SÄNGER. Ueber Leukämie bei Schwangeren. Archiv f. Gyn., xxxiii, 161–210, 1888.

SARWEY. Ein Fall von spätgeborener Missgeburt mit congenitaler Tuberculose. Archiv f. Gyn., xliii, 162–180, 1893.

SAVORY. Quoted by Preyer.

SCHALLER. Ueber Phloridzin-diabetes Schwangerer, etc. Archiv f. Gyn., lvii, 548–565, 1899.

SCHENK. Einfluss auf das Geschlechtsverhältniss, II. Aufl., Magdeburg, 1898.

SCHMORL und KOCKEL. Die Tuberculose der menschlichen Placenta, etc. Ziegler's Beiträge, xvi, 313.

SCHROEDER. Lehrbuch der Geburtshülfe, XIII. Aufl., 67, 1899.

Physiologie des Fötus. Lehrbuch der Geb., XIII. Aufl., 75, 1899.

SPEIER. Zur Casuistik des placentären Ueberganges der Typhusbacillen von der Mutter auf die Frucht. D. I., Breslau, 1897.

SPIEGELBERG. Fruchtwasser. Monatsschr. f. Geburtskunde, xviii, 374–400, 1861.

VARNIER. Les gros œufs. L'Obstétrique journalière, 185–191, 1900.

VICARELLI. La température du fœtus dans l'utérus. Ref. l'Obstétrique, v, 533, 534, 1900.

WINCKEL. Neue Untersuchungen über die Dauer des menschlichen Schwangerschaft. Volkmann's Sammlung klin. Vorträge, N. F., Nr. 292, 293, 1901.

WURSTER. Beiträge zur Tocothermometrie. D. I., Zurich, 1870.

ZWEIFEL. Untersuchungen über das Meconium. Archiv f. Gyn., vii, 474–490, 1875.

Die Respiration des Fötus. Archiv f. Gyn., ix, 291–305, 1876.

Der Uebergang von Chloroform und Salicylsäure in die Placenta. Archiv f. Gyn., xii, 235–257, 1877.

PHYSIOLOGY OF PREGNANCY

CHAPTER VI

CHANGES IN THE MATERNAL ORGANISM RESULTING FROM PREGNANCY

Uterus.—The maternal organism reacts to a greater or lesser extent under the influence of pregnancy, but naturally the most characteristic changes are observed in the generative tract, and especially in the uterus, which undergoes a very marked increase in size. Thus, it is converted from a small, almost solid organ, 6.5 centimetres long, into a thin-walled, muscular sac, capable of containing the fœtus, placenta, and a large quantity of amniotic fluid, and at the end of pregnancy is about 36 centimetres long, 25 centimetres wide, and 24 centimetres deep. Krause estimated that its capacity is increased 519 times. A corresponding increase in weight is also observed, the uterus at full term weighing in the neighbourhood of 1,000 grammes (2 pounds), as compared with 30 grammes (1 ounce) in the virginal condition.

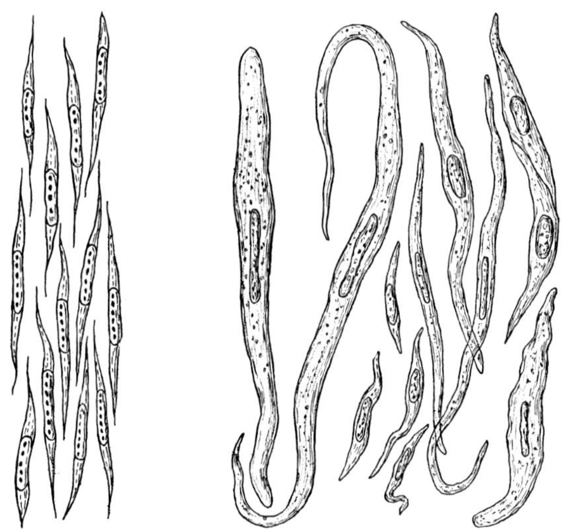

Fig. 156.—Muscle Fibres from Non-pregnant and Pregnant Uterus (Sappey).

This enlargement is due principally to the hypertrophy of pre-existing muscle cells, but partly also to the formation of new ones during the earlier months of pregnancy. The fully developed muscle fibres are from 2 to 7 times wider and from 7 to 11 times longer than those observed in the non-pregnant uterus, measuring 0.009 to 0.014 × 0.2 to 0.52 millimetre in the former, as compared with 0.005 × 0.05 to 0.07 millimetre in the latter. According to the researches of Luschka and Veit, the formation of new muscular fibres is limited to the first three or four months of pregnancy.

With the increase in the number and size of the muscle fibres is associated a marked development affecting the blood-vessels, especially the veins, which, in the neighbourhood of the placental site, become converted into large spaces, the so-called placental sinuses. Marked hypertrophy of the lymphatic and nervous supply of the uterus also takes place, of the extent of which some idea may be gained from the statement of Frankenhäuser that the cervical ganglion increases in size from 2×2.5 to 6×4.5 centimetres.

During the first few months, the hypertrophy of the uterus results from general systematic changes induced by the pregnancy itself. That it is not directly due to the presence of the ovum in the cavity itself is shown by the occurrence of precisely similar changes in cases of extra-uterine pregnancy, when the ovum is implanted in the tube or ovary. After the third month, however, the increase in size is mechanical to some extent, and is due directly to the pressure exerted by the growing ovum.

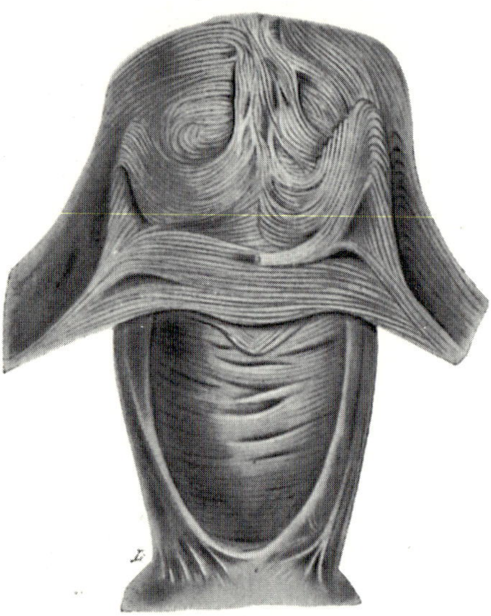

Fig. 157.—External Muscular Layer of Pregnant Uterus (Hélie).

During the first few months of pregnancy the uterine walls are considerably thicker than in the non-pregnant condition, but as gestation advances they gradually become thinner, so that at the end of the fifth month they are from 3 to 5 millimetres in thickness. This measurement is retained throughout the succeeding months, so that at term the uterus is represented by a muscular sac whose walls are rarely above 5, and never more than 10 millimetres thick. Occasionally they are found to measure considerably under 5 millimetres. The enlargement of the uterus is not symmetrical, but is most marked in the fundal region. This can readily be appreciated by observing the relative positions of the insertions of the tubes and ovarian ligaments, which in the early months of pregnancy are almost on a level with the fundus; whereas in the later months their attachments are found at points slightly above the middle of the organ.

The position of the placenta also exerts a determining influence upon the extent of the hypertrophy, the portion of the uterus to which it is attached enlarging more rapidly than the others, as is clearly shown by the position of the uterine ends of the round ligaments, which are close together when the placenta is inserted upon the posterior, and far apart when it is upon the anterior wall.

Arrangement of the Muscle Fibres.—Ever since the time of Vesalius, considerable attention has been devoted to the arrangement of the muscle fibres in the pregnant uterus. Among the numerous investigators whose careful studies on this subject deserve special mention are William Hunter in England; Madame Boivin, Deville, and Hélie in France; Roederer, Luschka, Henle, Hoffmann, Bayer, Hofmeier, and others in Germany. Unfortunately their investigations have not led to uniform results.

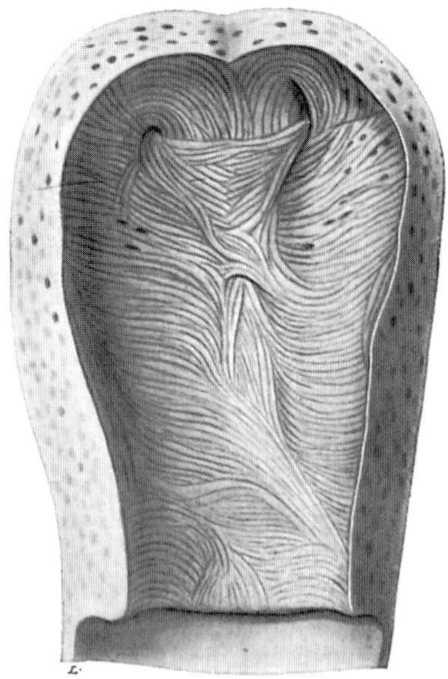

FIG. 158.—INTERNAL MUSCULAR LAYER OF PREGNANT UTERUS (Hélie).

According to Luschka and Henle, the musculature of the pregnant uterus is arranged in three strata: an external hood-like layer, which arches over the fundus and extends into the various ligaments; an internal layer, consisting of sphincter-like fibres around the orifices of the tubes and the internal os; while lying between the two is a dense network of muscle fibres perforated in all directions by blood-vessels.

The most important contributions, however, we owe to Hélie, Bayer, and Ruge. In the preface to his monograph, Hélie tells us that he had devoted twelve years to his investigations, and Bayer has been an indefatigable worker upon the subject since 1886.

According to Hélie, the uterine musculature consists of 3 main layers, each of which is made up of several subsidiary divisions. The external layer is composed of 2 longitudinal or ansiform portions, between which lies a transverse layer. The internal layer is composed of 2 triangular portions running along the inner surface of the anterior and posterior walls of the uterus respectively, and connected by an archiform layer at the fundus, an obicular portion around each tubal opening, and an annular layer around the internal os. The main portion of the uterine wall is formed by the middle layer, which consists of an interlacing network of muscle fibres, between which extend the blood-vessels.

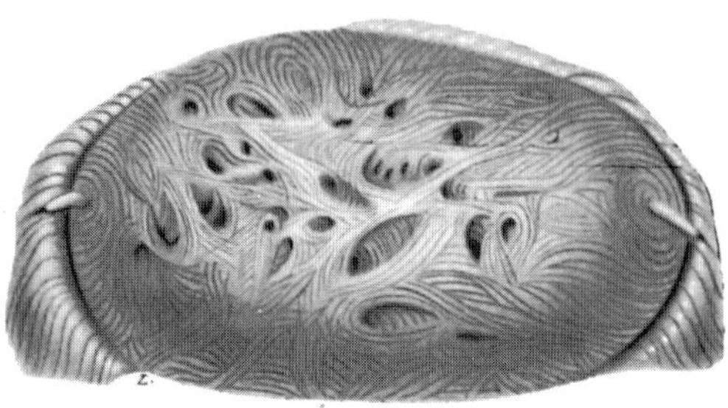

FIG. 159.—MEDIAN MUSCULAR LAYER OF PREGNANT UTERUS (Hélie).

Each fibre comprising this layer has a double curve, so that the interlacement of any two gives approximately the form of the figure "8." As a result of such an arrangement it happens that when the fibres contract they constrict the vessels and thus act as living ligatures. Bayer's work is extremely complicated, and those who desire particulars concerning it are referred to his monographs upon the subject.

Ruge pointed out that many of the layers which had been described by previous observers do not exist as such in the pregnant uterus, the appearances having resulted from the manner in which the dissections had been made. He showed that the muscle fibres composing the uterine wall, specially in its lower portion, overlap one another and are arranged more or less like shingles on a roof, one end of each fibre arising beneath the peritoneal covering of the uterus, and extending obliquely downward and inward, to be inserted into the decidua, thus giving rise to a large number of muscular lamellæ. The various lamellæ are connected with one another by short muscular processes, so that when the tissue is slightly spread apart it presents a sieve-like appearance, which on closer examination is seen to be due to the presence of innumerable rhomboidal spaces. Ruge attaches great importance to this arrangement of the muscle fibres, and believes that it explains very satisfactorily the mechanism of the uterine contractions and the manner in which the felt-like structure of the puerperal uterus is brought about.

Changes in Size and Shape of the Uterus.—As the uterus increases in size, it also undergoes important modifications in shape. For the first few weeks its original pyriform outlines are retained, but the body and fundus soon assume a more globular form, which at the third or fourth month becomes almost spherical. After this period, however, the organ increases more rapidly in length than in width, and assumes an oval form, which persists until the end of pregnancy.

The increase in the size of the uterus is limited almost entirely to its body, the cervix remaining practically unchanged until the onset of labour, so that throughout the course of pregnancy it appears as a mere appendage to the enlarged body. Its most characteristic change consists in a marked softening, which is readily appreciated by the examining finger, and constitutes one of the physical signs of pregnancy. The slight increase in size which can be noted is due in great part to increased vascularity, and depends only to a small extent upon hypertrophy of its muscle fibres. As a result, the secretion of the cervical glands becomes more copious and the cervical canal becomes filled with a plug of mucus. The changes occurring in it in the latter part of pregnancy will be considered in detail when we take up the physiology of labour.

As the body of the uterus becomes larger, the angle which it forms with the cervix becomes smaller—in other words, its physiological anteflexion is increased. As pregnancy advances the organ soon becomes too large to be contained in the pelvic cavity, and by the fourth month forms a tumour, the upper border of which reaches to a point midway between the symphysis pubis and the umbilicus. As it becomes still larger, it comes in contact with the anterior abdominal wall, displacing the intestines to the sides of the abdomen, and gradually rises up until it almost impinges upon the diaphragm. As the uterus leaves the pelvis for the abdominal cavity, considerable tension is exerted upon the broad ligaments, which then become more or less unfolded at their uterine ends.

The pregnant uterus possesses a considerable degree of mobility. Since its upper portion projects into and lies free in the abdominal cavity, and its lower portion is held somewhat in check by the lax broad ligaments, it readily changes its position. With the woman in a standing posture its longitudinal axis corresponds closely with that of the superior strait, the organ resting in great part upon the anterior abdominal wall. In this position the portion projecting above the symphysis has somewhat more breadth than height. With the woman lying on her back, however, the uterus falls backward and rests upon the vertebral column, its length being now greater than its breadth. Figs. 160 and 161 represent the same woman in the upright and horizontal positions respectively, and give a good idea of the changes in contour of the uterus and abdomen.

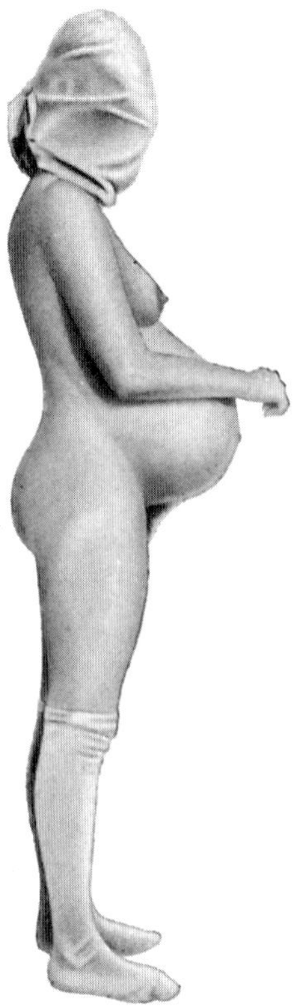

Fig. 160.

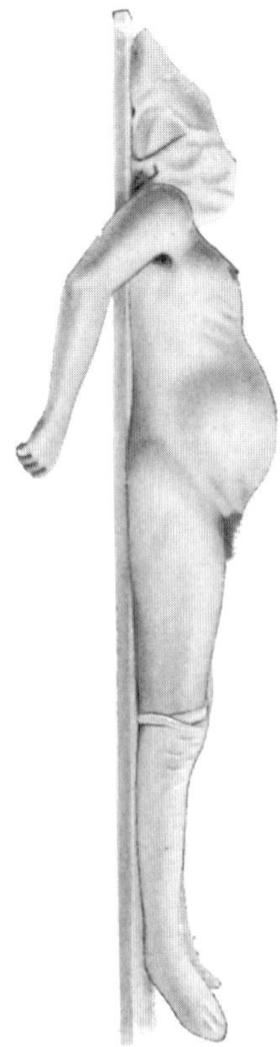

Fig. 161.

FIGS. 160, 161.—SAME FULL-TERM I-PARA IN VERTICAL AND HORIZONTAL POSITION.

As the uterus grows out of the pelvic cavity, it usually becomes slightly twisted to the right, so that its left margin is directed more anteriorly than the right. Occasionally the torsion may be in the opposite direction, statistics showing that it occurs to the right in 80 per cent and to the left in 20 per cent of the cases. The torsion is due in great part to the presence of the rectum, which usually occupies the left side, and only occasionally the right side, of the pelvis; though possibly, in a certain number of instances, the condition represents merely an exaggeration of the original position of the non-pregnant uterus, which, as is well known, is not always perfectly symmetrical. From my own observations, I am inclined to agree with Webster, that the frequency with which torsion of the uterus occurs has been somewhat exaggerated.

With the advance of pregnancy the uterus loses the firm, almost cartilaginous consistence which is characteristic of the non-pregnant condition, and becomes converted into a sac having very thin, soft walls, which are readily compressible. This is well demonstrated by the ease with which the fœtus can be palpated in some cases, and by the fact that not infrequently it is possible at operation to observe shallow depressions upon the surface of the uterus, which have resulted from the pressure of the intestines upon it. Again, it is noteworthy with what readiness the uterine walls yield to the movements of the fœtal extremities.

Tubes and Ovaries.—As has already been mentioned, the tubes and ovaries undergo marked changes in position with the advance of pregnancy, so that instead of extending outward almost at right angles with the cornua, their long axes become nearly parallel to the margins of the uterus. Of special importance, moreover, is their increase in vascularity, to which the large size of the corpus luteum of pregnancy is in great part due. Except in rare instances, ovulation ceases during pregnancy, so that new follicles do not ripen, and, accordingly, only the single large corpus luteum of pregnancy can be found upon the surface of one of the ovaries.

Most authors believe that the muscular fibres of the tubes undergo considerable hypertrophy under the influence of pregnancy, but this has recently been denied by Mandl, and it must be admitted that, if it occurs at all, it is very slight in extent. It is possible for a decidua to develop in the tubes while the pregnancy is situated in the uterus. Such observations have been made by Webster, Mandl, and Veit, but are of extreme rarity. In the microscopic study of the tubes from 10 or 12 cases of uterine pregnancy I have not met with such an occurrence.

Vagina.—Increased vascularity is the most marked change in the vagina, and to it is due the more copious secretion and the characteristic violet coloration of pregnancy. At the same time there is considerable hypertrophy of the elements composing the vaginal walls, the latter not infrequently increasing in length to such an extent that the lower portion of the anterior wall prolapses slightly through the vulval opening.

The papillæ of the vaginal mucosa also undergo considerable hypertrophy, whence results an increased roughness of the membrane, which in occasional instances feels almost like a calf's tongue. Owing to the increased vascularity, the vaginal secretion is considerably augmented, and in the majority of cases is represented by a thick, white, crumbly substance, somewhat like cottage cheese. Döderlein, who was the first to direct attention to its characteristic appearance, showed that the material consisted of epithelial cells and a large number of long, tolerably thin bacilli. The same authority states that under normal conditions it does not contain leucocytes or pathogenic micro-organisms.

The increased vascularity attending pregnancy is not confined to the genitalia, but extends to the various organs in their vicinity, and as a consequence there is a slight relaxation of the various pelvic joints, which is accompanied by an increase in their motility, as was conclusively shown by Budin.

Abdominal Walls.—With the enlargement of the uterus the skin covering the anterior abdominal walls and the adjoining portions of the thighs is subjected to considerable tension, which, according to Marie Schlee.

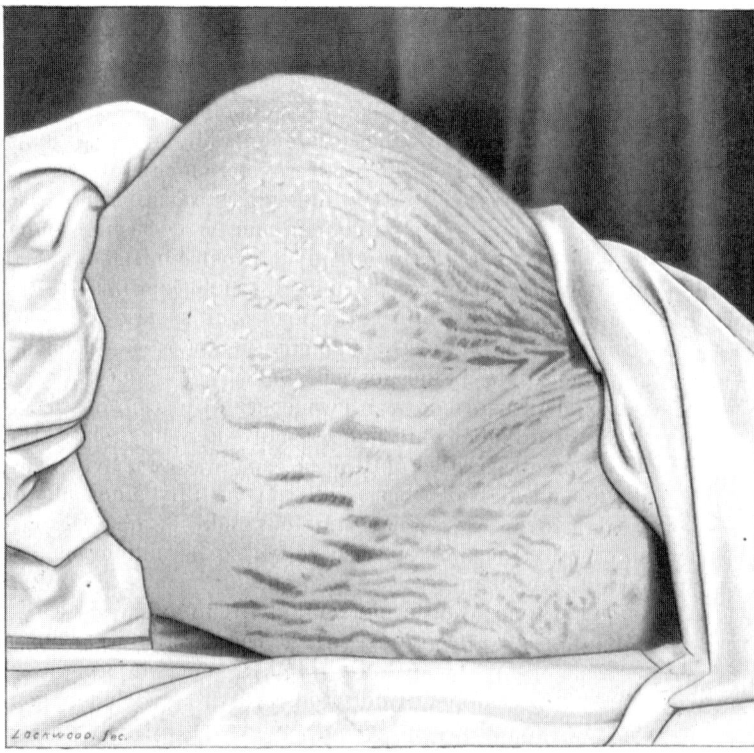

Fig. 162.—Abdomen of Primipara at Term, showing Striæ.

results in the stretching and distortion of the connective-tissue spaces of the cutis, and the formation of depressed areas which are known as the *striæ of pregnancy.* In primiparæ these present a pinkish or slightly bluish appearance, as is well illustrated in Fig. 162, whereas in multiparæ two varieties are observed, some resembling those of primiparous women, while others present a glistening silvery appearance, the former resulting from the present condition, and the latter representing cicatrices from previous pregnancies.

The formation of striæ is not characteristic of pregnancy, as it is lacking, according to Credé, in about 10 per cent of the cases and is not infrequently observed in non-pregnant women and occasionally in men, in whom there has been a rapid increase in the size of the abdomen, either from the presence of a tumour or ascites, or the rapid development of fat.

Not infrequently the abdominal walls are unable to withstand the tension to which they are subjected, and the recti muscles become separated in the middle line, giving rise to a *diastasis* of greater or less extent. Where the process is exaggerated, a considerable portion of the anterior wall of the uterus is covered by nothing beyond a thin layer of tissue consisting only of skin, fascia, and peritonæum. In rare instances the separation is sufficiently extensive to admit of a hernial protrusion of the gravid uterus.

The enlarged pregnant uterus occasionally presses upon the venous trunks, which return the blood from the lower extremities, the obstruction being sometimes sufficient to cause varicose veins or *œdema*. The latter is most commonly observed about the ankles and feet, but occasionally occurs to a marked degree in the neighbourhood of the vulva, when the labia majora may become immensely distended. Budin some years ago made an exhaustive study as to the frequency and mode of production of varicose veins in pregnancy, and to his monograph the reader is referred for further information.

Breasts.—Under the influence of pregnancy marked changes occur in the breasts, and in the early weeks the woman not infrequently complains of a sense of tenseness and pricking in these regions. After the second month the breasts begin to increase in size and offer a somewhat nodular sensation on palpation, which is due to the hypertrophy of the mammary alveoli, and as they become still larger a delicate tracery of bluish veins appears just beneath the skin. The most characteristic changes, however, are afforded by the nipples and the tissue in their vicinity. The nipples themselves soon become considerably larger, more deeply pigmented, and more erectile, and after the first few months a thin, yellowish fluid—*colostrum*—may be expressed from them by gentle massage. At the same time the areola surrounding the nipple becomes considerably broader and much more deeply pigmented, the degree of pigmentation varying according to the complexion of the individual. In blondes the areolæ and nipples assume a pinkish appearance, while in brunettes they become dark brown and occasionally almost black. Scattered through the areola are a number of small roundish elevations, the so-called *glands of Montgomery*, which result from the hypertrophy of the sebaceous glands. In a small number of cases similar structures make their appearance around the periphery of the areola, and are then designated as the *secondary areola*. If the increase in the size of the breasts be very marked, the skin not infrequently presents striations similar to those observed on the abdomen.

Changes in the Rest of the Body.—The changes resulting from pregnancy are not limited to the generative tract, but extend to other portions of the body as well, and in many cases the general condition of the patient differs markedly from what it was before conception. Many women suffer numerous inconveniences during this period, while others enjoy better health than at any other time.

Heart.—Owing to the upward pressure upon the diaphragm, the heart becomes displaced in such a way that its area of dulness undergoes a considerable increase in size. Basing his opinion upon this fact, Larcher in 1827 promulgated the doctrine that considerable cardiac hypertrophy was a constant concomitant of pregnancy. His views obtained rapid acceptance in France, but were received with scepticism in Germany. Gerhardt, Löhlein, Fellner, and others stated that actual weighing of the pregnant heart showed that hypertrophy did not occur.

It is apparent that the heart must perform a greater amount of work during this period than at other times, so that *a priori* the occurrence of hypertrophy would not be surprising. Moreover, the recent researches of Dreysel would appear to indicate that it does take place, as he found that the hearts of 76 pregnant and puerperal women weighed 8.8 per cent more than those of non-pregnant individuals. The question, however, cannot be regarded as definitely settled, and offers an attractive field for future work.

Blood.—In former times it was generally believed that the changes incident to the placental circulation demanded an increase in the amount of maternal blood, and all the earlier writers and most of the text-books stated that under the influence of pregnancy an increased hydræmia and a diminution in hæmoglobin and red corpuscles took place, while at the same time an abnormal amount of fibrin could be noted. These observations were based upon antiquated methods of research, and it was not until 1886 that Fehling, by the aid of modern appliances for examining the blood, came to the conclusion that it underwent little if any change.

Since then a number of articles have appeared upon the subject, the most important being those of Richard Schroeder in 1891, and Wild in 1897. Both of these writers proved that in the later months of pregnancy there was a slight increase in the amount of hæmoglobin and red corpuscles, instead of a decrease, as was formerly believed. The latter investigator also showed that there was a slight increase in the number of white corpuscles, which became markedly accentuated during the first few days of the puerperium. This leucocytosis he attributed to the changes associated with the healing of the wound at the placental site.

Blumreich, in 1899, apparently demonstrated a considerable increase in the alkalinity of the blood in pregnancy, both for human beings and also for rabbits, but advanced no theory as to its significance.

Kidneys.—During pregnancy the urine is considerably increased in quantity, though otherwise it should be perfectly normal and contain the usual amounts of urea and other excrementitious substances. From statements which have appeared at various times it would seem that considerable misapprehension exists concerning the daily amount of urea excreted by pregnant women. The examination of the urine passed in twenty-four hours by a considerable number of patients at the Johns Hopkins Hospital has led us to believe that from 20 to 24 grammes a day is the average quantity, instead of the larger amount generally given.

Albumin is not infrequently observed in the urine, and is often due to its admixture with vaginal secretion. Its occurrence in catheterized specimens, however, should always be regarded as pathological. The significance of albuminuria is of extreme importance, and will be considered in the chapter dealing with the diseases incident to the pregnant state.

Throughout pregnancy there is a marked tendency to disturbances in the renal function, and slight degrees of nephritis are so common that they are assigned by the Germans to "the kidney of pregnancy" (Schwangerschaftsniere). The condition is not normal, and is nearly always connected with disturbances of metabolism, which give rise to various forms of auto-intoxication.

Bladder.—As the uterus rises up into the abdominal cavity it carries with it the bladder, which in the later months of pregnancy becomes an abdominal instead of a pelvic organ, and when distended can be felt as a fluctuant tumour just above the symphysis pubis.

Lungs.—Owing to the upward displacement of the diaphragm in the last few months of pregnancy, it would seem as though the capacity of the lungs would be decreased. Nevertheless, the researches of Dohrn have shown that such is not the case, since the diminished height of the pleural cavities is compensated for by an increase in width, except in elderly primiparæ in whom the costal articulations have become ossified.

Normally, the patient gains in weight during the last three months of gestation. This is not entirely due to the increased size of the uterus and its contents, but to a considerable extent results from an additional deposit of fat in the other portions of the body. According to Gassner, the normal increase for the last three months is from 1,600 to 2,500 grammes a month (3 to 5 pounds).

Under the influence of pregnancy abnormalities of pigmentation are not infrequently noted. One of the most common, after those which appear in the breasts, is increased pigmentation along the linea alba. Again, in pregnant women irregularly shaped yellowish patches of varying size occasionally appear on the face and neck, the condition being known as *cloasma*.

In a small number of cases the thyroid increases markedly in size, though we are ignorant as to its significance.

We have already referred to the occurrence of œdema and varicose veins as a result of pressure exerted by the pregnant uterus upon the veins passing through the pelvis. Not infrequently disturbances of urination and defecation are due to the same factor, although, as a rule, the constipation is caused by the pregnant uterus interfering with the contraction of the muscles of the abdominal wall.

Functional disturbances of the nervous system are not infrequently observed during the course of pregnancy, the most frequent being the nausea and vomiting, to which we shall refer later. In a small number of cases varying degrees of salivation may also be observed, and some patients display a longing for abnormal articles of diet. Again, in women of neuropathic tendencies, the mental equilibrium may be overthrown to a greater or less degree, the patient becoming excitable or morbid and morose, and in rare instances developing a true psychosis.

LITERATURE

BAYER. Zur physiol. u. path. Morphologie der Gebärmutter. Freund's Gynäkologische Klinik, i, 369–662, 1885.

Weitere Beiträge zur Lehre vom unteren Uterinsegment. Hegar's Beiträge zur Geb. u. Gyn., i, 167, 1898.

BLUMREICH. Der Einfluss der Gravidität auf die Blutalkalescenz. Archiv f. Gyn., lix, 699, 1899.

BOIVIN et DUGÈS. Traité pratique des maladies de l'utérus, etc., 2me éd., Bruxelles, 1834.

BUDIN. Des varices chez la femme enceinte. Paris, 1880.

CREDÉ. Ueber die narbenähnlichen Streifen in der Haut, etc., bei Schwangeren u. Entbundenen. Monatsschr. f. Geburtskunde, xiv, 321–333, 1859.

DEVILLE. Bull. de la Soc. anatomique, 1844, quoted *in extenso* by Cazeaux, Traité de l'art des accouchements, 3me éd., 107–111, 1850.

DÖDERLEIN. Das Scheidensekret, etc. Leipzig, 1892.

DOHRN. Zur Kenntniss des Einflusses von Schwangerschaft etc. auf die vitale Capacität der Lungen. Monatsschr. f. Geburtskunde, xxviii, 457, 1866.

DREYSEL. Ueber Herzhypertrophie bei Schwangeren und Wöchnerinnen. D. I., München, 1891.

FEHLING. Ueber Blutbeschaffenheit und Fruchtwassermenge bei Schwangeren, etc. Archiv f. Gyn., xxviii, 453, 1886.

FELLNER. Herz und Schwangerschaft. Monatsschr. f. Geb. u. Gyn., xiv, 370–417, 1901.

FRANKENHÄUSER. Die Nerven der Gebärmutter. Jena, 1867.

GASSNER. Ueber die Veränderungen des Körpergewichtes bei Schwangeren. Monatsschr. f. Geburtskunde, xix, 1, 1862.

GERHARDT. De situ et magnitudine cordis gravidarum. Jena, 1862.

HÉLIE. Recherches sur la disposition des fibres musculaires de l'utérus developpés par la grossesse. Paris, 1864.

HENLE. Eingeweidelehre, II. Aufl., 476, 1873.

HOFFMANN. Morphologische Utersuchungen über die Muskulatur des Gebärmutterkörpers. Zeitschr. f. Geb. u. Frauenkrankheiten, 1876, i, 448–473.

HOFMEIER. Das untere Uterinsegment in anat. u. physiol. Beziehung. Der schwangere und kreissende Uterus, Bonn, 1886, 21–74.

HUNTER. The Anatomy of the Gravid Uterus, 1774.

JOESSEL und WALDEYER. Das Becken, 781. Bonn, 1899.

KRAUSE. Quoted by Spiegelberg-Wiener, Lehrbuch der Geburtshülfe, III. Aufl., 53, 1891.

LARCHER. Quoted from Ribemont-Dessaignes and Lepage, Précis d'obstétrique. Paris, 1894.

LÖHLEIN. Ueber das Verhalten des Herzens bei Schwangeren, etc. Zeitschr. f. Geb. u. Frauenkrankheiten, 1876, i, 482–516.

LUSCHKA. Die Anatomie des menschlichen Beckens, 365, Tübingen, 1864.

MANDL. Ueber den feineren Bau der Eileiter, etc. Monatsschr. f. Geb. u. Gyn., v (Ergänzungsheft, 130–140), 1897.

ROEDERER. Icones uteri humani, 7. Göttingen, 1759.

RUGE. Ueber die Contraction des Uterus in anat. u. klin. Beziehung. Zeitschr. f. Geb. u. Gyn., v, 149–157, 1880.

SCHLEE. Ueber die Dehnung der Bauchwand während der Schwangerschaft. Zeitschr. f. Geb. u. Gyn., xiii, 1–14, 1886.

SCHROEDER, R. Untersuchungen über die Beschaffenheit des Blutes von Schwangeren und Wöchnerinnen. Archiv f. Gyn., xxxix, 306–352, 1891.

VEIT. Anatomie des schwangeren Uterus. Müller's Handbuch der Geburtshülfe, i, 193, 1888.

Decidual Formation in Tube in a Case of Uterine Pregnancy. Schroeder's Lehrbuch der Geburtshülfe, XIII. Aufl., 101, 1899.

WEBSTER. Ectopic Pregnancy. Edinburgh, 1895.

A Criticism of Recent Views regarding the Lateral Deviation and Rotation of the Uterus. Edinburgh Med. Jour., September, 1897, 254–261.

WILD. Untersuchungen über den Hämoglobingehalt und die Anzahl der rothen und weissen Blutkörperchen bei Schwangeren und Wöchnerinnen. Archiv f. Gyn., liii, 363–381, 1897.

CHAPTER VII

DIAGNOSIS OF PREGNANCY—DURATION OF PREGNANCY—ESTIMATION OF DATE OF CONFINEMENT

Ordinarily, the diagnosis of pregnancy offers little or no difficulty, and the patient is usually aware of the true condition before she consults a physician. In a small minority of cases, however, the task is by no means easy, and despite every known method at our command we are occasionally unable to decide with absolute certainty.

Mistakes in diagnosis are most frequently made in the first few months, while the uterus is still a pelvic organ; although it is by no means impossible to confound a pregnancy, even at full term, with a tumour of some other nature. Such errors are usually the result of hasty or imperfect examination, but a false conclusion may sometimes be arrived at, even after the most conscientious exploration of the patient. Some idea of the frequency of such mistakes may be realized when it is stated that there is hardly a gynecologist of experience who has not opened the abdomen on one or more occasions, with the expectation of removing a tumour of the uterus or its appendages, and been surprised to find himself in the presence of a normal pregnancy.

It is often a matter of considerable importance that a diagnosis be made in the early months of pregnancy; but, unfortunately, it is just at this period that our diagnostic ability is most restricted, as the absolutely positive signs do not as a rule become available until the fifth month. Hence it follows that in cases in which the existence of such a condition might affect the reputation or interests of the patient, an expression of opinion should be deferred until the diagnosis is beyond all doubt.

Signs and Symptoms of Pregnancy.—The diagnosis is based upon the presence of certain symptoms and signs. The former are chiefly subjective and are appreciated by the patient; while the latter are made out by the physician after a careful physical examination, in which the senses of sight, hearing, and touch are employed.

The signs and symptoms are usually classified into three groups: positive, probable, and presumptive. The *positive signs* cannot usually be detected until after the fourth month, and are three in number: (1) hearing and counting the fœtal heart-beat; (2) perception of the active and passive movements of the fœtus; and (3) the ability to map out its outlines. The *probable signs* can be appreciated at a much earlier period, and are: (1) changes in the shape and consistency of the body of the uterus;

(2) changes in the cervix; (3) the detection of intermittent uterine contractions; and (4) increase in the size of the abdomen and uterus. The *presumptive evidences,* with a few exceptions, are subjective, and may be experienced at varying periods. They are: (1) cessation of the menses; (2) changes in the breasts; (3) morning sickness; (4) quickening; (5) Chadwick's sign; (6) disturbances in urination; (7) abnormalities in pigmentation; (8) abnormal cravings; and (9) mental disturbances.

Positive Signs of Pregnancy.—*The Fœtal Heart.*—Whenever we can hear and count the pulsations of the fœtal heart, we know that we have a characteristic and absolute sign of pregnancy; unfortunately, it is one that cannot usually be appreciated until the eighteenth or twentieth week, though occasionally the sounds can be heard at an earlier period, and on one occasion I was able to detect them as early as the fourteenth week.

The fœtal heart was first heard by Mayor, of Geneva, in 1818, in a few cases. The sign was also discovered independently by Lejumeau de Kegaradec in 1821, to whom we are indebted for most of our information upon the subject; indeed, so complete is his monograph that subsequent investigations have revealed but little with which he was not familiar. He made his discovery quite accidentally, while attempting to hear the sounds which the fœtus made by splashing in the liquor amnii. On auscultating the abdomen of a pregnant woman through her clothing, including the corset, he heard a double sound, which varied in frequency from 143 to 148 beats to the minute, and closely resembled the ticking of a watch under a pillow. He concluded that it could be produced only by the fœtal heart, as the pulse of the mother did not exceed 70. For further details concerning the history and earlier work upon the subject, the reader is referred to the works of Kegaradec, Kennedy, Depaul, and Montgomery.

As has already been said, the *fœtal heart-beat* cannot usually be heard until the eighteenth or twentieth week of pregnancy, but from then on it should be detected without difficulty. Ordinarily it varies in frequency from 120 to 140 beats to the minute, and is a double sound, closely resembling the tick of a watch under a pillow. In order to hear it the abdomen should be bared, or at most covered by a thin cloth. In the earlier months it is best detected by means of a stethoscope, but at a later period the direct application of the ear gives satisfactory results. It is advisable for the student to perfect himself in the latter method of auscultation, as he always has his ears with him, but occasionally may be without his stethoscope. One should not be content with merely hearing the fœtal heart, but should always attempt to count its rate and compare it with that of the maternal pulse.

In the early months of pregnancy the heart should be sought just over the symphysis pubis; but in the later months the situation at which it is best heard varies according to the position and presentation of the fœtus, details concerning which will be given when we consider the methods of obstetrical examination.

The rate of the fœtal heart is subject to considerable variations, which afford us a fairly reliable means of judging as to the well-being of the child. As a general rule, its life should be considered in danger when the heart-beats fall below 100 or exceed 160.

In women possessing very thin abdominal and uterine walls, the impulse of the fœtal heart may occasionally be appreciated by direct palpation, especially when the child is lying in the right mento-iliac position. Such observations have been reported by Fischel, Duval, and others.

Frankenhäuser stated that there was a marked difference in the rapidity of the heart-beat in the two sexes, and believed that a rate of 124 or less indicated a boy, and 144 or more a girl. Further investigation, however, has failed to confirm his conclusions, as the diagnosis of sex can be made by this means in only about 50 per cent of the cases. Indeed, there is no method by which the sex can be definitely determined before birth, except in a few cases of breech presentation, in which the genitalia can be differentiated by the examining finger.

Other Sounds which may be Heard on Auscultation.—In addition to hearing and counting the fœtal heart, auscultation of the abdomen of the woman in the later months of pregnancy often reveals other sounds, the most important of which are the funic souffle, the uterine or placental souffle, those due to movements of the fœtus, fœtal heart murmurs, the maternal pulse, and the gurgling of gas in the intestines of the mother.

The *funic souffle* is a sharp, whistling sound, synchronous with the fœtal pulse, which can be heard in about 15 per cent of all cases. It is very inconstant in its appearance, as it may be recognised distinctly at one examination and be absent on succeeding occasions. It was first described by Evory Kennedy, who supposed that it was due to some interference with the circulation of the blood through the umbilical arteries, and subsequent investigations have served to confirm his conclusions. Occasionally, in very thin women, the umbilical cord can be palpated between the body of the child and the uterine wall, and on making pressure upon it with the stethoscope a distant souffle can occasionally be elicited. This is not, however, a sign of very great importance, although, when heard, it is distinctly characteristic of pregnancy.

In rare instances, abnormalities of the fœtal heart have been diagnosed by auscultation during pregnancy. Such cases have been reported by Fochier, Cordell, and others, and have been confirmed at autopsy after birth.

The *uterine souffle* is a soft, blowing sound, synchronous with the maternal pulse, and is usually most distinctly heard upon auscultating the lower portion of the uterus. It is due to the passage of blood through the dilated uterine vessels. This sound was first described by Kegaradec, who considered that it was produced by the circulation of the blood through the placenta, and he therefore designated it as the *placental souffle,* and believed that it was of value in determining the situation of that organ. Subsequent investigations, however, have shown that such is not the case, and that the sound originates as I have indicated, and should therefore be designated as the uterine souffle. As stated by Rotter and others, it may occasionally be appreciated by the palpating finger. This sign is not characteristic of pregnancy, as it may be present in any condition in which the blood supply to the genitalia becomes markedly increased, and accordingly is not infrequently heard in non-pregnant women presenting tumours of the uterus or ovaries.

Certain *movements of the fœtus* may likewise be recognised on auscultation. According to Ahlfeld, it is impossible to hear the movements of the extremities, and he considers that the sounds which are usually so interpreted are produced by spasmodic contractions of the diaphragm, and are analogous to singultus.

Not infrequently the *maternal pulse* can be distinctly heard on auscultating the abdomen, and in some instances the pulsation of the aorta is so violent as to communicate a distinct throb to the ear.

In addition to the sounds just mentioned, it is not unusual to hear certain others produced by the passage of gases or fluids through the intestines of the mother.

Mapping out the Outlines of the Fœtus.—In the latter half of pregnancy it is possible to distinguish the outlines of the fœtus by palpation through the abdominal walls, and this becomes easier the nearer term is approached. When we desire to map out the fœtus we should go about the examination in a methodical manner, and follow the rules for palpation which will be given later.

A diagnosis of pregnancy should not be made from this sign alone, unless one is able to feel distinctly the various portions of the fœtus and distinguish its head, breech, back, and extremities. Subserous myomata occasionally simulate the head or small parts, or both, and their presence has occasionally given rise to serious diagnostic errors.

Movements of the Fœtus.—The third positive sign of pregnancy is present whenever the physician is able to feel the movements of the fœtus. These are active or passive, according as they are made spontaneously by the fœtus, or are imparted to it by the examining hand.

After the fifth month, *active movements* may be felt on placing the hand over the abdomen. These vary from a faint flutter in the early months to quite violent motions at a later period, which not infrequently are visible as well. Occasionally, somewhat similar sensations may be produced by contractions of the intestines or the muscles of the abdominal wall, though these should not deceive an experienced observer.

The *passive movements*, obtained by *ballottement*, consist in the rebound of a fœtal extremity when displaced from its position by the examining finger, whereby a sensation is afforded similar to that produced when a sudden motion is given to a piece of ice in a glass of water, so that at first it sinks and then slowly comes back to the finger. This sign is available from the early part of the fourth month, and may be obtained through either the vagina or the abdominal walls. To obtain vaginal ballottement the patient should be on her back; the physician then introduces two fingers into the vagina and carries them up to the anterior fornix, to which he imparts a sudden motion with his finger-tips, afterward retaining them in the same position. After a moment the extremity of the child which occupies the lower segment of the uterus, usually the head, drops down upon them again.

External ballottement can be obtained by imparting a sudden motion to the portion of the abdominal wall covering the uterus; in a few seconds the rebound of one of the extremities of the fœtus can be felt. This sign is of very considerable value, and can only be simulated by a pedunculated tumour swimming in ascitic fluid. When any one of the three positive signs is obtained, the diagnosis of pregnancy is established beyond doubt.

Probable Signs of Pregnancy.—*Enlargement of the Abdomen.*—From the third month onward the uterus can be felt through the abdominal walls as

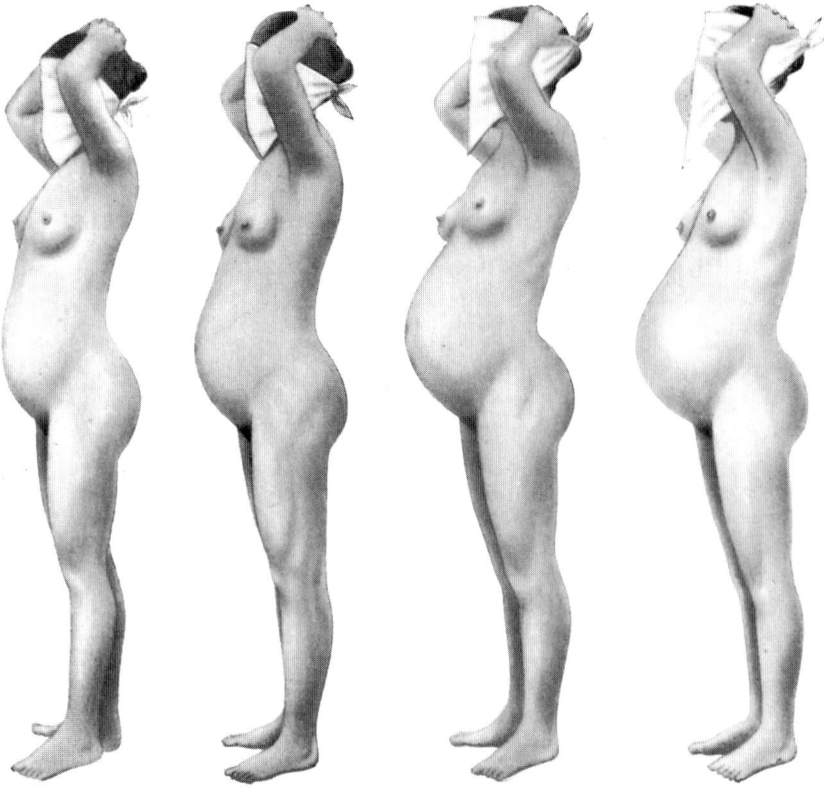

Fig. 163. Fig. 164. Fig. 165. Fig. 166.

Figs. 163–166.—Showing Relative Abdominal Enlargement at Third, Sixth, Ninth, and Tenth Month of Pregnancy.

a tumour, which gradually increases in size up to the end of pregnancy. Generally speaking, any enlargement of the abdomen during the childbearing period should be regarded as *prima facie* evidence of the existence of pregnancy. Figs. 163, 164, 165, and 166 give a good idea of the changes in the shape of the abdomen at the various months.

The abdominal enlargement is far less pronounced in primiparæ than in multiparæ, for the reason that in the latter the abdominal walls have lost a great part of their tonicity and are sometimes so flaccid that they afford little or no support to the uterus, which then becomes markedly anteflexed and sags forward and downward, giving rise to a *pendulous abdomen.* It should also be borne in mind that the abdomen changes its shape materially according as the woman is in the upright or horizontal position, being much less prominent when she is lying down. (See Figs. 160 and 161.)

Changes in Size, Shape, and Consistency of Uterus.—In the first three months these are the only physical signs available, and *the existence of an enlarged uterus at any time during the childbearing period should be regarded as presumptive evidence of pregnancy, until such a possibility has been conclusively eliminated.*

During the first few weeks the increase in size is limited almost entirely to the antero-posterior diameter; but at a little later period the body of the uterus becomes almost globular in shape, and at the third month attains the size of an orange. During the first two months the pregnant uterus still continues to be entirely a pelvic organ, whereas during the third month it begins to rise above the symphysis. At the same time the angle between the body and cervix becomes markedly accentuated—in other words, the physiological anteflexion is increased.

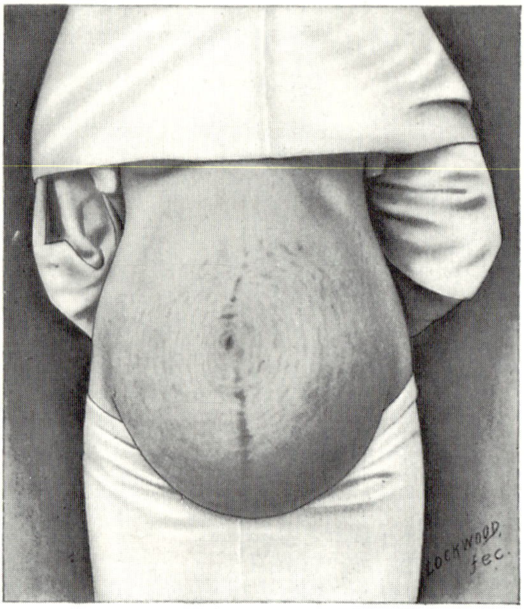

Fig. 167.—Pendulous Abdomen of a Multiparous Woman with Normal Pelvis.

More characteristic than the changes in shape are those affecting its consistency. On bimanual examination the uterine body offers a doughy or elastic sensation, and in many instances becomes so soft as to be hardly distinguishable. Dickinson has pointed out that these changes can be noted at a very early period, and states that he was able to differentiate a symmetrical elastic area in the body of the uterus in the latter part of the first week of pregnancy, which he considered almost pathognomonic.

According to R. von Braun, it would appear that the earliest evidence of pregnancy is afforded by the appearance of a more or less longitudinal furrow upon either the anterior or posterior surface of the uterus. Its presence he attributes to changes in consistence and the alteration between contraction and relaxation of the portion of the organ in which the ovum is situated. Von Braun claims that this sign enables him to diagnose the existence of pregnancy as early as the first week.

At about the sixth week another sign of considerable value—the so-called *Hegar's sign*—becomes available. On careful bimanual examination with one hand upon the abdomen and two fingers of the other hand in the vagina, or with a finger in the rectum and the thumb in the vagina, the

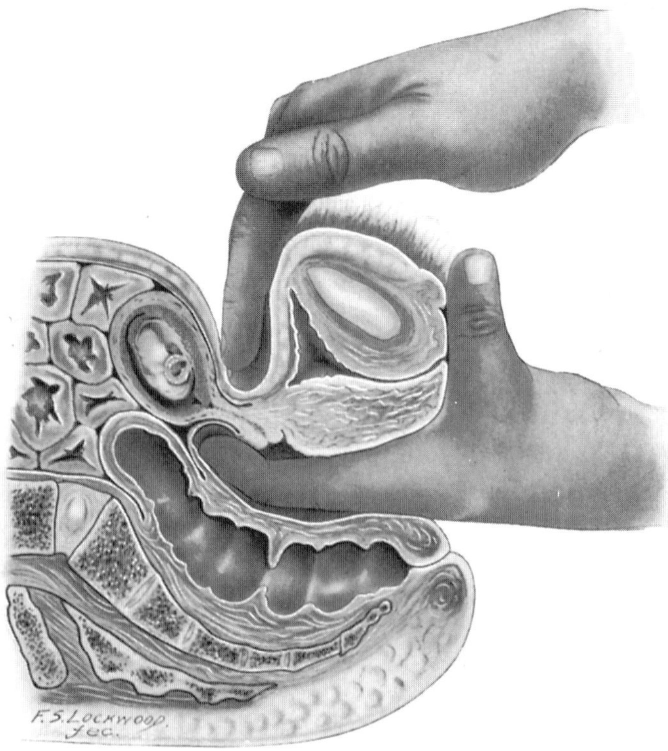

FIG. 168.—METHOD OF DETECTING HEGAR'S SIGN.

firm, hard cervix is felt, while above it is the elastic body of the uterus, and between the two quite a soft compressible area. Occasionally the change in consistence of the lower segment of the uterus is so marked that no connection between the cervix and body appears to exist, and in not a few instances inexperienced observers have mistaken the cervix for the uterus, and the softened body for a tumour of the uterine appendages.

This sign, first described by Reinl in 1884, was verified later by Sonntag and others, and its value is now universally admitted. Its production probably depends upon the forcing of the part of the ovum occupying the lower uterine segment into the upper part of the body of the uterus, so that the empty and softened lower uterine segment can then be readily compressed between the fingers. Fig. 168 gives a good idea of the sensation to be obtained on bimanual examination; and Figs. 169 and 170 show the condition of the uterus which makes it possible. This sign is of very considerable value, and its presence leaves but little doubt as to the diagnosis.

Cervix.—Beginning with the second month of pregnancy, the cervix becomes considerably softened, and in primiparous women the os externum offers to the finger a sensation similar to that obtained by pressing upon the more yielding lips instead of the harder cartilage of the nose, as at other times. In some cases, however, this sign does not become available, as in certain inflammatory conditions of the uterus, as well as in carcinoma, the cervix may remain firm and hard throughout the entire duration of pregnancy.

Intermittent Contractions of the Uterus.—From the third month on, at intervals of from five to ten minutes, the pregnant uterus undergoes painless contractions, which in the early months can be appreciated by bimanual examination, and later by the hand upon the abdomen, when

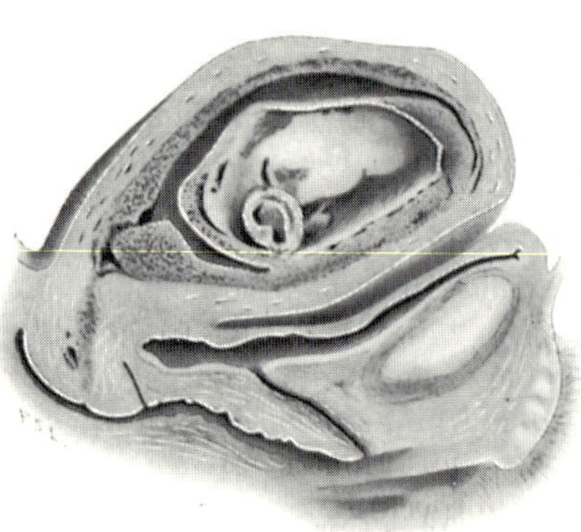

Fig. 169.—Ten-weeks' Pregnant Uterus (Pinard). × ½.

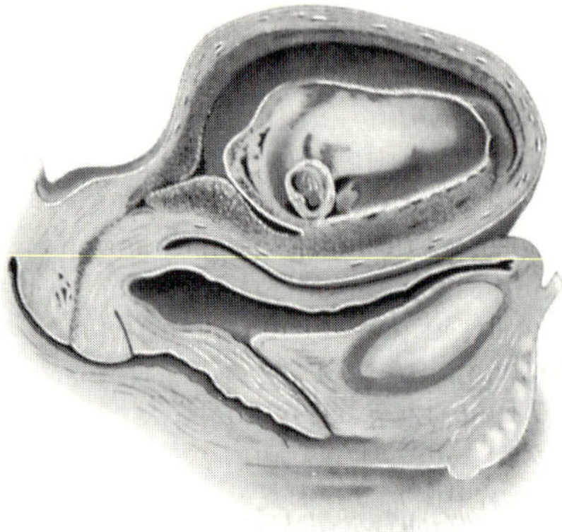

Fig. 170.—Showing Mode of Production of Hegar's Sign.

the previously relaxed organ is felt to become firm and hard, remaining so for a few moments, and then returning to its original condition. Attention was first called to this phenomenon by Braxton Hicks, and the sign has since been known by his name. It is not, however, infallible, as similar contractions are sometimes observed in hæmatometra, and occasionally in cases of submucous myomata.

Whenever one or several of these probable signs of pregnancy are detected the evidence becomes very strong. Nevertheless, if there is any possibility of wronging our patient we are not justified in making a positive assertion, even though we may feel morally sure of our diagnosis.

Presumptive Signs of Pregnancy.—The presumptive evidences of pregnancy are afforded in great part by subjective symptoms, which are appreciated by the patient herself.

Cessation of the Menses.—Most important is the cessation of the menstrual flow. In women exposed to the possibility of pregnancy, and whose menses have previously been regular, a sudden cessation is a most characteristic sign; and from it alone the majority of married women do not hesitate to diagnose their condition. But in patients presenting an irregular menstrual history this symptom does not possess the same diagnostic value, and we also know that certain diseases may give rise to amenorrhœa of many months' duration, in the course of which conception occasionally occurs.

Not infrequently a single menstrual period may be missed by women who fear the possibility of pregnancy; and false statements are often made in the hope of misleading the physician and inducing him to introduce a sound or some other instrument into the uterus, and thereby provoke an abortion.

In not a few instances menstruation may appear once after the commencement of pregnancy, though the flow is usually less profuse than at other times. In many of these cases it is probable that conception has occurred shortly before the period, although this rule by no means universally holds good. Only very rarely, however, does the menstrual flow appear more than once, and its regular recurrence should always arouse suspicion as to the existence of disease of the endometrium, carcinoma of the cervix, or some other pathological condition.

One occasionally hears of women who menstruate regularly throughout pregnancy, but the majority of these accounts are apocryphal, or else the condition is associated with uterine disease. At the same time it must be admitted that very exceptionally authentic cases are observed, and in a patient recently under my charge, the most careful examination revealed no other source for the hæmorrhage. Such an occurrence, however, should never be taken for granted, and all other possibilities must be carefully excluded.

Changes in the Breasts.—In the chapter upon the Physiology of Pregnancy reference has already been made to the changes which occur in the breasts. Generally speaking, in primiparæ these are quite characteristic, but are of less value in multiparæ, since the breasts of the latter not infrequently contain a small amount of milk or colostrum for months, and even for years, following the last labour. Occasionally, changes in the breasts similar to those produced by pregnancy may be observed in women suffering with ovarian or uterine tumours. Nor is the possibility of their occurrence excluded in instances of spurious or imaginary pregnancy.

Nausea and Vomiting.—The establishment of pregnancy is not infrequently marked by disturbances of the digestive system, more particularly manifested by nausea and vomiting. This "*morning sickness,*" as the name implies, usually comes on in the earlier part of the day, and passes off in a few hours, although it occasionally persists longer or may occur at other times. It usually appears about the end of the first month, and lasts for six or eight weeks, although some patients suffer from it for a much longer period.

There is considerable discrepancy of opinion as to the frequency with which these symptoms are observed. According to Gardner, they occur in only about 15 per cent of the cases, but my experience is that probably one half of pregnant women suffer from them to a greater or lesser degree. In many it amounts to nothing more than an occasional sensation of nausea; others have considerable vomiting, while in rare instances the nausea and vomiting may be so persistent and constant as to seriously interfere with nutrition. Occasionally, similar symptoms result from nervousness or from the fear of an illegitimate pregnancy, as well as in certain cases of pseudocyesis.

Quickening.—About the eighteenth or twentieth week, the woman becomes conscious of slight, fluttering movements in her abdomen, which gradually increase in intensity. These are usually due to movements of the fœtus, and their first appearance is designated as "quickening" or the perception of life. Occasionally fœtal movements may be perceived as early as the tenth week, while, on the other hand, in rare instances they may not be experienced at all.

This sign offers only corroborative evidence of pregnancy, and is of no value unless confirmed by the hand of the physician, as in many nervous women similar sensations are experienced in its absence.

Discoloration of the Mucous Membrane of Vagina and Vulva.—Under the influence of pregnancy the margins of the vaginal opening and the lower portion of the anterior vaginal wall frequently take on a somewhat dark bluish or purplish, congested appearance. Attention was first called to this condition by Jacquemier and Kluge, but particular stress was laid upon its significance by Dr. James R. Chadwick, of Boston, so that in this country it is known as *Chadwick's sign.* Its presence supplies valuable presumptive evidence, but is not conclusive, as it may likewise be observed in any condition leading to intense congestion of the pelvic organs.

Pigmentation of the Skin and Abdominal Striæ.—These manifestations, which have already been referred to in the chapter upon the physiology of pregnancy, are usually observed in this condition, but are not absolutely characteristic of it, as they are sometimes associated with tumours of other origin.

Urinary Disturbances.—In the early weeks of pregnancy the enlarging uterus, by exerting pressure on the bladder, causes a desire for frequent micturition. This is most marked in the first few months, and gradually passes off as the uterus rises up into the abdomen, to reappear when the head descends into the pelvis a few weeks before term.

Cravings—Mental and Emotional Changes.—Occasionally the appetite of the pregnant woman becomes very capricious, and she may evince an almost unconquerable desire for peculiar and sometimes revolting articles of food. I recall one patient who subsisted almost exclusively upon devilled crabs throughout the entire duration of pregnancy, and another who could retain nothing for the first four months except broiled lobster and Bass's ale.

We have already referred to the mental and emotional changes which sometimes characterize pregnancy, and occasionally we meet with women who diagnose their condition mainly from the occurrence of changes in their own temperament with which they have become familiar in previous pregnancies.

Synopsis of Signs and Symptoms of Pregnancy.—For convenience of reference, we give a synopsis of the signs and symptoms of pregnancy, dividing them into three groups corresponding to three different periods.

The first belongs to the first three months, the second to the fourth and fifth months, and the third to the last five months of pregnancy.

In the first period the symptoms are: (*a*) cessation of the menses; (*b*) changes in the breasts; (*c*) morning sickness; (*d*) urinary disturbances. The signs are: (1) enlargement of the body of the uterus and increased anteflexion; (2) changes in the consistency of the body of the uterus; (3) Hegar's sign; (4) changes in the cervix; (5) Chadwick's sign; (6) the abdomen is not prominent, the navel is depressed; (7) auscultation is negative.

Second period. Symptoms: (*a*) menses still absent; (*b*) more marked changes in the breasts; (*c*) disappearance or subsidence of gastric and urinary disturbances; (*d*) quickening. Signs: (1) the fundus is felt several fingers above the symphysis at the fourth month, and midway between the symphysis and umbilicus at the fifth month; (2) the cervix is soft; (3) ballottement is obtainable; (4) intermittent uterine contractions are recognisable; (5) at the very end of the period the fœtal heart sounds can be distinguished.

Third period. Symptoms: (*a*) menses still absent; (*b*) changes in the breasts more marked; (*c*) in the last month frequent urination reappears, often with neuralgic pains in the lower extremities. Signs: (1) progressive enlargement of the abdomen; (2) umbilicus smooth and later protruding; (3) the fœtal heart can be heard; (4) the different parts of the child can be palpated; (5) fœtal movements are perceptible.

In the first period the diagnosis is usually very probable, but never absolute; in the second, very rarely doubtful, and in the third absolute.

Differential Diagnosis of Pregnancy.—The pregnant uterus is often mistaken for other tumours occupying the pelvic or abdominal cavities, and *vice versa*, though, as a rule, the former mistake is more frequently made. The early periods of pregnancy may be simulated by enlargement of the uterus due to interstitial or submucous myomata, sarcomata, hæmatometra, and conditions resulting from inflammatory disturbances. As a rule, the uterus under these circumstances is harder and firmer than in pregnancy, and does not present its characteristic elastic or boggy consistency. Moreover, such conditions are not, as a rule, attended by cessation of the menses, except in hæmatometra. If, however, there is any possibility of a mistake, a delay of a few weeks will usually clear up the diagnosis.

The pregnant uterus is occasionally mistaken for small ovarian or tubal cysts, though this error should not occur if the patient be carefully examined bimanually and the pelvic contents isolated, if necessary under an anæsthetic. As the tumour becomes larger and rises up into the abdomen, other points become available for differential diagnosis, notably the intermittent contractions of Braxton Hicks and the positive signs of pregnancy.

The diagnosis of pregnancy in a myomatous uterus often presents serious difficulties, and for a time may be impossible. But a short delay will show a more rapid increase in the size of the tumour than is consistent with the existence of an uncomplicated myoma, and variations in the consistency of different parts should also serve to direct one's attention to the pregnant condition.

Occasionally, an ovarian cystoma may be complicated by pregnancy. In the early stages the diagnosis, as a rule, can be easily made, as careful bimanual examination should enable one to differentiate between the two tumours; but in the later months it may become extremely difficult and sometimes impossible, owing to the increased distention of the abdomen. Furthermore, if the positive signs of pregnancy cannot be elicited, its existence is usually overlooked and a simple cystoma diagnosed; whereas, if the heart sounds are heard, the cystoma may escape recognition and the excessive abdominal enlargement be attributed to a hydramnios.

In rare instances hypertrophy of the supravaginal portion of the cervix may seriously increase the difficulties of diagnosis, as the enlarged and hard cervix may be mistaken for the entire uterus, the soft and elastic body being either overlooked or regarded as a tumour of the uterine appendages. Careful bimanual examination under anæsthesia should do away with the possibility of this error.

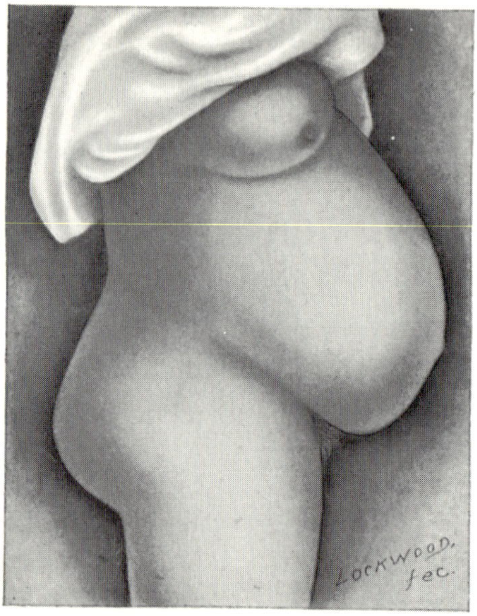

FIG. 171.—ABDOMINAL ENLARGEMENT DUE TO FAT, THE PATIENT IMAGINING HERSELF TO BE IN THE LAST MONTH OF PREGNANCY.

Irregular development of the pregnant uterus, associated with a sacculation of its anterior or posterior wall, may seriously complicate the diagnosis, especially if the fœtus be dead; as even after the most careful examination the existence of pregnancy may remain unrecognised and the sacculation be mistaken for an ovarian cyst. This is especially apt to occur when the pregnancy develops in the posterior wall, as the anterior wall may remain practically unchanged, and when, under anæsthesia, one can feel the fundus with both tubes extending from it, it is almost a pardonable error to conclude that the fluctuant tumour lying posterior to it is an ovarian cyst.

Spurious Pregnancy.—Imaginary pregnancy, or *pseudocyesis,* is a condition with which almost every practitioner, sooner or later, will meet. It is usually observed in patients nearing the menopause or in young women who intensely desire offspring. Such patients may present all the subjective symptoms of pregnancy, associated with a marked increase in the size of the abdomen, which is due either to an abnormal and rapid deposition of fat or to the existence of tympanites and occasionally of ascites. When it occurs in the earlier years of life the menses do not, as a rule, disappear, but may present certain abnormalities which the patient considers are due to her condition.

In many instances the woman may imagine that she detects fœtal movements, which are sometimes so violent as to make her fearful that they may be visible to onlookers. I recently saw a patient who imagined herself in the last month of pregnancy, and who, while talking to me, exclaimed at the violence of the movements, but on examination I found that her uterus was normal in size, and that her enlarged abdomen was due to a rapidly increasing deposit of fat.

The supposed fœtal movements usually result from contractions of the intestines or the muscles of the abdominal wall, and occasionally are so marked as to deceive even physicians. Careful examination of the patient usually enables one to arrive at a correct diagnosis without great difficulty, as the small uterus can be demonstrated on bimanual examination, made, if necessary, under anæsthesia. The greatest difficulty in these cases is to persuade the patient as to the correctness of the diagnosis.

Distinction between First and Subsequent Pregnancies.—Occasionally it is a matter of practical importance to decide whether a patient is pregnant for the first time or has previously borne children. Ordinarily childbearing leaves indelible traces behind it, which are readily appreciated; but very exceptionally such signs are lacking, as in a case reported by Budin. (See Fig. 33.) Again, in very rare instances, all the signs indicating a previous labour may result from the previous existence of a large tumour which has been removed through the vagina.

In a pregnant woman who has never borne children the abdomen is usually tense and firm, and the uterus is felt through it only with difficulty. The characteristic pinkish bluish striæ and the distinctive changes in the breasts are readily observed. The labia majora are usually in close apposition, the frenulum is intact, and the hymen torn in several places. The vagina is usually narrow and marked by well-developed rugæ. The cervix is softened, but does not usually admit the tip of the finger until the very end of pregnancy; and during the last four to six weeks of pregnancy the presenting part is found engaged in the superior strait, unless some disproportion exists.

In multiparous women, on the other hand, the abdominal walls are usually lax, flabby, and frequently pendulous, and the uterus is readily palpated through them. In addition to the pinkish striæ due to the present condition, the silvery cicatrices of past pregnancies may also be noted. The breasts are usually not as firm as in the first pregnancy, and frequently present striæ similar to those observed on the abdomen. The vulva is usually more or less gaping, the frenulum has disappeared, and the hymen is replaced by the *carunculæ myrtiformes*. The external os, even in the early months of pregnancy, usually shows signs of laceration, and at a little later period readily admits the tip of the finger, which can be carried up to the internal os. Furthermore, in the majority of cases the presenting part does not engage in the superior strait until the onset of labour.

Diagnosis of the Life or Death of the Fœtus.—Generally speaking, the fœtus should be considered to be alive unless definite evidence to the contrary can be adduced. In the early months of pregnancy the diagnosis of its death offers considerable difficulty, and can only be made after repeated examinations have demonstrated that the uterus has remained stationary in size for a number of weeks.

In the later months of pregnancy, the disappearance of fœtal movements usually directs the attention of the patient to this possibility, after which she suffers from ill-defined sensations, such as chilliness, languor, a sensation of weight in the abdomen, and perhaps a foul taste in the mouth. Careful investigation shows that the uterus does not correspond in size with the estimated duration of pregnancy, and perhaps has become smaller than previously; while at the same time retrogressive changes have occurred in the breasts, which have become soft and flabby. The diagnosis of the condition, however, can be considered absolute only after repeated examinations, when in addition to the signs just mentioned one has failed to hear the fœtal heart or perceive the movements of the child.

Positive information is occasionally afforded when it is possible to recognise by palpation the macerated skull through the partially dilated cervix; whenever one can feel that the bones of the head are loose and present a sensation as if they were contained in a flabby bag, the diagnosis can be made at once without hesitation.

Duration of Pregnancy.—As we have no means of ascertaining the exact date at which fertilization occurs, it is apparent that absolutely accurate statements as to the duration of pregnancy cannot be made; although, as has already been pointed out, conception usually occurs either soon after the last appearance of the menses, or shortly before the first period which is missed. In rare instances it takes place in the middle of the inter-menstrual period. These views have been confirmed, not only from the study of the condition of the ovaries, but also by the experience of embryologists, as it is not unusual for young embryos, which should be of the same age when we calculate from the last menstrual period, to present marked variations in development.

Usually labour ensues about two hundred and eighty days (ten lunar months) after the beginning of the last menstrual period, so that the approximate duration of pregnancy is two hundred and seventy days, supposing that conception has occurred within the few days immediately following the menstrual flow. This rule, however, is subject to many exceptions, as apparently well-developed children may be born as early as the two hundred and fortieth, and as late as the three hundred and twentieth day after the last menstrual period, and there is no doubt that in exceptional instances the actual duration of pregnancy may equal, if not exceed, three hundred days.

Every one practising obstetrics occasionally meets with cases in which the patient believes that she has passed a month beyond term; or, in other words, that the pregnancy has lasted eleven instead of ten lunar months. This belief, however, is usually erroneous, as in the majority of such cases conception has not occurred until just before the first period which was missed. Exceptionally, however, pregnancy may last for an abnormally long period, and I recall a patient who on two occasions did not fall into labour until considerably over eleven months after the last period. In both instances she had typical labour pains at the end of the tenth month, which after lasting a short time subsided, and did not return for more than four weeks. Both children weighed over 12 pounds, and were 55 to 56 centimetres in length, besides presenting markedly increased thoracic measurements.

Even when we know the date of the coitus from which the pregnancy has resulted, we are in no better position to estimate the actual length of pregnancy, inasmuch as Löwenhardt has pointed out that two women may have fruitful coitus on the same day, and yet the date of their deliveries may vary markedly. Ahlfeld analyzed 425 cases in which the date of coitus was supposed to be known, and found the average duration of pregnancy to be 269.91 days; but individual cases in the series presented marked differences, varying from two hundred and thirty-one to three hundred and twenty-nine days.

Similar differences are reported by veterinarians, who usually date the beginning of pregnancy from a single coitus. According to Franck-Albrecht-Göring, the average duration of pregnancy in the mare is three hundred and sixty-six days, but in a large series of cases individual variations between three hundred and seven and four hundred and twelve days were noted. In the cow the normal duration is placed at two hundred and eighty days, with extremes of two hundred and forty and three hundred and eleven days.

In view of these facts we must conclude that the duration of pregnancy varies within certain limits, which probably depend upon individual peculiarities, just as happens in the case of mares and cows of different races. Again, as Mme. Laurié has recently shown, it also depends upon the extent to which the patient can spare herself in the last three months of pregnancy. This observer found that it was twenty days longer in 1,550 women who lived comfortably in a hospital for several months prior to delivery, as compared with the same number of women who entered at the onset of labour. Her figures, then, go to show that hard work in poorly nourished women predisposes somewhat to the premature ending of pregnancy.

It must also be admitted that the duration of pregnancy not infrequently exceeds two hundred and eighty days from the last menstrual period, and that when it lasts much longer large children are developed, which are frequently delivered only after great difficulty. Thus, whenever the menstrual history of the patient indicates that she has passed much beyond the tenth and is approaching the eleventh lunar month, we should consider the propriety of the induction of labour, provided that careful examination shows that the child is larger than usual.

Estimation of the Probable Date of Confinement.—Unfortunately for the comfort of the physician, as well as of the patient, we possess no reliable means of estimating the exact date, but are obliged to content ourselves with the method proposed by Naegele, which is based upon the belief that labour occurs two hundred and eighty days from the beginning of the last menstrual period. The calculation is readily made by adding seven days to the date at which the last menstrual period first appeared, and then counting back three months. For example, if the last period began on January 10, 1902, we add seven days, making January 17th, and count back three months, thus fixing upon October 17, 1902, as the probable date of confinement.

In a small number of cases the patient will be confined on the precise day estimated, and in the great majority of cases within a few days of this date; but occasionally a period of several weeks may elapse before labour occurs. This marked difference is probably due to the fact that in the one case conception had occurred soon after the last period, and in the latter just before the first period which was missed. Accordingly, the physician should hesitate to predict a definite day for the confinement, and should always allow a margin of two to three weeks in his calculations.

Löwenhardt believed that the duration of pregnancy was not ten lunar months, but ten menstrual periods, and considered the labour as likely to occur when the tenth menstrual period following conception fell due. According to this calculation, in patients menstruating at intervals of twenty-six and thirty days, for example, the duration of pregnancy would be two hundred and sixty and three hundred days respectively. In the long run, however, this method of calculation does not give more accurate results than that of Naegele.

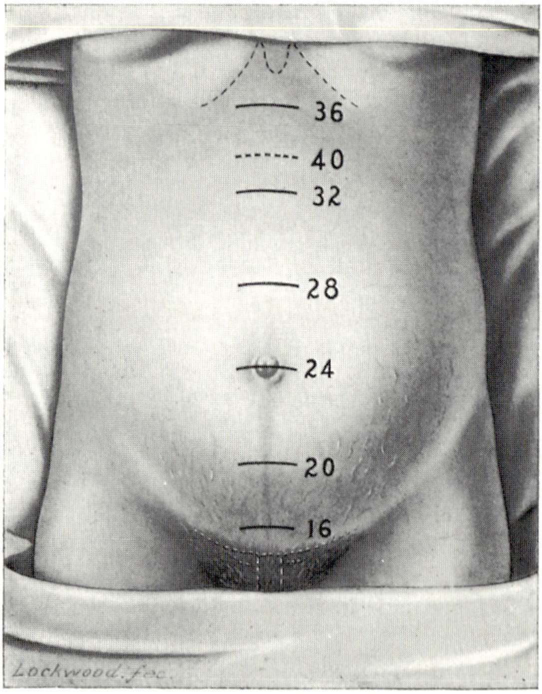

Fig. 172.—Relative Height of the Fundus at the Various Weeks of Pregnancy.

Occasionally the patient believes that she can date her pregnancy from a single coitus, and prefers to estimate the approaching date of confinement from that rather than from the beginning of the last period. This method is also subject to considerable error, as we have no means of ascertaining how long the spermatozoa may remain in the genital tract before conception occurs.

In not a few instances, especially in nursing women, conception may take place during a period of amenorrhœa, and the patient is often surprised by the enlargement of her abdomen or by the perception of fœtal movements; while occasionally the first intimation that she is pregnant is given by the fact that her milk, which has previously agreed very well with the infant, suddenly becomes indigestible. Under such circumstances, the usual methods of calculation are of no value, and we have to depend upon other means, which, unfortunately, are extremely unsatisfactory.

Frequent attempts have been made to estimate the date of confinement, by adding twenty or twenty-one weeks to the date upon which the patient first perceived fœtal movements. This method is founded on the belief that quickening is first experienced at the eighteenth or twentieth week of pregnancy. Unfortunately, this assumption is erroneous, as the symptom not infrequently occurs at a much earlier period, and sometimes not until considerably later.

In other cases, our calculations are based upon the enlargement of the abdomen and the height to which the fundus of the uterus has risen. Generally speaking, we find that the fundus at the fourth month is several fingers'-breadths above the symphysis pubis; at the fifth month midway between it and the umbilicus; at the sixth month at the level of the umbilicus; at the seventh month three fingers'-breadths above the umbilicus; at the eighth month an equal distance above its position at the seventh month; at the ninth month just below the xiphoid; whereas in the last month, particularly in primiparous women, it sinks downward and assumes almost the position it occupied at the eighth month.

This method, however, gives only approximate results, as the position of the umbilicus is subject to marked variations. Thus, according to Spiegelberg, its situation varies from 13 to 28 centimetres above the symphysis, so that if this author's figures are correct, there may be a difference of 6 inches in its position. On this account it has been thought preferable by some authors to estimate the distance of the fundus from the symphysis pubis with a tape measure, the average results obtained by Spiegelberg being as follows:

22d to 28th week	24 to 24.5 centimetres.
28th week	26.7 centimetres.
30th "	28.4 "
32d "	29.5 to 30 centimetres.
34th "	31 centimetres.
36th "	32 "
38th "	33.1 centimetres.
40th "	33.7 "

These measurements, however, are subject to considerable variations, as they are dependent not only upon the size of the fœtus contained within the uterus, but also upon the degree of distention of the abdominal contents. Nevertheless, in cases in which we possess no other data, they occasionally afford us information of very considerable value.

LITERATURE

Ahlfeld. Beobachtungen über die Dauer der Schwangerschaft. Monatsschr. f. Geburtsk., 1869, xxxiv, 180–225.

Die wahrnehmbaren kindlichen Bewegungen. Lehrbuch der Geburtshülfe, II. Aufl., 1898, 56.

von Braun. Ueber Frühdiagnose der Gravidität. Centralbl. f. Gyn., 1899, 488, 489.

Budin. Femmes en couches et nouveau-nés. Paris, 1897, 1–4.

Chadwick. Value of the Bluish Coloration of the Vaginal Entrance as a Sign of Pregnancy. Trans. Amer. Gyn. Soc., 1886, xi, 399.

Cordell. Congenital Anomaly of the Fœtal Heart, etc., in which a Systolic Murmur was heard before Birth. Trans. Med. and Chirurg. Faculty of Maryland, 1884, 218–222.

Depaul. Traité d'auscultation obstétricale. Paris, 1847.

Dickinson. The Diagnosis of Pregnancy between the Second and Seventh Weeks by Bimanual Examination. Amer. Gyn. and Obst. Journal, 1892, ii, 544–555.

Duval. Palpation of the Fœtal Heart Impulse in Pregnancy. Johns Hopkins Hospital Bulletin, 1897, viii, p. 207.

Fischel. Ueber ein bisher nicht beobachtetes Phänomen bei Deflexionslagen. Prager med. Wochenschr., 1881, Nr. 12, 13; 1882, Nr. 28.

Zur intrauterinen Tastbarkeit des fötalen Herzimpulses bei Deflexionslagen. Centralbl. f. Gyn., 1885, 769–771.

Fochier. Sur le bruit de souffle d'origine fœtale. L'Obstétrique, 1896, i, 279.

Franck-Albrecht-Göring. Die Trächtigkeitsdauer, Thierärztliche Geburtshülfe, IV. Aufl., 1901, 153–159.

Frankenhäuser. Ueber die Herztöne der Frucht und ihre Benutzung zur Diagnose des Geschlechts derselben, etc. Monatsschr. f. Geburtskunde, 1859, xiv, 161–174.

Gardner. The Diagnosis of Early Pregnancy. Amer. Jour. of Obst., 1897, xxxv, 54–63.

Hicks. On the Contraction of the Uterus throughout Pregnancy. Trans. London Obst. Soc., 1872, xiii, 216–231.

Kegaradec. Mémoire sur l'auscultation appliquée à l'étude de la grossesse. Paris, 1822.

Kennedy. Observations on Obstetric Auscultation. New York, 1847.

Lourié. De l'influence du repos sur la durée de la grossesse. Thèse de Paris, 1899.

Löwenhardt. Die Berechnung und die Dauer der Schwangerschaft. Archiv f. Gyn., 1872, iii, 456–491.

Mayor. Quoted in Bibliothèque universelle de Genève, November, 1818, ix.

Montgomery. An Exposition of the Signs and Symptoms of Pregnancy, 2d ed., London, 1863.

Reinl. Prager med. Wochenschr., 1884, Nr. 26.

Rotter. Fühlbares Uteringeräusch. Archiv f. Gyn., 1873, v, 539–546.

Sonntag. Hegar's Sign of Pregnancy. Amer. Jour. Obst., 1892, xxvi, 145–157.

Spiegelberg. Lehrbuch der Geburtshülfe, III. Aufl., 1891, 126, 127.

CHAPTER VIII

THE MANAGEMENT OF NORMAL PREGNANCY

From a biological point of view pregnancy and labour represent the highest functions of the female productive system, and *a priori* should be considered as normal processes. But when we recall the manifold changes which occur in the maternal organism, it is apparent that the border-line between health and disease is less distinctly marked during gestation than at other times, and derangements, so slight as to be of but little consequence under ordinary circumstances, may readily give rise to pathological conditions which seriously threaten the life of the mother or the child, or both.

It accordingly becomes necessary to keep pregnant patients under strict supervision, and to be constantly on the alert for the appearance of untoward symptoms. Ordinarily the services of an obstetrician are engaged some months before the expected date of confinement, so that upon him devolves the duty of advising the patient as to her mode of life during the intervening months. Any one who has a moderately extensive obstetrical practice can save himself some little trouble by having cards printed, which briefly outline what the patient is expected to do, and in which are enumerated the various abnormal symptoms which may occur and to which the physician's attention should be immediately called.

Unless it be found upon inquiry that the patient has been leading an ill-ordered existence, very little change should be made in her mode of living, and she should be encouraged to go on much as usual, care being taken that she receives the proper amount of amusement and diversion. It is the duty of the physician to gain the confidence of his patient and encourage her to come to him whenever anything occurs to worry her, instead of taking advice from her women friends. A woman in her first pregnancy generally stands in need of a certain amount of reassurance with regard to the dangers of parturition, and the knowledge that she is in the hands of a competent and careful physician will contribute largely to her peace of mind as well as to her physical well-being.

Exercise.—During pregnancy the woman should be encouraged to take as much outdoor exercise as possible, though in individual cases it is often difficult to specify the exact amount—a safe rule being to instruct her to desist while still feeling that she could do more without tiring herself. Exercise should consist of walking or driving, but the ordinary sports should be interdicted, though sea-bathing in many instances is very beneficial. When for various reasons outdoor exercise cannot be taken, massage in the hands of a skilful person is to be recommended. In the later months, long journeys should not be undertaken unless absolutely necessary, and driving over rough roads should be avoided.

Diet.—The diet should be abundant and nourishing, and ordinarily the patient should be allowed to continue her usual customs, but should be warned to abstain from very highly seasoned or indigestible articles of food. In slight degrees of pelvic contraction, or in patients who have previously given birth to excessively heavy children, a restricted diet may be advisable during the last two or three months. Prochownick pointed out, and his experience has been confirmed by Florschütz and others, that a diet poor in carbohydrates and fluids exerts a marked influence upon the weight of the child without otherwise affecting it, and in not a few cases these precautionary measures may obviate a difficult delivery, or even do away with the necessity for the induction of premature labour.

The Bowels.—In the later months of pregnancy the enlarged uterus sometimes interferes with the normal intestinal peristalsis, and gives rise to more or less marked constipation. Under such circumstances care should be taken that the bowels are moved daily, which is best accomplished by the administration of cascara sagrada or pills containing aloin, belladonna, and strychnine. The use of active cathartics is inadvisable, unless their employment be especially indicated in certain morbid conditions. In some instances, however, the judicious administration of an occasional dose of calomel is followed by marked beneficial results.

Clothing.—The physician is frequently asked concerning the clothing which is best adapted to the pregnant state, and especially whether corsets should be worn or not. Generally speaking, the clothing should be loose and so arranged as to exert as little pressure upon the waist as possible; and in the later months of pregnancy, at least, the corset should either be entirely dispensed with or replaced by a loosely fitting corset-waist. In multiparous women, when the abdomen is markedly relaxed from previous childbearing, the wearing of an abdominal support, either an ordinary Scultetus bandage, or one made of elastic material, adds materially to their comfort. When varicose veins of the extremities are present, the legs should be bandaged or encased in elastic stockings, and when large varices exist about the vulva the patient should be cautioned concerning the possibility of their rupture.

Sexual Intercourse.—In healthy persons sexual intercourse in moderation usually does no harm, as long as the abdominal enlargement is not too great to make it inconvenient for the patient. But where there is a tendency to abortion it should be strictly interdicted. It should also be positively forbidden in the last month of pregnancy, as I know of at least one case in which a severe puerperal infection has followed coitus during that period.

The Breasts.—In the last three months of pregnancy attention should be devoted to the condition of the breasts, and more particularly to the nipples, as by appropriate preliminary treatment nursing may be rendered easier, and the occurrence of fissures and the consequent danger of mammary infection in great part prevented. For this purpose the patient, during the last two months, should bathe her nipples night and morning with a lotion which tends to make the skin covering them more resistant. A saturated solution of borax or boric acid in 50 per cent alcohol will answer the purpose very well. Where the nipples are small it is advisable to attempt to lengthen them by making a few tractions upon them night and morning; and where they are but slightly prominent good results not infrequently follow the wearing of a wooden nipple shield (Fig. 173) for a few hours of each day. I know of no means, however, by which deeply retracted nipples can be made serviceable.

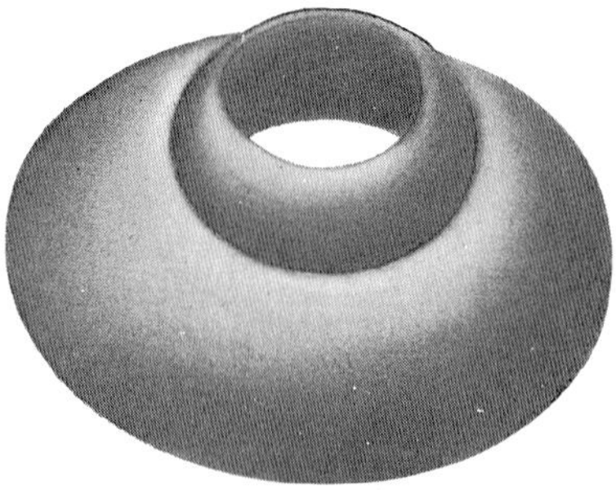

FIG. 173.—WOODEN NIPPLE SHIELD.

Urine.—Owing to the frequency of renal disturbances and the serious consequences which not infrequently result from them, the urine should be carefully examined at regular intervals: once a month for the first seven months, and at least twice a month, and preferably every week, during the last three months of pregnancy. It is advisable that the physician should not only arrange definite periods at which specimens are to be sent, but that he should himself make a note of these dates, so that in case the patient becomes careless in the matter and neglects to carry out his directions, he can remind her. Of course it may be very plausibly argued that the patient incurs the main risk from such neglect; but the prevention of a single death from eclampsia will amply repay the conscientious physician for much self-imposed labour.

The urine should be examined not only for the presence of albumin and sugar, but also microscopically. In certain cases also the estimation of the total urea excreted in twenty-four hours is of extreme importance. (See Chapter XXVI.)

In addition to giving the patient the advice above mentioned, the physician should also impress upon her the importance of informing him at once in case any of the following symptoms be noted: a scanty flow of urine, persistent headache, disturbances of vision, swelling of the feet and face, any loss of blood no matter how slight, and persistent constipation. In the majority of cases these symptoms are of secondary importance, but occasionally they serve to warn us of the imminence of some serious affection, which may be aborted or alleviated by appropriate treatment.

Preliminary Examination.—Four to six weeks before the expected date of confinement a careful examination is indispensable, and to neglect in this respect can be attributed the deaths of untold numbers of women and children. Usually this can be made much more conveniently with the patient in her own home and in bed than at the physician's office. At this time the general condition should be carefully noted, particular attention being also paid to the measurements of the pelvis as well as to the presentation and position of the child.

But unless the physician fully appreciates the importance of this examination, and has learned to look upon the making of it as a bounden duty, he may sometimes be deterred by feeling that it is repugnant to the patient, and that she may object to it or even refuse it. My experience, however, has always been that a few words of kindly explanation soon smooth away all such difficulties; and when, as happens fortunately in the vast majority of cases, after the examination we can reassure the woman as to the prospects of a simple and safe delivery, she will feel amply repaid for any inconvenience to which she may have been subjected. On the other hand, if any abnormality is present, it is highly desirable for the physician to know of its existence in advance, and even although he may not always deem it advisable to communicate his conclusions to the patient herself, he will generally do well to inform the husband or some other responsible member of her family of the existing condition. If, however, it should happen that, despite the exercise of the greatest tact on the part of the physician, and his insistence that such an examination is a necessity for her own sake, the patient persists in her refusal, the former has no alternative but to decline absolutely to attend the case.

The first point in the preliminary examination is careful *pelvic mensuration*, and Dohrn has well said that the physician who neglects pelvimetry is comparable to one who attempts to treat pulmonary diseases without the aid of auscultation and percussion. In the majority of instances the external measurements are quite sufficient, unless they indicate the possibility of some pelvic abnormality. Generally speaking, if the measurements between the iliac spines and crests bear an approximately normal relation to one another, internal pelvimetry is not necessary unless Baudelocque's diameter is 18.5 centimetres or less, or unless the head is not engaged in primiparous women, or the patient limps or presents signs of some spinal deformity. In the latter cases, however, the pelvis should be measured internally, if necessary with the woman under the influence of an anæsthetic; otherwise the physician will be unable to obtain any intelligent idea of the existing conditions and the probable outcome of the labour. Armed with this foreknowledge, in extreme cases he will be prepared at the proper time to suggest the induction of premature labour, or to keep the patient within reach of a competent operator who will be ready to perform Cæsarean section. It is an indisputable fact that the generally poor results obtained in this country from both of these operations are directly attributable to the neglect of pelvic mensuration.

After measuring the pelvis, the abdomen should be carefully examined, the duration of pregnancy estimated, and the existence of any abnormality, as hydramnios or twins, noted; after which the position and presentation of the child should be determined by *external palpation*, according to the rules which will be given later. An internal examination is necessary only in those cases in which palpation gives uncertain or unsatisfactory results, or when the head is not engaged in primiparous women. The physician who knows how to utilize all the resources of external palpation and manipulation, will find that by these means he can usually not only recognise normal and abnormal presentations in advance, but can also convert breech, transverse, or face presentations into those of the vertex.

In the rare cases in which *vaginal exploration* is necessary at the preliminary examination, when undertaken prior to the end of the ninth lunar month, rigorous hand disinfection is not necessary, and the physician may content himself with the use of a nail-brush, soap, and hot water. In the last month of pregnancy, however, the hands should be as carefully disinfected as at the time of delivery, for we have no means of knowing exactly when labour may supervene, and our neglect may occasionally give rise to puerperal infection.

The various abnormalities occurring in the course of pregnancy will be considered in a separate chapter.

LITERATURE

Dohrn. Ueber Beckenmessung. Volkmann's Sammlung klin. Vorträge, Nr. 11.

Florschütz. Kritik der Versuche durch eine bestimmte Diät der Mütter die Gefahren der Beckenenge zu umgehen. D. I., Giessen, 1895.

Prochownick. Ein Versuch zum Ersatze der künstlichen Frühgeburt. Centralbl. f. Gyn., 1889, 577–581.

CHAPTER IX

PRESENTATION AND POSITION OF THE FŒTUS—METHODS OF DIAGNOSIS

Irrespective of the relation which it may bear to the mother, the fœtus in the later months of pregnancy assumes a characteristic posture, which is described as its *attitude* or *habitus*; and, as a general rule, it may be said to form an ovoid mass, which roughly corresponds with the shape of the uterine cavity. Thus, it is folded or bent upon itself in such a way that the back becomes markedly convex, the head is sharply flexed so that the chin is almost in contact with the breast, the thighs are flexed over the abdomen, the legs are bent at the knee-joints, and the arches of the feet rest upon the anterior surfaces of the legs. The arms are usually crossed over the thorax or are parallel to the sides, while the umbilical cord lies in the space between them and the lower extremities.

This attitude is usually retained throughout pregnancy, though it is frequently modified somewhat by the movements of the extremities, and in rare instances the head may become extended, when a totally different posture is assumed. The characteristic attitude results partly from the mode of growth of the fœtus, and partly from a process of accommodation between it and the outlines of the uterine cavity.

Presentation.—By this term is understood the relation which the long axis of the fœtus bears to that of the mother, and we accordingly distinguish between longitudinal and transverse presentations. Not infrequently during pregnancy the fœtal may cross the maternal axis at an angle, and thus give rise to oblique presentations; but, as these always become longitudinal or transverse during the course of labour, they are not considered as distinct varieties. *Longitudinal presentations* are by far the most frequent, occurring in 99.5 per cent of all cases.

Considerable confusion has resulted from confounding the terms *presentation* and *presenting part.* By the latter we understand the portion of the fœtus which is felt through the cervix on vaginal examination, or which engages at the superior strait. Accordingly, when the long axes of both mother and fœtus are in the same direction, the presenting part may be either the head or the breech, and we speak of *cephalic* or *breech presentations* respectively. When the fœtus lies with its long axis transversely the shoulder is the presenting part, and we speak of *shoulder presentations.*

Longitudinal presentations are broadly classified as normal, and transverse as abnormal, inasmuch as with the former the child is usually delivered by the unaided efforts of Nature; whereas if the latter persist it cannot be born spontaneously, but always requires the aid of the obstetrician. These abnormal presentations will be considered in a separate chapter.

Cephalic presentations are divided into several groups, according to the relation which the head bears to the body of the child. Usually the head

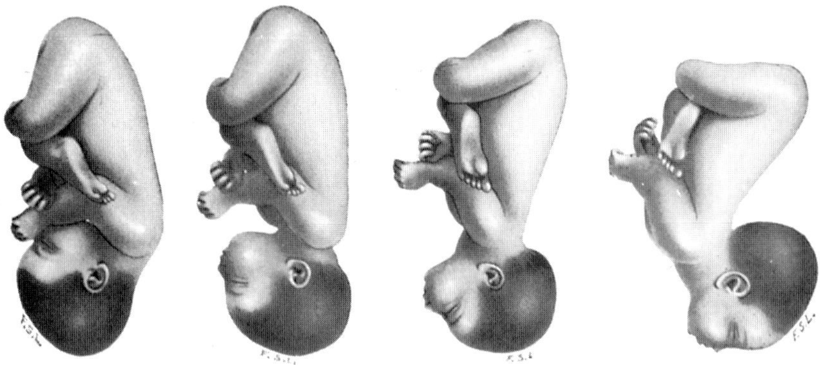

Fig. 174. Fig. 175. Fig. 176. Fig. 177.

FIGS. 174–177.—SHOWING DIFFERENCE IN ATTITUDE OF FŒTUS IN VERTEX, SINCIPUT, BROW, AND FACE PRESENTATIONS.

is sharply flexed, so that the chin is in contact with the thorax. Under these circumstances the vertex is the presenting part—*vertex presentation.* More rarely the neck may be overextended, so that the occiput and back come in contact and the face is felt through the cervix—*face presentation.* Again, the head may assume an intermediate position between the extremes of flexion and extension, being partially flexed in some cases, when the large fontanelle presents—*sincipital presentation*; or partially

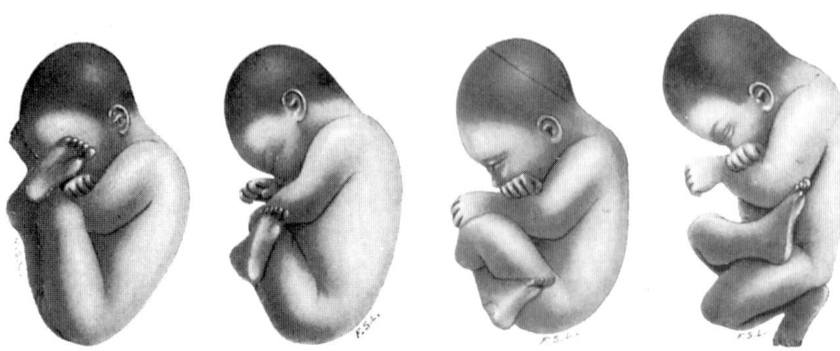

Fig. 178. Fig. 179. Fig. 180. Fig. 181.

FIGS. 178–181.—SHOWING DIFFERENCE IN ATTITUDE OF FŒTUS IN FRANK BREECH, FULL BREECH, FOOT, AND KNEE PRESENTATIONS.

extended in other cases, so that the brow becomes the presenting part—*brow presentation.* The last two are not usually classified as distinct varieties, as they are usually transient, and become converted into vertex or face presentations as labour progresses.

When the child presents by its pelvic extremity, the thighs are flexed and the legs may be extended over the anterior surface of the body—*frank breech presentation*; again, the thighs may be flexed on the abdomen and the legs upon the thighs—*breech presentation*; or the feet may be the lowest part—*foot* or *footling presentation*. Occasionally one leg may assume the position which is typical of one of the above-mentioned presentations, while the other foot or knee may present—*incomplete foot* or *knee presentation*. As the mechanism of labour, however, is essentially the same in all modifications of pelvic presentations, the several varieties need not be considered separately.

Position.—By this term we designate the relation of some arbitrarily chosen portion of the child to the right or left side of the mother. Accordingly, with each presentation we have one or other of two positions—right or left. With us and in France, the occiput, chin, and sacrum are the determining points in vertex, face, and breech presentations respectively; while in Germany the objective point is the child's back.

Variety.—Furthermore, for the purpose of still more accurate description, we take into consideration the relationship of some given portion of the presenting part to different portions of the mother's pelvis. Thus, in each position, the determining portion of the presenting part may be directed towards the anterior, transverse, or posterior portion of either side of the pelvis, making in all six varieties for each presentation. But as the transverse varieties are not persistent, and represent only a phase in the mechanism of labour, they need not be taken into account.

Nomenclature.—Unfortunately, a universal nomenclature for designating the various presentations and positions has not as yet been agreed upon, and the methods employed vary in different countries and even in different parts of the same country, though of late there has arisen a greater tendency towards uniformity.

In the earlier works upon obstetrics, as in Roesslin's Rosengarten (1513), it was believed that the child might assume any imaginable position *in utero*, and the number of presentations and positions was limited only by the ingenuity of the writer. More accurate observation gradually did away with the fanciful forms, but even as late as 1775 Baudelocque distinguished 94 different presentations. Mme. La Chapelle (1821) materially simplified the subject, and the classification which she suggested differs but little from that employed in France to-day, which has been best described by Farabeuf and Varnier.

According to the French method, vertex, face, and breech presentations are designated as occipito-iliac (O. I.), mento-iliac (M. I.), and sacro-iliac (S. I.). As the presenting part in any presentation may be either in the left or right position, we have left and right occipito-iliac, left and right mento-iliac, and left and right sacro-iliac presentations, which in an abbreviated form may be written L. O. I. and R. O. I.; L. M. I. and R. M. I.; L. S. I. and R. S. I. Again, as the presenting part in each position may be directed anteriorly, transversely, or posteriorly, we may have six varieties of each presentation, though the transverse modifications are frequently omitted. Thus we have the following classification:

	Position.	Presentation.	Variety.	Abbreviation.
Vertex presentations ..	Left.	Occipito-iliac.	Anterior.	(L. O. I. A.)
	"	"	Transverse.	(L. O. I. T.)
	"	"	Posterior.	(L. O. I. P.)
	Right.	"	Anterior.	(R. O. I. A.)
	"	"	Transverse.	(R. O. I. T.)
	"	"	Posterior.	(R. O. I. P.)

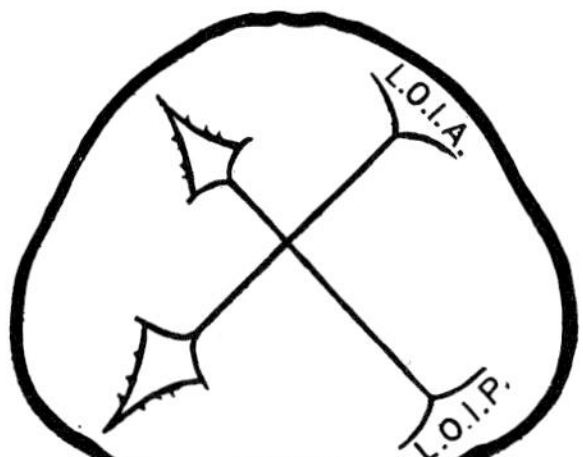

Fig. 182.

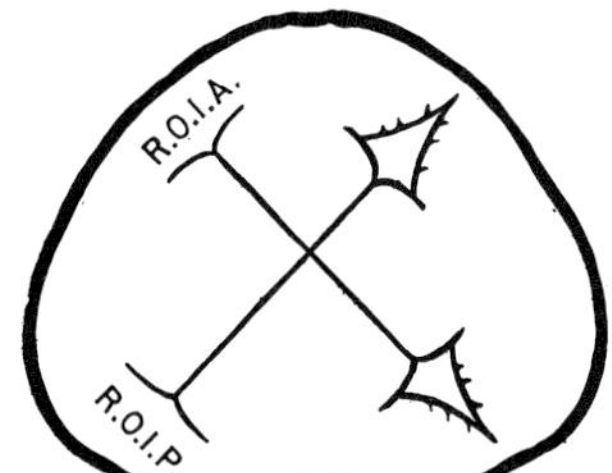

Fig. 183.

FIGS. 182, 183.—SHOWING VARIETIES OF VERTEX PRESENTATIONS.

	Position.	Presentation.	Variety.	Abbreviation.
Face presentations.....	Left.	Mento-iliac.	Anterior.	(L. M. I. A.)
	"	"	Transverse.	(L. M. I. T.)
	"	"	Posterior.	(L. M. I. P.)
	Right.	"	Anterior.	(R. M. I. A.)
	"	"	Transverse.	(R. M. I. T.)
	"	"	Posterior.	(R. M. I. P.)

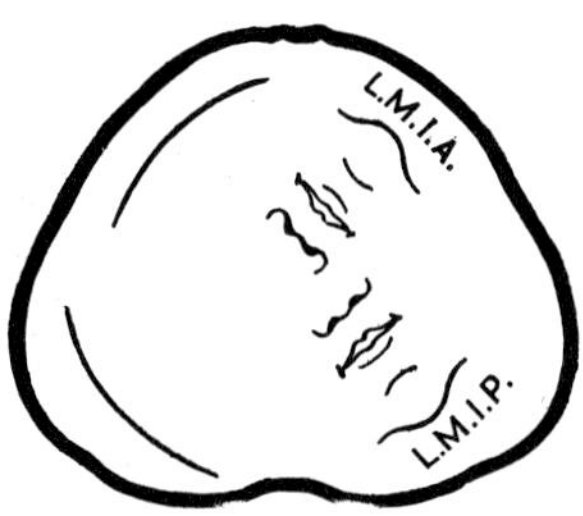

Fig. 184.

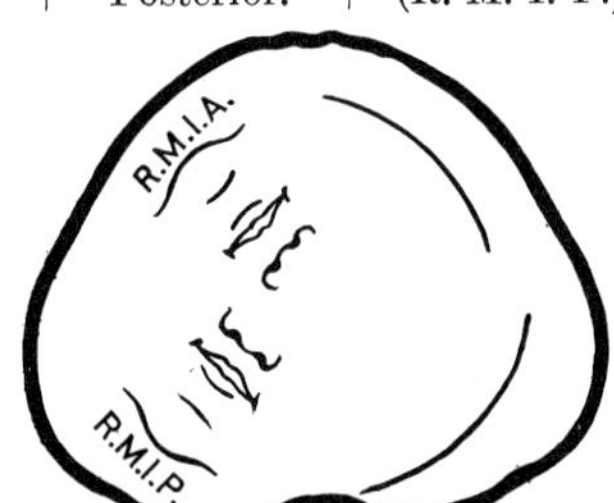

Fig. 185.

FIGS. 184, 185.—SHOWING VARIETIES OF FACE PRESENTATIONS.

	Position.	Presentation.	Variety.	Abbreviation.
Breech presentations...	Left.	Sacro-iliac.	Anterior.	(L. S. I. A.)
	"	"	Transverse.	(L. S. I. T.)
	"	"	Posterior.	(L. S. I. P.)
	Right.	"	Anterior.	(R. S. I. A.)
	"	"	Transverse.	(R. S. I. T.)
	"	"	Posterior.	(R. S. I. P.)

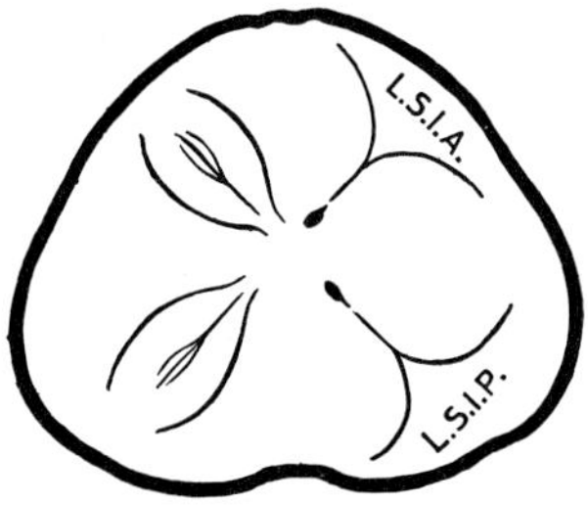

Fig. 186.

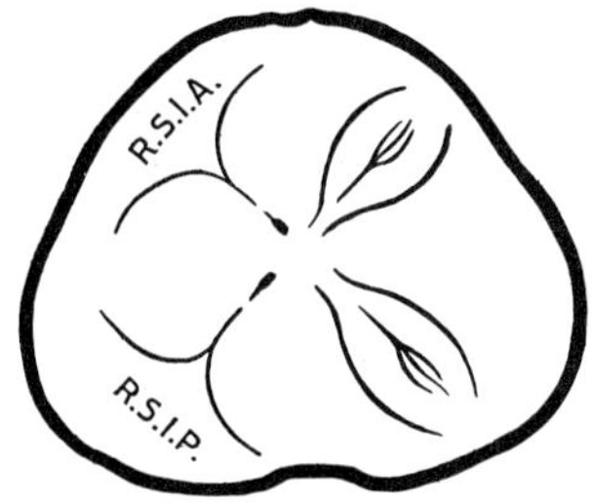

Fig. 187.

FIGS. 186, 187.—SHOWING VARIETIES OF BREECH PRESENTATIONS.

At the International Medical Congress which met in Washington in 1887, an attempt was made to secure greater uniformity in nomenclature. It was suggested that the denomination "iliac" be omitted and the various presentations designated as occipito, mento, and sacro respectively, preceded, as the case might be, by the word left or right to denote the position, and followed by anterior, transverse, or posterior to indicate the variety, the following abbreviations being employed: L. O. A., L. O. P., R. O. A., R. O. P.; L. M. A., L. M. P., R. M. A., R. M. P.; L. S. A., L. S. P.; R. S. A., R. S. P. The suggestion was quite generally adopted in this country, but failed to find favour abroad.

The older nomenclature, however, seems to be preferable and is more accurate. For example, when one speaks of a left occipito-iliac-anterior position, there is absolutely no doubt as to what is meant; whereas, on the other hand, the term left occipito-anterior simply describes the position of the head, and could be employed equally well to a breech or vertex presentation, were it not arbitrarily agreed that it applied only to the latter.

In Germany considerable confusion exists, as the various authorities still employ different classifications. Thus Schroeder, Olshausen and Veit do not distinguish variety at all, and designate the position according to the situation of the back of the child, speaking of first and second positions according as the back is directed to the left or right side of the mother respectively. Ahlfeld, Döderlein, and others employ a different nomenclature, and designate our L. O. I. A., R. O. I. A., R. O. I. P., and L. O. I. P., as first, second, third, and fourth positions respectively. The recent exhaustive article of Arthur Müller deals fully with this subject.

The nomenclature which we have adopted presents many advantages over the German, as it is based upon the relation of the presenting part to the maternal pelvis, and enables us to describe with accuracy the situation of the former at any period of labour.

Frequency of the Various Presentations and Positions.—According to the statistics collected by Schroeder, based upon several hundred thousand cases, the vertex presents in 95 per cent, the face in 0.6 per cent, and the breech in 3.11 per cent, transverse presentations occurring in only 0.56 per cent of all cases. Pinard gives 95.5, 0.4, 3.3 and 0.8 per cent respectively. These figures apply to all periods of pregnancy. But when the conditions at full term alone are considered, the predominance of vertex presentations becomes still more marked, as they are met with in 96.97 per cent of all cases; while breech presentations become less frequent, and occur only once in 62, as compared with once in 30 labours (1.77 and 3.3 per cent) respectively.

It is usually stated that about 70 per cent of all vertex presentations occur in the left, and only 30 per cent in the right position. Hecker estimated their relative frequency at 61.39 and 38.61 per cent respectively. Naegele first pointed out that the vertex was usually directed anteriorly in left, and posteriorly in right positions; so that the presenting part is usually found at one or other extremity of the right oblique diameter of the pelvis, owing to the fact that the left oblique diameter is materially encroached upon at its posterior extremity by the rectum.

Reasons for the Predominance of Head Presentations.—Hippocrates recognised the overwhelming frequency of head presentations at the end of pregnancy, but believed that the child presented by the breech up to the seventh month, when it suddenly turned and presented by the head, the process being often expressed by the French term *culbute*.

As a result of the more frequent examination of pregnant women, the error of the Hippocratic teachings was gradually demonstrated, so that from the time of Smellie and Baudelocque it was generally believed that head presentations predominated throughout all periods of pregnancy, but became more frequent in the later months. For many years it was taught that the presentation remained constant throughout pregnancy, and it was not until 1861 that Hecker and others demonstrated that it was not unusual for changes of position to occur even in the later months. Finally, it is now universally admitted that the presentation does not become definitely established until the presenting part enters the pelvic canal.

The theories put forward to account for the prevalence of head presentations are divided into two groups, the one being based upon gravitation, the other supposing a process of accommodation between the fœtus and the uterine cavity.

The *gravitation theory* was especially advocated by Matthews Duncan and G. Veit, both of whom showed that a fœtus recently dead, when placed in a vessel containing a solution of salt having about the same specific gravity as itself (1.050–1.055), floated with its head and right side downward. This result they attributed to the greater specific gravity of the head, together with the presence of the liver on the right side. Veit also showed that head presentations increase in frequency with the advance of pregnancy, but that breech presentations were noted much more frequently when the child was dead. This he attributed to the fact that the specific gravity of the head became diminished after death.

Furthermore, it was pointed out that since the axis of the uterus, with the woman in the upright position, forms an angle of about 35 degrees with the horizon, provided the experiments of Duncan and Veit held good, the head would necessarily sink downward, and the convex back of the fœtus would adapt itself to the concave anterior wall of the uterus; then, since the left margin of the latter would usually be directed somewhat forward, the frequency of the left anterior presentations could be readily explained.

Doubt has recently been cast upon the conclusions of Duncan and Veit by Schatz, who maintains that although their results were perfectly correct when experimenting with a medium of the same specific gravity as the fœtus, it has yet to be demonstrated that they hold good for the amniotic fluid, which, it must be remembered, possesses a specific gravity of between 1.008 and 1.009, or considerably less than that of the fœtus. Schatz suspended a recently dead fœtus from the pans of a balance in a solution of salt of the same specific gravity as the amniotic fluid, and found that the breech had a greater tendency to sink down than the head. He therefore concluded that some force other than gravity must be invoked to explain the frequency of head presentations.

We have been able to confirm Schatz's experiments, and found that the head sank downward, as described by Duncan and Veit, when the specific gravity of the medium in which it was suspended was in the neighbourhood of 1.050. But on gradually lowering it, by the addition of more water, the head slowly rose until the long axis of the child became horizontal, and as the specific gravity approached 1.008–1.010, the breech sank downward, thus showing that gravity does not account for the production of head presentations; for if it were the most important factor concerned, breech presentations would predominate at the end of pregnancy. As this is not the case, some other influence must be invoked to explain the prevalence of head presentations. This is supplied by the *theory of accommodation*, advanced by Dubois, Simpson, and Scanzoni, according to which they are brought about by a process of accommodation between the fœtal ovoid and the interior of the uterine cavity, the shape of the latter being such that the fœtus is most comfortable and fits it more accurately when presenting by the head. They held, therefore, that as soon as the fœtus came to occupy any other position, its cutaneous surface became irritated, whence resulted reflex movements of the extremities, giving rise in turn to uterine contractions, which tended to restore the head presentation. Pinard is an enthusiastic advocate of this theory.

The frequency of abnormal presentations in the early months of pregnancy, and in all conditions in which the uterus is abnormally distended by an excess of amniotic fluid, tends to substantiate this theory; for in such cases the body of the child does not come in contact with the uterine walls, and accordingly the conditions necessary for the production of the reflex movements, which give rise to accommodation, are entirely lacking, and gravity alone comes into play.

An exhaustive consideration of the various older theories can be found in the excellent monograph of Cohnstein published in 1868.

Methods of Diagnosing Position and Presentation of Fœtus.—The diagnostic methods at our disposal are fourfold: abdominal palpation, vaginal touch, combined examination, and auscultation.

Obstetrical Palpation.—Under ordinary circumstances external or abdominal palpation is the most reliable and valuable, and I should unhesitatingly choose it were I restricted to the employment of a single method of examination. In trained hands it enables one to make a satisfactory diagnosis without danger of infection and with the least possible discomfort to the patient, and it is not going too far to say that its popularization forms one of the greatest advances in modern obstetrics. Under these circumstances it behooves the student to become thoroughly familiar with the proper technique, and to avail himself of every opportunity to become proficient in the various manipulations.

Although crude forms of abdominal palpation had no doubt been practised from the earliest antiquity, just as they are still employed by many of the aboriginal peoples, its advantages were first pointed out by Roederer, Wigand, and Hohl, as late as the latter part of the seventeenth and the early part of the eighteenth century. Its practical importance, however, was not generally recognised until 1878, when Pinard published his work upon the subject, after which the method became popularized in France, but was not employed systematically in Germany and this country until Credé and Leopold had repeatedly urged its value.

In order to obtain satisfactory results, the examination should be made systematically by following the four manœuvres suggested by Leopold. The patient should be on a hard bed or sofa, with the abdomen bared, or at most covered with a thin chemise. During the first three manœuvres, the examiner stands at the side of the bed which is most convenient to him, and faces the patient, but reverses his position and faces her feet for the last manœuvre. (See Plates X, XI, XII, and XIII.)

First Manœuvre.—After ascertaining the outlines of the uterus, the fundus is gently palpated with the tips of the fingers of the two hands, and the fœtal pole occupying it differentiated, the breech giving the sensation of a large irregularly shaped, nodular body, and the head that of a hard, round object, which is freely movable and ballottable.

Second Manœuvre.—Having determined which pole of the fœtus lies at the fundus, the examiner places the palmar surface of his hands on either side of the abdomen and makes gentle but deep pressure. On one side he feels a hard resistant plane—the back—and on the other numerous nodulations—the small parts. In women with thin abdominal walls the legs and arms can readily be differentiated, but in fat persons only irregular nodulations can be felt. In the latter case, or when a considerable quantity of amniotic fluid is present, the appreciation of the back can be facilitated by making deep pressure with one hand while palpating with the other. After determining upon which side the back is situated, we next note whether it is directed anteriorly, transversely, or posteriorly, and thereby arrive at the position and variety of the presentation.

Third Manœuvre.—The examiner grasps the lower portion of the abdomen, just above the symphysis pubis, between the thumb and fingers of one hand, and tries to decide what is between them. If the presenting part be not engaged, a movable body will be felt, which is usually the head. The differentiation between it and the breech is made as at the fundus, the former being appreciated as a hard, round, ballottable body. If the presenting part be not engaged, this practically completes the examination, as we now know the situation of the head, breech, back, and extremities, and all that remains is to determine the attitude of the head. If careful palpation shows that the greatest cephalic prominence is on the same side as the small parts, we know that the head is flexed and that the vertex is the presenting part; but when the reverse is the case, we know that the head is extended and that we have a face presentation. On the other hand, if the presenting part be engaged, this manœuvre simply shows that the lower pole of the fœtus is fixed in the pelvis, and the details concerning it are ascertained as follows:

Fourth Manœuvre.—The examiner faces the patient's feet, and with the tips of the first three fingers of each hand makes deep pressure in the direction of the axis of the superior strait. If the head presents, he finds that one hand is arrested sooner than the other by a round body—the cephalic prominence; while the other hand descends deeper into the pelvis.

In vertex presentations, the prominence is on the same side as the small parts, and in face presentations on the same side as the back. Again, the degree of ease with which the prominence is felt indicates the extent to which descent has occurred. In breech presentations, the information obtained from this manœuvre is not so definite as in head presentations. In many instances, when the head has descended into the pelvis, the anterior shoulder of the child can be readily differentiated by the third manœuvre.

This method of examination is available throughout the later months of pregnancy, and in the intervals between the pains at the time of labour. By its use we cannot only determine the presentation and position of the child, but also obtain important information as to the extent to which the presenting part has descended into the pelvis. At the same time the size of the child can be roughly estimated and the second fœtus mapped out in twin pregnancy.

During uterine contractions, on carefully palpating in the region of the internal abdominal ring, one can often distinguish a rounded cord on either side—the *round ligaments*—from which important information may be obtained. In the first place, the intensity of their contraction gives us some idea of the manner in which the uterus is acting; and secondly, by noting their course, as pointed out by Palm and Leopold, we are enabled to diagnose the situation of the placenta in about 88 per cent of all cases. When the round ligaments are found converging towards the fundus of the uterus, the placenta is usually situated upon the posterior wall, whereas it is upon the anterior wall when they are parallel or diverging.

During labour, palpation also gives us valuable information concerning the *lower uterine segment*; when there exists some obstruction to the passage of the child, the *contraction ring* may be felt as a transverse ridge extending across the lower portion of the uterus. Moreover, in normal cases, we can differentiate by palpation between the contracting body of the uterus and the passive lower uterine segment; for during a pain the former presents a firm, hard sensation, while the latter appears elastic and almost fluctuant.

Vaginal Examination.—During pregnancy the results arrived at by vaginal examination, concerning the presentation and position of the child, are necessarily somewhat inconclusive, as one is obliged to palpate the presenting part through the lower uterine segment. During labour, on the other hand, after more or less complete dilatation of the cervix, important information may be obtained. In vertex presentations, the position and variety are determined by the differentiation of the various sutures and fontanelles; in face presentations, by the differentiation of the various portions of the face; and in breech presentations, by the palpation of the sacrum and ischial tuberosities.

Under the most favourable circumstances, the information to be derived from vaginal touch alone is not more accurate than that obtained by abdominal palpation, and in vertex presentations the fontanelles are not infrequently mistaken for one another, and occasionally face and breech presentations escape differentiation. Moreover, in the latter part of labour, after the formation of a fluid tumour beneath the skin covering the presenting part—the *caput succedaneum*—detection of the various diagnostic points often becomes impossible.

A much more serious objection, however, is the danger of puerperal infection, no matter how carefully the obstetrician may have attempted to disinfect his hands, for it is now generally admitted that absolute hand disinfection cannot always be accomplished; and even granting that the use of rubber gloves overcomes this difficulty, the gloved fingers may still carry pathogenic micro-organisms from the margins of the vulva up into the vagina, and thus infect the patient. Moreover, vaginal examination necessitates exposure of the patient, and subjects her to more or less serious inconvenience.

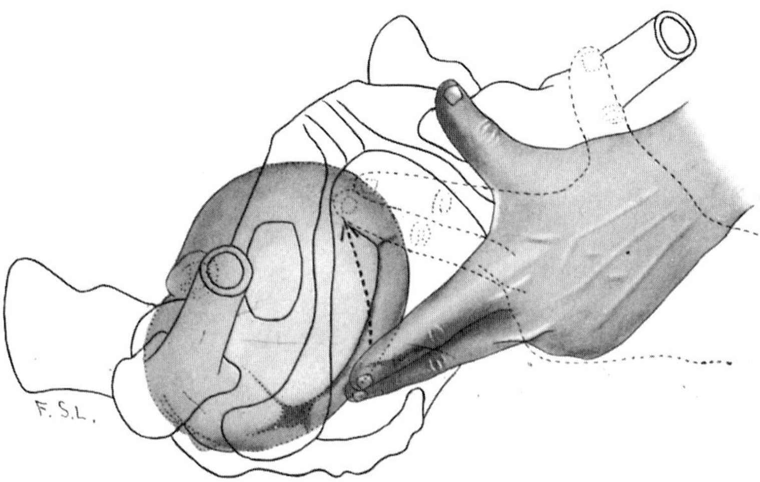

FIG. 188.—DIAGRAM SHOWING METHOD OF LOCATING SAGITTAL SUTURE ON VAGINAL EXAMINATION.

Accordingly, it is advisable to limit its employment as much as possible, and in normal cases to do away with it altogether. For if the patient has a normal pelvis, and we find by the fourth manœuvre that the head is deeply engaged, all that we gain by vaginal examination is information as to the degree of dilatation of the cervix, and this does not counterbalance the possible danger of infection. Accordingly, vaginal examination becomes absolutely necessary only in the few cases in which palpation does not give satisfactory results, or in those presenting some abnormality, or in which the course of labour is unduly delayed. Personally, I conduct more than 50 per cent of my private cases by palpation alone, and do not make a vaginal examination until about to discharge the patient.

In attempting to diagnose presentation and position by vaginal examination, it is advisable to pursue a definite routine, which is readily accomplished by three manœuvres.

First Manœuvre.—After most careful hand disinfection and appropriate preparation of the patient, two fingers of either the right or left hand, as best suits the examiner, are introduced into the vagina and carried up to the presenting part. A few moments suffice to determine whether it is a vertex, face, or breech.

Second Manœuvre.—If the vertex be presenting, the fingers are carried up behind the symphysis pubis, and are then swept backward over the head towards the sacrum. During this movement they necessarily cross the sagittal suture. When it is felt, its course is outlined, and we know that the small fontanelle lies at one, and the large fontanelle at the other end of it.

Third Manœuvre.—We then attempt to determine the position of the two fontanelles. For this purpose the fingers are passed to the anterior extremity of the sagittal suture, and the fontanelle there encountered is carefully examined and identified; then, by a circular motion, the fingers are passed around the side of the head until the other fontanelle is felt and differentiated. By this means the various sutures and fontanelles are

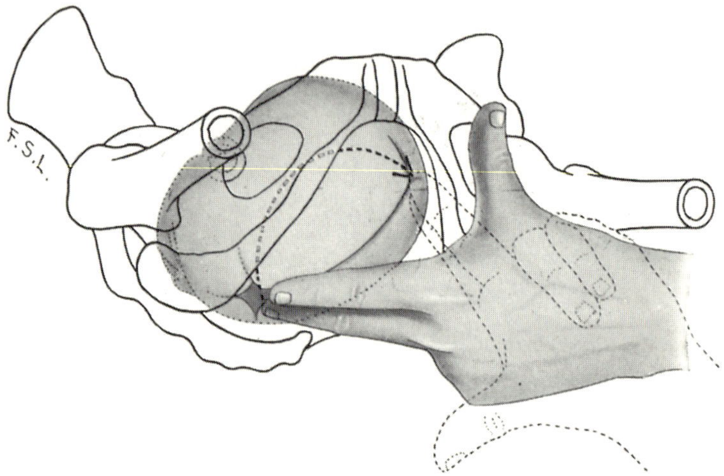

Fig. 189.—Diagram showing Method of Differentiating between the Fontanelles.

readily located, and the possibility of error is considerably lessened. In face and breech presentations it is still further minimized, as the various parts are more readily distinguished.

Combined Examination.—By combined examination we understand the introduction of two fingers of one hand into the vagina, and the application of the other hand over the lower portion of the abdomen. This method is rarely employed except when the presenting part is not engaged, and the external hand is used to fix it so as to permit the internal fingers to explore it satisfactorily.

Auscultation.—By itself, auscultation does not give very important information as to the presentation and position of the child, but it not infrequently re-enforces the results obtained by palpation. Ordinarily the heart sounds are transmitted through the convex portion of the fœtus, which lies in intimate contact with the uterine wall. Accordingly they are heard loudest through the back in the cervix and breech, and through the thorax in face presentations. The region of the woman's abdomen in which the fœtal heart is heard most plainly varies according to the presentation. In head presentations the point of maximum intensity is usually midway between the umbilicus and the anterior superior spine of the ilium, while in breech presentations it is usually about on a level with the umbilicus.

Auscultation frequently gives us not a little supplementary aid in determining the position of the child. Thus, in occipito-anterior presentations the heart is usually best heard a short distance from the middle line; in the transverse varieties it is heard more laterally, and in the posterior varieties well back in the patient's flank. Occasionally, however, in right occipito-posterior presentations, the information gained from the position of the fœtal heart is misleading, and may give rise to serious diagnostic errors, for if the flexion of the head be imperfect, the thorax may become convex, and the heart sounds being transmitted through it would apparently indicate a left anterior position.

LITERATURE

Ahlfeld. Lehrbuch der Geburtshülfe, II. Aufl., Leipzig, 1898.

Baudelocque. L'art des accouchements. Paris, 1789, 2me éd.

Cohnstein. Die Aetiologie der normalen Kinderlage. Monatsschr. f. Geburtsk., 1868, xxxi, 141–193.

Credé. Gesunde und kranke Wöchnerinnen. Leipzig, 1886, 80–81.

Credé und Leopold. Die geburtshülfliche Untersuchung. Leipzig, 1892.

Döderlein. Leitfaden für den geburtshülflichen Operationskurs. Leipzig, 1893.

Dubois. Mémoire sur la cause des présentations de la tête. Mém. de l'Acad. de Méd., 1833, ii.

Duncan. The Position of the Fœtus. Researches in Obstetrics, Edinburgh, 1868, 14–37; also Edinburgh Med. and Surg. Jour., 1855.

Farabeuf et Varnier. Introduction à l'étude clinique et à la pratique des accouchements. Paris.

Hecker. Klinik der Geburtshülfe, Leipzig, 1861, i, 17.

Statistisches aus der Gebäranstalt München. Archiv f. Gyn., 1882, xx, 378–398.

Hohl. Die geburtshülfliche Exploration, Halle, 1834, ii, 144–166.

International Medical Congress. Uniformity in Obstetrical Nomenclature. American Jour. Obst., 1889, xx, 1084–1086.

La Chapelle, Madame. Pratique des accouchements, Paris, 1821, i, 17–25.

Leopold. Die Diagnose des Placentarsitzes in der Schwangerschaft und während der Geburt. Arbeiten aus der Dresdener Frauenklinik, 1895, ii, 151–166.

Leopold und Goldberg. Ueber die Entbehrlichkeit der Scheiden-Ausspülungen, etc., und über die grösstmögliche Verwerthung der äusseren Untersuchung in der Geburtshülfe. Archiv f. Gyn., 1891, xl, 439–473.

Leopold und Orb. Die Leitung normaler Geburten nur durch äussere Untersuchung. Archiv f. Gyn., 1895, xlix, 304–323.

Leopold und Pantzer. Die Beschränkung der inneren und die grösstmögliche Verwerthung der äusseren Untersuchung in der Geburtshülfe. Archiv f. Gyn., 1890, xxxviii, 330–366.

Leopold und Spörlin. Die Leitung der regelmässigen Geburten nur durch äussere Untersuchung. Archiv f. Gyn., 1894, xlv, 337–368.

Müller, A. Ueber die Ursachen der Ungleichheit und Unklarheit in der Benennung und Eintheilung der Kindeslagen. Monatsschr. f. Geb. u. Gyn., 1900, xii, 161–181, 266–291.

Naegele. Die Lehre vom Mechanismus der Geburt, Mainz, 1838, 10.

PALM. Ueber die Diagnose des Placentarsitzes in der Schwangerschaft, etc. Zeitschr. f. Geb. u. Gyn., 1893, xxv, 317–350.

PINARD. L'accommodation fœtale. Traité du palper abdominal. Paris, 1878; 2me ed., 1889.

ROEDERER. Elementa artis obstetriciae. Goettingae, 1766.

SCANZONI. Lage und Haltung des Kindes in der Gebärmutter. Lehrbuch der Geb., II. Aufl., Wien, 1853, 89–93.

SCHATZ. Ueber den Schwerpunkt der Frucht. Centralbl. f. Gyn., 1900, Nr. 40, 1033–1036.

SCHROEDER, OLSHAUSEN und VEIT. Lehrbuch der Geburtshülfe, XIII. Aufl., 1899.

SIMPSON. Attitude and Positions of the Fœtus *in utero.* Monthly Journal of Med. Sciences, ix, 1848–'49.

SMELLIE. A Treatise on the Theory and Practice of Midwifery, 8th ed., London, 1774.

VEIT, G. Die Lagenverhältnisse bei Früh- und Zwillingsgeburten. Scanzoni's Beiträge, 1860, iv, 279–292.

WIGAND. Die Geburt des Menschen. Berlin, 1820, ii, 99.

PHYSIOLOGY OF LABOUR

CHAPTER X

THE PHYSIOLOGY AND CLINICAL COURSE OF LABOUR

By labour we understand the process which brings about the separation of the mature or nearly mature product of conception from the interior of the uterus, and its extrusion from the maternal organism, whether the birth occurs spontaneously or requires external aid.

Cause of the Onset of Labour.—From time immemorial inquiring minds have sought an explanation for the fact that labour usually ensues about two hundred and eighty days after the appearance of the last menstrual period, but thus far no satisfactory universal cause has been discovered. The following are among the most important theories which have been advanced as to its causation:

1. The growing irritability of the uterus, associated with an increase in the frequency and strength of the intermittent contractions.
2. Increasing distention of the uterus.
3. Dilatation of the cervix by the presenting part.
4. Increasing distention of the lower uterine segment, with pressure upon the neighbouring nervous structures.
5. Changes in the decidua—loosening, thinning, and thrombosis.
6. Excess of carbon dioxide or lack of oxygen in the placental blood, acting on a centre in the medulla.
7. The circulation of fœtal metabolic products acting upon a centre in the medulla.
8. Menstrual periodicity.
9. Heredity and habit.
10. Senility of the placenta.
11. Physical and emotional causes.

1. The increasing readiness with which the uterus reacts to stimulation during the later months of pregnancy affords abundant evidence of its growing irritability. The intermittent contractions, which occur at intervals throughout pregnancy, come on more frequently at this time, and with so much greater intensity that it is ofttimes difficult, in the last few weeks before delivery, to distinguish between them and actual labour pains.

2. Since the time of Mauriceau it has been believed that the uterus, when distended up to a certain point, must begin to contract and attempt to empty itself, just as happens in the case of any other hollow viscus. This presumption is supported by the frequency with which premature

labour occurs in hydramnios or twin pregnancies. On the other hand, even an extreme distention does not necessarily give rise to labour, as is shown by the cases of prolonged pregnancy which are associated with large children.

3. Galen supposed that labour resulted from gradual dilatation of the cervix, which was brought about by the pressure of the presenting part, and the view has had numerous adherents ever since. That the condition of the cervix is not the sole factor is shown by the fact that in a certain number of instances, especially in twin pregnancies, considerable dilatation may exist for days or even weeks before the onset of labour.

4. Keilmann (1891) and Knüpffer advanced the theory that the onset of labour was the result of the gradual formation of the lower uterine segment, with consequent pressure upon the surrounding nervous ganglia. Their work was done upon the bat and was quite convincing, so far as that animal is concerned. But inasmuch as their conclusions are based upon the assumption that the lower uterine segment is formed from the upper portion of the cervix, it cannot be accepted for human beings without hesitation.

5. Naegele, Simpson, Scanzoni, and others believed that the decidua in the latter weeks of pregnancy underwent fatty degeneration, which resulted in the partial separation of the ovum and its practical conversion into a foreign body, which then gave rise to uterine contractions. More recent investigations, however, have shown that such changes occur rarely, if at all.

It has also been stated that the septa, by which the glandular spaces of the compact layer of the decidua are bounded, become progressively thinner in the later months of pregnancy, so that in the last few weeks very slight movements suffice to bring about more or less extensive separation of the ovum from the uterine wall. No doubt the septa are considerably thinner in the later than in the earlier months of pregnancy, but they are not torn through, as a rule, until after the expulsion of the fœtus.

6. Brown-Séquard, in 1853, demonstrated that an excess of carbon dioxide in the blood led to energetic uterine contractions, and his results have been confirmed by all subsequent investigators (Keiffer). In spite of this fact, however, it is difficult to explain why there should be a marked and sudden increase in the amount of carbon dioxide in the blood sufficient to give rise to labour at the appointed time.

Friedländer, Leopold, and others have described giant cells in the depths of the decidua. These, they claimed, were associated with the production of thrombosis in many of its vessels, in consequence of which the placental blood became loaded with carbon dioxide, which in turn stimulated a centre in the medulla. More recent work, however, has shown that the giant cells play little if any part in the production of the thrombosis.

7. Spiegelberg advanced the view that the onset of labour was due to fœtal rather than maternal changes. He considered that the mature fœtus needed materials for its sustenance other than those furnished by the placenta, and that as a result of insufficient nutrition certain excrementitious substances gained access to the maternal circulation, and in some way stimulated the uterine centre.

8. Mende, Tyler-Smith, Löwenhardt, Beard, and others believe that there is an increased tendency towards uterine contractions at the periods at which the menstrual flow should appear if the patient were not pregnant, and that these reach their acme at about the date of the tenth menstrual period and give rise to labour.

9. Geyl and others are inclined to attribute the onset of labour at the usual time to the fact that Nature, after ages of experiment, has found the end of the tenth month to be the most suitable time. For when labour occurs at a later period it is usually very difficult and results in dead children, while at an earlier period puny children are born which usually perish soon after birth.

10. Eden and the writer have pointed out that the frequent occurrence of infarct formation in the placenta at term must be regarded as evidence of its senility, and that this change is analogous to the obliteration and atrophy of the chorion læve at an earlier period. Where these changes are marked the nutrition of the fœtus must be interfered with, and it is possible that certain of its metabolic products may result in stimulation of the uterine centre.

11. It is also a well-known fact that excessive physical exercise, sudden jars or violence, as well as extreme mental emotion, such as grief and anger, may lead to the termination of pregnancy.

While, then, there is no lack of theories upon the subject, at the same time it is manifest that most of them are extremely unsatisfactory, and that none are of universal application. It is probable, therefore, that in the majority of cases the onset of labour is due to the combination of a number of the above-mentioned causes, and that only some slight stimulus or irritant is needed to set it in progress. On the other hand, it is possible that some law may be discovered in the future which will explain the rhythm of the various sexual functions in women—menstruation, as well as the onset of labour.

Nearly all of the theories to which reference has been made require the intervention of the nervous system for the ultimate production of labour. It is generally admitted that there exists in the medulla a centre for uterine contractions, which can be stimulated by an excess of carbon dioxide in the blood, by anæmia and the presence of various toxic substances; and it seems highly probable that the frequency of premature labour in cases of renal insufficiency and eclampsia may be due to the action of metabolic poisons upon this centre. Furthermore, it seems likely that another centre exists in the lower portion of the lumbar cord, which, however, is subsidiary in character, inasmuch as labour may ensue without its intervention, as is demonstrated by the fact that normal but painless deliveries have occurred following the severance of the cord above the lumbar region.

According to Keiffer the uterus has a threefold nervous supply, which is derived principally from the sympathetic system, partly from branches of the lumbar cord, and partly from its intrinsic nerves, and that contractions may result from the stimulation of all or any one of them.

Reflex contractions of the uterus can be induced by the stimulation of the central end of any spinal nerve, and it is evident, therefore, that the reflex impulses must be transmitted through the cord. The only exception to this rule, so far as I am aware, is the observation of Keiffer concerning the inhibitory effect of stimulation of the crural nerve. But, on the other hand, it has been shown by the experimental work of Rein that the transmission of impulses through the cord is not absolutely necessary to the production of labour. He isolated the uterus in rabbits from all connection with the cerebro-spinal system, and found that labour proceeded without difficulty. Similar observations have been made upon human beings after injuries to the lower portion of the cord (Routh, Benicke, Lusk, and others).

Oser and Schlesinger, on the other hand, showed that pregnancy and labour might go on without interruption and end with normal labour after complete severance of the sympathetic fibres which supply the uterus. Moreover, Kehrer has demonstrated that the organ can continue to contract after its removal from the body, provided it be kept moist and sufficiently warm. In view of these facts, therefore, it must be admitted that the uterus contains an intrinsic nerve supply, more or less similar to that found in the heart and other organs.

Labour Pains.—With the onset of labour, the painless intermittent contractions which have persisted throughout pregnancy are replaced by others of increasing intensity, giving rise to severe pain, and bringing about the dilatation of the cervix and the expulsion of the child and placenta.

The uterine contractions, just as those of all other non-striated muscles, are independent of the will of the patient, and can neither be increased nor diminished in frequency by her volition. But at the same time they may be affected by the emotions, and any sudden excitement may either check them or cause them to become more violent. Thus, it is a matter of common observation that the entrance of the obstetrician may be followed by a marked lull in the intensity and frequency of the pains.

The contractions begin slowly, gradually reach an acme, and then gradually diminish in intensity, the active process being followed by a pause of some length. The tracings of Schatz and Polaillon show that the period of increase occupies the greater portion of the pain, and that its acme is of very short duration. In the lower animals which possess bicornuate uteri, the contractions are distinctly peristaltic in character; but the appearance of the uterus at Cæsarean sections does not appear to indicate that such is the case in human beings, although Schatz believes that a certain amount of peristalsis may be observed. It is important to bear in mind that labour pains are effective only during the period of increase, and that the tightly contracted organ is worthless from a mechanical standpoint.

These uterine contractions are nearly always accompanied by painful sensations, whence the term "labour pains," although the amount of suffering varies markedly in different individuals. The pain usually begins in the sacral region and then slowly passes to the abdomen and down the thighs. In the early stages of labour it is due almost exclusively to pressure upon the nerve endings between the muscle fibres; but in the later stages it is augmented by the overstretching and dilatation of the soft parts, and becomes most marked when the head distends the vulva just before its birth. Occasionally the suffering experienced during labour is very slight, and in rare instances the process may be almost entirely painless, even though the patient be perfectly conscious. A considerable number of such cases have been collected by Coliez in a recent thesis. Usually, however, the pains are very severe, and not infrequently are almost insupportable.

At the onset of labour the pains come on at intervals of from fifteen to thirty minutes; as it advances they gradually become more frequent, and eventually occur every two or three minutes. Their average duration is about one minute—thirty to ninety seconds—though suffering is not experienced during the entire contraction, as the hand placed over the abdomen may feel the uterus becoming hard for several seconds before the patient perceives the slightest pain.

Force exerted by Labour Pains.—On this point there has been a good deal of misconception, and a marked tendency towards exaggeration appears in the writings of not a few authors. Thus Sterne, in Tristram Shandy, estimated that the force exerted at each pain during labour amounted to 470 pounds, while Professor Haughton put it at 577 pounds. Poppel, Duncan, Ribemont, and others have attempted to approximate it by trying to determine the force necessary to cause the rupture of the membranes outside of the body. This, they found, varied markedly, the extremes being 2,134 and 17,301 grammes. In 100 experiments Duncan placed the extremes at 4 and 37.58 pounds respectively, with an average of 16.73 pounds.

Joulin and other observers have attempted to solve the problem by calculating the force exerted in forceps deliveries. Thus, on interpolating a dynamometer between the operator and the ends of the instrument, it was found that the tractile force rarely exceeded 80, though in some cases it reached 100 pounds. A greater force than this cannot come into play, as it has been shown that one of 120 pounds is sufficient to tear the child's head from its body.

Schatz approached the subject in a more accurate manner, and inserted into the uterus a rubber bag which was connected with a manometer. In this way he found that the intra-uterine pressure, in the intervals between the contractions, was represented by a column of mercury 20 millimetres high, 5 of which were due to the tonicity of the uterine walls and 15 to its contents. During the pains, however, the mercury rose considerably, reaching a height of from 80 to 250 millimetres, which corresponds to a force of $8\frac{1}{2}$ to $27\frac{1}{2}$ pounds. He also showed that the force exerted by the uterus increases markedly when the fœtus is partially expelled from it.

A rough idea may also be gained by estimating the expenditure of energy necessary to restrain the head as it emerges from the vulva. This rarely exceeds 50 pounds, although the obstetrician not infrequently finds it impossible to hold it back at the acme of a pain. This inability is in great part due to the disadvantageous manner in which one is obliged to exert one's energy, rather than to the actual force exerted by the uterine and abdominal contractions.

Physical Changes during Uterine Contractions.—During contraction the uterus undergoes marked changes in shape. With the patient on her back, the organ in the flaccid state rests upon the vertebral column, and its transverse equals or exceeds its vertical diameter. But when it contracts the uterus leaves the vertebral column, becomes more erect, and pushes the anterior abdominal wall forward. At the same time the vertical increases at the expense of the transverse diameter (Fig. 190).

The dilatation of the cervix is usually brought about solely by the action of the uterine muscles, whereas during the expulsion of the child those of the abdominal wall also come into play. During the second stage the patient braces her body against some fixed object, takes a deep inspiration, closes the glottis, and makes forcible straining movements with the

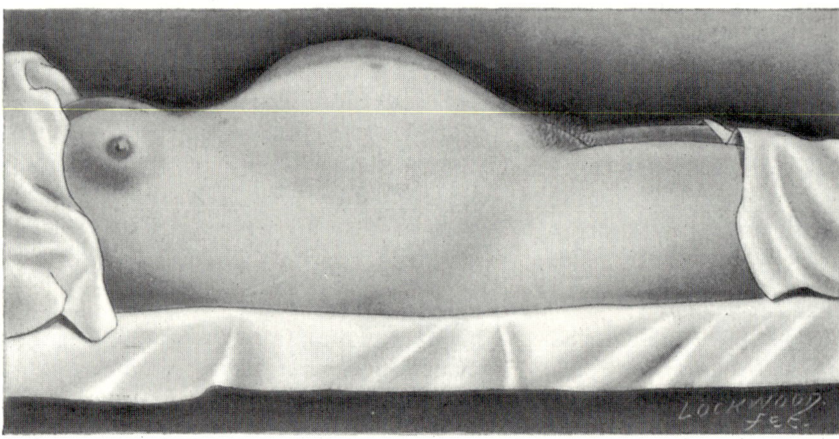

Fig. 190.—Composite Picture, showing Change in Shape of Abdomen before and during a Uterine Contraction, the Darker Outlines indicating Contraction.

abdominal and respiratory muscles. By these means the intra-abdominal pressure is markedly increased, and is transmitted directly to the uterus. At first these movements are voluntary, but as labour advances they pass beyond the control of the will, and may occur even with the patient under profound anæsthesia.

The abdominal muscles, therefore, play an important part in the expulsion of the child, which in many instances makes no progress without their aid. The fact that spontaneous labours occasionally occur in women who are paralyzed from the waist down shows that their action is not indispensable in every case; but, on the other hand, the application of low forceps is frequently rendered necessary by the inability of the abdominal muscles to do their work, or to the unwillingness of the patient to bear the pain associated with their employment.

The various ligamentary structures connected with the uterus also take part in the contractions. Of these the most important are the round ligaments, which in contracting tend to draw the fundus of the uterus forward and to fix it in position. They can be readily palpated through the abdominal wall, and some idea of the intensity of the uterine contractions may be gained from their consistency.

The part played by the vagina during labour is almost entirely passive, and it is only after the expulsion of the child that the contraction of the muscular elements in its walls comes into play.

The general arterial tension is raised during the labour pains, as is indicated by the flushed look of the patient. The pulse becomes accelerated during, and slower in the intervals between the pains. It is also stated that the temperature rises a fraction of a degree during each pain, though its detection requires the employment of very accurate thermometers. Respiration becomes slower during the contractions, more rapid in the interval between them, and is totally abolished during the expulsive pains of the second stage of labour.

Clinical Course of Labour.—Before taking up the consideration of the forces concerned in the expulsion of the fœtus and the mechanism by which it is accomplished, it is advisable for the student to follow as a spectator the course of parturition in a primiparous woman.

Several weeks before the onset of labour the abdomen undergoes a marked change in shape, its lower portion becoming more pendulous; whereas in the neighbourhood of the costal margin it looks decidedly flatter. This change is perceived by the woman herself, who feels that her waist has become lower; and occasionally it occurs so suddenly as to cause her to fear that something has given way inside her abdomen.

Abdominal palpation at this period shows that the fundus of the uterus has descended from the position which it occupied at the ninth month, and resumed that of the eighth; while the third manœuvre shows that the head, which was previously freely movable, has become fixed in the superior strait. These changes are most marked in primiparæ, and frequently do not occur in multiparæ until the onset of labour.

After this the patient experiences considerable relief from the respiratory disturbances from which she may have suffered; but at the same time locomotion may become more difficult, and she may suffer from severe cramp-like pains in the lower extremities and a more frequent desire to urinate.

During the last few weeks of pregnancy the vaginal secretion is increased in amount, the labia become more swollen and succulent, gape more or less widely, and not infrequently the patient may experience a few transient pains for a number of days before confinement.

For purposes of description, labour is divided into three stages: The first, or period of dilatation, extends from the commencement of labour until the cervix is completely dilated. The second, or period of expulsion, extends from the complete dilatation of the cervix to the birth of the child; while the third stage, or placental period, lasts from the birth of the child to the extrusion of the placenta.

First Stage.—About the end of the tenth lunar month the primiparous patient begins to experience cramp-like pains in the lower portion of her abdomen, which she frequently mistakes for intestinal colic. At first these sensations recur only at long intervals, but soon are felt more frequently. They are most marked in the lumbar region and gradually extend towards

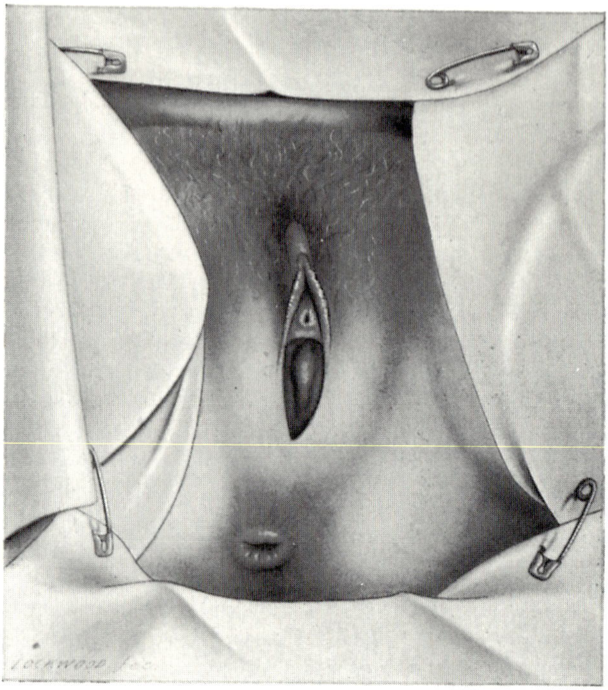

Fig. 191.—Birth of Head, Scalp appearing at Vulva.

the abdomen and down the thighs. As the pains become more frequent they likewise increase in severity, and in the latter part of the first stage the patient may complain bitterly, and often seeks to ease herself by making pressure over the sacral region.

The result of the pains in this stage of labour is to bring about the dilatation of the cervix, and as it slowly yields to the pressure of the amniotic fluid contained in the membranes, slight lesions occur about its margins, which are manifested by a small admixture of blood with the vaginal discharge—the "*show.*" During this period the patient is perfectly comfortable between the pains, and for a time can attend to her ordinary avocations; but as they become more severe, she assumes a sitting or leaning posture, and frequently gives utterance to short, sharp, querulous cries.

After the pains have continued for from twelve to fifteen hours, more or less, there is a sudden gush of clear fluid from the vagina, which in the majority of cases indicates that the cervix has become completely dilated, and that the membranes, having fulfilled their function as a hydrostatic wedge, have ruptured. The amount of fluid which escapes varies according to the situation of the point of rupture and the position of the presenting part. In vertex presentations, where the pelvis is normal, the cervix is tamponed, so to speak, by the rounded head, and only the portion of liquor amnii which lies in front of it escapes. On the other hand, if the head be not engaged, or there be some disproportion between it and the presenting part, the entire amount of amniotic fluid may escape. But even in perfectly normal cases a small quantity gushes out with each pain.

Not infrequently the membranes may rupture before complete dilatation of the cervix, and occasionally even before the onset of labour. Under such circumstances the presenting part has to act as a dilating wedge, and as it fills out the cervix less completely and accurately than the unruptured membranes, dilatation proceeds more slowly. These are instances of what are commonly known as *dry labours.*

Second Stage.—For a short time after rupture of the membranes there is a lull in the labour pains, after which they recur with increasing frequency and vigour, and compel the patient to take to her bed, where if left to herself she assumes a crouching or squatting posture. During this period the abdominal muscles are brought into play. At first the patient, with each uterine pain, may cause them to contract by an effort of her will. Later, however, this act becomes involuntary, and she is usually unable to resist bearing down. At the onset of the pain she braces her feet against

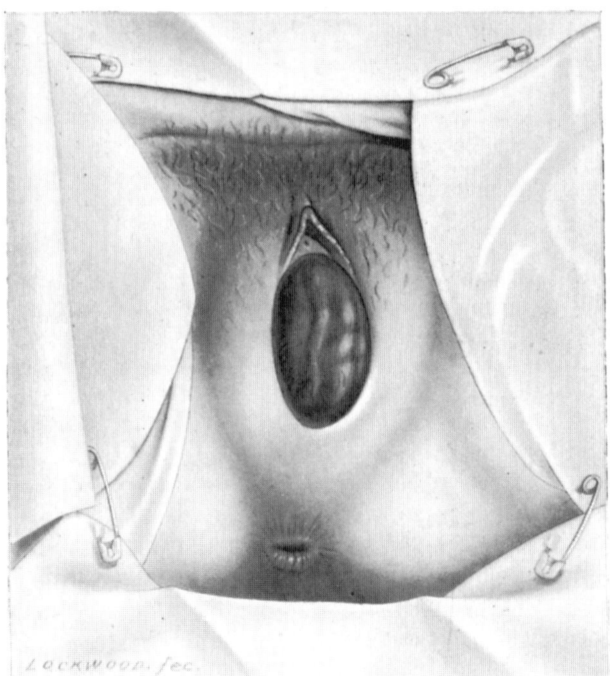

Fig. 192.—Birth of Head, Vulva partially Distended.

some solid object, takes a deep inspiration, and brings her abdominal and respiratory muscles into active play, her efforts being accompanied by a characteristic grunting sound. At the same time her face becomes markedly congested, and in the later stages of labour covered with sweat. As the pain passes off, the glottis is opened and respiration re-established, the same phenomena being repeated as soon as another contraction comes on.

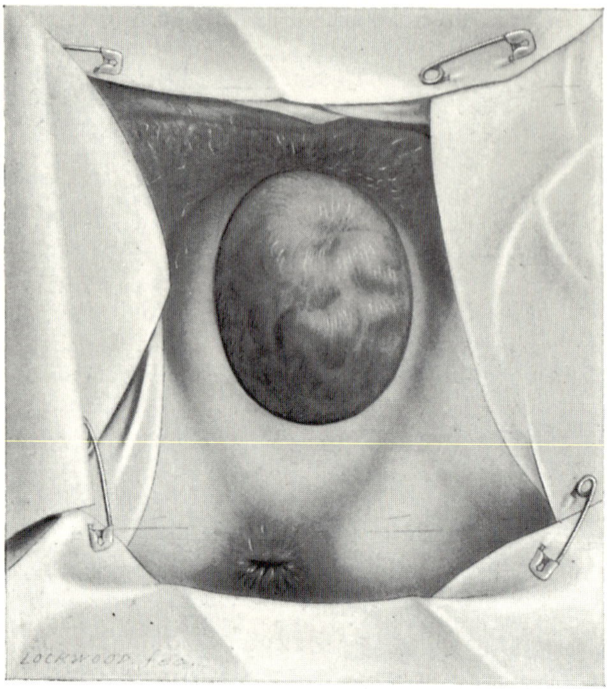

Fig. 193.—Birth of Head, Vulva completely Distended.

It is during this period that the child descends through the pelvis. After expulsive pains have continued for about an hour the patient experiences a marked desire to go to stool, which indicates that the head has passed into the pelvic cavity and is pressing upon the rectum. In a short time the pelvic floor may be seen to bulge with each pain, and a little later the scalp of the fœtus may be detected through the slit-like vulval opening. With each subsequent pain the perinæum bulges more and more, and the vulva becomes more and more dilated and distended by the head, being gradually converted into an ovoid, and at last into an almost circular opening. With the subsidence of each contraction, it becomes smaller and the head recedes from it, to advance again with the next pain.

As labour progresses the perinæum becomes still more distended and thinner, especially in its anterior portion; so that eventually its frenulum does not exceed a piece of paper in thickness, and looks as if it would rupture with each pain. At the same time the anus becomes markedly stretched and protuberant, and the anterior wall of the rectum protrudes through it. By this time the perinæum has become converted into a deep gutter, 6 to 7 centimetres long, at the end of which is the vulval opening, which looks almost directly upward and is distended by the head of the child, the occiput being pressed firmly against the symphysis pubis. The distention of the vulva is most marked at its perineal margin, and only slight at its lateral portions.

The head advances a little with each pain and recedes in the intervals between them. This continues until the parietal bosses become engaged in the vulva, when further recession becomes impossible, and with the next two or three pains it is rapidly expelled by a movement of extension, the base of the occiput rotating around the lower margin of the symphysis pubis as a fulcrum, while the bregma, brow, and face successively pass over the frenulum. In the majority of cases the perinæum is unable to withstand the strain to which it is subjected, and tears in its anterior portion, though usually only to a slight extent.

Immediately after its birth the head falls backward, so that the face comes almost in contact with the anus. In a few moments the occiput turns towards the one or other thigh, and eventually the entire head assumes a transverse position. This is known as external rotation or restitution, and serves to bring the bisacromial diameter of the child into relation with the antero-posterior diameter of the pelvic outlet.

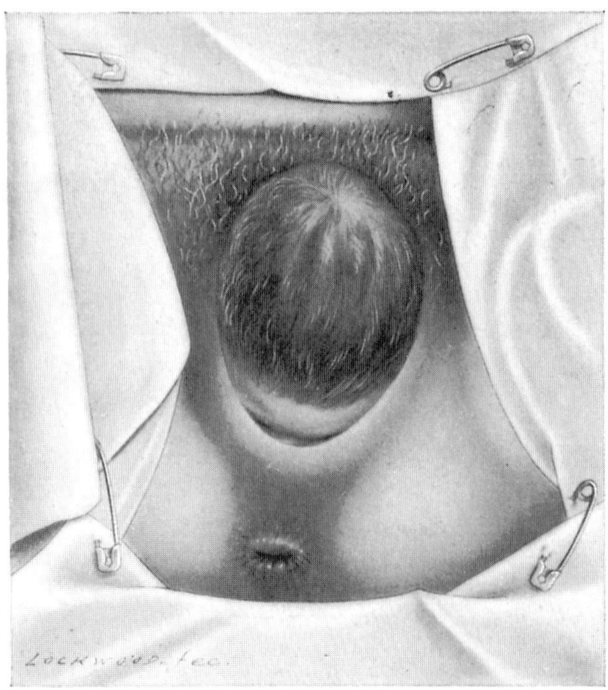

Fig. 194.—Birth of Head, showing Delivery by Extension.

At this time the perinæum is quite tightly retracted around the neck of the infant, whose face in consequence becomes markedly congested, so that the inexperienced obstetrician often has an almost uncontrollable desire to seize the head and to extract the child by traction upon it. This, however, is usually unnecessary, for the next pain forces the anterior shoulder down under the symphysis pubis, where it becomes fixed; while the posterior shoulder emerges over the anterior margin of the perinæum, after which the body of the child is rapidly expelled by a movement of lateral curvature, corresponding to the axis of the birth canal.

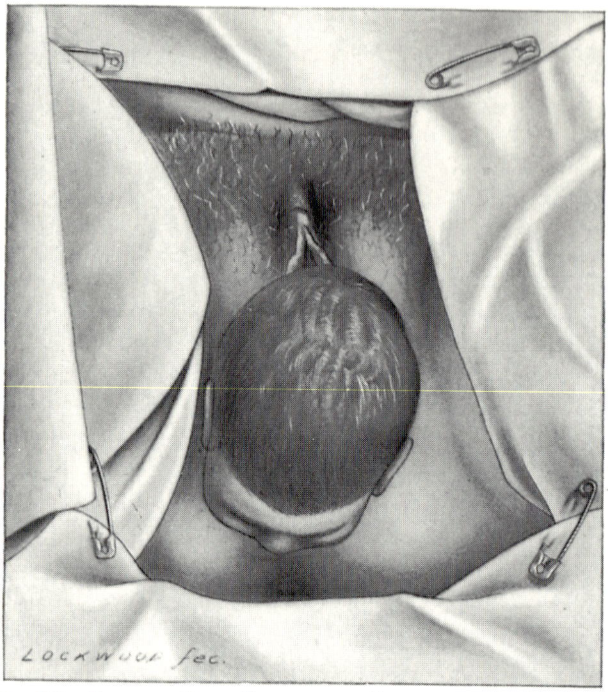

FIG. 195.—BIRTH OF HEAD, FACE FALLING BACKWARD TOWARDS ANUS.

Immediately following the child comes a gush of amniotic fluid, which represents the portion which did not escape at the time of rupture of the membranes, and is more or less tinged with blood.

In primiparous women the second stage of labour usually lasts about two hours, and a much shorter period in multiparous women, in whom two or three pains not infrequently suffice for the completion of the period of expulsion.

Third Stage.—For a few minutes after the birth of the child there is a cessation of the uterine contractions, and the patient experiences a marked sense of relief. On glancing at the abdomen it is seen that the uterus has become much smaller and forms a solid tumour which barely reaches the umbilicus. After a longer or shorter period the uterine contractions commence once more and the woman begins to bear down; a few moments later the fundus of the uterus may be seen to rise up for several centimetres, and a slight tumefaction appears immediately above the symphysis pubis. (See Figs. 284 and 285.) This indicates that the placenta has become separated from the interior of the uterus and is now in the lower uterine segment or the upper portion of the vagina. From this position it is expelled by the action of the abdominal muscles, the time varying according to the efficiency of their contraction. In some women the entire placental period may be terminated spontaneously within a few minutes after the birth of the child, while in others the placenta may remain in the lower uterine segment for hours unless forced from it by proper manipulation on the part of the obstetrician.

During the third stage there is nearly always a slight amount of hæmorrhage, which in normal cases amounts to 300 or 400 cubic centimetres. Not infrequently the patient may have a chill during this period, or immediately after its completion. This, although it may appear somewhat alarming, in itself has no significance, as it is merely a vaso-motor phenomenon.

Duration of Labour.—The duration of labour presents considerable individual variations, and is usually about six hours longer in primiparæ than in multiparæ. Generally speaking, the average for the former is about eighteen hours, of which sixteen are occupied by the first, one and

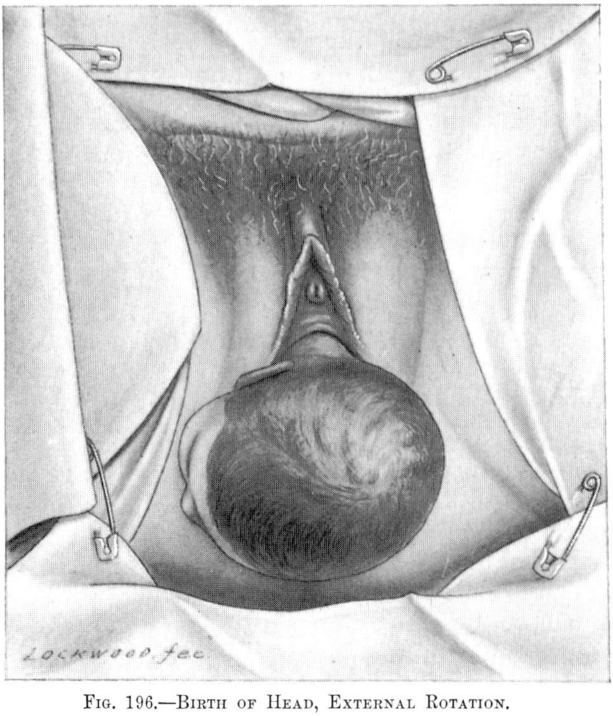

FIG. 196.—BIRTH OF HEAD, EXTERNAL ROTATION.

three quarters to two by the second, and a quarter to a half hour by the third stage of labour; for the latter it is about twelve hours, eleven of which are occupied by the first, and one by the second stage.

According to G. Veit, the average duration of labour is twenty hours for primiparæ and twelve for multiparæ; according to Spiegelberg, seventeen and twelve hours respectively; while Varnier, from the records of 2,000 cases, one half of which were primiparæ, estimates it at thirteen and a half and seven and a half hours respectively; the second stage lasting seventy-five minutes in the former, and thirty-five minutes in the latter.

The slower course of labour in primiparæ is due to the resistance offered by the soft parts. Occasionally labour may be extremely rapid, and even in primiparæ the entire process is not very infrequently completed within a few hours; while, on the other hand, a duration of twenty-four to thirty-six hours or even longer is not unusual.

Labour is usually more prolonged in elderly than in young primiparæ—that is, after the thirtieth year. According to Ahlfeld, it averages seven hours longer in the former, though Varnier states that the difference is very much less. At the same time the latter author points out that forceps are much more frequently required in older primiparæ, being applied in 25 per cent and 1.6 per cent of the cases respectively, thus indicating that labour would have lasted much longer had it not been terminated by operative means.

It is generally stated that the majority of women fall into labour in the early evening, and that delivery occurs most frequently between the hours of 2 and 4 A. M.

LITERATURE

AHLFELD. Die Geburten älterer Erstgeschwängerten. Archiv f. Gyn., 1872, iv, 510–520.

BEARD. The Span of Gestation and the Cause of Birth. Jena, 1897.

BENICKE. Vier Fälle von Geburtscomplication durch seltene Erkrankungen der Mutter. Zeitschr. f. Geb. u. Gyn., 1877, i, 24–72.

BROWN-SÉQUARD. Experimental Researches applied to Physiology and Pathology, 1853, 117.

COLIEZ. Quelques considérations médico-légales sur les accouchements inconscients et sans douleur. Thèse de Paris, 1899.

DUNCAN. A Contribution to the Dynamics of Labour. Researches in Obstetrics, Edinburgh, 1868, 229–333.

EDEN. A Study of the Human Placenta. Jour. Path. and Bacteriology, 1897, iv, 265–282.

GEYL. Ueber die Ursache des Geburtseintrittes. Archiv f. Gyn., 1881, xvii, 1–18.

JOULIN. Mémoire sur l'emploi de la force en obstétrique. Arch. gén. de méd., fév. et mars, 1867.

KEHRER. Die Zusammenziehungen der glatten Genitalmuskulatur, etc. Beiträge zur vergleich. und exp. Geburtskunde, 1867, Heft II, 41–50.

KEIFFER. Recherches sur la physiologie de l'utérus, Bruxelles, 1896.

KEILMANN. Zur Klärung der Cervixfrage. Zeitschr. f. Geb. u. Gyn., 1891, xxii, 106–178.

KNÜPFFER. Ueber die Ursache des Geburtseintrittes, etc. D. I., Dorpat, 1892.

LEOPOLD. Studien über die Uterusschleimhaut, etc. Archiv f. Gyn., 1877, xi, 443–500.

LÖWENHARDT. Die Berechnung und die Dauer der Schwangerschaft. Archiv f. Gyn., 1872, iii, 356–391.

LUSK. The Science and Art of Midwifery. New edition, 1895, 126.

MAURICEAU. Traité des maladies des femmes grosses, etc., 6me éd., 1721, 203.

MENDE. Handbuch der gerichtlichen Medicin, 1821, ii, 303.

NAEGELE. Versuche eines Systems der Geburtshülfe, 1812, 97.

OSER und SCHLESINGER. Exper. Untersuchungen über Uterusbewegungen. Stricker's med. Jahrbücher, 1872, 57.

POLAILLON. Recherches sur la physiologie de l'utérus gravide. Paris, 1880.

POPPEL. Ueber die Resistenz der Eihäute. Monatsschr. f. Geburtskunde, 1863, xxii, 1–15.

REIN. Beitrag zur Lehre von der Innervation des Uterus. Pflüger's Archiv, xxiii, 68.

ROUTH. Parturition during Paraplegia. Trans. London Obst. Soc., 1897, xxxix, 191–200.

SCANZONI. Ursache der Geburt. Lehrbuch der Geburtshülfe, II. Aufl., 1853, 165–167.

SCHATZ. Beiträge zur physiologischen Geburtskunde. Archiv f. Gyn., 1872, iii, 58–144.

Ueber die Formen der Wehencurve und über die Peristaltik des menschlichen Uterus. Archiv f. Gyn., 1886, xxvii, 284–292.

Ueber die Entwickelung der Kraft des Uterus im Verlaufe der Geburt. Verh. d. deutschen Gesell. für Gyn., 1895, 531–542.

SPIEGELBERG. Die Dauer der Geburt. Lehrbuch der Geburtshülfe, II. Aufl., 1891, 146.

SPIEGELBERG-WIENER. Lehrbuch der Geburtshülfe, II. Aufl., 1891, 134–137.

TYLER-SMITH. The Principles and Practice of Obstetrics. London, 1849.

VARNIER. Combien de temps dure l'accouchement. L'Obstétrique journalière, 1900, 174–181.

VEIT. Beiträge zur geburtshülflichen Statistik. Monatsschr. f. Geburtskunde, 1854, v, 344–381; 1855, vi, 101–132.

WILLIAMS, J. WHITRIDGE. The Frequency and Significance of Infarcts of the Placenta. Amer. Jour. of Obst., 1900, xli, No. 6.

CHAPTER XI

PHYSIOLOGY OF LABOUR (Continued)

THE FORCES CONCERNED IN LABOUR

The Cervix in the Later Part of Pregnancy.—On vaginal examination in the later months of pregnancy, the cervix is found to be much softer and somewhat broader than in the non-pregnant condition. At the same time it usually gives the impression of being considerably shortened, especially in its anterior portion. This condition led Mauriceau, Roederer, and nearly all of the earlier authorities to believe that from the fifth month onward the upper portion of the cervix gradually became obliterated and contributed to the enlargement of the uterine cavity, that which was left at the end of pregnancy representing merely its inferior end.

Stoltz, in 1826, demonstrated the incorrectness of this doctrine, and stated that the shortening was only apparent, and was brought about by a fusiform dilatation of the cervical canal which resulted in the approach of the internal to the external os. He believed that the cervix retained its integrity until about two weeks before the onset of labour, when the canal slowly became obliterated and came to form part of the uterine cavity. Matthews Duncan accepted these views, but pointed out that they had been anticipated by the anatomical work of Verhegen, De Graaf, and Weitbrecht (1710–'50). At the same time he insisted upon certain modifications, holding that the cervical canal remained practically unchanged until the onset of labour. His statements soon received abundant confirmation from the observations of Holst, Müller, Lott, Taylor, Lusk, and many other investigators.

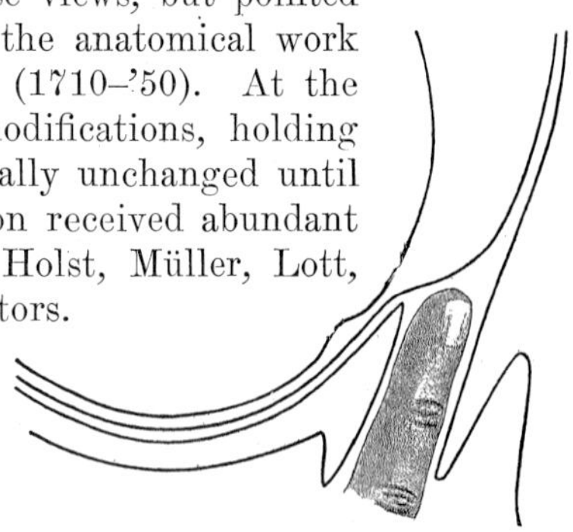

Fig. 197.—Diagram showing Condition of Cervix at End of Pregnancy (Müller).

Müller pointed out that the apparent shortening of the cervix was due to the marked anteflexion of the uterus and the depression of the anterior fornix of the vagina by the presenting part, to which should be added the increased succulence of the entire genital tract. He also stated that the finger, at the end of pregnancy, could be introduced into the canal for a distance of 2.5 to 3 centimetres before it was arrested by the internal os. His conclusions were verified by further clinical observation, so that it is now generally admitted that in the great majority of cases the canal remains practically unaltered until the onset of labour, and that it may even be slightly longer than in the non-pregnant condition, thus indicating that the cervix shares somewhat in the general hypertrophy of the uterus.

In recent years the results obtained by examination during life have received additional confirmation from the study of frozen sections made through the bodies of women dying late in pregnancy. Valuable contributions along these lines have been made by Waldeyer, Schroeder, Braune and Zweifel, Pinard and Varnier, Leopold, and others.

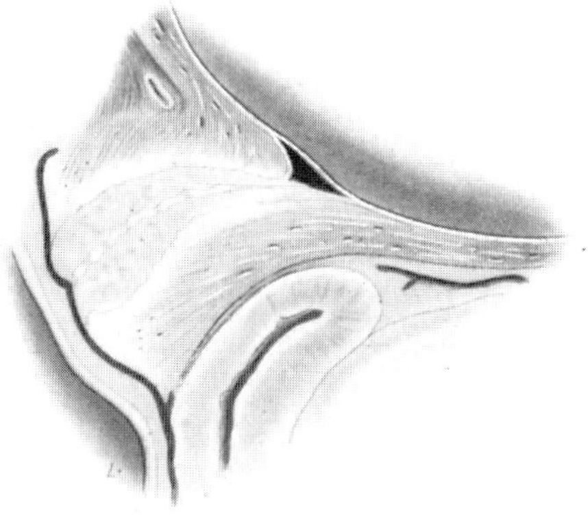

FIG. 198.—CERVIX AT THE END OF PREGNANCY (Waldeyer). × ½.

Lower Uterine Segment.—For a short time after the appearance of Müller's work in 1868, the question concerning the behaviour of the cervix was regarded as practically settled; but these hopes were rudely shattered in 1872 by the studies of Braune upon frozen sections made through a woman who had died during the second stage of labour. His specimen showed distinctly that the interior of the uterus was divided into two parts by a projecting circular ridge, which was 10 and 11 centimetres above the margins of the dilated external os, its situation being marked by a large vein and by the deflection of the peritonæum from the anterior surface of the uterus (Fig. 201). The portion above it possessed thick walls, while the remainder appeared as a simple, thin-walled, muscular tube through which the head had partially passed. Braune identified this ring or ridge with the internal os, and concluded that everything below it had been derived from the cervix; nor did he think it remarkable that the small canal which had ex-

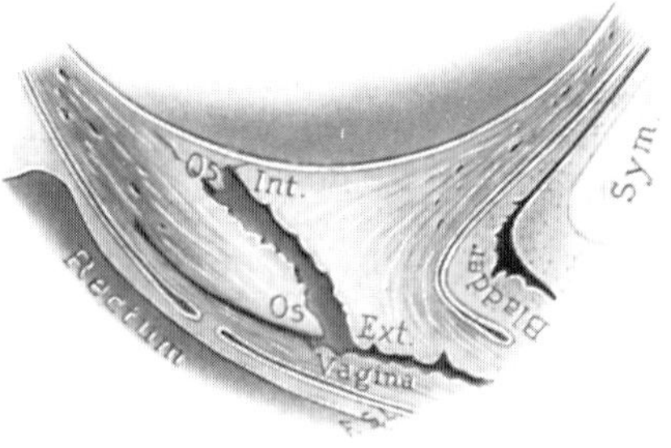

FIG. 199.—CERVIX AT THE END OF PREGNANCY (Braune and Zweifel). × ½.

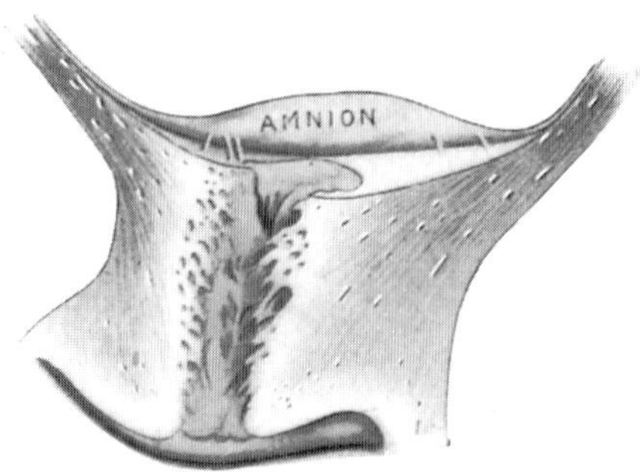

FIG. 200.—CERVIX AT THE END OF PREGNANCY, SHOWING PRESERVATION OF CANAL (Leopold). × ½.

isted up to the time of labour should have been converted into a structure of such dimensions.

Bandl, in his work upon rupture of the uterus, which appeared in 1875, pointed out that when such an accident occurs, the point of rupture is nearly always situated below Braune's ring—namely, in the *lower uterine segment.* The next year he took up the subject again, and considered it inconceivable that the cervical canal, which was only 2.5 to 3.5 centimetres long at the end of pregnancy, could be converted in a few hours into the structure described by Braune. He therefore concluded that, if the upper boundary of the latter really represented the internal os, certain preparatory modifications must have taken place during the latter part of pregnancy in order to make such a remarkable change possible. He believed that the tissue forming the outer portion of the cervix was gradually shifted during the last few weeks of pregnancy, so that it became incorporated with the musculature of the lower portion of the body of the uterus, while the cervical mucous membrane retained its original position. According to his view, then, the true internal os was situated not at the upper termination of the cervical mucosa, but much higher, and at a level corresponding to that of Braune's ring.

Although Bandl's complicated explanation is no longer accepted, his name will always have a place in the literature of the subject. Nor should

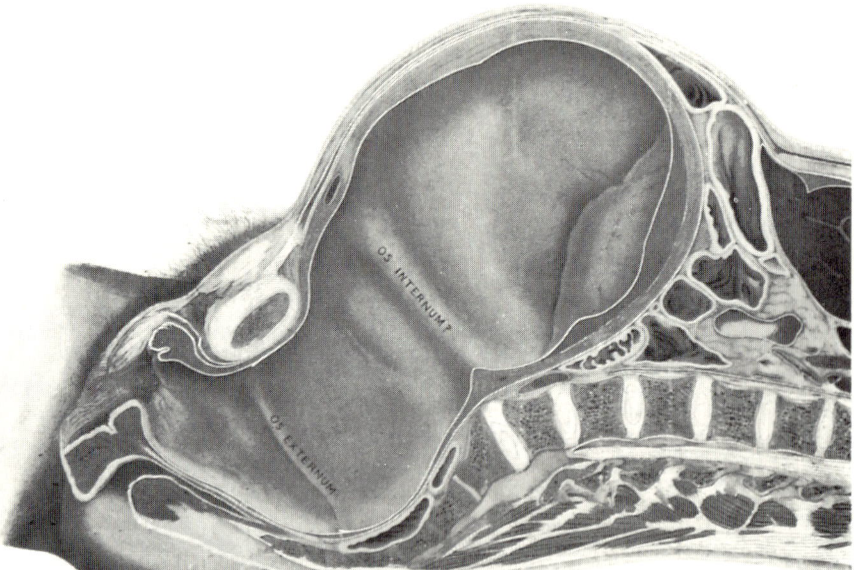

FIG. 201.—FROZEN SECTION THROUGH WOMAN DYING DURING SECOND STAGE OF LABOUR, SHOWING CONTRACTION RING (Braune).

the fact be lost sight of that to him we are indebted for our clinical conception concerning the lower uterine segment, inasmuch as he was the first to distinguish clearly between the function of the upper contractile and active, and the lower passive segments of the uterus, as well as the relation which they bear to the occurrence of rupture.

The discussion started by Bandl has been responsible for an immense literature, and even now the question cannot be regarded as definitely settled. Two main views have been advanced concerning the nature and origin of the lower uterine segment. According to the first, it is derived partly from the cervix, the internal os being supposed to be situated 3 or 4 centimetres above the external, while the rest of the structure is formed by the lower portion of the body of the uterus. According to the second view, the entire structure, from Braune's ring to the external os, is derived from the cervix. The first view has received the indorsement of such authorities as Schroeder, Ruge, von Franqué, Dittel, and Veit, while the correctness of the second explanation is upheld by Bandl, Küstner, Bayer, Zweifel, and others.

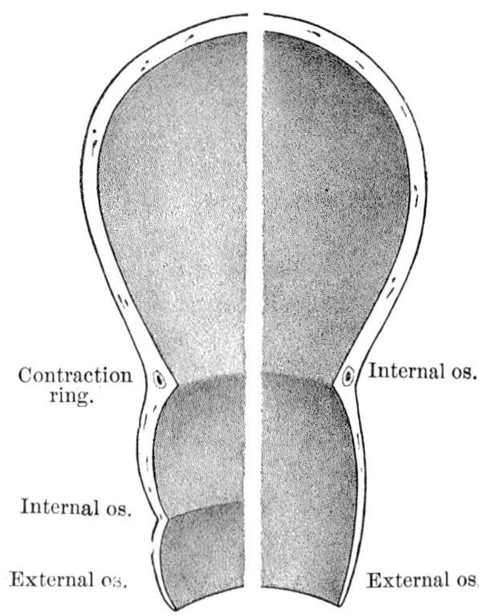

FIG. 202.—DIAGRAM ILLUSTRATING MAIN VIEWS AS TO NATURE OF LOWER UTERINE SEGMENT (American Text-Book).

At first glance it might appear strange that the question has given rise to such divergence of opinion, as it would seem a very simple matter to demonstrate the structure of the parts by microscopical examination. If the first view be correct, the inner surface of the portion which is supposed to be derived from the uterus should be lined by decidua, and the portion below it, corresponding to the cervical canal, by the characteristic cervical mucosa. On the other hand, if the second explanation is to be accepted, the entire structure below Braune's ring—*the contraction ring*, as it is generally designated—should be lined by cervical epithelium.

Unfortunately, the question is not so easily solved. In the first place, the formation of the contraction ring and the lower uterine segment is in great part a clinical phenomenon; and while its situation can usually be definitely made out by the examining finger during labour, it is not so clearly marked after the removal of the uterus from the dead body. Again, the majority of the specimens which have been relied upon to settle the question were frozen before being subjected to microscopical examination, so that the finer histological details had become obliterated. In spite of these obstacles, however, the question has gradually approached a solution, so that the majority of investigators are inclined to accept the first view, which is generally known by Schroeder's name; and the recent monographs of von Franqué and Dittel practically settle the matter beyond all doubt. To these the reader is referred for the full literature upon the subject.

Plate IX represents a vertical mesial section through the uterus of a woman seven months pregnant, who died at the Johns Hopkins Hospital during premature labour. In this it is clearly seen that the external os is not dilated, but that the cervical canal has become obliterated and a distinct lower uterine segment has been formed. Careful examination shows that the latter is lined with a typical cervical mucous membrane for a distance of 3.5 to 4 centimetres from the margins of the external os, whereas above this point the tissue is distinctly uterine in appearance and is covered by decidua.

Fig. 203 represents part of a frozen section through a pregnant cadaver, shown in Plate I, which was kindly placed at my disposal by Drs. J. Holmes

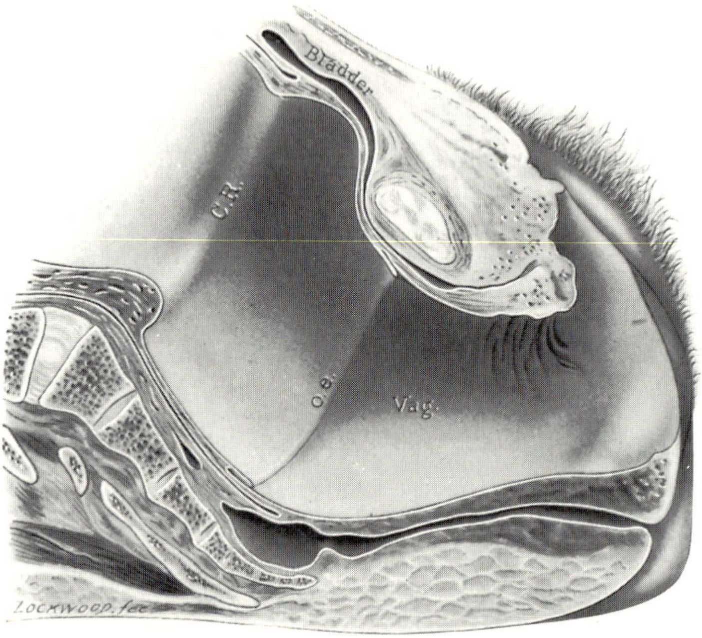

Fig. 203.—Frozen Section, showing Condition of the Birth Canal in First Part of Second Stage of Labour. × ½.

C.R., contraction ring; *o.e.*, external os.

Smith and L. E. Neale. The woman, who had a slightly generally contracted rhachitic pelvis, died in labour with the membranes protruding from the vulva. The child presented by the breech, which had not yet become engaged. The cervical canal was obliterated and the external os fully dilated, its margins being 1 millimetre thick. There was no trace of the internal os. Seven centimetres above the external os was a well-marked contraction ring. Unfortunately, the specimen was so badly macerated that the lining membrane of the cervical canal and lower uterine segment had disappeared. Microscopical examination revealed only a few cervical glands in the neighbourhood of the external os, and gave no information as to whether the portion below the contraction ring was lined by decidua or cervical epithelium.

PLATE IX.

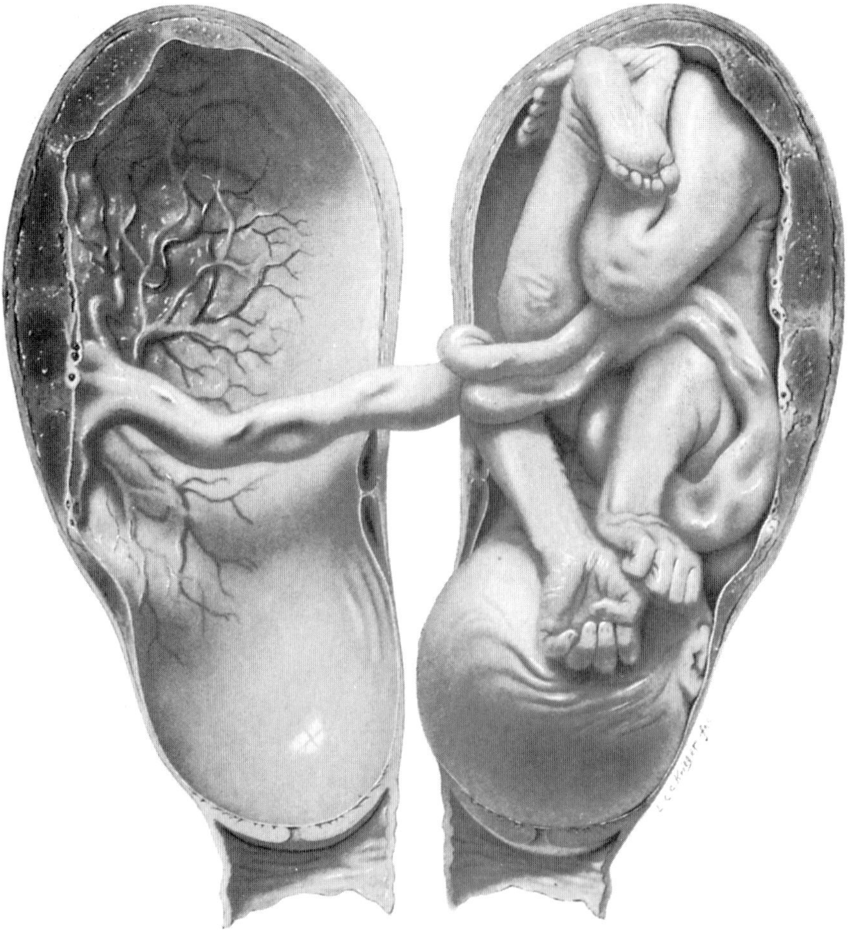

SEVEN AND A HALF MONTHS' PREGNANT UTERUS FROM WOMAN DYING IN THE FIRST STAGE OF LABOUR. $\times$ 1/2.

Veit has lately pointed out that the portion of the uterus from which the lower uterine segment is to develop is clearly indicated even in the non-pregnant condition. He demonstrated that for several millimetres above the internal os the lower part of the uterine cavity is represented by a small canal, which he designated as the "Engpass" (narrow passage), and from which he believes the structure in question is developed. Fig. 128, representing a six- to seven-weeks' pregnant uterus in my possession, clearly shows a similar condition.

It is possible that the cervix may occasionally take a larger share in the formation of the lower uterine segment than is here indicated, but what we have said undoubtedly holds good for the vast majority of cases.

Hofmeier, in 1886, demonstrated that the structure of the lower uterine segment is not homogeneous, and that the portion which corresponds to the cervix is composed of dense connective tissue rich in elastic fibres, while its upper part is made up of muscular lamellæ which pursue an almost parallel course, whereas as soon as the contraction ring is reached the uterine musculature takes on its characteristic appearance.

Changes in the Uterus during the First Stage of Labour.—Passing from these more or less theoretical considerations to the condition of the uterus at the onset of labour, we find that the organ is made up of two parts: a large, thin-walled, muscular sac—the body—to the lower end of which the small cervix is attached. The wall of the former rarely exceeds 5 millimetres in thickness. It is lined by decidua and the fœtal membranes, inside of which are the amniotic fluid and the fœtus. The cervix is softened and very succulent. It presents a more or less fusiform canal, 3 to 4 centimetres long, which is bounded at its upper and lower ends by the internal and external os respectively; its walls rarely exceed 1.5 centimetre in thickness. The condition of the external os varies considerably, according as the patient is a primiparous or multiparous woman. In the former it is quite tightly closed and barely admits the tip of the little finger; while in the latter it is widely gaping, so that the index finger can be readily passed into it, and can frequently be carried up to the internal os.

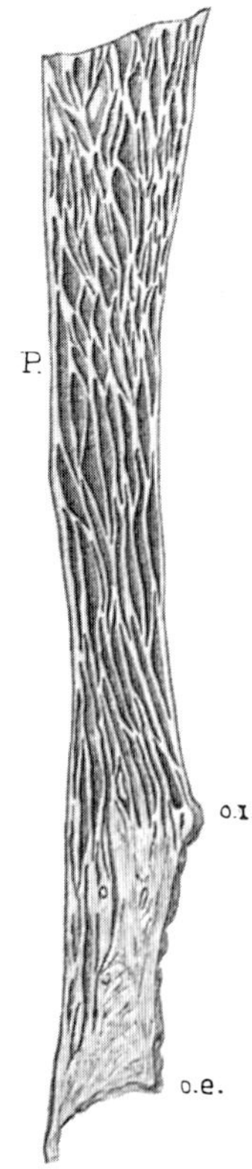

Fig. 204.—Section through Lower Uterine Segment and Cervix, showing Rhomboidal Arrangement of Muscle Fibres in Former and Dense Structure in Latter (Hofmeier).

P., peritoneal covering of uterus; *o.e.*, os externum; *o.i.*, os internum.

During labour, under the influence of the uterine contractions, the uterus becomes differentiated into two distinct portions, which are separated from one another by the contraction ring. The upper is the active contractile portion and becomes thicker as labour advances, while the lower plays a merely passive part, becoming converted into a muscular tube for the transmission of the fœtus (Fig. 206).

With the onset of labour pains the fluid contents of the uterus are subjected to pressure. As the lower uterine segment and the cervix will naturally constitute a point of least resistance, the fluid pressure, which is transmitted equally in all directions by the amniotic fluid, consequently gives rise to an increased tension and distention of these portions of the uterus. On abdominal palpation, before the rupture of the membranes, two zones can readily be differentiated, the upper one of which is firm and hard during a contraction, while the lower affords a semifluctuant sensation. The former represents the contractile portion of the uterus, the latter the passive lower uterine segment and cervix.

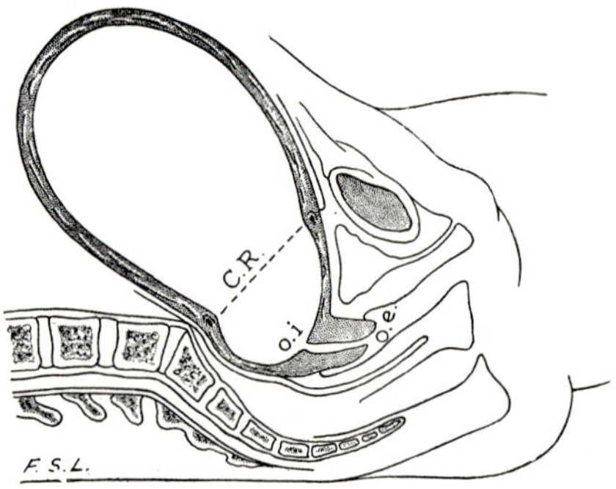

Fig. 205.

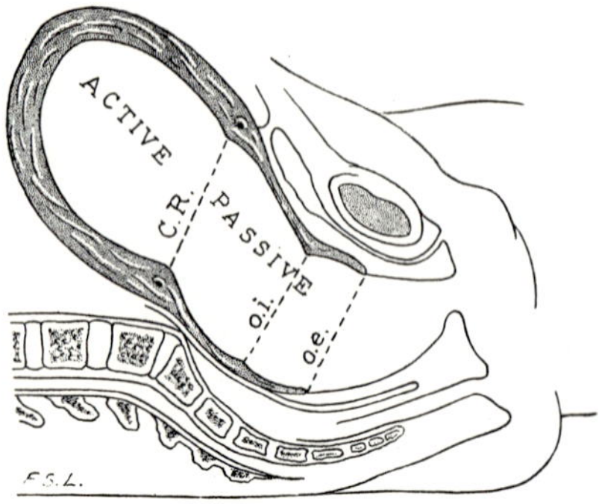

Fig. 206.

FIGS. 205, 206.—DIAGRAMS OF BIRTH CANAL AT END OF PREGNANCY AND DURING SECOND STAGE OF LABOUR, SHOWING FORMATION OF BIRTH CANAL (Schroeder).

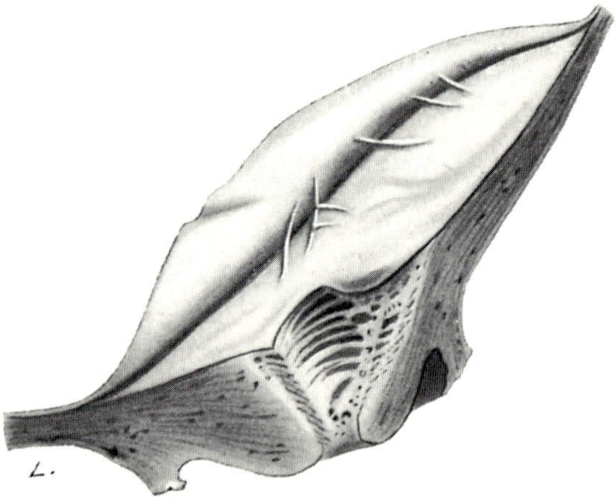

FIG. 207.—DILATATION OF CERVIX, FUNNEL-SHAPED OBLITERATION OF INTERNAL OS AND CERVICAL CANAL (Leopold).

Again, since the cervix is perforated by its canal, the fluid pressure exerted by the bag of waters tends to cause its obliteration and final dilatation, which is aided by the traction exerted upon its margins by the contracting fibres of the lower portion of the uterus. When complete dilatation has been effected, the margins of the external os lie 10 to 11 centimetres below the contraction ring, and no trace of the internal os can be

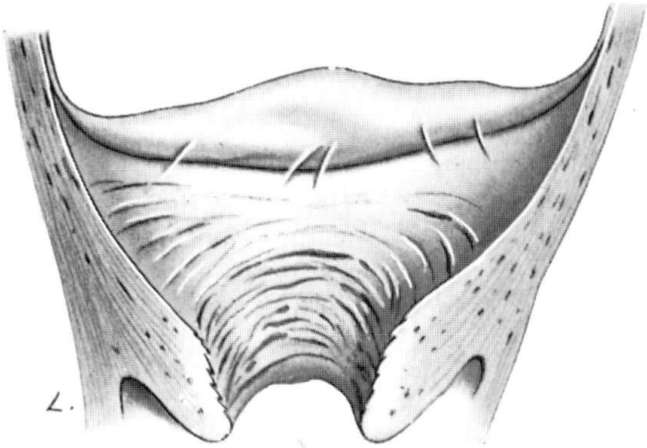

FIG. 208.—DILATATION OF CERVIX FURTHER ADVANCED THAN IN FIG. 207 (Leopold). × 1.

found. At the same time the bladder is gradually drawn up in front of the lower uterine segment until it becomes almost entirely an abdominal organ.

The *dilatation of the cervix* may be regarded as consisting of two stages: first, obliteration of the canal; and second, dilatation of the external os. The obliteration occurs from above downward, the beginning being indicated by a funnel-shaped depression at the region of the internal os, which gradually increases in extent and depth until the entire canal has disappeared, when the uterine cavity is separated from the vagina merely by

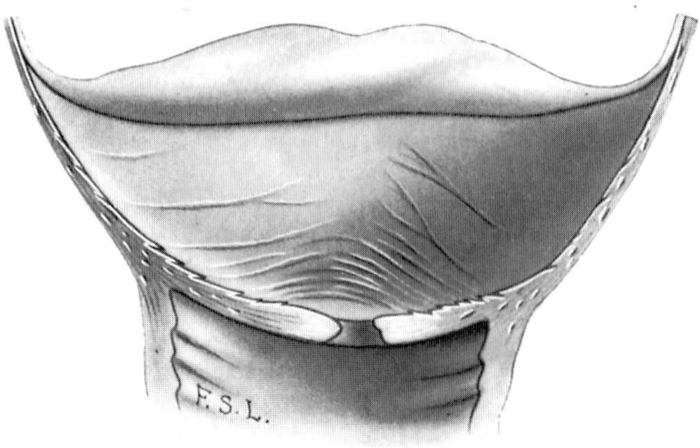

FIG. 209.—CERVICAL CANAL COMPLETELY OBLITERATED, EXTERNAL OS INTACT. × 1.

the external os. This is clearly shown in Figs. 207, 208, and 209, and also in Figs. 210, 211, 212, and 213, which represent reconstructions from the frozen sections of Schroeder, Winter, Säxinger, and Tibone, all of which were made through women who died during the first stage of labour.

After the cervical canal has become obliterated, dilatation of the external os occurs. In many instances its margins become extremely thin, and occasionally give a sensation as if they would cut the examining finger. This change is brought about almost entirely by the force exerted by the bag of waters, or when that has ruptured prematurely, by the pressure of the presenting part itself.

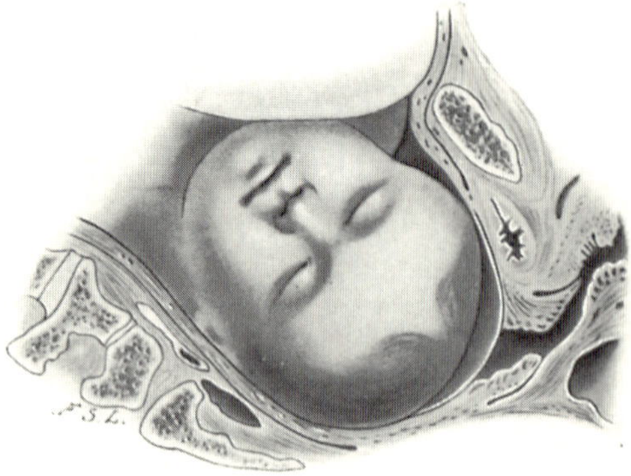

Fig. 210.—Dilatation of Cervix, Funnel-shaped Obliteration of Internal Os; Canal 2 Centimetres Long (Schroeder). × ⅛.

The course of events differs considerably according as the woman is in her first or a subsequent pregnancy. In the former case marked resistance is offered by the external os, and a considerable time must elapse before complete dilatation is accomplished; while in the latter, the os is gaping and very little force is required for its complete dilatation after the cervical canal has become obliterated.

Changes in the Uterus during the Second Stage of Labour.—During the first stage of labour the contractions of the uterus have resulted in its differentiation into two parts, which are separated from one another by the

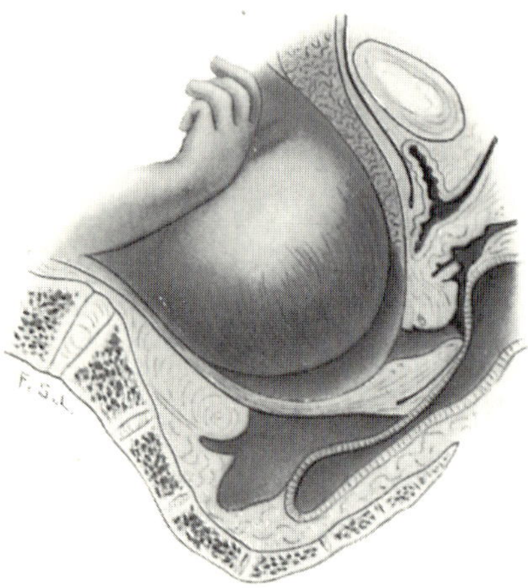

Fig. 211.—Dilatation of Cervix, all but Lower 10 Millimetres of Canal obliterated; External Os Unchanged (Winter). × ⅛.

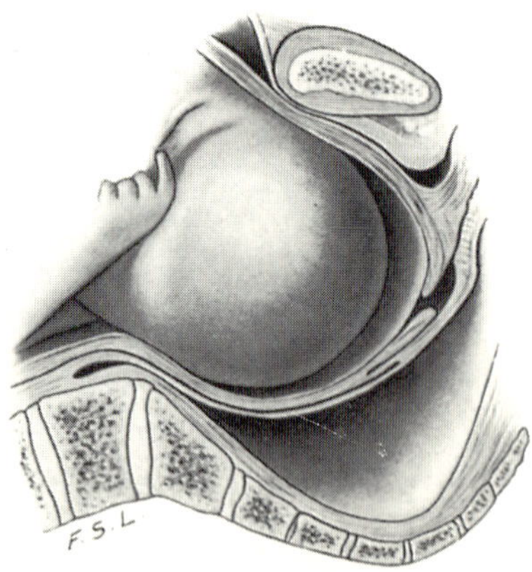

Fig. 212.—Dilatation of Cervix, all but Lower 3 Millimetres of Canal obliterated; External Os Unchanged (Säxinger). × ⅛.

contraction ring. Above is the active, contractile portion, which becomes thicker as labour advances, while below we have the thin-walled, passive, lower uterine segment and cervix (Fig. 206).

While these changes are being effected, there has been no advance on the part of the fœtus, and as a rule the presenting part occupies the same position from the onset of labour until complete dilatation of the cervix. With the commencement of the second stage, however, descent begins, and under normal conditions continues slowly but steadily until delivery is accomplished. Naturally, the differentiation into stages is more or less arbitrary, so that it occasionally happens that the presenting part begins to descend during the latter part of the first stage.

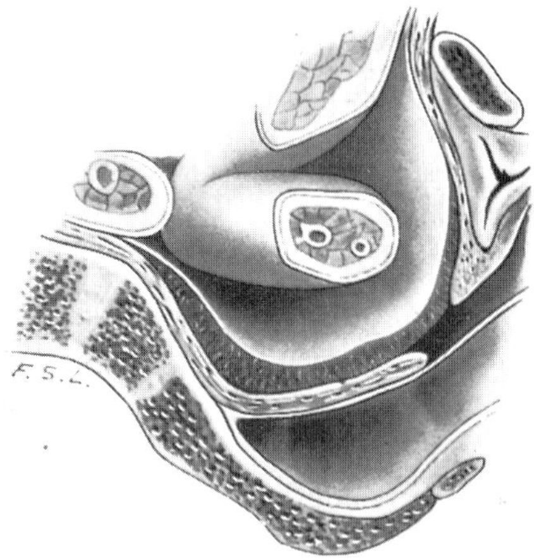

Fig. 213.—Dilatation of Cervix, Canal obliterated; External Os 1.5 Centimetre in Diameter. Placenta Prævia. (Tibone). × ⅛.

After it has brought about complete dilatation of the cervix, the bag of waters has subserved its function, and rupture usually now occurs, which is manifested by a sudden rush of a greater or lesser quantity of a tolerably clear fluid from the vagina. Occasionally the membranes give way some time before complete dilatation of the cervix has been brought about; whereas, on the other hand, in rare instances they may retain their integrity until the completion of labour, so that the fœtus is born surrounded by them, the portion covering its head being designated as a *caul.*

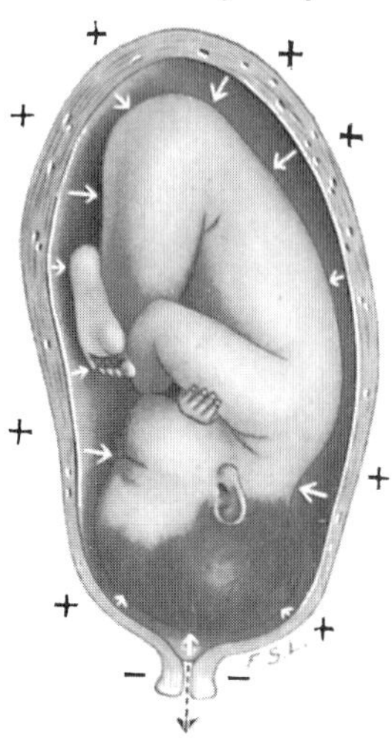

Fig. 214.—Diagram showing Action of Intra-uterine Pressure, Membranes not Ruptured.

We have already directed attention to the changes in shape which the uterus presents during contraction. These may be noticed in the first, but more especially in the second stage, when the organ increases considerably in length, and at the same time diminishes in its transverse and antero-posterior diameters with each contraction. The increase in length is due almost entirely to the stretching of the lower uterine segment: but we are unable to make definite statements as to its extent, for at present we possess no means of ascertaining how far the retraction of the upper portion of the uterus may serve to counterbalance the stretching of its lower segment. In obstructed labours, in which marked disproportion exists between the size of the presenting part and the pelvic canal, the lower uterine segment is subjected to excessive stretching, and consequently the contraction ring assumes a much higher level, and not infrequently can be palpated as a distinct transverse ridge a short distance below the umbilicus. With the formation of the lower uterine segment, the upper portion of the uterus increases markedly in thickness, and, as labour proceeds, covers a progressively decreasing portion of the child. Thus, when the head is upon the perinæum less than one half of the fœtus is in the upper segment.

Forces Concerned in Labour.—As long as the membranes are unruptured —that is, during the entire first stage of labour, and in the rare instances in which they remain intact in the second stage—whatever force is exerted by the contracting uterus is transmitted to the liquor amnii, and by it to the fœtus. In accordance with the laws of fluid pressure, therefore, it is applied with equal intensity to all portions of the child, and were it not that the lower uterine segment and cervix represent the point of least resistance in the uterus, all its effect would be wasted; whereas, under the circumstances, it gives rise to the formation of the lower uterine segment and the dilatation of the cervix, but plays no part in causing the descent of the child. Attention was first directed to this point by Schatz and Lahs, and all subsequent authorities have accepted their conclusions.

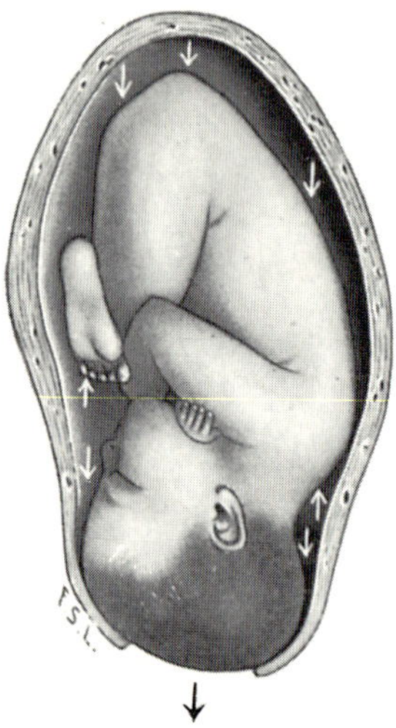

Fig. 215.—Diagram showing Action of Intra-uterine Pressure after Rupture of the Membranes.

After rupture of the membranes, a greater or lesser portion of the amniotic fluid escapes, but in vertex presentations the presenting part usually acts as a fairly efficient tampon and causes the retention of a considerable quantity of it in the uterus, where it fills out the interstices between the fœtus and the uterine walls. Lahs believed the amount retained was usually sufficient to prevent actual contact with the surface of the fœtus, and that therefore extrusion of the latter was brought about by fluid pressure alone. He argued that under such circumstances (Fig. 215) the entire surface of the fœtus, except the portion projecting through the cervix, would be subjected to fluid pressure, which, as it is equal in all directions, would exert no effect upon the fœtus, except in a line passing through the centre of the portion not subjected to it, thus manifesting itself as a downward force bringing about descent.

On the other hand, Lahs held that in all other presentations, as well as in those of the vertex when the amniotic fluid has almost completely drained off, other factors come into play which he regarded as distinctly pathological. In such cases the contracting uterus would come in direct contact with the surface of the fœtus, and the force exerted by the fundus would be directly transmitted to the presenting part by way of the vertebral column.

Most recent writers have not hesitated to accept Lahs's interpretation, but Olshausen has lately directed attention to the fact that the latter force comes into play even in normal vertex presentations. He pointed out that only four frozen sections, through women dying in the second stage of labour, are available for the study of the question—namely, two of Braune and those of Chiari and Barbour—and that in three of them the fundus was in direct contact with the breech of the child. He then estimated that at least 300 cubic centimetres of amniotic fluid were required to fill out the interstices between the surface of the fœtus and the uterine wall, and stated that it was out of the question that the child could be expelled solely by fluid pressure unless a greater quantity than this were present.

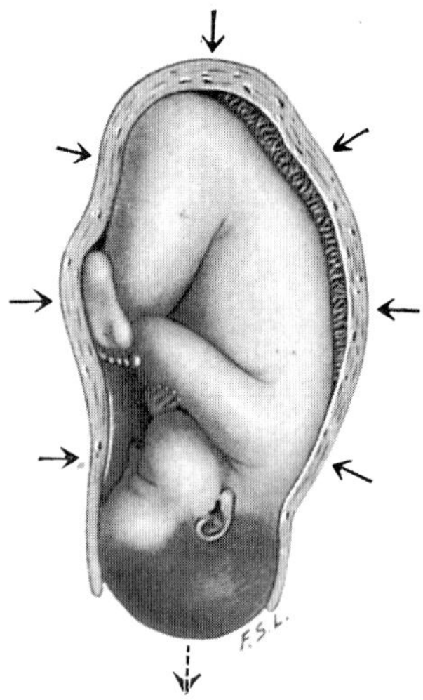

FIG. 216.—DIAGRAM SHOWING DIRECT PRESSURE EXERTED BY FUNDUS AFTER RUPTURE OF THE MEMBRANES.

In 200 cases he measured the amount of amniotic fluid escaping when the child was born, which practically represents the quantity remaining in the uterus after rupture of the membranes, and found that in 80 per cent of the primiparæ it did not exceed 300 cubic centimetres; while in 60 per cent it was not over 200 cubic centimetres, an amount by no means sufficient to fill out the interstices, let alone to bring about the separation of the breech from the fundus, which is absolutely essential for the proper action of fluid pressure. He therefore concluded that under such circumstances direct pressure must be exerted by the contracting uterus upon the breech, whence it is transmitted through the vertebral column to the head, and that this is rendered possible by the diminution in the transverse and antero-posterior diameter of the uterus, which results in an extension of the child and its conversion for the time being into a comparatively rigid object.

In addition to these factors, the contractions of the abdominal muscles of the woman also play no mean part in effecting the extrusion of the child; indeed, according to Schroeder, they alone bring it about. Olshausen, on the other hand, while not denying their importance, does not consider that they are the sole factors concerned. It is apparent, however, in most cases, that their action is absolutely essential for the birth of the fœtus, for when it is entirely absent, or only partially comes into play, labour is delayed, and a resort to forceps frequently becomes necessary.

The descent of the child is no doubt partly due to the fact that it becomes straightened out by the action of the pains during the second stage. According to Schroeder, its length from vertex to breech is increased by 5.5 centimetres as a result of this extension; while Olshausen considers that the increase is considerably greater, and estimates that it varies from 7.25 to 13 centimetres in 70 per cent of the cases. Part of this, it is true, is counterbalanced by the greater length of the uterus, but the remainder is accounted for by the descent of the presenting part.

When the head has descended through the pelvis and is resting on the pelvic floor, more than half of the entire length of the child lies beneath the contraction ring; moreover, as the upper portion of the uterus becomes smaller and smaller, it necessarily exerts a diminished effect upon the child, so that in the majority of cases it becomes essential that the abdominal contractions should participate in the work.

Immediately after the birth of the child a marked change occurs in the position and size of the uterus, and on palpation it can be distinguished as a firm, rounded body which reaches to the umbilicus. At this time its contracted and retracted body is freely movable above the collapsed lower uterine segment, and can readily be displaced in any desired direction.

Changes in the Vagina and Pelvic Floor during Labour.—The outlet of the pelvis is closed by a number of layers of tissue, which together constitute what is known as the pelvic floor. Beginning from within outward

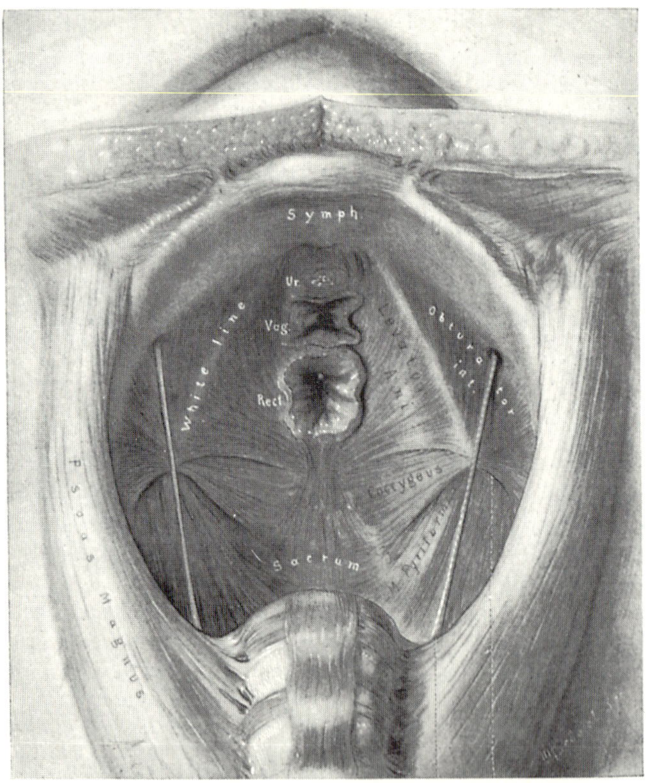

Fig. 217.—The Pelvic Floor seen from above (Kelly).

one meets successively with the peritonæum, the subperitoneal connective tissue, the internal pelvic fascia, the levator ani and coccygeus muscles, the external pelvic and perineal fascia, and, included between the latter, the superficial muscles of the perinæum, external to which are the subcutaneous tissue and the cutaneous covering of the perineal and vulvar regions.

Of these structures the most important are the levator ani muscle and the fascia covering its upper and lower surfaces, which for practical obstetrical purposes may be considered as constituting the pelvic floor. This muscle

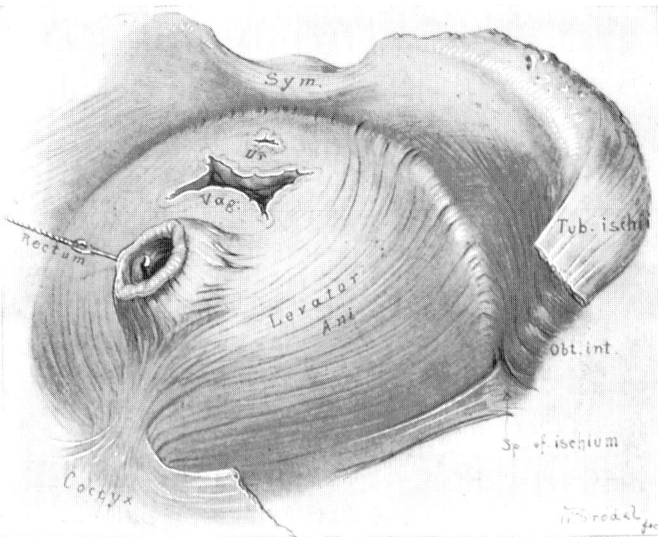

FIG. 218.—THE PELVIC FLOOR SEEN FROM BELOW (Kelly).

closes the lower end of the pelvic cavity as a diaphragm, and presents a concave upper and a convex lower surface. On either side it consists of a pubic and iliac portion; the former is a band 2 to 2.5 centimetres in width, which arises from the horizontal ramus of the pubis 3 to 4 centimetres below its upper margin, and 1 to 1.5 centimetre from the symphysis pubis. Its fibres pass backward and encircle the rectum, giving off a few fibres which pass behind the vagina. The greater or iliac portion of the muscle arises on either side from the white line, the tendinous arch of the pelvic fascia, and from the ischial spine, at a distance of about 5 centimetres below the margin of the superior strait. Its fibres do not possess a uniform arrangement, but, according to the researches of Dickinson, the following portions can be distinguished: Passing from before backward, there is a narrow band which crosses the pubic portion and descends to the recto-vaginal septum. The greater part of the muscle passes backward and unites with that from the other side of the rectum, while the posterior portions meet together in a tendinous rhaphe in front of the coccyx, the most posterior fibres being attached to the bone itself. The muscle fails to fill out the posterior and lateral portions of the pelvic floor, which are occupied by the pyriformis and coccygeus muscles on either side.

The levator ani muscle varies from 3 to 5 millimetres in thickness, though its margins, which encircle the rectum and vagina, are somewhat thicker. On contraction it serves to draw both the rectum and vagina forward and upward in the direction of the symphysis pubis, and is to be regarded as the real closer of the vagina, since the constrictor cunni, one of the superficial muscles of the perinæum, is too delicate in structure to have more than an accessory function.

The muscles forming the pelvic floor would not be sufficiently strong to afford support to the pelvic contents were they not re-enforced by the strong pelvic fascia. The internal pelvic fascia, which forms the upper covering of the levator ani, is attached to the margin of the superior strait, where it is joined by the fascia lining the iliac fossæ, as well as the transverse fascia of the abdominal walls. It passes down over the pyriformis and the upper half of the obturator internus muscle, and is firmly attached to the periosteum covering the lateral wall of the pelvis, the white line indicating its point of deflexion from the latter, whence it spreads out over the upper surface of the levator ani and coccygeus muscles.

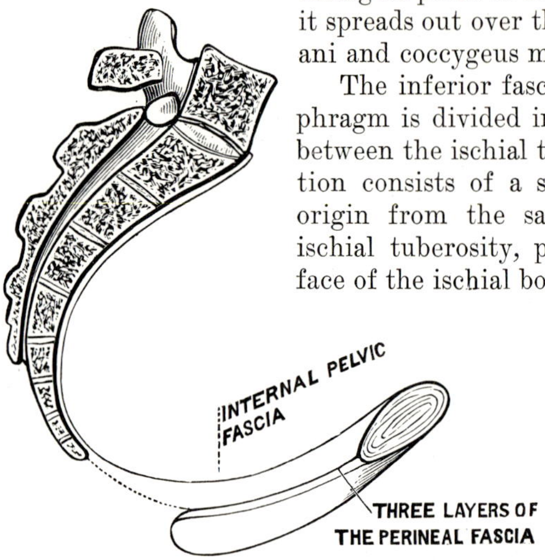

Fig. 219.—Diagram showing Arrangement of Pelvic and Perineal Fascia (Tarnier).

The inferior fascial covering of the pelvic diaphragm is divided into two parts by a line drawn between the ischial tuberosities. Its posterior portion consists of a single layer which, taking its origin from the sacro-sciatic ligament and the ischial tuberosity, passes up over the inner surface of the ischial bones and the obturator internus muscles to the white line, in whose formation it takes part. From this tendinous structure it is reflected at an acute angle over upon the inferior surface of the levator ani, the space included between the latter and the lateral pelvic wall being designated as the ischio-rectal fossa. The anterior portion, or the perineal fascia proper, fills out the space between the line joining the ischial tuberosities and the pubic arch. It is made up of three layers: (1) The deep perineal fascia which covers the anterior portion of the inferior surface of the levator ani muscle and is continuous with the fascia just described; (2) the middle perineal fascia which is separated from the former by a narrow space in which are situated the pudic vessels and nerves; (3) the superficial perineal fascia which, together with the layer just described, form a compartment in which lie the superficial perineal muscles, the rami of the clitoris, the vaginal bulbs, and the vulvovaginal glands.

The superficial perineal muscles consist of the constrictor cunni, the ischio-cavernosi, and the transversus perinei muscles. These structures are delicately formed and possess no obstetrical significance, except the last-named muscles, which are always torn through in perineal lacerations, when they serve in great part to bring about gaping of the wound.

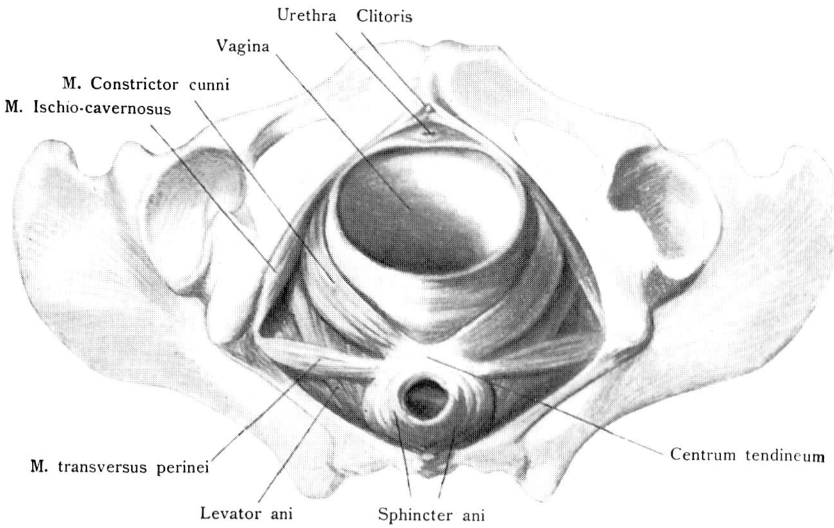

FIG. 220.—PELVIC FLOOR DISTENDED BY PRESENTING PART, SHOWING SUPERFICIAL MUSCLES OF PERINÆUM (Bumm).

From a practical point of view, Hart has divided the pelvic floor into two segments—pubic and sacral—which are separated from one another by the vagina. Their condition remains practically unchanged throughout the

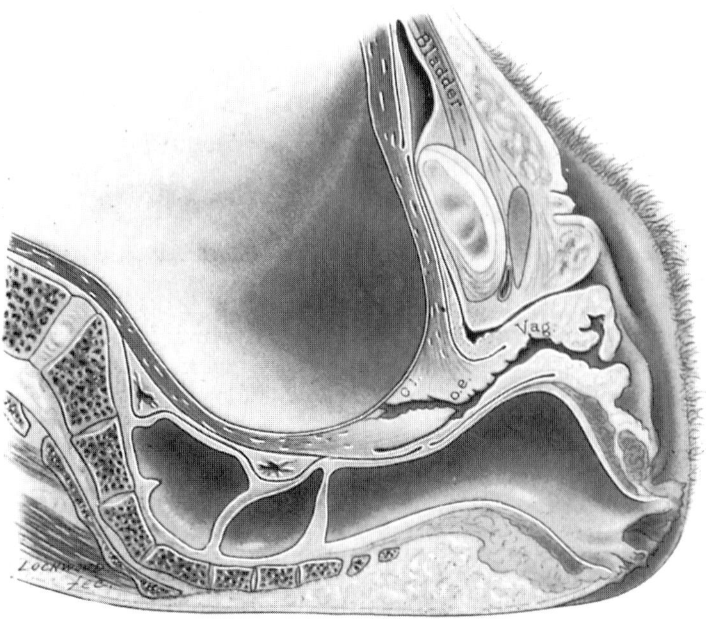

FIG. 221.—FROZEN SECTION, SHOWING CONDITION OF BIRTH CANAL IN LAST MONTH OF PREGNANCY (Braune and Zweifel). × ½.

entire duration of pregnancy, except that towards the end they become more relaxed, owing to the greater succulence and some œdema of the tissues, which are manifested by a slight increase in thickness and a certain amount of drooping.

In the first stage of labour the bag of waters takes part in the dilatation and distention of the upper portion of the vagina, but after its rupture the changes occurring in the pelvic floor are due entirely to the pressure exerted by the presenting part. As this descends, the pubic segment becomes slightly drawn up and forced against the inferior and posterior portions of the symphysis. On the other hand, the sacral segment

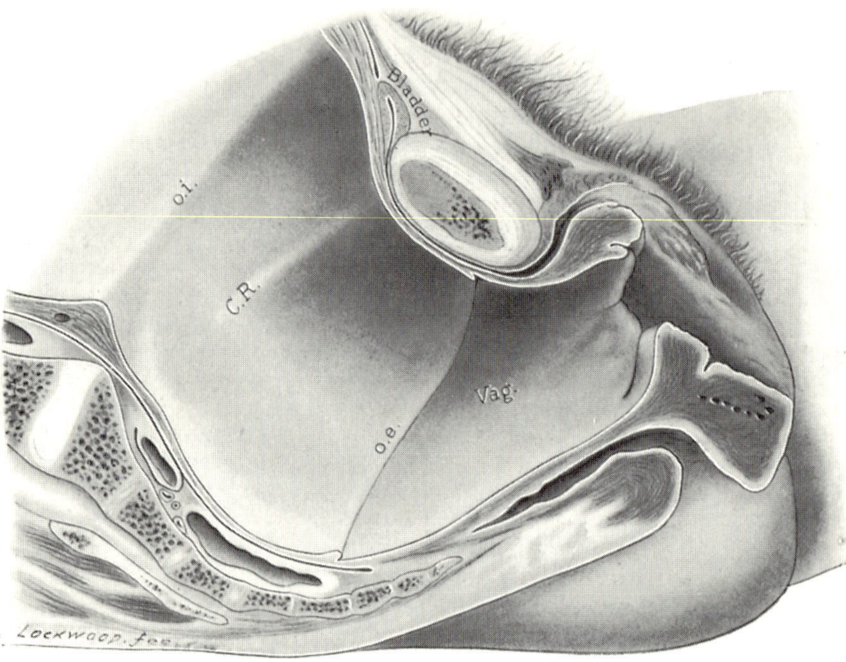

Fig. 222.—Frozen Section, showing Condition of the Birth Canal in First Part of Second Stage of Labour (Braune). × ½.

undergoes marked changes, becoming pushed downward and forward, and subjected to great stretching, eventually being converted into a thin-walled, tubular structure—the perineal gutter. Fig. 220 gives a good idea of the changes occurring in the pelvic floor, and demonstrates the important part played by the levator ani and the altogether insignificant function of the superficial perineal muscles. When the head distends the vulva, its opening looks upward and forward, and the course of the birth canal along the pelvic floor follows the curve indicated in Figs. 203 and 222.

Webster has pointed out that the most marked change consists in the stretching of the fibres of the levator ani muscle and the thinning of the central portion of the perinæum, which becomes transformed from a wedge-shaped mass of tissue 5 centimetres in thickness to a thin, almost transparent membranous structure 2 to 4 millimetres thick. At the same time it is pushed down about 2.5 centimetres from its original position.

When the perinæum is distended to the utmost, the anus becomes markedly dilated, and presents an opening which varies from 2 to 2.5 centimetres in diameter, through which the anterior wall of the rectum is seen to bulge. Westphalen has recently called attention to the fact that these changes may be accompanied by slight lesions in continuity. They were noted in 13 per cent of the 100 cases studied by this author, and were sometimes sufficiently marked to be accompanied by slight hæmorrhage.

LITERATURE

Bandl. Ueber Ruptur der Gebärmutter. Wien, 1875.
Ueber das Verhalten des Uterus und Cervix, etc. Stuttgart, 1876.
Barbour. Atlas of the Anatomy of Labour Exhibited in Frozen Sections. Third edition, Edinburgh, 1896.
Bayer. Zur physiol. und path. Morphologie der Gebärmutter, in Freund's Gyn. Klinik. Stuttgart, 1885.
Uterus und unteres Uterinsegment. Archiv f. Gyn., 1897, liv, 13–71.
Braune. Die Lage des Uterus und Fötus am Ende der Schwangerschaft. Leipzig, 1872.
Braune und Zweifel. Gefrierdurchschnitte durch den Körper einer Hochschwangeren. Leipzig, 1890.
Chiari. Ueber die topographischen Verhältnisse des Genitales einer intrapartum verstorbenen Primipara. Wien, 1885.
Dickinson. Studies of the Levator Ani Muscle. Amer. Jour. Obstet., 1889, xxii, 897–917.
Dittel. Die Dehnungszone des schwangeren und kreissenden Uterus. Leipzig, 1898.
Duncan. On the Length of the Cervix Uteri in Advanced Pregnancy. Researches in Obstetrics, Edinburgh, 1868, 243–273.
von Franqué. Cervix und unteres Uterinsegment. Stuttgart, 1897.
Untersuchungen und Erörterungen zur Cervixfrage. Würzburg, 1899.
Hart. The Structural Anatomy of the Pelvic Floor. Edinburgh, 1880.
Hofmeier. Das untere Uterinsegment in anat. und klin. Beziehung, in Schroeder's Der schwangere und kreissende Uterus. Bonn, 1886, 21–74.
Holst. Beiträge zur Geburtshülfe u. Gynäkologie, Heft I, 130–169, 1865.
Küstner. Das untere Uterinsegment und die Decidua cervicalis. Jena, 1882.
Lahs. Zur Mechanik der Geburt. Marburg, 1869; Berlin, 1872.
Die Theorie der Geburt. Bonn, 1877.
Langhans und Müller. Weiterer anat. Beitrag zur Frage vom Verhalten der Cervix während der Schwangerschaft. Archiv f. Gyn., 1879, xiv, 184–189.
Leopold. Uterus und Kind. Leipzig, 1897.
Lott. Zur Anatomie u. Physiologie der Cervix uteri. Erlangen, 1872.
Lusk. The Science and Art of Midwifery, 82, new edition, 1895.
Mauriceau. Traité des maladies des femmes grosses, etc. 6me éd., 1721, t. i, 97.
Müller. Untersuchungen über die Verkürzung der Vaginalportion, etc. Scanzoni's Beiträge, 1868, v, 191–346.
Olshausen. Beitrag zur Lehre vom Mechanismus der Geburt. Stuttgart, 1901.
Pinard et Varnier. Études d'anatomie obstétricale normale et pathologique. Paris, 1892.
Roederer. Elementa Artis Obstetriciae. Gottingae, 1766, 26.
Ruge. Ueber die Contraction des Uterus in anat. u. klin. Beziehung. Zeitschr. f. Geb. u. Gyn., 1880, 141–148.
Säxinger. Gefrierdurchschnitt einer Kreissenden. Tübingen, 1888.

SCHATZ. Der Geburtsmechanismus der Kopfendlagen. Leipzig, 1868.
Beiträge zur physiologischen Geburtskunde, 1871.

SCHROEDER. Der schwangere und kreissende Uterus. Bonn, 1886.
Lehrbuch der Geburtshülfe, XIII. Aufl., 173, 1899.

STOLTZ. Considérations sur quelques points relatifs à l'art des accouchements. Thèse de Strasbourg, 1826.

TAYLOR. On the Cervix Uteri. Amer. Med. Times, June 21, 1862.

TIBONE. Sulla placenta praevia tavole omolografiche preparate sopra il cadavere congelato. Turin, 1394.

VARNIER. Le col et le segment inférieur à la fin de la grossesse, etc. Paris, 1888.

VEIT. Unteres Uterinsegment und Cervixfrage. Verh. der deutschen Gesell. f. Gyn., 1899, viii, 430–449.

WALDEYER. Medianschnitt einer Hochschwangeren bei Steisslage des Fötus. Bonn, 1886.

WEBSTER. The Female Pelvic Floor. Researches in Female Pelvic Anatomy, 93–112. Edinburgh, 1892.

VON WESTPHALEN. Ueber das Verhalten des Mastdarms während der Geburt. D. I., Strassburg, 1900.

WINTER. Zwei Medianschnitte durch Gebärende. Berlin, 1889.

ZWEIFEL. Zwei neue Gefrierschnitte Gebärender. Leipzig, 1893.

CHAPTER XII

PHYSIOLOGY OF LABOUR (*Continued*)

MECHANISM OF LABOUR IN VERTEX PRESENTATIONS

Vertex presentations occur in from 96 to 97 per cent of all cases, and in them, as was first pointed out by Naegele, the sagittal suture nearly always occupies the right oblique diameter of the pelvis. In other words, one usually has to deal with a left occipito-iliac anterior, or a right occipito-iliac posterior presentation. That this is so, and that the first-mentioned presentation is the one most frequently observed, practically all the authorities are agreed; but that wide differences of opinion exist as to the relative frequency of the several other varieties is clearly shown by the following table:

	Dubois in 1,913 cases.	Pinard in 500 cases.	The author in 1,687 cases.
L. O. I. A.	71 per cent.	52.6 per cent.	60.9 per cent.
L. O. I. P.	.63 "	11 "	2.6 "
R. O. I. A.	2.87 "	.2 "	22.3 "
R. O. I. P.	25.6 "	38.8 "	14.2 "

Mechanism of Left and Right Occipito-iliac Anterior Presentations.—We shall consider in the first place the mechanism of labour in the anterior

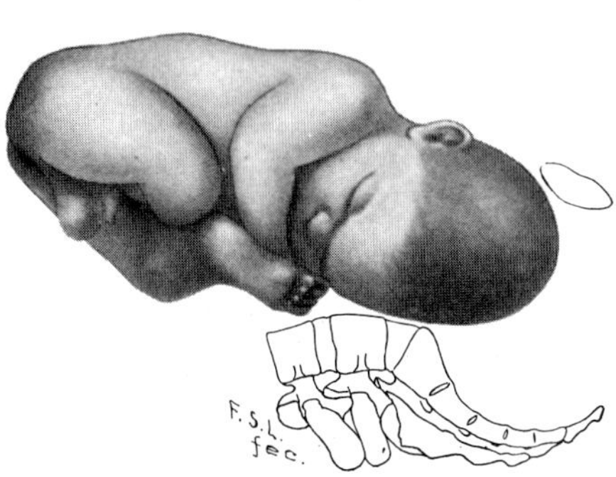

Fig. 223.—Diagram showing Child in L. O. I. A.

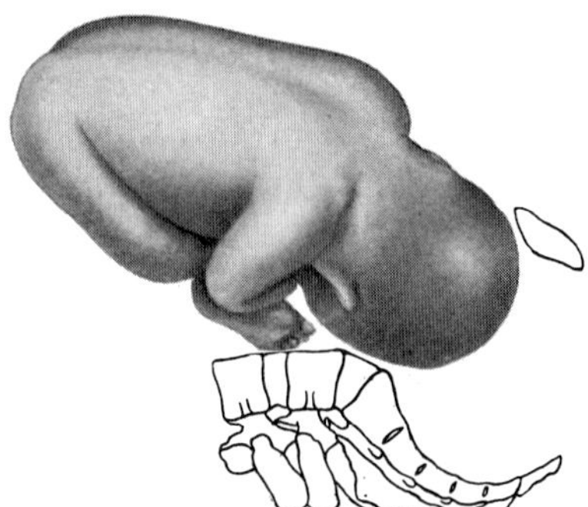

Fig. 224.—Diagram showing Child in R. O. I. A.

varieties of vertex presentations—namely, the left and right occipito-iliac anterior.

Diagnosis.—The way in which the fœtus is presenting is most reliably determined by abdominal palpation, which can be utilized not only during pregnancy but also at the time of labour, provided it be practised in the intervals between the pains. Its accuracy, however, is markedly impaired

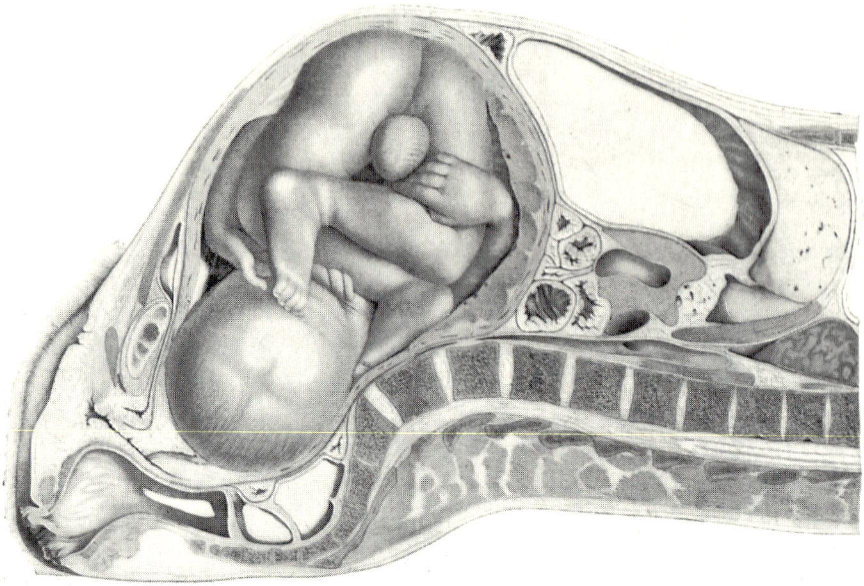

FIG. 225.—FROZEN SECTION THROUGH WOMAN AT END OF PREGNANCY, CHILD IN R. O. I. T. (Zweifel).

in patients with very fat abdominal walls, or in whom the uterus is unduly distended by an excessive amount of amniotic fluid, or deformed by subperitoneal or intramural myomata, which may occasionally be mistaken for portions of the child.

For purposes of diagnosis we employ the manœuvres already described, and with the fœtus in the left occipito-iliac position obtain the following data:

First manœuvre: Irregular breech at fundus.
Second manœuvre: Resistant plane of back in the left and anterior portion of the abdomen, with the small parts on the right side.
Third manœuvre: If the head be not engaged, it is felt as a freely movable body over the superior strait; but if the head is fixed, the anterior shoulder may be detected.
Fourth manœuvre: Negative if the head be not engaged; otherwise the cephalic prominence is felt on the right side (Plate X).

For the right occipito-iliac anterior position we obtain the following:

First manœuvre: Irregular breech at fundus.
Second manœuvre: Resistant plane of back in the right and anterior portion of the abdomen, with the small parts on the left side.
Third manœuvre: As in L. O. I. A.
Fourth manœuvre: Cephalic prominence on the left side.

PLATE X.

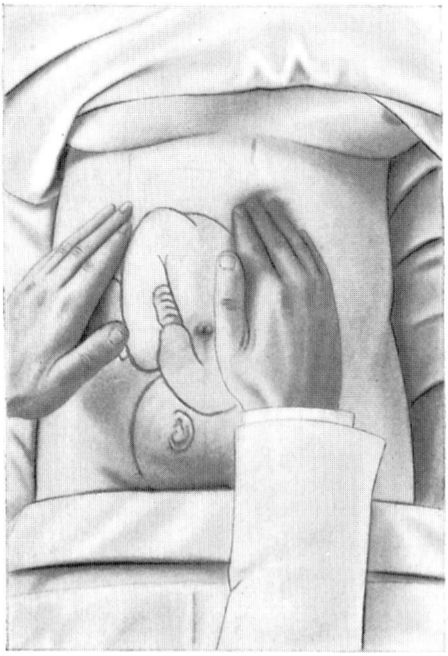

First manœuvre.

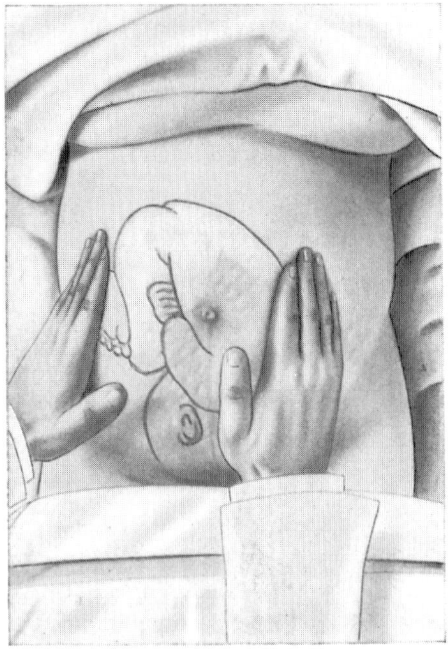

Second manœuvre.

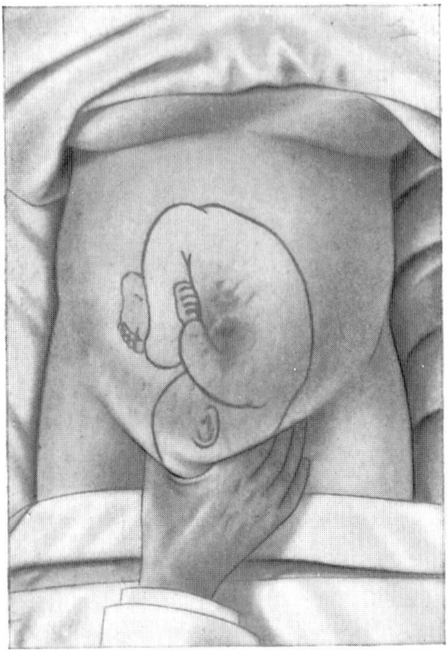

Third manœuvre.

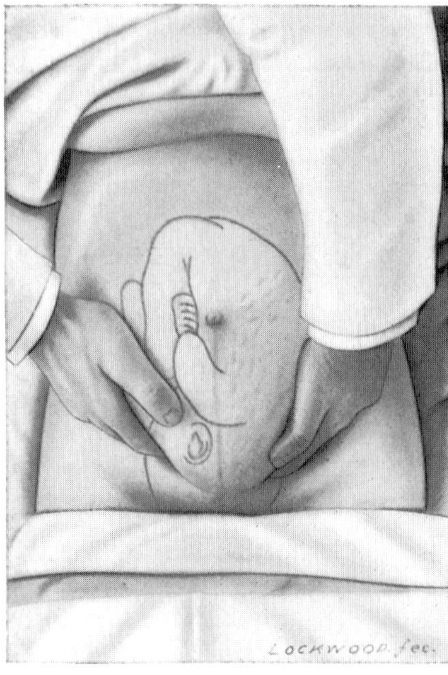

Fourth manœuvre.

PALPATION IN LEFT OCCIPITO-ILIAC-ANTERIOR PRESENTATION.

Until the head has become engaged the information obtained by vaginal examination is extremely meagre; and even after engagement satisfactory results cannot be obtained until the cervix is sufficiently dilated to permit the finger to distinguish the various sutures and fontanelles.

In the left anterior variety, the sagittal suture occupies the right oblique diameter of the pelvis, with the small fontanelle in the neighbourhood of the left ilio-pectineal eminence and the large fontanelle directed towards the right sacro-iliac synchondrosis. In the right anterior variety, the sagittal suture occupies the left oblique diameter, the small fontanelle lying in the neighbourhood of the right ilio-pectineal eminence, while the large fontanelle looks towards the left iliac synchondrosis.

The diagnostic value of vaginal examination is further impaired by the fact that the presence of a marked *caput succedaneum* may make it impossible to feel the sutures and fontanelles, not to speak of differentiating between them.

In the left anterior positions, the fœtal heart sounds are usually heard on the left side of the abdomen along a line joining the umbilicus and the left anterior superior spine of the ilium; and in right positions at a corresponding point on the right side.

Mechanism.—Owing to the relatively small size and irregular shape of the pelvic canal and the large dimensions of the mature fœtal head, it is apparent that any portion of the latter, chosen at random, cannot necessarily pass through every plane of the former; hence it follows that some process of adaptation or accommodation of suitable portions of the head to the various pelvic planes is necessary to insure the completion of childbirth. This is brought about by certain movements of the presenting part, which belong to what is termed the mechanism of labour.

For purposes of instruction, we are obliged to describe the various movements as if they occurred separately and independently of one another; whereas in reality the mechanism of labour consists of a combination of movements, several of which are going on at the same time, it being extremely rare for any individual one to take place totally irrespective of the others. These movements are divided into two classes, according as they are absolutely essential to the completion of labour, or as they merely facilitate its progress. To the first group belong the cardinal movements—*descent*, *internal rotation*, and *extension*; to the second the accessory movements—*flexion* and *external rotation.*

Engagement.—The mechanism by which the presenting part enters the superior strait is designated as engagement. This is best studied in women who have borne one or more children, for the following reason: In primiparæ the head descends into the pelvic canal some weeks before the onset of labour, and when there is no disproportion between the two, the most dependent portion of the presenting part lies just above a line joining the ischial spines; whereas in multiparous women this frequently does not occur until the commencement of labour pains.

In most multiparæ at the end of pregnancy the head is freely movable above the superior strait, or rests upon one or other iliac fossa, and occupies a position midway between flexion and extension. Accordingly, when the uterus begins to contract and to force it towards the pelvic opening, the cephalic circumference which first reaches it is the one that passes through the extremities of the fronto-occipital diameter, which normally measures 11.5 centimetres. Now, as the conjugata vera is only 11 centimetres in length, it is apparent that a normal-sized head cannot engage with its sagittal suture directed antero-posteriorly. It is true that Sentex, Müller, and McKerron have recently revived the old teachings as to the possibility of such an occurrence, and have reported cases of moderately contracted pelves in which the head engaged in this manner, with the small fontanelle situated either just behind the symphysis pubis or just in front of the promontory of the sacrum; but inasmuch as in all of these cases the labour proved to be extremely difficult, it is evident that such conditions must be considered as distinctly pathological.

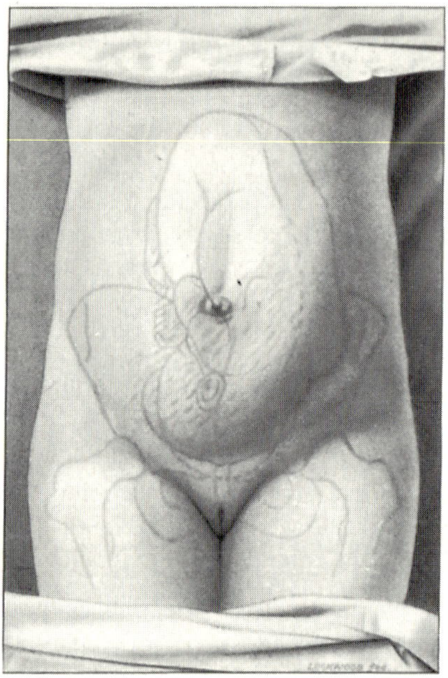

Fig. 226.—Position of Fœtus before Engagement.

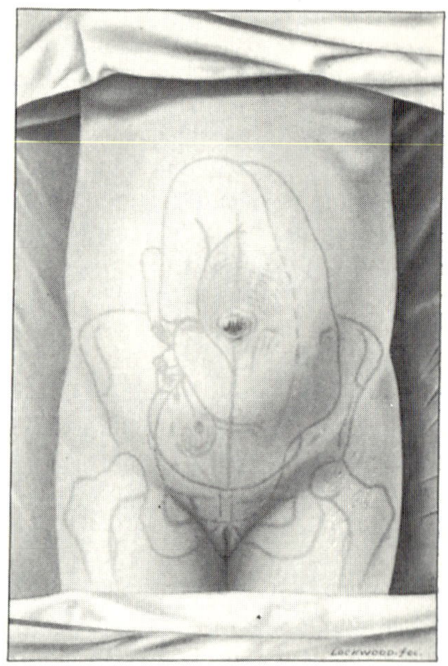

Fig. 227.—Position of Fœtus after Engagement.

As has already been said, the head usually enters the superior strait in one of its oblique diameters (12.75 centimetres), usually the right, with one end of the sagittal suture directed towards the left ilio-pectineal eminence, and the other towards the right sacro-iliac synchondrosis. This is brought about by two factors. In the first place, the fœtus, in the later months of pregnancy, usually assumes this position spontaneously; and secondly, the posterior end of the left oblique diameter is encroached upon by the rectum; so that, for practical purposes, it is shorter than the right.

At first glance it may appear strange that the head does not engage in the transverse diameter of the pelvis, which measures 13.5 centimetres;

but when one recalls the normal outlines of the superior strait (Figs. 228 and 229), it is seen that the promontory of the sacrum juts forward in such a manner as to make it impossible for engagement to occur in this way, as the available transverse diameter is considerably shorter than the oblique.

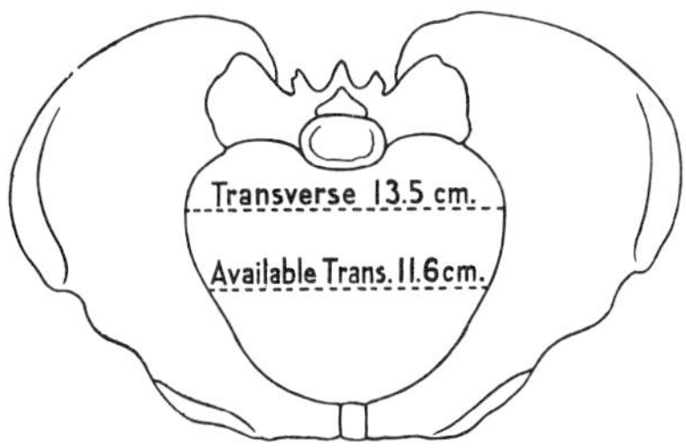

Fig. 228.

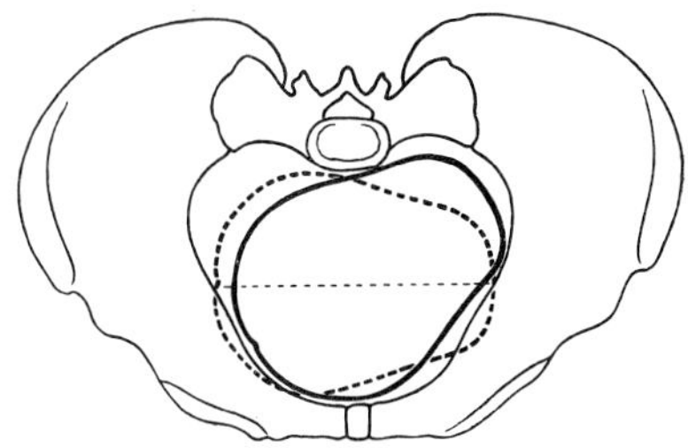

Fig. 229.

FIGS. 228, 229.—DIAGRAMS SHOWING WHY THE HEAD DOES NOT ENGAGE IN THE TRANSVERSE DIAMETER OF THE SUPERIOR STRAIT.

The mechanism of engagement has given rise to a great deal of discussion. Naegele believed that it took place in such a way that the sagittal suture assumed an eccentric position, being nearer the promontory of the sacrum than the symphysis, and that therefore the anterior parietal bone of the fœtus was first felt on vaginal examination—*Naegele's obliquity.* Varnier, on the other hand, from the study of the various frozen sections at his disposal, concluded that the head entered the pelvis in an exactly opposite direction—namely, with its sagittal suture nearer the symphysis pubis, so that the posterior parietal bone was first felt on examination.

Neither of these views are quite correct when the pelvis is normal and the uterus not pendulous. The first presupposes that the axis of the uterus is to be found somewhat in front of that of the superior strait, and the second, that it lies posterior to it. It would seem that Varnier overlooked the fact that the cadavers, upon which his conclusions were based, were frozen in the horizontal position, with the flaccid uterus resting upon the vertebral column; and while his observations were perfectly correct under the circumstances, they do not apply to the living woman, in whom the uterus rises with each contraction, so that its long axis corresponds more or less closely with that of the superior strait. Moreover, careful vaginal examination reveals the fact that the head usually engages in such a manner that its sagittal suture lies either in the middle of the pelvis or approaches the promontory of the sacrum, but only slightly and not by any means to the extent that Naegele had supposed. On the other hand, the condition of affairs noted by Varnier obtains only in those cases in which considerable disproportion exists between the size of the head and the pelvis.

Descent.—The first requisite for the birth of the child is descent, which occurs continuously, though slowly, throughout labour, from the time the head engages until its expulsion from the vagina. With it are associated the various movements to which reference has already been made. Descent is brought about by four forces: (1) Intra-uterine fluid pressure; (2) direct pressure of the fundus upon the breech; (3) contraction of the abdominal muscles; and (4) extension and straightening of the child's body.

As the anterior surface of the sacrum and the posterior surface of the symphysis measure 12 and 5 centimetres respectively, it is apparent that if all parts of a body passing through the pelvic cavity are to reach the inferior strait at the same time, the one lying posteriorly must descend much more rapidly than the anterior portion. This compensatory difference in the rate of descent of the portions of the presenting part occupying the anterior and posterior segments of the pelvis is known as *synclytism,* and is clearly illustrated in Fig. 230.

Flexion.—As soon as the descending head meets with resistance, whether it be from the margins of the superior strait or the cervix, the walls of the pelvis or the pelvic floor, flexion results. By this is meant that the head rotates about its transverse axis in such a manner as to bring the chin into more intimate contact with the thorax, thereby substituting the suboccipito-bregmatic for the fronto-occipital diameter.

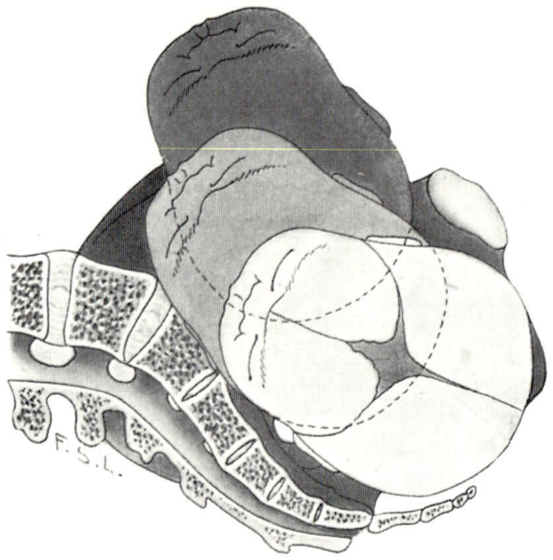

Fig. 230.—Diagram illustrating Synclitism (Ahlfeld).

This is a purely mechanical phenomenon, and is due to the manner in which the head is articulated with the vertebral column, whereby the former becomes converted into a two-armed lever, the short arm extending from the occipital condyles to the occipital protuberance, and the long arm from the same point to the chin (Fig. 234). It is therefore apparent that when resistance is encountered the long arm of the lever, following the ordinary laws of mechanics, must ascend, while the short arm descends, and thus flexion is brought about.

The point of the birth canal at which this movement occurs varies greatly. If descent begins before the external os is fully dilated, especially if its margins are resistant, flexion may be completed before the head has left the uterus. In generally contracted pelves, flexion takes place in an exaggerated manner while engagement is going on; but, as a rule, when there is no disproportion between the presenting part and the pelvic canal, it does not occur until the resistance of the pelvic floor is encountered.

Internal Rotation.—By this we understand a turning of the head about its vertical axis in such a manner that the occiput gradually moves from the position which it originally occupied towards the symphysis pubis.

In left positions the motion is from left to right, and in the reverse direction in right positions (Figs. 235 and 236).

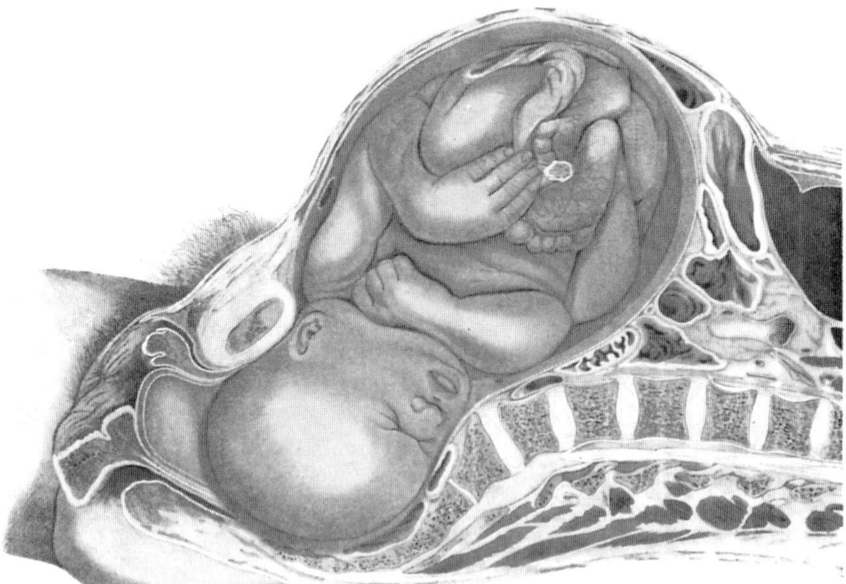

FIG. 231.—FROZEN SECTION, SECOND STAGE OF LABOUR, CHILD IN R. O. I. A., MEMBRANES UNRUPTURED (Braune). Compare with Fig. 225.

Internal rotation is absolutely essential for the completion of labour, except when the child is abnormally small, and in the anterior positions

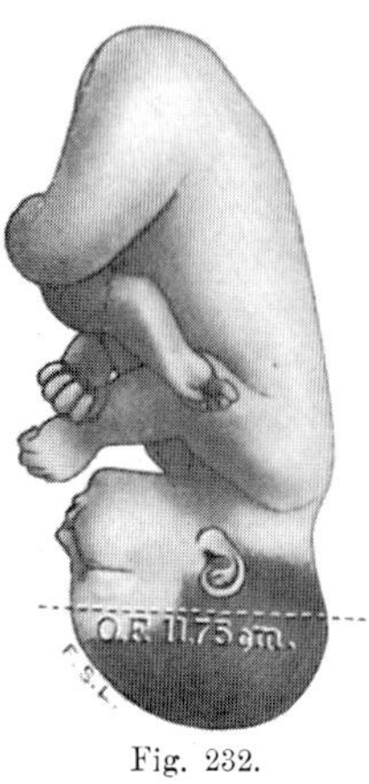

Fig. 232.

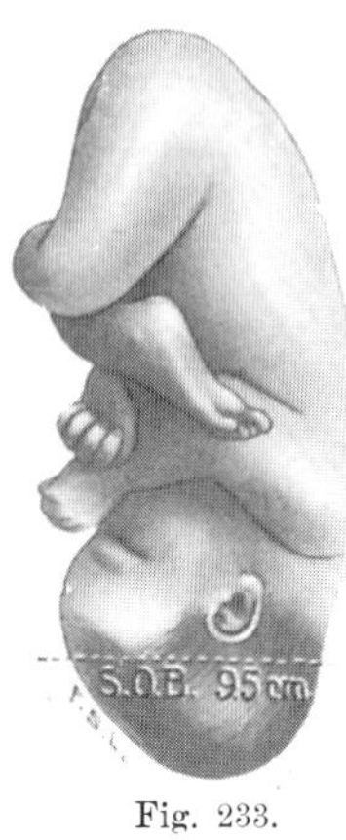

Fig. 233.

FIGS. 232, 233.—DIAGRAMS SHOWING EFFECT OF FLEXION, CONVERSION OF OCCIPITO-FRONTAL INTO SUBOCCIPITO-BREGMATIC DIAMETER.

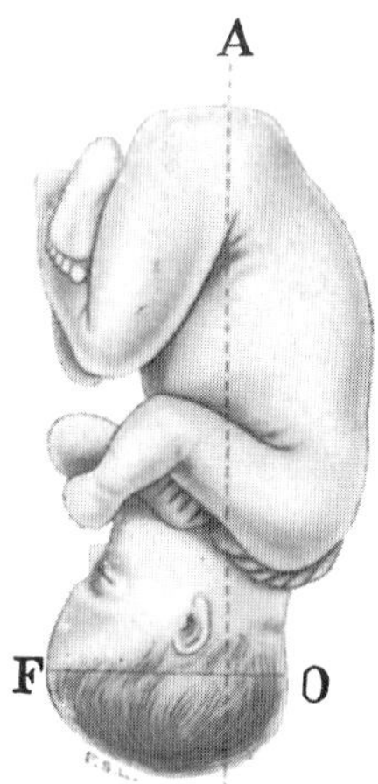

FIG. 234.—DIAGRAM SHOWING HEAD LEVER (American Text-Book).

always occurs in the direction indicated. Indeed, no matter what the original position of the head may be, the occiput usually rotates to the front, although exceptionally, in occipito-posterior presentations, it may turn towards the hollow of the sacrum. It should be remembered that

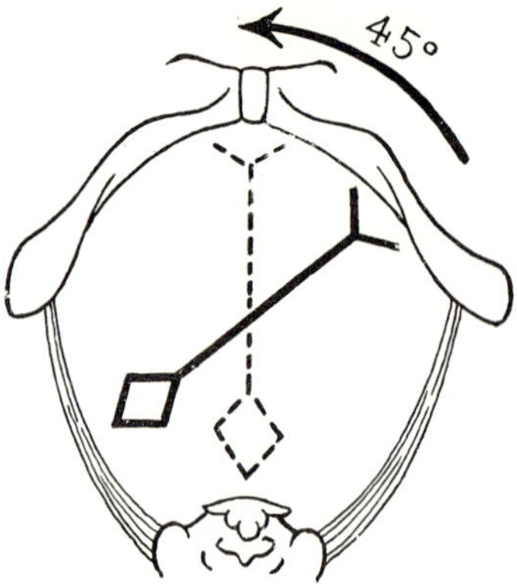

Fig. 235.—Diagram showing Anterior Rotation from L. O. I. A.

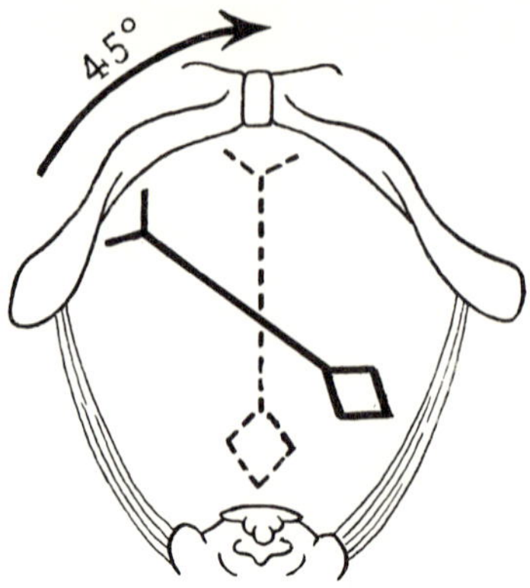

Fig. 236.—Diagram showing Anterior Rotation from R. O. I. A.

internal rotation does not occur by itself, but is always associated with the descent of the presenting part.

Various theories have been advanced in the attempt to explain the manner in which internal rotation is brought about, and a vast literature has accumulated upon the subject. The general belief has been that it is rendered necessary by the shape of the pelvic canal, it having been formerly taught that the superior strait represented an ellipse whose long axis lay transversely, and the inferior strait one whose long axis was antero-posterior; so that for the head to descend it was necessary that its sagittal suture be directed transversely or obliquely to pass through the former, and antero-posteriorly to pass through the latter. A little consideration, however, will show that this is not the case, for the inferior strait presents an almost circular opening, its transverse diameter being 11 and its antero-posterior 9.5 centimetres, when the coccyx is in its usual position, and 11.5 centimetres when it is displaced backward during labour. Varnier is therefore justified in concluding that the shape of the pelvis alone does not necessarily explain the production of this movement; and, moreover, when we recall the fact that the diameter of the head, which passes through it during expulsion, is not the fronto-occipital, as is usually stated, but the suboccipito-frontal, which measures 10.5 centimetres (Fig. 237), it is evident that unless some other factor rendered it necessary, the head could be born without internal rotation.

This factor is to be found in the structure of the pelvic floor, and particularly in the levator ani muscle. The latter is perforated by a narrow slit, through which the head must pass. This opening, even when markedly distended, still retains an oval outline, its transverse diameter always remaining considerably less than its antero-posterior, and to this shape the head must adapt itself in order to be born. Furthermore, the curved walls of the perineal gutter offer a concave inclined plane over which the rounded head readily glides in its downward course.

This explanation, although satisfactory when the occiput is originally situated in the anterior portion of the pelvis, would not necessarily seem to apply with equal force to those cases in which it occupies a posterior position. But the following account of Dubois's experiment clearly demonstrates that even under such circumstances the pelvic floor exerts a predominating influence in the production of this movement. "In a woman who had died a short time previously in childbed, the uterus, which had remained flaccid and of large size, was opened up as far as the cervical orifice and held by assistants in a suitable position above the superior strait. The fœtus of the woman was then placed in the soft and dilated uterus in the right occipito-posterior position. Several pupil-midwives pushing the fœtus from above, readily caused it to enter the cavity of the pelvis. Much greater force was needed to make the head travel over the perinæum and clear the vulva, and it was not without astonishment that we saw, in three successive attempts, that when the head had traversed the external genital organs, the occiput had turned to the right anterior position, while the face was turned to the left and to the rear. In a word, rotation had taken place as in natural labour. We repeated the experiment a fourth time, but as the head cleared the vulva the occiput remained posterior. We then took a dead-born fœtus of the previous night, but of much larger size than the preceding, and placed it in the same position as the first, and twice in succession witnessed the head clear the vulva after having executed the movement of rotation. Upon the third and following essays delivery was accomplished without the occurrence of rotation. Thus the movement only ceased after the perinæum and vulva had lost the resistance which had made it necessary, or at least had been the inciting cause of its accomplishment."

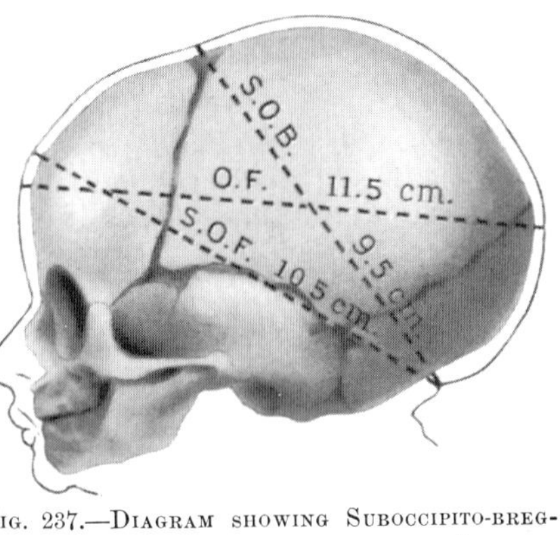

FIG. 237.—DIAGRAM SHOWING SUBOCCIPITO-BREGMATIC, SUBOCCIPITO-FRONTAL, AND OCCIPITO-FRONTAL DIAMETERS.

From Solayrès de Renhac (1771) to the present time, many authors, among whom may be mentioned Scanzoni, Hodge, and Reynolds, have sought to explain the production of rotation by calling attention to the shape of the pelvic canal, and pointing out that the inclination of its walls —the *inclined planes of the pelvis*—served to direct the occiput anteriorly. By others it was thought that the projecting ischial spines also played a similar part by interposing an obstacle to posterior rotation.

Schroeder believed that the movement was inaugurated by the body of the child rotating in such a way as to bring its back more to the front, and that the head followed it. He considered that this was brought about by an attempt on the part of the uterus to assume its normal flattened shape, as its contents were expelled. He did not believe that the shoulders were rotated until the bisacromial diameter was directly transverse, but considered that they remained somewhat behind the occiput—30 degrees according to Schatz—and that the movement of the body merely inaugurated that of the head, which was still further accentuated by accessory causes.

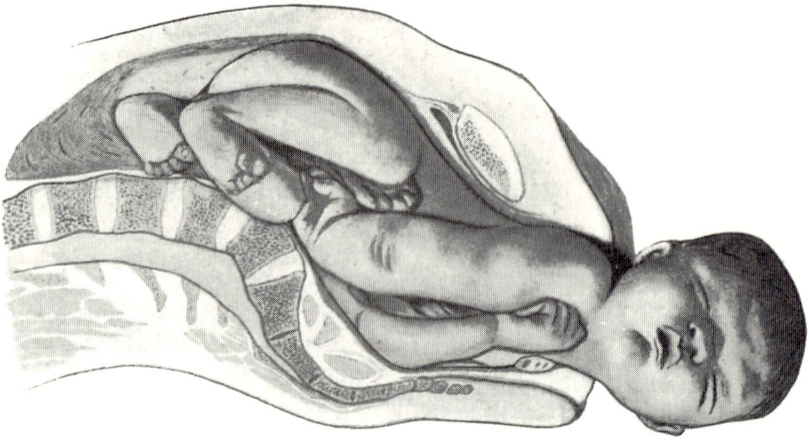

FIG. 238.—FROZEN SECTION THROUGH WOMAN IN LABOUR WITH CHILD PARTLY DELIVERED, SHOWING THAT EXTERNAL ROTATION OF THE HEAD IS NOT DEPENDENT UPON ROTATION OF THE SHOULDERS (Zweifel).

Olshausen has recently argued in favour of this theory, but does not seem to have adduced any additional evidence in its support. On the other hand, the recent frozen section of Zweifel, through a woman who had died just after the birth of the child's head, shows that the latter had undergone a complete rotation, while the shoulders had hardly rotated at all, and to my mind offers convincing evidence against the views of Schroeder and Olshausen.

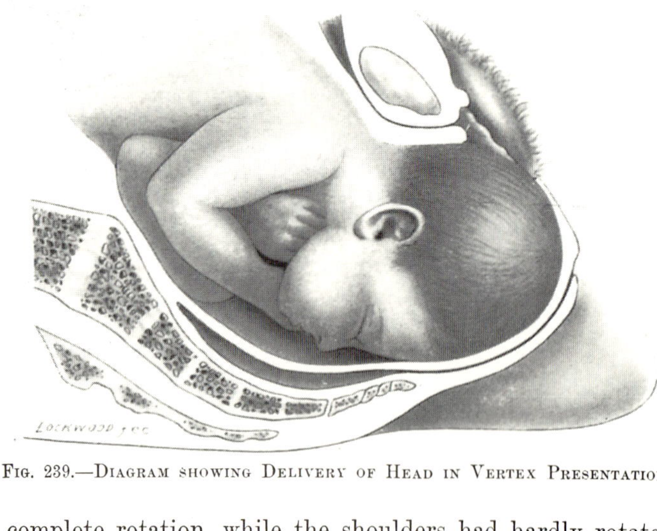

FIG. 239.—DIAGRAM SHOWING DELIVERY OF HEAD IN VERTEX PRESENTATION.

Extension.—When, after internal rotation, the sharply flexed head reaches the vulva, it undergoes another movement which is absolutely essential to its birth—namely, it becomes extended so that the base of the occiput comes in direct contact with the inferior margin of the symphysis pubis. This movement is brought about by two factors. In the first place, as the vulval outlet looks upward and forward, extension must occur before the head can pass through it. For if the sharply flexed head, on reaching the pelvic floor, continued to be driven downward in the same direction as heretofore—in the axis of the superior strait—it would impinge upon the end of the coccyx and the posterior portion of the perinæum, and if the *vis a tergo* were sufficiently strong, would eventually be forced through the perineal tissues. But when the head presses upon this structure, two forces come into play, the first acting downward, exerted by the uterus, and the second upward, supplied by the resistant pelvic floor, the resultant force

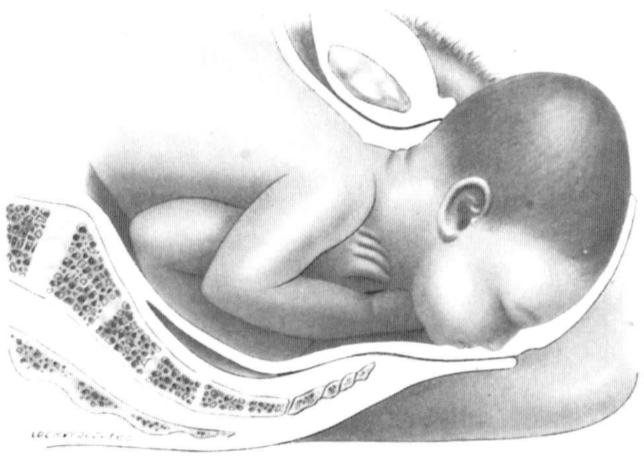

FIG. 240.—DIAGRAM SHOWING DELIVERY OF HEAD IN VERTEX PRESENTATION.

being one directed forward and somewhat upward in the direction of the vulval opening, thereby giving rise to extension.

After the suboccipital region has come in contact with the inferior margin of the symphysis pubis, the head is no longer to be regarded as a two-armed, but simply as a one-armed lever, the occiput being the fulcrum with the arm extending from it to the chin, so that any force exerted upon the head must necessarily lead to farther extension. As this becomes marked, the vulval opening gradually dilates and the scalp of the child soon becomes apparent through it. Now, if we mark the point which first appears, and carefully examine the child after its birth, we find in left occipito-anterior presentations that it was the upper and posterior margin of the right parietal bone that first came into view, while the reverse holds good in right occipito-anterior positions.

With increasing distention of the perinæum and vaginal opening, a larger and larger portion of the occiput gradually appears, and the head is born by further extension, the occiput, bregma, forehead, nose, mouth, and finally the chin, successively passing over the anterior margin of the perinæum. Immediately after its birth the head falls downward and the chin comes in contact with the region of the anus.

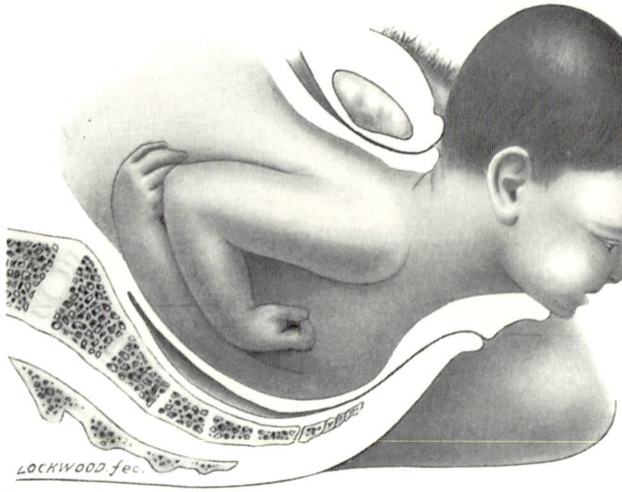

FIG. 241.—DIAGRAM SHOWING DELIVERY OF HEAD IN VERTEX PRESENTATION.

External Rotation.—A few moments after its birth the head undergoes another movement, and, when the occiput has been originally directed towards the left, it rotates towards the left tuber ischii, and in the opposite direction when it has been originally towards the right. This is known as external rotation or restitution, and is simply the index of a corresponding rotation of the body of the child, which serves to bring its bisacromial diameter into relation with the antero-posterior diameter of the pelvic outlet. This movement is brought about by essentially the same factors which produce the internal rotation of the head.

Expulsion.—Almost immediately after the occurrence of external rotation, the anterior shoulder appears under the symphysis pubis, and in a short time the anterior portion of the perinæum becomes distended by the posterior shoulder, which is first born, being rapidly followed by the other. Finally, the body of the child is quickly extruded along a curved line corresponding to the axis of the lower part of the birth canal—that is, with its upper side markedly concave and its lower convex.

Mechanism of Right and Left Occipito-iliac Posterior Presentations.—In 1,687 cases of labour at the Johns Hopkins Hospital we observed 283 occipito-posterior presentations (16.8 per cent), the occiput being directed to the right in 239 cases, and to the left in 44 cases, a proportion of about 1 to 5. From our figures it would appear that these presentations occur less frequently than is usually stated, a result probably due to the fact that many of our patients were not examined until well advanced in labour; so that in not a few the occiput, which was originally directed posteriorly, had undergone anterior rotation.

Diagnosis.—Palpation in a right occipito-iliac posterior presentation gives the following data:

First manœuvre:	The fundus is occupied by the breech.
Second manœuvre:	The resistant plane of the back is felt well back in the right flank, the small parts being on the left side and much more readily palpable than in anterior presentations.
Third manœuvre:	Negative if the head is engaged; otherwise the movable head is detected above the superior strait.
Fourth manœuvre:	Cephalic prominence on the left side (Plate XI).

Whenever the back of the child is felt on the right side of the mother, the possibility of a right posterior position should always be borne in mind, as it occurs nearly or quite as frequently as the right anterior variety. It should also be remembered, whenever the small parts are distinctly felt in the anterior portion of the abdomen, that one has in all probability to deal with a posterior position, more especially in the rare instances in which the occiput occupies the hollow of the sacrum. In the less frequent left posterior positions, palpation gives similar results, except that the back is felt in the left flank and the small parts and cephalic prominence are found on the right side of the abdomen.

On vaginal touch in the right posterior position, the sagittal suture occupies the right oblique diameter, the small fontanelle is felt opposite the right sacro-iliac synchondrosis, the large fontanelle being directed towards the left ilio-pectineal eminence, while in the left position the reverse obtains. In many cases, in the early part of labour, owing to imperfect flexion of the head, the large fontanelle lies at a lower level than in anterior positions, and is more readily felt.

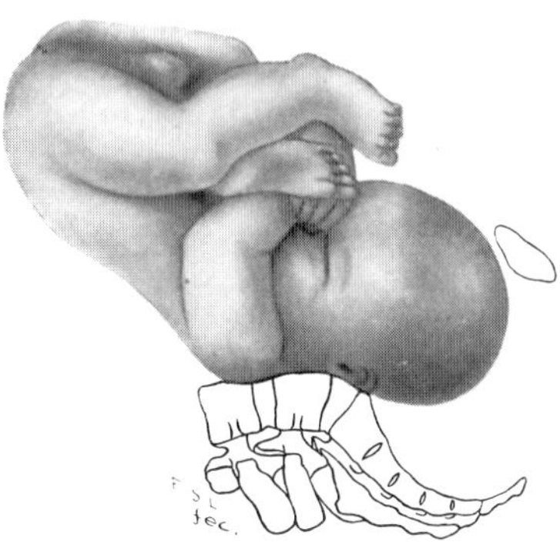

FIG. 242.—DIAGRAM SHOWING CHILD IN L. O. I. P.

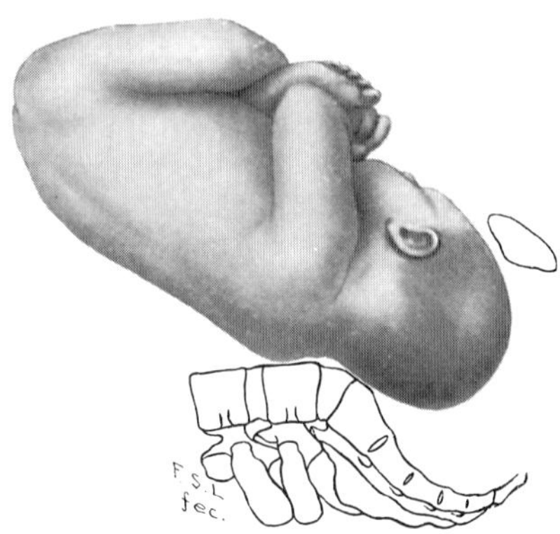

FIG. 243.—DIAGRAM SHOWING CHILD IN R. O. I. P.

On auscultation the heart is heard in the right or left flank of the mother, according as one has to deal with a right or left position. But it should be remembered that in the right posterior position the heart sounds are occasionally transmitted through the thorax of the child, and are best heard either in the middle line or slightly to the left of it. This is due to a partial extension of the head and the altered relation of the body of the child, whereby the thorax comes in contact with the anterior uterine wall.

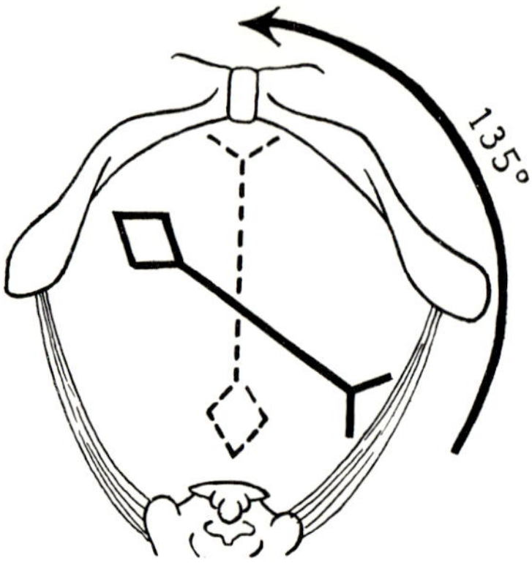

Fig. 244.—Diagram showing Anterior Rotation from L. O. I. P.

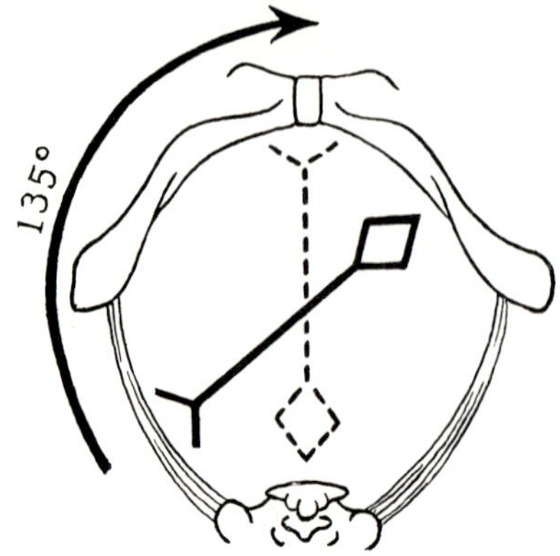

Fig. 245.—Diagram showing Anterior Rotation from R. O. I. P.

Mechanism.—In the vast majority of occipito-posterior presentations the mechanism of labour is identical with that observed in the anterior varieties, except that the occiput has to rotate from the region of the sacro-iliac synchondrosis to the symphysis pubis, instead of from the ilio-pectineal eminence—through 135 degrees instead of 45 degrees.

Not infrequently internal rotation does not take place until the perinæum begins to bulge, and occasionally does not occur at all, spontaneous labour being then out of the question unless the child is very small. This movement usually requires considerable time for its completion, so that there results a not inconsiderable prolongation of labour. Varnier has compared the duration of labour in 400 cases of occiput posterior with

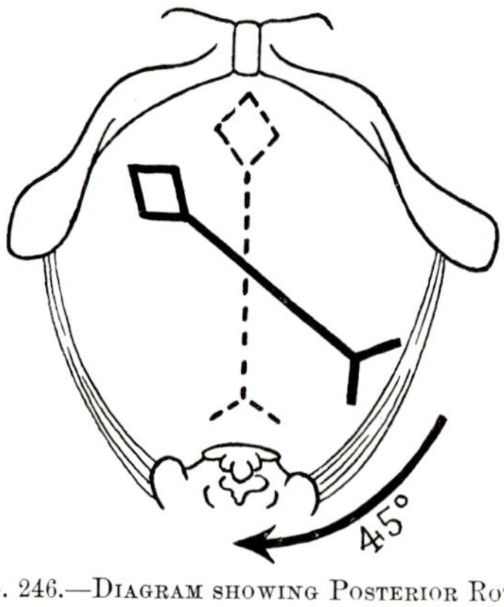

Fig. 246.—Diagram showing Posterior Rotation from L. O. I. P.

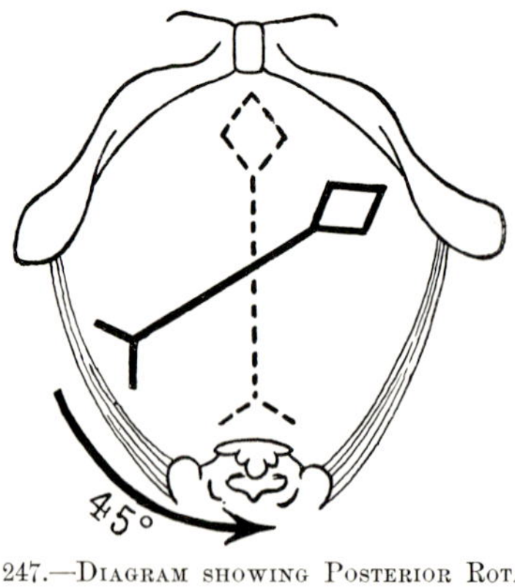

Fig. 247.—Diagram showing Posterior Rotation from R. O. I. P.

that of 660 cases of occiput anterior presentation, and found that it averaged three hours and sixteen minutes to one hour and fifty minutes longer, according as the patient was a primiparous or multiparous woman.

PLATE XI.

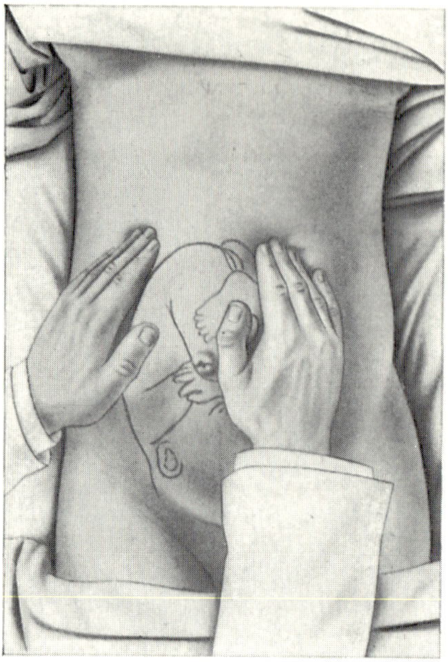

First manœuvre.

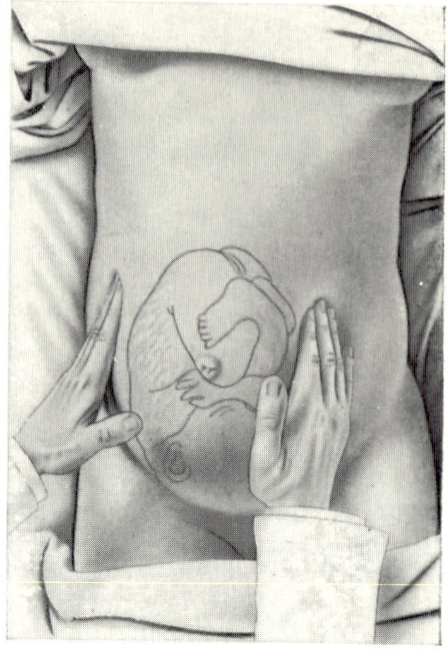

Second manœuvre.

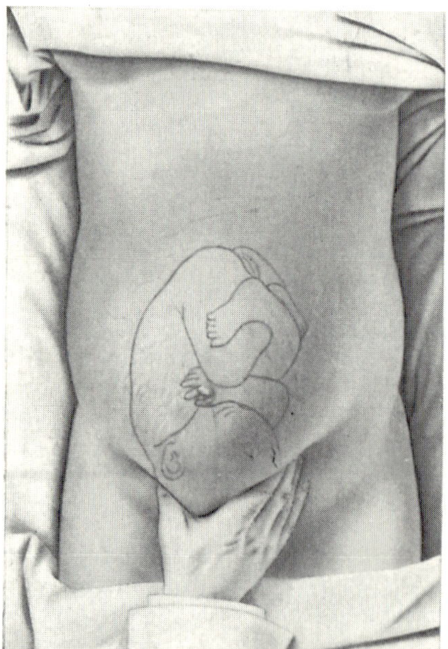

Third manœuvre.

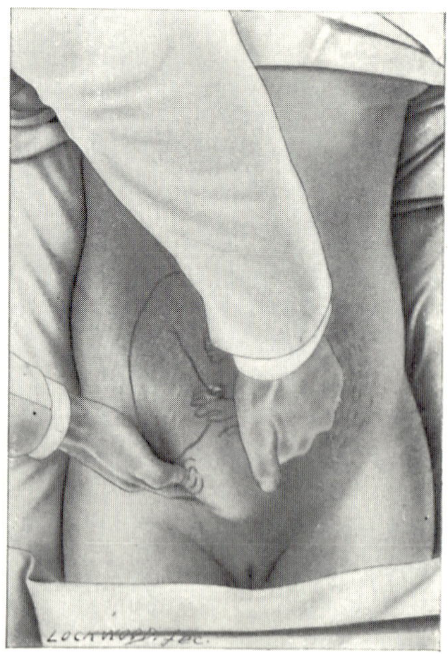

Fourth manœuvre.

PALPATION IN RIGHT OCCIPITO-ILIAC-POSTERIOR PRESENTATION.

In a small percentage of cases the occiput, instead of rotating anteriorly, turns towards the sacrum, so that it eventually occupies its concavity. According to West this occurs in 3 per cent of the cases, while Varnier and the writer have noted it in 2 per cent and 8.79 per cent respectively. In many instances it is difficult to explain why posterior rotation occurs; but when the head is imperfectly flexed, the large fontanelle occupies a lower level than the small, whence it would appear that the portion of the head which remains lowest is the one which rotates anteriorly.

After the occiput has rotated into the hollow of the sacrum, the child may be born in one of two ways. Ordinarily the head becomes markedly flexed and lengthened in its mento-occipital diameter and eventually the region just anterior to the large fontanelle impinges upon the lower margin of the symphysis pubis, after which the occiput is slowly pushed over the anterior margin of the perinæum. Then by a movement of extension

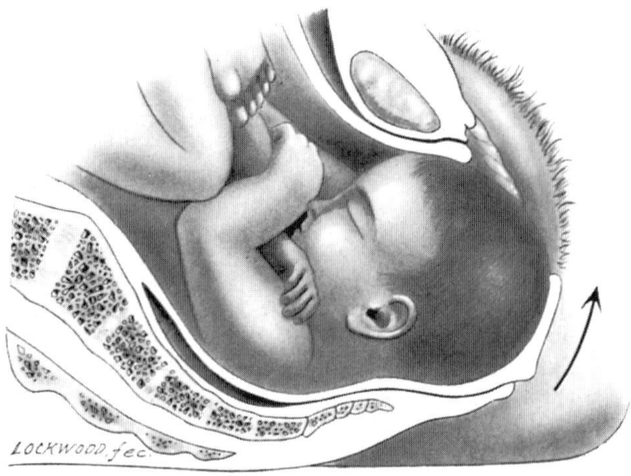

FIG. 248.—USUAL MECHANISM OF DELIVERY OF HEAD WITH OCCIPUT IN HOLLOW OF SACRUM.

the occiput falls backward, and the brow, nose, mouth, and chin appear successively under the symphysis. After the birth of the head, external rotation and expulsion of the body occur in the usual manner.

According to Sentex, Winckel, Weiss, and Müller, the head is occasionally born by another mechanism, which comes into play in those cases in which partial extension persists. Under such circumstances the brow appears at the vulva, and while the root of the nose impinges upon the symphysis, by a movement of flexion the brow, bregma, and occiput successively pass over the perinæum, until finally the face slips out from under the symphysis pubis. This mechanism approaches closely to that observed in brow presentations, and is much more difficult than the one just considered, and is more liable to lead to tears of the maternal soft parts, since it is evident that in the first instance the vulva is distended by the suboccipito-frontal diameter of the head, and in the second by the occipito-frontal, which measure respectively 10.5 and 11.75 centimetres.

Prognosis.—It is generally believed that occipito-posterior offer a much more gloomy prognosis than occipito-anterior presentations. This is probably due to the fact that Mauriceau, Smellie, and all the early authorities taught that in such cases the occiput always rotated into the hollow of the sacrum. It is true that Naegele showed that posterior rotation was only of exceptional occurrence, and that in the vast majority of cases the occiput rotated anteriorly. But in spite of his teachings, the older views still prevailed. Thus Capuron, in 1833, taught that spontaneous delivery could not take place; and Tarnier, while admitting the correctness of Naegele's conclusions, nevertheless taught that the prognosis was always serious, for even when anterior rotation occurred, the duration of labour was markedly increased and the maternal and fœtal mortality augmented.

A comparatively large experience with this class of cases has led me to discount somewhat these gloomy views, and to regard the occurrence

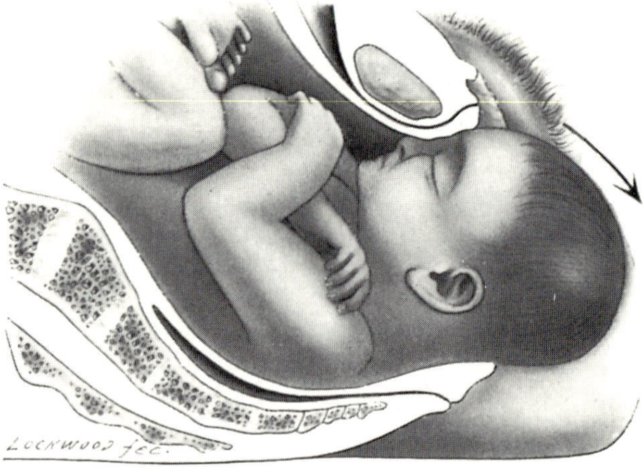

Fig. 249.—Usual Mechanism of Delivery of Head with Occiput in Hollow of Sacrum.

of posterior presentations with equanimity. Moreover, in view of our uniformly good results, I do not consider it advisable to attempt to convert them into other positions during the course of labour, except when the forceps is to be applied. It is true that labour is somewhat prolonged in these cases, and instrumental interference is required more frequently—in 10 per cent of the cases, according to Varnier, as compared with 3.6 per cent in anterior presentations. In 281 cases in which delivery occurred spontaneously or was aided by forceps, we had no maternal mortality directly attributable to the posterior position, and only one child was lost.

Even when the occiput rotates into the hollow of the sacrum, the prognosis is not so very bad, as in the majority of cases spontaneous delivery occurs, being noted by Varnier in 30 out of 35 cases. No doubt when the occiput remains posterior there is an increased tendency towards perineal tears, which is particularly marked when the head is born by the less frequent mechanism. But to my mind the main cause of the dread in which posterior presentations are held is the fact that they frequently escape recognition, and accordingly, when for any reason operative delivery becomes necessary, the forceps is applied improperly—that is, as in occipito-anterior presentations.

When occipito-posterior presentations have descended into the pelvis, it is my practice to leave them to Nature as long as possible, and to interfere only when absolutely necessary. But when convinced that the best interests of the mother and child will be subserved by prompt delivery, forceps should be applied according to the directions which will be given in the appropriate chapter. On the other hand, when the head is arrested at the superior strait in a posterior position, version should be resorted to as soon as one is convinced that spontaneous advance will not occur, provided, of course, that the operation is feasible and is not contra-indicated by disproportion between the size of the head and the pelvis.

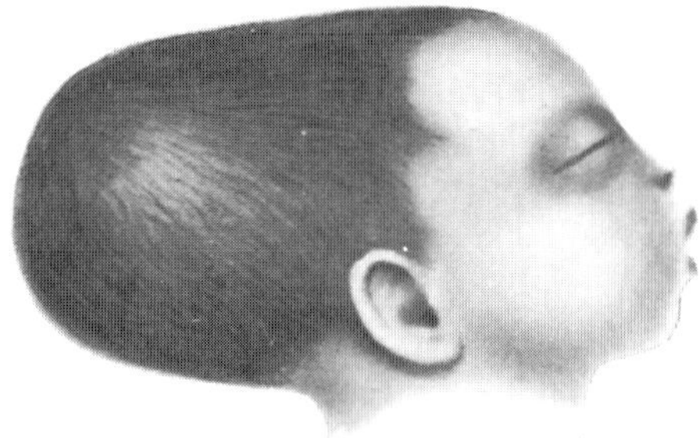

Fig. 250.

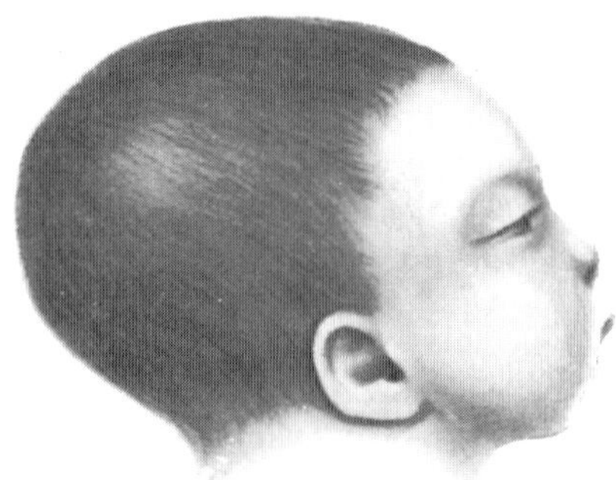

Fig. 251.

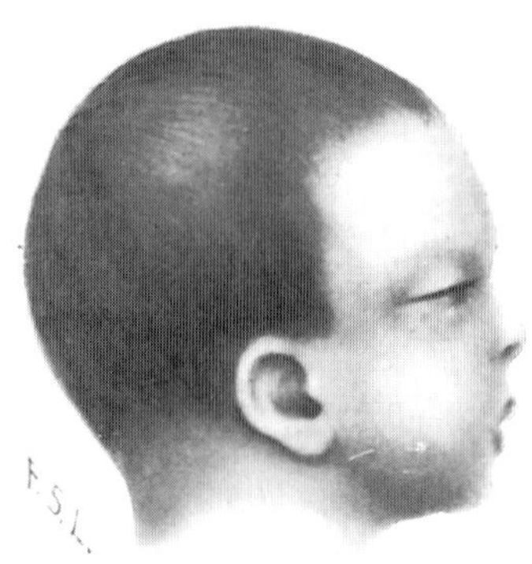

Fig. 252.

Figs. 250–252.—Disappearance of Caput Succedaneum; Same Head at Birth, Three and Ten Days respectively after Labour.

Changes in the Shape of the Head.—In vertex presentations the child's head undergoes important and characteristic changes in shape, as the result of the pressure to which it is subjected during labour. In prolonged labours in which the membranes have ruptured before complete dilatation of the cervix, the portion of the head immediately over the os is relieved from the general pressure existing in the uterus, and as a consequence a serous exudate occurs under the scalp at this point, giving rise to a soft swelling which is known as the *caput succedaneum*. In most cases this attains a thickness of only a few millimetres, but in prolonged labours, under the circumstances named, it may become very considerable and effectually prevent the examining finger from distinguishing the various sutures and fontanelles. More usually the caput is formed when the head is in the lower portion of the birth canal, and not infrequently only after the resistance of a rigid vaginal outlet is encountered. It occurs upon the most dependent portion of the head, and therefore in left occipito-iliac positions is found over the upper and posterior extremity of the right parietal bone, and in right positions over the corresponding area of the left parietal bone. Hence it follows that in many instances after labour we are enabled to diagnose the original presentation by the situation of the caput succedaneum.

More important, however, are the plastic changes which the head undergoes. Owing to the fact that the various bones of the skull are not firmly united, movement may occur at the various sutures. Ordinarily the margins of the occipital bone, and more rarely those of the frontal bone, are pushed under those of the parietal bones; and in many cases one parietal bone may overlap the other, the rule being that the one occupying the posterior position is overlapped by the anterior. These changes are of marked significance, especially in contracted pelves, when the ability of the child's head to become moulded may make the difference between a spontaneous labour and a major obstetrical operation.

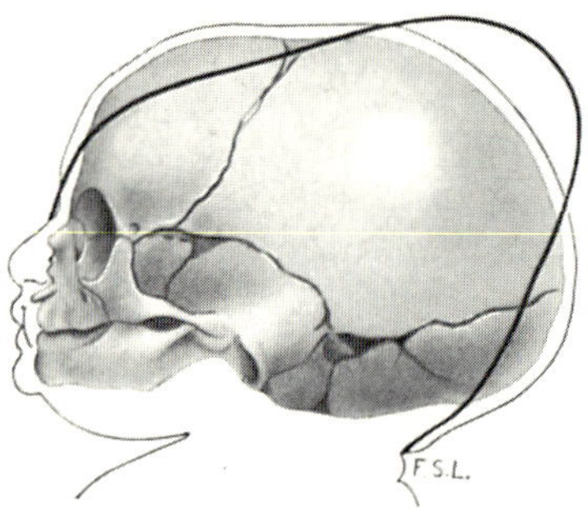

Fig. 253.—Diagram showing Configuration of Head in Vertex Presentation (American Text-Book).

As a result of pressure the head also undergoes a marked change in shape, which consists in a diminution of its suboccipito-mental and occipito-frontal diameters. In other words, it becomes lengthened from chin to occiput and compressed in other directions. This is clearly shown in Fig. 253.

In occipito-posterior presentations, when the occiput has rotated into the hollow of the sacrum, the frontal bone is markedly overlapped by the anterior margins of the parietal bones, which leads to a distinct depression of that part of the head, and gives some idea of the force with which the region of the large fontanelle has been pressed against the lower margin of the symphysis.

LITERATURE

Capuron. Mémoire sur l'impossibilité de l'accouchement naturel et la nécessité du forceps dans les positions occipito-postérieures. Bulletin de l'Acad. de Médecine, Nov. 2, 1833.

Dubois. Quoted by Pinard.

Quoted by Lusk. The Science and Art of Midwifery. New edition, 1895, 175.

Hodge. The Principles and Practice of Obstetrics. Philadelphia, 1866, 159–160.

Mauriceau. Traité des maladies des femmes grosses, etc., 6me éd., Paris, 1721.

McKerron. Antero-posterior Position of the Head as a Cause of Difficult Labour. Trans. London Obst. Soc., 1900, xli, 142–150.

Müller, A. Ueber Hinterhauptslagen und Scheitellagen. Monatsschr. f. Geb. u. Gyn., 1898, vii, 382–399 and 534–550.

Naegele. Die Lehre vom Mechanismus der Geburt. Mainz, 1838.

Olshausen. Beitrag zur Lehre vom Mechanismus der Geburt. Stuttgart, 1901.
Pinard. Traité du palper abdominal, 2me éd., Paris, 1889, 27 and 37–44.
Reynolds. Mechanism of Labour. Amer. Text-Book of Obstetrics, 1897, 384–492.
Scanzoni. Lehrbuch der Geburtshülfe, II. Aufl., Wien, 1853, 219.
Schroeder. Lehrbuch der Geburtshülfe, XIII. Aufl., 1899, 187–188.
Sentex. Étude statistique et clinique sur les positions occipito-postérieures. Paris, 1872.
Smellie. A Treatise on the Theory and Practice of Midwifery. Eighth edition, 1774.
Solayrès de Renhac. Dissertatio de partu viribus maternis absoluto. Paris, 1771.
Tarnier. De l'accouchement dans les occipito-postérieures. Semaine méd., Paris, 1889.
Varnier. De l'attitude de la tête au détroit supérieur et du mechanisme de son engagement. Annales d'Obst. et de Gyn., 1897, xlviii, 442–444.
Accommodation de la tête fœtale au bassin maternel. Obstétrique journalière, Paris, 1900, 131–149.
Les occipito-postérieures. Obstétrique journalière, 1900, 181–184.
Weiss. Zur Behandlung der Vorderscheitellagen. Volkmann's Sammlung klin. Vorträge, N. F. Nr. 60, 1892.
West. Cranial Presentations, etc. Glasgow, 1857.
Winckel. Lehrbuch der Geburtshülfe, II. Aufl., 1893, 147–150.
Zweifel. Zwei neue Gefrierschnitte Gebärender. Leipzig, 1893.

CHAPTER XIII

PHYSIOLOGY OF LABOUR (Continued)

MECHANISM OF LABOUR IN FACE, BROW, AND BREECH PRESENTATIONS

Face Presentations.—In mento-iliac presentations the head is markedly extended, so that the occiput is in contact with the back, while the face looks downward. Pinard, in an analysis of 92,026 cases of labour, found 374 face presentations, a percentage of 0.4 per cent—that is, 1 in every 250 cases.

The face most frequently occupies the right oblique diameter of the pelvis, so that the chin is directed either towards the left ilio-pectineal

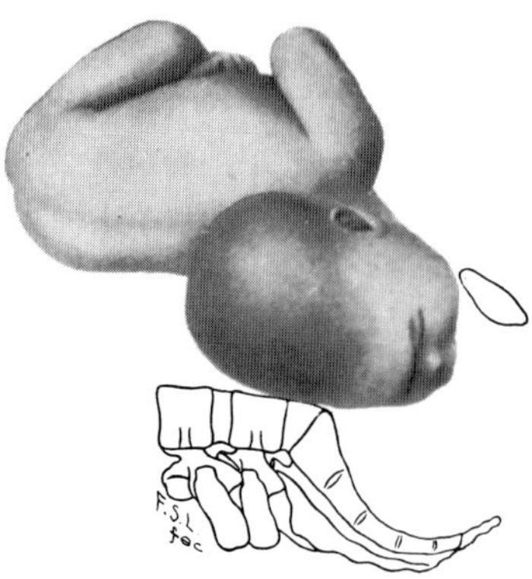

Fig. 254.—Diagram showing Position of Child in L. M. I. A.

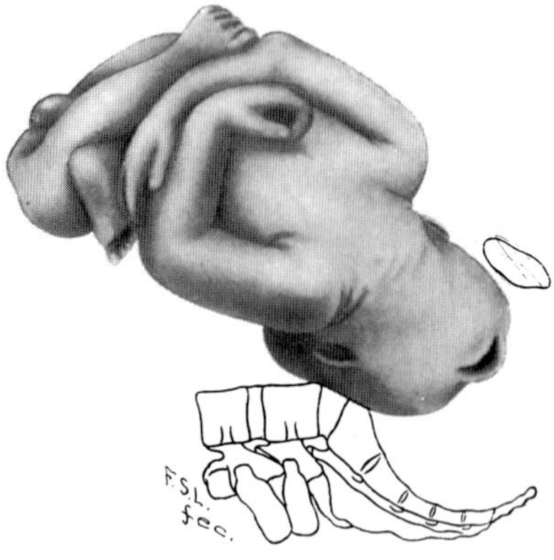

Fig. 255.—Diagram showing Position of Child in R. M. I. A.

eminence or the right sacro-iliac synchondrosis. Accordingly, the left mento-iliac anterior and right mento-iliac posterior are the varieties usually observed.

It is generally stated that face presentations do not exist during pregnancy, but owe their origin to extension of the head at the superior strait at the onset of labour, although Mme. La Chapelle, Naegele, Spiegelberg, Ribemont-Dessaignes, Fieux, and others have described instances in which they were diagnosed during pregnancy. These are designated as primary, in contradistinction to the much more frequent secondary face presentations.

Diagnosis.—In the left mento-iliac anterior variety, palpation gives the following data:

First manœuvre:	Breech in fundus.
Second manœuvre:	Back in the right and posterior portion of the abdomen, and distinctly felt only in its upper portion; small parts in left and anterior portion of the abdomen.
Third manœuvre:	Marked cephalic prominence on right side.
Fourth manœuvre:	Marked cephalic prominence on right side; fingers can be depressed deeply on left (Plate XII).

The reverse holds good in the right posterior variety. The characteristic sign is that the cephalic prominence can be palpated on the same side as the back, the latter being distinctly felt only in the neighbourhood of the breech.

On vaginal touch the face is found in the birth canal, and the variety of presentation is diagnosed by the differentiation of the various features, the mouth and nose, malar bones and orbital ridges being the distinctive points. In the left anterior variety, the chin occupies the anterior and the brow the posterior extremity of the right oblique diameter of the pelvis, while in right posterior positions the reverse obtains.

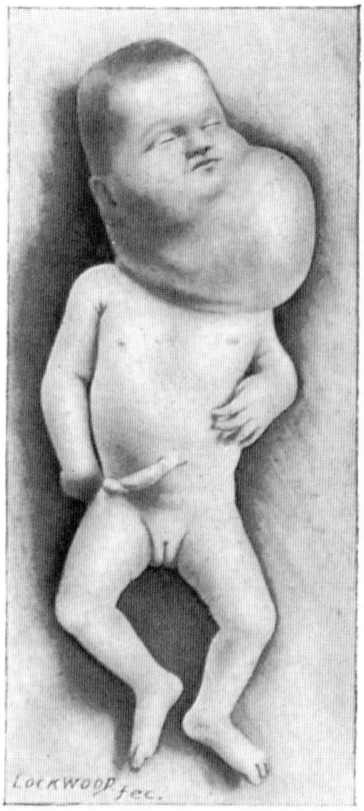

FIG. 256.—TUMOUR OF NECK CAUSING FACE PRESENTATION.

On auscultation the heart sounds are heard below the umbilicus on the side of the abdomen over which the small parts are felt; in other words, they are transmitted through the thorax. The only other condition in which this observation obtains is in brow presentations, and in the rare cases of occipito-posterior presentations in which the head is partially extended.

Causation.—The causes of face presentations are manifold, and, roughly speaking, are afforded by any factor tending to bring about extension or to prevent flexion of the head. Thus, marked enlargement of the neck or thorax, coils of cord about the neck, or spastic contraction of the cervical muscles, may act in this way. Again, it is well known that hemicephalic children usually present by the face, as the result of the faulty development of the cranial vault.

Hecker pointed out that face presentations were occasionally due to an elongation of the occipital portion of the head—*dolichocephalus.* There is no doubt that most children that are born by the face have heads of this character, but the fact that they usually resume their normal shape a few days after labour shows beyond question that the deformity is the result rather than the cause of the presentation. Zweifel delivered by Cæsarean section a dolichocephalic child, which had presented by the breech before operation, and considered that this case demonstrated the possibility of the existence of a primary dolichocephalus; but Fritsch and most observers contend that the peculiar shape of the head resulted from pressure exerted upon it by the fundus of the uterus. On the other hand, Jellinghaus and Gessner have recently reported cases which they believe support the original theory of Hecker; and, on the whole, it would seem probable that such a condition may occasionally bear a causal relation to face presentations.

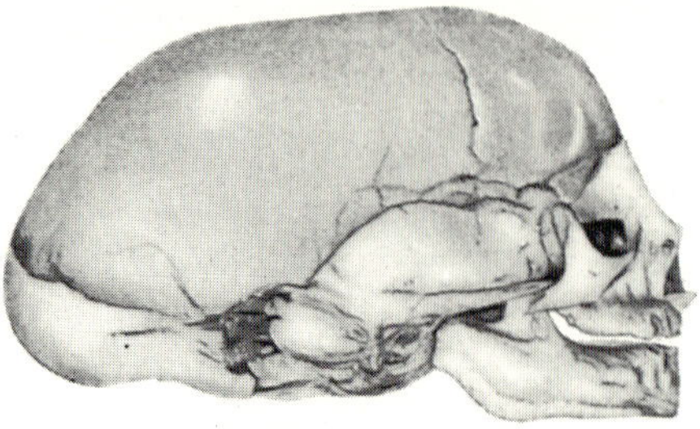

Fig. 257.—Dolichocephalic Head from Breech Presentation (Jellinghaus).

Any factor which interferes with engagement of the head favours the production of face presentations, and accordingly we find that they occur more frequently when the pelvis is contracted or the child very large. It is therefore an excellent practical rule to bear this latter possibility in mind whenever one meets with lack of engagement in a normal pelvis.

Matthews Duncan directed attention to the most frequent cause of face presentations—namely, an oblique position of the uterus, which permits the child's back to sag towards the side to which the vertex lies. He pointed out that under such circumstances

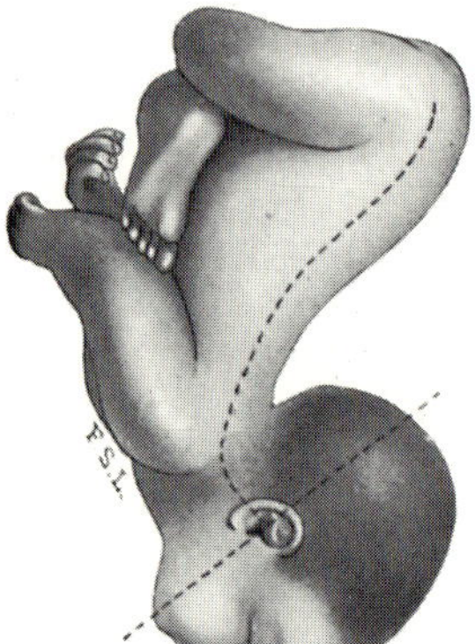

Fig. 258.—Diagram showing that in Face Presentations the Occiput is the Long End of Head Lever.

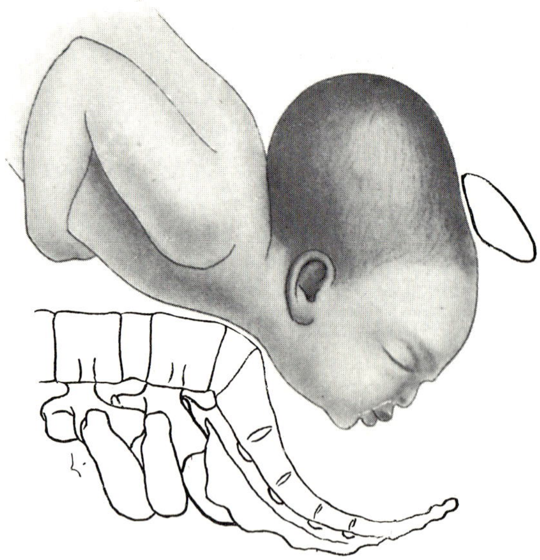

Fig. 259.—Diagram illustrating Impossibility of Labour in Face Presentations when the Chin is directly Posterior.

PLATE XII.

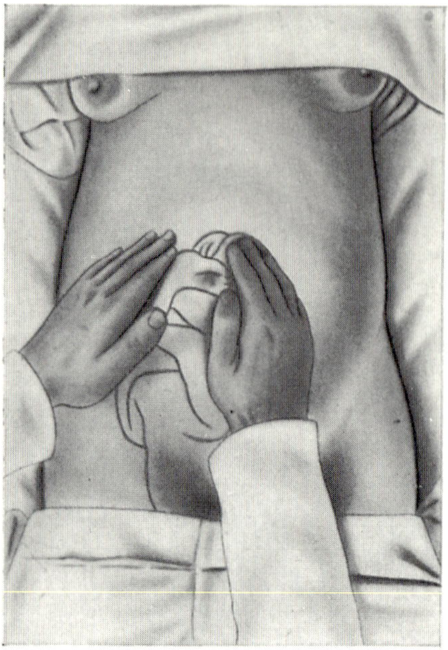

First manœuvre.

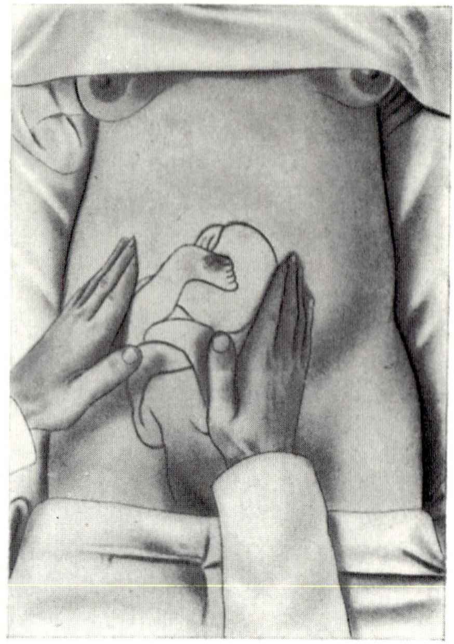

Second manœuvre.

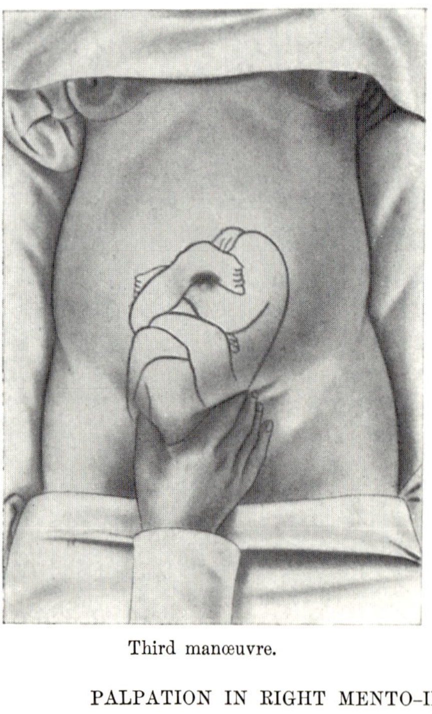

Third manœuvre.

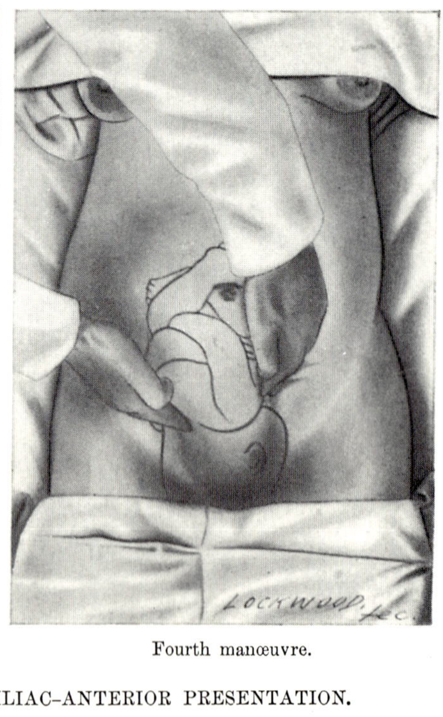

Fourth manœuvre.

PALPATION IN RIGHT MENTO-ILIAC-ANTERIOR PRESENTATION.

the attitude of the fœtus becomes distorted and abnormal, so that a slight obstacle to the descent of the posterior portion of the head will result in its

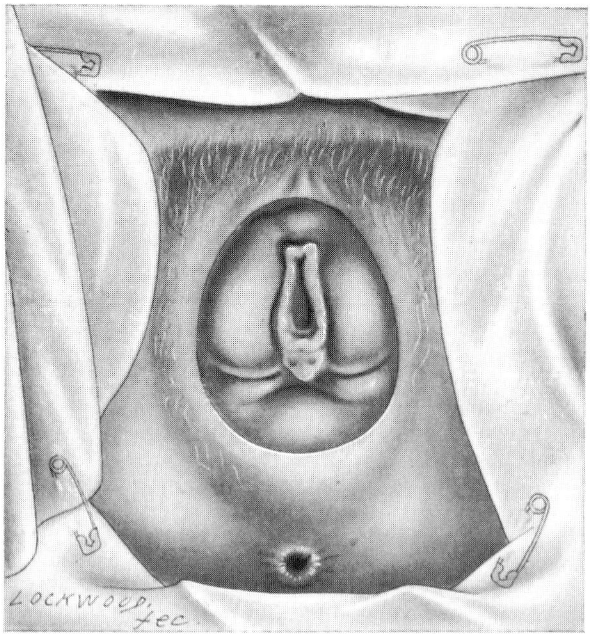

FIG. 260.—DISTENTION OF VULVA IN FACE PRESENTATION (modified from Ahlfeld).

extension. This occurs most frequently in right occipito-iliac posterior presentations, as is shown by the fact that while left occipito-anterior are

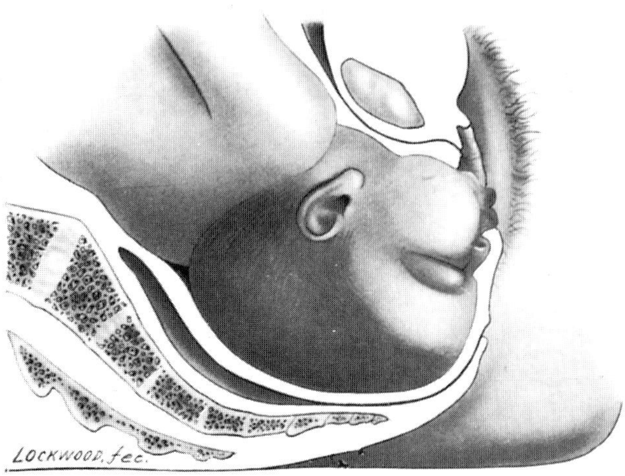

FIG. 261.—DIAGRAM SHOWING DELIVERY OF HEAD IN FACE PRESENTATION.

four times more frequent than right occipito-posterior presentations, the same two varieties of face presentation occur with almost equal frequency.

That multiparity would naturally favour the production of this condition is evident, since lax abdominal walls allow the uterus to assume an oblique position. Thus Pinard and Winckel state that 60 per cent of their cases occurred in multiparous, and only 40 per cent in primiparous women.

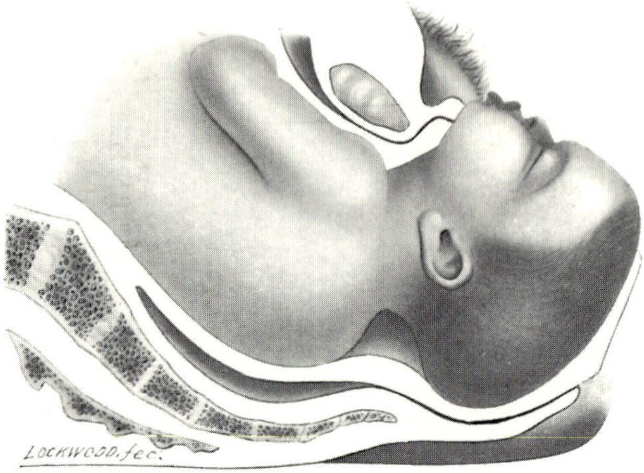

FIG. 262.—DIAGRAM SHOWING DELIVERY OF HEAD IN FACE PRESENTATION.

Mechanism.—As face are usually derived from vertex presentations, it is apparent that the former are but rarely observed in a fully developed state at the superior strait, where the brow generally engages, while the face descends only after further extension.

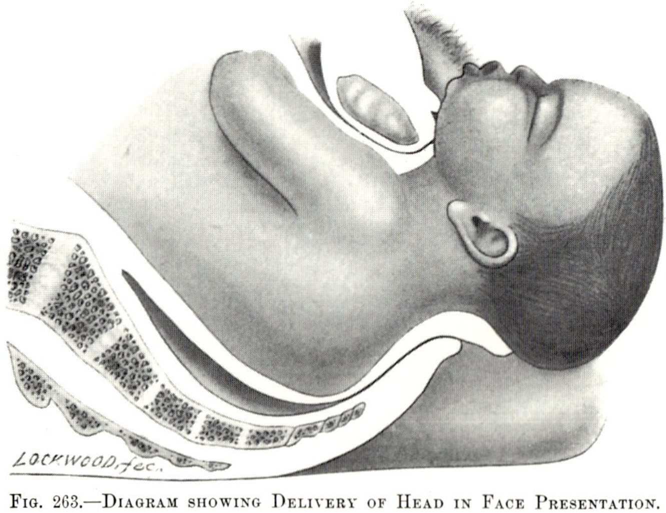

FIG. 263.—DIAGRAM SHOWING DELIVERY OF HEAD IN FACE PRESENTATION.

The mechanism in these cases consists of the *cardinal movements*—descent, internal rotation and flexion; and the *accessory movements*—extension and external rotation. *Descent* is brought about by the same factors as in vertex presentations, while *extension* results from the relation which the body of the child bears to its head, the latter being converted as it were into a two-armed lever, the longer arm of which extends from the occipital condyles to the occiput; so that when resistance is encountered the latter is pushed upward, while the chin descends (Fig. 258).

Internal rotation has for its object the rotation of the face in such a manner as to bring the chin under the symphysis pubis, since otherwise natural delivery cannot be accomplished. Only in this way can the neck subtend the posterior surface of the symphysis pubis; whereas, if the chin be directed posteriorly, the short neck must subtend the anterior surface of the sacrum, which measures 12 centimetres in length, when the birth of the head is manifestly impossible unless the shoulders can enter the pelvis at the same time, which is possible only with very small or premature children (Fig. 259).

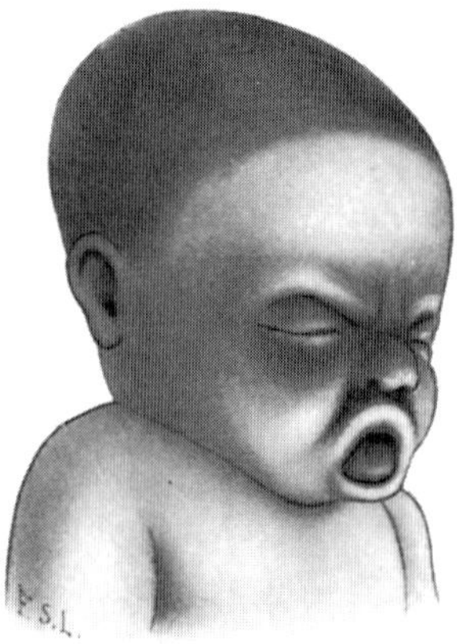

Fig. 264.—Showing Distortion of Face after Delivery in Face Presentation.

After anterior rotation the chin and mouth appear at the vulva; the under surface of the chin becomes stemmed against the symphysis, and the head is delivered by a movement of *flexion*, the nose, eyes, brow, bregma, and occiput appearing in succession over the anterior margin of the perinæum (Figs. 261, 262, and 263). After the birth of the head the occiput sags backward towards the anus, and in a few moments *external rotation* occurs, the shoulders being born as in vertex presentations.

In a small number of cases internal rotation, instead of occurring anteriorly, may take place towards the hollow of the sacrum. Under such circumstances, for the reasons given above, the birth of a normal-sized child is impossible.

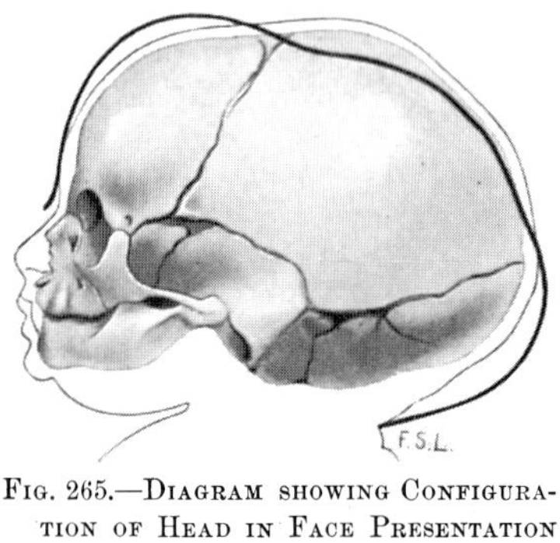

Fig. 265.—Diagram showing Configuration of Head in Face Presentation (American Text-Book).

In mento-iliac presentations the face becomes distorted owing to the effusion of serum beneath the skin, which when marked completely obliterates the features and is very likely to cause confusion with a breech presentation. At the same time the skull undergoes considerable moulding, which is manifested by an increase in length of the mento-occipital diameter and a diminution in the vertical diameters of the head.

Prognosis.—Until the latter part of the eighteenth century face presentations were considered extremely unfavourable, and most authorities advised their conversion into some other variety. But about that time Deleurye, in France, and Zeller and Boer, in Austria, pointed out that most of them would end spontaneously if left alone, the latter author stating that he had observed spontaneous labour in 79 out of 80 cases, and had applied forceps in only a single instance.

Owing to the excessive distention of the vulval outlet by the greatest circumference of the head—the mento-occipital—deep tears of the perinæum are of frequent occurrence; and owing to the prolongation of labour the fœtal mortality is markedly increased, being usually estimated at about 14 per cent, though Weiss lost only 4 out of 78 children (5.1 per cent).

In dealing with face presentations it should always be borne in mind that internal rotation does not occur until the pelvic floor is well distended by the advancing face; and frequently, when the chin is obliquely posterior, it does not take place until the obstetrician has almost abandoned hope of its occurrence. Nor should it be forgotten that the face must occupy a lower level than the vertex before one can feel assured that the greatest circumference of the head has passed through the superior strait. This can be readily appreciated from a study of Figs. 266 and 267, in which it is seen that the distance from the parietal boss to the vertex is only 3 centimetres, whereas a line drawn from the same point to the face will measure 7 centimetres.

Treatment.—In the anterior varieties spontaneous delivery is the rule, and even when the chin is obliquely posterior, anterior rotation usually occurs, although often not until a very late period. In view of the serious prognosis attending its failure, and particularly when the face rotates into the hollow of the sacrum, in appropriate cases an attempt should be made

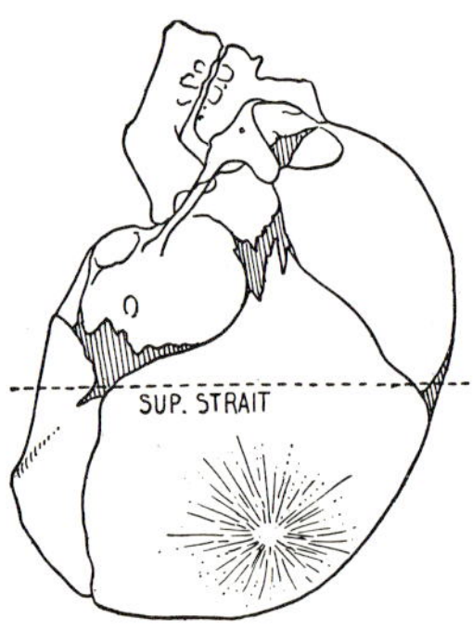

Fig. 266.—Diagram showing that when the Vertex is on the Line joining the Ischial Spines, the greatest Diameter of the Head has passed the Superior Strait.

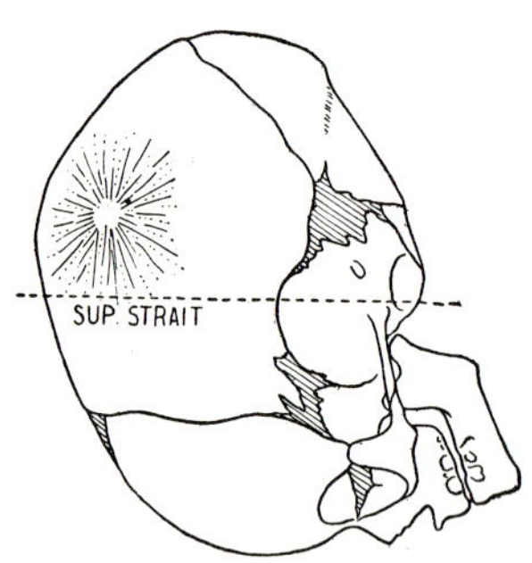

Fig. 267.—Diagram showing that when the Face is on the Level of the Ischial Spines, the Greatest Diameter of the Head is still Above the Superior Strait.

to substitute a vertex presentation. When the face is not deeply engaged this can be readily accomplished, either by pushing up the chin or by making traction upon the occiput.

When the chin is directed anteriorly, attempts at conversion are not advisable, as they would merely substitute an occipito-posterior position, which is but slightly more favourable than the original face presentation, not to speak of the increased danger of sepsis to which the woman must necessarily be subjected during the manœuvre. In obliquely posterior positions, on the other hand, conversion is urgently indicated, and should be attempted as soon as the condition is recognised and the degree of dilatation of the cervix permits. Under these circumstances the unfavourable mento-posterior is converted into a favourable occipito-anterior presentation.

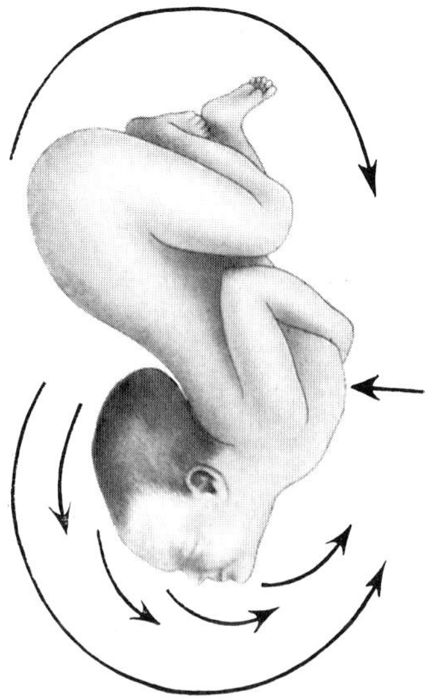

Fig. 268.—Diagram showing Direction of Pressure in Conversion of a Face into a Vertex Presentation by Thorn's Manœuvre.

From time to time numerous methods have been suggested for this purpose, the oldest and most effectual being the following, advocated by Baudelocque and revived by Thorn, Weiss, and others: Attempts are made to push up the chin by two fingers introduced into the vagina; if this does not succeed the patient is anæsthetized, the whole hand introduced, and the head dislodged, after which the vertex is grasped and drawn down. At the same time the external hand of the operator or the assistant carries the back in the opposite direction, so as to facilitate flexion. Very excellent results have been obtained by this manœuvre, and its adoption in suitable cases cannot be too strongly recommended.

Schatz suggested the method of external manipulation pictured in most text-books, by which the vertex is substituted for a presenting face. This, however, is rarely available, inasmuch as the presentation does not become well developed until after engagement has occurred.

If the face be too deeply engaged in the pelvis to admit of the Baudelocque manœuvre, the patient should be let alone and descent allowed to take place, in the hope that external rotation will occur when the face reaches the pelvic floor. If, however, this does not take place after a reasonable delay, forceps should be applied in the manner to be described later, and an attempt made to rotate the chin to an anterior position; finally, if this fails, the only resource lies in craniotomy; although symphyseotomy has been suggested by Davis in such cases.

When the chin is situated directly posteriorly, and attempts at conversion have failed, podalic version should be performed as soon as the condition of the cervix will permit; but if the face be so firmly engaged that it cannot be pushed up under anæsthesia, craniotomy or symphyseotomy must be resorted to as soon as the patient's condition calls for delivery. The former has been repeatedly practised, but so far as I know no one has as yet performed symphysiotomy under the circumstances.

Brow Presentations.—In brow presentations the head occupies a position midway between flexion and extension; hence the portion situated between the orbital ridge and large fontanelle presents at the superior strait.

As nearly every child which is born by the face has gone through a preliminary stage of brow presentation, the latter must occur quite as frequently as that of the face, later undergoing spontaneous conversion into

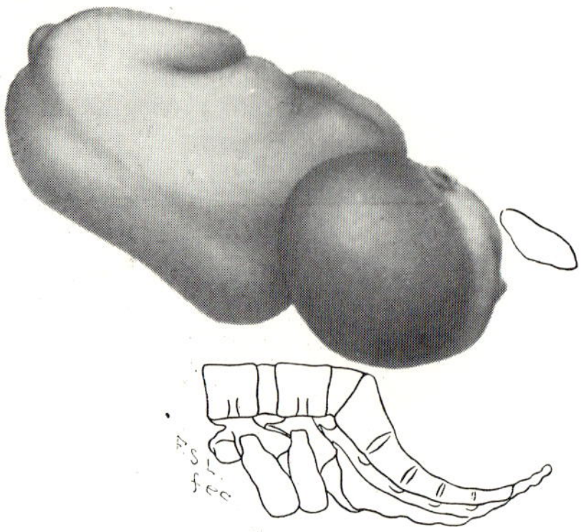

Fig. 269.—Diagram showing Position of Child in Left Anterior Brow Presentation.

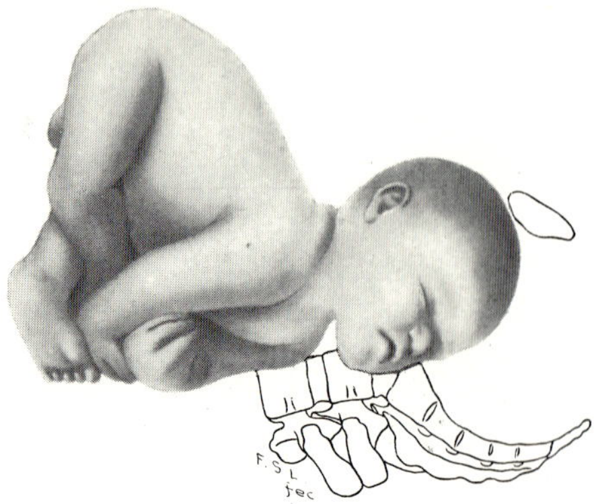

Fig. 270.—Diagram showing Position of Child in Right Posterior Brow Presentation.

either a face or a vertex presentation. It is generally stated that persistent brow presentations occur once in every 1,500 to 1,750 cases, though von Weiss observed one example in every 1,000 cases.

The causes of this presentation, which have been carefully studied by Ahlfeld, are practically identical with those giving rise to face presentations, and depend upon any factor which interferes with flexion or promotes extension of the head. In twin pregnancies not infrequently one or both children may present in this manner, and Ahlfeld maintains that the anterior surfaces of the two fœtuses coming in contact mutually disturb the normal flexed attitude, so that extension is facilitated. Usually the brow is directed towards one or other extremity of the right oblique diameter of the superior strait, and accordingly the left anterior and right posterior varieties are the ones most frequently encountered.

Diagnosis.—The presentation can be recognised by palpation and vaginal touch, though the data obtainable from the first are not so characteristic as in the more common presentations. The condition of affairs is found to be very similar to that observed in face presentations, except that the cephalic prominence is less marked on the side of the back, while the resistance offered by the chin can be felt on the same side as the small parts. On vaginal touch the frontal and the anterior portion of the sagittal suture are encountered in one of the oblique diameters, at one end of which the large fontanelle or the portion of the skull just posterior to it may be felt; while at the other the orbital ridges, the root of the nose, and the eyes may be distinguished. Ordinarily it is not possible to palpate the mouth or chin, for when these are within reach we have to deal with a face presentation.

Mechanism.—The mechanism of labour in brow presentations differs materially with the size of the fœtus. Ahlfeld and most observers have stated that this is most frequently below the normal; whereas Weiss maintains that large children are the rule. In the former case the course of labour as a rule is quite easy, while in the latter it is usually very difficult. The cause of the difficulty is apparent when we consider that the diameter of the head which must engage at the superior strait is the mento-occipital, and that engagement is therefore impossible, unless the child is of small size, until after marked moulding has taken place, by which the mento-occipital diameter has become diminished and the fronto-occipital increased in length.

After moulding and descent have occurred the brow usually rotates anteriorly, and the forehead, orbital ridges, and root of the nose appear at the vulva. One of the superior maxillary bones then becomes stemmed against the inferior margin of the symphysis, and the rest of the head is born by a movement of extreme flexion, the brow, bregma, and occiput appearing in succession over the anterior margin of the perinæum. After the birth of the occiput, the mouth and chin descend from behind the pubic arch by a movement of extension. In other words, we have a mechanism somewhat similar to that observed in the less frequent mode of delivery in the case of posterior occiput presentations, which have rotated into the hollow of the sacrum.

As has already been pointed out, a large child cannot enter the birth canal without considerable moulding of the head. This adds materially to the length of labour and results in the birth of children with characteristically deformed heads. The caput is found over the forehead and extends from the orbital ridges to the large fontanelle, and in many cases is so marked as to render diagnosis by vaginal touch almost impossible. In these cases, as is shown in Fig. 271, the forehead is very prominent and square, the mento-occipital diameter being diminished and the fronto-occipital diameter increased in length.

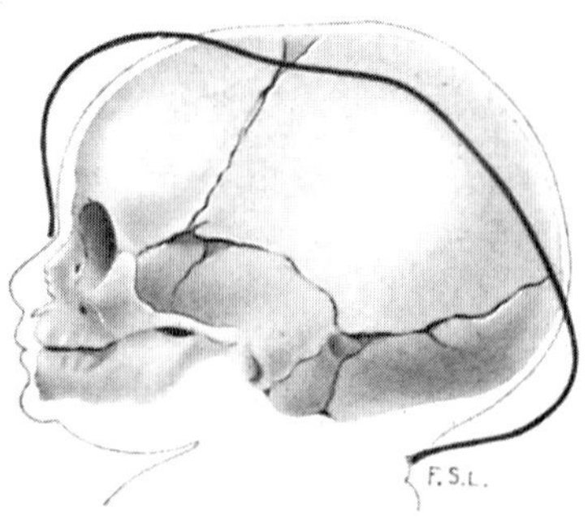

Fig. 271.—Diagram showing Configuration of Head in Brow Presentation (American Text-Book).

Prognosis.—The outlook in persistent forms of brow presentation is generally considered to be bad, unless the fœtus be small. In the transient varieties, of course, it depends upon the presentation which ultimately results, and whether the face or vertex enters the birth canal.

Rational methods of treatment, and more particularly stricter attention to aseptic technique, have led to a marked improvement in the prognosis. Thus Ahlfeld, Fritsch, and Budin (1873–'76) collected 34 cases with 2 maternal and 7 fœtal deaths, 4 of which were directly due to the presentation. Weiss, on the other hand, has recently reported 29 cases from Braun's clinic in Vienna, without a death of fœtus or mother.

Treatment.—If the brow be recognised at the superior strait, the treatment will vary according as the presentation promises to be transient or persistent. The former should be left alone if the brow be anterior, as it will become converted into a mento-anterior presentation, and the child will probably be born spontaneously. On the other hand, if the presentation appears to be persistent, and even in transient cases with the brow posterior, attempts at conversion should be made before the head has undergone any great degree of moulding—that is, as soon as the first stage of labour is completed. If the brow be directed posteriorly it is occasionally possible to substitute an occipito-anterior presentation by pushing up the presenting part with the fingers in the vagina, while at the same time attempts are made to flex the child's body with the external hand. If these manipulations are not successful, version should be performed, as recommended in face presentations. If the brow be directed anteriorly, we have the choice between conversion into a face presentation by vaginal manœuvres, or internal podalic version followed by immediate extraction. Personally I am in favour of the latter procedure, which should always be employed when attempts at manual conversion fail. If the brow be well engaged and firmly fixed, conversion should not be attempted unless one is able to push the presenting part up to the level of the superior strait, when the treatment is identical with that outlined above. But if this cannot be accomplished, the case should be left to nature, and forceps applied when indicated by the condition of the mother or child. It should be remembered, however, that delivery under these circumstances is nearly always associated with considerable injury to the maternal soft parts, owing to the large circumference of the fœtal head by which they are distended. Wallich has made an earnest plea for the performance of symphysiotomy in persistent brow presentations, and has reported 7 operations with no maternal and only 2 fœtal deaths.

Breech Presentations.—As has already been pointed out, the relation between the lower extremities and buttocks of the child is not always the

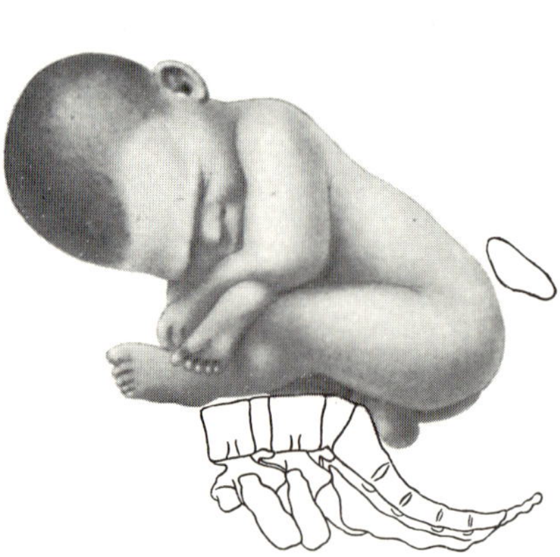

Fig. 272.—Diagram showing Position of Child in L. S. I. A.

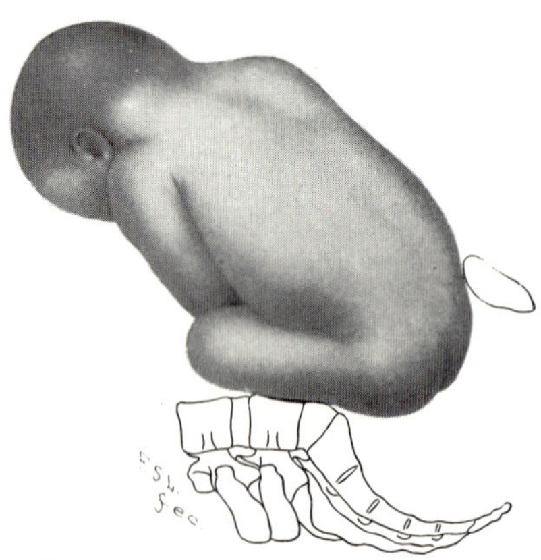

Fig. 273.—Diagram showing Position of Child in R. S. I. A.

same in sacro-iliac presentations, and we therefore distinguish between frank breech, complete breech, foot and knee presentations. In all these varieties, however, the mechanism of labour is essentially the same, so that they need not be considered separately.

Normally the breech engages in such a manner that the bitrochanteric diameter occupies the right oblique diameter of the superior strait, and

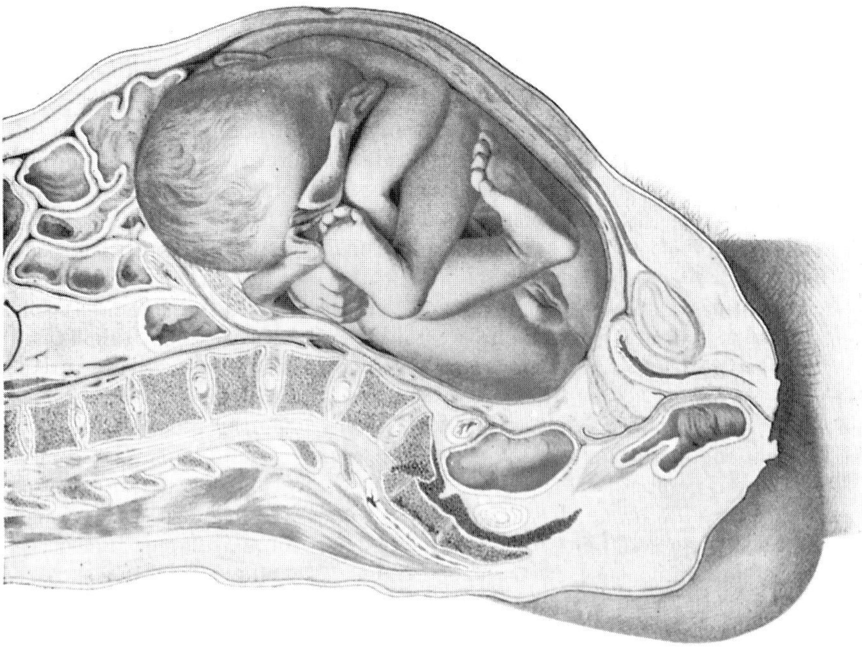

FIG. 274.—FROZEN SECTION, LATTER PART OF PREGNANCY, CHILD IN L. S. I. T. (Waldeyer).

accordingly the right sacro-iliac anterior and left sacro-iliac posterior are the presentations most frequently observed.

In 100,000 cases of labour, Pinard observed 3,301 breech presentations—about 3.33 per cent. These statistics include premature as well as full-term labours, but if the latter alone are considered, we find one in 62 cases.

Diagnosis.—On palpation, the first manœuvre reveals a hard, round, ballottable body occupying the fundus of the uterus, and when the abdominal walls are very thin one can occasionally obtain a characteristic crackling sensation offered by the bones of the skull. By the second manœuvre the back is found to occupy one side of the abdomen and the small parts the other, position and variety being determined by the location of the former. On the third manœuvre, if engagement has not occurred, the irregular breech is freely movable above the superior strait; while, if it has already occurred, the fourth manœuvre shows that the pelvis is filled by a soft mass which interferes with the penetration of the fingers into its cavity (Plate XIII).

On vaginal examination the diagnosis is made by recognising the characteristic portions of the breech. Generally speaking, one can feel both tubera ischii, the sacrum with its spines and the anus, and when further descent has occurred the external genitalia may be distinguished. In many cases, especially where labour is prolonged, the buttocks become markedly swollen, so that differentiation between the face and breech may be rendered very difficult, as the anus may be mistaken for the mouth, and the ischial tuberosities for the malar bones. Care in examination, however, should prevent this error, for when the finger is introduced into the anus it experiences a muscular resistance, whereas in the mouth the firmer, more unyielding jaws would be felt. Again, on removing the finger, it is not infrequently found to be stained with meconium, which could never occur with a face presentation. The most accurate information, however, is obtained from the sacrum and its spines, for when these are felt the diagnosis of position and variety is established.

In complete breech presentations, the feet may be felt alongside of the buttocks, and in footling presentations one or both feet may hang down into the vagina. In the latter case, one can readily determine which foot is encountered by bearing in mind the relation of the great toe. When the breech has descended deeper into the pelvic cavity, the genitalia may be felt, and if these are not deformed by an effusion of serum, it is possible to diagnose the sex of the fœtus. Only under such circumstances can we feel certain as to this point before delivery.

The fœtal heart sounds are heard through the back of the child, usually at the level of the umbilicus or slightly above it.

Ætiology.—The causes of breech presentations are manifold. According to the experiments of Schatz the fœtus, when suspended in liquor amnii, always sinks by its buttocks, so that if gravity were the only factor concerned, breech presentations would be the most frequent of all. As a matter of fact, however, this is by no means the case.

In the later months of pregnancy head presentations result from a process of accommodation between the fœtal ovoid and the uterus; but in the earlier months these factors do not so readily come into play, and breech presentations are accordingly much more common than at term. They also occur very frequently in twin pregnancies and in cases of hydramnios, inasmuch as the increased distention of the uterus interferes with accommodation, when gravity causes the breech to descend. According to Pinard's statistics, 59 per cent of all breech presentations occur in multiparæ, in whom the flaccidity of the uterine and abdominal walls plays a part in their production. Their occurrence is also favoured by the presence of any obstacle which opposes the engagement of the head, as in contracted pelves, excessive size of the normal head, or hydrocephalus.

Mechanism.—Unless there be some disproportion between the size of the child and the pelvis, *engagement* and *descent* readily occur in one of the oblique diameters of the pelvis, the anterior hip being directed toward one ilio-pectineal eminence, and the posterior hip towards the opposite sacro-iliac synchondrosis. When the latter encounters the resistance of the pelvic floor, *internal rotation* usually occurs and brings the anterior hip to the pubic arch, the bitrochanteric diameter of the child coming into relation with the antero-posterior diameter of the pelvic outlet. Rotation

PLATE XIII.

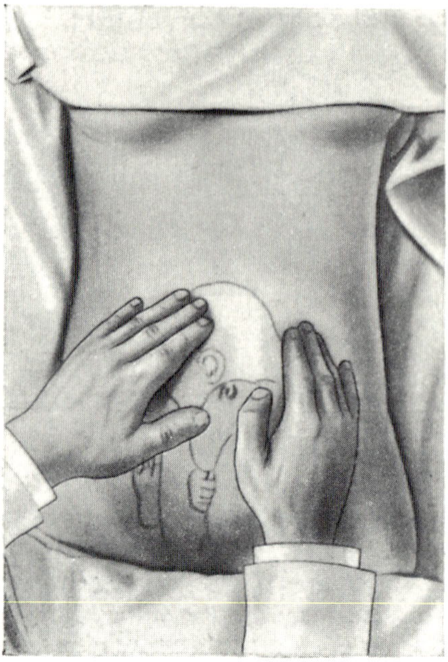
First manœuvre.

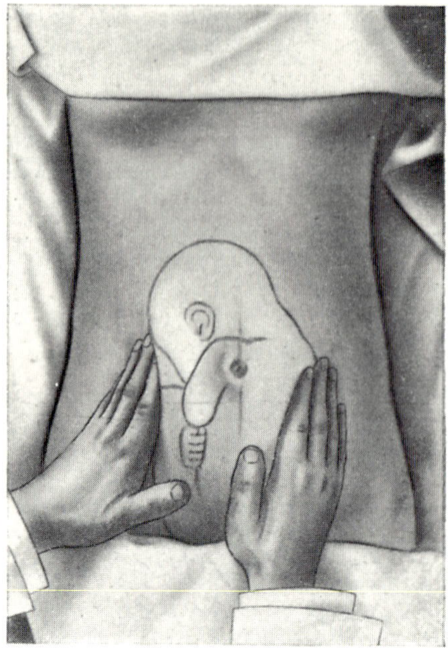
Second manœuvre.

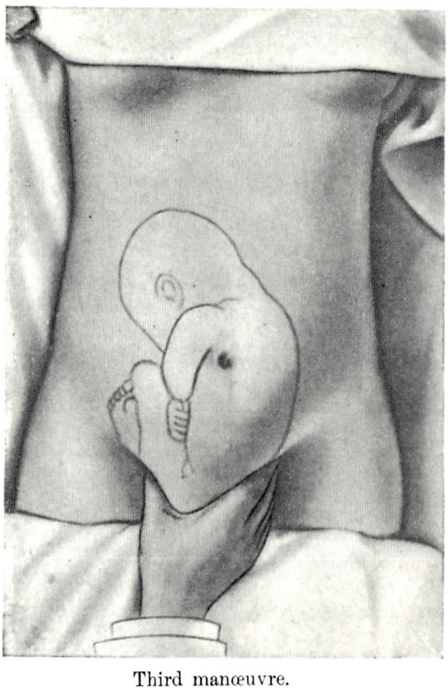
Third manœuvre.

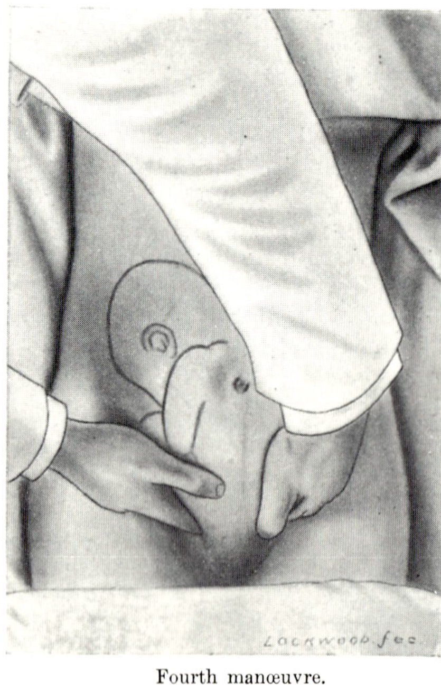

Fourth manœuvre.

PALPATION IN LEFT SACRO-ILIAC-ANTERIOR PRESENTATION.

usually takes place from the ilio-pectineal eminence to the pubis through an arc of 45 degrees; but in a small proportion of cases, particularly when the posterior extremity is prolapsed, it may occur in the opposite direction, the posterior hip rotating past the sacrum and through the opposite half of the pelvis—i. e., through an arc of 225 degrees.

After rotation, descent continues until the perinæum is distended by the advancing breech, while the anterior hip appears at the vulva and is stemmed against the pubic arch. By a movement of *lateral flexion* of the body, the posterior hip is then forced over the anterior margin of the perinæum, which retracts upward over the child, thus allowing its body to straighten out, when the anterior hip is born. The legs and feet follow the breech and may be born spontaneously, although not infrequently the aid of the obstetrician is required. After the birth of the breech a move-

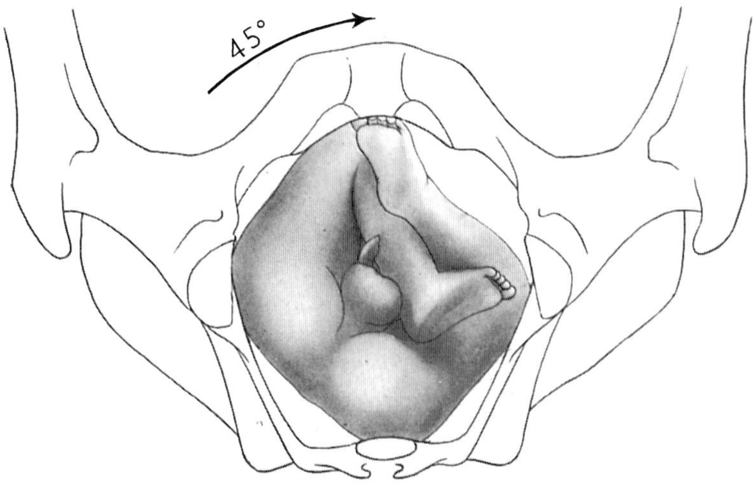

Fig. 275.—Diagram showing Direction of Internal Rotation in R. S. I. P. Position.

ment of *external rotation* occurs, as a result of which the shoulders are brought into relation with one of the oblique diameters of the pelvis. They then descend rapidly and undergo internal rotation, the bisacromial diameter now corresponding with the antero-posterior diameter of the inferior strait. The shoulders are followed by the head, which descends sharply flexed upon the thorax. Immediately following their birth a second movement of external rotation occurs, which serves to bring the neck under the symphysis pubis, after which the head is born in a position of flexion, the chin, mouth, nose, forehead, bregma, and occiput appearing in succession over the perinæum (Figs. 276 and 277).

In a small number of cases rotation occurs in such a manner that the back of the child is directed towards the vertebral column, instead of towards the abdomen of the mother. Under such circumstances the face appears under the symphysis pubis, and the head is born, the face, brow, and finally the occiput slipping down under it. It is of the utmost importance to remember that if premature traction be employed the head

18

may become extended, when its delivery can only be accomplished by the operation of extraction.

Prognosis.—So far as the life of the mother is concerned, the prognosis differs but slightly in breech and vertex presentations, except that with the former labour is slower and more liable to be complicated by perineal

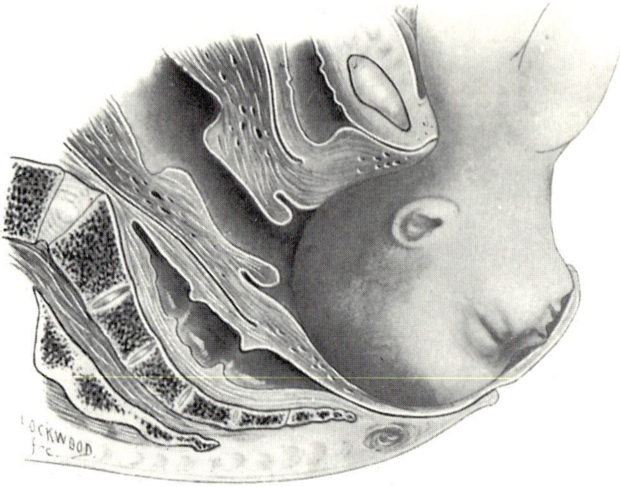

Fig. 276.—Birth of Head in Breech Presentation.

tears, which not infrequently extend through the sphincter ani muscle. The prognosis for the child, on the other hand, is considerably worse than in vertex presentations, the fœtal mortality being generally estimated at about 10 per cent. This figure applies to primiparous women, but a somewhat lower percentage obtains when all classes of cases are taken into consideration. It is not so high in multiparous women, for owing to the greater relaxation of the soft parts the child is more readily expelled spontaneously, and when extraction becomes necessary it is more readily accomplished. Porak states that 1 child in 9 succumbs in the former class of cases, and only 1 in 30 in the latter.

The sombre prognosis for the child is due to several factors. In the first place, after the breech is born as far as the umbilicus, the cord is exposed to a greater or lesser degree of compression between the head and the pelvic brim. It is usually stated that not more than eight minutes can elapse between the birth of the umbilicus and the delivery of the head, if the child is to be born alive, while asphyxiation may occasionally occur at an earlier period.

Not infrequently fœtal death is due to the premature separation of the placenta, for if the delivery is not promptly effected after the head has passed into the lower part of the birth canal, the partially emptied uterus may retract to such an extent as to separate the placenta from its walls, and thus put a stop to the utero-placental circulation.

In primiparous women, where considerable resistance is offered by the pelvic soft parts, spontaneous delivery of the head is often unavoidably delayed and fœtal death results, unless the child be extracted manually. In all cases of breech presentation, therefore, the obstetrician should be prepared to render prompt assistance if Nature shows herself unable to fulfil her task.

Treatment.—In view of the serious fœtal prognosis attending breech presentations, the obstetrician should aim to prevent their occurrence as far as possible, and whenever they are diagnosed in the later weeks of pregnancy, an attempt should be made to substitute a vertex presentation by means of *external version.* This is readily accomplished in multiparæ with lax abdominal walls, but is much more difficult in primiparæ. After the substitution has been effected, the child should be held in its new position by a properly fitting bandage until engagement of the head occurs, for if this precaution be not taken it is not unusual for the child to revert to its original position. External version may also be attempted in the first stage of labour, provided the breech has not descended deeply into the pelvis; but when it has once become fixed, all such efforts are unavailing, and it is best to leave the case to nature and be prepared to interfere when necessary.

In many cases spontaneous delivery occurs, and the attitude of the obstetrician is merely one of expectancy; nevertheless, he should always hold himself in readiness to intervene at a moment's notice. For this

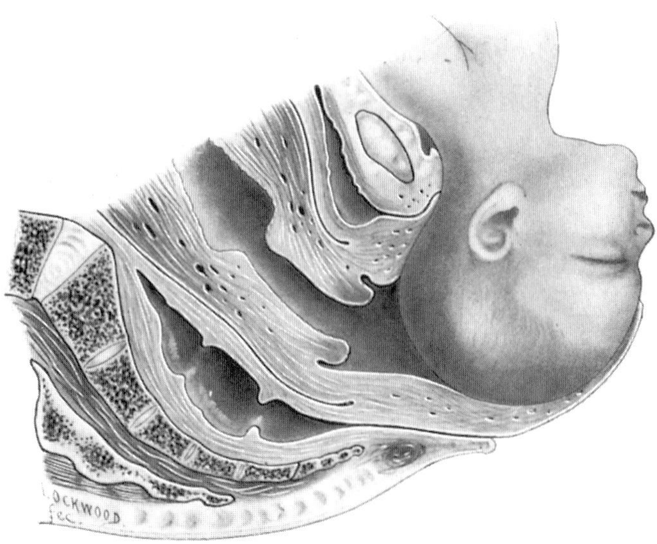

FIG. 277.—BIRTH OF HEAD IN BREECH PRESENTATION.

reason, as soon as the breech appears at the vulva, the patient should be brought to the edge of the bed in order that not a moment may be lost in performing extraction should it become necessary. At the same time everything required for the resuscitation of the asphyxiated child should be ready for instant use. It is most important to remember that labour is materially facilitated by the arms retaining their normal crossed position over the thorax, as well as by sharp flexion of the head. This is best attained by firm downward pressure upon the fundus, which should be maintained by the nurse or an assistant, so that the obstetrician can keep his hands clean for any emergency.

Owing to the fact that the breech forms a less efficient dilating wedge than the head, care should be taken to prevent premature rupture of the membranes and the escape of the amniotic fluid. For this reason among others, as few internal examinations as possible should be made. Generally speaking, the frank breech forms a better dilating wedge than the complete breech, inasmuch as it allows a closer application to the margins of the partially dilated os. On the other hand, if interference becomes necessary, the complete breech offers more satisfactory conditions for immediate delivery, as a foot can readily be brought down and used as a tractor, so that the question arises whether it might not be better in the former class of cases to make it a rule to bring down one or both feet prophylactically. Usually this is not advisable, unless some abnormality exists on the part of the mother or child which renders it probable that prompt delivery may be called for. In such cases a foot should be brought down by Pinard's manœuvre as soon as the membranes rupture. The technique of this manipulation, as well as the rules for extraction, will be considered in Chapter XXI.

LITERATURE

Ahlfeld. Die Entstehung von Stirn- und Gesichtslagen. Leipzig, 1873.

Baudelocque. L'art des accouchemens, 1789, t. ii, 36–40.

Boer. Sieben Bücher über natürliche Geburtshülfe, Wien, 1834, 96.

Budin. De la tête du fœtus au point de vue de l'obstétrique. Paris, 1876.

Davis. The Management of Face Presentations. Medical News, July 14, 1894.

Deleurye. Traité des accouchemens, etc. Paris, 1770.

Duncan. On the Production of Presentation of the Face. Mechanism of Natural and Morbid Parturition. Edinburgh, 1875, 218–231.

Fieux. Une observation de présentation primitive de la face. Comptes rendus de la Soc. d'Obst., de Gyn. et de Pæd., 1900, ii, 225–231.

Fritsch. Klinik der geburtshülflichen Operationen. Halle, 1894, 142.

Gessner. Zur Aetiologie der Gesichtslagen. Zeitschr. f. Geb. u. Gyn., 1897, xxxvii, 302.

Hecker. Ueber die Schädelform bei Gesichtslagen. Berlin, 1869.

Jellinghaus. Ueber fötale Schädelformen, etc. Archiv f. Gyn., 1896, li, 33–48.

Lachapelle. Pratique des accouchemens, 1821, t. i, 382.

Pinard. Traité du palper abdominal, 2me éd., Paris, 1889, 32–50.

Ribemont-Dessaignes. Précis d'obstétrique, 1894, 427.

Schatz. Die Umwandlung von Gesichtslagen zu Hinterhauptslagen durch alleinigen äusseren Handgriff. Archiv f. Gyn., 1873, v, 306–331.

Ueber den Schwerpunkt der Frucht. Centralbl. f. Gyn., 1900, Nr. 40, 1033–1036.

Spiegelberg-Wiener. Lehrbuch der Geburtshülfe, II. Aufl., 1891, 172.

Thorn. Zur manuellen Umwandlung der Gesichtslagen in Hinterhauptslagen. Zeitschr. f. Geb. u. Gyn., 1886, xiii, 186–220.

Die Stellung der manuellen Umwandlung in der Therapie der Gesichts- und Stirnlagen. Volkmann's Sammlung klin. Vorträge, 1902, Nr. 339.

Wallich. De la symphyséotomie dans les présentations persistantes du front. Comptes rendus de la Soc. d'Obst., de Gyn. et de Pæd., 1902, iv, 18–34.

WEISS. Zur Behandlung der Gesichts- und Stirnlagen. Volkmann's Sammlung klin. Vorträge, N. F., Nr. 74.

WINCKEL. Zur Lehre von den Gesichtslagen. Klinische Beobachtungen zur Pathologie der Geburt. Rostock, 1869, 59–65.

ZELLER. Bemerkungen über einige Gegenstände aus der praktischen Entbindungskunst. Wien, 1797.

ZWEIFEL. Lehrbuch der Geburtshülfe. III. Aufl., 177.

CHAPTER XIV

PHYSIOLOGY OF LABOUR (Continued)

PHYSIOLOGY AND MANAGEMENT OF THE THIRD STAGE OF LABOUR

Situation of the Placenta in Utero.—The older authors believed that the placenta was usually implanted at or in the immediate neighbourhood of the fundus. The researches of Schroeder, Pinard, Ahlfeld, Leopold, Holzapfel, and others, however, have shown that this is by no means the rule, but that the most common situation is on the anterior or posterior wall of the uterus, occasionally on its lateral wall, and only in exceptional instances upon the fundus. Fig. 278, which represents a vertical section through the uterus at term, shows the usual mode of attachment. As a rule the lower margin of the placenta lies somewhat above the internal os, for when it impinges upon or overlaps the latter we have to deal with a pathological condition—placenta prævia.

Mechanism of Separation of the Placenta.—Under normal conditions the placenta remains fixed to the uterine wall until after the birth of the child, and becomes separated from it only during the third stage of labour. While the first and second stages are proceeding, the uterine contractions bring about a slight decrease in area of the surface to which it is attached, and in its attempt at accommodation the placenta becomes slightly folded upon itself, its margins being somewhat rounded and prominent. At the same time, however, it is pressed firmly against the uterine wall by the amniotic fluid, through which the intra-uterine pressure is transmitted; otherwise it is probable that premature separation would be the rule and not the exception.

After the expulsion of the child, the contraction and retraction of the uterus leads to a considerable thickening of its walls, with a corresponding decrease in the size of its cavity, as well as to a rapid lessening in the area of the placental site. Eventually the disproportion becomes so great that the inner portion of the glandular layer of the decidua is torn through, and the placenta and membranes are separated from the walls of the uterus and come to lie free in its cavity, whence they are expelled by further contractions into the lower uterine segment or the upper portion of the vagina.

After its extrusion, the maternal surface of the placenta still retains a thin covering of decidua, which represents the atrophic compact layer and the innermost portion of the spongy layer of the decidua serotina, which must be stripped off in order to reach the chorionic villi.

Mode of Extrusion of the Placenta.—As early as 1789 Baudelocque had described two ways in which the placenta could be extruded from the uterus. Thus, separation from the uterine wall could commence either at the centre of the placenta or at a point in its circumference. "In the first case, the middle of the placenta being pushed forward by an effusion of blood beneath it, the organ becomes inverted upon itself in such a manner that it presents by its fœtal surface, which is covered by the membranes and vessels. . . . But when the placenta becomes detached below, particularly if the loosening begins at a point in the neighbourhood of the internal os, the mechanism is entirely different, for the afterbirth becomes rolled upon itself in the form of a cylinder, whose long axis corresponds to that of the uterus, in such a manner that it presents its detached maternal surface to the examining finger, and its exit is always preceded by a small amount of fluid blood."

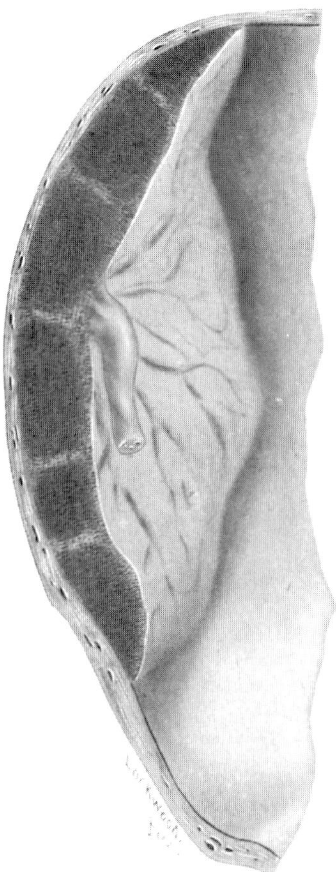

FIG. 278.—DIAGRAM SHOWING RELATION OF PLACENTA TO UTERINE WALL IN LATTER PART OF PREGNANCY. × ½.

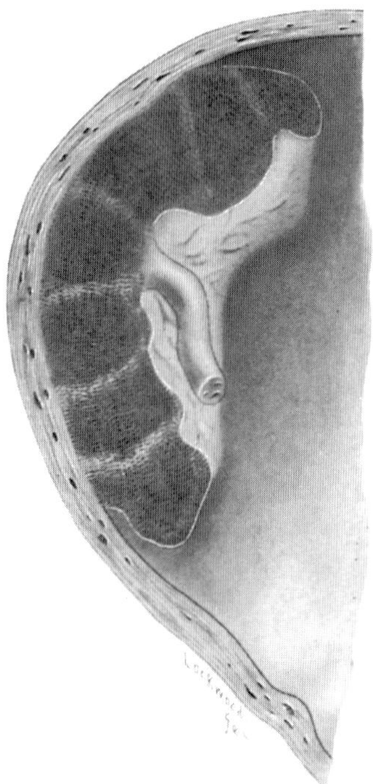

FIG. 279.—DIAGRAM SHOWING RELATION OF PLACENTA TO UTERINE WALL IN SECOND STAGE OF LABOUR (modified from Schroeder). × ½.

These ideas seem to have excited but little interest until 1865, when

Schultze advanced the opinion that the placenta was usually expelled by the first method described by Baudelocque. This belief remained practically undisputed until 1871, when Matthews Duncan contended that the second was the more frequent and normal mechanism. The active discussion aroused by this statement, although it led to no final settlement of the question, had the effect of directing more earnest attention to the physiology of this stage of labour.

The two methods are now designated by the names of Schultze and Duncan respectively. In the former, separation begins first at the central portion of the placenta, between which and the uterine wall more or less blood is poured out, which gradually increases in amount until a retro-placental hæmatoma of considerable size is formed, which eventually

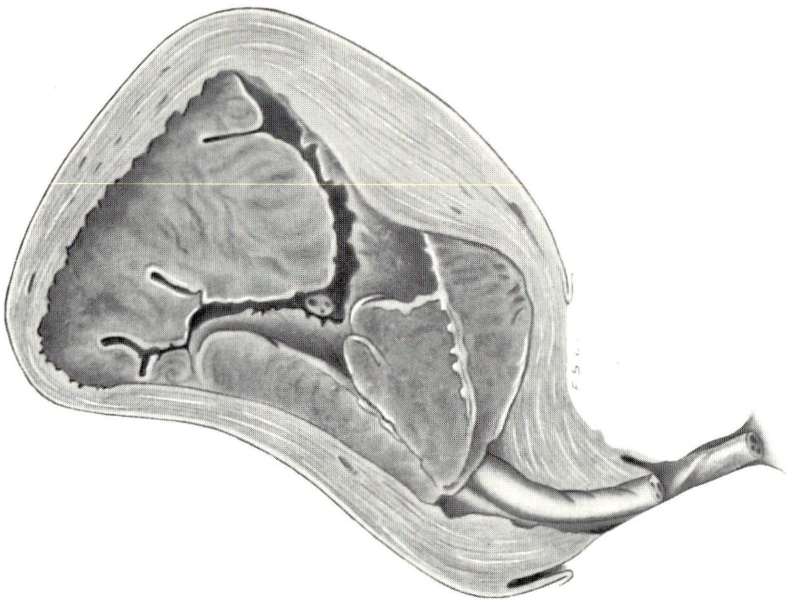

Fig. 280.—Frozen Section, Third Stage of Labour, showing Twin Placentæ in Utero (Pestalozza). × ½.

brings about the complete separation of the organ from its site of attachment, while the membranes still remain adherent. The placenta then presents at the internal os by its fœtal surface and passes through the opening in the membranes, dragging them after it; it is then expelled from the vulva, its fœtal or amniotic surface first, and the now inverted membranes following after. In this mechanism there is no escape of blood until after the extrusion of the placenta (Figs. 281 and 282).

In Duncan's method, on the other hand, the placenta, after its separation from the uterine wall, becomes folded upon itself and its lower margin presents at the internal os. It then traverses the vagina and emerges from the vulva by one margin, the membranes being sometimes, but by no means always, inverted. When expulsion occurs in this manner, there is slight but continuous hæmorrhage from the birth of the child until the placenta is delivered (Fig. 283).

With respect to the relative frequency with which these two mechan-

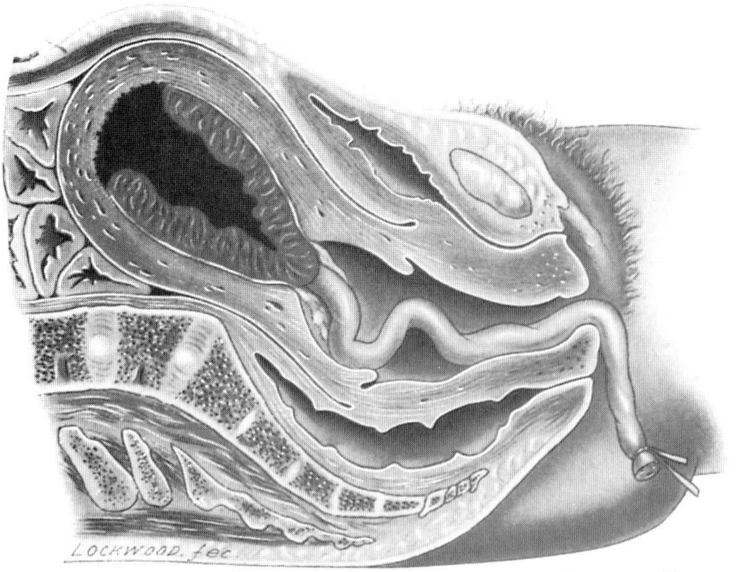

FIG. 281.—DIAGRAM ILLUSTRATING EXTRUSION OF PLACENTA BY SCHULTZE'S MECHANISM.

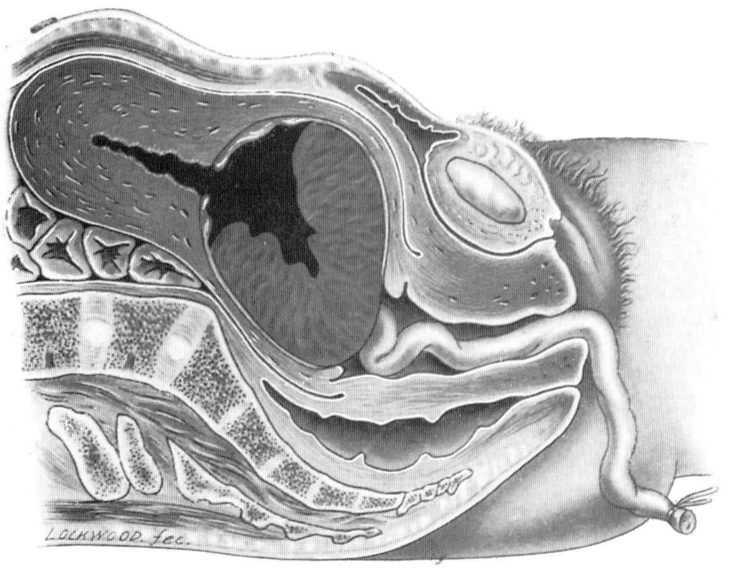

FIG. 282.—DIAGRAM ILLUSTRATING LATER STAGE IN THE EXTRUSION OF THE PLACENTA BY SCHULTZE'S MECHANISM.

isms occur, there has been much discussion. In this country and in England, Duncan's views are commonly accepted, and it is generally held that

Schultze's method borders on the abnormal. In Germany the opinions are still very conflicting, Olshausen and Veit stating that Duncan's method occurs in the majority of cases, whereas Schroeder held that the reverse was the case. Moreover, the statistics brought forward by various authors would seem to render the matter still more uncertain. Thus Zeigler, writing under the inspiration of Fehling, states that he observed Duncan's mechanism in 83.6 per cent of his cases, whereas in 79.76 per cent of Ahlfeld's cases that of Schultze was noted.

Holzapfel, in a recent monograph, has given details and a full literature dealing with the present status of the question, and, as the result of very interesting experiments and observations, concludes that the placenta

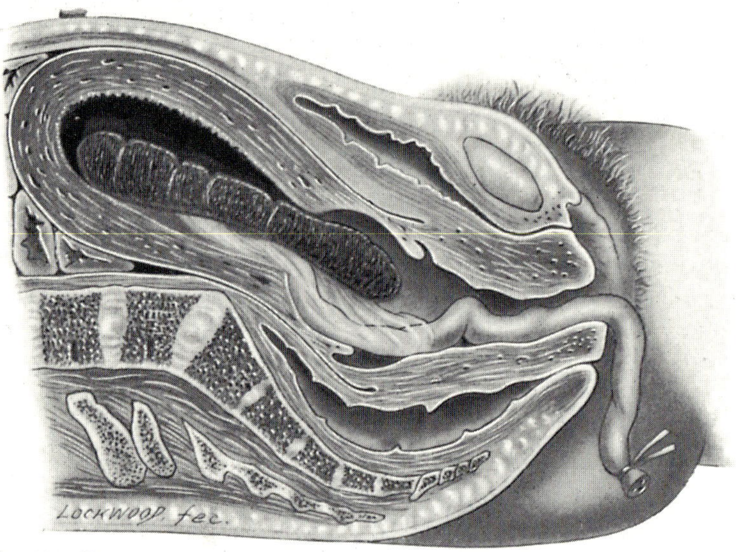

FIG. 283.—DIAGRAM ILLUSTRATING EXTRUSION OF PLACENTA BY DUNCAN'S MECHANISM.

nearly always presents at the internal os by Duncan's, but leaves the uterus by Schultze's mechanism.

Although it is difficult to reconcile the contradictory statements of the various observers, it would appear justifiable to class both mechanisms as perfectly normal, that of Duncan occurring most often when the placenta is situated in the lower portion of the uterus, that of Schultze when it is situated in the upper portion.

Clinical Picture of the Third Stage of Labour.—Immediately following the birth of the child, the remainder of the amniotic fluid escapes, after which there is usually a slight flow of blood. The uterus can now be felt as a firm, hard mass, the fundus lying a few centimetres below the umbilicus. For a short time the patient experiences no pain, but after a few minutes uterine contractions begin again and recur at regular intervals, until the placenta becomes separated and is expelled into the lower uterine segment.

At some time, varying between five and thirty minutes after the birth of the child, careful palpation shows that the fundus of the uterus has risen 3 to 5 centimetres above its original position, while simultaneously

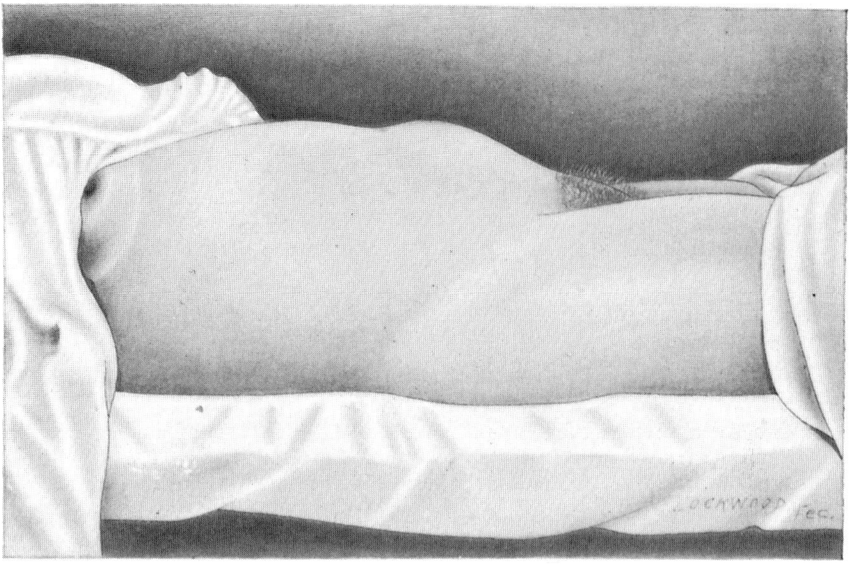

FIG. 284.—ABDOMEN IMMEDIATELY AFTER BIRTH OF CHILD.

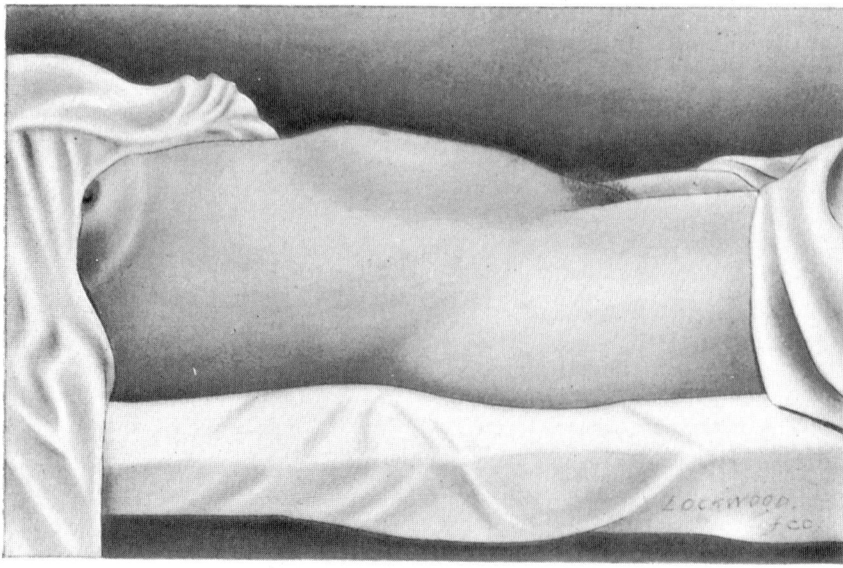

FIG. 285.—ABDOMEN OF SAME PATIENT, SHOWING RISING UP OF FUNDUS FOLLOWING EXTRUSION OF THE PLACENTA INTO THE LOWER UTERINE SEGMENT.

a slight prominence has appeared immediately above the symphysis pubis (Figs. 284 and 285). This change indicates that the placenta has become detached and has been extruded from the uterine cavity proper into the lower uterine segment, or even into the upper part of the vagina. In rare cases the placenta is born almost immediately after the child, but as a rule not until fifteen to thirty minutes later, while occasionally hours may pass before it appears at the vulva. The possibility of wide divergence in this respect can readily be appreciated when we remember that the action of the uterus ceases after the placenta has been extruded from its cavity, so that its further descent depends partly upon gravity, but principally upon the contractions of the abdominal muscles. But owing to the great distention to which the latter have been subjected, their tonicity is frequently so impaired that they can no longer exert sufficient force to expel the afterbirth from the vagina, so that in many cases it will not be born for hours unless the patient assumes a sitting position or assistance is rendered by the physician. Ahlfeld has stated that spontaneous termination of the placental period occurred in only 13.6 per cent of his cases, even when he waited for one and a half to two hours after the birth of the child.

The average loss of blood during the third stage of labour is estimated at about 400 cubic centimetres, a constant but slight flow occurring throughout the entire period when the placenta is delivered by Duncan's mechanism, and a sudden gush of blood immediately following its expulsion by Schultze's mechanism.

Management of the Third Stage of Labour.—Up to 1861 the management of the third stage of labour varied greatly, and delivery of the placenta was effected either by traction upon the cord or by passing the hand into the vagina or uterus, as the case might be, and bringing it away. Both of these methods, but more particularly the latter, as will be explained later, are necessarily attended by grave dangers.

In 1861, Credé described what he considered the ideal method of delivering the placenta, which was somewhat as follows: Immediately after the exit of the child, the obstetrician grasps the uterus with his hand, and after waiting from five to ten minutes, gently kneads it, thereby stimulating it to contract. The hand is then applied to the abdomen in such a manner that the thumb rests upon the anterior and the fingers upon the posterior surface of the uterus, and as soon as a contraction occurs, firm and steady pressure should be made downward in the axis of the superior strait.

The introduction and routine employment of Credé's method of expression undoubtedly marked a most important advance, inasmuch as by doing away with the necessity for traction upon the cord and the frequent manual removal of the placenta, it has saved the lives of thousands of women. With certain modifications it is now generally employed throughout the world. As a matter of history, Jellett has noted that the method, while usually ascribed to Credé, had been practised for many years previously at the Rotunda Hospital in Dublin.

In opposition to the expression of the placenta immediately after the birth of the child, Dohrn, Ahlfeld, and others stated that a greater amount of blood is lost during the third stage, and that there is a greater tendency to post-partum hæmorrhage than when the extrusion of the placenta is left to Nature, or expression is resorted to only after an interval of several hours. But, while it must be recognised as incontrovertible that too early a resort to Créde's method is harmful, inasmuch as it defeats the very purpose for which it is employed and interferes with the physiological separation of the placenta, the arguments adduced in favour of waiting so long a time appear to be neither satisfactory nor rational. It is difficult to see what advantages are to be gained by delaying expres-

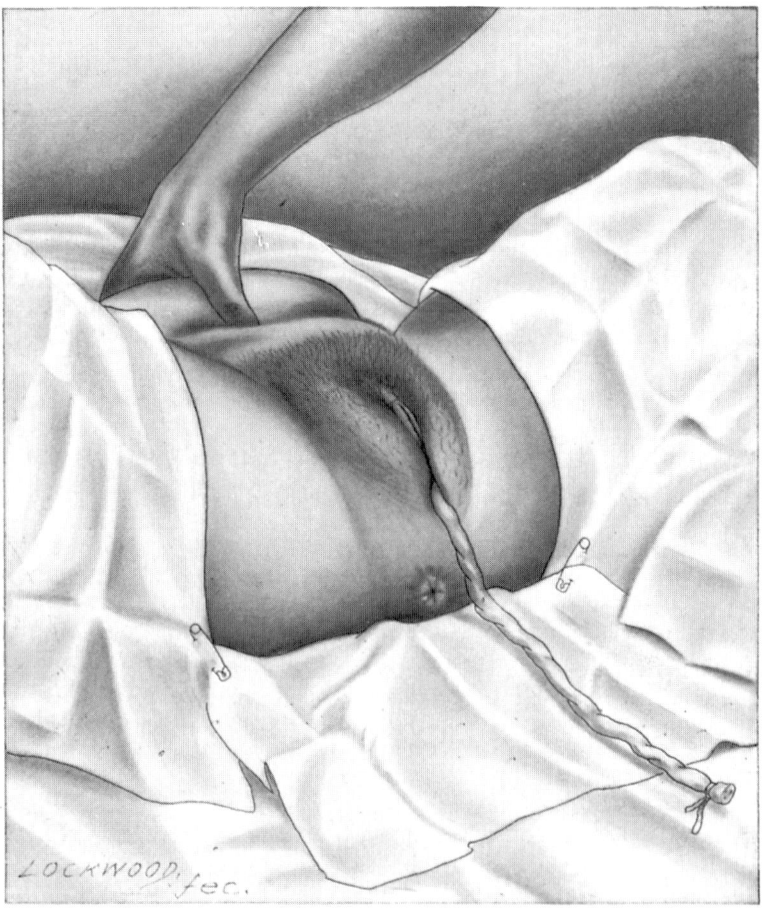

Fig. 286.—Expression of Placenta.

sion after the placenta has once become detached from its original site and lies in the lower uterine segment, especially if Ahlfeld's statement is correct that spontaneous delivery will occur only in 13 to 14 per cent of the cases at the end of two hours. On the other hand, there are certainly very obvious objections to any unnecessary prolongation of the third stage of labour. For the patient a delay of several hours between the birth of the child and the completion of labour, means much additional discomfort and an increased risk of infection; while the busy physician can ill afford the expenditure of valuable time, unless he be convinced that by such personal sacrifice he can better insure the well-being of his patient.

In normal cases, therefore, attempts at expression should not be made until the placenta has been spontaneously expelled into the lower uterine segment or upper portion of the vagina; but as soon as this has taken place there is no reason why the process should not be hastened. In my own clinic the following procedure has been adopted with most satisfactory results: As soon as the child is born the hand is laid upon the abdomen, and if the uterus can be felt as a firm, hard, globular mass it is left alone. On the other hand, if it appears to be soft and flaccid, it is gently kneaded until firm contractions are induced. The condition of the uterus is then carefully watched, the hand being applied to it at frequent intervals, but kneading is carried out only when necessary. In the majority of cases, after a lapse of ten or fifteen minutes, it is noticed that the fundus rises up 4 to 5 centimetres above the position which it has just occupied, but at the same time remains firm and hard. This change indicates that the placenta has become separated from the uterine wall and has been expelled into the lower uterine segment or the upper portion of the vagina. Attention was first directed to this point by Pinard, Schroeder, and Cohn, but its importance has not been generally recognised. The placenta is now expelled by grasping the uterus and making downward pressure in the axis of the superior strait, using the uterus merely as a piston to shove the placenta downward and outward. When the latter appears at the vulva it should be grasped by the hand and the membranes gently twisted into a cord, so as to prevent their being torn off from the margins of the placenta, after which they are slowly extracted.

In most cases the placenta can be expressed in this manner within half an hour after the birth of the child; but if the fundus does not rise up spontaneously by the end of that period, the typical Credé method should be resorted to. The modification of the original procedure, here recommended, leaves the separation of the placenta from the uterine wall absolutely to Nature, and simply expresses it after it has been spontaneously expelled from the uterine cavity.

Not infrequently small portions of the membranes may be left behind *in utero* or in the vagina. If the ends be outside the vulva, they should be seized and the remnants delivered by gentle traction; but otherwise it is advisable to leave them alone and to allow them to be cast off with the lochia, rather than to introduce the fingers into the vagina or uterus in the attempt to remove them.

Immediately following the birth of the placenta, the uterus should be palpated again; normally it is found firmly contracted and retracted, and if it remains so, there is no danger of hæmorrhage. But, on the other hand, if it shows any tendency towards relaxation, it should be kneaded until it contracts. There is usually no danger of relaxation and consequent hæmorrhage, provided no signs of it appear during the first hour after the extrusion of the placenta. Accordingly, the condition of the uterus should be carefully watched during this period by the physician or nurse. But, even when this duty is delegated to the latter, the physician should remain at the house of the patient for one hour, so as to be on hand in case an emergency should arise.

Occasionally, the amount of blood lost immediately following the birth of the child may be so great as to render imperative the prompt delivery of the placenta, and under such circumstances expression should be employed at once. Under all other conditions, however, we should watch for the rising up of the fundus before resorting to this procedure.

As soon as the placenta and membranes are born they should be carefully inspected for the purpose of ascertaining whether the structures have been expelled entire, or whether portions have been left behind in the uterus. If they are perfectly intact, all is well; but if the maternal surface of the placenta shows defects which are not due to mere tears of its substance, but which appear to indicate that a considerable part has been left behind, the hand should be carefully redisinfected, a sterile rubber glove put on, and the retained portion removed manually, since if allowed to remain in the uterus it nearly always gives rise to hæmorrhage.

In rare cases it may be found impossible at the end of half an hour to expel the placenta by means of Credé's method, and under such circumstances, unless the condition of the patient be serious, or there be free hæmorrhage, the obstetrician should wait patiently and repeat his attempts at expression at intervals, and should not despair of eventual success until at least two hours have elapsed. Under such circumstances, it is probable that abnormal adhesions exist between the placenta and the uterine wall which require a longer time than usual for their separation. In any case, manual removal of the organ must never be undertaken unless absolutely necessary, as it is a more serious procedure than the application of forceps or the performance of version. In the former the hand, which is rarely perfectly sterile, is introduced between the placenta and the uterine wall, and comes in direct contact with the freshly wounded placental site, through which are scattered numerous thrombosed vessels which afford a most excellent culture medium for bacteria; whereas in the latter, the hands or instruments are introduced into the amniotic cavity, so that whatever micro-organisms may have been carried up by them are likely to be cast off with the afterbirth.

For particulars concerning the technique of manual removal of the placenta, the reader is referred to the section on obstetrical operations.

LITERATURE

Ahlfeld. Abwartende Methode oder Credé'scher Handgriff? Leipzig, 1888.

Ueber die ersten Vorgänge bei der physiologischen Lösung der Placenta. Zeitschr. f. Geb. u. Gyn., 1895, xxxiii, 418–442.

Weitere Untersuchungen über die physiolog. Vorgänge der Nachgeburtsperiode. Zeitschr. f. Geb. u. Gyn., 1897, xxxvi, 443–466.

Baudelocque. De la délivrance naturelle. L'art des accouchemens, 1789, t. i, 413–415.

Cohn. Zur Physiologie und Diätetik der Nachgeburtsperiode. Zeitschr. f. Geb. u. Gyn., 1886, xii, 381–417.

Credé. Ueber die zweckmässigste Methode der Entfernung der Nachgeburt. Monatsschr. f. Geburtskunde, 1861, xvii, 274–292.

Ueber die zweckmässigste Methode der Entfernung der Nachgeburt. Archiv f. Gyn., 1881, xvii, 260–280.

Dohrn. Zur Behandlung der Nachgeburtsperiode. Deutsche med. Wochenschr., 1880, Nr. 41.

Die Behandlung des Nachgeburtszeitraumes. Jena, 1898.

Duncan. The Expulsion of the Placenta. (Read to the Edinburgh Obstetrical Society, March 22, 1871.) Mechanism of Natural and Morbid Parturition. Edinburgh, 1875, 246–256.

Holzapfel. Ueber den Placentarsitz. Hegar's Beiträge zur Geb. u. Gyn., 1898, i, 286–337.

Ueber die Lösung und Ausstossung der Nachgeburt. Hegar's Beiträge zur Geb. u. Gyn., 1899, ii, 413–481.

Jellett. The Dublin Method of Effecting the Delivery of the Placenta. Dublin Jour. Med. Science, June, 1900.

Leopold. Die Diagnose des Placentarsitzes in der Schwangerschaft und während der Geburt. Arbeiten aus der königlichen Frauenklinik in Dresden, 1895, ii, 151–166.

Olshausen-Veit. Schroeder's Lehrbuch der Geburtshülfe, XIII. Aufl., 1899, 175.

Pinard. Du palper pendant la délivrance normale. Traité du palper abdominal, 2me éd., Paris, 1884, 241–253.

Pinard et Varnier. Études d'anatomie obstétricale normale et pathologique. Paris, 1892.

Schroeder. Beiträge zur Physiologie der Austreibungs- und Nachgeburtsperiode, Der Zeitschr. f. Geb. u. Gyn., 1885, xi, 421.

Schroeder und Stratz. Zur Physiologie der Austreibungs- und Nachgeburtsperiode. schwangere und kreissende Uterus, Berlin, 1886, 75–112.

Schultze. Wandtafeln zur Schwangerschaft und Geburtskunde. Leipzig, 1865.

Ueber den Mechanismus der spontanen Ausscheidung der Nachgeburt, etc. Deutsche med. Wochenschr., 1880, Nr. 51, 252.

Ziegler. Beiträge zum Mechanismus der physiologischen Placentarlösung. D. I., Halle. 1895.

CHAPTER XV

CONDUCT OF NORMAL LABOUR

As a rule the services of the obstetrician are engaged some time before the expected date of confinement, in order that the patient may be under medical supervision for at least the last few months of pregnancy.

The importance of a careful *preliminary examination*, not later than four to six weeks before term, has already been insisted upon. This can be more conveniently carried out with the patient at home and in bed, when the obstetrician should take careful measurements of the pelvis, determine the presentation and position of the child, and acquaint himself, not only with any abnormality which may exist in the generative tract, but also with the general physical condition. At the time of this visit also it is well to give the patient a list of such articles as may be needed at the time of labour and during the puerperium, and which she is expected to supply. The physician should also communicate with the nurse in order to make sure that she understands the preparations which fall to her share. Experience has taught me that the only way by which mistakes can be avoided is to have all necessary directions written down in black and white, or preferably to use printed cards containing definite and concise instructions for the patient and nurse.

Preparations for Labour on the Part of the Patient and Nurse.—At the time of the preliminary examination, the physician should inspect the room which is to be used for the confinement and make necessary suggestions as to its arrangement. He should also inquire as to the number of wash-basins which are available; for with the increasing perfection of plumbing the ordinary wash-basin and pitcher are often replaced by permanent wash-stands, so that in the homes of the well-to-do it is sometimes difficult to find a sufficient number for disinfecting the hands and cleansing the patient. Five basins will be needed: four for the use of the physician and one for the patient; and if so many are not already in the house, a sufficient number, made of plain agate-ware and measuring 10 inches across the top, should be procured.

The patient should also be instructed to provide herself with a bed-pan, a 2-quart fountain syringe for rectal enemata, 15 yards of non-sterilized gauze and 2 pounds of cotton batting, for making bed-pads, or 6 prepared sanitary bed-pads and 2 pieces of rubber sheeting, one 1×2 yards and the other $\frac{3}{4} \times 1$ yard. The following articles should be obtained from the druggist at least one month before the expected date of confinement, so that they may be in readiness in case labour should occur unexpectedly:

100 cubic centimetres Squibb's chloroform,
4 ounces potassium permanganate,
8 " oxalic acid,
4 " boric acid,
1 ounce tube of green soap,
1 " tube of vaseline,
100 Bernays's bichloride tablets,
8 ounces alcohol,
2 drams ergotol,
1 nail-brush,
2 pounds absorbent cotton.

If one has a large obstetrical practice, it is advisable to have some reputable druggist arrange and keep in stock a box containing the above-mentioned articles, so that the patient can be told simply to buy an obstetrical outfit.

The nurse should see that a sufficient number of bed and vulval pads are prepared in advance. A week or ten days before the expected date of confinement she should sterilize a portion of them, together with 5 packages containing the following articles: Six towels or diapers (2 packages), 1 sheet, half a pound of absorbent cotton, and cotton pledgets or gauze sponges. At the commencement of labour she should prepare 2 large pitchers of boiled water, one of which should be kept hot, while the other is allowed to cool, the top being carefully covered with a sterile towel.

Preparations on the Part of the Physician.—When the physician expects to be called to an obstetrical case, he should hold himself in readiness to respond promptly at any hour within two weeks of the expected date of confinement. If he is obliged to leave town about that time, he should notify the patient and arrange for a competent substitute to take his place if necessary. He should also remember that the proper care of such cases requires a great deal of time, and frequently no small sacrifice of personal convenience, and if he is not willing to place himself at the disposal of his patients, as far as may be necessary, he should refuse to attend them. Undue haste is one of the most frequent causes of unsatisfactory results in this branch of medicine.

The physician should provide himself with an *obstetrical outfit*, which should be neatly packed in an appropriate box or valise and be kept ready for immediate use. It should contain not only the instruments which he may need, but also the various drugs required for hand disinfection, anæsthesia, and the usual emergencies, as well as a certain number of sterile towels and dressings, in case the patient has failed to provide herself with such materials, and for sudden calls or consultations. The obstetrical valise should contain a pelvimeter, a pair of nail-clippers and a nail-cleaner, chloroform, permanganate of potash, oxalic acid, bichloride tablets, green soap, and a nail-brush, 1 ounce of ergotol or fluid extract of ergot, tablets of sodium chloride for preparing normal salt solution, and a hypodermic syringe with the usual tablets. There should also be a chloroform inhaler, a suit of white clothes, three packages containing respectively 6 sterile towels and a sheet, sterilized absorbent cotton, and several sterilized roller gauze bandages for packing the uterus and vagina, as well as a small jar of sterile vaseline. Glass tubes containing sterile catheters, silk and silkworm-gut sutures, and bobbin for tying the cord are also needed, as well as a Kelly obstetrical pad and a leg-holder.

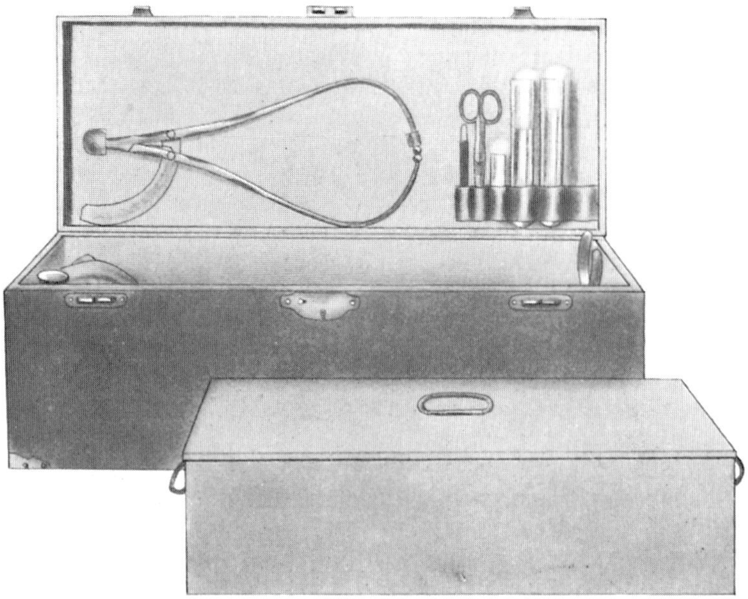

FIG. 287.—OBSTETRICAL BAG.

The following instruments for repairing perineal and cervical lacerations should be sterilized and wrapped in a package ready for instant use: A pair of scissors, a needle-holder, 4 artery clamps, dissecting forceps, long dressing forceps, bullet forceps, a three-bladed or a Simon speculum, and an assortment of needles. The valise should also contain a tin box, 40 × 13 × 10 centimetres, provided with a lid and wooden handles. In this the various instruments can be packed when not in use, and at operation it serves as a boiler and as a receptacle for them after sterilization. A Tarnier axis-traction, or an ordinary Simpson forceps, should be carried, according as the physician has become accustomed to the one or other instrument, as well as a 3-quart fountain syringe with a glass nozzle for intra-uterine, and a hollow needle for subcutaneous injections of salt solution. The latter should be sterilized in advance and wrapped in a sterile towel, so as to be ready for immediate use.

This list does not include the instruments required for the destructive operations, as they are not usually carried by the general practitioner. Everything mentioned in the above list may be packed into a box 21 × $8\frac{1}{2}$ × 8 inches.

Conduct of the First Stage of Labour.—The physician should instruct the patient as to the best method of communicating with him without delay; but generally speaking, should direct the nurse not to send for him if the labour commences at night, between 11 P. M. and 7 A. M., unless it seems necessary that he should see the patient at once. On the other hand, when the pains begin between 7 A. M. and 11 P. M., the physician should be notified immediately, so that he may make his plans accordingly.

As soon as the nature and severity of the pains indicate that labour has set in, the patient should receive a full bath and a rectal enema. When the physician arrives he should make a careful external examination, map out the presentation and position of the child, and listen to the fœtal heart. In primiparæ, if the pelvis be normal, and the child present by the vertex, which is firmly engaged, there is no necessity for making an internal examination, provided that the heart sounds are in good condition, as all that can be gained therefrom is information concerning the degree of dilatation of the cervix. On this point one can usually form a fairly accurate idea from the behaviour of the patient and the extent to which the head has descended into the pelvis, which can usually be determined by external palpation. Again, the rupture of the membranes and the onset of bearing-down pains usually indicate the beginning of the second stage, after which, as a rule, there is ample time in primiparæ for the arrival of the physician.

In general, then, it may be said that in primiparæ, if no abnormality be suspected, an internal examination is unnecessary and should not be made unless the first stage is unduly prolonged. On the other hand, in view of the fact that in multiparous women the first stage is frequently very short, and the second occasionally terminating with a few expulsive pains, unless the physician is prepared to remain in the house indefinitely, it may be desirable to ascertain the condition of the cervix by vaginal touch, as the patient should not be left after the external os is two thirds dilated.

Frequent internal examinations should be avoided for two reasons: to minimize the possibility of infection and to save the feelings of the patient as far as possible.

Hand Disinfection.—Recent experimental work has conclusively demonstrated that it is impossible, in a large proportion of cases, at any rate, to render the hands absolutely sterile, no matter what method of disinfection may be employed. Even after the most rigorous directions have been scrupulously followed, there still remains a not inconsiderable danger of infection. For details concerning the latest work upon the subject the reader is referred to Haegler's monograph.

With the view of still further minimizing these risks, the use of rubber gloves has been introduced. These can be rendered perfectly sterile by boiling, and when drawn over the carefully disinfected hands afford the greatest safety possible. Since, however, they are liable to tear occasionally, the necessity for disinfecting the hands before putting them on is apparent. But that their employment, even in conjunction with all our other precautions, does not entirely do away with the possibility of introducing bacteria into the genital tract, is evident, since I have shown that pathogenic organisms are present upon the inner surfaces of the labia and the margins of the hymen in at least 60 per cent of pregnant women, and that the mere introduction of a sterilized glass speculum 2 centimetres in diameter, which is no larger than the two fingers employed for examination, carries micro-organisms into the vagina in at least one half of such cases. Moreover, inasmuch as the delicate structure of the parts renders their thorough disinfection out of the question, and as the examining fingers necessarily come in contact with them, it must be admitted that vaginal examinations during labour can never be entirely devoid of danger, and they should therefore be avoided so far as is consistent with the welfare of the patient. While these considerations should not deter us from making as many examinations as may be necessary in abnormal cases, it should always be borne in mind that the best results are obtained by the least possible employment of the vaginal touch and the widest possible utilization of external methods of examination.

If the hands of the physician have recently come in contact with infectious material at operation or autopsy, labour should be conducted by external examinations alone, vaginal examinations being made only in the presence of some abnormality, and then only after most careful disinfection and the use of gloves.

In all cases, before making an internal examination, the hands should be disinfected as carefully as for a major surgical operation. The best method for this purpose, introduced by Dr. Halsted some years ago, and described by Dr. Kelly in 1891, consists of the following steps:

1. Cut the finger-nails with clippers or scissors to 1 millimetre in length.

2. Scrub the hands and forearms up to the elbows vigorously with nail-brush, green soap, and hot water, for at least five minutes by the clock, and longer if they are not macroscopically clean, paying particular attention to the nails and palmar surface of the fingers. The water must be changed at least once. After changing it, remove dirt from beneath the finger-nails with nail-cleaner or knife and renew the washing.

3. Rinse the hands in fresh water and then soak them in a hot saturated solution of potassium permanganate until they take on a deep mahogany-brown colour.

4. Dissolve this off in a hot saturated solution of oxalic acid.

5. Then soak the hands and forearms in a 1-to-1,000 bichloride solution for at least three minutes by the clock.

6. Touch nothing until ready to examine the patient, going directly from the bichloride to her.

The only objection which can be made to this method of hand disinfection is the length of time which it requires and the roughness of the hands which sometimes follows it. The first objection cannot be overcome, as I do not believe that the hands can be thoroughly disinfected in less than ten minutes by any method. The second can be obviated to a great extent by anointing the hands with glycerin or some emollient after the examination has been made.

The rapid method of disinfection introduced by Fürbringer, by which he believed that the hands could be rendered absolutely sterile in three minutes, has been shown by later experimental work to be absolutely unreliable. Nor have the recent methods of disinfection by means of alcohol substantiated the claims which have been made for them, inasmuch as Krönig has shown that they are based upon a fallacy, and that alcohol does not possess a markedly germicidal action, but simply produces conditions in the skin which for the time being render it difficult to remove the organisms from its surface.

Preparation of Patient for Examination.—While the physician is disinfecting his hands, the nurse should be making her preparations for the internal examination. The patient should lie on the right or left side of the bed, according as the physician prefers to examine with his right or left hand. She should then be covered with a sheet, which is pulled up from the foot of the bed and its ends wrapped about the legs in such a manner as to leave the external genitalia free with the least possible exposure of the rest of the person. The bedclothes should not be thrown back so as to leave the legs of the patient exposed. Nor should the physician be expected to examine under any covering. The vulva and the inner surfaces of the thighs are then thoroughly washed with soap and hot water, particular attention being paid to the regions about the anus and clitoris. If the pubic hairs are very long they should be cut short with scissors or shaved. After a thorough cleansing the parts should be rinsed with fresh water

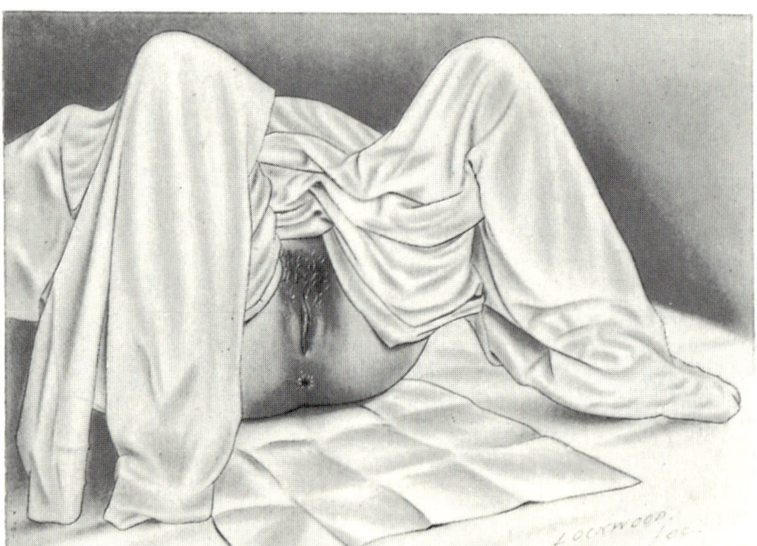

Fig. 288.—Showing proper Method of covering Patient with Sheet before making a Vaginal Examination.

and then sponged with a 1-to-2,000 bichloride solution, after which they should be covered with a towel soaked in the same solution, which remains in place until the physician is ready to commence his examination. Finally, a sterile towel should be placed under the patient's buttocks, so as to prevent the examining hand from coming in contact with the bed.

Method of making a Vaginal Examination.—After thorough disinfection, the thumb and forefinger of one hand distend the labia widely, so as to stretch the vaginal opening and prevent the examining fingers from coming in contact with the inner surface of the labia and the margins of

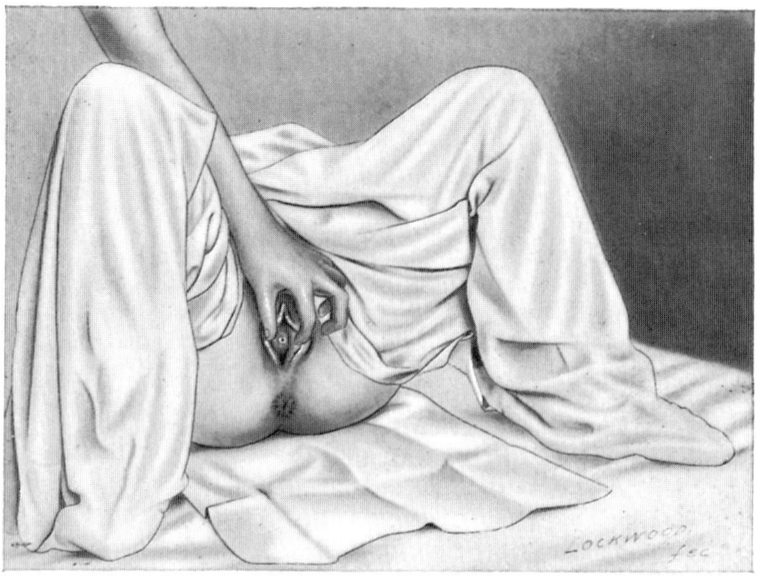

FIG. 289.—ILLUSTRATING SPREADING APART THE LABIA BEFORE MAKING A VAGINAL EXAMINATION

the hymen, while the index and second fingers of the other hand are anointed with sterile vaseline and introduced into the vagina.

In making the examination a definite routine should be followed: 1. The fingers should be introduced along the anterior surface of the vaginal wall, and the shape and size of the pubic arch and the height of the symphysis noted. 2. The cervix should then be examined in order to determine whether its canal is obliterated, the degree to which the external os is dilated, and the character of its margins. Next we observe whether the membranes are intact or not, great care being taken to avoid rupturing them if the patient is in the first stage of labour. 3. The presenting part should be felt for, and, if the os be dilated, the presentation and position of the child should be made out. It is also important to determine its relation to the superior strait and to the line connecting the ischial spines. 4. After having decided these points, the palmar surface of the fingers should be directed posteriorly, and the perinæum palpated between the two fingers in the vagina and the thumb outside, with special reference to its consistency, thickness, and resistance. 5. The mobility of the coccyx should then be tested, after which the fingers should be passed upward over the anterior surface of the sacrum and its vertical and lateral curvature noted. If the presenting part is not low down, the three lower sacral vertebræ are readily palpable in normal women, whereas the first and second can be felt only in contracted pelves. 6. If the presenting part is not deeply engaged, the diagonal conjugate should be measured.

If it becomes necessary to repeat the examination, exactly the same rigorous preparation is imperative, it being important to remember that a single disinfection of the hands is efficient only for a comparatively short period.

After completing the examination, the physician is usually expected to express an opinion as to the probable course of events. If everything is normal, he should assure the patient that all will be well, but should guard against making any very definite statement as to the probable duration of labour, and content himself with saying that under such circumstances the average time is only a certain number of hours, and that her suffering will probably be ended within that period. The obstetrician who ventures to make more precise statements will speedily find that his predictions are often very faulty, even when the head is on the perinæum. If some abnormality be present, it is not always wise to inform the patient of the fact, but the physician should be careful to impart his knowledge to some responsible member of the family for his own protection, in case an emergency should arise.

During the first stage of labour the patient usually prefers to move about her room, and frequently is more comfortable when occupying a sitting position. During this period, therefore, she should not be compelled to take to her bed unless she feels so inclined, and when she does so she should be cautioned against attempting to hasten labour by voluntarily bringing her abdominal muscles into play, for they have little or no effect upon the dilatation of the cervix, and the effort will only serve to exhaust her strength.

Conduct of the Second Stage of Labour.—The beginning of the second stage of labour is usually indicated by the rupture of the membranes and the onset of bearing-down pains, though these signs are not absolutely characteristic, as in a small number of cases rupture may occur at an early period, or the patient may attempt to hasten the course of labour by making premature use of her abdominal muscles. On the other hand, the membranes sometimes remain intact until they protrude from the vulva. In still rarer cases they do not rupture at all, the child coming into the world surrounded by them, or, as it is popularly termed, being born with a *caul.*

In the latter part of the first stage the pains generally become so severe that the patient naturally seeks the recumbent position; but if she is still moving about the room or sitting up, she should go to bed immediately upon the rupture of the membranes and the beginning of bearing-down pains.

Preparation of the Bed.—The bed should be prepared as soon as the pains become severe, since in the case of a multiparous woman the second stage of labour is often extremely short, and delivery occasionally occurs while the patient is being moved from a chair or sofa to the bed. A high single iron bedstead is preferable, but in private practice one usually has to be content with the ordinary double bed. Under such circumstances one side of it should be prepared for the patient; whether the right or left depends upon which hand the physician expects to use for vaginal examination and the conduct of labour. A large piece of rubber sheeting, 1 × 2 yards, should be placed over the centre of the mattress, covering its entire width, and over this a sheet is spread. A second piece of rubber sheeting, $\frac{3}{4}$ × 1 yard, is placed upon the side of the bed upon which the patient is to lie, in such a position that it will come directly under her buttocks. The entire bed is then covered by a draw-sheet; over this is placed a sterile bed-pad upon which the buttocks rest, or a Kelly obstetrical rubber pad may be used. With this arrangement, the upper sheet and the small piece of rubber cloth can be removed at the completion of labour, leaving the mattress protected by a large piece of rubber sheeting and the under sheet. To avoid exposure the legs should be encased in long leggings which reach to the thighs and are pinned to the rolled-up nightgown. In winter these should be made of canton flannel and in summer of thin muslin.

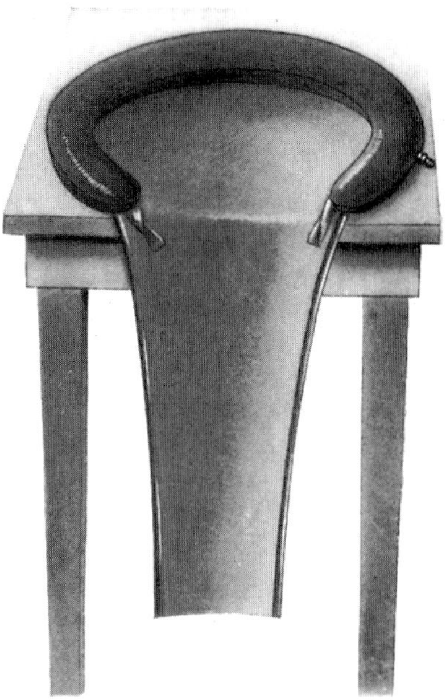

FIG. 290.—KELLY'S RUBBER PAD.

Examination in the Second Stage.—After the patient has been put to bed, the question arises whether or not a vaginal examination should be made, and this is determined by the condition of affairs in each case. If the head has become engaged in the first stage of labour, it can be omitted; but if the presenting part is not engaged, or any abnormality is present or suspected, an internal examination is absolutely necessary in order to ascertain whether the cord has prolapsed, or if everything is as it should be.

If the patient has apparently been in the second stage of labour for some time without rupture of the membranes, an examination is advisable in order to determine the condition of the cervix; for, after it has become completely dilated, the membranes have served their purpose and retard rather than hasten the birth of the child, so that it may be advisable to rupture them artificially. This is usually readily accomplished by sawing through them with the finger-nail, or pinching them between the two examining fingers. In rare instances, however, they are so resistant that it becomes necessary to resort to instrumental means. For this purpose a sterilized bullet forceps is admirably suited, but if it is not available, a hat-pin, previously heated in the flame of an alcohol lamp, is a convenient substitute. The membranes should not be ruptured during the acme of a pain, particularly when the head is not deeply engaged, as occasionally the rush of amniotic fluid may be so great as to carry the cord along with it, and thus bring about its prolapse. The beginner should always be careful to differentiate between the distended membranes and a tense caput succedaneum.

When vaginal examinations are made in the second stage of labour, the same stringent precautions as to disinfection of the hands and the patient's genitalia should be observed. When the head is deeply engaged

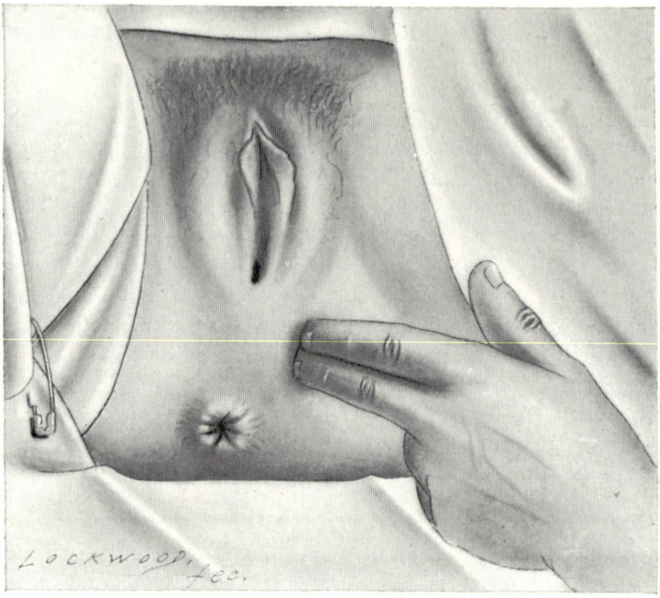

Fig. 291.—Palpating Head through Perinæum.

in the pelvis, internal examinations are quite unnecessary, as its descent can readily be traced by the increasing difficulty with which the cephalic prominence is felt on employment of the fourth manœuvre. Moreover, when it can no longer be felt from above, if the legs are widely separated and the tips of the fingers applied to the perinæum, to the side of and in front of the anus, and pressed firmly inward and upward, the presenting part can be felt as a firm, rounded body. Generally speaking, this manœuvre becomes available as soon as the head has passed below the level of the ischial spines.

During the entire second stage, auscultation should be practised at frequent intervals, particularly when the head has reached the pelvic floor, for occasionally the cord is pressed upon tightly, and the child may be asphyxiated at this period and be lost, if not delivered promptly.

Delivery.—As soon as the head can be palpated through the perinæum, preparations should be made for delivery. A table should be placed in a convenient position at the side of the bed, and upon it a basin of boiled water and another of 1-to-2,000 bichloride solution, as well as sterilized cotton pledgets or gauze sponges, a certain number of sterile towels, and the material for tying the cord. The instruments needed for the repair of the perinæum should also be within easy reach.

The patient should then be placed in position upon the bed. In this country it is customary for her to lie upon her back with the legs drawn up, though in England and many places on the Continent the lateral position is preferred. If the leggings have not been used, they should now be drawn up and pinned to the night-gown, which has been rolled up beneath the patient's back, so that it may not be soiled. The genitalia should again be washed with soap and water, and bathed with a bichloride solution.

After having carefully disinfected his hands so that he may make an immediate vaginal examination if necessary, the physician should place a sterile towel beneath the patient's buttocks, a second over her abdomen, and others over her legs, and pin them in place so as to cover everything in the neighbourhood of the genitalia with which his hands may come in contact, leaving only the vulva and perinæum exposed.

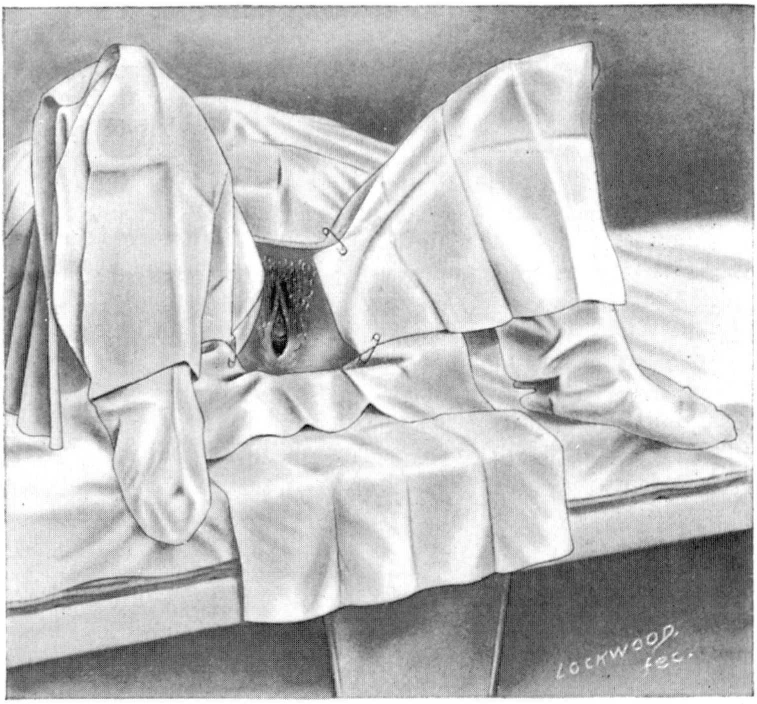

FIG. 292.—SHOWING PATIENT IN PROPER POSITION FOR DELIVERY, AND COVERED BY STERILE DRESSINGS.

As the head passes down into the pelvis, small particles of fæces are frequently expelled, and as they appear at the anus they should be wiped away with a piece of cotton, after which the parts should be sponged off with fresh pledgets soaked in bichloride solution.

As soon as the head begins to distend the vulva the patient's sufferings become greatly increased, and are frequently excruciating. At this stage it is advisable to begin to use chloroform, partly to relieve the pain, and partly to aid in protecting the perinæum. If the nurse be competent, its administration should be intrusted to her. The patient having been instructed to give notice as soon as she feels a pain beginning, several drops of chloroform are poured upon an Esmarch inhaler, and she is told to inspire deeply. This is repeated with each pain, the inhaler being removed immediately after its cessation. In this manner, after a short time the sensation of pain becomes markedly diminished, while the patient retains consciousness and is generally able to talk rationally. But when the head begins to emerge from the vulva, the chloroform should be pushed to complete anæsthesia, during which the head is born. This degree, however, should last only for a few moments.

Protection of the Perinæum.—As soon as the perinæum shows signs of bulging, the physician should make preparations for its protection, placing himself in such a position as to be able effectually to check the progress of the head if necessary.

Injuries to the perinæum are of very frequent occurrence, and cannot always be avoided even under the most skilful treatment. The statements as to their frequency vary considerably, but all authorities agree that they occur much oftener in primiparous than in multiparous women. Thus, Schroeder observed them in 34.5 and 9 per cent of his cases respectively; Balandin in 25.99 and 4.19 per cent; and Olshausen in 21.1 and 4.7 per cent. These figures would seem to be rather too conservative, as slight tears implicating the fourchette occur in from one half to two thirds of all primiparæ, and in 10 per cent of multiparæ. Occasionally one meets with physicians who state that they have delivered several thousand women with one or two, or possibly without a single perineal tear. Such statements, however, are always erroneous, and merely indicate that the physician has not inspected the parts after labour, and designates as torn only those cases in which the vagina and rectum have been converted into a cloaca, to the existence of which his attention would assuredly be called by the patient.

In the greatest number of cases the fourchette alone suffers, but not uncommonly the tear extends through a greater or lesser portion of the perineal body and is usually associated with another extending some distance up one or both vaginal sulci, while in rare cases the entire perinæum is torn through and the rectum opened up. The first two varieties are frequently unavoidable, but the common occurrence of complete tears is an indication of ignorance or negligence.

Generally speaking, the causes of rupture are threefold: disproportion between the head and the vulva, too rapid expulsion, and abnormalities in the mechanism of labour. Where the head is excessively large or the vulva excessively small, the mechanical conditions are such that birth cannot take place without a certain amount of laceration. In not a few cases the tearing is due not so much to absolute disproportion between the head and the vulva as to the lack of elasticity of the perinæum, which is particularly marked in elderly primiparæ. Too rapid expulsion, however, is a much more frequent cause of rupture, and when the head is suddenly and forcibly extruded through the imperfectly distended vulva, its mode of production is manifest.

Various abnormalities in the mechanism of labour favour rupture of the perinæum. The most frequent of these is imperfect extension of the head, so that the vulva is distended by the occipito-frontal, instead of the suboccipito-bregmatic or suboccipito-frontal circumference. In a certain number of cases the presenting part may be directed too far backward—in other words, extension does not occur—and under the influence of the uterine contractions the presenting part is forced directly downward upon the perineal body, instead of being guided upward and forward towards the vulval opening. Occasionally a similar condition is observed in women having a pelvis which approaches the male type, and in which the pubic arch is long and narrow, whereby the head is prevented from engaging directly under the symphysis pubis. Again, in rare instances, an abnormal inclination of the pelvis, by causing the vulval opening to look more upward than usual, may bring about a similar condition. In considering the mechanism of labour we directed attention to the factors which predispose to perineal rupture, when the head is delivered in persistent occipito-posterior positions, or when the child presents by the brow, face, or breech.

Giffard, in 1733, was the first to direct attention to the advisability of attempting to prevent perineal tears. Numerous devices have since been suggested having the same object in view, but their very multiplicity argues that they are not uniformly satisfactory. In most of the older methods pressure was applied directly to the perinæum, or various attempts were made to relieve the tension to which it was subjected, so that the physician was said to support the perinæum. An excellent *résumé* of the early literature upon the subject will be found in Goodell's scholarly article, published in 1871.

In the method which has stood me in best stead no attempt is made to support the perinæum by pressure, but the obstetrician simply endeavours to favour extension of the head and prevent it from being suddenly extruded during the acme of a pain. For this purpose, when the vertex begins to distend the vulva, it should be seized between the thumb and three fingers of one hand, and forcible pressure made against it during each pain. At the same time the pressure should be directed in such a manner as to bring the occiput, and later the nape of the neck, directly in contact with the inferior margin of the symphysis, and thus increase extension. Accordingly, as soon as the head appears at the vulva the physician should be ready to restrain its progress. He should hold his hand in such a manner as to be able to bring it immediately into action, for in many instances the resistance of the vulva is unexpectedly overcome, and a single pain may be sufficient to push the head suddenly through it with a resulting perineal tear. After the head is so far born that the vulva is distended by the perietal bosses, it may be advisable to attempt to express it by *Ritgen's method* in an interval between the pains. For this purpose, the patient having been instructed to open her mouth and not to attempt to

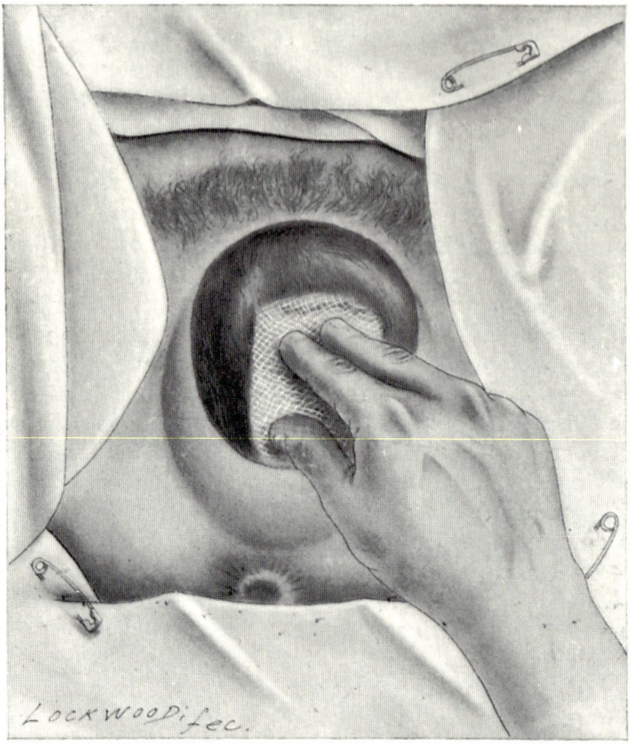

FIG. 293.—METHOD OF HOLDING BACK HEAD TO PROTECT PERINÆUM.

bear down, the anæsthesia is deepened. At the same time two fingers are applied just behind the anus, and forward and upward pressure is made upon the brow through the perinæum.

The student is warned from attempting to protect the perinæum by any method which aims at stripping it back over the presenting part. Such a procedure is useless, even if carried out successfully, and not infrequently, while it is being attempted, the head will suddenly shoot past the hand and cause a more or less severe laceration. The same may be said of the introduction of the finger into the anus, for the purpose of drawing the perinæum up over the head, as suggested by Dr. Goodell. In fact, all such procedures are not only of questionable utility, so far as the protection of the perinæum is concerned, but are dangerous in that they contaminate the hand and throw it out of function in case an emergency should arise which calls for its prompt introduction into the genital tract.

Many obstetricians introduce one or two fingers into the vagina as soon as the head appears at the vulval opening, so that it may not surprise them by a sudden advance. Such a practice is extremely reprehensible, as it markedly increases the possibility of contamination and infection.

Many authorities, when rupture of the perinæum seems imminent, advise the performance of *episiotomy*. In this operation a strong pair of scissors is introduced between the head and the perinæum, and an oblique incision made downward and backward on either side between the anus and the tuber ischii. The operation is practised in the belief that the vulval opening, if sufficiently enlarged by the incisions, will not tear farther, or that in any case the laceration will occur in the continuation of the incisions, whose clean-cut edges will heal more readily than the irregular spontaneous tears. Personally, I see no advantage in the procedure, as my experience is that ordinary perineal tears will heal almost uniformly if properly sutured and cared for.

Coils of Cord about the Neck.—Immediately after the birth of the head the finger should be passed to the neck of the child in order to ascertain whether it is encircled by one or more coils of the umbilical cord. This complication occurs in about every fourth case, and the vessels are sometimes pressed upon so tightly that asphyxiation results. If such a coil be felt, it should be drawn down between the fingers, and, if loose enough, slipped over the child's head; but if the cord be too tightly applied to permit of this procedure, and the head appears congested and suffused, the former should be seized and cut between two artery clamps, and the child immediately extracted.

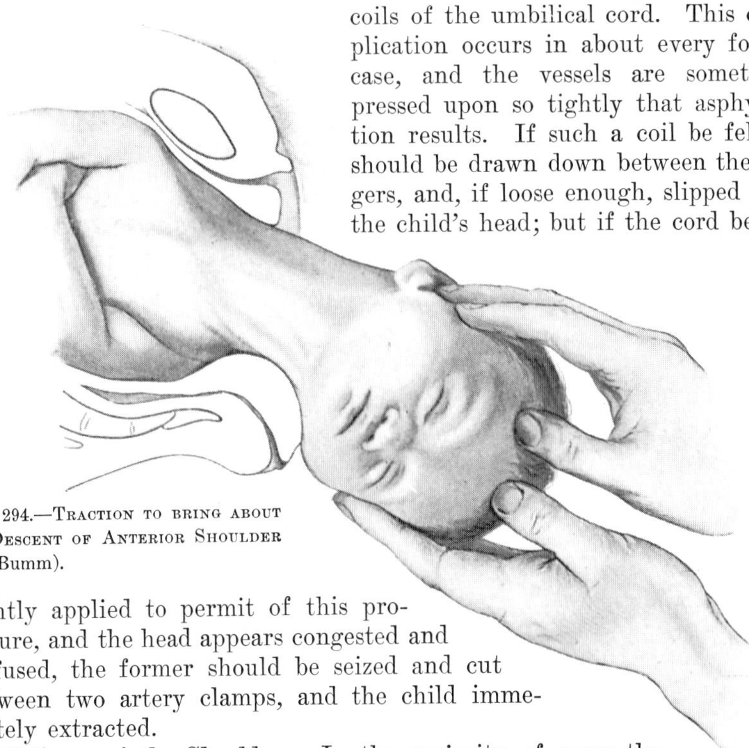

Fig. 294.—Traction to bring about Descent of Anterior Shoulder (Bumm).

Delivery of the Shoulders.—In the majority of cases the shoulders appear at the vulva just after the occurrence of external rotation, and are born without difficulty. Occasionally, however, a delay occurs and immediate extraction may appear advisable. To accomplish this the occiput and chin should be seized by the two hands, and downward traction made until the anterior shoulder appears under the pubic arch; next, by an upward movement, the posterior shoulder should be delivered, after which the other will usually drop from beneath the symphysis.

The body almost always follows the shoulders without difficulty, but in case of prolonged delay its birth may be hastened by traction upon the head, but not by hooking the fingers in the axillæ, since by the latter procedure the nerves of the arm may be injured and transient or permanent paralysis result. Indeed, even the former method of extraction is not devoid of danger, for occasionally the oblique traction employed may cause excessive stretching of the brachial plexus, with subsequent paralysis.

Tying the Cord.—Immediately after its birth the child usually makes an inspiratory movement and then begins to cry. Under such circumstances it should be placed between the patient's legs in such a manner as to leave the cord lax and thus avoid traction upon it. If, however, the child does not begin to breathe immediately, the cord should be seized and cut between two artery clamps, and efforts at resuscitation commenced at once.

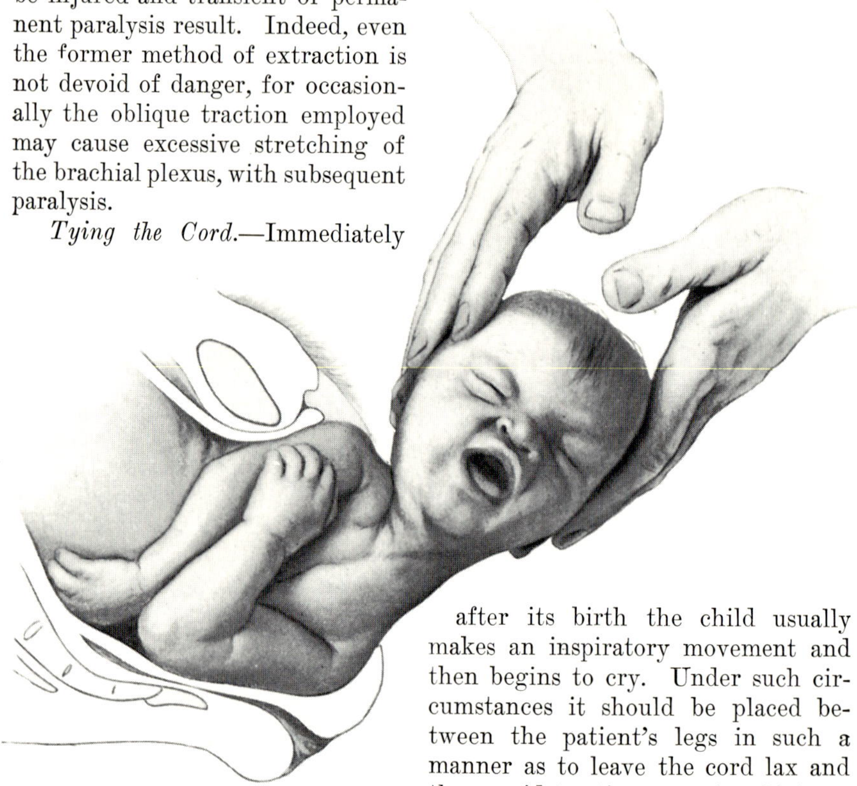

FIG. 295.—DELIVERY OF POSTERIOR SHOULDER (Bumm).

Normally, the cord should not be ligated until it has ceased to pulsate. In securing it, a ligature of sterilized bobbin should be applied 2 centimetres from the abdomen of the child and tightly tied; a second ligature is placed several centimetres above the first, and the cord cut between the two. Usually ligation of the maternal end merely serves to avoid soiling the bedclothes by blood escaping from it; but in twin pregnancies double ligation is essential, for when the two fœtuses are derived from a single ovum there is marked anastomosis in the placental circulation, so that the second child, while still in the uterus, may bleed to death from the maternal end of the cord of the first.

The question as to the proper time for tying the cord has given rise to a great deal of discussion. Formerly it was the custom to ligate it immediately after the birth of the child; but Budin showed that 92 cubic centimetres more blood escaped from the maternal end of the cord after early than after late ligation, thus indicating that that amount was lost to the fœtus by early, and saved for it by late ligation. Schücking also demonstrated the same fact by weighing the child just after birth and again after the cord had ceased to pulsate, and was able to demonstrate a corresponding increase in weight in the latter case. Budin believed that this amount of blood was drawn into the circulatory system of the fœtus by thoracic aspiration, while Schücking held that it was driven into it as a result of the compression of the placenta by the contracting uterus. Hofmeier, Zweifel, and Ribemont have also shown that the initial loss of weight in the first few days after birth is usually less after late than after early ligation.

I have always practised late ligation of the cord and have seen no injurious effects following it, and therefore recommend its employment unless some emergency arises which calls for earlier interference.

After ligation of the cord, the child should be wrapped in a piece of flannel or blanket prepared for the purpose, and laid in a safe place until the placenta is born and the mother has been cleaned up and made comfortable.

Anæsthesia.—We are indebted to Sir James Y. Simpson, the discoverer of chloroform, for the introduction of anæsthesia into obstetrical practice. He employed ether for this purpose in the year 1847, and replaced it by chloroform after the discovery of the latter drug. Every one agrees as to the marked benefits derived from anæsthesia when operative procedures are to be undertaken, but there is still considerable difference of opinion as to the advisability of its routine employment in normal labour.

The most popular anæsthetics are ether and chloroform, and when obstetrical operations are to be performed it makes very little difference which is employed, as it is well known that the dangers incident to chloroform are markedly reduced at the time of labour, and that only a very few deaths have followed its use under such circumstances. Exactly why the parturient woman should enjoy this immunity is a question which has not yet been definitely settled, but it is nevertheless a fact which has been established beyond peradventure.

On the other hand, chloroform is far preferable in normal labour, for by its use obstetrical anæsthesia can be rapidly and safely produced; whereas ether, owing to its slower action, does not lend itself so readily to this method of employment. As the result of my experience, I believe that chloroform, when properly administered, is practically devoid of danger in such cases, and should be used whenever there is time for its administration. Of course it is contra-indicated when the patient has religious objections to its use, as well as in those cases in which labour is almost painless.

The choice of the time for its administration, however, is of great importance, nor should it be used before the latter part of the second stage, when the head becomes visible at the vulva, or at least until the perinæum begins to bulge. A few drops of chloroform should then be poured upon the inhaler, and with the beginning of a pain the patient should be instructed to breathe in the fumes vigorously; but as soon as the contraction has ceased the inhaler should be removed, to be used again when the patient makes a sign that she feels the first indication that another is beginning. When the distention of the vulva is at its maximum, obstetrical anæsthesia is not sufficient to abolish the pain, and it is my practice, as the head emerges, to render my patient completely unconscious for the moment by increasing the dose of the drug.

By this procedure the woman is saved an immense amount of unnecessary pain, and at the same time the danger of perineal laceration is diminished. For, if the suffering is minimized, and done away with entirely at the critical moment, the patient will lie still instead of tossing in her bed, and there will not be the same danger of the head being suddenly expelled at the acme of a contraction, while the physician is employing his energies in persuading the patient to keep quiet, or may even be forcing her legs apart so that he may be able to protect the perinæum. The amount of chloroform required for this purpose is very small, and rarely exceeds 2 or 3 drams.

For various reasons, the administration of chloroform should be deferred as long as possible in the second and never resorted to in the first stage, unless exceptional indications call for its employment. Leaving out of consideration its possible influence upon the efficiency of the uterine contractions, it is only natural that as soon as the patient has experienced the soothing effects of the drug she is extremely loath to do without it, and, once having begun, the physician may find himself forced to continue its administration for a considerable length of time, unless he possesses more fortitude than is generally the case.

Against the employment of anæsthetics in labour it has been urged that they diminish the force of the uterine contractions. This statement is partially correct, for when administered for any great length of time they undoubtedly lead to a shortening of the uterine contractions and to a prolongation of the interval between them, as was clearly demonstrated by the experiments of Dönhoff and Hensen. On the other hand, when exhibited only at the proper time and in no excessive amount, this objection does not hold good, and in many instances small doses appear to stimulate the uterine contractions, and by diminishing the sensation of pain enable the patient to bring her abdominal muscles into full play, which she previously may have been unwilling to do, and thus hasten the completion of labour.

Again, it has been taught that anæsthesia predisposes to relaxation of the uterus after the expulsion of the placenta, and thus increases the danger of post-partum hæmorrhage. So far as my own experience goes, such sequelæ are not likely to occur provided the drug has been properly administered. At the same time it must be admitted that its prolonged administration certainly tends towards uterine inertia, and is not without a deleterious influence upon the child.

In exceptional cases chloroform, while diminishing the pain, appears to excite the patient. Under such conditions it should not be employed unless complete anæsthesia is necessary. It should never be used in the first stage of prolonged labours in the hope of hastening the dilatation of the cervix, as this object is better attained by the proper administration of chloral or morphia.

Ordinarily the patient is allowed to come from under the influence of the anæsthetic as soon as the child is born, as its exhibition is not necessary in the third stage of labour, except when the placenta is to be removed manually or an extensive perineal laceration is to be repaired. Moreover, it should be remembered that after the birth of the child the patient does not appear to enjoy the same immunity as when in active labour.

Cocaine Anæsthesia.—Following the rehabilitation by Bier of the subarachnoidal injection of cocaine for the production of anæsthesia of the lower portion of the body, and its popularization by the work of Tuffier, it was but natural that its efficiency should be tested upon the parturient woman.

The first publication concerning its employment at the time of labour was made in August, 1900, by Kreis, who reported the results obtained in 6 cases in Bumm's clinic in Bâle. It would appear, however, that Doléris was working simultaneously upon the same lines. Since then a number of observers, notably Marx, Stone, Demelin, and Doléris and Malartic have reported series of cases treated in this manner. From their reports, as well as from observations made in my clinic, there is no doubt that most striking results are obtained in a certain proportion of cases.

In favourable cases, the patient being in the second stage of labour, the injection into the lumbar portion of the vertebral canal of 10 to 15 minims of a 1-per-cent solution of cocaine ($\frac{1}{10}$–$\frac{1}{6}$ grain) is followed within a few minutes by complete abolition of painful sensations. At the same time, the patient continues to make visible expulsive efforts with great regularity and ofttimes with increased frequency, so that if the effects of the drug do not wear off too rapidly, the child may be expelled without pain and almost without the knowledge of the patient. Likewise, various operative procedures, such as manual dilatation of the cervix, version, or forceps, may be painlessly performed.

Notwithstanding these very wonderful results, I do not hesitate to advise strongly against the employment of the method in obstetrical practice, and therefore shall not enter into the details of the technique of making the injection. In the first place, the results are not always uniform, a certain number of patients appearing to be absolutely refractory to the influence of the drug when administered in doses consistent with safety. Again, its effects are sometimes very transient and fade away just when most needed. More serious, however, are the after-effects, the majority of patients suffering severely from headache and nausea, and frequently from an alarming but transient elevation of temperature. In view of their comparatively short duration, these symptoms are usually regarded as a manifestation of intoxication rather than of infection.

The most serious objection to the method is the fact that Hahn, in 1901, reported 8 deaths in 1,708 cases in which its use has been recorded in the literature (1–200). No doubt, in several instances the fatal issue could not be fairly attributed to the method, but in several others the autopsy showed lesions of the spinal or cerebral meninges which could be due only to infection.

In view, therefore, of its various shortcomings and dangers, I see no reason to recommend the employment of spinal anæsthesia in obstetrics, being convinced that more uniform and satisfactory results may be obtained by the proper administration of chloroform with far greater safety to the patient. Moreover, were spinal anæsthesia to come into more extended use, under the adverse conditions frequently encountered in private practice, I feel sure that many women would perish from meningitis, the result of the imperfect application of the rules of aseptic technique.

Hypnotism.—Numerous observers, among whom may be mentioned Leichstein, Cocke, and others, have reported instances in which labour was painlessly conducted under the influence of hypnotism. Personally I have seen it employed successfully in only a single instance. As a rule, its field of usefulness in obstetrics is very limited, for the reason that the patient must be a susceptible subject, and one who has already been hypnotized on previous occasions.

The Use of Ergot.—Many authorities recommend the administration of a dram of fluid extract of ergot by the mouth immediately after the expulsion of the placenta, as a prophylactic measure against post-partum hæmorrhage. This is usually unnecessary, as the drug is called for only in those cases in which the uterus remains soft and flabby, instead of forming a hard tumour beneath the umbilicus. Personally, I always prefer to administer it hypodermically, and have found the ergotol prepared by Sharp and Dohme much better than the officinal fluid extract, inasmuch as it is less likely to produce an abscess at the point of injection. Instead of being inserted just under and parallel to the skin, the needle is plunged deeply into the muscle of the thigh, and from 30 to 40 minims are injected, the dose being repeated if necessary. It should be remembered that such injections usually give rise to a slight but painful induration, which persists for several days, but only exceptionally eventuates in abscess formation.

I must insist once more that this is the only time at which ergot should be employed in labour, as its administration before the completion of the third stage has led to untold harm. Formerly, even well-trained physicians used it in large quantities during the second stage to stimulate uterine contractions, but at the present time it is so employed only by ignorant midwives. The danger lies in the fact that the premature use of the drug readily leads to tetanic contractions of the uterus, which in the presence of any marked disproportion between the size of the child and pelvis are likely to bring about rupture of the uterus and the death of the patient. Moreover, its administration in the third stage of labour, before the expulsion of the placenta, cannot be too strongly deprecated, as the resulting tetanic contraction tends rather to produce a further retention of the organ, so that not infrequently its manual removal becomes imperative.

Conduct of the Third Stage of Labour.—This subject has already been considered in the preceding chapter.

Repair of the Lacerated Perinæum.—Strictly speaking, this subject should be deferred until the obstetrical operations are dealt with; but as perineal tears are of such frequent occurrence, and as they are best repaired in the interval between the birth of the child and the expulsion of the placenta, the proper method of procedure will be considered at this time.

For convenience in description, perineal tears are divided into three groups, those of the first, second, and third degrees. To the first belong

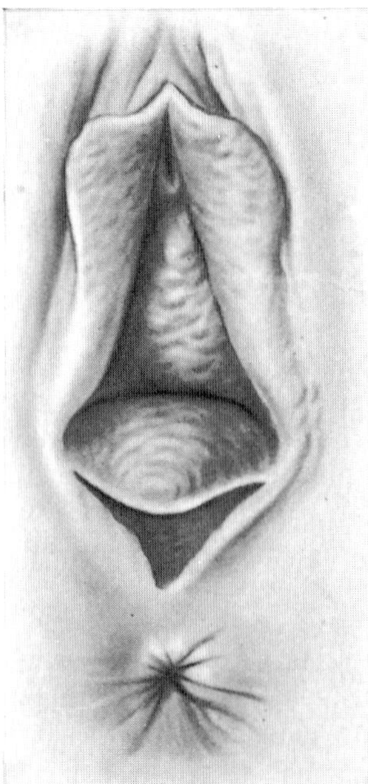

FIG. 296.—SUPERFICIAL PERINEAL TEAR.

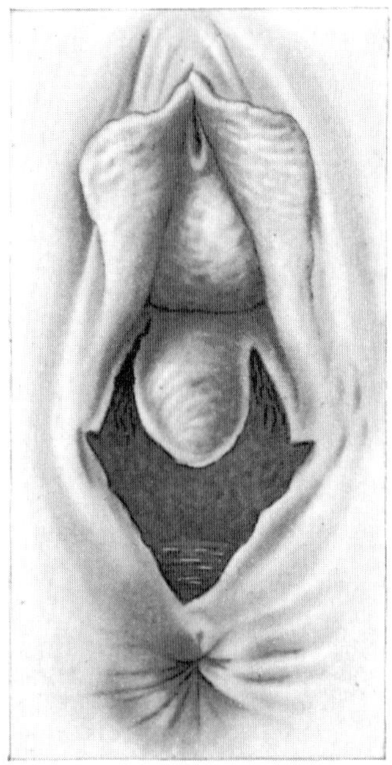

FIG. 297.—DEEP PERINEAL TEAR.

those which involve simply the fourchette and anterior margin of the perinæum, giving rise to a small, triangular wounded surface which is rarely more than 1.5 centimetre deep.

In the second, the laceration extends through a greater or lesser portion of the perineal body, and not infrequently exposes the sphincter ani muscle. Usually its course does not quite follow the median line, but is directed obliquely downward and outward from the posterior margin of the vulva. In many of these cases there are also lesions of the vagina. The latter usually involve the sulcus on the same side as the perineal tear, but frequently that on the other side as well, so that a triangular portion of the vaginal mucosa, which represents the inferior extremity of the posterior column, may become separated from the rest of the canal.

In the third degree, the tear extends completely through the perineal body and the sphincter ani muscle, and for a certain distance up the anterior wall of the rectum, thus giving rise to a cloaca, into which both vagina and rectum open. These are designated as complete, in contradistinction to those of the first and second degrees—the incomplete tears—in which the rectum is not involved. Incomplete tears are encountered very often, even in the practice of the most competent obstetricians, no matter what precautions may be taken to prevent them; but the frequent occurrence of the complete varieties indicates that the method employed for protecting the perinæum has been at fault in spontaneous, or that the extraction has been too forcible or hasty in operative deliveries.

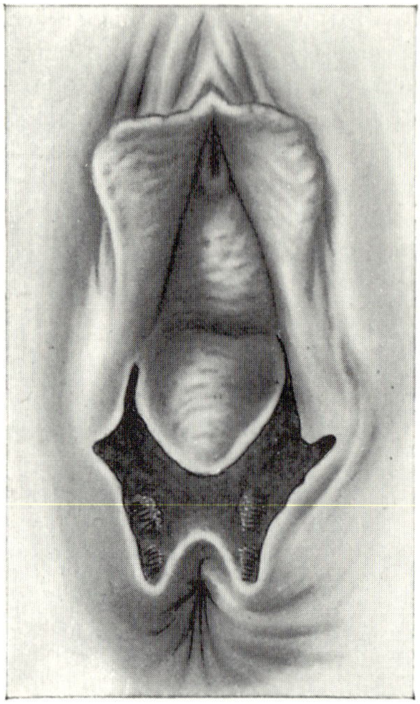

Fig. 298.—Complete Perineal Tear.

In tears of the first degree, the mucous membrane of the fourchette and the skin covering the upper portion of the perinæum and the subcutaneous tissue are implicated; in those of the second degree, the skin surface of the perinæum, the various perineal muscles, particularly the constrictor vaginæ and transversus perinei, are torn through, and the wide gaping wound is due in great part to the laceration of the last-named muscles. When the tear extends up the vagina, certain fibres of the levator ani muscle are likewise involved; while in lacerations of the third degree, the sphincter ani muscle and the anterior surface of the rectum are implicated in addition to the structures above named.

As has been said, the perineal tear commences, as a rule, at the fourchette and extends obliquely downward and outward from it. But in the very rare cases in which the vulval outlet looks markedly upward, or in which the perinæum is extremely resistant and the mechanism of expulsion faulty, the laceration may begin in the central portion of the perinæum, and the head appear in an opening which is surrounded on all sides by skin. This is known as a *central tear*, and is of extremely infrequent occurrence. Ordinarily, as the head is forced down still farther, the tear extends towards the fourchette or towards the anus, or even in both directions, and thus gives rise to a deep, incomplete, or complete laceration as the case may be.

In not a few cases, where the vaginal opening is very resistant, and when the head has remained a long time upon the pelvic floor, even although there may be no external wound or appreciable lesion of the vagina, there may nevertheless have occurred a submucous tear or separation of certain fibres of the levator ani muscle, which will later give rise to a marked relaxation of the vaginal outlet. Not infrequently the condition, although unrecognized at the time, later gives rise to such aggravated symptoms as to call for operation years after the birth of the child.

No matter what the degree, the *immediate closure of perineal lacerations* by suture is urgently indicated. Even slight tears through the fourchette are better repaired than left alone, for if not united by suture they are often extremely painful, and furnish an excellent nidus for infection in case the nurse is lax in her care of the patient. In more extensive tears immediate repair is always necessary, unless the condition of the patient be so serious as to contra-indicate further operative procedures.

For these operations, the patient should be brought to the edge of the bed and placed in the lithotomy position, and the sutures introduced while waiting for the expulsion of the placenta. They should not be tied until the completion of the third stage, as the distention of the vulva by the placenta may subject the repaired wound to undue strain. By introducing the sutures during this period a good deal of time is saved, and the temptation to hasty expression of the placenta is diminished, since the physician has plenty to do while waiting for the fundus to rise up.

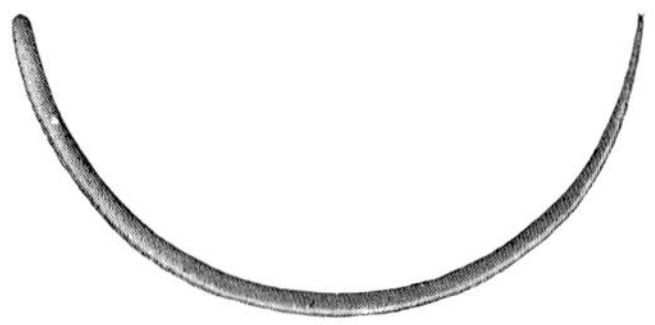

FIG. 299.—NEEDLE FOR REPAIRING PERINEAL TEARS.

The mode of repairing the wounded perinæum differs according as the tear extends only through the perineal body or is complicated by lacerations of the vagina or rectum. In the first case, the wound should be closed by deep sutures of silkworm gut, which are introduced at least 0.5 centimetre from one margin and carried well down under its base, being then brought out through the skin surface on the opposite side. It is important that the sutures should be inserted and emerge at a considerable distance from the edges of the wound, for, owing to the marked œdema which frequently follows their introduction, they are very prone to tear through unless this precaution be taken. They should be placed at intervals of about 1 centimetre, and if accurate approximation is not secured in this way superficial sutures should be employed between them. Large curved needles, which can make the entire sweep at a single movement, should be used, as they render much better service than small needles which require several bites. The sutures should be tied very loosely from below upward, and not cut off short, their long ends being twisted together into a cord and brought together into a loose knot, so as not to irritate the patient.

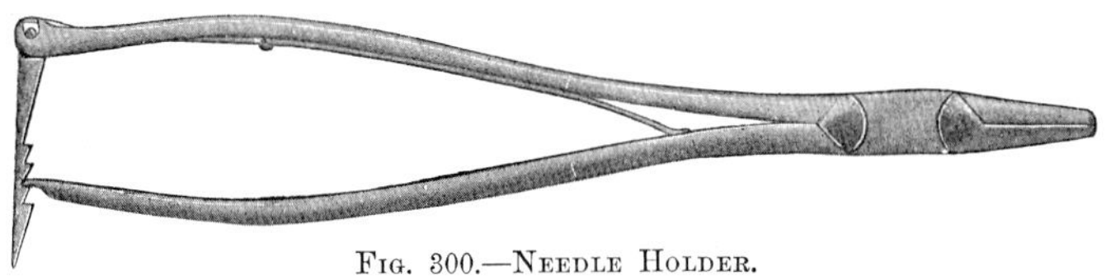

FIG. 300.—NEEDLE HOLDER.

As a suture material, silkworm gut is preferable to silver wire, since it can be more readily handled. Silk sutures are objectionable, as they readily become impregnated with the lochial secretion and are more likely to favour infection of the wound. Ordinary catgut is not satisfactory for deep sutures, as it is too rapidly absorbed, owing to the fact that the exposed portions are kept moist by the lochia. It is very useful, however, for superficial sutures, which are only required to remain for a short time.

When the perineal tear is complicated by laceration of the vagina, the edges of the latter should be brought together by deep silkworm and superficial catgut sutures, just as in Emmet's relaxed outlet operation, after which the perineal wound should be repaired in the usual manner.

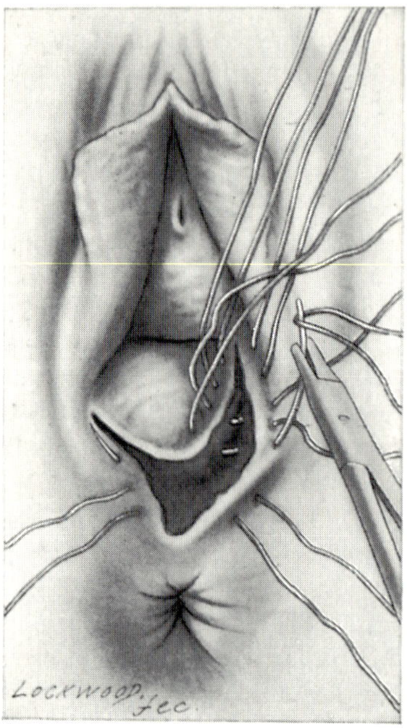

Fig. 301.—Repair of Perineal Tear extending up the Vagina.

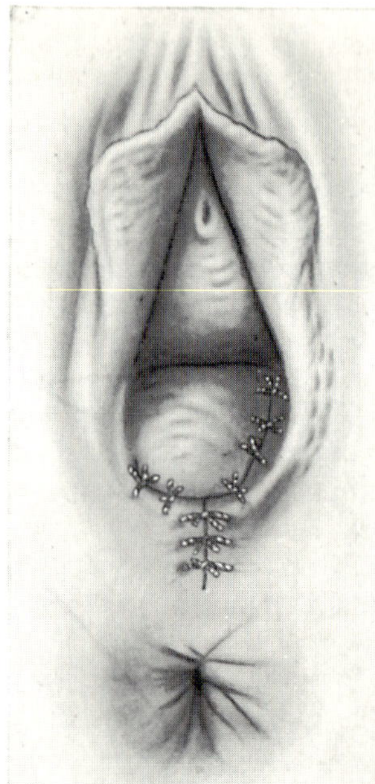

Fig. 302.—Same, Sutures Tied.

In complete tears, attention should first be given to the wounded rectum and its ruptured mucosa united by fine silk sutures, which are knotted into the rectum, the ends being allowed to protrude from the anus. When the rectum has been repaired, the ends of the sphincter ani should be isolated and firmly sutured by catgut or fine silk sutures, after which the vaginal and perineal tears should be dealt with in the manner indicated above.

The after-treatment of all degrees of tears is comparatively simple, and consists in keeping the wound clean and covered by sterile dressings. Whenever the latter are changed, the wounded surface should be washed with a 1-to-5,000 bichloride solution for a few days, and later with one of boric acid. The continuous use of antiseptic powders, such as iodoform or boric acid, is not indicated, as the wounds heal equally well without them. Nor is there any necessity for binding the legs together, unless the patient is very unruly and refuses to keep still. Catheterization may also be dispensed with, except in cases of retention, as the flow of urine over the wound does no harm, provided it is followed by proper cleansing. Generally speaking, the external sutures should be removed on the tenth day, and the vaginal stitches a few days later. In tears of the first and second degrees the bowels should be moved daily, but in complete lacerations it is advisable to prevent an action for the first two or three days, after which a large high enema of sweet oil should be given, followed by calomel or castor-oil by the mouth.

The results following these operations are usually very satisfactory, and when the parts have been correctly approximated, primary union is the rule, provided the sutures have been introduced far enough from the margins of the wound and not tied too tightly. This is a point to which too much attention can hardly be paid, for too often there is a tendency to attempt to make a neat-looking operation by introducing the sutures close to the margins of the wound and tying them snugly. As a result of this short-sighted policy, however, owing to the œdema which usually follows, the majority of the stitches cut through and become useless, so that union by primary intention becomes impossible. On the other hand, when less attention is paid to the first appearance of the wound, the sutures being introduced far from its margins and tied somewhat loosely, excellent results almost always follow.

Unfortunately, operations for complete tears are by no means so satisfactory, and as a general rule not more than one half of the cases heal by first intention. In the cases of complete or partial failure, a secondary operation is indicated before the patient is discharged from treatment.

LITERATURE

BALANDIN. Ueber den Mechanismus der Dammrisse und der verschiedenen Dammschutzverfahren. Klinische Vorträge, 1883, Heft I, St. Petersburg, 95–127.

BIER. Versuche über Cocainisirung des Rückenmarkes. Deutsche Zeitschr. f. Chirurgie, 1899, li, 361.

BUDIN. A quel moment doit-on opérer la ligature du cordon ombilical? Le Progrès Médical, 1875, decembre; 1876, janvier. (Obstétrique et Gynécologie, 1886, 1–35.)

DEMELIN. De la cocaine en obstétrique. L'Obstétrique, 1901, vi, 122–130.

DOLÉRIS et MALARTIC. Analgésie obstétricale par injections de cocaine. Comptes rendus de la soc. d'obst., de gyn. et de pæd. de Paris, 1900, ii, 279–289.

DÖNHOFF. Ueber die Einwirkung des Chloroforms auf den normalen Geburtsverlauf, etc. Archiv f. Gyn., 1892, xlii, 305–328.

FÜRBRINGER. Untersuchungen und Vorschriften über die Desinfection der Hände des Arztes, nebst Bemerkungen über den bakteriologischen Character des Nagelschmutzes. Wiesbaden, 1888.

GIFFARD. Cases in Midwifery. London, 1734, 396–398.

GOODELL. A Critical Inquiry into the Management of the Perinæum during Labour. Amer. Jour. Med. Sciences, 1871, lxi, 53–79.

HAEGLER. Händereinigung, Händedesinfection und Händeschutz. Basel, 1900.

HAHN. Ueber subarachnoideale Cocaininjectionen nach Bier. Centralbl. f. d. Grenzgebiete der Med. u. Chirurgie, 1901, iv, 304–317 und 340–354.

HENSEN. Ueber den Einfluss des Morphiums und des Aethers auf die Wehenthätigkeit des Uterus. Archiv f. Gyn., 1898, lv, 129–177.

HOFMEIER. Der Zeitpunkt der Abnabelung in seinem Einfluss auf die ersten Lebenstage des Kindes. Zeitschr. f. Geb. u. Gyn., 1879, iv, 114–132.

KELLY. Hand Disinfection. Amer. Jour. Obst., 1891, xxiv, 1414–1419.

KREIS. Ueber Medullarnarkose bei Gebärenden. Centralbl. f. Gyn., 1900, 724–729.

KRÖNIG. Versuche über Spiritusdesinfection der Hände. Centralbl. f. Gyn., 1894, 1346–1353.

MARX. Analgesia in Obstetrics produced by Medullary Injection of Cocaine. Phila. Med. Jour., 1900, vi, 857–859.

OLSHAUSEN. Ueber Dammverletzung und Dammschutz. Volkmann's Sammlung klin. Vorträge, 1872, Nr. 44.

RIBEMONT. Recherches sur la tension du sang dans les vaisseaux du fœtus et du nouveau-né. Archives de Tocologie, octobre, 1897.

RITGEN. Ueber ein Dammschutzverfahren. Monatsschr. f. Geburtsk., 1855, vi, 321–347.

SCHROEDER. Lehrbuch der Geburtshülfe, VII. Aufl., 681.

SCHÜCKING. Zur Physiologie der Nachgeburtsperiode. Berlin. klin. Wochenschr., 1877, Nr. 182.

SIMPSON. On the Employment of the Inhalation of Sulphuric Ether in the Practice of Midwifery. Monthly Jour. of Med. Sciences, 1847, 728.

Anæsthesia. Philadelphia, 1849, 248.

STONE. Cocainization of the Spinal Cord by Means of Lumbar Puncture during Labour. Amer. Jour. Obstet., 1901, xliii, 145–154.

TUFFIER. L'anesthésie medullaire en gynécologie. Revue de gyn. et de chir. abd., 1900, iv, 683–692.

WILLIAMS, J. WHITRIDGE. The Cause of the Conflicting Statements concerning the Bacterial Contents of the Vaginal Secretion of the Pregnant Woman. Amer. Jour. Obst., 1898, xxxviii, 807–817.

ZWEIFEL. Wann sollen die Neugeborenen abgenabelt werden? Centralbl. f. Gyn., 1878, 1–3.

CHAPTER XVI

THE PUERPERIUM

THE puerperium or puerperal state comprises the five or six weeks following labour which are required for the return of the generative tract to its normal condition. Although the changes occurring during this period are considered as physiological, they border very closely upon the pathological, inasmuch as under no other circumstances does such marked and rapid tissue metabolism occur without a departure from a condition of health.

Anatomical Changes in the Puerperium.—*Involution of the Uterus.*—Immediately following the expulsion of the placenta, the contracted and retracted body of the uterus forms a hard muscular tumour, the apex of which lies about midway between the umbilicus and symphysis, usually 12 centimetres ($4\frac{3}{4}$ inches) above the latter. During the next few days the uterus decreases so rapidly in size that by the tenth day it has descended once more into the cavity of the true pelvis, and can no longer be felt above the symphysis. It reaches its normal size by the end of five or six weeks. Some idea of the rapidity with which the process goes on may be gained by recalling the fact that the freshly delivered uterus weighs about 1,000 grammes, one week later 500 grammes, at the end of the second week 375 grammes, and at the end of the puerperium only 60 grammes.

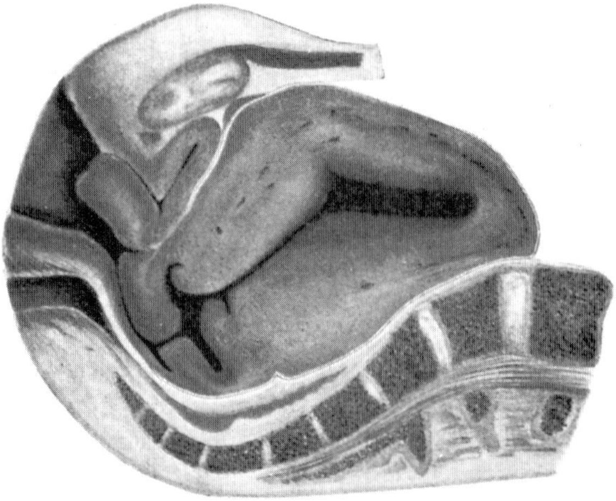

FIG. 303.—FROZEN SECTION, SHOWING UTERUS IMMEDIATELY AFTER DELIVERY (Webster).

This rapid decrease in size is due to what is designated as *involution,* and is brought about mainly by changes occurring in the muscular layer. On examining the uterus of a woman dying immediately after labour, one is struck with its markedly anæmic appearance as compared with that of the pregnant organ. This is due, according to Webster, to compression of its vessels by the contracting and retracting muscular fibres, and represents the first stage of its involution. At the same time a considerable portion of the tissue juices is expressed from it by the same mechanism.

It was formerly believed that the muscle cells underwent fatty degeneration during the puerperium, and that large numbers of them completely disappeared. The researches of Sänger have shown, however, that only the excess of protoplasm is so removed, and that the actual number of individual cells is not materially diminished. In other words, they undergo marked atrophy, but are not destroyed. Sänger estimated that their average length in the full-term uterus was 208.7 microns, as compared with 24.4 microns five weeks after labour.

As has been said before, the separation of the placenta and its membranes occurs in the inner portion of the spongy layer of the decidua, and accordingly the greater part of this layer remains in the uterus after their expulsion. It presents an irregular, jagged appearance, and is markedly infiltrated with blood, especially at the placental site. As the result of hyalin and fatty degeneration, the greater portion of this tissue is cast off in the lochia, leaving behind only the fundi of the glands of the spongy layer and a minimal amount of connective tissue, from which the new endometrium is regenerated.

The processes concerned in its regeneration have been carefully studied by Friedländer, Kundrat and Engelmann, Leopold, Krönig, and others, and it has been definitely shown that the epithelium of the new endometrium results from the proliferation of the epithelial cells of the fundi of the glands of the decidua, whereas the connective tissue is derived from the interglandular stroma. Except at the placental site, the process is ordinarily completed by the end of four to six weeks.

Pels Leusden has recently advanced the view that the syncytial tissue lying in the deeper portions of the decidua and the upper layers of the muscularis plays an important part in the process, and that the greater portion of the new epithelium is derived from it. This theory was formulated at a time when it was believed that the syncytium was of maternal origin, but since it has been shown that it represents fœtal ectoderm, such a view is no longer tenable.

Changes in the Uterine Vessels.—Immediately after the completion of the third stage of labour, the placental site is represented by an irregular, nodular, elevated area of about the size of the palm of the hand, the elevations being due to the presence of thrombosed vessels. This area decreases rapidly in size, so that it measures 3 or 4 centimetres in diameter at the end of the second week, and only 1 to 2 centimetres at the completion of the puerperium, although it still remains elevated above the general surface of the interior of the uterus and is tinged with blood pigment. Its original position remains recognisable for quite a long period, and even six months after childbirth appears as a slightly elevated pigmented area.

In the last month of pregnancy some of the sinuses at the placental site undergo thrombosis, but the process becomes more marked in the latter portion of the second and particularly after the completion of the third stage of labour, although many sinuses never become thrombosed, but are simply compressed by the contracting uterine muscle. The thrombi become organized by the proliferation of the intima of the vessels, and eventually are converted into typical connective tissue.

As the non-pregnant uterus requires a much less abundant blood supply than the pregnant organ, it is apparent that the lumina of its various arteries must undergo a certain amount of constriction. This is brought about by a *compensatory endarteritis,* which is not infrequently associated with hyalin changes in the tunica media. The latter persist for years, and under the microscope offer a ready means of differentiating between the uteri of women who have and of those who have not borne children.

Changes in the Cervix, Vagina, and Vaginal Outlet.—Immediately after the completion of the third stage, the cervix is represented by a soft, muscular tube, whose boundaries can be made out only with difficulty.

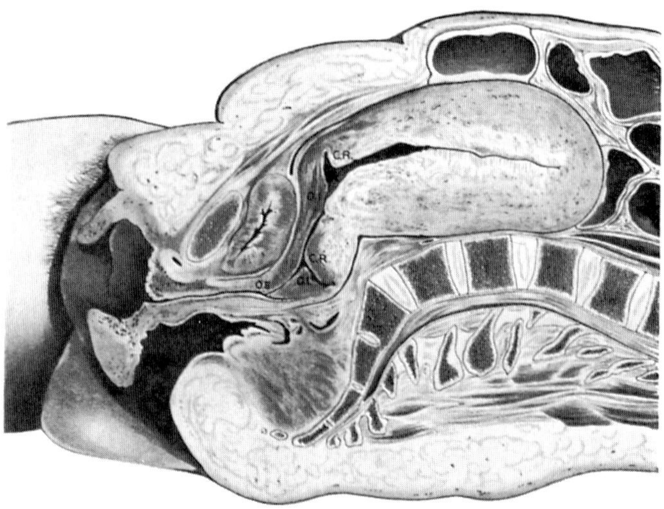

FIG. 304.—FROZEN SECTION JUST AFTER COMPLETION OF THIRD STAGE OF LABOUR, SHOWING COLLAPSE OF LOWER UTERINE SEGMENT AND CERVIX (Benckiser).

C.R., contraction ring; *O.E.*, external os; *O.I.*, internal os.

The margins of the external os are soft and flabby, and are usually marked by depressions indicating the seat of lacerations. Its opening contracts slowly. For the first few days immediately following labour it readily admits two fingers, but by the end of the first week it has become so narrow as to render difficult the introduction of one finger. At the same time the lower uterine segment collapses, and what remains of the contraction ring comes in contact with the upper portion of the cervical canal. As Webster has pointed out, there is no doubt that the structure which is usually taken for the internal os on digital examination, really represents the lower margin of the contraction ring (Fig. 304). The changes in this portion of the uterus readily explain the production of the marked anteflexion which occasionally characterizes this period.

The vagina requires some time to recover from the distention to which it has been subjected. In the first part of the puerperium, it is represented by a large, smooth-walled passage, which gradually diminishes in size, though it rarely returns to its virginal condition. The rugæ begin to reappear about the third week. The vaginal outlet is also markedly distended, and usually bears signs of more or less extensive laceration. The hymen, as such, has disappeared, and its place is taken by a number of small tags of tissue, which, as the process of cicatrization goes on, become converted into the *carunculæ myrtiformes,* which are characteristic of the vaginal opening of parous women. The labia majora and minora become flabby and atrophic, as compared with their condition before childbirth.

Changes in the Peritonæum and Abdominal Wall.—While these changes are taking place in the uterus and vagina, the pelvic peritonæum and the structures of the broad ligaments are accommodating themselves to the changed condition of affairs. For the first few days after labour the peritonæum covering the uterus is arranged in folds, which soon disappear. The broad ligament is much more lax than in the non-pregnant condition, and requires a considerable time to recover from the stretching and loosening to which it has been subjected.

As a result of prolonged distention due to the presence of the enlarged pregnant uterus, the abdominal walls remain soft and flabby for some time. Except for the presence of silvery striæ, they gradually return to their normal condition if the abdominal muscles have retained their tonicity; but when this is markedly impaired they never regain their original consistency, but remain lax and flabby. In not a few instances, particularly in women who have borne a number of children in rapid succession, there may be a marked separation or *diastasis of the recti muscles,* so that a considerable portion of the abdominal contents is covered simply by peritonæum, thinned-out fascia, and skin.

The changes occurring in the breasts are very characteristic, and will be considered in Chapter XVII.

Clinical Aspects of the Puerperium.—*Post-partum Chill.*—Not infrequently the patient may have a more or less violent rigor coming on shortly after the completion of the third stage of labour. This is purely a nervous or vaso-motor phenomenon, and is without prognostic significance. In this respect it stands in marked contrast to a chill occurring later in the puerperium, which nearly always indicates the onset of an acute infectious process or the recrudescence of a malarial attack.

Temperature.—Generally speaking, the temperature remains practically normal during the puerperium; hence any considerable rise should always be considered as a sign of infection, until convincing evidence to the contrary can be adduced. Not infrequently the temperature may become slightly elevated towards the end or just after the completion of a difficult labour. Under such circumstances it rarely goes above 100.4° (38° C.), usually falls to normal within twelve hours, and does not rise again. A higher temperature during labour in all probability indicates infection of the liquor amnii.

Owing to the fact that slight rises of temperature occur frequently during the puerperium without apparent cause, 100.4° F. (38° C.) has arbitrarily been chosen as the upper temperature limit for the normal puerperium, any rise above it being regarded as pathological.

It was formerly believed that the establishment of the lacteal secretion on the third or fourth day of the puerperium was naturally attended by a slight rise in temperature. Indeed, so prevalent was this idea that in pre-antiseptic times the so-called *milk fever* was regarded as a normal phenomenon. But at present we no longer believe in the existence of such a pathological entity, and whenever the temperature exceeds the normal limit at this time, the conscientious obstetrician should fear the beginning of an infection and begin to look for the errors of technique which may have led to it.

Pulse.—During the puerperium the pulse is usually somewhat slower than at other times, averaging between 60 and 70. In nervous women, however, and in those who have had difficult labours or have suffered any considerable loss of blood, a more rapid rate than normal is not infrequent. In a certain number of cases, a day or two after the birth of the child, the pulse becomes markedly slower, and not infrequently falls to 50, 40, or even fewer beats to the minute. Fehling has reported a case in which the rate was only 36.

Ordinarily this phenomenon becomes most marked on the second or third day, after which the pulse becomes quicker and attains its normal rate by the end of the first week or ten days. The slow pulse is usually regarded as a favourable prognostic sign, whereas a rapid heart action, unless it can be accounted for by hæmorrhage or cardiac disease, should be looked upon with suspicion.

This puerperal slowing of the pulse is usually regarded as a physiological phenomenon. Heil, however, in 1898, stated that the belief was based upon faulty observation. He affirmed that if the pulse be carefully counted in the same patient for some days before as well as after labour, it will be found slightly quicker in the puerperium than during pregnancy. He noted the puerperal slow pulse in only 12 per cent of his cases. Similar investigations undertaken by Varnier failed to confirm Heil's conclusions, since they showed that the puerperal slow pulse occurred in 72 per cent of the cases. My own observations show that the condition occurs more frequently than noted by Heil and less frequently than by Varnier, since the rate was subnormal in 32 out of 71 cases (45 per cent) observed in my clinic.

Numerous theories have been advanced from time to time in the attempt to explain its mode of production, but none of them are wholly satisfactory. It is not impossible that the solution is quite simple, and that the condition may depend upon two factors: the absolute rest of the patient in bed, together with the great diminution in work which the heart is called upon to perform after the elimination of the utero-placental circulation. Kehrer attributed the slowing in great part to the lowering of the blood pressure following delivery; Schroeder, to the sudden diminution of the vascular area after the utero-placental circulation is thrown out of function; Fritsch, to the horizontal position and rest in bed; Löhlein, to stimulation of the vagus or other nervous influences; and Olshausen, to the absorption of various products set free in the blood during the involution of the uterus.

Changes in the Blood.—It is usually stated that there is a slight decrease in the number of red corpuscles and the amount of hæmoglobin immediately after delivery. This is attributable to the loss of blood at the time, and is usually compensated for within the first week, after which the normal condition is restored.

Hofbauer has directed attention to the occurrence of a marked leucocytosis occurring during and just after labour. He showed that the leucocytes gradually increase in number from the onset of labour and reach a maximum ten or twelve hours after its conclusion, at which time they are nearly twice as abundant as during pregnancy. Having attained their acme, they promptly fall to normal, rising again slightly on the third or fourth day, with the establishment of the lacteal secretion, after which they remain at the normal level.

After-pains.—In primiparous women the uterus remains in a state of tonic contraction and retraction during the puerperium, unless it has been subjected to unusual distention, or blood-clots or other foreign bodies have been retained in its cavity, as a consequence of which active contractions occur in the effort to expel them. In multiparous women, on the other hand, the uterus has lost part of its initial tonicity, so that persistent contraction and retraction cannot be maintained, and it therefore contracts and relaxes at intervals, the contractions giving rise to painful sensations, which are known as after-pains. In many patients these are particularly noticeable when the child is put to the breast, and may last for many days, but ordinarily they lose their intensity and become quite bearable after the twenty-four hours immediately following delivery.

Lochia.—During the first part of the puerperium there occurs normally a variable amount of vaginal discharge—the lochia. For the first few days after delivery it consists in great part of blood—*lochia rubra*; after three or four days it becomes paler—*lochia serosa*; and after the tenth day, owing to a marked admixture with leucocytes, it assumes a whitish or yellowish-white colour—*lochia alba.* It is alkaline in reaction, and has a peculiar fleshy odour, suggesting fresh blood. Foul-smelling lochia indicate infection with putrefactive bacteria. In many instances the reddish colour is preserved for several weeks, but when it persists for a longer period, it indicates imperfect involution of the uterus or the retention of portions of the after-birth. When examined under the microscope during the first few days, the lochia consist of red blood-corpuscles, leucocytes, fatty epithelial cells, and shreds of degenerated decidual tissue.

Micro-organisms can always be demonstrated in the discharge gathered at the vulva, but are not always present when it is obtained from other portions of the generative tract. The investigations of Döderlein, Krönig, Döderlein and Winternitz, myself, and others have shown that the lochia obtained directly from the uterine cavity do not contain bacteria, except in cases of infection, whereas micro-organisms are always present in large numbers in the vaginal discharge. The early work of Kehrer, Karewski, and others, appeared to indicate that the vaginal lochia nearly always contained pyogenic bacteria, since small quantities of the discharge, when injected under the patient's skin, gave rise to abscess formation. The more recent investigations of Krönig, however, have demonstrated that these conclusions were erroneous, and that the vaginal lochia, although rich in harmless parasites, do not contain pyogenic organisms, with the exception of gonococci, unless the uterus is the seat of infectious processes. The same investigator also showed that the bacterial flora of the vagina undergoes a marked change during the puerperium. During pregnancy bacilli predominate, but are in great part replaced by cocci during the puerperium. This change is probably due to the altered reaction of the secretion, which is markedly acid before, and alkaline after labour.

The amount of lochial discharge varies in different individuals. Gassner estimated its average quantity at 1,485 cubic centimetres, but in many cases it is less, and occasionally much more profuse. In practice an approximate idea of its amount may be gained from the frequency with which it is necessary to change the dressings during the twenty-four hours.

General Functions.—The function of the skin is markedly accentuated during the puerperium, as is demonstrated by the profuse sweating which frequently characterizes this period. It is most marked at night, and it is not unusual for the patient to awake from a sound sleep to find her night-gown drenched with perspiration.

The appetite is usually diminished during the first few days after labour, and the patient experiences very little desire for nutritious food. At the same time, owing to the marked diaphoresis and the quantity of fluid lost through the lochial discharge, thirst is considerably increased.

The bowels are nearly always constipated during the first part of the puerperium. This is due partly to the fact that the patient eats but little solid food, but principally to the marked relaxation of the abdominal walls and their consequent inability to aid in evacuating the intestinal contents.

Urine.—The urine is generally somewhat increased in amount during the first few days of the puerperium, but in normal cases the quantity of urea is slightly less than at other times.

In the majority of cases the examination of specimens of urine, removed by catheterization immediately after the completion of the third stage of labour, shows a slight amount of albumin and numerous hyalin casts, even though both may have been absent throughout pregnancy. In 1,000 of my own cases which were studied with this point in view, albumin was noted in 62.9 per cent and casts in 19.46 per cent, and similar results have been obtained by Temesvary and others. This is a transient phenomenon resulting from the systemic strain caused by labour, and has no prognostic significance.

Occasionally a small amount of sugar may be found in the urine on the second or third day of the puerperium, coincidently with the establishment of the lacteal secretion. Careful investigation shows that the reaction is due to the presence of lactose, or milk-sugar, which is supposed to be absorbed from the mammary glands, so that the condition has nothing to do with diabetes. Ney observed it in 77 per cent of his cases, while McCann and Turner detected it in small quantities in every case which they examined. In my own clinic it was present in only a small proportion of the cases—2.6 per cent. For a full discussion of the question the reader is referred to the dissertation of Gusnar.

Couvelaire and Scholten have recently demonstrated that there is a marked increase in the amount of acetone in the urine immediately after labour, which disappears within the next three days. The last-named investigator noted it in 94 per cent of his cases, and found that it was most abundant after difficult and prolonged labours. He attributes its production to the excessive breaking up of carbohydrates resulting from the increased muscular activity incident to parturition.

Not infrequently there is a marked tendency towards retention of the urine during the first few days of the puerperium, and the distended bladder can frequently be distinguished as a fluctuant tumour above the umbilicus. The retention may result from numerous causes, but is particularly apt to follow operative or difficult labours; and under such circumstances may be attributable to contusions or other slight lesions of the urethra. In other cases it is probably caused by the diminished intra-abdominal pressure which allows a greater quantity of urine to accumulate in the bladder than under other conditions, as well as by the flaccidity of the abdominal walls and the consequent difficulty of bringing them into play during urination. In not a few cases it is due to the fact that possibly at any time the patient is unable to evacuate the bladder in the recumbent position.

Loss of Weight.—In addition to the loss of 6 to 6½ kilos, which results from the evacuation of the contents of the uterus, it is generally stated that there is a still further loss of body weight during the puerperium, which according to Gassner amounts to 4,500 grammes in the first week. Heil estimates it at 2,000, and Klemmer at only 900 grammes. This apparent contradiction is due to the fact that Gassner's results were obtained at a time when the diet was greatly restricted, but at present, when it is more liberal, the loss of weight is much less, and in many instances does not occur at all if sufficient food be taken. In normal cases it is nearly always regained by the end of the puerperium.

Care of the Patient during the Puerperium.—*Attention immediately after Labour.*—After carefully examining the placenta immediately after its expulsion, to make sure that it is intact, the physician should devote his attention to watching the condition of the uterus. At this time it should form a hard, round, resistant tumour, whose upper margin lies below the umbilicus. As long as it resembles a cricket-ball in consistence there is no danger of post-partum hæmorrhage. But if it becomes soft and flabby there is imminent danger of such an occurrence, unless proper measures are taken at once to guard against it. For this purpose the uterus should be palpated through the abdominal walls immediately after the conclusion of the third stage, and if it is found to be firmly contracted, the same manœuvre should be repeated at intervals of a few minutes. If, however, any tendency towards relaxation is detected, the organ should be grasped through the abdominal walls and vigorously kneaded until it remains persistently contracted; at the same time ergot should be administered hypodermically.

In normal cases, even although there may be no tendency towards hæmorrhage, the uterus should be palpated at intervals for the first hour after the expulsion of the placenta; but if satisfactory contractions do not occur at once, its behaviour should be carefully watched for at least an hour after these have been induced. The physician should never leave the patient immediately after the completion of labour, even if it has been perfectly normal, but should remain within call for at least an hour, so as to be ready should any complication arise. If the patient has a competent trained nurse, the duty of watching the uterus may be delegated to her; but the physician should not leave the house until he has made a final examination and is satisfied that all reasonable danger of hæmorrhage has passed.

Toilet of the Vulva.—Immediately after the birth of the placenta, the soiled linen having been removed from beneath the patient, the buttocks and external genitalia are cleansed with hot water and soap and bathed with a 1-to-2,000 bichloride solution. A sterilized vulval pad, made of cotton wrapped in gauze, is then applied over the genitalia and held in place by a "T" bandage, being replaced by a clean one whenever necessary. The number of pads required in the twenty-four hours varies according to the amount of lochial discharge, and affords a fairly accurate means of estimating its quantity. Each time the pads are changed, and after each movement of the bowels, the genitalia should be washed with cotton pledgets soaked in bichloride solution. Ordinary sponges should never be used for this purpose. The parts should be washed from above downward, so as to avoid contamination from the rectum.

The vulval pad not only absorbs the lochia and prevents contamination of the vulva from without, but also makes it difficult for the patient to touch her genitalia, a practice very common among the uneducated classes, and one that occasionally gives rise to infection.

Binder.—Many authorities recommend that a tightly fitting binder of unbleached muslin, reaching from the trochanters to above the umbilicus, be applied immediately after delivery, since they hold that it exerts a beneficial effect upon the involution of the uterus, makes the patient more comfortable, and tends to restore her figure to its original condition. Personally, I am not in favour of its employment, and do not believe that it serves any of the purposes for which it is recommended. On the other hand, I am strongly of the opinion that it occasionally gives rise to retroversion or retroflexion of the enlarged and soft uterus, especially if it be applied sufficiently snugly to exert compression. This objection, however, does not hold good after the organ has descended into the pelvic cavity—that is, after the tenth day. From this time on a well-fitting bandage can do no harm, and some patients find that it adds considerably to their comfort by supporting the lax abdominal walls when they first begin to sit up. Nor can I find any evidence of its value in restoring the figure, which will gradually return without its use, provided the tonicity of the abdominal muscles be retained; but when this is seriously impaired I know nothing that will bring about the desired result, although gentle massage applied later may do something towards it.

After-pains.—As after-pains usually occur in multiparæ, but only in primiparæ when the uterus has been subjected to undue distention, it is not usually necessary to provide for their treatment after the birth of the first child. On the other hand, after the delivery of a multiparous patient, it is advisable to leave with the nurse several tablets of $\frac{1}{4}$ grain of morphine and $\frac{1}{150}$ grain of atropine, with instructions to administer them by the mouth at intervals of four or six hours, if the pains be severe.

Rest and Quiet.—As soon as the patient has been made comfortable, the room should be darkened and she should be encouraged to go to sleep. The relatives should be excluded, and the nurse should bathe and dress the baby in an adjoining apartment, if there is one at her disposal. The patient should be kept as quiet as possible for the first ten days, and during this period, as a rule, only the immediate members of the family should be admitted to see her. Moreover, if these are numerous, strict instructions should be given the nurse as to the number of visitors each day.

Diet.—Formerly it was the custom to restrict to a minimum the diet of the puerperal woman, and as has already been said, this limitation goes far to explain the loss of weight which was frequently observed during the first few days. At present, however, a more liberal allowance is customary, and the patient is encouraged to take plenty of plain nourishing food.

If not nauseated, she should be given a glass of milk or a cup of tea soon after labour. For the first few days the appetite is not vigorous, but small quantities of easily digested food may be taken at frequent intervals. I usually give the nurse the following directions: For the first twenty-four hours, water, milk, coffee, tea, or cocoa, and buttered or soft toast. On the second and third days the same, with the addition of simple soups or bouillon, boiled or poached eggs, raw or stewed oysters, and wine jelly. On the fourth and fifth days as above, with the addition of chicken, baked potatoes, and rice, after which the ordinary diet should be gradually resumed.

Temperature.—The temperature should be carefully watched during the first week of the puerperium, as fever is usually the first symptom of the onset of an infectious process. If the patient be in charge of a trained nurse, it should be taken four times daily—at 8 A. M., 12 M., 4 P. M., and 8 P. M., and recorded upon a suitable chart. The physician should be immediately notified if it rises above 100°. But when the nurse is ignorant, the temperature should be taken by the physician himself, morning and evening, for the first five days. This, of course, means that during that time he must visit the patient twice a day, once a day for the following two or three days, and afterward at less frequent intervals. But when the nurse is competent, a single visit a day will suffice, unless untoward symptoms develop, as the physician can rely upon being notified promptly of any change. It is always better, however, whenever possible, that the patient should be seen within the first twelve hours following delivery.

Urination.—The patient should be encouraged to urinate within the first six hours. When she is unable to do so, the catheter should not be employed until the bladder forms a marked tumour above the symphysis, and not even then until the patient has attempted to urinate in a sitting position; inasmuch as many women are unable to use a bed-pan. I consider the change in position much less dangerous than catheterization, as the latter, no matter how carefully performed, always carries with it some risk of infection and of a consequent cystitis. Moreover, in not a few cases, the procedure, when once commenced, must be continued for a number of days, a condition of affairs which, leaving out of account the danger of infection, becomes very onerous to the physician, unless he has a competent nurse in charge.

When, however, catheterization becomes absolutely necessary, the genitalia having been first exposed and bathed with a bichloride or boric solution, a glass catheter, which has been sterilized by boiling, should be introduced by carefully disinfected fingers; or, better still, it should be grasped with a piece of freshly boiled cotton, so as to prevent its coming in contact with the fingers at all. At the present day, to catheterize a woman under a sheet or by the sense of touch is not justifiable.

Bowels.—In view of the sluggishness of the bowels in the puerperium, a mild cathartic should be administered on the morning of the second day, unless they have previously been evacuated spontaneously. For this purpose I generally employ half an ounce of Rochelle salts in a small quantity of water, half a bottle of the effervescent citrate of magnesia, or, if the patient will consent to take it, half an ounce of castor-oil.

After the preliminary cathartic, the bowels should be moved once daily. If a spontaneous action does not occur, the administration of the fluid extract of cascara at bedtime, in 20- to 60-minim doses, or 1 or 2 drams of the aromatic elixir, according to the susceptibility of the patient, is indicated. Sometimes a pill containing aloin, belladonna, and strychnine proves very satisfactory.

Care of the Nipples.—Details concerning the care of the nipples will be given in Chapter XVII, but the physician should be careful to impress upon the nurse the necessity of observing aseptic precautions in dealing with them; and she should be directed to report immediately the appearance of fissures, as their proper treatment will usually prevent mammary infection and the consequent danger of mastitis.

Time for Getting Up.—It is a time-honoured custom to allow the puerperal woman to sit up on the tenth day. This rule, however, should not be slavishly followed, and every patient should be kept in bed until the fundus of the uterus has disappeared behind the symphysis pubis. This frequently occurs by the tenth day, occasionally a day or so earlier, but very often not until some days later. Generally speaking, a two-weeks' rest in bed is not excessive.

Küstner has lately advocated the practice of allowing the patient to get up on the third or fourth day, and states that he has seen no ill consequences follow such a procedure. His suggestion was promulgated before the German Gynæcological Congress in 1899, but was not favourably received, no one who spoke upon the subject indorsing his views.

It is also advisable to give rigid directions as to the length of time the patient should remain out of bed. I have found it a convenient rule to direct that she should sit up for one hour on the first day, two hours on the second, and to increase the time by an hour each day until she is able to be up all the time. She should be kept in her room until the expiration of the third week, and allowed to move about on the floor on which she was confined during the fourth week. She should not be permitted to go downstairs until the expiration of this period, as it is a matter of experience that the average woman cannot be prevented from assuming the ordinary duties of her household after she has once gone downstairs; whereas as long as she is kept on one floor she is usually amenable to the direction of her physician.

Final Examination.—At the end of the third or the beginning of the fourth week the patient should be subjected to an internal examination, and the condition of the perinæum, uterus, and appendages carefully investigated. Not infrequently the uterus will be found displaced, when the introduction of a properly fitting pessary may lead to a prompt cure; whereas if treatment be deferred until symptoms appear, the condition may not be relieved so readily. In other cases, various abnormalities may be noted, which should be treated before the patient is discharged, and occasionally it may be necessary to warn her or her husband that operative procedures will be required in the future. If everything is perfectly normal, it is a great comfort to the patient to be assured of the fact; whereas if any abnormality is noted and the attention of some responsible member of the family be directed to it, the physician may save himself from censure if a subsequent examination be made by some one else.

LITERATURE

COUVELAIRE. De l'acetónurie transitoire du travail de l'accouchement. Annales de Gyn. et d'Obst., 1899, li, 353–367.

DÖDERLEIN. Untersuchungen über das Vorkommen von Spaltpilzen in den Lochien des Uterus und der Vagina, etc. Arch. f. Gyn., 1887, xxxi, 412–447.

Das Scheidensekret. Leipzig, 1892.

DÖDERLEIN und WINTERNITZ. Die Bakteriologie der puerperalen Sekrete. Hegar's Beiträge zur Geb. u. Gyn., 1900, iii, 161–175.

FEHLING. Physiologie und Pathologie des Wochenbetts. Stuttgart, 1890.

FRIEDLÄNDER. Physiol.-anat. Untersuchungen über den Uterus. Leipzig, 1870.

FRITSCH. Die puerperale Pulsverlangsamung. Archiv f. Gyn., 1875, viii, 383–390.

GASSNER. Ueber die Veränderungen des Körpergewichtes bei Schwangeren, Gebärenden u. Wöchnerinnen. Monatsschr. f. Geburtskunde, 1862, xv, 1–68.

GUSNAR. Beiträge zur Lactosurie der Wöchnerinnen. D. I., Halle, 1895.

HEIL. Untersuchungen über die Körpergewichtsverhältnisse normaler Wöchnerinnen. Arch. f. Gyn., 1896, li, 18–32.

Giebt es eine physiologische Pulsverlangsamung im Wochenbette? Archiv f. Gyn., 1898, liv, 265–280.

HOFBAUER. Zur Physiologie des Puerperiums. Monatsschr. f. Geb. u. Gyn., 1897, v, Ergänzungsheft, 52–57.

KAREWSKI. Exp. Untersuchungen über die Einwirkungen der puerperalen Sekrete auf dem thierischen Organismus. Zeitschr. f. Geb. u. Gyn., 1882, vii, 331.

KEHRER. Ueber die Veränderungen der Pulscurve im Puerperium. Heidelberg, 1886.

Wirkung der Lochien auf lebendes Gewebe. Müller's Handbuch der Geb., i, 545, 1888.

KLEMMER. Untersuchungen über den Stoffwechsel der Wöchnerinnen und die zweckmässigste Diät derselben. Winckel's Berichte und Arbeiten, 1876, ii, 155–186.

KRÖNIG. Bakteriologie des Genitalkanales der schwangeren, kreissenden und puerperalen Frau. Leipzig, 1897, 54–64 und 196–201.

Beitrag zum anat. Verhalten der Schleimhaut der Cervix und des Uterus während der Schwangerschaft und im Frühwochenbett. Arch. f. Gyn., 1901, lxiii, 26–38.

KUNDRAT und ENGELMANN. Untersuchungen über die Uterusschleimhaut. Stricker's med. Jahrb., 1873.

KÜSTNER. Ist einer gesunden Wöchnerin eine protrahirte Bettruhe dienlich? Verh. der deutschen Gesellsch. f. Gyn., 1899, viii, 525–535.

LEOPOLD. Studien über die Uterusschleimhaut, etc. Berlin, 1878. (Archiv f. Gyn., xi und xii.)

LÖHLEIN. Ueber das Verhalten des Herzens bei Schwangeren und Wöchnerinnen. Berliner Zeitschr. f. Geb. u. Frauenkr., 1876, i, 482–516.

MCCANN and TURNER. On the Occurrence of Sugar in the Urine during the Puerperal State. Trans. London Obst. Soc., 1892, xxxiv, 473–490.

NEY. Ueber das Vorkommen von Zucker im Harne der Schwangeren, etc. Archiv f. Geb. u. Gyn., 1889, xxxv, 239–256.

OLSHAUSEN. Ueber die Pulsverlangsamung im Wochenbette und ihre Ursache. Centralbl. f. Gyn., 1881, 49–53.

PELS LEUSDEN. Ueber die serotinalen Riesenzellen, etc. Zeitschr. f. Geb. u. Gyn., 1897, xxxvi, 1–61.

SÄNGER. Die Rückbildung der Muscularis des puerperalen Uterus. Beiträge zur path. Anat. und klin. Med., von Wagner's Schülern, 1887, 134.

SCHOLTEN. Ueber puerperale Acetonurie. Hegar's Beiträge zur Geb. u. Gyn., 1900, iii, 439–451.

SCHROEDER. Lehrbuch der Geburtshülfe, XIII. Aufl., 1889, 268.

TEMESVARY. Physiologie des Wochenbettes. Sänger-Herff Encyklopädie der Geb. u. Gyn., 1900, 498–502.

VARNIER. Du ralentissement du pouls pendant les suites des couches. Annales de Gyn. et d'Obst., 1899, li, 30–47.

WEBSTER. The Anatomy of the Female Pelvis during the Puerperium. Researches in Female Pelvic Anatomy, Edinburgh, 1892, 1–55.

CHAPTER XVII

THE NEWLY BORN CHILD

NORMALLY the newly born child begins to cry almost immediately after its exit from the vulva. This act indicates the establishment of respiration, which is accompanied by important modifications in the circulatory system.

Circulatory Changes.—As soon as the lungs begin to function, the blood which is brought by the inferior vena cava to the right auricle no longer passes through the foramen ovale, but makes its way directly into the right ventricle, whence it is carried to the lungs by means of the pulmonary arteries. Coincident with the establishment of the pulmonary circulation, there ensues a marked increase in the pressure in the left auricle. This in turn brings about the closure of the valve of the foramen ovale, which after a few months fuses with the periphery of the opening. At the same time the blood ceases to flow through the ductus Botalli into the aorta, and the canal itself gradually becomes obliterated. According to Strassmann, the primary cause for this change is to be found in the fact that the ductus traverses the wall of the aorta in an oblique direction, so that as soon as the pressure in the aortic arch is increased, its wall acts as a valve and occludes the distal end.

The circulation through the umbilical arteries ceases a few minutes after birth, when, owing to the contraction of their thick muscular walls, the lumina become practically obliterated. It is usually stated that after the establishment of the pulmonary circulation the general arterial pressure is diminished to such an extent that it is insufficient to force the blood through them. The investigations of Ahlfeld have shown that this is not the case, and would rather indicate that the contraction of the arteries is brought about by the stimulation resulting from the cooling of the cord immediately after birth. That this explanation is correct is demonstrated by the fact that the circulation can be re-established by immersing the child in a warm bath and thus doing away with this factor.

This point is of practical importance in view of the fact that occasionally, when the cord has not been ligated sufficiently tightly, secondary hæmorrhage occurs from its fœtal end after the child has been placed in a warm bed. To guard against such an occurrence the cord should always be reinspected within an hour after delivery.

The child passes urine almost immediately after birth, and not infrequently while in the act of being born. In a considerable number of cases a certain amount of meconium is also discharged. As a result of the cooling of the surface of the child on coming into the world, its temperature becomes reduced by a few degrees, which, however, are promptly regained after it has been bathed and placed in a warm bed. For the first few days of life the temperature is in very unstable equilibrium, and a very slight cause may give rise to a considerable elevation.

Care of the Umbilical Cord.—As has already been said, the umbilical cord should not be ligated until it has ceased to pulsate, unless there is some urgent reason to the contrary. Two ligatures of sterilized bobbin should be placed about it and tightly tied, one about 1 centimetre from the surface of the abdomen, and the other 2 centimetres beyond the first, the cord being then cut between them with a pair of sterile scissors.

Owing to the absence of circulation, what is left of the cord undergoes mummification, and gradually a line of demarcation appears just beyond the skin surface of the abdomen, until in a few days the stump sloughs off, leaving behind a small, granulating wound, which, after healing, forms the umbilicus.

The separation of the cord usually takes place within the first week after birth, but it is not unusual for it to require a longer time, and occasionally several weeks may elapse before it occurs. In the very rare instances in which the stump is still adherent at the end of the puerperium, it may become necessary to clip it off with a pair of scissors.

Formerly the care of the cord was considered a very trivial matter, and the midwife, as a rule, would wrap it in a piece of greased or singed linen, after which little or no attention was paid to it. This practice, however, and the total neglect of aseptic precautions, frequently resulted in an infection which was transmitted through the umbilical vessels, and from which in times past large numbers of children have perished. Even now, when the necessity for proper treatment is generally recognised, umbilical infections are not of infrequent occurrence, as is shown by the monograph of Eröss. Moreover, it may be stated as a general rule that, whenever children die without any appreciable cause within a few weeks after birth, such an infection should be suspected, and the examination of the intra-abdominal portion of the umbilical vessels will usually show that they are filled with purulent thrombi, in which pyogenic micro-organisms can be demonstrated. In view, therefore, of the not inconsiderable danger of infection from this source, strict aseptic precautions should be observed in caring for the cord. The reader is referred to Ploss's work for interesting details concerning its treatment in various countries and by aboriginal peoples.

After making the mother comfortable the nurse should devote her attention to the child. It should first be anointed with vaseline or olive oil, and then placed in a warm bath and thoroughly washed with Castile soap. Experience has shown that the vernix caseosa is much more readily removed when some oleaginous substance is first employed than by the use of soap and water alone. After the bath, the stump of the cord should be thickly sprinkled with powdered boric acid and covered with a pad of sterile absorbent cotton, which should be held in place by a flannel bandage tightly pinned about the abdomen. If the child is doing well this dressing need not be changed for some days unless it becomes moist or soiled. On removing it, the cord will usually be found to have become completely separated, otherwise a similar dressing should be reapplied. I have obtained very satisfactory results with this method of treatment, although in some cases it appears to prolong unduly the separation of the cord.

After the cord has sloughed off the granulating umbilicus should be treated in the same manner, and the child should not receive another full bath until it has completely healed. During this period it should be bathed in the lap of the nurse and not in a tub, care being taken not to contaminate the umbilical dressings.

In the winter of 1900 Dr. W. M. Dabney, one of my assistants, performed a series of experiments in the hope of determining the best method of dealing with the cord. He treated several series of cases, respectively, with the following dressings: boric acid, salicylic acid, a mixture of salicylic acid and starch, and a wrapping of silver foil. So far as he could see it made no difference which method was employed, provided the dressings were sterile. In still another series of cases, he applied an occlusive dressing of liquid celloidin and absorbent cotton, but found that under such circumstances the cord was kept unduly moist, and separation was perceptibly delayed.

During the past few years this question has given rise to a great deal of discussion. Dickinson, at the meeting of the American Gynæcological Society in 1899, read a paper entitled, Is the Sloughing Process at the Child's Navel consistent with Asepsis in Child-bed? and answered the question in the negative. As the result of his observations, he recommended that the cord be completely excised where it joins the abdomen, its vessels ligated, and the wound closed by sutures. Possibly this may be the ideal method of treatment in hospital practice, but it is a question whether it is advisable to adopt it as yet in private practice, as it is probable that, should the child die within a few weeks after such a procedure, the physician would be severely criticised by members of the family who have become accustomed to the time-honoured treatment.

In 1900 Martin recommended that the cord be ligated close to the abdomen and cut through with a pair of red-hot scissors. But although his student, Reick, reported very excellent results from this method of treatment, Martin himself has since abandoned it. Porak and others advocate compression of the cord by powerful forceps, as in the recently introduced methods of angiotripsy. But to my mind these procedures offer no advantages over those already in use; the important point in the treatment being not so much the method employed as the avoidance of infection by the most rigid adherence to the principles of asepsis.

Care of the Eyes.—In view of the frequency with which the eyes of the newly born child become infected when passing through the birth canal of women suffering from gonorrhœa, Credé introduced the practice of instilling into each eye immediately after birth one drop of a 1-per-cent solution of nitrate of silver, which was afterward washed out with salt solution. This procedure has led to a marked decrease in the frequency of gonorrhœal ophthalmia and the cases of blindness resulting from it, and should be followed as a matter of routine in lying-in hospitals. In private practice, on the other hand, a boric-acid solution should be employed instead, although if there is any reason for believing that the mother has gonorrhœa, Credé's method should be followed.

The prophylactic value of silver nitrate was strikingly demonstrated by Haab, whose statistics showed that its employment in hospital practice reduced the frequency of ophthalmia neonatorum from 9 to 1 per cent. If, however, the disease should appear in spite of the precautions taken, it should be promptly and vigorously treated, inasmuch as when neglected it almost invariably leads to clouding of the cornea and often to complete blindness. Cohn estimated in 1876 that 30 per cent of the patients in the blind asylums of Germany, Austria, Holland, and Switzerland owed their trouble to ophthalmia neonatorum, while twenty years later these figures had become reduced to 19 per cent.

Zweifel has recently advocated substituting a 1-per-cent solution of silver acetate for the nitrate, and reports that, in a series of 5,222 children so treated, ophthalmia was observed in only 0.23 of 1 per cent, and that not a single case ended in blindness.

Stools and Urine.—For the first few days after birth the intestinal contents are represented by a brownish or brownish-green, soft material—the meconium. It is made up of cast-off epithelial cells from various portions of the intestinal tract, a few epidermal cells and lanugo hairs which have been swallowed with the amniotic fluid. Its peculiar colour is due to the presence of bile pigments. During pregnancy and for a few hours after birth, the intestinal contents are sterile, but bacteria soon gain access to them and are afterward present throughout life.

After the third or fourth day, with the establishment of the mammary secretion, the meconium disappears, and its place is taken by fæces, which are light yellow in colour, homogeneous in consistence, and possess a characteristic odour. For the first few days the stools are not formed, but after a short time they take on the characteristic cylindrical shape. The bowels, as a rule, move twice daily, but a single large dejection is sufficient.

The child usually urinates almost immediately after birth, and continues to do so at frequent intervals for the first few months of its life. The physician should impress upon mother and nurse the necessity of attempting to train the child to regular habits as to urination and defecation, and it is surprising how soon these may be formed if proper care is taken. For this purpose the napkins should be changed before each feeding, and after the first few weeks the child should be held over a small chamber at these times. It should also be encouraged to defecate at regular intervals. To accomplish this, it should be laid upon the bed at the same hour each day with a napkin under its buttocks, and its abdomen should be stroked along the course of the colon. The physician should make it a rule to inspect the stools at each visit, and instruct the nurse to save a napkin in anticipation of his arrival, as in this way important information may be gained concerning the digestion of the child.

Icterus.—Not infrequently on the third or fourth day after birth the skin and conjunctivæ of the child take on a yellowish hue, which may vary from a hardly visible discoloration to an intense jaundice. Kehrer concluded that icterus occurred in 75 per cent of all children, and although this estimate is probably too high, there is no doubt that it is very common. According to Hofmeier, the condition is hæmatogenous in origin, and is due to the breaking-down of large numbers of red corpuscles soon after birth. Ordinarily it possesses no clinical significance, and passes off in a few days without treatment.

Initial Loss of Weight.—Owing to the fact that the child receives little or no nutriment, and at the same time casts off considerable quantities of urine, fæces, and sweat, it progressively loses weight for the first four or five days of its life, the total loss usually aggregating 250 grammes (8 ounces). If the child is nourished properly, this is usually regained by the end of the tenth day, after which the weight should increase steadily at the rate of about 25 grammes (6 drams) a day for the first few months.

The initial loss is usually much greater when the child is excessively large, as well as in premature infants and those who receive an insufficient supply of food.

Anatomy of the Breasts and Lactation.—Each breast is made up of from 15 to 24 lobes, which are arranged more or less radially, and separated from one another by a varying amount of fat, to which the size and shape of the organ is in great part due. Each lobe consists of several lobules, which in turn are made up of large numbers of acini. These last are composed of a single layer of epithelium, beneath which is a small amount of connective tissue richly supplied with capillaries. Every lobule is provided with a small duct, which, meeting others, unites to form a single larger canal for each lobe. These so-called *lactiferous ducts* make their way to the nipple and open separately upon its surface, where they may be distinguished as minute isolated orifices.

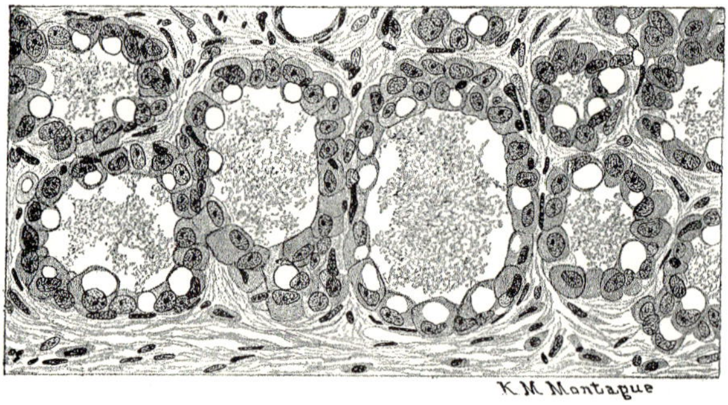

FIG. 305.—LACTATING BREAST (Zeiss, DD–4).

The acini represent the functioning portion of the breasts, and it is from their epithelium that the various constituents of the milk are formed. This fact was first demonstrated by Heidenhain.

We have already referred to the changes occurring in the breasts during pregnancy, and their condition remains much the same for the first two days after labour. At this time they do not contain milk, but a small amount of *colostrum* can be expressed from the nipples. This is a thin, yellowish fluid, which owes its colour to the presence of a pigment which is soluble in ether and, according to Kühne, analogous to the colouring matter contained in the cells of the corpus luteum.

When examined under the microscope, colostrum is seen to consist of a fluid in which are suspended numerous round bodies, 0.001 to 0.025 millimetres in diameter—the so-called *colostrum corpuscles*—which represent cast-off epithelial cells which have undergone fatty degeneration. The fluid portion is a transudate which consists in great part of serum

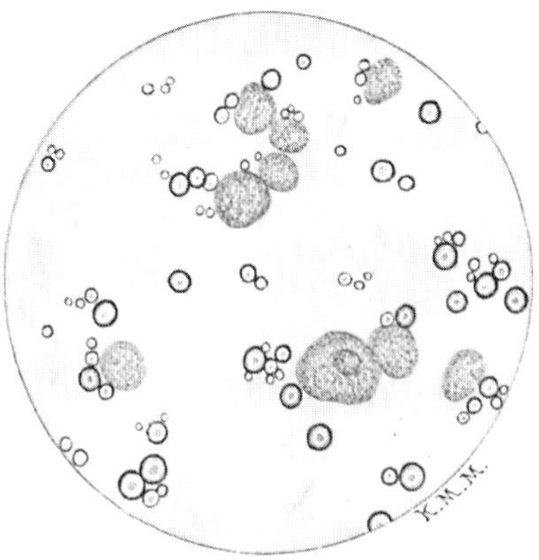

Fig. 306.—Human Colostrum (Zeiss, DD-4).

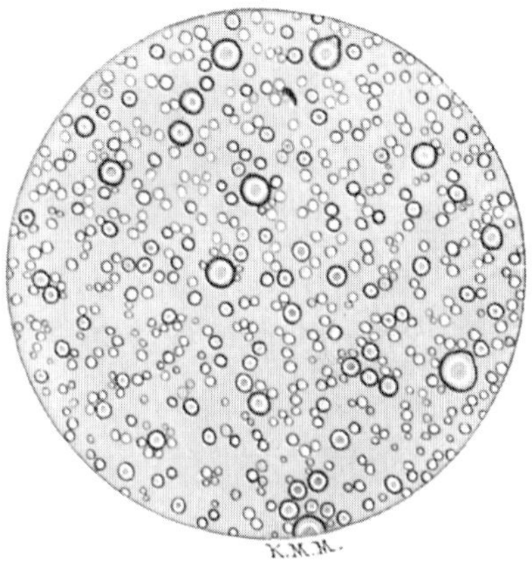

Fig. 307.—Human Milk (Zeiss, DD-4).

albumin and coagulates on heating. It is generally stated that colostrum contains more fat, sugar, and salts, but less proteid material, than normal milk. It possesses but slightly nutritive properties, and is generally believed to act as a mild cathartic, thus aiding in ridding the bowels of the meconium.

Milk.—On the third or fourth day after labour and occasionally on the second, the breasts suddenly become larger, firmer, and more painful. This indicates the establishment of the lacteal secretion, and on pressure a small amount of bluish-white fluid—the *milk*—will exude from the nipples. Coincident with these changes, the patient experiences more or less lassitude, and may suffer from headache. At the same time she has throbbing pains in the breasts, which may extend into the axillæ, and the pulse becomes slightly accelerated. There is rarely any elevation of temperature. It was formerly believed that the establishment of the milk flow was associated with marked constitutional disturbances, which were regarded as manifestations of the so-called milk fever. As has already been said, a rise in temperature from this cause is very exceptional, and in the vast majority of cases is indicative of infection.

Mother's milk is usually bluish-white in colour, though it sometimes has a yellowish tinge. It is slightly alkaline in reaction, and has a specific gravity of from 1.028 to 1.034. Under the microscope it appears as a clear fluid in which are suspended large numbers of small round bodies, 0.008 millimetres in diameter—the so-called *milk corpuscles*. These consist of minute drops of fat surrounded by a membrane. Chemical examination shows that they are made up of the triglycerides of olein, palmatin, and stearin. The fluid portion of the milk is a transudate, and consists of proteid material, milk sugar, salts, and water. Milk, therefore, represents an emulsion of fine fat droplets in a fluid medium.

The proteid material in milk serum consists of casein or caseinogen, which is a direct metabolic product of the mammary epithelium, and differs from serum albumin in that it does not coagulate on heating. The fat and lactose, or milk sugar, are also products of the epithelial cells. The milk serum contains a considerable amount of mineral matter, which, according to the investigations of Rotch, consists principally of calcium phosphate, 28.87 per cent, potassium carbonate, 23.47 per cent, sodium chloride, 21.77 per cent, potassium chloride, 12.05 per cent, potassium sulphate, 8.33 per cent, magnesium carbonate, 3.97 per cent, and minute quantities of several other salts.

The average composition of milk is as follows: Proteids, 1 to 2 per cent; fats, 3 to 4 per cent; sugar, 6 to 7 per cent; salts, 0.1 to 0.2 per cent, the rest being water. Milk also contains a not inconsiderable number of bacteria, which, according to the researches of Köstlin, are derived from the terminal ends of the lactiferous ducts and the surface of the nipples; it is questionable whether they are present in the deeper portions of the breast.

Nutritious mother's milk varies markedly in its composition, not only in different individuals, but also in the same individual at various times. It is not unusual to find that the milk of one woman, which agrees perfectly with her own child, will prove indigestible when given to the healthy child of another woman. The variation in the composition of the milk of the same woman at different times is dependent upon various factors, principally the diet, the amount of exercise, and the mental condition. The quantity of milk varies to a large extent with the amount of fluid ingested by the patient, and a diet rich in cow's milk conduces to increased mammary activity.

There are large numbers of preparations in the market which are known as *galactagogues*, and are vaunted as increasing the amount of milk; but whatever virtue they may possess is due in great part to the quantity of fluid taken with them. Exercise in the open air also increases the milk flow, and it is frequently observed that a woman who has but a small quantity so long as she is confined to her room, will secrete an abundant supply as soon as she begins to take outdoor exercise.

The quality of the milk is likewise dependent in great part upon the food and the amount of exercise taken by the mother. It is a matter of experience that a diet rich in proteids increases the ratio of the fats, while excessive exercise diminishes the amount of proteid material. Marked alterations in the quality and quantity of the milk not infrequently result from nervous and mental influences, and it is not unusual for some profound emotion to lead to almost complete suppression of the lacteal secretion, or to so change its quality as to render it unfit for the use of the infant. Certain drugs also exert a marked influence upon the milk flow, and it is well known that the use of belladonna or atropine markedly diminishes it.

Many substances ingested by the mother may be transmitted through the milk, and thus exert their physiological influence upon the child. This is particularly true of the various cathartics and alcoholic liquors.

The occurrence of menstruation, or the onset of another pregnancy during lactation, not infrequently exerts a very deleterious effect upon the quality of the milk, in some cases rendering it necessary to wean the child.

Nursing.—The ideal food for the newly born child is the milk of its mother, and unless lactation be contra-indicated by some physical defect, it is the physician's duty to insist that every woman should at least attempt to nurse her child. In many instances where the supply of milk at first appears insufficient, it becomes increased in amount if nursing be persisted in. The act itself usually exerts a beneficial influence upon the patient, as it is well known that the repeated irritation of the nipples results in reflex stimulation of the uterus and hastens its involution. This fact should be urged upon women who are unwilling to nurse their children, and it not infrequently happens that, although they may have commenced it from selfish motives, they will continue it as long as is necessary.

Unless it be otherwise arranged, the physician who conducts the labour should hold himself responsible for the well-being of the child during the first few weeks of its life, and should remember that he has not only the mother but also the child to care for. He should accordingly give minute directions as to the way in which it should be fed, and see that they are accurately carried out.

Frequency of Feeding.—As the nutritive properties of colostrum are very limited, the child should be put to the breast only three times a day until the milk flow becomes established, but after that time it should be fed at frequent and regular intervals. Definite hours should be set for each feeding, and if necessary the child should be awakened from a sound sleep at stated times to take its nourishment, for only by this means can its habits be made regular. I do not consider that a nurse has fulfilled her whole duty unless she leaves the patient with a child properly trained in the matter of taking its food.

A definite hour should be arranged for the child's bath, which should be taken as a starting-point in arranging the schedule for feeding. Ordinarily the most convenient time is between 9 and 10 A. M. If the former hour be chosen, the first feeding should be at 7 A. M., and the next immediately after the bath; while if the latter be chosen the child should be fed at 6 and 8 A. M., and again shortly after ten. After the feeding immediately following the bath the baby should be allowed to sleep as long as it will, which will usually be about three hours, after which it should be given nourishment at intervals of two hours until bedtime. By this arrangement it will receive eight or nine feedings during the twenty-four hours. The last should be timed for the usual bedtime of the parents, and only one feeding should be given during the night—that is, between 11 P. M. and 6 or 7 A. M.—and not infrequently the child may be trained to sleep the entire night without awakening. This, however, can only be accomplished by feeding it at regular intervals during the day, so as to insure that it receives the proper amount of nutriment in the twenty-four hours.

Just before each feeding the napkin should be changed and the child encouraged to urinate, but as soon as it is taken from the breast it should be placed in bed and not disturbed. It should not be allowed to sleep at its mother's breast, nor should it be rocked or fondled after feeding. If these regulations be persisted in, the child will usually go to sleep within a few minutes after being put to bed, and if it wakes before the next feeding is due it will remain quiet. The importance of following these directions cannot be overestimated, for it is only by rigid adherence to such details that the child can be given regular habits, and the care of it prevented from becoming a strain upon all concerned.

After the fourth or fifth week, one or two of the breast feedings should be replaced by a bottle, no matter how much milk the mother may have. By so doing the slavery of nursing is greatly reduced, and many a woman is induced to continue to nurse her child when she would otherwise wean it. When a mother is obliged to return home every two or three hours to nurse her child, it is apparent that her time is so broken in upon as to render it impossible for her to obtain any real relaxation; whereas if a single bottle be interpolated between any two feedings a free space of four to six hours will be afforded.

Duration of Feeding.—Definite rules cannot be given concerning the proper length of each feeding, as this point is dependent upon several factors—the quantity of milk, the readiness with which it can be obtained from the breast, and the avidity with which the child nurses. Generally speaking, it is advisable to allow the child to remain at the breast for ten minutes at first, and to lengthen or decrease the time according to circumstances, three or four minutes being sufficient for some children, while fifteen or twenty minutes will be required by others. There is a universal tendency towards overfeeding, so that at first it is better to err in giving too little than too much milk. Crying is not always a symptom of hunger, but much more frequently indicates that the baby is suffering from indigestion, resulting from an overloaded stomach. A child which is receiving the proper amount of nourishment should not spit up its food, should increase steadily in weight, and should have normal yellow homogeneous passages. The occurrence of regurgitation, or the presence of curds in the stools, is a sure sign that it is being nursed too long. On the other hand, loss of weight, associated with normal stools and the absence of regurgitation, indicates insufficient feeding.

The child should be weighed daily, or at least twice a week, upon a fairly accurate pair of scales, and its actions inspected daily by the physician. As has already been said, it should regain its birth weight by the end of the tenth day, and from then on it should gain regularly 25 grammes a day, or, roughly speaking, 5 ounces a week. After the first few months the increase is more gradual, the average child doubling its weight at the fifth and trebling it at the fifteenth month.

Where practicable, if the child is doing well, an analysis of the mother's milk should be made, so that definite information may be at hand as to the quality of the food upon which it thrives, in case artificial feeding should at any time become necessary.

Care of the Breasts.—Before and after each feeding the nipples should be carefully washed with a boric-acid solution, so as to avoid the possibility of bacteria being ground into them during the nursing. In many cases, particularly if preliminary precautions have not been taken to harden them, the nipples become very sore during the first few days of nursing, and little cracks or fissures appear upon them. These are extremely painful to the mother, and in some cases render the act of nursing agonizing. In addition to the suffering which they cause, they are also a source of considerable danger, as it is through them that bacteria usually gain access to the interior of the breast. The nurse should therefore be instructed to be on the lookout for them, and to warn the physician at once of their appearance, as prompt treatment will usually lead to their speedy cure. On the other hand, neglect of these premonitory signs is not infrequently followed by a mammary abscess, for the occurrence of which the physician and nurse are usually more or less justly blamed.

The fact that large numbers of remedies are recommended for the cure of such conditions is abundant evidence that they are not always readily relieved. They are best treated by rest, and if the infant could be kept from the breast for twenty-four hours they would heal without further treatment. As this is out of the question, some other means of securing rest must be adopted, and this is best attained by the use of nipple shields, those of the ordinary English type being the most suitable. Many women claim that they are unable to use such a contrivance, but the difficulty is usually due to the fact that the holes in the rubber nipple are too small, and if they are enlarged by passing a red-hot hairpin through them a quantity of milk sufficient for the child can usually be obtained without much difficulty. In the intervals between the feedings the nipples should be covered by compresses soaked with boric-acid solution. Particular attention should be devoted to the care of the shield, which should be carefully washed after each feeding and kept in a vessel containing a saturated solution of boric acid.

In rare cases the nipples may be so depressed below the surface of the breast as to render nursing out of the question. Under such circumstances it is useless to attempt it, and steps should be promptly taken to arrest the mammary secretion.

The child's mouth should be scrupulously cleansed before each feeding. This is best accomplished by washing it out with a clean piece of linen dipped in boric-acid solution. The recent investigations of Kneise, which have shown that bacteria are present in the buccal cavity of 98 per cent of newly born children, and that streptococci and staphylococci are not infrequently observed, emphasize the necessity for care in this direction.

Artificial Feeding.—When the supply of mother's milk is defective, or when abnormalities of the nipples or constitutional diseases render nursing inadvisable, artificial feeding must be resorted to. Numerous so-called infant foods are advertised for this purpose, but most of them are very defective, so that for practical purposes *cow's milk* in some form is the only available substitute for the mother's milk. Unfortunately, however, it differs markedly from the latter in composition, and under the most favourable circumstances is only an imperfect substitute for it. It is usually slightly acid in reaction, and has a specific gravity of 1.029 to 1.033. Its average composition is: proteids, 4 per cent, fats, 4 per cent, sugar, 4.5 per cent, and salts, 0.7 per cent. It is apparent, therefore, that it contains less fat and sugar, and more proteid material and salts than mother's milk, and consequently cannot be used in its natural form, but must first be modified in some way.

If the child is healthy, satisfactory results are frequently obtained by diluting cow's milk with various proportions of water and adding sugar. Such preparations contain approximately the normal amount of proteid material and sugar, but are lacking in fat. In hot weather the mixture should be sterilized, but in cool weather this procedure is unnecessary.

Modified milk, in which the various constituents of cow's milk can be altered at will, so that theoretically, at least, it closely approximates mother's milk in composition, promised to supply us with an ideal artificial food, and in many respects is the best substitute for breast milk. But at the same time it differs from it in the fact that its proteid material is far less digestible, and, when coagulated by the gastric juice, forms a thick, dense coagulum, contrasting unfavourably with the fine curd formed from human milk. In employing it, therefore, smaller quantities of proteid material must be prescribed than are normally present in breast milk.

The space at our disposal is too limited to permit us to take up the many and complicated problems connected with artificial feeding. For extended information upon this subject the reader is referred to the various treatises upon Pædiatrics. There are, nevertheless, two points to which we must refer—namely, the capacity of the stomach and the necessity for training the child to regular habits, no matter what method of feeding is employed. It should be remembered that the stomach of the newly born child is very small, and that 1 ounce will fill it to repletion for the first few days after birth. That amount of fluid, therefore, should not be exceeded for the first few days, after which it should be increased very gradually. The instructions as to the frequency and manner of feeding, which we have already given, apply equally well whether the child is fed from the breast or the bottle, and too great stress cannot be laid upon their rigid observance.

LITERATURE

Ahlfeld. Lehrbuch der Geburtshülfe. II. Aufl., 1897, 179.

Cohn. Ueber Verbreitung und Verhütung der Augeneiterung der Neugeborenen. Berlin, 1896.

Credé. Die Verhütung der Augenentzündung beim Neugeborenen. Berlin, 1884.

Dickinson. Is a Sloughing Process at the Child's Navel Consistent with Asepsis in Childbed? Amer. Jour. Obst., 1899, xl, 14–66.

Eröss. Beobachtungen an 1000 Neugeborenen über Nabelerkrankungen, etc. Archiv f. Gyn., 1891, xli, 409–449.

Haab. Die Mikrokokken der Blenorrhoea neonatorum. Festschrift zu Horner, Wiesbaden, 1881.

Hofmeier. Die Gelbsucht der Neugeborenen. Zeitschr. f. Geb. u. Gyn., 1882, viii, 287–353.

Kehrer. Studien über den Icterus neonatorum. Jahrbuch für Pädiatrik, 1871, ii, 71.

Kneise. Die Bakterienflora der Mundhöhle des Neugeborenen, etc. Hegar's Beiträge f. Geb. u. Gyn., 1901, iv, 130–148.

Köstlin. Beiträge zur Frage des Keimgehaltes der Frauenmilch. Archiv f. Gyn., 1897, liii, 201–277.

Martin. Die Versorgung des Nabels der Neugeborenen. Zeitschr. f. Geb. u. Gyn., 1900, 42, 593–596.

Zur Nabelschnurversorgung bei Neugeborenen. Monatsschr. f. Geb. u Gyn., 1900, xii, 762–763.

Ploss. Das Weib in der Natur- und Völker-kunde. IV. Aufl., 1895, Bd. II, 182–198.

Porak. De l'omphalotripsie. Annales de Gyn. et d'Obst., 1900, liv, 112–113.

Rieck. Die Versorgung des Nabels der Neugeborenen. Monatsschr. f. Geb. u. Gyn., 1900, xi, 918–933.

Strassmann. Anat. u. physiol. Untersuchungen über den Blutkreislauf beim Neugeborenen. Archiv f. Gyn., 1894, xlv, 393–445.

Der Verschluss des Ductus arteriosus. Hegar's Beiträge zur Geb. u. Gyn., 1902, vi, 98–117.

Zweifel. Die Verhütung der Augeneiterung Neugeborenen. Centralbl. f. Gyn., 1900, 1361–1380.

CHAPTER XVIII

MULTIPLE PREGNANCY

THE uterus occasionally contains two or more embryos; thus, according to the number present we have a twin, triplet, quadruplet, or quintuplet pregnancy.

Vassalli has recorded the only credible instance of sextuplet pregnancy, but even his case has been subjected to considerable criticism. On the whole, it may be said that reports of the birth of more than six children at a single labour are to be regarded as apocryphal, although many such are to be found in the older literature, the most remarkable being the Rhine legend, according to which the Countess Hagenau was delivered of 365 embryos at a single labour—manifestly an hydatidiform mole.

Frequency.—Wappaeus found that more than one child was born in 1.17 per cent of 20,000,000 cases of labour which he analyzed. The statistics of G. Veit, which were based upon 13,000,000 cases occurring in Prussia, showed that twins occurred once in 89, triplets once in 7,910, and quadruplets once in 371,125 labours. According to Mirabeau, triplets occur more frequently—once in 6,500 cases.

It would appear that multiple pregnancy is more common in cold than in warm climates. This statement is borne out by the statistics of Bertillon and Mirabeau, the latter stating that they occur once in 41.8 labours in Russia, as compared with once in 113.6 labours in Spain. According to Duncan, twin pregnancy is noted most frequently in multiparæ, especially between the twenty-fifth and twenty-ninth years.

It has been estimated that in 64 per cent of the cases only one, and in 36 per cent both sexes are represented. Thus Pinard, in 150 observations, found that both children were males in 46, females in 46, and of different sexes in 58 cases.

Ætiology.—Certain individuals appear to be predisposed towards multiple pregnancy, since it is not unusual for the same woman to give birth to twins or triplets upon several occasions. Thus Peuch, upon analyzing 1,262 cases of twin pregnancy, found that 48 of the mothers had had twins twice, 3 thrice, and 1 upon 4 occasions. In some instances multiple pregnancy has been known to occur in all the females of a family throughout several generations. Mirabeau has pointed out that an hereditary tendency towards triplet pregnancies was recorded in 13 out of the 75 cases collected by him. This was particularly marked in one family, in which triplets, not to mention twins, had occurred one or more times in five successive generations.

In rare instances, however, this tendency appears to come through the father, and reference is frequently made to the somewhat apocryphal case of the Russian peasant, Wasilef, who had 87 children by 2 wives, the first having had 4 quadruplet, 7 triplet, and 16 twin pregnancies; and the second 2 triplet and 6 twin pregnancies.

According to Hellin, Patellani, and Larger, multiple pregnancy should be regarded as a sign of degeneration, and represents an atavistic reversion. The first-mentioned authority states that the ovaries of women who have had a number of multiple pregnancies contain an excessive number of ova, but that individual ova with double nuclei are very rarely noted. According to this view, the condition is probably due to the maturation each month of several ova, instead of one, as is generally the rule.

Twin pregnancy may result either from the fertilization of two separate ova or of a single ovum, the first giving rise to *double*, and the second to *single ovum twins*. In the former case, the ova may come from the same ovary, or one from each ovary; while in rare instances both may originate in a single follicle. In the latter, the ovum may present two distinct germinal vesicles, each of which becomes converted into a female pronucleus and undergoes fertilization; or the twins may result from the cleavage or division of a single embryonic area, or from double gastrulazation of the blastodermic vesicle. Saniter states that in triplet pregnancy the children are usually derived from two ova—one from one and two from the other—while in rare cases, one of which he has studied personally, all three children are derived from a single ovum.

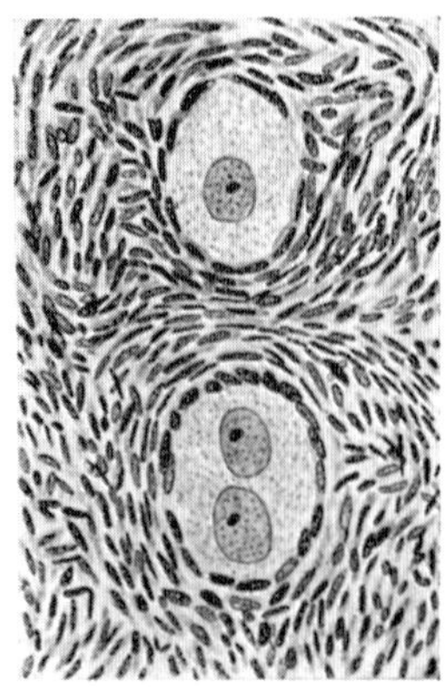

FIG. 308.—OVUM WITH DOUBLE GERMINAL VESICLE.

The existence of ova with double nuclei is indisputable, Franqué, Herff, Klien, and others having reported undoubted examples of such a condition. Fig. 308 represents an ovum of this character observed by the author. Whether, however, single ovum twins are derived from such ova, or whether they are due to cleavage of an ordinary blastodermic vesicle, are questions that as yet have not been decided, and whose solution offers great difficulties. Years ago Ahlfeld advanced the latter view, which has lately (1901) been revived by Sobotta.

It is well known that cleavage of the embryonic area can be produced experimentally in many of the lower animals, and Ahlfeld and Sobotta believe that similar changes may occur in human beings. According to this view, single-ovum twins are closely related to the so-called double monsters. Sobotta is inclined to believe that this is the only mode of origin of this class of twins, as he considers it impossible for two spermatozoa to enter the same ovum and unite with two female pronuclei.

Of 1,159 instances of twin pregnancy analyzed by Ahlfeld, 977 were derived from two ova and 180 from a single ovum. In the former case the children may or may not be of the same sex, while in the latter they are always of the same sex, and often closely resemble one another.

Relation of Placenta and Membranes.—The examination of the placenta and fœtal membranes after labour usually enables one to determine the mode of origin of the twins. When they are derived from a single ovum there is a single large placenta from which the two umbilical cords come off; but when they are developed from two ova there are usually two separate placentæ, although occasionally, when these were originally inserted near one another, their contiguous edges may fuse together, thus giving rise to an apparently single large placenta, in which, however, there is no connection between the circulation of the two twins.

In double-ovum twins, no matter whether the placentæ are separate or fused together, there are two chorions and two amnions, each child being enveloped in its own membranes. Single-ovum twins possess only a single chorion, but, as a rule, two amnions, for the reason that the former represents the wall of the original blastodermic vesicle, while the amnion is more directly connected with the embryo itself. In rare instances a

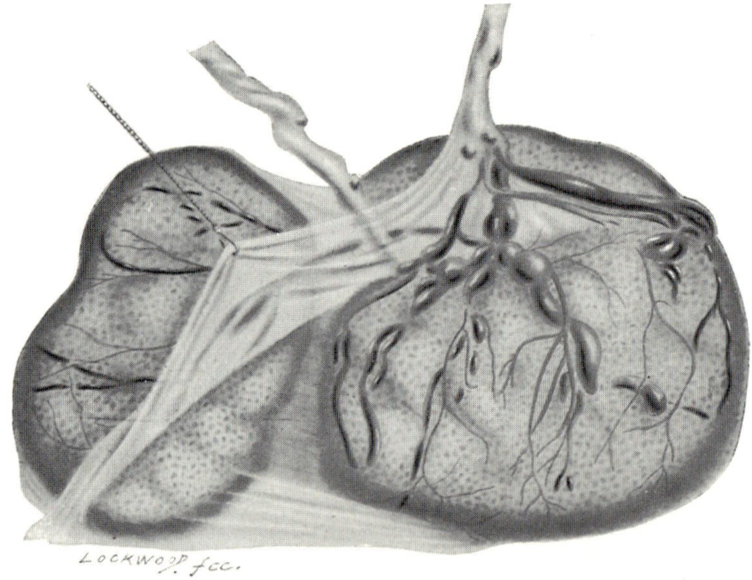

FIG. 309.—PLACENTA, DOUBLE-OVUM TWINS, VELAMENTOUS INSERTION OF CORD.

single amnion is found. This condition, which was noted in 3 of Ahlfeld's 1,157 cases, is not primary, but results from perforation of the partition wall between the two original amniotic cavities.

This arrangement of the membranes was known to Viardel in the seventeenth century, who stated that when the children were of the same sex they were usually inclosed in a single amnion; whereas twins of different sexes were separated by a partition wall. He expressed the belief that

Providence took this means of guarding their morals *in utero*. Saniter (1901), in a very interesting article, has carefully studied the relation of the fœtal membranes in triplet pregnancy.

In single-ovum twins there is always a certain area of the placenta in which there is anastomosis between the two vascular systems, which is never present in the fused placenta of double-ovum twins. This condition has been exhaustively studied by Schatz, and occasionally leads to serious consequences. Thus, if at an early period the heart of one embryo is considerably stronger than that of the other, a gradually increasing area of the communicating portion of the placenta is monopolized by the former, so that its heart increases rapidly in size, while that of the latter receives less and less blood and eventually atrophies. Herein is to be found the explanation of the deformity known as *acardia*. In such cases almost the entire placental circulation is utilized by the normal embryo, while the deformed twin receives only enough blood to nourish its lower extremities.

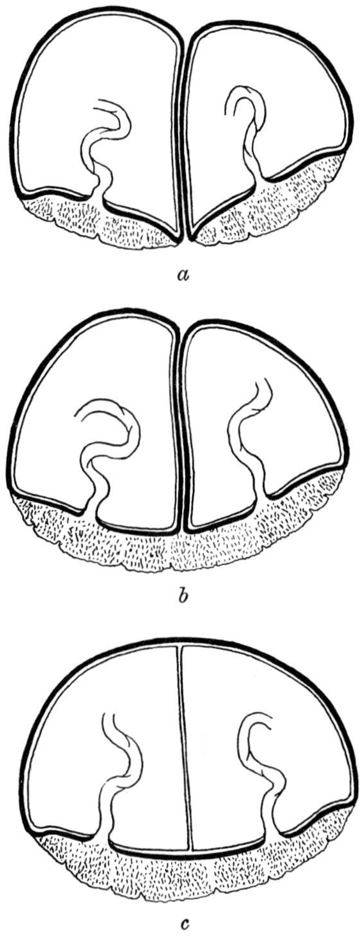

FIG. 310.—DIAGRAM SHOWING RELATION OF PLACENTA AND MEMBRANES IN DOUBLE- AND SINGLE-OVUM TWIN PREGNANCY.

a., double-ovum twins; *b.*, double-ovum twins, double membranes, single placenta; *c.*, single-ovum twins, one chorion, two amnions, and one placenta.

Not infrequently a difference in the strength of the two hearts leads to the production of hydramnios in one ovum. In such cases it is believed that the stronger heart appropriates an ever-increasing share of the blood from the placenta and undergoes hypertrophy, which is followed by an abnormal urinary secretion and a consequent increase in the quantity of amniotic fluid.

In the rare instances in which single-ovum twins are inclosed in a common amnion, their umbilical cords may become so twisted about one another as to interfere with the circulation through them, and thus lead to death and an early termination of pregnancy. Hermann, in 1891, collected 16 such cases from the literature.

Ordinarily in double-ovum twin pregnancies each ovum occupies, roughly speaking, one half of the uterus, the long axis being directed vertically. Occasionally, however, they run transversely, so that one fœtal sac comes to lie above the other. Under such circumstances the placenta and membranes of the first child must be expelled from the uterus before the second child can be born, unless the latter can make its way past them.

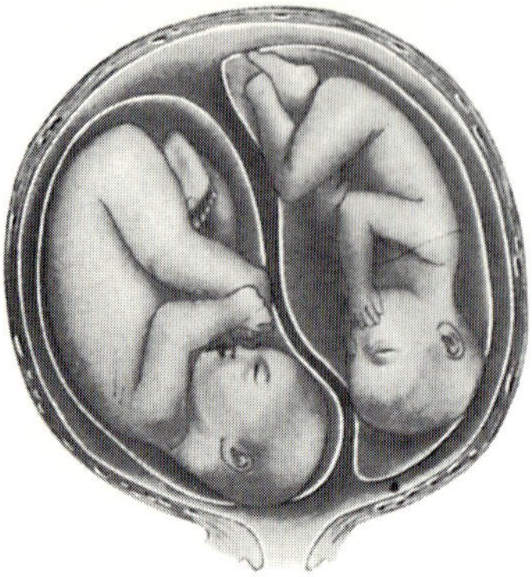

Fig. 311.

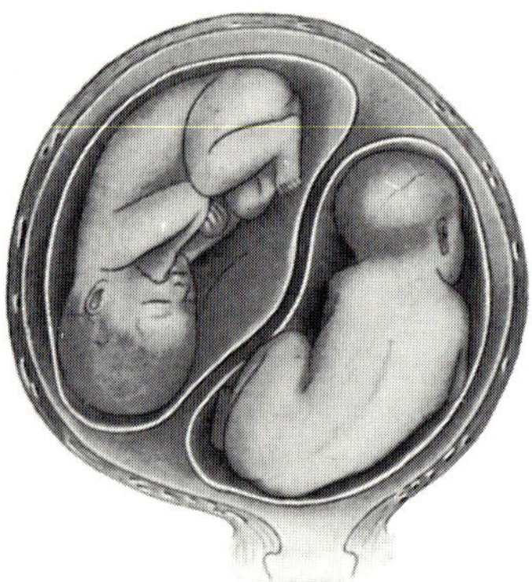

Fig. 312.

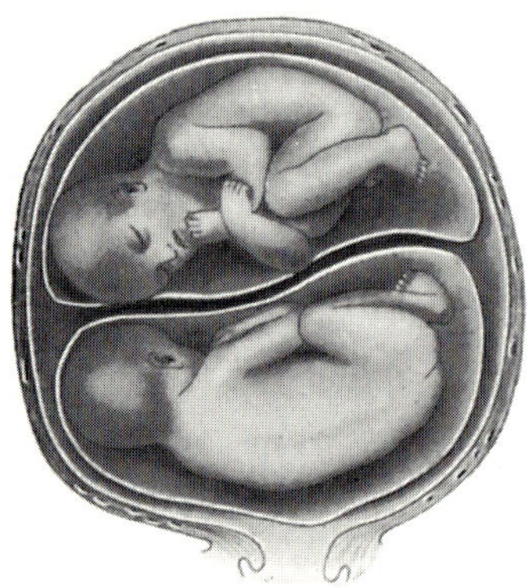

Fig. 313.

Figs. 311–313.—Diagrams showing Position of Twins in Utero.

Size of Children.—Generally speaking, twins are smaller and weigh less than children resulting from simple pregnancies, although their combined weight is usually greater than that of a single child. The smaller size may be considered normal, but in some instances is partially to be explained by the fact that the excessive distention of the uterus tends, more or less, to premature labour, so that the twins are often born several weeks before maturity. According to Ribemont-Dessaignes this occurs in 83 per cent of primiparæ and 75 per cent of multiparæ.

It is not unusual for twins to differ considerably in size and weight, especially when derived from a single ovum. Ahlfeld has reported three cases in which the twins weighed, respectively, 2,320 and 1,120, 2,700 and 1,650, and 1,920 and 790 grammes.

In double-ovum twin pregnancy it is not unusual for one child to die at an early period and be expelled from the uterus soon afterward, while the other may go on to full development. More frequently, however, the dead fœtus is retained until the end of pregnancy, and becomes flattened out and partially mummified, being compressed between the uterine wall and the membranes of the living child—*fœtus papyraceus* or *compressus* (Fig. 314).

Superfecundation and Superfœtation.—The consideration of the difference in the weight of twins, and the possibility of one being aborted while the other develops until full term, leads up to the question of superfecundation and superfœtation. By the former we understand the fertilization of two ova within a short period of one another, but not at the same coitus; whereas in the latter several months may intervene.

Superfecundation is a well-recognised occurrence in the lower animals, and undoubtedly occurs in human beings, although it is impossible to determine its frequency. It is probable that in many cases the two ova are not fertilized at the same coitus, but this can be demonstrated only under exceptional circumstances. In a case observed at the Lariboisière, in Paris, the woman had had connection with a white and a coloured man respectively within a short period, and was delivered of twins, one of which was white and the other a mulatto. At the Johns Hopkins Hospital a coloured woman gave birth to twins, one being born dead and the other perfectly healthy. Distinct evidences of syphilis were present in the first child and its placenta, while the second remained perfectly well some months after its delivery. On questioning the patient it was ascertained that she had had connection with her husband and another man within a period of a few days, and that the former was under treatment for syphilis at the time.

The occurrence of superfœtation has never yet been clearly demonstrated, though its theoretical possibility must be admitted. Generally speaking, the uterine cavity does not become completely obliterated until the decidua reflexa and vera fuse together at the end of the third month of pregnancy, after which superfœtation is out of the question; but prior to that period there is no theoretical objection to supposing that, if ovulation should occur, an ovum might find its way into the uterine cavity and there be fertilized. Still more favourable conditions would be afforded by a uterus duplex.

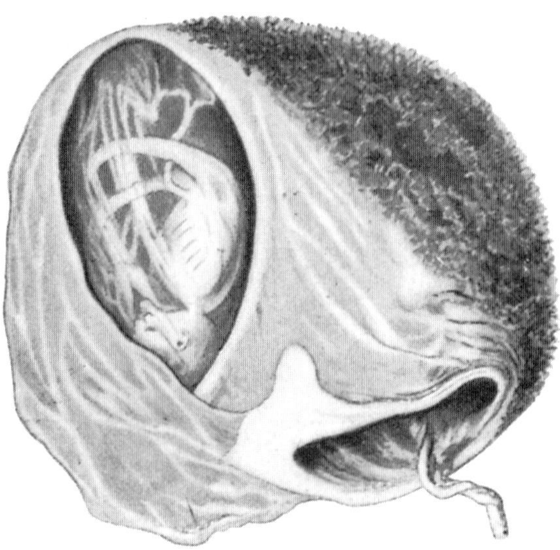

FIG. 314.—FŒTUS PAPYRACEUS (Ribemont-Dessaignes).

The French authorities consider that such an event has been conclusively demonstrated, and many of the arguments which have been advanced in its favour are given by Tarnier. On the other hand, most English and German authors are somewhat sceptical, and, while admitting its theoretical possibility, believe that the majority of instances put under this category, have been due either to the abortion of one twin or to marked inequality of development.

Diagnosis.—It often happens that the presence of twins in the uterus is unsuspected during pregnancy, and the first intimation which the physician has of the true condition is afforded by the unusually large size of the uterus after the expulsion of the first child. Despite this fact, however, it may be said that such surprises will rarely occur in the practice of those who take the trouble to make a thorough preliminary examination.

Excessive size of the abdomen during pregnancy frequently causes one to suspect the presence of twins, though usually it will be found to be due to some other condition. Thus, owing to the marked relaxation of the abdominal walls following the birth of the first child, women pregnant for a second time often think that they will give birth to twins, although, as a matter of fact, their fears are generally without foundation.

The diagnostic means at our disposal are palpation, auscultation, and touch. If a multiplicity of small parts is encountered on palpation, the possibility of a twin pregnancy should always be suspected and a further examination made with especial reference to this point. Positive evidence is afforded by the palpation of two heads, two breeches, and two backs; or at least of one back and four fœtal poles. The detection of three fœtal poles is not conclusive, for the reason that in rare instances a subperitoneal or intramural myoma may simulate the head of a child and thus give rise to serious diagnostic errors.

Auscultation occasionally gives most valuable information, and if one can distinguish two areas, considerably removed from one another, in which a fœtal heart can be heard, twins should be suspected; but a positive diagnosis should not be made unless there is a difference of at least 10 beats per minute in the rate of the two hearts, the sounds being counted for at least a minute in each location.

In rare instances vaginal touch may reveal important findings, as it is sometimes possible to distinguish through a macerated head the intact membranes, or a prolapsed and pulseless cord may be felt through the cervix, while auscultation gives positive evidence of the presence of a living child.

The presence of more than two children can be predicted with certainty only under very exceptional and favourable circumstances, although Ribemont-Dessaignes reports the diagnosis of triplets during pregnancy and its confirmation at the time of labour.

Course of Labour.—We have already referred to the abnormal size of the uterus resulting from the presence of twins, which may be still further increased by hydramnios of one ovum. This may give rise to considerable discomfort, the patient suffering markedly from dyspnœa, pressure symptoms, and œdema.

Occasionally the extreme stretching of the uterus may lead to an early dilatation of the cervix. Thus, in one instance, I found the cervical canal completely obliterated and the os externum dilated to 5 centimetres three weeks before the onset of labour. Reference has already been made to the frequency of premature expulsion in these cases; and when labour sets in, owing to the overdistention of the uterus, the pains usually occur at long intervals and are lacking in intensity, so that the birth of the first child is often markedly prolonged. The cord of this child should be cut between double ligatures, as failure to ligate its maternal end may lead to the death of the second child from hæmorrhage if the twins are derived from a single ovum.

Generally speaking, the membranes of the second child appear at the cervix immediately after the first is born and soon rupture. Its expulsion usually follows the first within half an hour, 75 per cent of the cases collected by Kleinwächter occurring within this period; while in the remainder a longer time elapsed—as much as twelve hours in 7 of his cases. As a rule it may be said that if spontaneous delivery of the second child does not occur within half an hour interference is indicated.

Changes in position of the second child not infrequently occur during and just after the birth of the first, so that at this time a renewed examination is necessary in order that any abnormality may be detected and the proper measures taken. The condition of the fœtal heart should also be carefully watched, and delivery immediately effected if it becomes abnormal. In most cases both twins present by the vertex, though not very rarely one descends by the breech. In 316 cases analyzed by Depaul and Tarnier, the following were noted: Both vertices in 131 cases; vertex and breech in 81 cases; breech and vertex in 47 cases; both breeches in 29 cases; breech and shoulder in 4 cases; vertex and face in 4 cases; other combinations occurring in a small number of cases.

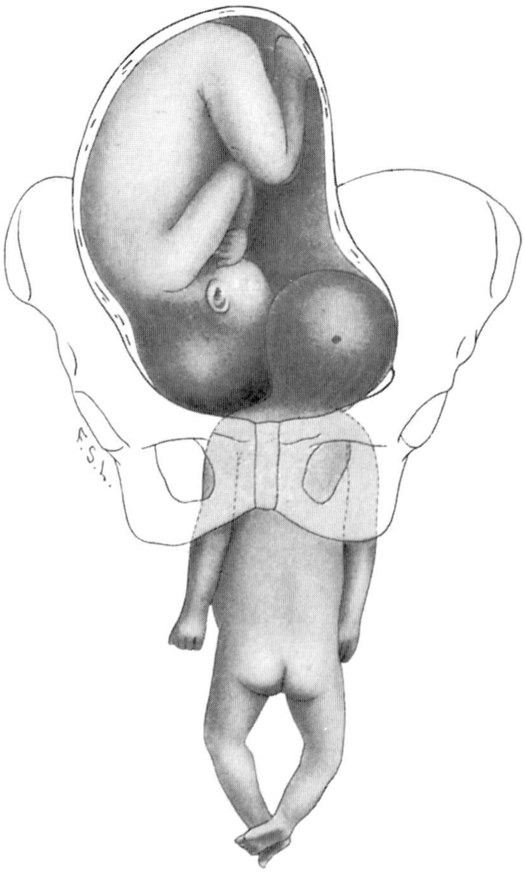

FIG. 315.—DIAGRAM SHOWING COLLISION BETWEEN HEADS OF TWINS.

As a rule the placenta of the first child remains *in situ* until the completion of labour, but in rare instances it may become partly or completely separated and give rise to hæmorrhage. Under these circumstances the second child should be delivered at once.

Owing to previous overdistention, the uterus not infrequently fails to contract and retract satisfactorily during the third stage of labour, so that abnormalities in the placental period are not infrequent. If there is any tendency toward an excessive loss of blood, the obstetrician should immediately express the placenta by Credé's method, instead of waiting for the fundus to rise up. Occasionally the area of placental attachment may be so large that abnormalities in its detachment may render necessary its manual removal. This operation, however, should not be resorted to unless urgently indicated.

The danger of hæmorrhage does not end with the expulsion of the placenta, as the uterus sometimes relaxes during the hour immediately following. Accordingly, the physician should remain in the house for some time after the completion of labour and give his personal supervision to the condition of the uterus, kneading it upon the first indication of relaxation, and re-enforcing it by the hypodermic administration of ergot. Neglect in this direction has sometimes led to the death of the patient from post-partum hæmorrhage.

Owing to the small size of the children, their presenting parts may both attempt to enter the superior strait at the same time and thus mutually interfere with one another. This complication is known as *collision,* and may occur when both children present by the vertex, or when one presents by the head and the other by the breech. In the first case an attempt should be made to push up the presenting part, which is less distinctly engaged, and then deliver the other child rapidly. If this is not possible, the whole hand should be introduced into the uterus and the condition of affairs carefully studied. Occasionally it will be found advisable to apply forceps to the uppermost child and attempt to drag it past the other. In rare instances craniotomy upon one child may be indicated.

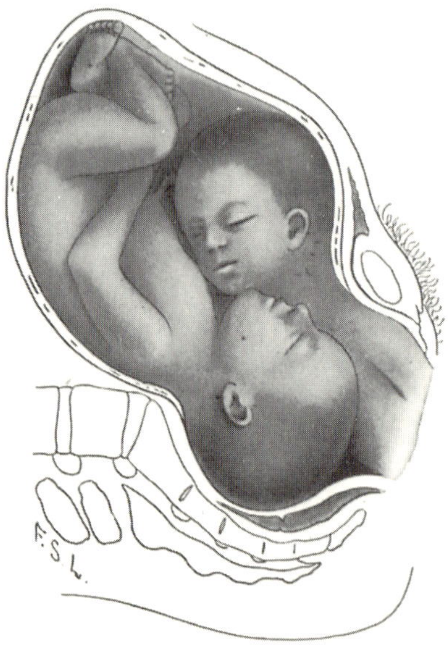

Fig. 316.—Diagram illustrating Locked Twins (American Text-Book).

Now and again during extraction, when the first child presents by the breech and the second by the vertex, the two heads may become locked just above the superior strait, that of the second fitting into the neck of the first child and making its delivery impossible. Under such circumstances, if the head of the second child cannot be displaced, the first child should be decapitated, as it must inevitably perish during any attempt at extraction; after this the body should be brought away and the second child then delivered by forceps.

In rare instances the first child may present transversely and be straddled by the second in such a manner that the legs of the latter protrude from the cervix. Traction upon them will serve only to wedge the shoulder of the other child more firmly into the pelvis and give rise to insuperable difficulties. The proper treatment can only be determined after most careful examination under anæsthesia with the entire hand in the uterus, as the second child cannot be born until the delivery of the first has been effected. The condition may call for version or decapitation, according to the exigencies of the individual case.

LITERATURE

AHLFELD. Die Entstehung der Doppelbildungen und der homologen Zwillinge. Archiv f. Gyn., 1876, ix, 196–251.

Lehrbuch der Geburtshülfe, II. Aufl., 1898, 356–362.

BERTILLON. Bulletin de la Soc. d'Anthropologie de Paris, 1874, ix, 267–290.

DEPAUL. Leçons de clinique obstétricale. Paris, 1876.

DUNCAN. On Some Laws of the Production of Twins. Edinburgh Med. Jour., March, 1865.

VON FRANQUÉ. Beschreibung einiger seltener Eierstockspräparate. Zeitschr. f. Geb. u. Gyn., 1898, xxxix, 326–346.

HELLIN. Die Ursache der Multiparität der uniparen Tiere, etc. München, 1895.

HERMANN. Ueber Verschlingungen der Nabelschnür bei Zwillingen. Archiv f. Gyn.- 1891, xl, 253–260.

KLEINWÄCHTER. Die Lehre von den Zwillingen. Prag, 1871.

KLIEN. Ueber mehreiige Graaf'sche Follikel beim Menschen. Münchener med. Abhand, lungen, 1898, IV. Reihe, Heft 4.

LARGER. Les stimates obstétricaux de la dégénérescence. Thèse de Paris, 1901.

MIRABEAU. Ueber Drillingsgeburten. Munchener med. Abhandlungen, 1894, IV. Reihe, Heft 5.

PATELLANI. Die mehrfachen Schwangerschaften, etc. Zeitschr. f. Geb. u. Gyn., 1896, xxxv, 373–413.

PINARD. Quoted by Ribemont-Dessaignes.

PUECH. Des grossesses multiples, etc. Paris, 1873.

RIBEMONT-DESSAIGNES et LEPAGE. Précis d'Obstétrique, 1894, 864–897. (Grossesse gémellaire.)

SANITER. Drillingsgeburten. Eineiige Drillinge. Zeitschr. f. Geb. u. Gyn., 1901, xlvi, 347–385.

SCHATZ. Die Gefässverbindungen der Placentakreisläufe eineiiger Zwillinge, ihre Entwickelung und ihre Folgen. Archiv f. Gyn., 1882–1900, Bde. xix, xxiv, xxvii, xxix, xxx, liii, lv, lviii und lx.

SOBOTTA. Neuere Anschauungen über die Entstehung der Doppel-(miss)-bildungen, etc. Würzburger Abhandlungen, 1901, Bd. 1, Heft 4.

TARNIER et CHANTREUIL. Des grossesses multiples. Traité de l'art des accouchements, Paris, 1888, t. i, 543–563.

VASSALLI. Caso di gravidanza sesquilgemellare. Gazette medica Italiano-Lombardia, 1888, Nr. 38, 216.

VEIT, G. Beiträge zur geburtshülflichen Statistik. Monatsschr. f. Geburtsk., 1855, vi, 126–132.

VIARDEL. Anmerkungen von der weiblichen Geburt. Frankfurt, 1676, 21.

WAPPAEUS. Allg. Bevölkerungsstatistik. Leipzig, 1859.

OBSTETRIC SURGERY

CHAPTER XIX

INDUCTION OF ABORTION AND PREMATURE LABOUR—ACCOUCHEMENT FORCÉ

Preparations for Obstetrical Operations.—Owing to the increased manipulation within the generative tract incident to an obstetrical operation, any lack of cleanliness entails even more risk than in the case of normal labour. Accordingly, the maintenance of a rigid aseptic technique is absolutely imperative.

The hands of the operator and his assistants should be thoroughly prepared by prolonged scrubbing with a nail-brush, plenty of hot water and

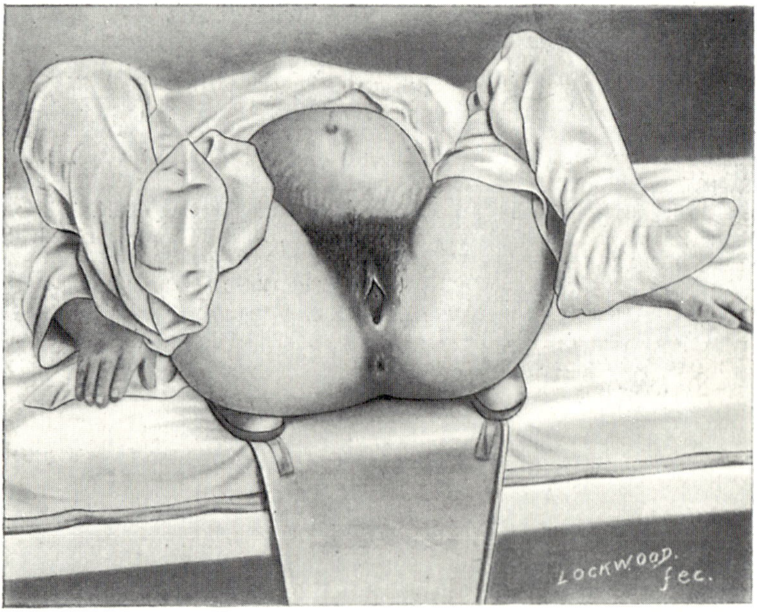

Fig. 317.—Showing Patient at Edge of the Bed, with Legs held in Position by Leg-Holder.

green soap being used, after which they should be passed successively through permanganate of potassium, oxalic acid, and bichloride solutions, as described when considering the conduct of a normal labour. If the hands have recently come in contact with septic material, or if the patient be infected, or present syphilitic lesions about the vulva, thin rubber gloves are necessary. Under other circumstances they may be employed or not, according to the practice of the operator.

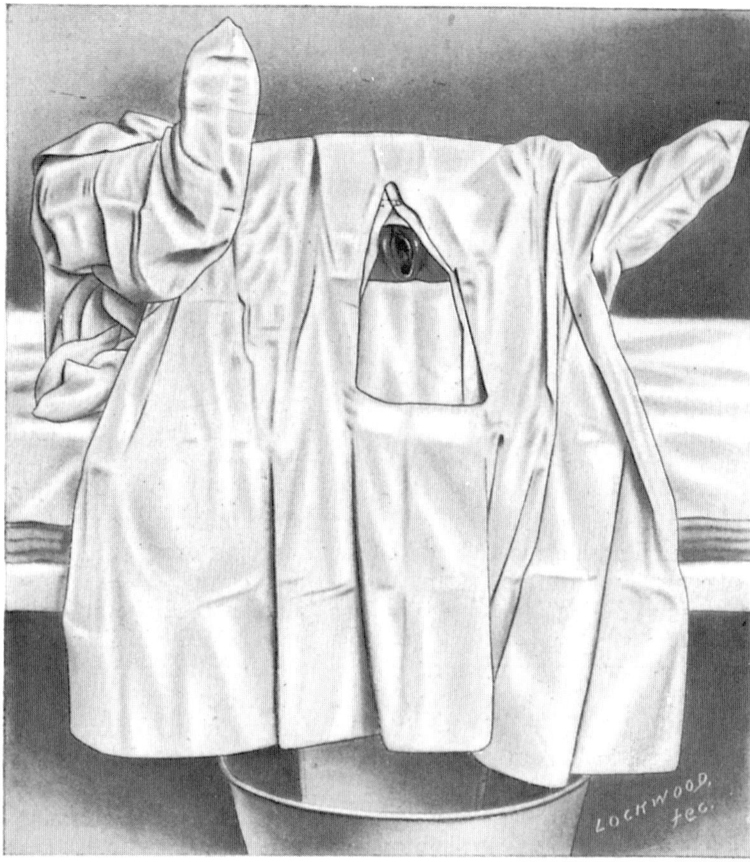

FIG. 318.—SHOWING PATIENT COVERED WITH STERILE DRESSINGS PREPARATORY TO OPERATION.

A sufficient quantity of dressings, towels, gauze, absorbent cotton, and ligatures, carefully sterilized beforehand, should be in readiness. All instruments should be rendered sterile by boiling immediately before the operation. As an emollient, vaseline, which has beeen sterilized by boiling in small jars, will serve every purpose.

The external genitalia are thoroughly cleansed with green soap and hot water, rinsed off with sterile water, freely irrigated with a 1-to-2,000 bichloride solution, and finally covered with a towel soaked in the same, which should remain in place until the operation is begun. If the pubic hairs are long and abundant they should be cut short with scissors or removed entirely with a razor.

If the woman is uninfected, it is not necessary to attempt to disinfect the vagina by means of antiseptic irrigations or other manipulations. But if the temperature is elevated, or the patient has been subjected to repeated examinations or attempts at delivery, a vaginal douche of a 1-to-5,000 bichloride solution may be given.

Obstetrical operations, with the exception of Cæsarean section and symphyseotomy, are usually undertaken with the patient in the lithotomy position. As the ordinary low beds now in use are very inconvenient for the performance of an operation, it is advisable, as a rule, even in private practice, to place the patient upon a narrow table: one that will answer the purpose quite satisfactorily is usually to be found in every kitchen. Anæsthesia is indispensable for all but the simplest operative procedures, and as soon as the patient is fully under its influence her buttocks should be brought to the edge of the table and her legs held in place by a leg-holder. If a table is not available, the patient should be placed crosswise in bed with her buttocks protruding over its edge. The nightgown should be rolled up above the hips to avoid soiling, and as soon as the external genitalia have been prepared, the patient's legs should be encased in sterile stockings made especially for this purpose, and her abdomen and buttocks covered with sterile towels in such a manner as to leave only the genitalia exposed. To avoid the possibility of contamination from the rectum, it is advisable to first empty the lower bowel by means of an enema, and then cover the anus with a folded sterilized towel, which can be held in place by a strip of adhesive plaster passed over the buttocks, after which a specially prepared sterile sheet should cover everything except the immediate field of operation.

Induction of Abortion.—By this term is understood the artificial termination of pregnancy before the fœtus has attained viability—namely, prior to the twenty-eighth week. The operation dates from the most remote antiquity, and more or less accurate directions for its performance are to be found in the earliest writings upon medicine. It was so extensively practised in Rome that we find it repeatedly referred to by Plautus, Juvenal, and other secular writers as a matter of every-day occurrence. With the spread of Christianity, however, it came to be considered as criminal, except when undertaken as a last resort in order to save the life of the mother; and we now draw a sharp distinction between criminal and therapeutic abortion. For full historical details the reader is referred to the works of Levin and Brenning, Brouardel and Kleinwächter.

Indications.—Three groups of cases may offer an indication for the operation. Thus we may think it our duty to induce an abortion: (1) As a direct means of saving the life of the mother; (2) to do away with a condition which may threaten her life if gestation continues; and (3) to avoid certain dangers which may supervene if pregnancy is allowed to progress to full term.

Under no circumstances should the operation be undertaken unless a careful and thorough examination has demonstrated that the patient is in a most serious condition. Her statements are entitled to but little weight, and the decision to interfere should be based entirely upon objective symptoms and conditions. Moreover, the operation should never be undertaken without a consultation with a second physician, who assumes his share of the responsibility. This precaution, besides securing for the patient additional advice, will protect the physician from a possible blackmailing on the part of unscrupulous persons.

In the first group, the best-recognised indication for the operation is present when the *vomiting of pregnancy* is uncontrollable. In most cases this symptom amounts to nothing more than a serious annoyance, and can be relieved by appropriate medical and dietetic measures, more particularly by the temporary employment of rectal feeding; but now and again every attempt will prove unavailing, and the condition becomes so serious that the patient is in danger of starvation unless promptly relieved.

Owing to the fact that the vomiting of pregnancy usually ceases spontaneously, or becomes better under treatment, there is a natural hesitancy on the part of the physician to interfere. For this reason the operation is not infrequently postponed until the condition of the patient has become so serious that death is the inevitable consequence whether abortion be induced or not. Accordingly, when all food is vomited, the patient is rapidly becoming emaciated, and the pulse is very rapid, there should be no hesitation as to the propriety of interference, and radical measures should be resorted to while they still offer a reasonable chance of saving the woman's life. Almost every year I see one or more cases in which procrastination has led to the death of the patient.

The induction of abortion is likewise urgently indicated when the uterine contents have become infected, a condition which frequently follows attempts at *criminal abortion*. Under such circumstances, if the fœtus has not already succumbed it will almost certainly die, and the only chance of saving the woman's life lies in promptly emptying the uterus and cleansing its cavity.

Formerly it was believed that abortion should be induced for incarceration of the *retroflexed pregnant uterus*, as well as in the rare cases of hernia of that organ, inasmuch as death is the usual result if the patient be left to herself. At present, however, better results are obtained in the former condition by performing laparotomy, freeing the uterus from adhesions and replacing it in a normal position, after which pregnancy not infrequently pursues an uninterrupted course.

In the second group, marked *renal insufficiency* or acute nephritis may necessitate the operation. But inasmuch as such conditions usually make their appearance only when pregnancy is well advanced, they will be considered when we take up the induction of premature labour.

Diseases of the ovum, such as hydatidiform mole and hydramnios, occasionally afford an indication for the operation. Whenever the former condition is diagnosticated the uterus should be emptied at once, no matter what be the period of pregnancy, as under such circumstances the fœtus is either dead or very imperfectly developed, and if the diseased chorion be allowed to remain in the uterus, a deciduoma malignum—a chorio-epithelioma—may develop.

Uterine hæmorrhage in the early months of pregnancy is generally a sign of beginning spontaneous abortion, but if the loss of blood continues for some time and is not followed by expulsion of the ovum, the uterus should be emptied by operative means. Later in pregnancy the most frequent cause of hæmorrhage is a faulty implantation of the placenta, particularly placenta prævia, and under such circumstances delivery should be effected as soon as possible. The rare cases of *missed abortion,* in which the ovum is retained for weeks or months after the death of the embryo, demand that the uterus should be emptied as soon as serious symptoms appear.

The indications in the third group are afforded by markedly *contracted pelves* or tumour formations. Formerly, the induction of abortion at an early period was considered justifiable when the pelvis was so contracted as to present an absolute indication for Cæsarean section; but at present, in view of the excellent results which attend the latter operation, this view has been modified. The same applies when pregnancy is complicated by the presence of *uterine myomata* or ovarian cysts. In the former class of cases, if the symptoms are urgent, hysterectomy should be promptly performed without regard to the existence of pregnancy; but if the tumour promises to act merely as a mechanical obstacle to labour, pregnancy should be allowed to go on to term, and Cæsarean section then performed, followed by removal of the uterus.

Ovarian tumours complicating pregnancy should be removed by laparotomy as soon as the diagnosis is made. In many such cases this can be done without causing interruption of the pregnancy, and spontaneous delivery will occur at term.

The induction of abortion is not indicated in *malignant growths,* whether they affect the uterus or adjacent organs. In carcinoma of the cervix the treatment to be pursued differs according to circumstances. If the case be operable, immediate hysterectomy is indicated without regard to the presence of pregnancy; but if the disease has progressed too far to offer a prospect of permanent cure after operation, gestation should be allowed to continue in the interests of the child, which should be delivered at term by the procedure most appropriate to the particular case.

Methods of Inducing Abortion.—Generally speaking, the methods of inducing abortion vary according to the duration of pregnancy. In the first four months the operation can usually be completed at a single sitting, whereas between this period and the seventh month the methods employed for the induction of premature labour are more appropriate.

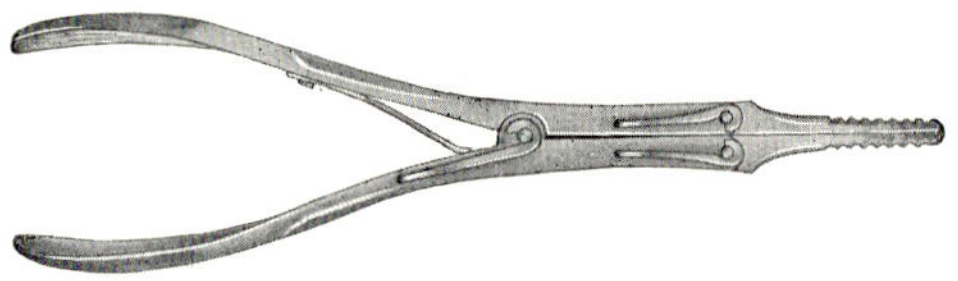

Fig. 319.—Goodell's Dilator.

In the first period, the cervix should be dilated sufficiently to admit at least one finger. For this purpose Goodell's or Hegar's dilators will be found very convenient. The entire hand, anointed with sterile vaseline, is then introduced into the vagina and the index finger carried up into the uterine cavity; while the other hand, placed upon the abdomen, forces the uterus downward. With the finger within the uterus the placenta is separated from its attachments, after which, according to the duration of pregnancy, the product of conception is removed entire or is broken up into small pieces, which can be removed by means of an abortion or ovum forceps.

To attempt to empty the uterus blindly by means of a curette and ovum forceps is an unwise procedure, inasmuch as many cases are reported in which such operations have caused perforation. Still more frequently larger or smaller portions of the placenta are left behind in the uterus, giving rise by their presence to serious hæmorrhage and occasionally to infection. Accordingly, one can never feel sure that the operation is complete unless one or more fingers have been introduced into the uterus and carefully palpated its interior.

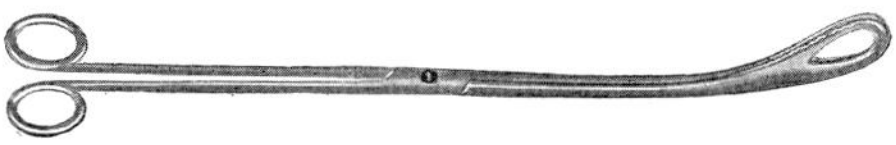

Fig. 320.—Ovum Forceps.

In rare cases the cervix may be so resistant as to render rapid dilatation impossible. Under such circumstances a strip of sterile gauze should be tightly packed into the canal and the vagina firmly tamponed with the same material. Half-drachm doses of ergot should then be administered every four hours. When the pack is removed at the end of twenty-four hours the entire ovum will frequently follow it; while in other cases the cervix will be sufficiently softened to permit the introduction of the finger, or at least of its dilatation with a suitable instrument. The employment of a laminaria tent has been recommended by many authorities in place of the pack, but in my opinion its use adds somewhat to the risk of infection.

Abortion is sometimes induced by perforating the membranes with a sterile sound and allowing the liquor amnii to drain off. The desired result, however, does not always follow this manœuvre, and it frequently becomes necessary to supplement it by one of the procedures just described.

Prognosis.—The prognosis varies according to the indication for which the operation is undertaken, but with the patient in fairly good condition satisfactory results should always follow, provided a rigid aseptic technique is observed.

Induction of Premature Labour.—By this term we designate the artificial termination of pregnancy after the child has reached the period of viability—that is, after the twenty-eighth week. The operation was performed by Guillemeau, Mauriceau, Justine Siegemundin, and others in isolated cases for hæmorrhage, but, according to Denman, it was not generally advocated until 1756, when a conference of physicians was held in London to devise means for doing away with the frightful mortality following Cæsarean section for contracted pelves.

Indications.—The indications for the operation are twofold: to obviate the dangers attending delivery at term through a contracted pelvis, and to save the life of the mother when seriously threatened by some disease from which she may be suffering, or on account of some pathological condition existing in the ovum.

In *contracted pelves* premature labour is induced with the idea that the imperfectly developed child will be born more readily than at term. This view is undoubtedly correct, and if the welfare of the mother alone were concerned the operation should be undertaken in all cases. On the other hand, the interests of the child are entitled to some consideration. We know that labour will be easier the earlier the operation is performed, but it must be remembered that the child will be less liable to survive it, and even if born alive its chances of succumbing to accidental causes after its birth will be proportionately greater. Inasmuch, then, as the later the operation the better the outlook so far as the child is concerned, the induction of premature labour should not be attempted before the thirty-fourth, and preferably not before the thirty-sixth, week of pregnancy.

The question as to the propriety of the operation has given rise to an extensive literature. At the International Medical Congress of 1890, held in Berlin, it was one of the chief subjects under discussion. On that occasion Parvin, Macan, Calderini, Dohrn, Leopold, Löhlein, and others spoke upon the subject, and in the end it was agreed, Sänger only dissenting, that the operation was indicated in generally contracted pelves with a conjugata vera varying from 7.5 to 9 centimetres, and in flat pelves with a conjugata vera of 7 centimetres or more, and should be performed as late in pregnancy as possible, preferably about the thirty-sixth week.

The principal difficulty connected with the operation is to choose the correct time for its performance, since we are unable to determine accurately the size of the child's head. The methods of Müller, Ahlfeld, and others, to which reference will be made in the chapter upon the treatment of contracted pelves, do not lead to very accurate results, so that owing to the desire of postponing the operation until the latest possible moment, it is frequently not undertaken until the child's head has attained such proportions as to render its passage through the pelvis difficult or impossible.

The results obtained are extremely satisfactory so far as the mother is concerned, the maternal mortality being only 1.03 per cent in 391 operations performed by Ahlfeld, Bar, Leopold, and Pinard. On the other hand, the fœtal mortality is relatively high, varying from 45 to 12 per cent, according to the statistics from various lying-in hospitals. Kleinwächter, after an exhaustive study of the subject, concludes that 78.3 per cent of the children are born alive, but that many of them die soon after birth, and only 60.4 per cent leave the hospital in good condition. According to these figures, then, the net mortality would be 39.6 per cent; but when we consider that most careful nursing and appropriate feeding are afterward necessary, it is apparent that no inconsiderable portion of the children dismissed from the hospital in good condition must inevitably perish within the first year, and it is hardly an exaggeration to state that hardly one third of those born survive that period. It would therefore appear that the ultimate results, so far as the children are concerned, are so poor as not to commend the operation to favourable consideration.

In this connection, it is important not to lose sight of the fact that practically 70 per cent of all labours occurring in contracted pelves end without artificial aid, and that it is extremely difficult in the degrees of contraction under consideration to foretell in a given case whether spontaneous delivery will occur or not. Personally I have had a gross fœtal mortality of only 13 per cent in a series of 278 cases of contracted pelves in which premature labour was not induced, and these figures, when taken in connection with those of others, are certainly not in favour of the operation. Moreover, if the rules laid down in the chapter on the treatment of labour complicated by contracted pelves be followed, and Cæsarean section promptly performed when indicated, the fœtal mortality should be practically nothing, or at least not much greater than with normal pelves.

At present Pinard considers the induction of labour no longer justifiable, and advocates allowing all cases to go on to term, when symphyseotomy is performed if necessary. Bar, who has had a large experience with the induction of premature labour, has likewise abandoned it, and recommends the performance of Cæsarean section at term if spontaneous delivery does not occur. So far as my own experience goes, I am heartily in accord with this last authority, and believe that this practice would effect the saving of nearly all the children; whereas by the induction of premature labour a much smaller number will be brought into the world alive, many of whom are doomed to certain death or to lifelong afflictions.

At the present time, then, it seems to me that the only rational indication for the induction of premature labour, so far as concerns the existence of disproportion between the size of the head and the pelvis, is afforded by the rare cases in which the pelvis is normal but the child abnormally large, owing either to excessive development or to an undue prolongation of pregnancy. If such a condition be diagnosed some weeks before labour, the operation is clearly indicated, particularly in multiparous women who have repeatedly given birth to very large dead children.

The most usual indication for the operation, however, is afforded by diseases which threaten the life of the mother, while at the same time there exists a probability of cure after the termination of gestation. This is particularly true in those cases of *toxæmia* or *acute nephritis* complicating pregnancy, which show no tendency to subside in spite of appropriate treatment. Experience teaches that under such circumstances, even if pregnancy be allowed to continue, premature labour frequently occurs spontaneously, when a large proportion of the children are born dead, or, if alive, very imperfectly developed. Moreover, one should also take into consideration the possibility that the renal changes may become chronic. Accordingly, if alarming symptoms supervene, labour should be induced at any period of pregnancy without too conservative a regard for the life of the child.

In patients presenting nephritic symptoms, the total amount of albumin and urea contained in the twenty-four hours' urine should be determined daily, and whenever there is a steady increase in the amount of albumin and a corresponding decrease in the amount of urea, in spite of appropriate treatment, labour should be induced in the hope of preventing the onset of eclampsia. If eclampsia supervenes, pregnancy should be terminated as soon as possible by *accouchement forcé*, if the condition of the cervix permits; but if this procedure promises to be very difficult delivery should be effected by slower and less violent means.

Cardiac lesions occasionally demand the induction of premature labour, but this should be resorted to only in cases of broken compensation which do not yield to appropriate treatment.

From the time of D'Outrepont (1828), it has been recommended that the operation be undertaken in the interests of the child in the rare cases of *tuberculosis* in which the condition of the mother is so serious as to make it probable that she will not live until term.

Spontaneous interruption of pregnancy frequently occurs during the course of the acute infectious diseases—pneumonia, typhoid fever, etc.—but inasmuch as experience has shown that it materially increases the risks to the mother, the induction of premature labour is contra-indicated.

In rare instances a general peripheral *neuritis* may so endanger the life of the mother as to call for interference. Lepage and Sainton (1901) reported a case of alcoholic origin in which the induction of labour was followed by most happy results.

The milder forms of *chorea* complicating pregnancy are usually readily amenable to treatment, but when the disease assumes a grave type it is attended with great danger, the maternal mortality, according to Fehling, being 36 per cent. Therefore, if the patient appears to be in serious danger, premature delivery should be brought about, as experience has shown that the emptying of the uterus is usually followed by marked improvement.

In patients suffering from *diabetes*, gestation sometimes exerts a very deleterious influence upon the course of the disease. Accordingly, if the patient's condition becomes alarming, labour should be induced. In the majority of cases, however, the so-called diabetes of pregnancy is merely a lactosuria which is not likely to be attended by serious symptoms, the patients being spontaneously delivered of healthy children at term.

According to Graefe and others, the occurrence of pregnancy in patients suffering from *pernicious anæmia* or leukæmia adds markedly to the gravity of the condition, so that in occasional cases the induction of premature labour may be indicated.

In rare instances in patients suffering from pyelitis, the pregnant uterus may so compress the ureter as to cause a damming back of the purulent discharge, and thus give rise to a *pyelo-nephritis*. Under such circumstances the induction of premature labour is indicated. In two cases recently under my care, interference was followed by surprisingly good results, the patients recovering without further treatment.

Many authors recommend the induction of premature labour when pregnancy is complicated by *uterine* or *ovarian tumours*, or by malignant disease of the uterus or rectum which would offer an insuperable obstacle to the birth of a full-term child. At the present day, however, the operation can hardly be considered justifiable. What has already been said in connection with the induction of abortion under similar conditions, also holds good here.

In *hydramnios*, when the abdomen is so distended as to seriously threaten the life of the patient, pregnancy should be terminated without too much regard for the preservation of the child, as in many cases it is so poorly developed as to have but little chance of living, even if born at full term.

In cases of *hydatidiform mole* alarming symptoms usually come on before the fœtus is viable; but even should the twenty-eighth week be safely passed the immediate termination of pregnancy is imperatively demanded.

Whenever *placenta prævia* is positively diagnosed, the termination of pregnancy is urgently indicated, as it is impossible to predict at what moment uterine contractions may come on and give rise to profuse or even fatal hæmorrhage.

In rare cases of *habitual death of the fœtus* in the later months of pregnancy, when not due to syphilis or renal disease, the induction of premature labour has been recommended at a time slightly anterior to that at which fœtal death has occurred in previous pregnancies, in the hope that a living child may be obtained. In such cases the operation may be undertaken if the parents are extremely anxious for a living child, although in no instance should a positive assurance of success be held out to them.

Prognosis.—As far as the mother is concerned, the prognosis of the induction of premature labour is excellent, provided a rigorous aseptic technique is observed and her physical condition is not critical at the time of the operation.

The prognosis for the child depends, of course, upon the degree of its development, as well as upon the pathological condition for which the operation is undertaken. Generally speaking, in the case of children born before the thirty-second week the chances of surviving are very small, especially when nephritis or hydramnios affords the indication for interference.

Methods of Inducing Premature Labour.—The simplest method—that of Scheele—consists in perforating the membranes with a sharp instrument and allowing the amniotic fluid to drain off. The results, however, are uncertain, so that the procedure is applicable only in a very limited number of cases, more especially in hydramnios and occasionally in placenta prævia.

In the method most usually employed—that of Krause—a bougie is introduced between the membranes and the uterine wall. In carrying out this procedure the patient is placed in the dorsal or Sims's position, and the external genitalia carefully disinfected. The cervix is then brought into view by means of a speculum, and a sterilized bougie passed through it and gently carried high up into the uterine cavity, between the membranes and the uterine wall. In place of the bougie, I prefer a thick-walled, rubber catheter, 8 to 10 millimetres in diameter, which can be readily sterilized by boiling. It should be introduced by means of a copper stylet, which is withdrawn after the catheter is in place.

The only objection to Krause's method is its uncertainty. In many cases the introduction of a single catheter is followed by uterine contractions within a few hours, which lead to the expulsion of the fœtus after a longer or shorter period. Not infrequently, however, twenty-four hours or more may elapse without the appearance of pains. Under such circumstances a second catheter should be introduced, to be followed by a third if necessary, after the lapse of a similar period. In rare instances even then the desired result is not accomplished, and it becomes necessary to terminate pregnancy in some other manner. But for the general practitioner, when haste is not essential, this is the safest and best method of procedure.

More certain and rapid results are obtained by the use of the balloon of Champetier de Ribes. This is a conical rubber bag with a capacity of 400 or 500 cubic centimetres, from one end of which extends a thick rubber tube provided with a stop-cock. The patient having been placed in the dorsal or Sims's position, the cervix is brought into view. If its lumen is 1.5 centimetre in diameter the bag can be passed through it without difficulty, but if smaller it should be dilated up to that size by means of a Goodell or other suitable dilator. The bag, which has been sterilized by boiling, is then tightly rolled into a cylinder, seized with an appropriately shaped forceps, thickly smeared with sterile vaseline, introduced into the lower uterine segment, and then pumped full of sterile salt solution. Within a few hours it usually so irritates the uterus as to induce contractions which soon lead to dilatation of the cervix and the expulsion of the bag, after which the child can be extracted or labour allowed to end spontaneously, according to the exigencies of the case. Where great haste is necessary, the dilatation may be accelerated by attaching a weight to the end of the tube and allowing it to hang over the foot of the bed. This method gives very satisfactory results, though it is evident that the introduction of the large bag into the lower uterine segment must displace the presenting part, and occasionally give rise to malpresentations.

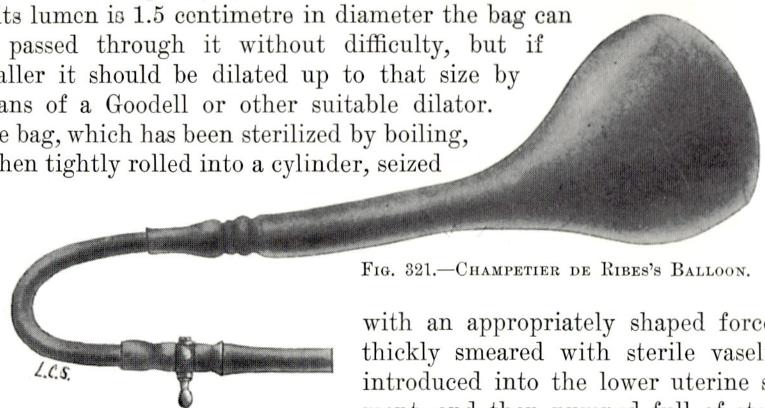

FIG. 321.—CHAMPETIER DE RIBES'S BALLOON. × ⅓.

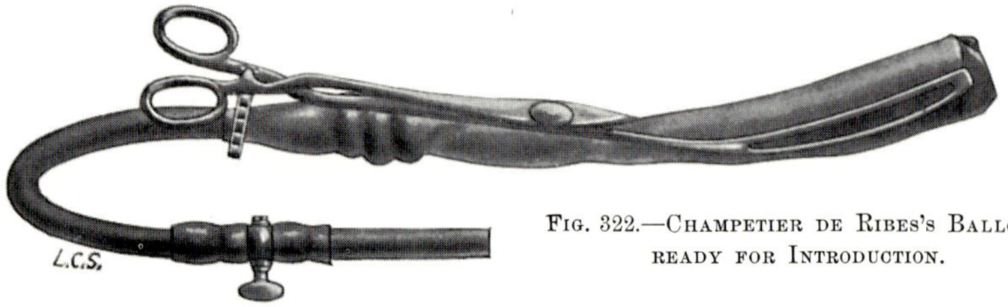

FIG. 322.—CHAMPETIER DE RIBES'S BALLOON READY FOR INTRODUCTION.

Tarnier's *excitateur utérin*—a thin-walled rubber bag 3 or 4 centimetres in diameter—and Barnes's fiddle-bags are based upon the same principle, but their smaller size renders them much less efficient irritants.

In placenta prævia, more particularly when the cervix is but slightly dilated, the use of a sterile tampon may be attended by most excellent results. In such cases, under the most rigid aseptic precautions, the end of a sterilized 4-inch roller gauze bandage is tightly packed into the cervical canal by means of a uterine dressing forceps, after which the vagina is firmly and tightly packed with the same material. The pack should not be allowed to remain in place for more than twelve or at most twenty-four hours, and on its removal at the expiration of that period the cervix will be found completely dilated, or at least sufficiently so to permit of other manœuvres.

Numerous other methods for the induction of premature labour have been suggested from time to time, among which may be mentioned that of Cohen. This consisted in the injection of 200 to 300 cubic centimetres of aqua picis between the uterine wall and the membranes. Other writers have substituted various fluids. Thus, in 1891, Pelzer suggested the use of 100 cubic centimetres of sterile glycerine, which promptly gives rise to uterine contractions. Its employment, however, is not to be recommended, as it is occasionally followed by serious symptoms of intoxication, hæmoglobinuria, albuminuria, elevation of temperature, cyanosis, and occasionally by death. Pfannenstiel was the first to call attention to these dangers,

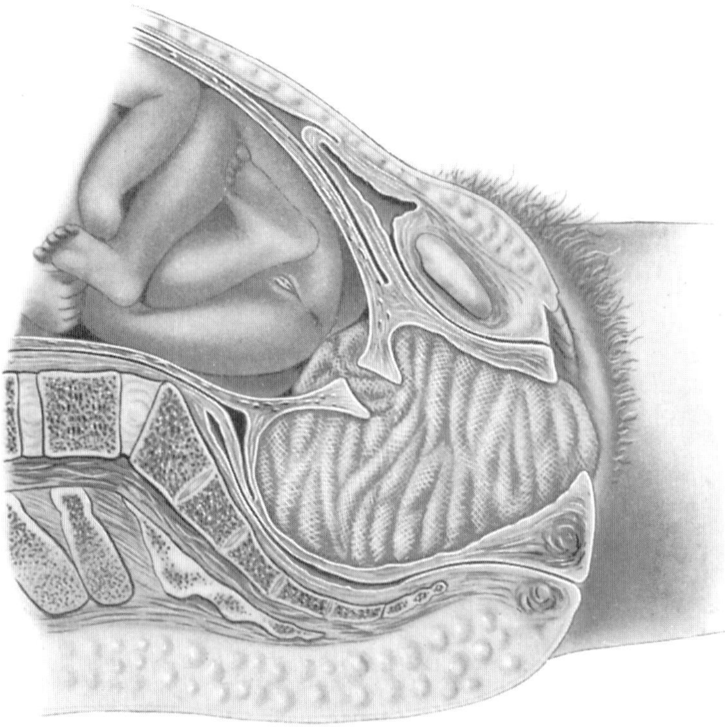

FIG. 323.—VAGINAL AND CERVICAL PACK IN POSITION.

and his warning has been re-enforced by similar experiences in the practice of other writers. Full details respecting the various other methods suggested for the induction of premature labour will be found in the monographs of Kleinwächter and Fieux.

Accouchement Forcé.—By this term is understood the forcible dilatation of the intact or partially dilated cervix, followed by version and extraction of the child. In pre-antiseptic times the operation was so universally followed by infection that it fell into deserved disrepute; but at the present day it has been rehabilitated, and when properly performed under suitable conditions has been the means of saving many lives.

Generally speaking, if the cervix be firm and hard and the canal not obliterated, the operation is apt to be very difficult and occasionally impossible, while at the same time it is attended with considerable risk to the mother. On the other hand, when the cervix is soft and the internal os partially dilated, the operation is readily performed, and is followed by most satisfactory results. As a general rule, it is more difficult in primiparous than in multiparous women.

Indications.—In this country the most usual indication for *accouchement forcé* is threatened or actual eclampsia. Occasionally it becomes necessary in concealed or accidental hæmorrhage, and also in the rare cases of acute œdema of the lungs, or broken cardiac compensation complicating pregnancy, as well as in certain cases of placenta prævia.

Methods.—If labour has already begun and the upper portion of the cervical canal is obliterated, most excellent results are obtained by the

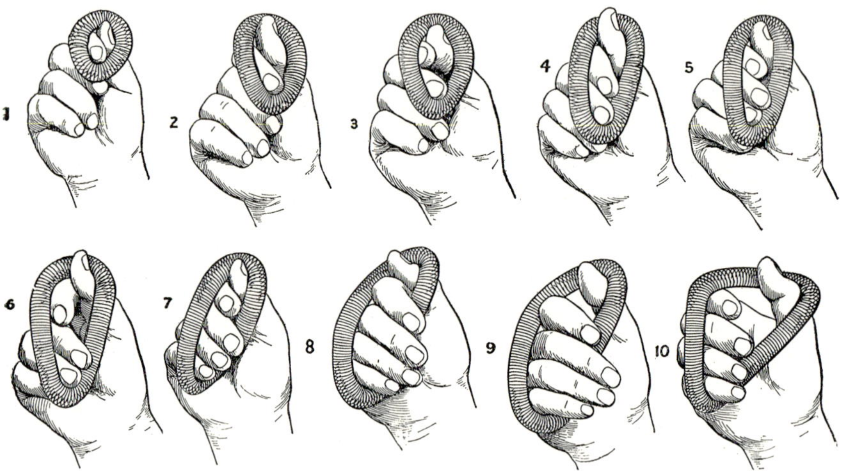

FIG. 324.—DIAGRAMS ILLUSTRATING MANUAL DILATATION OF CERVIX (Harris).

method of manual dilatation suggested by Philander A. Harris. But if labour has not set in, and the cervix is hard and rigid, the operation may be extremely difficult; and if dilatation be effected by brute force it is frequently accompanied by deep tears through the cervix, and occasionally through the lower uterine segment, which may lead to the death of the patient from hæmorrhage or infection.

Generally speaking, if the index finger can be carried through the internal os, dilatation can be readily accomplished by this method. Moreover, if the cervical canal is soft and yielding, although too narrow to admit the finger, the first stage of dilatation may be effected by means of a steel dilator and completed by Harris's method. On the other hand, if the cervix be cartilaginous in consistency, or instrumental dilatation proves more difficult than was expected, the operation should be abandoned as presenting more danger than does expectant treatment.

At the time of operation, the patient should be profoundly anæsthetized and the aseptic technique most rigorous. The danger of contamination from the fæces can be minimized by moving the bowels freely by means of a rectal enema, and then applying over the anus a sterile towel, which is held in place by strips of adhesive plaster until the completion of the various manipulations. One hand, thoroughly anointed with sterile vaseline, is then introduced into the vagina, and the index finger carried up the cervical canal and slowly forced through the internal os, after which the tips of the index and second fingers are passed into the cervical canal, gradually dilating it as well as the internal os. When this has been accomplished, completion of the dilatation is usually comparatively easy. The thumb is pushed past the index finger with much the same motion as is employed in snapping one's fingers; then, as dilatation progresses, past two, three, and finally all four fingers. These manœuvres are clearly shown in Fig. 324.

When the internal os is obliterated, complete dilatation of the cervix can be effected in a very few minutes by Harris's method, and in appropriate cases when the internal os will admit only the tip of the index finger, satisfactory results can usually be obtained within half an hour. Personally I have found this method very effective, and am able to confirm all that Harris has claimed for it. It would certainly seem to be far superior to the procedures advocated by Edgar and Bonnaire, in which both hands are employed simultaneously. Furthermore, since they come into intimate contact with the anus, the risk of infection from the rectal contents is greatly increased.

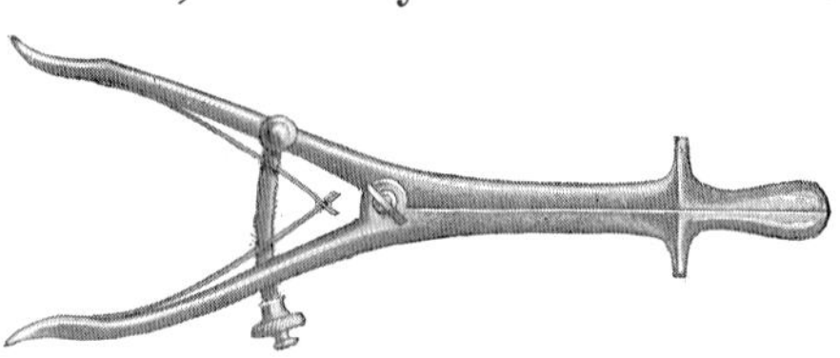

FIG. 325.—REYNOLDS'S CERVICAL DILATOR.

Various instruments have been devised to effect the rapid and complete dilatation of the cervical canal, but none of these are as satisfactory as manual dilatation. Occasionally, when the cervical canal is completely obliterated, and the resistance is offered only by the external os, excellent results may be obtained with Reynolds's instrument.

When rapid delivery is urgently indicated, Dührssen recommends that deep incisions be made through several portions of the cervical canal, which are united by sutures after the completion of labour. This manipulation, however, requires considerable surgical skill, and is not to be recommended save under exceptional circumstances. It is occasionally indicated in concealed hæmorrhage, when prompt evacuation of the uterine contents is imperative in order to save the life of the patient, in whom the consistence of the cervix is such that rapid manual or instrumental dilatation appears impossible. Under other conditions, however, it cannot be looked upon as a justifiable procedure, a remark which also applies to Dührssen's so-called vaginal Cæsarean section.

LITERATURE

AHLFELD. 118 Fälle von Einleitung der künstlichen Frühgeburt. Centralb. f. Gyn., 1890, 529–534.

Lehrbuch der Geburtshülfe, II. Aufl., 1898, 498.

Bar. Contribution à l'étude des indications de l'accouchement prématuré artificiel, etc. L'Obstétrique, 1899, iv, 471.

Leçons de pathologie obstétricale. Paris, 1900.

Bonnaire. Tarnier et Budin, Traité de l'art des accouchements, 1901, t. iv, 444.

Brouardel. L'avortement. Paris, 1901.

Calderini. See Parvin.

Champetier de Ribes. De l'accouchement provoqué. Annales de gyn. et d'obst., 1888, xxx, 401–438.

Davis. Puerperal Pernicious Anæmia. Trans. Amer. Gyn. Soc., 1891, xviii, 173.

Denman. An Introduction to the Practice of Midwifery. 7th ed., London, 1823, 318.

Dohrn. See Parvin.

D'Outrepont. Beobachtungen u. Bemerkungen. Gemeinsame Zeitschr. f. Geburtsk., 1828, ii, 549.

Dührssen. Ueber den Werth der tiefen Cervix- und Scheiden-Damm Einschnitte in der Geburtshülfe. Archiv f. Gyn., 1890, xxxvii, 27–66.

Ueber vaginalen Kaiserschnitt. Volkmann's Sammlung klin. Vorträge, N. F., Nr. 232.

Edgar. Methods and Aids in Obstetric Teaching. N. Y. Med. Jour., 1896, November 14th, 21st, 28th, and December 5th.

Fehling. Ein Fall von Chorea gravidarum. Archiv f. Gyn., 1874, vi, 137–139.

Fieux. Procédés de provocation et de la terminaison artificielle rapide de l'accouchement. Annales d'obst. et de gyn., 1901, lv, 409–450.

Graefe. Ueber den Zusammenhang der perniciösen Anaemie mit der Gravidität. D. I., Halle, 1880.

Guillemeau. De l'heureux accouchement des femmes. Paris, 1594.

Harris. A Method of performing Rapid Dilatation of the Os Uteri, etc. Amer. Jour. Obst., 1894, xxix, 37–49.

Kleinwächter. Die kunstliche Unterbrechung der Schwangerschaft, III. Aufl., 1902.

Krause. Die künstliche Frühgeburt. Breslau, 1855.

Leopold (Buschbeck). Beitrag zur künstl. Frühgeburt wegen Beckenenge. Arbeiten aus der königl. Frauenklinik in Dresden, 1893, i, 93–123. See Parvin.

Leopold (Schoedel). Erfahrungen über künstliche Frühgeburten, eingeleitet wegen Beckenenge. Archiv f. Gyn., 1901, lxiv, 151–164.

Lepage et Sainton. Accouchement provoqué pour un cas de névrite périphérique alcoholique. Comptes rendus de la Soc. d'Obst., de Gyn. et de Pæd. de Paris, 1901, iii, 93–99.

Levin und Brenning. Die Fruchtabtreibung durch Gifte. Berlin, 1899.

Löhlein. See Parvin.

Macan. See Parvin.

Mauriceau. Traité des maladies des femmes grosses, etc. 6me éd., 1721, 161.

Parvin et al. Artificial Premature Labour, its Indications and Methods. Verh. des X. Internat. med. Congresses, Berlin, 1891, Bd. iii, Abtheilung, viii, 107–149.

Pelzer. Ueber Einleitung der künstlichen Frühgeburt. Centralbl. f. Gyn., 1892, 35–36.

Pfannenstiel. Ueber die Gefährlichkeit der intraut. Glycerineinspritzung. Centralbl. f. Gyn., 1894, xxix, 37–49.

Pinard. De l'accouchement provoqué. Annales de Gyn. et d'Obst., 1891, xxxv, 1–16, 81–112.

Indication de l'opération Césarienne considerée en rapport avec celle de la symphyséotomie et de l'accouchement prématuré artificiel. Annales de Gyn. et d'Obst., 1899, lii, 81–117.

Sänger. See Parvin.

Siegemundin. Die königl. preussische und Chur-Brandenb. Hof-Wehe-Mutter. Berlin, 1756, 216.

CHAPTER XX

FORCEPS

THE obstetrical forceps is an instrument designed for the extraction, under certain conditions, of the child when it presents by the head. It consists of two branches which cross one another, being designated respectively right and left, according to the side of the pelvis to which each corresponds. They are introduced separately into the genital canal and are articulated after being placed in position. Each branch is made up of four portions—the handle, blade, shank, and lock.

The instruments vary considerably in size and shape, as will be seen when certain varieties of forceps are considered. The blades possess a double curvature—the cephalic and the pelvic—the former being adapted to the shape of the child's head, the latter to that of the birth canal. The blades are more or less elliptical in shape, tapering towards the shank, and are usually fenestrated so as to allow of a firm hold upon the head. Certain authorities, however, prefer solid blades in the belief that they can be made less bulky.

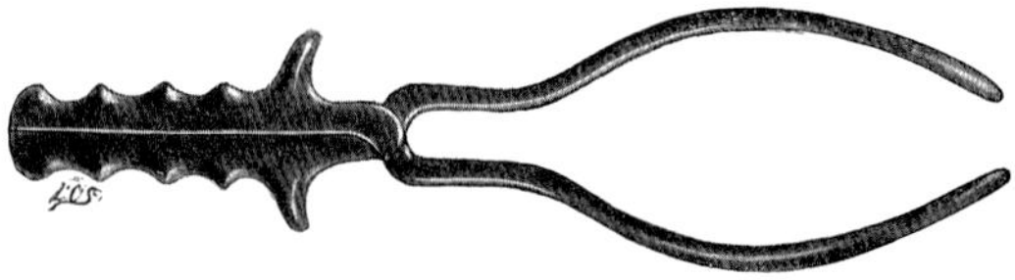

FIG. 326.—SIMPSON'S FORCEPS, CEPHALIC CURVE.

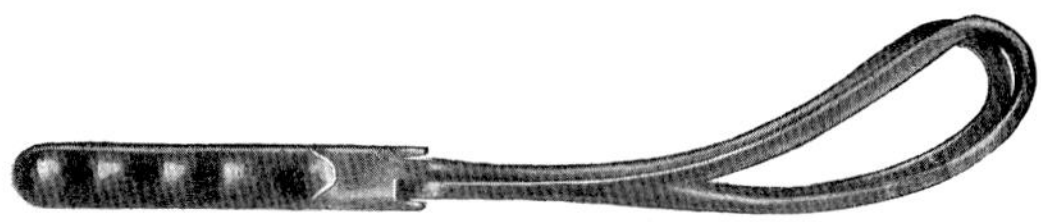

FIG. 327.—SIMPSON'S FORCEPS, PELVIC CURVE.

The cephalic curves should be such as to permit the head to be grasped firmly but without serious compression. The greatest distance between the two blades should not exceed 7.5 centimetres (3 inches) when they are articulated. The pelvic curve corresponds more or less to the axis of the birth canal, but varies considerably in different instruments. When the forceps is placed upon a plane surface, the tips of the blades should be about 8.8 centimetres ($3\frac{1}{2}$ inches) higher than the handles. The latter are connected with the blades by the shanks, which give the requisite length to the instrument.

The two branches articulate at the lock, which varies widely in different instruments. The English type consists of a socket upon each branch, into which fits the shank of the other half of the instrument. This arrangement permits of ready articulation, but does not hold the blades firmly together. In the French lock a pivot is screwed into the shank of the left branch, while the right presents an opening which can be adjusted to it, the screw being tightened after articulation. The German lock is a combination of the two, the shank of the left branch bearing a pivot with a broad, flat head, while the right is provided with a notch which corresponds to the pivot. When the instrument is properly articulated the handles should fall together in such a way as to be conveniently grasped by the operator with one hand.

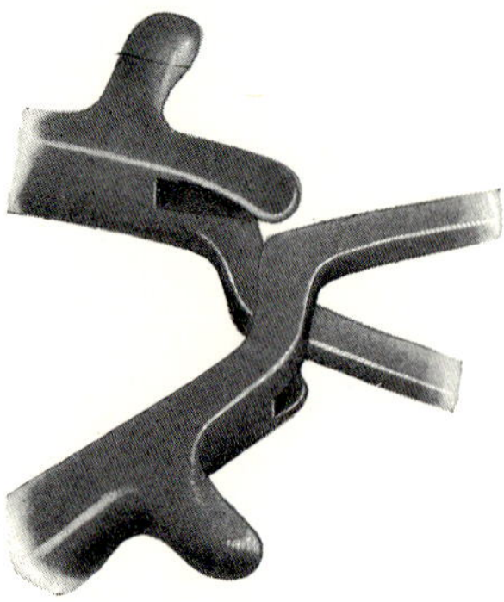

Fig. 328.—Lock of English Forceps.

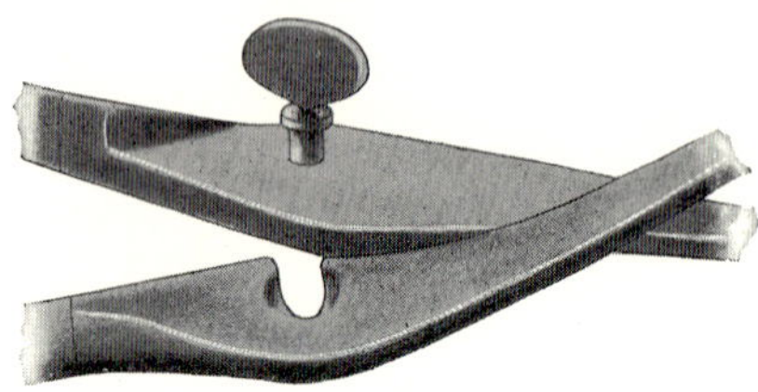

Fig. 329.—Lock of French Forceps.

History.—Crude forceps were in use from an early period, several varieties having been described by Albucasis, who died in 1112; but as their inner surfaces were provided with teeth intended to penetrate the head, it is evident that they were intended for use only upon dead children.

The true obstetrical forceps was devised in the latter part of the sixteenth or the beginning of the seventeenth century by a member of the Chamberlen family. The invention, however, was not made public at the time, but was preserved as a family secret through four generations, and did not become generally known until the early part of the eighteenth century. Prior to that time version had been the only method which permitted the artificial delivery of an unmutilated child, and, accordingly, when that operation was out of the question and delivery became imperative, it could be accomplished only by the destruction of the child, when delivery was effected by means of hooks and crotchets. Thus, before the invention of forceps, the use of instruments was synonymous with the death of the child, and frequently of the mother also, and tended to bring obstetrics into disrepute.

William Chamberlen, the founder of the family, was a French physician, who fled from France as a Huguenot refugee and landed at Southampton in 1569. He died in 1596, leaving a large family. Two of his sons, both of whom were named Peter, and designated as the elder and younger respectively, studied medicine and settled in London. They soon became successful practitioners, and devoted a large part of their attention to midwifery, in which they became very proficient. They attempted to control the instruction of midwives, and in justification of their pretensions claimed that they could successfully deliver patients when all others had failed.

The younger Peter died in 1626 and the elder in 1631. The latter left no male children, but the former was survived by several sons, one of whom, born in 1601, was likewise named Peter. To distinguish him from his father and uncle, he is usually spoken of as Dr. Peter, as the other two did not possess that title. He was well educated, having studied at Cambridge, Heidelberg, and Padua, and on his return to London was elected a Fellow of the Royal College of Physicians. He was most successful in the practice of his profession, and counted among his clients many of the royal family and nobility. Like his father and uncle, he attempted to monopolize the control of the midwives, but his pretensions were set aside by the authorities. These attempts gave rise to a great deal of discussion, and many pamphlets were written as to the morality of women in labour being attended by men, which he answered in a paper entitled "A Voice in Ramah, or the Cry of Women and Children as echoed Forth in the Compassions of Peter Chamberlen." He was a man of considerable ability, and united at the same time some of the virtues of a religious enthusiast with many of the devious qualities of a quack. He died at Woodham, Mortimer Hall, Essex, in 1683, the place remaining in the possession of his family until well into the succeeding century. Formerly he was considered the inventor of the forceps, but, as we now know, this view was incorrect.

He left a very large family, and three of his sons—Hugh, Paul, and John—became physicians, and devoted special attention to the practice of midwifery. Of these Hugh (1630–1706) was the most important and influential. Like his father, he possessed considerable ability, and at the same time took a practical interest in politics. Some of his views not being in favour, he was forced to leave England, and while in Paris in 1673 attempted to sell the family secret to Mauriceau for 10,000 livres, claiming that by its means he could deliver in a very few minutes the most difficult cases. Mauriceau placed at his disposal a rhachitic dwarf whom he had been unable to deliver, and Chamberlen, after several hours of strenuous effort, was likewise obliged to acknowledge his inability to do so. Notwithstanding his failure, however, he maintained friendly relations with Mauriceau, and on returning home translated the latter's book into English. In his preface he refers to the forceps in the following words: "My father, brothers, and myself (though none else in Europe as I know) have by God's blessing and our own industry attained to and long practised a way to deliver women in this case without prejudice to them or their infants."

Some years later he went to Holland and sold his secret to Roonhuysen. Shortly afterward the Medico-Pharmaceutical College of Amsterdam was given the sole privilege of licensing physicians to practise in Holland, to each of whom, under pledge of secrecy, was sold Chamberlen's invention for a large sum. This practice continued for a number of years, until Vischer and Van der Poll purchased the secret and made it public, when it was found that the device consisted of one blade only of the forceps. Whether this was all that Chamberlen sold to Roonhuysen, or whether the Medico-Pharmaceutical College had swindled the purchasers of the secret, is not known.

Hugh Chamberlen left a considerable family, and one of his sons—Hugh (1664–1728)—practised medicine. He was a highly educated, respected, and philanthropic physician, and numbered among his clients members of the best families in England. He was an intimate friend of the Duke of Buckingham, and when he died the latter caused a statue to be erected in his honour in Westminster Abbey. During the later years of his life he allowed the family secret to leak out, and the instrument soon came into general use.

For more than one hundred years it was believed that the forceps was the invention of Dr. Peter Chamberlen, but in the year 1813 Mrs. Kembell, the housekeeper of a rich brewer who had purchased Dr. Peter Chamberlen's country house, found in the garret a trunk containing numerous letters and instruments, among the latter being four pairs of forceps, together with several levers and fillets. As is evident from the drawings, the forceps were in different stages of development, one pair being hardly applicable to the living woman, while the others were useful instruments. Aveling, who has carefully investigated the matter, believes that the three pairs of available forceps were used respectively by the three Peters, and that in all probability the first was devised by the elder Peter, son of the original William. Probability is lent to this view by the fact that Dr. Peter, on one occasion, at least, spoke of the invention of his uncle. Sänger and Budin, who have also investigated the subject, incline to the same belief.

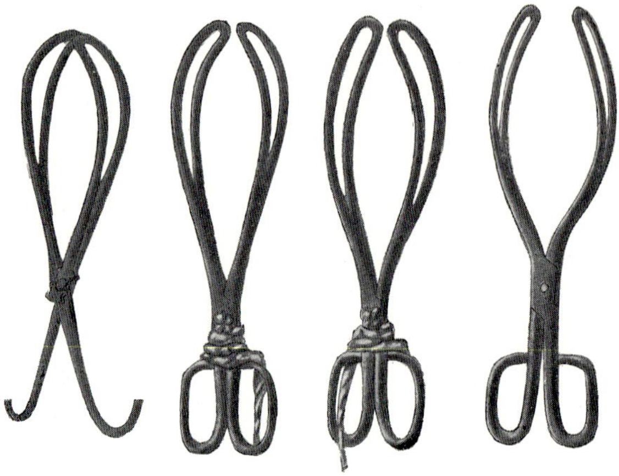

Fig. 330.—Chamberlen's Forceps.

The forceps came into general employment in England during the lifetime of Hugh Chamberlen, the younger. The instrument was used by Drinkwater, who died in 1728, and was well known to Chapman and Giffard. The former, writing in 1733, says: "The secret mentioned by Dr. Chamberlen was the use of the forceps, now well known by all the principal men of the profession, both in town and country."

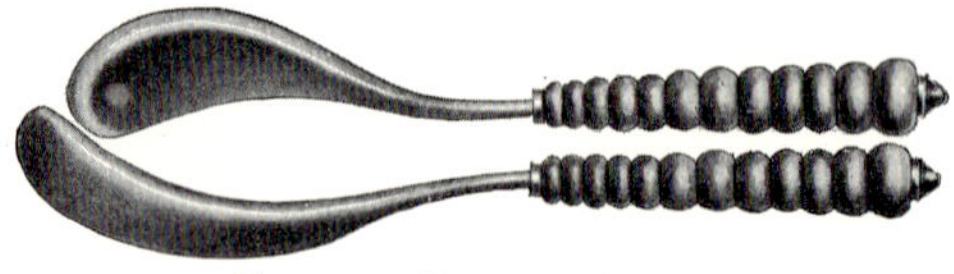

Fig. 331.—Palfyn's Forceps.

In 1723, Palfyn, a physician of Ghent, exhibited before the Paris Academy of Medicine a forceps which he designated as *mains de fer*. It was crude in shape and did not articulate. In the discussion following its presentation De la Motte stated that it would be impossible to apply it to the living woman, and added that if by chance any one should happen to invent an instrument which could be so used, and keep it secret for his own profit, he deserved to be exposed upon a barren rock and have his vitals plucked out by vultures, little knowing that at the time he spoke such an instrument had been in the possession of the Chamberlen family for nearly one hundred years.

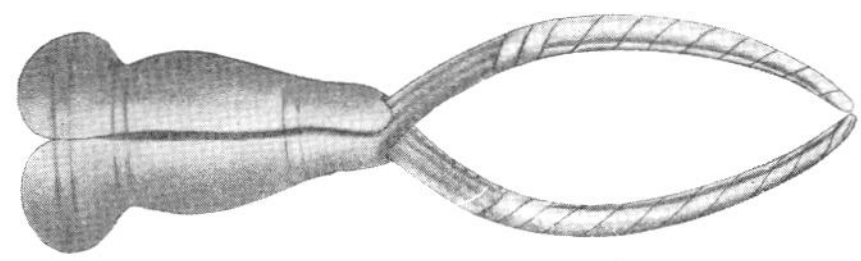

Fig. 332.—Smellie's Short Forceps.

The Chamberlen forceps was a short, straight instrument, which possessed only a cephalic curve, and is perpetuated in the short or low forceps of to-day. It was used exclusively, but with little modification, until the middle of the eighteenth century, when Levret, in 1747, and Smellie, in 1751, quite independently of one another, added the pelvic curve and increased the length of the instrument. Levret's forceps was longer and possessed a more decided pelvic curve than that of Smellie, and it is from these two instruments that the long forceps of the present day is descended—the long French forceps being the lineal descendant of the former, and that of Simpson of the latter.

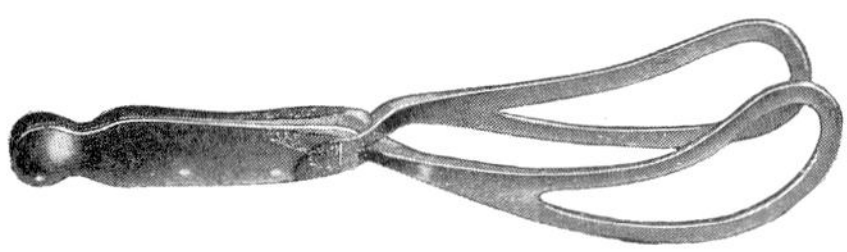

Fig. 333.—Short Forceps.

As soon as the forceps became public property it was subjected to various modifications, so that Mulder, in his atlas published in 1798, was able to give illustrations of nearly 100 varieties. Some idea of the desire to modify and improve the instrument may be gained by glancing at Witkowski's Obstetrical Arsenal, in which are pictured several hundred forceps, which, after all, constitute only a small portion of those devised. Poullet's interesting monograph contains an excellent historical sketch of the development of the instrument.

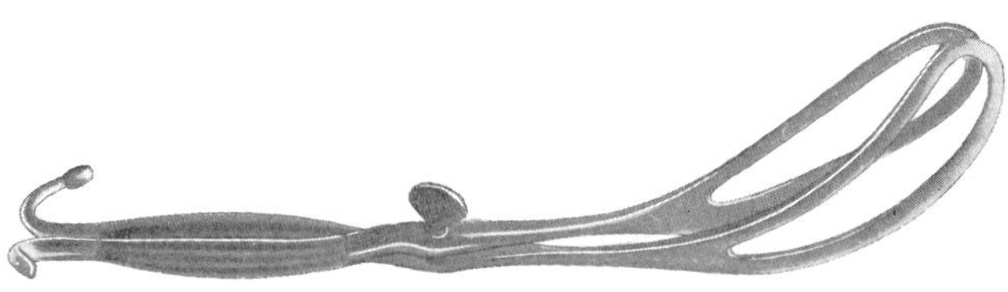

Fig. 334.—Long French Forceps (Levret).

But, considering all the work done, it is surprising how little advance was made over the instruments of Levret and Smellie until 1877, when Tarnier clearly enunciated the principle of axis traction which has since practically revolutionized our ideas upon the subject.

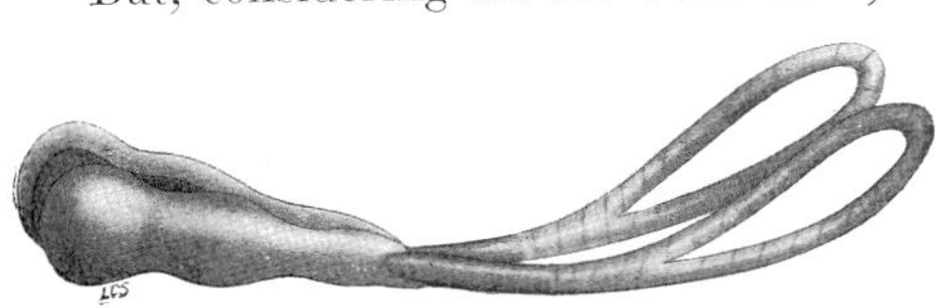

Fig. 335.—Smellie's Long Forceps.

The Choice of Forceps.—Inasmuch as it would appear that nearly every one interested in obstetrics has thought it necessary to attempt to modify the forceps and to have an instrument bearing his own name, the young physician is likely to be embarrassed by the multitude from which he has to choose. Any properly shaped instrument will give satisfactory results provided it be used intelligently, but for general purposes the ordinary Simpson forceps is probably the best, though, if one expects to do much obstetrical work, a Tarnier axis-traction forceps becomes essential. Personally I always employ the latter, using the traction rods or not, according to circumstances, as I believe it better to become thoroughly familiar with one instrument than to have several for use under different conditions.

The forceps should be entirely of metal, so that it can be readily sterilized by boiling.

Functions of the Forceps.—This subject has been considered in detail by Chassagny. The forceps may be used as a tractor, rotator, compressor, dilator, lever, or irritator.

Its most important function is traction exercised for the purpose of drawing the head through the genital tract. In not a few cases, however, particularly in occipito-posterior presentations, its employment as a rotator is attended by most happy results. It should never be used primarily as a compressor, though of course it is impossible to make traction without subjecting the head to a slight degree of compression; but when it is desired to bring about a diminution in its size other instruments are more appropriate.

Many authors, especially in this country, advocate applying the forceps through a partially obliterated cervix, and assisting dilatation by traction upon the head. Such a procedure, however, is unjustifiable, for when it becomes necessary to deliver the child under such conditions, the cervix should be stretched manually, and forceps not applied until dilatation is complete.

In rare instances, one blade of the forceps may be employed as a lever, although at present use is very seldom made of this function. Formerly great stress was laid on the so-called dynamic action of the forceps, by which is meant the irritation of the uterus which follows its introduction. Before the employment of anæsthetics, this function was of considerable importance in operative cases, but at the present day it possesses but little significance.

Indications for the Use of Forceps.—Strictly speaking, the termination of labour by forceps, provided it can be accomplished without too great danger, is indicated in any condition which threatens the life of the mother or child. On the part of the mother, such conditions are eclampsia, heart lesions attended by broken compensation, acute œdema of the lungs, hæmorrhage from premature separation of the placenta, intrapartum infection, or exhaustion. Whenever there is question of interference for the last-named condition, definite objective symptoms should be present, the condition of the pulse being of especial importance; whereas, on the other hand, but little weight should be attached to the statements of the patient.

As regards the child, the operation may be called for by prolapse of the umbilical cord, premature separation of the placenta, undue pressure exerted upon the head, and especially by changes in the rhythm of its heart-beat and the escape of meconium in vertex presentations. A fœtal pulse falling below 100, or exceeding 160 to the minute, indicates that the child is in danger and will perish if not promptly delivered. In vertex presentations the discharge of amniotic fluid tinged with meconium indicates interference with the placental circulation and imperfect oxygenation, manifesting itself by paralysis of the sphincter ani. In breech presentations, on the other hand, the presence of meconium is without significance, being due merely to pressure exerted upon the child's abdomen.

In practice, however, the maternal indications for the use of forceps may be considerably extended, and in many instances the operation may be advisable in the case of women suffering from acute infectious diseases, heart lesions, and diseases of the respiratory tract, who must be saved as far as possible from the exhaustion incident to an unaided second stage of labour. Occasionally also it may appear wise to relieve the strain upon a cicatrix resulting from a recent abdominal section.

One of the most frequent indications for the operation is afforded by faulty contraction of the uterine or abdominal muscles, the forceps being utilized merely to re-enforce the insufficient *vis-a-tergo*. In occasional instances, particularly in elderly primiparæ, the resistance offered by the perinæum and the vaginal outlet may be so great as to oppose a serious obstacle to the passage of the child, even when the expulsive forces are normal. In uncomplicated cases it is a good practical rule to apply forceps if advance does not occur after two hours of satisfactory second stage pains, but if the head is upon the perinæum and no progress has been made for one hour in spite of good pains, it is usually not advisable to wait much longer. At the same time it must be insisted upon that the operation should never be performed to save the physician's time, but only when distinctly indicated by the condition of the mother or child.

The following conditions must be fulfilled before forceps can be applied with safety: (1) The child must present correctly; (2) the cervix must be fully dilated or dilatable; (3) the membranes must be ruptured; (4) the head of the child must be neither too large nor too small; and (5) the pelvis must not be contracted.

The child should present by the vertex or face, and an accurate diagnosis be made as to the position and variety, forceps not being available when the chin is directly posterior. The forceps is not applicable to transverse or shoulder presentations, nor is it intended to be applied to the breech. It should not be employed in brow cases until after conversion into a vertex or face presentation has been brought about.

The cervix must always be completely dilated before the application of forceps, offering a diameter of from 9 to 10 centimetres. Of course it is possible to apply the blades through a canal measuring only 4 or 5 centimetres, but under such circumstances the cervical ring offers marked resistance, and if the head be dragged through it by brute force deep tears may result, which may implicate not only the cervix but also the lower uterine segment. Even if only gentle traction is made, the practice is not to be recommended, as it is difficult to know exactly when the cervix has become sufficiently wide to permit the passage of the head, and the operator is prone to attempt delivery before complete dilatation. Accordingly, if prompt delivery becomes imperative when the cervix is only partially dilated, its complete dilatation should be effected manually by Harris's method, after which delivery may be accomplished with forceps if the head is deeply engaged. On the other hand, if it is only partially engaged, or is floating above the superior strait, delivery is best effected after podalic version.

The membranes should always be ruptured before applying forceps, as the instrument is intended to be applied directly to the child's head. If the membranes intervene, the grasp is not so firm, and, what is still more important, traction upon them may bring about premature separation of the placenta.

Before applying forceps, particularly when engagement has not yet occurred, the size of the head should be determined as accurately as possible, for if it be unduly large, as in an excessively developed or hydrocephalic child, it cannot pass the superior strait. On the other hand, if it be abnormally small, it cannot be properly grasped, since the blades will slip off when traction is made. Accordingly, the employment of forceps is contra-indicated when the fœtus is premature or macerated.

Generally speaking, contracted pelves present an absolute contra-indication to the application of forceps; for if the contraction be marked it will be impossible to drag the head through the pelvis, and if brute force be employed it will result in the death of the child and severe injuries to the soft parts of the mother, and occasionally cause her death. On the other hand, when the contraction is but slight, and especially when the head is firmly engaged in the upper part of the pelvic cavity, the tentative application of forceps may be justifiable. Under such circumstances a few tractions of moderate intensity should be made; if the head follows them they should be continued, but if not the forceps should be removed and delivery effected in some other manner.

Preparations for Operation.—When the application of forceps becomes necessary, either in the interests of the mother or child, the physician should so inform a responsible member of the family. It is usually not

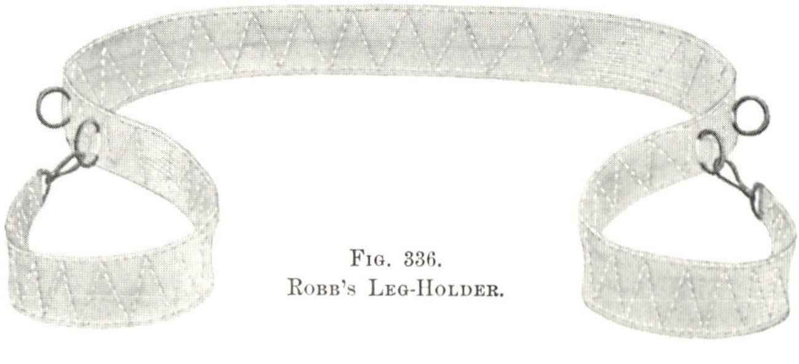

Fig. 336.
Robb's Leg-Holder.

advisable to consult the patient upon the subject, as she is not in a condition to make an intelligent decision.

If the operation promises to be easy it may be performed upon the bed, but in all other cases, whenever possible, the patient should be placed upon a table of suitable height. Anæsthesia should always be employed, and whenever practicable its administration should be intrusted to a competent assistant, rather than to the nurse or some member of the family, since in the latter case a large part of the obstetrician's attention must of necessity be devoted to watching the general condition instead of being concentrated upon the operation.

When anæsthesia is complete, the patient's buttocks should be brought to the edge of the bed or table, and her legs held in position by an appropriate leg-holder, which is particularly convenient in private practice, as it enables one to dispense with assistants for holding the legs. After the pubic hairs have been shaved, the genitalia should be thoroughly washed with soap and hot water, bathed with alcohol, and thoroughly soaked in a 1-to-1,000 bichloride solution. Disinfection of the vagina is not necessary unless the patient is infected or has been subjected to previous attempts at delivery. The legs and body should be covered with sterile towels in such a manner as to leave only the genitalia exposed, special attention being given to covering the anus so as to prevent contamination from the fæces. (See Figs. 317 and 318.)

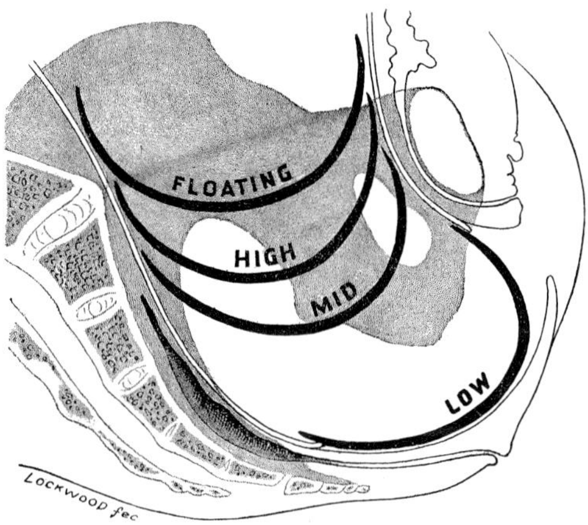

FIG. 337.—DIAGRAM SHOWING POSITION OF HEAD IN VARIOUS FORCEPS OPERATIONS.

If the outlet be small and rigid, it is advisable to dilate it by means of the hand before beginning the operation. For this purpose the fingers, anointed with sterile vaseline, are arranged in the form of a cone, and with a rotary motion slowly introduced through the vulva until the entire hand can readily be carried up into the vagina.

Application of Forceps.—Forceps operations are designated as low, mid, high, and floating, according to the position of the head. When the presenting part rests upon the perinæum, or lies below the line joining the ischial spines, we speak of *low forceps*; when it presents at or just above the ischial spines, *mid forceps*; when the head has partially descended into the pelvic canal, but its greatest circumference has not passed the superior strait, *high forceps*; and when it is freely movable above the pelvic brim the operation is termed *forceps upon the floating head.*

The low forceps operation usually offers but little difficulty, and may be undertaken upon comparatively slight indications. The mid operation is more difficult, but not often excessively so. On the other hand, the high operation is always difficult, and should not be attempted unless imperatively demanded by the condition of the mother or child. Forceps upon the floating head is a most serious procedure, and is very rarely indicated. Generally speaking, the fact that the head is not engaged indicates some disproportion between it and the superior strait, so that the operation should not be thought of until accurate information as to the size of both is available. Moreover, in those cases in which there is no serious disproportion, and in which the operation appears feasible, delivery can usually be accomplished more safely and rapidly by version.

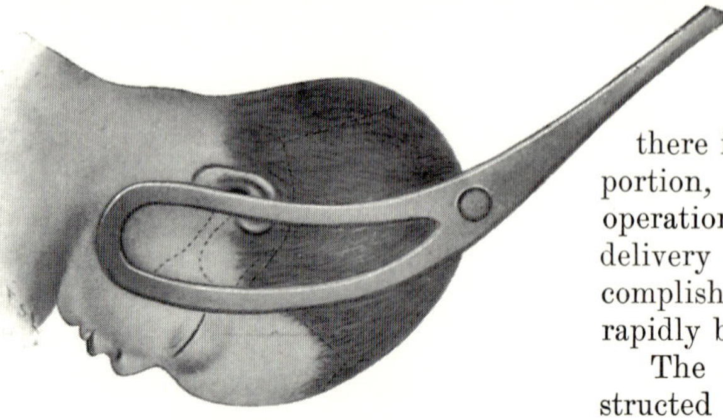

FIG. 338.—FORCEPS CORRECTLY APPLIED ALONG OCCIPITO-MENTAL DIAMETER, PELVIC CURVE TOWARDS OCCIPUT.

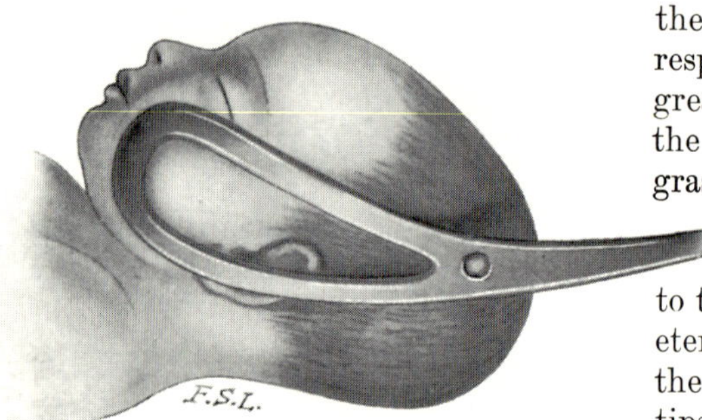

FIG. 339.—FORCEPS CORRECTLY APPLIED ALONG OCCIPITO-MENTAL DIAMETER, PELVIC CURVE TOWARDS FACE.

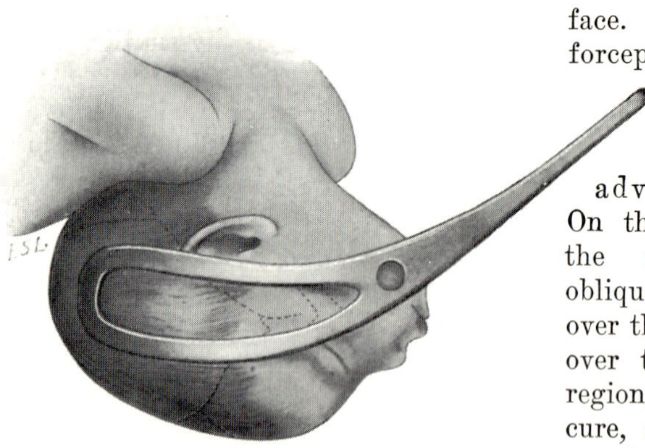

FIG. 340.—FORCEPS APPLIED TO FACE ALONG OCCIPITO-MENTAL DIAMETER.

The forceps is so constructed that its cephalic curve is best adapted to the sides of the child's head, the biparietal diameter corresponding to the line of greatest distance between the blades. The head is grasped in an ideal manner when the long axis of the blades corresponds to the occipito-mental diameter, the fenestra including the parietal bosses and the tips lying over the cheeks, while the concave margins of the blades look towards either the occiput or the face. With such a grasp the forceps obtains a firm hold and cannot slip off, and traction can be made in the most advantageous manner. On the other hand, when the forceps is applied obliquely with one blade over the brow and the other over the opposite mastoid region, the grasp is less secure, and the head is exposed to more injurious pressure. If one blade is accurately applied over the face and the other over the occiput, the instrument cannot be locked, while if the former is slipped down so as to lie only over the forehead, the grasp is very insecure, and each traction tends to extend the head (see Figs. 342 and 343).

For these reasons, then, the forceps should be applied, when possible, directly to the sides of the head along its *occipito-mental* or *jugo-parietal diameter*. This is known as the *cephalic*, in contra-distinction to the *pelvic application*. The former was recommended by Smellie and Baudelocque, but, as it

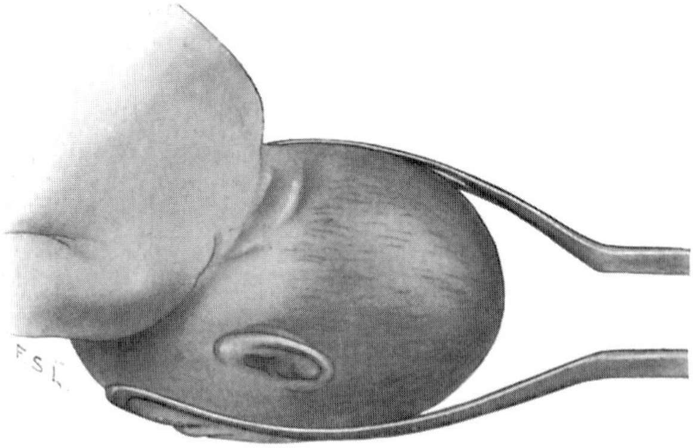

FIG. 341.—FORCEPS APPLIED OBLIQUELY OVER BROW AND MASTOID REGION.

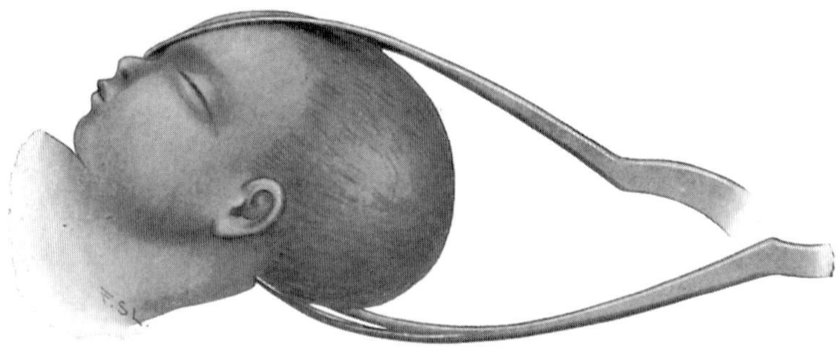

FIG. 342.—SHOWING THAT WHEN ONE BLADE IS APPLIED OVER OCCIPUT AND OTHER OVER THE FACE, FORCEPS CANNOT BE LOCKED.

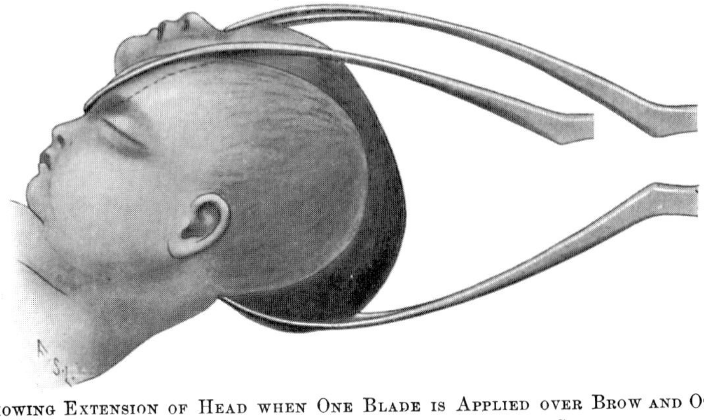

FIG. 343.—SHOWING EXTENSION OF HEAD WHEN ONE BLADE IS APPLIED OVER BROW AND OTHER OVER OCCIPUT, EXPLAINING TENDENCY OF THE INSTRUMENT TO SLIP OFF.

is more difficult than the latter, it fell into disuse, and was not generally practised until Pinard, Farabeuf and Varnier demonstrated the inestimable advantages which it possessed over the pelvic application. In the latter the left blade is applied to the left and the right blade to the right side of the mother's pelvis, no matter what the presentation, consequently the head is grasped obliquely, unless the sagittal suture is directed antero-posteriorly.

An accurate idea of the exact position of the head is absolutely essential to the cephalic application. With the head resting upon the perinæum this can usually be obtained by examining with two fingers; but when it is higher up an absolute diagnosis can be made only *by locating the posterior ear*, which usually necessitates the introduction of four fingers or the entire hand into the vagina. This, of course, requires profound anæsthesia, and is therefore practicable only just before introducing the forceps. Ordinarily, after locating the ear, the examining hand is not removed, but remains in place to serve as a guide for the introduction of the first blade, which should be applied over the posterior ear no matter whether it be the right or left. This rule admits of exception in two instances only—namely, when the head is resting upon the perinæum, when the sagittal suture usually extends antero-posteriorly, or when it is movable at the pelvic brim. Faulty diagnosis not infrequently gives rise to an improper application of forceps, and is one of the most frequent factors in converting what should be an extremely simple procedure into a serious and difficult operation.

Forceps Delivery with the Head at the Vulva.—With the head in this position, the obstacle to delivery is usually due to insufficient expulsive force or to abnormal resistance on the part of the perinæum. Under such circumstances the sagittal suture usually occupies the antero-posterior

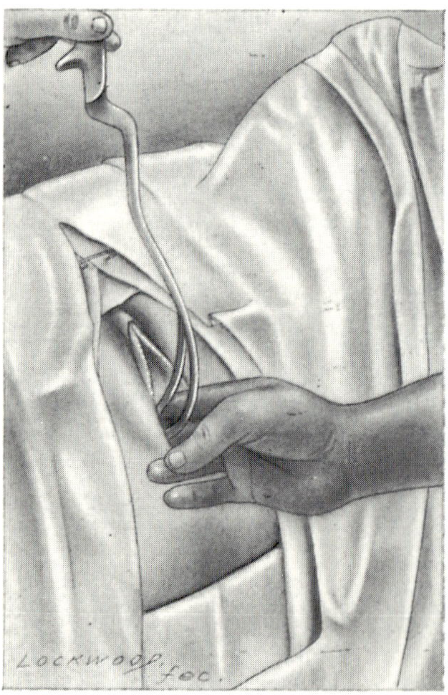

Fig. 344.—Low Forceps, Introduction of Left Blade to Left Side of Pelvis.

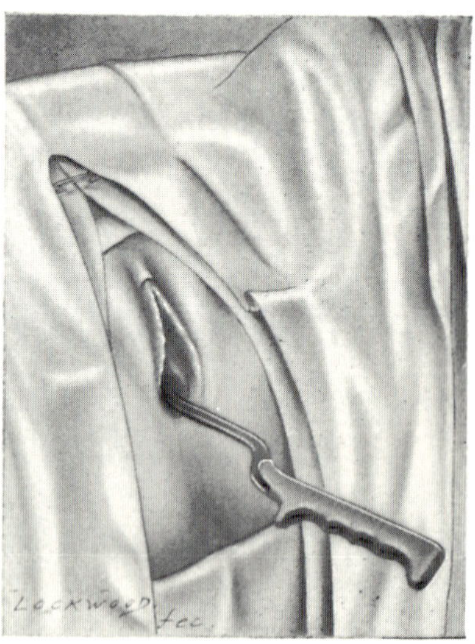

Fig. 345.—Low Forceps, Left Blade in Place.

diameter of the pelvic outlet, with the small fontanelle directed towards either the symphysis pubis or the concavity of the sacrum. In either event the forceps, if applied to the sides of the pelvis, will grasp the head in an ideal manner. Accordingly, the left blade is introduced to the left and the right blade to the right side of the pelvis, the mode of procedure being somewhat as follows: Two fingers of the right hand are passed into the left and posterior portion of the vulva and carried up the vagina to the region of the internal os. The handle of the left branch is then seized between the thumb and two fingers of the left hand—just as in holding a pen—and the tip of the blade is gently passed into the vagina along the fingers of the right hand which serve as a guide. As it is introduced the handle is held almost vertically at first, but as the blade adapts itself to the head it is depressed, so that it eventually takes a horizontal position. The guiding fingers are then withdrawn, and the handle is left to itself or held by an assistant. In the same manner, two fingers of the left hand are then introduced through the right and posterior portion of the vulva to serve as a guide for the right blade, which is held in the right hand and introduced into the vagina. The guiding fingers are now removed and all that remains to be done is to articulate the branches. Usually they lie in such a manner that they can be locked without difficulty; but when this cannot be done, first one and then the other blade should be gently moved until they are brought into such a position as to be articulated with ease.

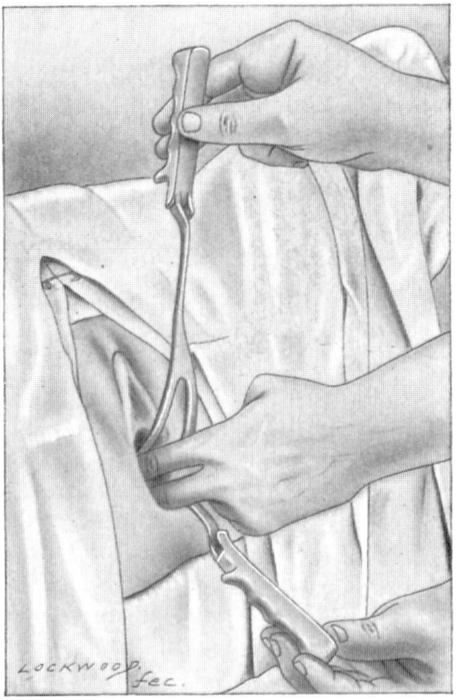

FIG. 346.—LOW FORCEPS, LEFT BLADE IN PLACE, INTRODUCTION OF RIGHT BLADE.

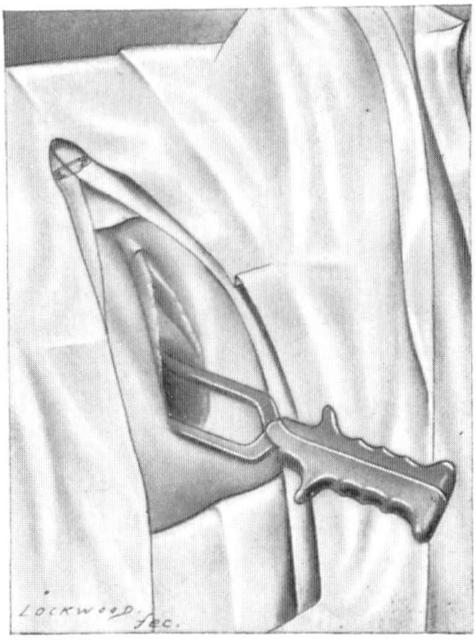

FIG. 347.—LOW FORCEPS; INSTRUMENT IN PLACE AND ARTICULATED.

When this has been accomplished, an examination is made to ascertain whether the blades have been correctly applied, or whether they inclose the lips of the cervix. In the latter case the forceps should be loosened and reapplied. When we are certain that the blades are satisfactorily placed, the handles are seized with one hand and gentle intermittent traction is made in a horizontal direction until the perinæum begins to bulge. As soon as the vulva becomes distended by the occiput, the handles are gradually elevated so that they come almost in contact with the abdomen of the patient as the parietal bosses emerge. During the latter manœuvre the four fingers should grasp the upper surface of the handles and shanks, while the thumb up their lower surface exerts the necessary force.

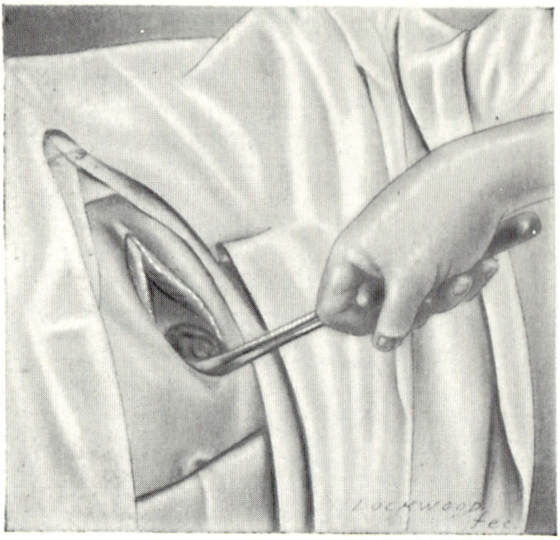

Fig. 348.—Low Forceps; Horizontal Traction.

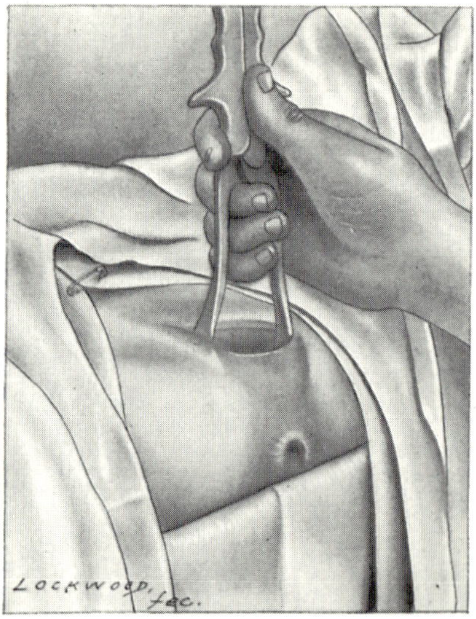

Fig. 349.—Low Forceps; Upward Traction.

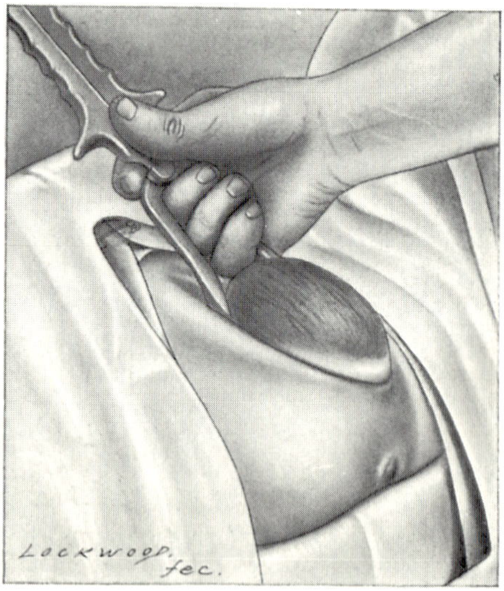

Fig. 350.—Low Forceps; Extreme Upward Traction.

In delivering the head nature's method should be simulated as closely as possible. Accordingly, traction should be made intermittently, the head being allowed to recede in the intervals, as in spontaneous labour. Except when urgently indicated, it should be extracted very slowly, so as to give time for proper stretching and dilatation of the perinæum, which in primiparous women cannot be satisfactorily accomplished in less than from fifteen to twenty minutes.

Many authors recommend removing the forceps as soon as the vulva is distended by the head, and slowly expressing it by pressure upon the posterior portion of the perinæum, in the belief that by so doing the liability to perineal rupture is diminished. It is my practice, however, to leave the forceps in place until the head is completely born, since in this way it is possible to exercise far more control over its advance, the increased distention of the vulva due to the thickness of the blades being so slight as to be without practical importance.

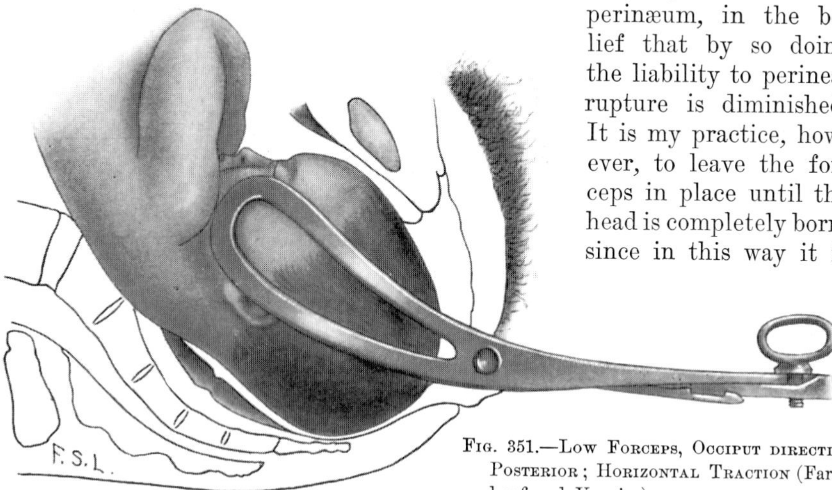

FIG. 351.—LOW FORCEPS, OCCIPUT DIRECTLY POSTERIOR; HORIZONTAL TRACTION (Farabeuf and Varnier).

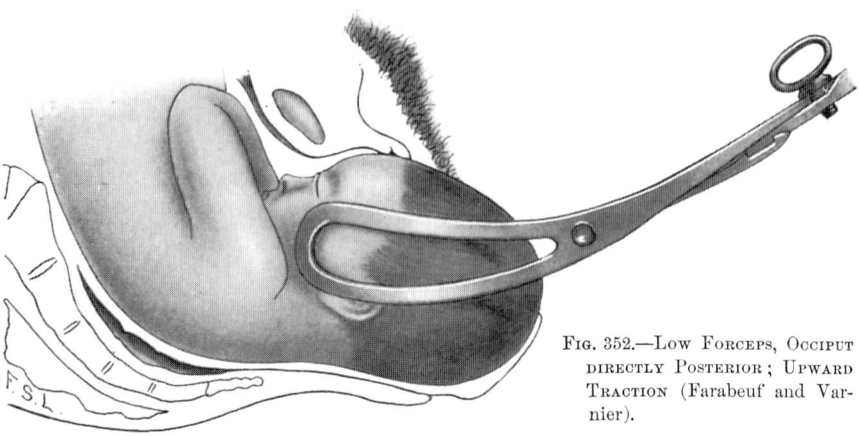

FIG. 352.—LOW FORCEPS, OCCIPUT DIRECTLY POSTERIOR; UPWARD TRACTION (Farabeuf and Varnier).

When the occiput is directed posteriorly, traction should be made in a downward direction until the forehead or root of the nose engages under the symphysis, after which the handles should be slowly elevated, when the bregma, followed by the occiput, slowly emerges over the anterior margin of the perinæum. In these cases extraction is more difficult than when the occiput is anterior, and owing to the larger circumference of the head, which distends the vulva, is more liable to give rise to perineal tears.

Mid Forceps Operations.—When the head lies above the perinæum, the sagittal suture usually occupies an oblique or transverse diameter of the pelvic canal. In such cases the forceps should be applied to the sides of the head. This is best accomplished by introducing two or more fingers into the vagina sufficiently deeply to feel the posterior ear, over which, no matter whether it be the right or left, the first blade should be applied.

In left occipito-anterior positions, the entire right hand introduced into the left posterior segment of the pelvis should locate the posterior ear, and at the same time serve as a guide for the introduction of the left branch of the forceps, which is held in the left hand and applied over the posterior

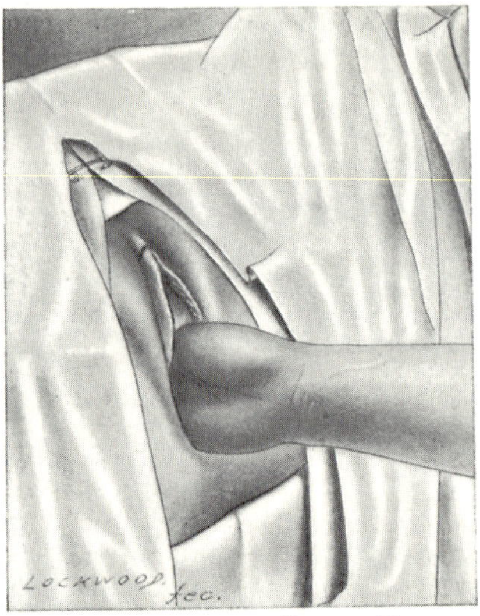

Fig. 353.—Mid Forceps, Hand in Vagina seeking Posterior Ear.

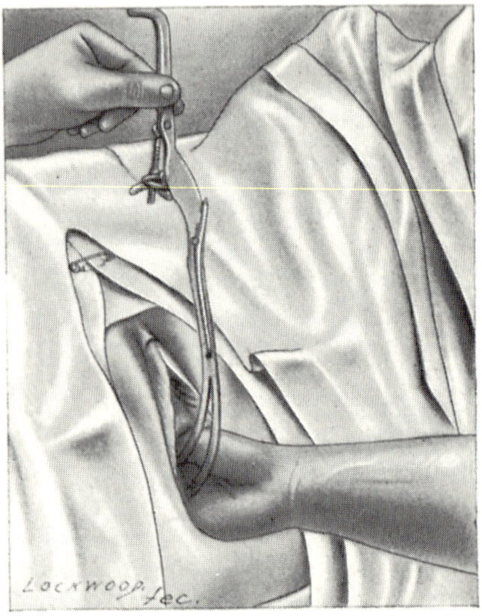

Fig. 354.—Mid Forceps, Introduction of First Blade.

ear. The guide hand is then withdrawn, when the handle of the forceps may be held by an assistant or left to itself, as it will usually retain its position without difficulty.

Two fingers of the left hand are then introduced into the right and posterior segment of the genital canal, no attempt being made to reach the anterior ear, which lies in the neighbourhood of the right ilio-pectineal eminence. The right branch of the forceps, held in the right hand, is then introduced along the left hand as a guide. After its introduction it still remains to apply it over the anterior ear of the child. This is accomplished by gently rotating it anteriorly until it comes to lie directly opposite the blade which was first introduced. The two branches being now articulated, one blade of the forceps occupies the posterior and the other the anterior extremity of the left oblique diameter (see Figs. 354 to 357).

If the head is in the left transverse position, the forceps is introduced in a similar manner, the first blade being applied over the posterior ear, and the second being rotated anteriorly until it comes to lie opposite the first. In this case one blade lies in front of the sacrum and the other behind the symphysis.

In the right positions, the blades are introduced in a similar manner but in opposite directions, for in this case the right is the posterior ear, over which the first blade must be applied (see Figs. 358 to 360).

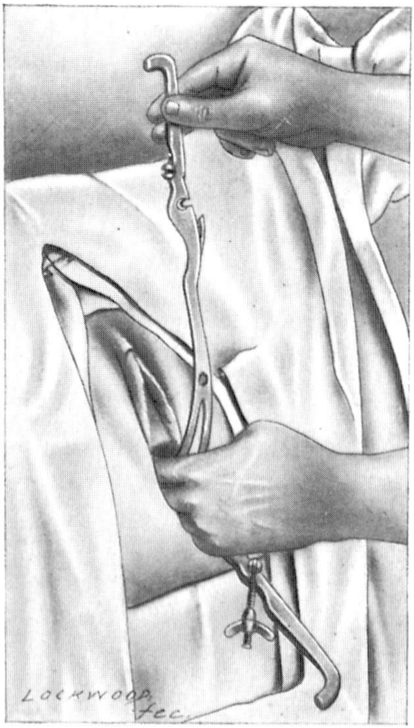

FIG. 355.—MID FORCEPS, INTRODUCTION OF SECOND BLADE.

Whatever the original position of the head may be, delivery is effected by making traction obliquely downward until the occiput appears at the vulva, the rest of the operation being completed in the manner already described. When the occiput is obliquely anterior it gradually rotates spontaneously to the symphysis pubis as traction is made. But when it is directed transversely, it is sometimes necessary to impart a rotary motion to the forceps while making traction in order to bring it to the front. The direction in which this is to be made varies, of course, according to the position of the occiput, rotation from the left side towards the middle line being necessary when the occiput is directed towards the left, and in the reverse direction when it is directed towards the right side of the pelvis (see Figs. 358 to 360).

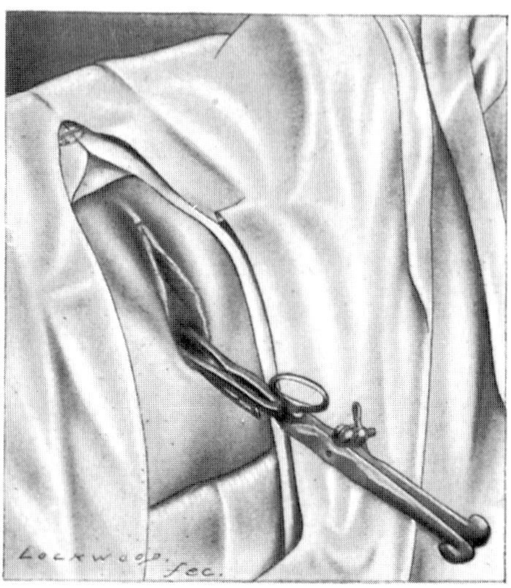

Fig. 356.

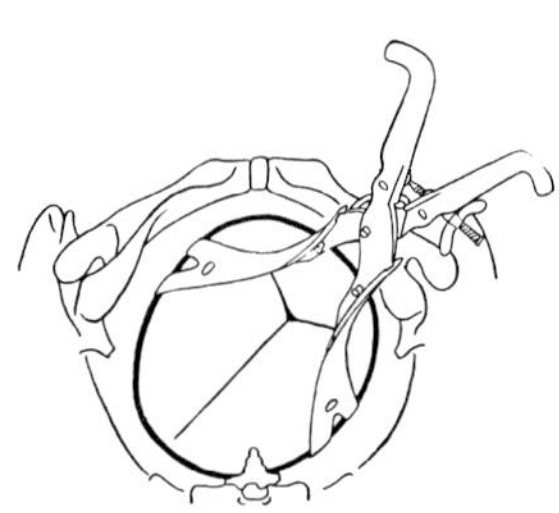

Fig. 357.

FIGS. 356, 357.—MID FORCEPS, INSTRUMENT APPLIED IN L. O. I. A.

In making traction, before the head appears at the vulva, one or both hands may be employed according to the amount of force required. In the latter case, when the Simpson forceps is used, one hand grasps the handles of the instrument, while the fingers of the other are hooked over the transverse projection at their upper ends. Care must be taken not to employ too much force. To avoid this error the operator should stand or sit with his arms flexed and the elbows held closely against the thorax, as it is not permissible to make use of the body weight, and still less to brace the feet against the side of the bed (Fig. 361).

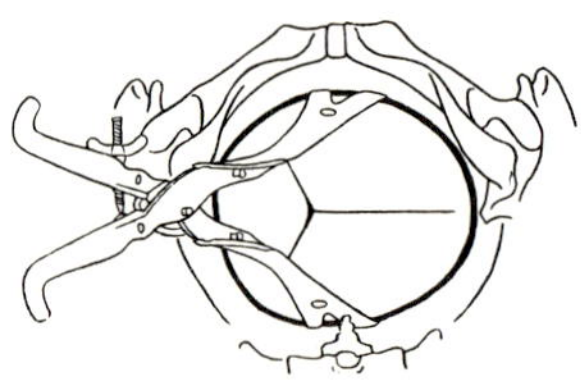

Fig. 358.

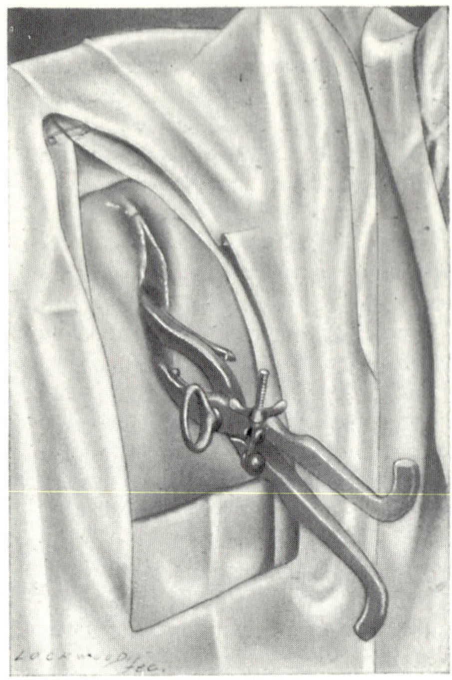

Fig. 359.

Figs. 358, 359.—Mid Forceps, Instrument Applied in R. O. I. T.

Application of Forceps in Obliquely Posterior Positions.—Prompt delivery frequently becomes necessary when the small fontanelle is directed towards one or other sacro-iliac synchondrosis—namely, in R. O. I. P. and L. O. I. P. presentations. When interference is required in either of these, the head usually lies at or below the level of the ischial spines, and is usually imperfectly flexed.

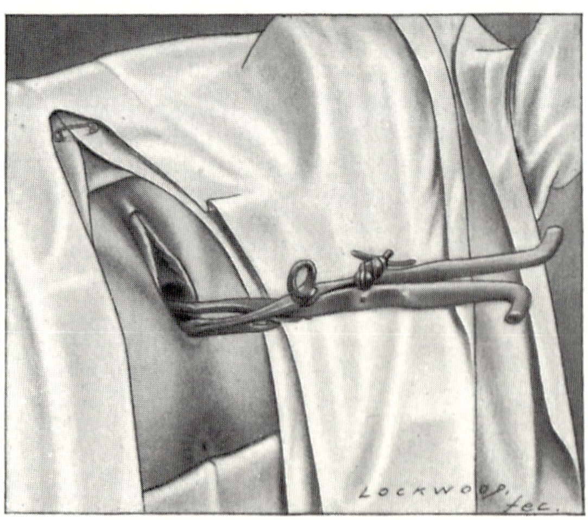

Fig. 360.—Mid Forceps, Rotation to R. O. I.

In many cases, when the hand is introduced to locate the posterior ear, the occiput will rotate spontaneously from a posterior to a transverse position, and delivery by forceps is then readily accomplished, as already described. If, however, rotation does not occur, the head should be seized, with four fingers over its posterior and the thumb over its anterior

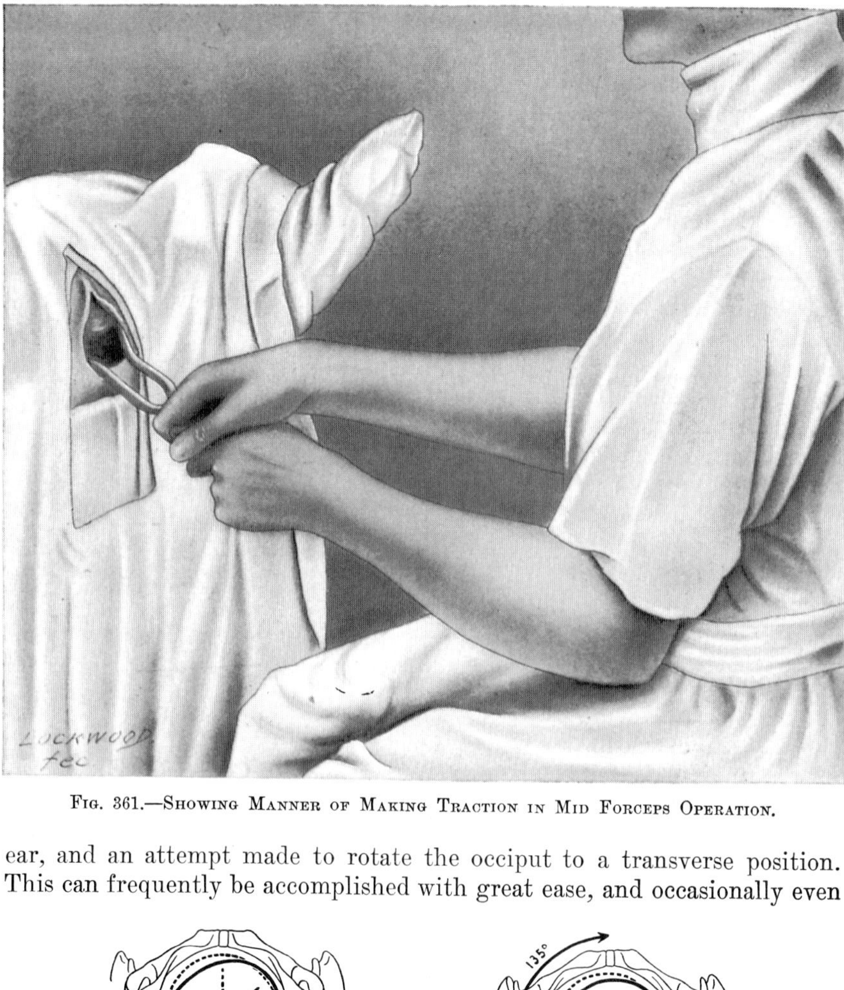

Fig. 361.—Showing Manner of Making Traction in Mid Forceps Operation.

ear, and an attempt made to rotate the occiput to a transverse position. This can frequently be accomplished with great ease, and occasionally even

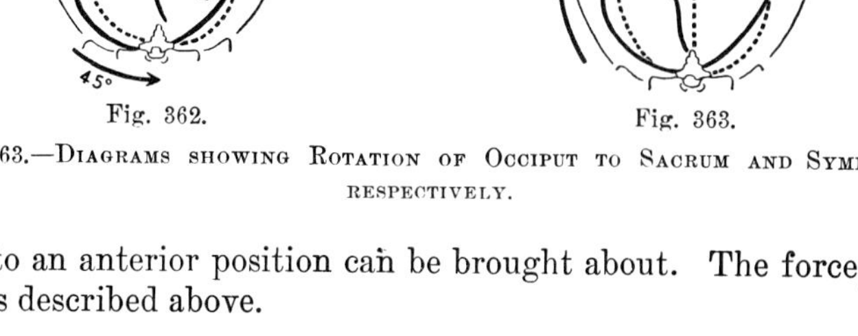

Fig. 362. Fig. 363.

Figs. 362, 363.—Diagrams showing Rotation of Occiput to Sacrum and Symphysis Pubis respectively.

rotation to an anterior position can be brought about. The forceps is then applied as described above.

In a certain number of cases, however, manual rotation cannot be effected, and the forceps must then be applied with the occiput still directed obliquely posterior. Under these circumstances, if the instrument be applied to the sides of the head, or even obliquely, and an attempt made to effect delivery by making traction in the usual manner, great difficulty is experienced and very powerful traction becomes necessary, which, nevertheless, usually fails to bring about the desired result. It is this experience which has given rise to the great dread in which these presentations are generally held, and it is a very good practical rule whenever unexpected difficulty is experienced in delivering what is apparently a simple anterior presentation, to think of the possibility of a mistake in diagnosis and to re-examine the patient. In the vast majority of such cases the small fontanelle will be found directed towards one or other sacro-iliac synchondrosis.

In order for delivery to occur the head must rotate so as to bring its sagittal suture into coincidence with the antero-posterior diameter of the pelvic outlet. This can be accomplished by rotating the occiput by means of the forceps, either through an arc of 45 degrees to the hollow of the sacrum, or through one of 135 degrees to the symphysis pubis. The latter is preferable, for the reason that delivery in the former position is more difficult and also more likely to give rise to deep perineal tears (Figs. 362 and 363).

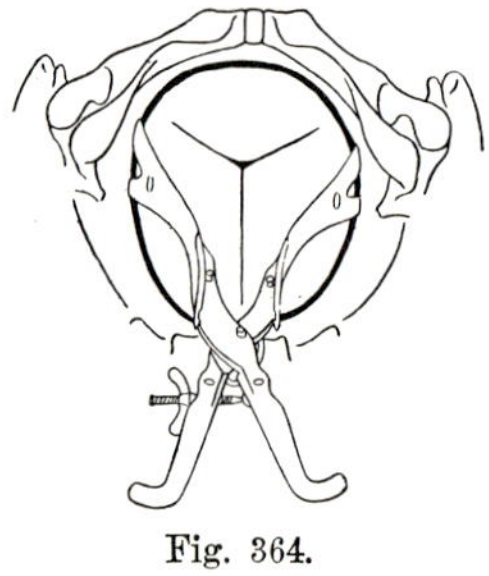

Fig. 364.

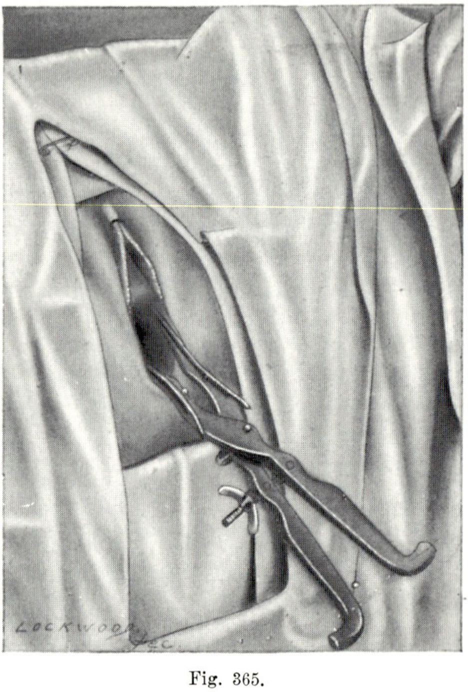

Fig. 365.

Figs. 364, 365.—Showing Inversion of Forceps when Anterior Rotation is attempted in an R. O. I. P. Position, without reapplying the Instrument.

Unfortunately, when it is desired to rotate the occiput forward, the forceps, if applied to the sides of the head in the usual manner, with the pelvic curvature directed forward, becomes inverted by the time rotation is completed, so that the pelvic curve looks posteriorly, and an attempted delivery with the instrument in this position is liable to cause serious injury to the maternal soft parts (Figs. 364 and 365). In order to avoid this, it is best to remove and reapply the instrument. If one wishes to avoid this double application, the head may be seized obliquely with one blade over the anterior brow and the other over the posterior mastoid region; but this procedure is much more difficult for the operator and far more dangerous for the child.

The *double application of forceps* in this class of cases was recommended by Scanzoni many

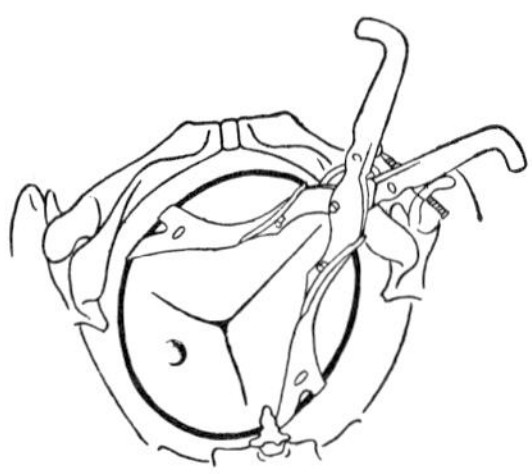

Fig. 366.

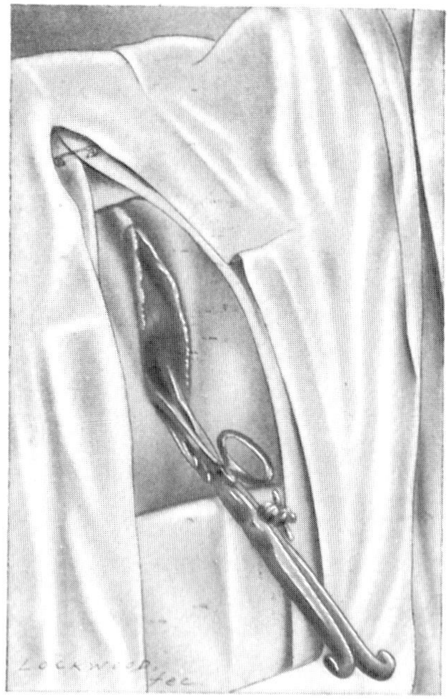

Fig. 367.

FIGS. 366, 367.—SCANZONI'S MANŒUVRE, FIRST APPLICATION OF FORCEPS.

years ago, and in my hands has given such excellent results that I employ it to the exclusion of all other methods. As the right occipito-iliac posterior occurs far more frequently than the left variety, I shall describe in detail the procedure indicated in the former.

In the first step of the operation, the blades are applied to the sides of the head with the pelvic curve looking towards the face of the child, whereas in the second manipulation it looks towards the occiput. For the

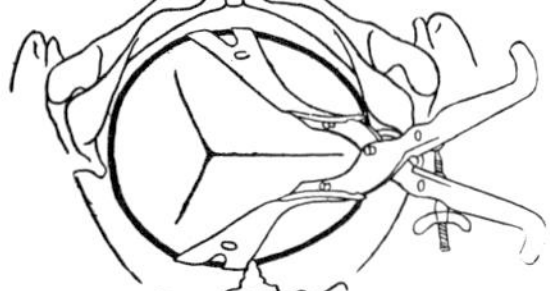

Fig. 368.

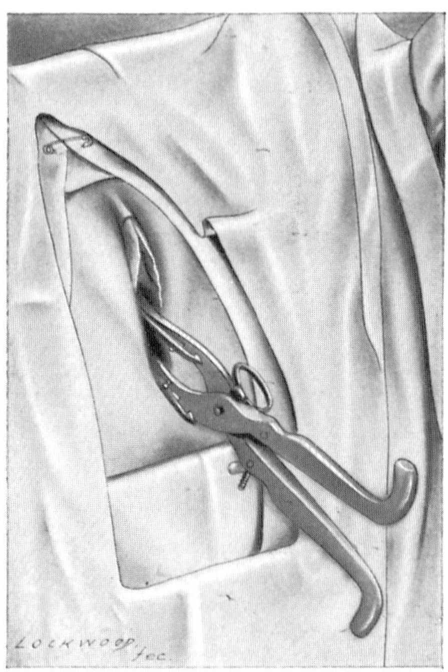

Fig. 369.

FIGS. 368, 369.—SCANZONI'S MANŒUVRE, SHOWING ROTATION TO TRANSVERSE POSITION.

first application (Figs. 366 and 367) the right hand is passed into the left posterior segment of the genital tract, and the posterior (right) ear sought for. Over it the left blade is applied. This is held in position by an assistant, while the operator's left hand is passed into the right side of the vagina and over it is introduced the right blade, which is then rotated anteriorly until it

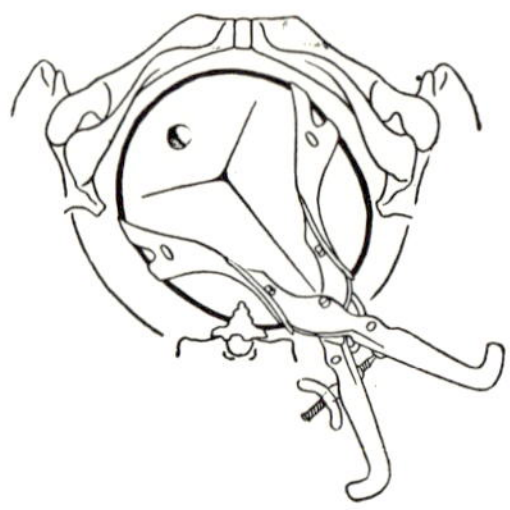

Fig. 370.

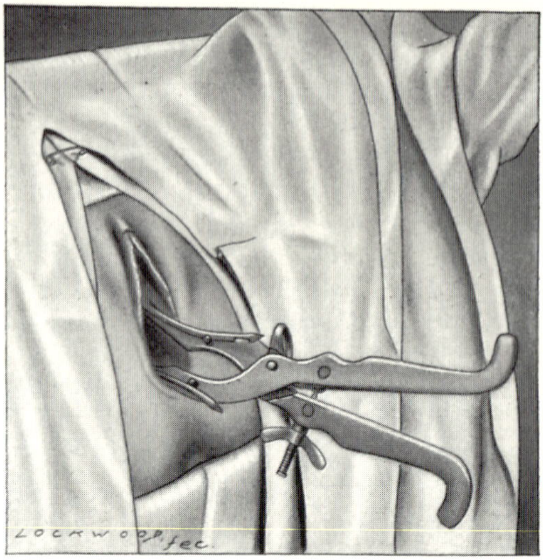

Fig. 371.

FIGS. 370, 371.—SCANZONI'S MANŒUVRE, SHOWING ROTATION TO ANTERIOR POSITION; FORCEPS INVERTED.

comes to lie opposite the blade first introduced. The forceps is then locked, its blades now occupying the left and the sagittal suture the right oblique diameter of the pelvis. Downward traction is then made until the head impinges upon the pelvic floor, when a rotary motion is imparted to the forceps by which the occiput is slowly rotated to a right transverse, and later on to an obliquely anterior position (see Figs. 368 and 370).

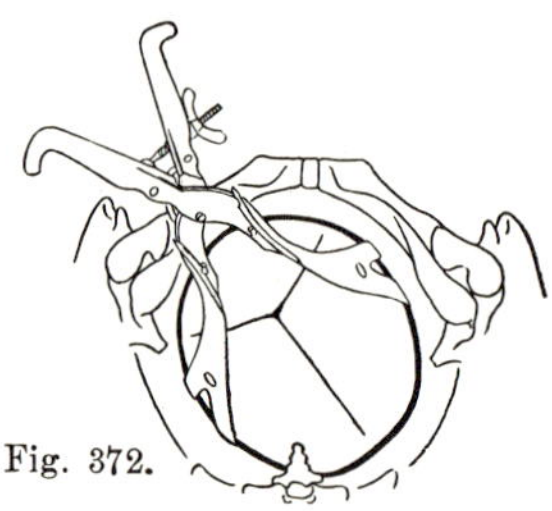

Fig. 372.

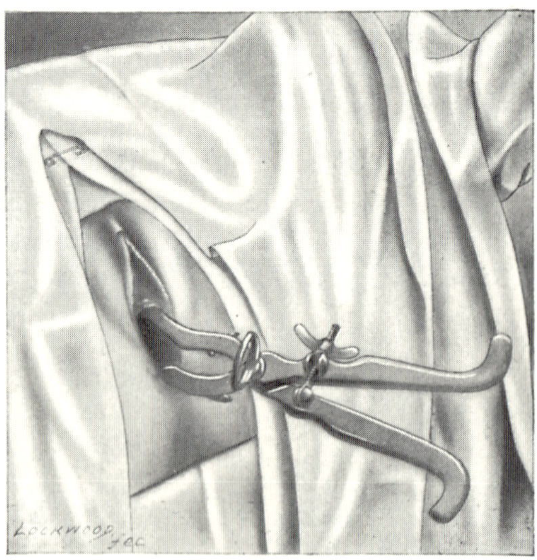

Fig. 373.

FIGS. 372, 373.—SCANZONI'S MANŒUVRE, SECOND APPLICATION OF FORCEPS.

The forceps having become inverted must be taken off, and reapplied in the usual manner to the head, which now occupies a right anterior position, when delivery is readily accomplished. Some difficulty may arise in bringing about proper articulation, since the handle of the left branch lying above the right cannot be locked, but this can be readily overcome by rotating the former around the latter so as to bring the lock into proper position (see Fig. 374). In left positions the blades are applied in a similar manner, but in the reverse direction.

By this method I have obtained most satisfactory results, and have been able to deliver many women with ease after the usual methods had failed. Indeed, my experience has been so satisfactory that I have ceased to dread occipito-posterior presentations, and now regard them with equanimity, feeling that delivery can be readily and safely effected when necessary.

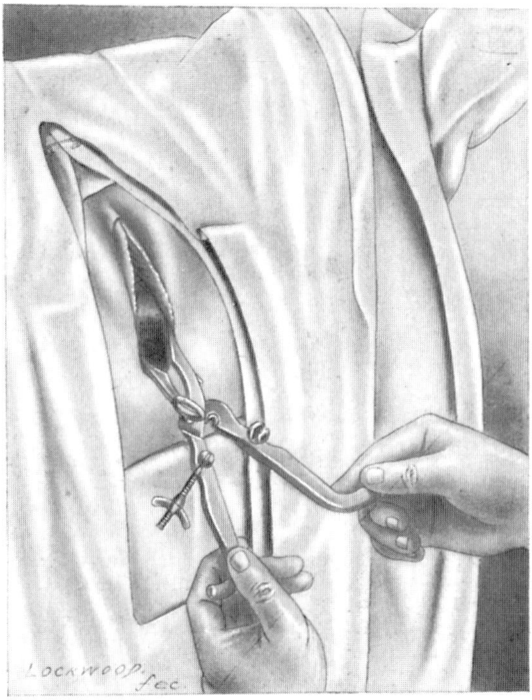

Fig. 374.—Scanzoni's Manœuvre, showing Difficulty in articulating Blades in Second Application of Forceps.

To avoid the necessity of constantly bearing in mind which is the left and which the right branch of the forceps, it is a good practical rule for a beginner, after having made an accurate diagnosis of the position of the head, to articulate the forceps and to hold them before the vulva of the patient. In this way he readily appreciates how they should be applied, and which blade is to go over the posterior ear.

High Forceps. — As has already been said, the high are much more difficult than the mid or low forceps operations, and should not be undertaken unless urgent indications are present. If the head be well engaged, the forceps should be applied as in the mid or low operation, except that, owing to the more elevated position of the head, the blades must be introduced for a greater distance into the genital tract.

On the other hand, if the entire head lies above the superior strait, or only a small segment of it is engaged, the use of forceps should be avoided if possible, as such a condition usually indicates considerable disproportion between the head and the pelvis. If, however, the operation appears to be called for, the forceps should be applied obliquely, one blade over the mastoid and the other over the opposite brow. To my mind this is the only condition in which the interests of the mother and child are not best subserved by applying the forceps directly to the sides of the head; but under these circumstances there are several contra-indications. In the first place, as the pelvis is usually contracted, the sagittal suture will generally lie transversely, and accordingly the blades of the forceps, if applied to the sides of the head, will occupy the extremities of the conjugata vera, and thus still further increase the disproportion. But more important still is the fact that, since the shape of the birth canal makes it impossible for the forceps to conform to its axis, the posterior blade bridges over the anterior

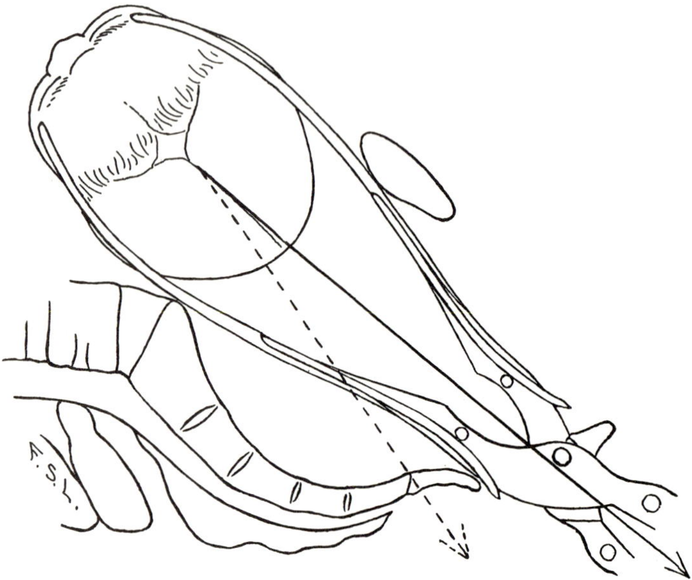

FIG. 375.—DIAGRAM SHOWING DEFECT OF CEPHALIC APPLICATION OF FORCEPS WHEN HEAD IS AT SUPERIOR STRAIT; BLACK LINE INDICATING DIRECTION OF ACTUAL AND DOTTED LINE THAT OF IDEAL TRACTION (Farabeuf and Varnier).

concavity of the sacrum and thus prevents the head from entering the pelvic cavity, and so defeats the very purpose for which the operation would be undertaken.

Axis-traction Forceps.—With the ordinary long forceps, the high and occasionally even the mid operation is comparatively difficult, strong traction being necessary to effect delivery. This is due to the fact that, owing to the shape of the birth canal and of the forceps, it is impossible to exert traction directly in the axis of the superior strait. The latter, as we know, would, if continued downward, pass through the lower portion of the sacrum; but, owing to the presence of the perinæum, the extremity of the sacrum and the coccyx, it is impossible to depress the handles of the forceps sufficiently to permit of traction in the desired direction. As a consequence, a very considerable part of the force exerted is wasted in dragging the head against the symphysis instead of bringing it downward. Thus, Tarnier pointed out that a force of 40 pounds employed in an ordinary high forceps operation would be resolved into two forces—one of 30 pounds and the other of 26 pounds—the former being in the axis of the superior strait and serving to bring about descent, whereas the latter would be directed against the symphysis pubis and would not only be wasted but would actually retard delivery.

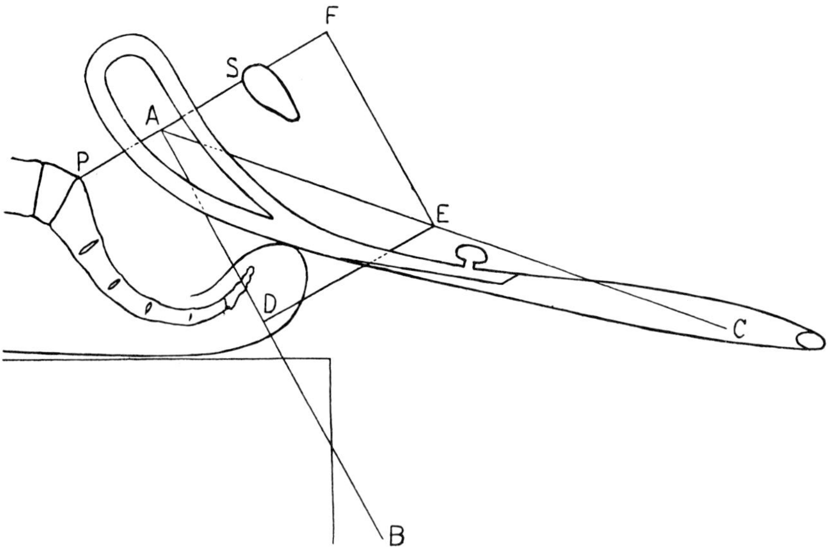

FIG. 376.—TARNIER'S DIAGRAM, SHOWING DEFECTS OF ORDINARY FORCEPS.
A E C, line of actual traction; *A D B*, line of desired traction; *A S F*, force wasted against symphysis pubis.

This defect in the forceps has long been recognised. Saxtorph, in 1772, suggested that delivery could be greatly facilitated by attaching a lac to the eye of each blade and making traction upon these, as well as

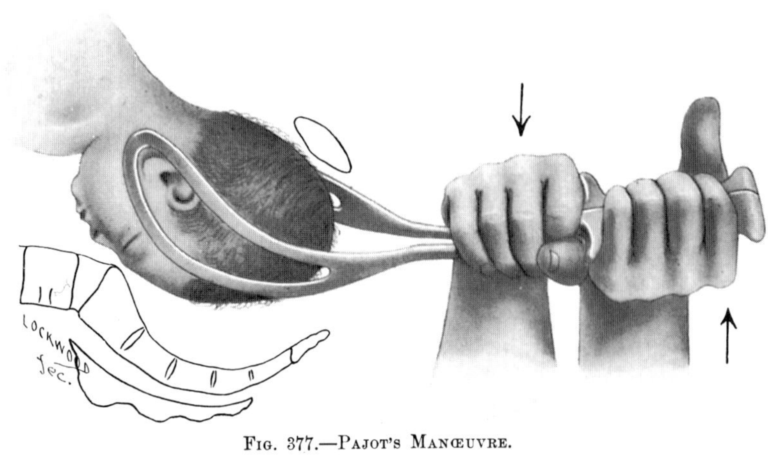

FIG. 377.—PAJOT'S MANŒUVRE.

with the handles. He also showed that a similar result might be attained by making strong downward pressure with one hand in the neighbourhood of the lock, while the other was used for traction. This manœuvre is usually attributed to Pajot, but was recommended by Saxtorph forty-four years before his birth.

Hermann, of Berne, in 1844, was the first to attempt to overcome the difficulty by devising an axis-traction forceps, his crude instrument being shown in Fig. 378. Hubert, of Louvaine (1860), found that in certain cases, by turning the handles downward, he could make traction along the axis of the superior strait, his instrument giving ideal results when the sagittal suture was directed antero-posteriorly, but being useless in all other positions. Moralès (1871) added a perineal curve to the forceps, but his invention possessed the same disadvantages as that of Hubert. None of these instruments were of much practical value, but they served to emphasize the faults of those in general use.

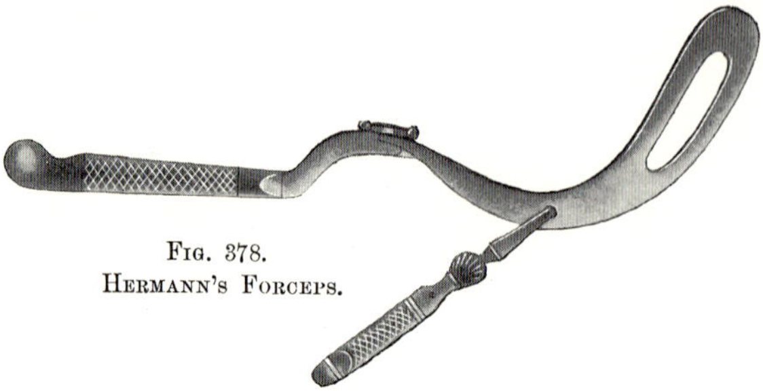

Fig. 378.
Hermann's Forceps.

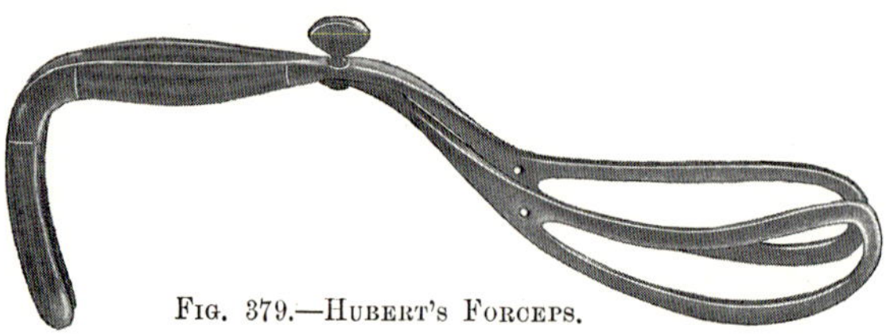

Fig. 379.—Hubert's Forceps.

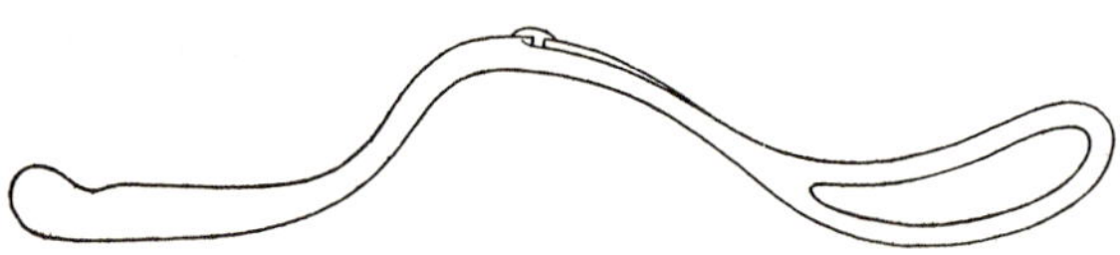

Fig. 380.—Moralès's Forceps.

Finally, in 1877, Tarnier solved the problem by attaching a traction-rod to each blade and fastening them to a handle. His original forceps possessed a definite perineal curve, and was very cumbersome. The importance of his invention was soon recognised, and obstetricians throughout the world promptly attempted to improve upon it; so that at present one or more modifications of axis-traction forceps, each designated by the name of the modifier, are to be found in every large city.

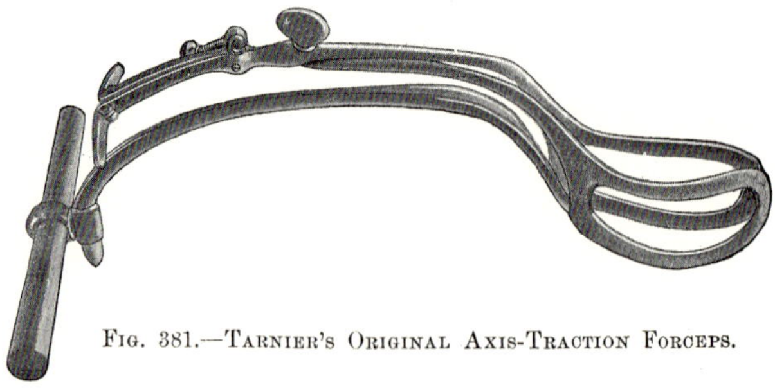

Fig. 381.—Tarnier's Original Axis-Traction Forceps.

Tarnier himself, not considering his original forceps satisfactory, continued to make changes and improvements, so that before his death he had devised an instrument which leaves little to be desired. It is practically a long French forceps without a perineal curve, provided with short, detachable traction-rods, one of which is inserted just beyond the eye of each blade. When not in use these are held in place by a pin upon the under surface of the shank, from which they can be readily freed, and attached by their free ends to a traction attachment which terminates in a handle-bar which can be grasped by one or both hands (see Figs. 382 and 383).

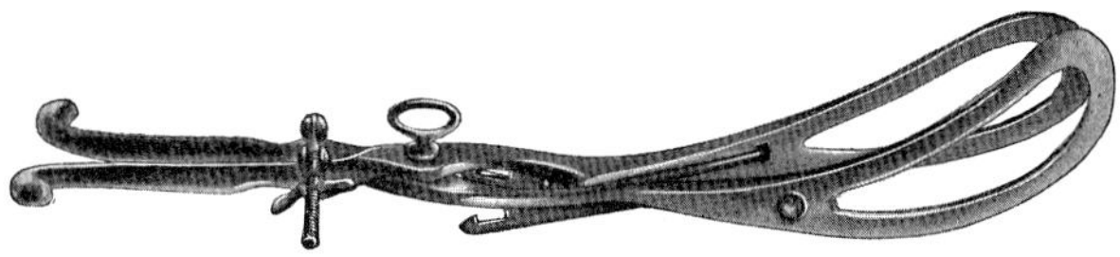

Fig. 382.—Tarnier's Forceps, Traction Rods in Place without Handle-Bar.

With this device, traction can be made almost in the axis of the superior strait, and, owing to the presence of numerous joints in the traction attachment, the instrument can be used in any position. The handles of the forceps merely serve to indicate the direction in which traction should be made, the force being applied to the handle-bar, which is held horizontally no matter what the position of the blades may be, the traction-rods being kept 1 centimetre beneath the handles (Fig. 384).

To my mind, this instrument is superior to all other axis-traction forceps, and with it most excellent results can be obtained with a minimum expenditure of energy, and by its aid a delivery can occasionally be effected which would have been impossible with the ordinary instruments. One of its best points is the joint between the horizontal and vertical portions of the traction attachment, as a result of which the handle-bar can be held horizontally, even though the forceps is applied at the ends of the antero-posterior diameter of the pelvis. I use this instrument in all cases, without the traction-rods in low and mid, and with them in high forceps operations.

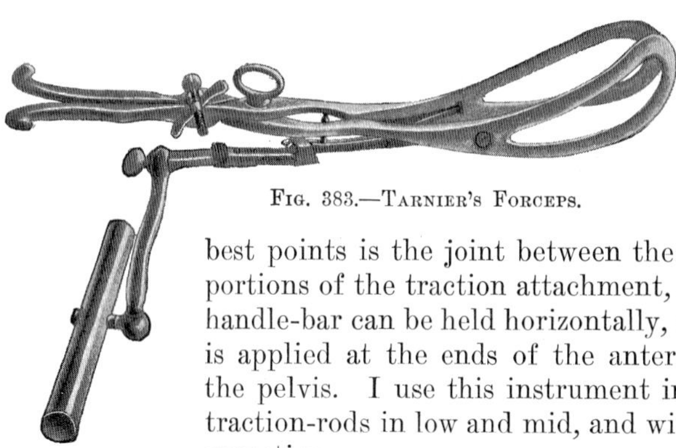

Fig. 383.—Tarnier's Forceps.

Application of Forceps in Face Presentations.—In face presentations the application of forceps occasionally becomes necessary, but should be attempted only in the transverse and anterior varieties, the blades being applied to the sides of the head along the mento-occipital diameter, with the pelvic curvature directed towards the neck. Traction is made in a downward direction until the chin appears under the symphysis; then by an upward movement the face is slowly extracted through the vulva, the nose, eyes, brow, and occiput appearing in succession over the anterior margin of the perinæum.

Forceps should not be applied when the chin is directed towards the hollow of the sacrum, as delivery cannot be effected in this position. In rare instances, however, an expert operator may endeavour to rotate the chin to a transverse and later to an anterior position, though such attempts are rarely successful, and are permissible only in exceptional cases.

Application of Forceps in Breech Presentations.—Occasionally, the application of forceps is recommended in frank breech presentations, the blades being applied over the trochanters. This is very rarely indicated, as delivery can usually be effected more satisfactorily by the methods to be mentioned in the following chapter.

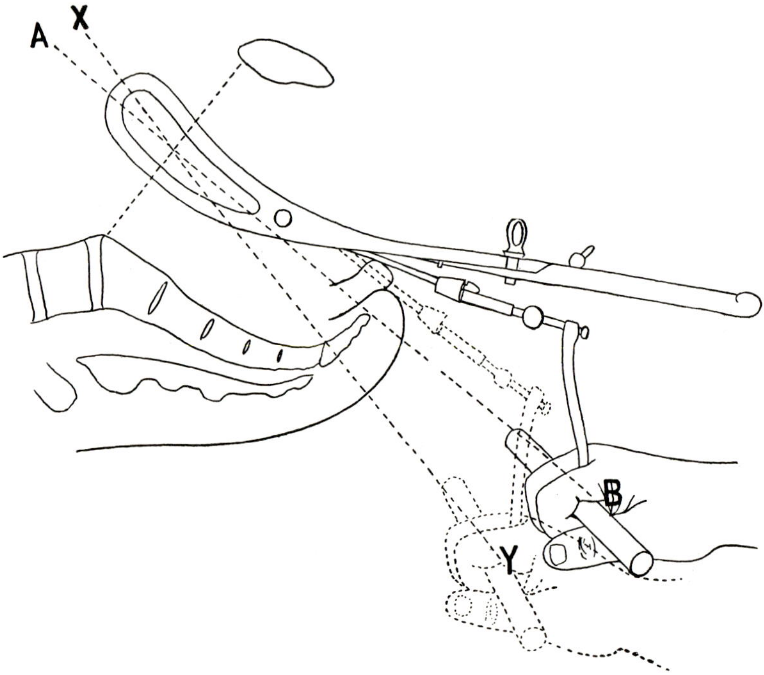

FIG. 384.—DIAGRAM SHOWING TRACTION WITH TARNIER'S FORCEPS.
A B in proper and *X Y* in improper manner (Ribemont-Dessaignes.)

From the time of Smellie, many authors have recommended the extraction of the *after-coming head* in breech presentations by means of the forceps. In such cases the body of the child is carried up over the abdomen of the mother, and the blades are introduced under it and applied to the sides of the head. As a matter of fact, it is never necessary to resort to the forceps under such conditions, so its employment is not to be recommended, since the more expert one becomes in the use of Mauriceau's method of extraction the less frequently will difficulty be experienced in delivering the after-coming head.

Prognosis.—Low and mid forceps operations, when intelligently performed upon healthy women under proper aseptic precautions, should not be followed by maternal mortality, the operation being undertaken to save maternal and fœtal life.

It is generally held that perineal tears occur more frequently in forceps than in spontaneous deliveries. This, however, should not be the case, provided that the head is extracted sufficiently slowly. Unfortunately, it would appear as though the average operator, as soon as the head appears at the vulva, is seized with an almost uncontrollable desire to effect its immediate delivery by brusque traction, instead of imitating nature and devoting from fifteen to twenty minutes to overcoming the resistance of the perinæum and vulval outlet. Leopold has stated that the forceps is the bloodiest of all obstetrical operations, and this is undoubtedly true if the child is rapidly dragged through a partially dilated birth canal by brute force. On the other hand, if properly employed, it is a means of saving instead of destroying the perinæum, inasmuch as the exit of the head can be controlled more effectively by means of the forceps than by any other procedure.

Attempts at delivery through an imperfectly dilated cervix are most dangerous, and frequently give rise to deep cervical tears, which may lead to the death of the patient from hæmorrhage or infection. Moreover, the application of forceps requires an accurate diagnosis as to the position and presentation of the child, and when this is lacking, as in certain occipito-posterior and brow presentations, and the forceps is incorrectly applied, delivery can be effected only by brute force, which can hardly fail to cause serious lesions for mother and child. Similar untoward results often follow an attempt to drag the head forcibly through a markedly contracted pelvic brim.

The fœtal mortality depends upon the position of the head and the general difficulty of the operation. It should be practically zero in low and mid operations, except in the rare cases in which a funnel-shaped pelvis is overlooked. In a comparatively large experience, I can recall only two children whose deaths could be directly attributed to the operation when properly performed. On the other hand, the high forceps operation is attended by a very serious fœtal mortality, which becomes greater the less deeply the head is engaged. In such cases the head may be subjected to injurious pressure, which may lead to the rupture of intracranial vessels and the subsequent death of the child. In rare instances actual fracture of the skull may occur, and occasionally the upper part of the occipital bone may become separated from its base.

Not infrequently the child may be born with *facial paralysis*, or the condition may develop shortly after birth. This is most frequently noted when the head has been seized obliquely, and is due to the pressure exerted by the posterior blade of the forceps upon the neighbourhood of the stylomastoid foramen, through which the nerve leaves the skull. Not every facial paralysis, however, following delivery by forceps, should be attributed to the operation, as such a condition is occasionally encountered after a spontaneous labour, and may be due to intracranial causes quite independent of the use of instruments. Full literature upon this subject will be found in Macé's article (1901).

LITERATURE

AVELING. The Chamberlens and the Midwifery Forceps. London, 1882.

BAUDELOCQUE. De la manière de se servir du forceps, etc. L'art des accouchements. Nouv. éd., Paris, 1789, t. ii, 300–343.

BUDIN. L'invention du forceps à double courbure. Progrès Médical, 1876, 779.

Les Chamberlens. Lequel d'entre eux imagina le forceps. Obstétrique et Gynécologie, 1886, 659–668.

CHAPMAN. An Essay on the Improvement of Midwifery, etc. London, 1733.

CHASSAGNY. Le forceps, etc. Paris, 1871.

Fonctions du forceps. Paris, 1891.

FARABEUF et VARNIER. Introduction à l'étude clinique et à la pratique des accouchements. Paris, 1891, 276–466.

GIFFARD. Cases in Midwifery. London, 1734.

HERMANN. Ueber eine neue Geburtszange. Berne, 1844.

HUBERT. Note sur l'équilibre du forceps et du levier. Mémoires de l'Acad. Royale de Belgique, 1860.

LEVRET. Observations sur les causes et les accidents de plusieurs accouchements laborieux. Paris, 1747.

MACÉ. Des paralysies faciales spontanées du nouveau-né. L'Obstétrique, 1901, vi, 517–526.

MORALÈS. Modification nouvelle du forceps. Jour. de Méd. de Bruxelles, 1871.

MULDER. Historia literaria et critica forcipum et vectium obstetriciorum, Lugd. Bat., 1794.

PALFYN. See Levret.

POULLET. Des diverses espèces du forceps. Paris, 1883.

SÄNGER. Die Chamberlens. Archiv f. Gyn., 1887, xxxi, 119–144.

SAXTORPH. Theoria de diverso partu, etc. Havniae and Lipsiae, 1772.

SCANZONI. Lehrbuch der Geburtshülfe, II. Aufl., 1853, 838–840.

SMELLIE. A Treatise on the Theory and Practice of Midwifery. London, 1852.

TARNIER. Description de deux nouveaux forceps.. Paris, 1877.

WITKOWSKI. L'arsenal obstétrical. Paris, Steinheil.

CHAPTER XXI

EXTRACTION AND VERSION

Extraction in Breech Presentations.—The delivery of the child by traction when the feet protrude from the vulva in breech presentations, was probably the earliest obstetrical operation.

From the time of Hippocrates up to the beginning of the sixteenth century head presentations alone were considered normal, and hence all the authorities, with the exception of Celsus, advised the conversion of breech into vertex presentations at any cost, even though it rendered necessary amputation of the limbs. After the resuscitation of podalic version by Ambroise Paré and Jacques Guillemeau, more rational views prevailed, so that in the seventeenth century we find Mauriceau advising the method of extraction which is in general use at the present time.

As the technique of the operation varies according as one has to deal with a complete breech or foot, or with a frank breech presentation, it will be necessary to consider the two conditions separately. In both, the essential prerequisite for the successful performance of extraction lies in the complete dilatation of the cervix and the absence of any serious mechanical obstacle. It is true that in a certain number of cases extraction through an imperfectly dilated cervix is possible, but this is usually effected only at the cost of deep cervical tears. Moreover, the additional resistance offered to the passage of the head will generally lead to its extension, the arms at the same time becoming elevated over it, thereby so complicating and delaying delivery that the child is almost invariably lost. For these reasons premature extraction is indicated but rarely, and then only in the interests of the mother.

Indications for Extraction.—It has already been pointed out that the fœtal mortality is considerably greater in breech than in vertex presentations, since in the former death from asphyxiation is almost inevitable if the head be not delivered in less than *eight minutes* after the appearance of the umbilicus at the vulva. In these cases the untoward result may be due to one or other of several causes. Thus, very often the cord is subjected to pressure between the pelvic brim and the head, which may be so severe as to completely check the circulation. Less frequently the rapid decrease in the size of the uterus following the extrusion of the body of the child results in premature separation of the placenta before the head is born, so that death becomes inevitable unless extraction is promptly effected.

In all breech presentations, preparations should be made for extraction as soon as the buttocks appear at the vulva, so that the operation can be promptly resorted to if, after the appearance of the umbilicus, the extrusion of the rest of the body does not rapidly follow. In a certain number of cases, no matter what the position of the breech, extraction may be called for by any condition which seriously threatens the life of the mother or child, just as in vertex presentations. When speaking of the latter, however, it was said that the passage of meconium indicated that the child was in danger, whereas in breech presentations such an occurrence is without significance, as it is simply the result of the compression to which the abdomen of the child is being subjected.

Extraction by One or Both Feet.—Before beginning the operation the patient should be brought to the edge of the bed and subjected to the usual preliminary preparations. Complete anæsthesia is necessary, except in those cases in which the body of the child has already been born and only the head remains to be extracted.

As a rule, extraction is an extremely simple operation when the breech has been born spontaneously, whereas it is less so when the feet are in the vagina, and very much more difficult when they are still within the uterus. In the latter case, one hand should be passed through the cervix and an attempt made to seize both feet, the ankles being grasped in such a manner that the second finger lies between them. They are then brought down into the vagina, and traction is made until they appear at the vulva. If, however, difficulty is experienced in seizing both feet, one should be grasped and extracted in a similar manner.

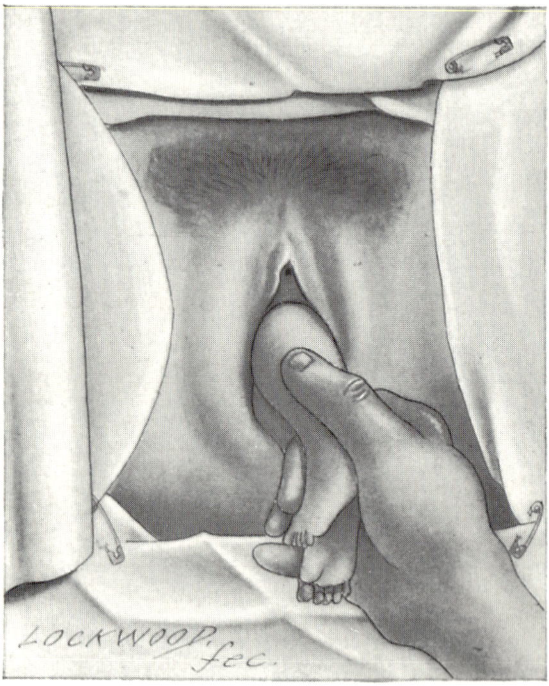

Fig. 385.—Breech Extraction, Traction upon Feet.

As soon as the feet emerge from the vulva they should be wrapped in a sterile towel so that a firmer grasp may be obtained; since the vernix caseosa renders them so slippery that they are very difficult to hold. Traction is then made in a downward direction, and as the legs protrude still farther they are grasped higher up, first by the calves and later by the thighs. When the breech appears at the vulva, traction is made in an upward direction until it is delivered. The thumbs are then applied over the sacrum and the fingers over the hips, and traction is continued in the same manner until the thorax is born, when the arms must be freed in order to effect delivery.

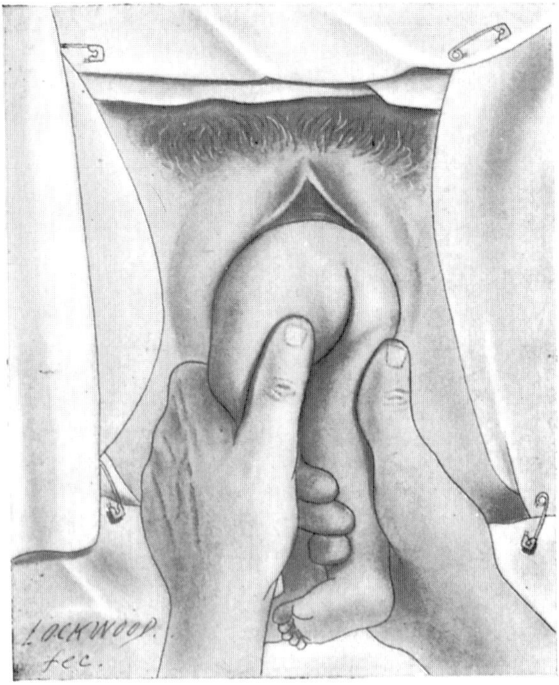

FIG. 386.—BREECH EXTRACTION, TRACTION UPON THIGHS.

If only one foot has been seized, traction should be made upon it until the buttocks appear at the vulva, when the index finger of the other hand is introduced into the posterior groin and aids in traction.

As soon as the operator begins to pull upon the legs, an assistant or the nurse should exert strong pressure upon the uterus in the axis of the superior strait, with the object of preserving the flexed attitude of the head and preventing the arms from becoming extended above it. Besides serving these purposes it also aids directly in the expulsion of the child, and thus renders necessary a smaller amount of force on the part of the operator.

In order *to free and deliver the arms*, the child should be seized with the thumbs over the scapulæ and the fingers over the sides of the thorax, and rotated until the bisacromial diameter occupies an oblique diameter of the pelvis (Fig. 387). The posterior arm should be freed first, since there is more available space in the posterior and lateral segments of the pelvis than elsewhere. To accomplish this, the feet should be seized by one hand and carried towards the groin of the mother opposite the posterior shoulder. In many cases this manœuvre causes the latter to emerge over the perineal margin, the hand and arm escaping spontaneously. If this does not occur two fingers are introduced beneath the shoulder and passed along the humerus until the elbow is reached (Fig. 388). The fingers are now applied in such a way as to serve as a splint to the arm, which is swept downward over the thorax and delivered from the vulva. To effect the delivery of the anterior arm, the body is seized as before and rotated so as to bring the undelivered shoulder into the neighbourhood of the nearest sacro-sciatic notch. The legs are then carried upward, so as to bring the body to the opposite groin of the mother, and if the arm be not born spontaneously it is delivered in the same manner as the other.

If pressure from above has not been made—and occasionally in spite of it—the arms may become extended over the head. Under such circumstances their delivery, although more difficult, can be accomplished by the manœuvres ordinarily employed. In doing this, particular care must be taken to carry the fingers up to the elbow and use them as a splint, for if the finger be merely hooked over the arm and strong traction made, the humerus or clavicle is exposed to great danger of fracture. Occasionally, the manœuvre may be rendered easier by pushing the child a short distance up the generative tract.

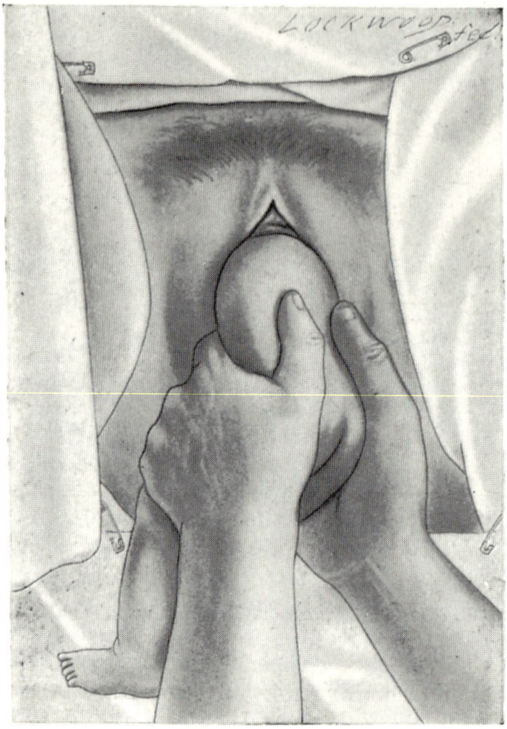

Fig. 387.—Breech Extraction, Posterior Rotation of Shoulder.

In other cases the arm is found around the back of the neck, when its delivery becomes still more difficult. If it cannot be freed in the manner just described, it must be forcibly extracted by hooking a finger over it. Unfortunately, fracture of the humerus is very common in such cases, and the dangers attending the procedure should be pointed out to some responsible member of the family; although, inasmuch as the life of the child can be saved only in this way, the risk is always justifiable.

After the shoulders have been born, the head usually occupies an oblique diameter of the pelvis with the chin directed posteriorly, when its extraction is best effected by *Mauriceau's manœuvre* (Figs. 389 and 390). For this purpose the index finger of one hand is introduced into the mouth of the child and applied over the superior maxilla, while the body rests upon the palm of the hand and the forearm, with the legs straddling the latter. Two fingers of the other hand are then hooked over the neck, and, grasping the shoulders, make downward traction until the occiput appears under the symphysis. The body of the child is now raised up towards the mother's abdomen, and the mouth, nose, brow, and eventually the occiput, successively emerge over the perinæum. Traction should be exerted only by the fingers over the shoulders, and not by the finger in the mouth, since in many cases the latter slips from the superior maxilla and comes to rest upon the inferior maxilla and base of the tongue, as a consequence of which serious injuries may be done to the child if energetic traction be employed.

This manœuvre was first practised by Mauriceau in the seventeenth century, but for some reason fell into disfavour. Nearly a hundred years later Smellie described a similar procedure, but rarely made use of it, as he preferred the employment of forceps. In the meantime other devices came into use, until G. Veit, in 1863, directed attention to the inestimable advantages which Mauriceau's method of extraction possessed over all others. For this reason in Germany the procedure is frequently called after Veit, or, when greater accuracy is desired, is designated as the Mauriceau-Smellie-Veit manœuvre. Litzmann, however, is certainly right in pointing out the

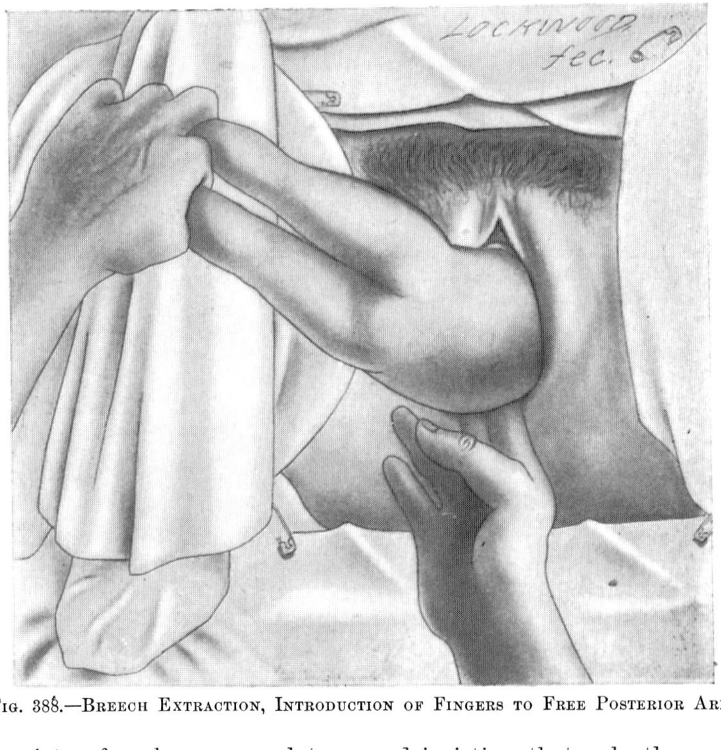

FIG. 388.—BREECH EXTRACTION, INTRODUCTION OF FINGERS TO FREE POSTERIOR ARM.

impropriety of such a nomenclature, and insisting that only the name of the original inventor (Mauriceau) should be used in describing it. Numerous other methods of extraction have been devised, Winckel being able in 1888 to collect 21 different procedures from the literature, although none has proved as serviceable as that of Mauriceau.

In the vast majority of cases the back of the child eventually rotates towards the front, no matter what its original position; but when it does not take place spontaneously the movement may be inaugurated by making stronger traction upon the leg, which would naturally rotate anteriorly.

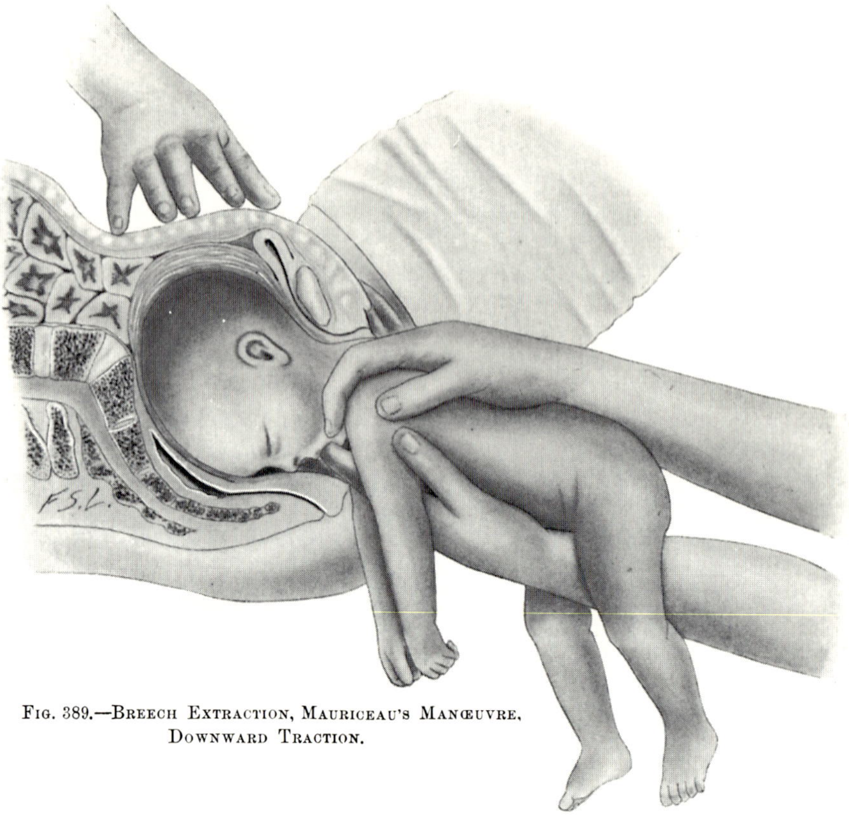

Fig. 389.—Breech Extraction, Mauriceau's Manœuvre, Downward Traction.

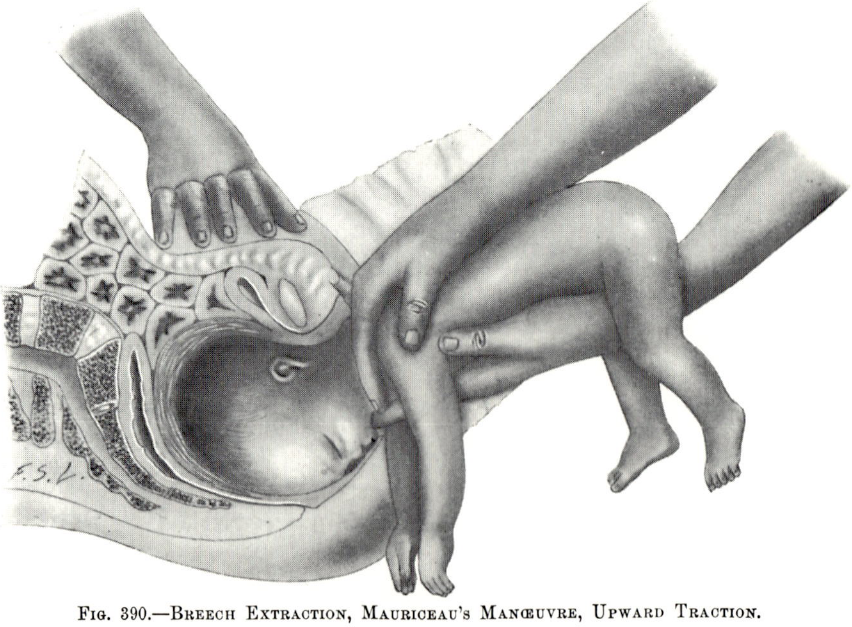

Fig. 390.—Breech Extraction, Mauriceau's Manœuvre, Upward Traction.

If this does not bring about the desired result, and the back remains posterior after the birth of the shoulders, extraction must be begun with the occiput posterior. As a rule, rotation can still be effected by means of the finger in the mouth, after which the head can be extracted by Mauriceau's manœuvre. When, however, this is impossible, delivery must be attempted, with the head in its abnormal position, by the employment of a modified *Prague manœuvre,* which is so called for the reason that its advantages were strongly urged and practised more particularly by Kiwisch, of that city, although it had been described by Pugh a century earlier. The procedure is somewhat as follows: Two fingers of one hand grasp the shoulders, while the other hand draws up the feet over the abdomen of

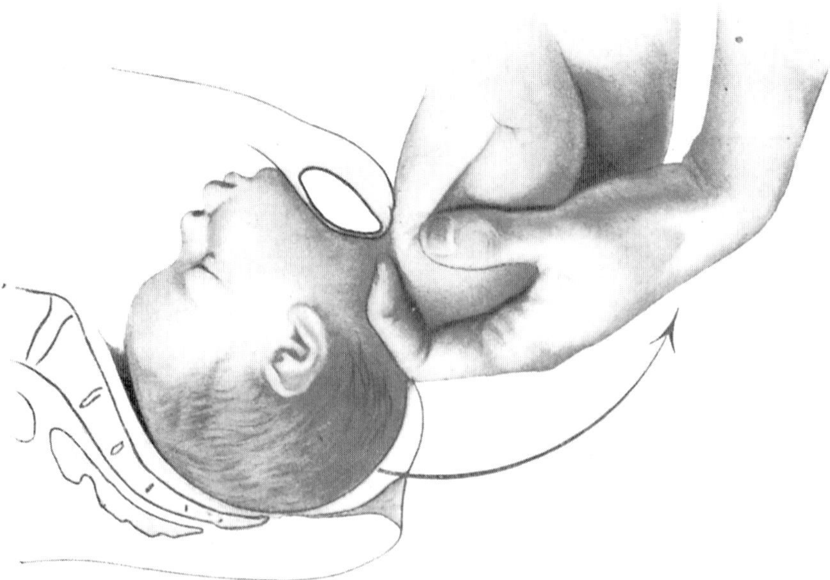

FIG. 391.—DELIVERY OF AFTER-COMING HEAD, BACK POSTERIOR (Bumm).

the mother. As a result the occiput of the child is born first and the perinæum is necessarily subjected to greater liability of rupture.

Prognosis.—The prognosis, so far as the mother is concerned, is very favourable, even when considerable disproportion exists between the child and the pelvis, since the pressure to which the maternal soft parts are subjected lasts but a few seconds, instead of being prolonged for hours, as in head presentations. Owing to the necessary intra-vaginal manipulations, there is a slightly increased danger of infection, and more particularly in the case of a primipara with a rigid vaginal outlet there is greater liability to laceration of the perinæum than in head presentations.

For the child, however, the outlook is not so favourable, and becomes more serious the higher the situation of the presenting part at the beginning of the operation. The fœtal mortality is in great part due to the dangers inherent to breech presentations, which are augmented by the greater liability to the occurrence of traumatism during extraction, particularly if there is marked disproportion between the head and the pelvis.

As has already been said, fractures of the humerus and clavicle cannot always be avoided, even in the hands of expert operators. Occasionally *hæmatomata of the sterno-cleido-mastoid muscle* are noted after the operation, though these are usually of but slight significance and disappear spontaneously within a short time. More serious results, however, may follow the *separation of the epiphyses* of the scapula or humerus. In exceptional cases *paralysis of the arm* results from pressure exerted upon the brachial plexus by the fingers in making traction, but more frequently is due to an overstretching of the neck in freeing the arms or in effecting extraction by the Prague manœuvre. As will be shown in Chapter XLV, the condition usually undergoes spontaneous cure, although in rare instances it persists throughout life.

When the child is forcibly extracted through a markedly contracted pelvis, spoon-shaped depressions or actual *fractures of the skull* may result, which generally prove fatal.

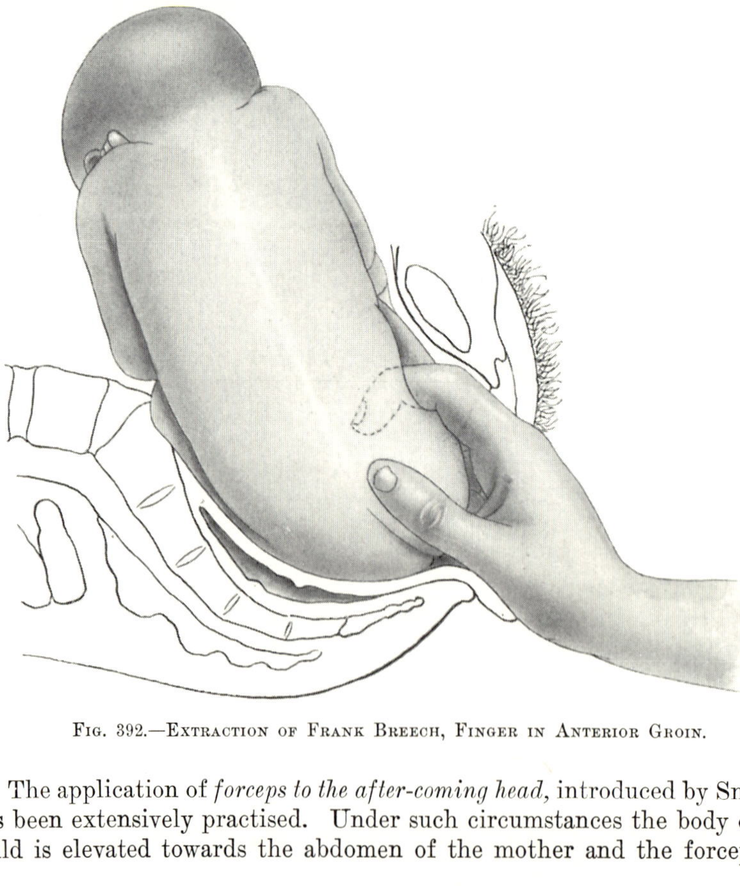

FIG. 392.—EXTRACTION OF FRANK BREECH, FINGER IN ANTERIOR GROIN.

The application of *forceps to the after-coming head*, introduced by Smellie, has been extensively practised. Under such circumstances the body of the child is elevated towards the abdomen of the mother and the forceps introduced under it, the blades being applied to the sides of the head. Personally, I have never found it necessary to resort to this procedure, and believe that it is but rarely called for if the obstetrician has made himself thoroughly familiar with Mauriceau's manœuvre.

Extraction of Frank Breech Presentations.—When indications for delivery arise after the breech has descended into the birth canal, its extraction can usually be effected without difficulty by hooking the index finger of one hand into the anterior groin and making traction until the buttocks appear at the vulva, the index finger of the other hand being then inserted into the posterior groin in order to furnish additional aid.

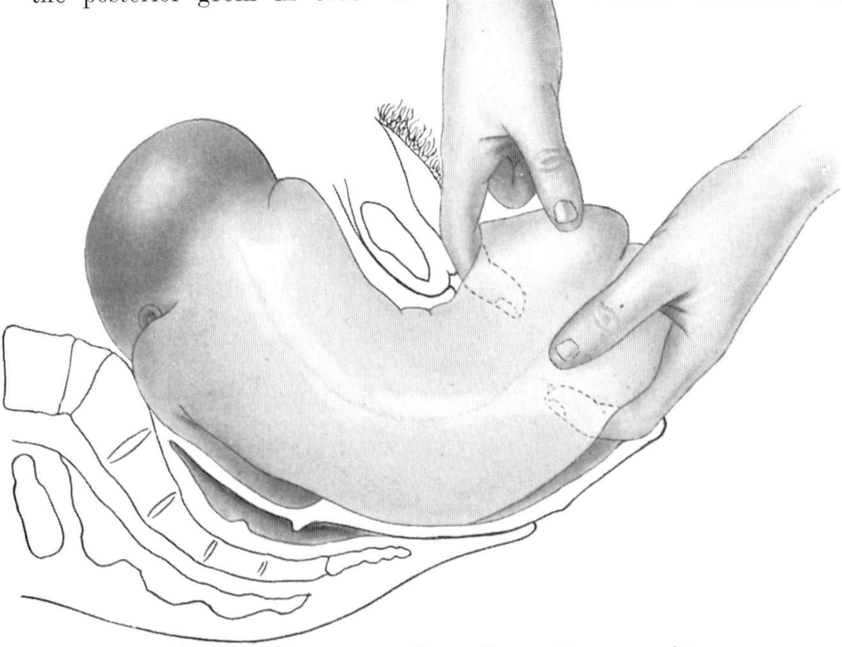

Fig. 393.—Extraction of Frank Breech, Fingers in Groins.

On the other hand, when the breech is at the superior strait delivery is much more difficult. In such cases it is advisable to try to decompose the wedge and bring down one or both feet, which can be readily accomplished if attempted shortly after rupture of the membranes, but becomes extremely difficult if a considerable time has been allowed to elapse after the escape of the liquor amnii and the uterus has become tightly contracted over the child.

In many cases the employment of the following manœuvre suggested by Pinard will often aid materially in bringing down the foot: Two fingers are carried up along one leg to the knee and push it away from the middle line. This procedure is usually followed by spontaneous flexion, and the foot of the child will be felt to impinge upon the back of the hand, when it can be readily seized (Fig. 394).

In view of the fact that it is often very difficult to seize and bring down a foot in the latter part of the second stage of labour, Ahlfeld and others have suggested the propriety of rupturing the membranes as soon as the cervix is fully dilated, and bringing down a foot prophylactically, so that a convenient handle may be available in case extraction becomes necessary. This can be readily accomplished, but is not advisable as a routine practice, since the frank breech forms a much better dilating wedge than the incomplete breech presentation. The procedure is justifiable, however, in those cases in which it is highly probable that rapid delivery will become imperative; for instance, in patients suffering from acute diseases and heart lesions.

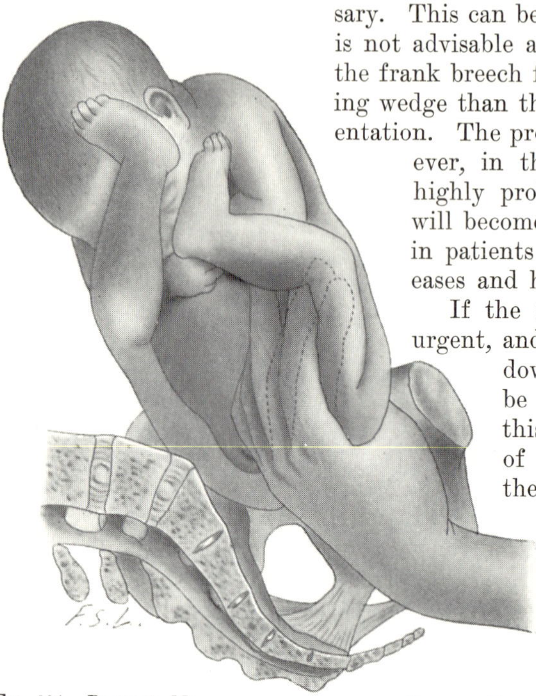

Fig. 394.—Pinard's Manœuvre for bringing Down a Foot in Frank Breech Presentation.

If the indication for delivery is urgent, and it is impossible to bring down a foot, the child must be extracted as it lies. For this purpose the index finger of one hand is hooked into the anterior groin, and strong downward traction made, supplemented, if necessary, by the use of the other hand which grasps the wrist. This procedure is continued until the posterior buttock has almost reached the pelvic floor, when the index finger of the other hand is hooked into the posterior groin and traction made with both hands. As soon as the latter becomes accessible, delivery can usually be readily effected, but, unfortunately, in a considerable number of cases one is unable to bring the breech low enough to offer this advantage. For this reason, when the breech is high up, its extraction should not be attempted unless imperatively demanded by the condition of the mother or child; otherwise it is far better to wait until it has descended lower before interfering.

As soon as the buttocks are born, first one leg and then the other is drawn out and extraction accomplished as described above. As was said before, traction must always be supplemented by pressure upon the abdomen from above. This precautionary measure should never be neglected, as delivery can frequently be accomplished by its aid when it would be impossible if traction by the fingers were alone relied upon. Indeed, it is not until one has attempted a difficult frank breech extraction that one learns how little force can be exerted by the fingers.

Prognosis.—The prognosis for both mother and child is less favourable in frank breech than in foot presentations. In the former the increased manipulation affords greater opportunity for infection; while the attempt to reach the posterior groin often gives rise to deep tears before the child has reached the perinæum. Again, in view of the longer time required to effect delivery, the child is exposed to more danger, and in addition to the accidents incident to extraction by the feet, fracture of the femur may follow the attempt to bring down a foot, especially when strong traction is made upon the groin.

Use of Forceps.—In view of the difficulty which sometimes attends the extraction of the frank breech when high up, Lusk, Budin, Reynolds, and other authorities have recommended the employment of forceps, the blades being applied obliquely, one over the sacrum and the other over the thigh. Up to the present time I have had no experience with this procedure, having been able to effect delivery in all my cases by traction exerted with a finger in the groin. When this fails the application of forceps is certainly justifiable, although when the breech is high up it should not be attempted except under pressing indications.

The Fillet.—In these cases it is sometimes convenient to make use of the fillet. This may consist of several thicknesses of sterile gauze bandage which are passed over the anterior groin. The fillet is a very efficient tractor, but its application offers considerable difficulty. Unless the operator has at his disposal a specially constructed instrument, a fairly satisfactory carrier may be improvised from a rubber catheter, through which a piece of stout thread is passed, a loop being allowed to protrude from the eye. A stylet is then introduced, and an appropriate curve having been given to the closed end of the catheter, the bent extremity is passed around the anterior groin until the fingers in the vagina can seize the loop, to which one end of the fillet is attached and then cautiously drawn up into place.

Aside from the difficulty encountered in applying it, the only disadvantage of the fillet is its liability to cut through the skin of the groin; but this accident can be avoided by employing several thicknesses of gauze and taking care that they do not become twisted into a cord.

The older authors advocated making traction upon the groin by means of a metallic hook. This instrument should never be employed upon living children on account of its liability to cause fracture of the femur. On the other hand, when the child is dead and such an accident is a matter of indifference, the hook affords a most convenient means of making traction.

Version.—Version, or turning, is an operation through which the presentation of the fœtus is artificially altered, one pole being substituted for the other, or an oblique or transverse being converted into a longitudinal presentation.

According as the head or breech is made the presenting part, the operation is spoken of as cephalic or podalic version respectively. It is also designated according to the method by which it is accomplished. Thus we speak of *external version* when the manipulations are made exclusively through the external abdominal wall; of *internal version* when the entire hand is introduced into the uterine cavity; and of *combined version* when one hand manipulates through the abdominal wall while two or more fingers of the other are introduced through the cervix.

Cephalic Version.—This operation was practised from the most remote antiquity, and only gradually fell into disfavour after the introduction of podalic version by Paré and his followers. After the discovery of Wigand (1807) that the position of the child could easily be altered by external manipulations, cephalic version came into more general use, and since the publications of Hubert and Pinard has become a well-recognised procedure in certain conditions.

The object of the operation is to substitute a vertex for a less favourable presentation. As it does not, however, afford a means for immediate delivery, its field of usefulness is comparatively limited, and its employment is still further restricted by various contra-indications.

Indications.—If a breech or transverse presentation is diagnosed in the last few weeks of pregnancy, its conversion into a vertex should be attempted by external manœuvres, provided there be no marked disproportion between the size of the child and the pelvis. If the breech be not engaged, cephalic version is indicated by reason of the increased fœtal mortality attending spontaneous delivery in that presentation; while if the child lies transversely a change of presentation is imperatively demanded, inasmuch as a natural labour is out of the question, and if appropriate measures are not adopted the lives of both mother and child will be lost.

Unfortunately, after the accomplishment of external cephalic version, the child tends to return to its original position, unless the new presentation can be retained until engagement occurs. Consequently, whenever this procedure is employed during pregnancy, the wearing of a suitable bandage is necessary. Moreover, the operation can be accomplished only under the following conditions: (1) The presenting part must not be engaged; (2) the abdominal wall must be sufficiently thin to admit of accurate palpation; (3) the abdominal and uterine walls must not be too irritable; (4) the uterus must contain a sufficient quantity of liquor amnii to permit the easy movement of the child. Given these essentials, external cephalic version should always be attempted, since it is absolutely harmless, and if the new position is maintained it may do away with the necessity for serious operative procedures at the time of labour.

In the early stages of labour, before the membranes have ruptured, the same indications hold good, and at this time may be extended to oblique presentations as well, though these usually right themselves spontaneously as labour progresses. On the other hand, external cephalic version is not indicated after the cervix has become fully dilated and the membranes have ruptured, except in occasional cases of shoulder presentations; since it can be effected but rarely, and better results are obtained from podalic version followed by immediate extraction. This is particularly true in cases complicated by prolapse of the cord or placenta prævia. Serious pelvic contraction is a decided contra-indication, since although it may be readily accomplished, the procedure is useless, and more serious operative measures will be necessary before delivery can be effected.

Methods.—Cephalic version may be brought about either by *external manipulations* alone, or by the combined method—with one hand on the abdomen and two or more fingers, or even the whole hand, in the uterus. During pregnancy the former is the only method applicable, and at the time of labour it should be employed whenever feasible. The technique has been carefully described by Pinard, and is somewhat as follows: The patient's abdomen having been bared, the presentation and position of the child are carefully mapped out. The fœtal poles are then seized with either hand and the one which we wish to present is gently stroked towards the superior strait, while the other is moved in the opposite direction. After version has been completed, the child must be held in its new position until engagement occurs. During pregnancy this is accomplished by appropriately fitting pads, which are held in place by a bandage; but at the time of labour the head may be pressed down into the superior strait and held firmly in position until it becomes fixed under the influence of the uterine contractions.

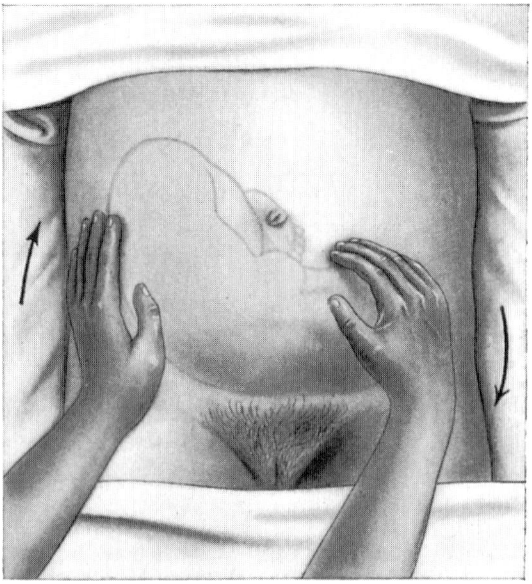

Fig. 395.—External Cephalic Version (Pinard).

At the time of labour, if external manipulations prove futile, cephalic version may be accomplished by the *combined method of Braxton Hicks* as soon as the cervix is sufficiently dilated to admit of two fingers. For carrying out this procedure Hicks gave the following directions:

"Introduce the left hand into the vagina as in podalic version. Place the right hand on the outside of the abdomen in order to make out the position of the fœtus and the direction of the head and feet. Should the shoulder, for instance, present, then push it with one or two fingers on the top in the direction of the feet. At the same time pressure by the other hand should be exerted upon the cephalic end of the child. This will bring the child close to the os. Then let the head be received upon the tips of the inside fingers. The head will then play like a ball between the hands, and can be placed at almost any part at will. . . . It is well, if the breech will not rise to the fundus readily and the head is fairly in the os, to withdraw the hand from the vagina and with it press up the breech from the exterior."

Busch, D'Outrepont, and others advocated attempting cephalic version after complete dilatation of the cervix, by introducing one hand into the uterus and seizing the head, while the other is employed for external manipulations. This is rarely if ever advisable, as under such circumstances it is preferable to perform internal version, which is no more dangerous, and at the same time permits immediate delivery if necessary.

Podalic Version.—By this is understood the seizure of one or both feet by two or more fingers, and drawing them through the cervix, the operation being usually followed by extraction. Podalic version was introduced and warmly advocated by Paré, and, until the invention of the forceps, afforded the only means of artificially delivering unmutilated children. It is interesting to note that Guillemeau, one of Paré's students, was enabled by this means to save his master's daughter from dying of hæmorrhage due to placenta prævia. The value of the operation was recognised and insisted upon by Louise Bourgeois, Mauriceau, and among many others by De la Motte, who employed it very frequently with most excellent results.

Indications.—Podalic version is indicated in two great groups of cases—namely, in transverse and oblique presentations and in head presentations in which it is believed that delivery can be more safely and more rapidly accomplished after version.

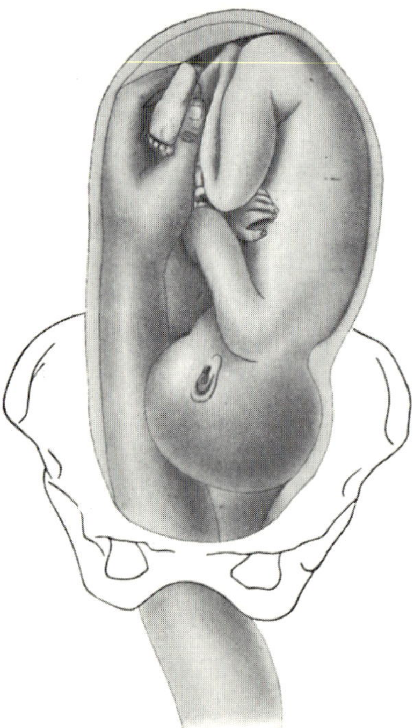

Fig. 396.—Seizure of Foot in Internal Podalic Version (Tarnier).

The necessity for version in transverse and oblique presentations is obvious. In abnormal head presentations, when the face, brow, or occiput is posterior and movable above the superior strait, delivery can frequently be more readily accomplished after version than by any other means. Podalic version is usually the operation of choice in prolapse of the extremities or umbilical cord, and in many cases of placenta prævia. Moreover, when the child presents some deformity delivery is sometimes very much facilitated after version. Generally speaking, the operation is indicated in all cases requiring prompt delivery when the head is floating at the superior strait or is but slightly engaged, provided there is no great disproportion between its size and that of the pelvis. Under such circumstances it is usually a much safer procedure than the application of high forceps.

One of its widest fields of usefulness is after the manual dilatation of the cervix in *accouchement forcé*, especially in eclampsia and hæmorrhage, when version and extraction supply the readiest and most conservative method of delivery.

Marked degrees of pelvic deformity contra-indicate the operation. It is true that version can be accomplished, but afterward it is frequently impossible to extract an unmutilated child. It should never be attempted when the child is suffering from *hydrocephalus*.

The most favourable time for the performance of the operation is immediately after the rupture of the membranes, before the amniotic fluid has drained off, and while the child is readily movable in any direction. Generally speaking, podalic version should not be attempted through an imperfectly dilated cervix, except in certain cases of placenta prævia.

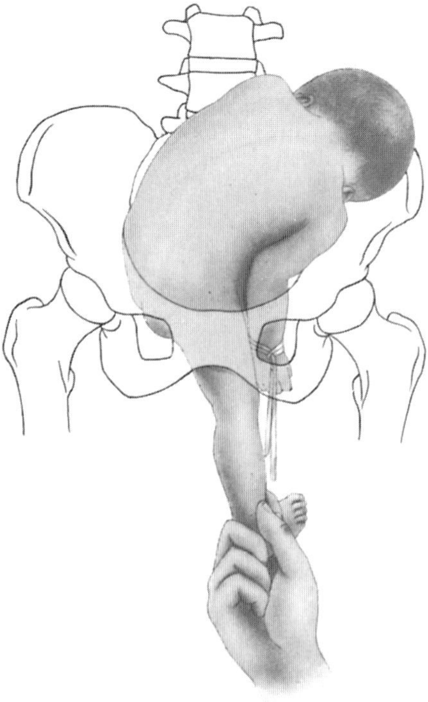

FIG. 397.—VERSION: TRANSVERSE PRESENTATION, BACK ANTERIOR, SEIZURE OF LOWER FOOT.

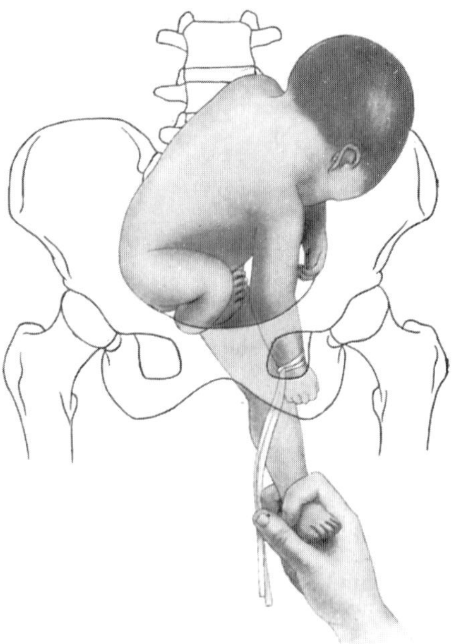

FIG. 398.—VERSION: TRANSVERSE PRESENTATION, BACK ANTERIOR, SEIZURE OF UPPER FOOT.

In many cases the patient is not seen until long after rupture of the membranes, and conditions may be present which render the operation extremely difficult or even impossible. For example, the uterus may be tetanically contracted and so tightly applied to the body of the child as to render even the introduction of the hand extremely difficult. In other cases, if a long interval has elapsed since the rupture of the membranes, the contraction ring may have risen to such an extent, and the lower uterine segment be so stretched as to render the operation dangerous in the highest degree, as the attempt at version will probably lead to rupture of the uterus.

Technique.—The patient should be anæsthetized and placed upon a table or brought to the edge of the bed, and the usual preparations for an operation made. Version should never be undertaken without an accurate diagnosis as to the presentation and position of the child. The abdomen should be covered by sterile towels so as to allow one hand to be applied over its lower portion without becoming infected.

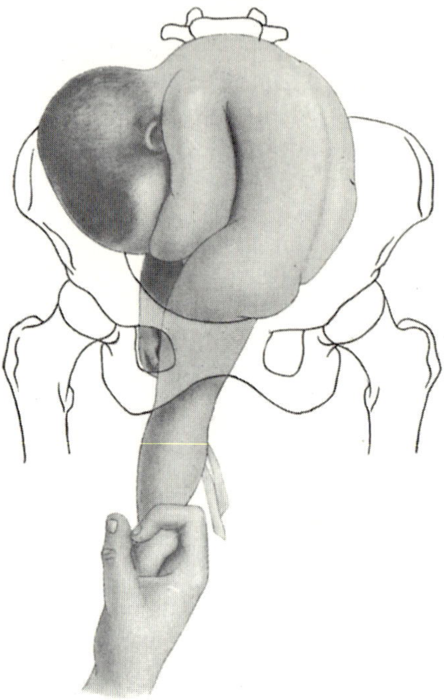

Fig. 399.—Version: Transverse Presentation, Back Posterior, Seizure of Upper Foot.

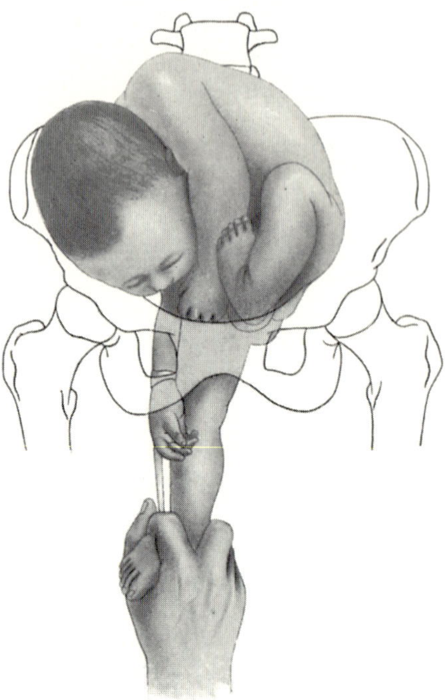

Fig. 400.—Version: Transverse Presentation, Back Posterior, Seizure of Lower Foot, showing Arrest of Buttocks at the Pelvic Brim.

Podalic version may be accomplished by one or two methods—internal or combined. In the former the entire hand is introduced into the uterus, while in the latter only two fingers are pressed through the cervix; but in both methods the other hand is applied over the abdomen and controls the movements of the fœtus.

Internal Podalic Version.—This should be attempted only after complete dilatation of the cervix. If the membranes are intact, they are ruptured and the hand is immediately introduced into the uterus; the feet are then seized and drawn through the cervix, the operation being usually, but not necessarily, followed by extraction. The method of procedure varies somewhat, according as one has to do primarily with a head or a transverse presentation. In the first instance the hand and arm must be introduced considerably farther into the genital canal than in the latter (Fig. 396).

If the child presents by the head, the choice of the hand which is to be passed into the uterus depends upon the location of the small parts. If the back be directed to the left, the feet can be seized most conveniently with the left hand, and *vice versa.* Generally speaking, it is advisable to attempt to grasp only one foot—if possible the anterior one—for when traction is made upon it the back will rotate to the front. The feet may be differentiated by tracing the course of the thigh and leg or by noting the relation of the great toe. Having found the proper foot, the ankle should be grasped between the index and second fingers, and slowly drawn through the cervix, while the external hand controls and guides the movements of the head.

In transverse presentations one foot is seized and version accomplished in the same manner. The choice of the foot, however, is a matter of very considerable importance. When the back is directed anteriorly, the lower one should be seized, as by so doing the back of the child is kept directed towards the symphysis; whereas, if the upper foot be seized the back may turn in the opposite direction. On the other hand, when the back looks posteriorly, the upper is the foot of choice, since traction upon it will cause the back to rotate to the front; while, if the lower foot be seized, although anterior rotation will usually occur, the upper buttock is liable to impinge upon the anterior portion of the pelvic brim, and great force may become necessary to effect its dislodgment (Figs. 397 to 400).

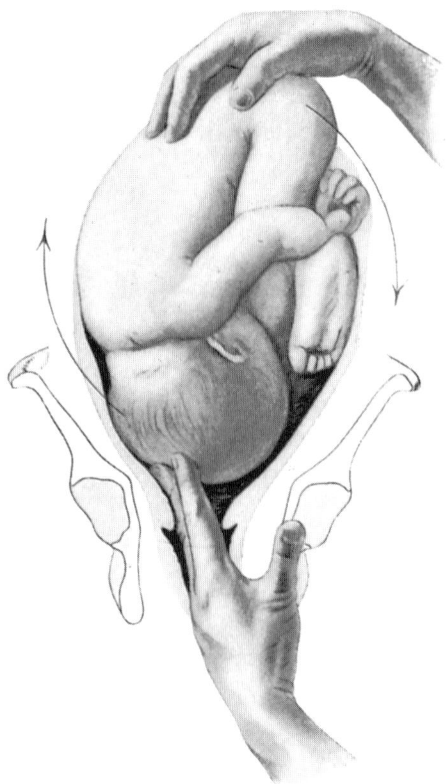

Fig. 401.—Bipolar Podalic Version (Bumm).

Not a few cases of transverse presentation are complicated by the prolapse of an arm into the vagina. Under such circumstances, a fillet should be applied around the wrist and held loosely by an assistant, while version is performed in the usual manner. In this way the arm is prevented from becoming extended over the head, and the necessity of freeing it during extraction is obviated.

Whatever may have been the original position of the child, firm pressure should be exerted upon the fundus of the uterus as soon as extraction is begun, in order to facilitate the delivery and at the same time prevent extension of the head or arms.

Combined Podalic Version.—In other instances, particularly in placenta prævia, version may be attempted by the combined or bipolar method as soon as the cervix is sufficiently dilated to admit two fingers. With these the presenting part is dislodged and pushed upward, while the external hand gradually brings the breech downward towards the external os. As soon as a foot can be felt it is seized by the two fingers and drawn through the cervix. For the time being this finishes the operation, as extraction should not be thought of until the cervix is fully dilated, for it is extremely difficult and can be effected only at the cost of deep cervical tears.

Prognosis.—For the mother, the prognosis following podalic version is excellent in properly selected cases, provided the patient be in good condition at the commencement of the operation. On the other hand, when attempted in the case of a tetanically contracted uterus, or when the lower uterine segment is overstretched, forcible attempts at version may lead to the rupture of the organ and death.

The prognosis for the child is fairly good, and depends upon the nature of the indication and the difficulty experienced in extraction. On the other hand, if the operation be undertaken through an imperfectly dilated cervix, and the child's head be arrested by the external os, the time required for its extraction is usually so great that death from asphyxiation is inevitable. Moreover, in cases of marked pelvic contraction, the fœtal mortality is very high. In many such cases forcible traction may enable one to deliver the child, but usually not until after the cord has been so long compressed as to have caused pronounced asphyxia and death, not to mention injuries to the head resulting from pressure.

LITERATURE

Ahlfeld. Ueber Behandlung gedoppelten Steisslagen, etc. Archiv f. Gyn., 1873, v, 174–176.

Bourgeois, Louise. Observations diverses, etc. Paris, 1609.

Budin. Tarnier et Budin, Traité de l'art des accouchements, 1901, t. iv, 296.

De la Motte. Traité complet des accouchements. Nouv. éd., Leiden, 1729.

D'Outrepont. Abh. und Beiträge, Würzburg, 1817, Theil I, 69.

Guillemeau. De l'heureux accouchement des femmes. Paris, 1609.

Hicks. On combined External and Internal Version. London, 1864.

Hubert. Quelques faits sur les présentations vicieuses du fœtus et sur la possibilité de les corriger par les manipulations extérieures. Annales de Gyn. et de Péd., 1843, août.

Kiwisch. Beiträge zur Geburtskunde, Würzburg, 1846, I. Abth., 69.

Litzmann. Der Mauriceau-Levret'sche Handgriff. Archiv f. Gyn., 1887, xxxi, 102–118.

Lusk. The Science and Art of Midwifery. New York, 1895, 338–391.

Mauriceau. Le moyen d'accoucher la femme, quand l'enfant présente un ou deux pieds les premiers. Traité des maladies des femmes grosses. 6me éd., 1721, 280–285.

Paré. Édition Malgaigne, 1840, t. ii, 623.

Pinard. De la version par les manœuvres externes. Traité du palper abdominal, Paris, 1889.

Quoted by Farabeuf and Varnier, Introduction à l'étude clinique des accouchements. Paris, 1891, 185–187.

Pugh. A Treatise on Midwifery chiefly with Regard to the Operation. London 1754.

Reynolds. The Value of Forceps in Complicated High Arrest of the Breech. Amer. Jour. Obst., 1892, xxvi, 586.

SMELLIE. The First Class of Preternatural Labours, when the Feet, Breech, or Lower Parts of the Fœtus Present. A Treatise on the Theory and Practice of Midwifery, eighth edition, 1774, 195–206.

VEIT, G. Ueber die beste Methode zur Extraction des nachfolgenden Kindeskopfes. Greifswalder med. Beiträge, 1863, ii, Heft I.

WIGAND. Ueber Wendung durch äussere Handgriffe. Hamburger med. Mag., 1807, i, 52.

WINCKEL. Zur Beförderung der Geburt des nachfolgenden Kopfes. Verh. d. deutschen Gesellsch. f. Gyn., 1888, ii, 19–32.

CHAPTER XXII

CÆSAREAN SECTION AND SYMPHYSEOTOMY

Cæsarean Section.—In this operation the child is removed from the uterus through an incision in the abdominal and uterine walls. The origin of the term has given rise to a great deal of discussion. It has been generally asserted that Julius Cæsar was brought into the world by this means, and obtained his name from the manner in which he was delivered (*a cæso matris utero*). This explanation, however, can hardly be correct, as his mother, Julia, lived many years after her son's birth; and, besides, Julius was not the first of his name, since there is mention of a priest named Cæsar who lived several generations before. The following view, however, would at least appear to be more plausible. In the Roman law, as codified by Numa Pompilius, it was ordered that the operation should be performed upon women dying in the last few weeks of pregnancy. This *lex regia*, as it was called at first, under the emperors became converted into the *lex cæsarea*, and the procedure itself became known as the *Cæsarean operation*.

History.—The history of Cæsarean section may be said to extend over three periods, the first lasting from the earliest times to the beginning of the sixteenth century. During this period the operation was occasionally resorted to after the death of the mother, in the hope of saving the child, but it is improbable that it was practised upon the living woman, although several authorities are inclined to believe that certain passages in the Talmud may be so interpreted. The fact that Dr. Felkin saw a Cæsarean section performed among the natives of Uganda renders it possible that it may have been employed upon the living woman at an early period by certain of the uncivilized races.

The second period extends from the year 1500 to 1876, when Porro described his method of amputating the pregnant uterus.

According to Caspar Bauhin, the first Cæsarean section upon a living woman was performed in 1500, when Jacob Nufer, a castrator of pigs at Sigerhausen, Switzerland, operated successfully upon his own wife after she had been given up by the midwives and barbers in attendance. The fact, however, that the woman had five spontaneous labours later would go to show that this was not a true Cæsarean section, but probably the simple removal of an extra-uterine child from the abdominal cavity.

François Rousset, a contemporary of Paré, wrote a treatise upon the subject in 1581, in which he gave the histories of a number of Cæsarean sections collected from various sources. Several of them were probably apocryphal, while others, in all probability, were operations for advanced extra-uterine pregnancy. His article, however, had the merit of directing attention to the operation and to the possibility of performing it upon the living woman. The first authentic Cæsarean section was probably done in 1610 by Trautmann, of Wittenberg. Following this, it was occasionally performed upon the living woman up to 1777, when it became temporarily eclipsed by symphyseotomy, to be taken up again after the latter operation fell into disrepute.

During this period the uterus was simply incised and the child extracted. The uterine walls were not sutured, the contraction and retraction of the organ being relied upon to check hæmorrhage. Most of the women perished from hæmorrhage or infection. Sutures were first employed by Lebas (1769), but did not come into general use until after the appearance of Sänger's epoch-making article upon the subject in 1882.

Before the work of Porro and Sänger, the mortality following the operation was appalling. Meyer (1867) collected 1,605 cases from the literature with a mortality of 54 per cent; while in 80 cases performed in the United States up to 1878, collected by Harris, 52.5 per cent of the women died. According to Budin, not a single successful Cæsarean section was performed in Paris between the years 1787 and 1876. Such poor results were obtained by physicians that Harris pointed out that the operation was more successful when performed by the patient herself, or when the abdomen was ripped open by the horn of an infuriated bull. He collected 9 such cases from the literature with 5 recoveries, and stated that out of 11 Cæsarean sections performed in the city of New York during the same period, only one patient recovered.

The third period began with the year 1876, when Porro advised amputating the body of the uterus and stitching the cervical stump into the lower angle of the abdominal wound in order to lessen the danger from hæmorrhage and infection. This procedure being followed by very satisfactory results, soon became quite popular, so that in 1890 Harris was able to collect 264 operations from the literature. Storer, of Boston, in 1868, performed a similar operation upon a pregnant myomatous uterus, with a fatal result, but inasmuch as he did not appear to recognise the importance of the innovation, the credit for proposing it undoubtedly belongs to Porro.

Sänger, in 1882, revolutionized the Cæsarean section by directing attention to the necessity for the employment of uterine sutures. As the uterus was not sacrificed in this operation, it was designated as the *conservative*, in contradistinction to the *Porro* Cæsarean section. With the increasing perfection of surgical technique more and more satisfactory results were obtained from the former operation, while the latter became less popular.

After the supravaginal amputation of the myomatous uterus had become more perfected, similar methods were applied to the Porro operation, the cervical stump being covered by a flap of peritonæum and dropped into the abdominal cavity; while in a small number of cases, particularly when the cervix was carcinomatous, the entire organ was removed. The latter procedure, which was first attempted by Bischoff, has a limited field of application.

Indications.—The most frequent and important indication for Cæsarean section is afforded by pelves which are so contracted as to offer a serious mechanical obstacle to labour. The pelvic indication may be either *absolute* or *relative,* the upper limits being a conjugata vera of 5 and 7.5 centimetres respectively. In the former the contraction is so pronounced that the birth of the child cannot be effected by any other means; while in the latter it is sufficiently marked to render spontaneous labour impossible, but permits delivery after craniotomy. When the conjugata vera measures not less than 6.5 centimetres, a living, not overlarge child may be delivered after symphyseotomy.

In view of the excellent results which now follow Cæsarean section, and the fact that the spontaneous delivery of an ordinary full-term child is out of the question when the conjugata vera is less than 7 centimetres, the upper limit for the absolute indication has been extended to that point, provided the patient is in good condition and amid suitable surroundings for a major operation. Otherwise the old limits are retained.

At the 1901 meeting of the American Gynæcological Society, I advocated that the relative indication be likewise broadened in appropriate cases, and its upper limit placed at a conjugata vera of 8.5 centimetres in flat, and 9 centimetres in generally contracted pelves.

In cases of this character, the course of labour will depend upon the size and consistency of the head and the character of the uterine contractions. Given two women with pelves of the same size, one may have a spontaneous and easy labour, while the other may require Cæsarean section for delivery. In such cases the operation is undertaken primarily in the interests of the child, instead of resorting to high forceps, version, or craniotomy. The patient is allowed to go into labour, to complete the first and enter the second stage. In most cases the head becomes engaged, and spontaneous delivery occurs. On the other hand, if signs of engagement are wanting after one hour of strong second-stage pains, the propriety of performing Cæsarean section should be considered, provided the patient has not been subjected to repeated vaginal examinations, is in good condition, and in the hands of a competent operator. By so doing nearly all the children will be saved, and quite as many mothers as after difficult high-forceps operations or craniotomy. If, however, these conditions cannot be fulfilled, Cæsarean section becomes a very dangerous procedure and should not be considered. In such cases the patient should be allowed to continue in labour until a definite indication for its termination arises, when high forceps, version, or craniotomy should be resorted to according to the exigencies of the particular case.

There is a general misconception as to the *innocuousness of craniotomy,* a somewhat general belief existing that it is unattended by maternal mortality. The results of Pinard and Bar, however, prove the contrary, as their mortality was 11.5 and 9.39 per cent respectively. At the same time, it must be admitted that many of their patients were infected and in bad condition when first seen, and consequently their results were infinitely worse than they would have been had all been clean cases. But when this fact has received full consideration, their figures still serve to show that the operation is not devoid of danger even when undertaken under favourable conditions.

Pelvic contraction involving the superior strait is not the only indication for Cæsarean section; in not a few cases abnormalities of the pelvic outlet likewise call for its performance. Under such circumstances a bis-ischial diameter of 7 centimetres or less is a positive indication for the operation. Other pelvic deformities which occasionally necessitate the operation will be considered in the chapter upon Contracted Pelves.

Obstruction to labour, due to conditions other than pelvic contraction, occasionally affords an indication for the operation. Thus, myomata in the lower segment of the uterus, as well as ovarian and other tumours which are prolapsed and cannot be replaced under anæsthesia, may so block the pelvic canal as to render Cæsarean section imperative. The same may be said of certain cicatricial contractions of the cervix or vagina.

Carcinoma of the cervix occasionally results in the formation of such dense and rigid tissue that dilatation becomes impossible. In such cases Cæsarean section is demanded in the interests of both the child and mother, and should be supplemented by total hysterectomy, if the disease be not too far advanced. In rare instances malignant tumours of the rectum may so obstruct the pelvic canal as to render Cæsarean section imperative. Holzapfel lately reported a case of this character and collected 6 others from the literature.

Halbertsma suggested Cæsarean section as the best method of delivery in certain cases of eclampsia complicated by an undilated and rigid cervix. Olshausen's experience also favours this view. In exceptional cases, in a well-regulated hospital, it is certainly a more conservative procedure than the forcible dilatation of a cartilaginous and rigid cervix.

Contra-indications.—Except in the presence of an absolute indication, Cæsarean section should never be performed when the child is dead or in serious danger. It is likewise contra-indicated when the mother is infected, in poor condition, or among surroundings which render an aseptic operation impracticable. Under such circumstances craniotomy is the operation of choice, and Cæsarean section should not be undertaken unless a living child is earnestly desired; and then only after the risks incident to it have been clearly explained to a responsible member of the family. Again, the operation is usually contra-indicated when the patient has been subjected to repeated vaginal examinations during labour by one whose technique is questionable, even though no signs of infection are apparent at the time. If, however, the operation should be decided upon in the presence of such risks, the entire uterus should be removed after delivery of the child.

Operative Technique: (*a*) *Conservative Cæsarean Section.*—When undertaken for the absolute or even for the relative indication, if previous labours have repeatedly ended in the birth of dead children, the operation, if possible, should be performed at an appointed time, a day or so prior to the expected onset of labour. In many cases, however, especially in hospital practice, this is out of the question, inasmuch as the patient is often not seen until she is well advanced in labour. Moreover, in the border line cases, with the broadened relative indication, the patient must be allowed to go into labour in order to afford Nature an opportunity of demonstrating what she can do. In such cases only one vaginal examination should be made, and that not until some time has elapsed after the rupture of the membranes. Then, if there appears to be no likelihood of spontaneous delivery, Cæsarean section should be promptly performed, as the prospects for recovery decrease in almost geometrical ratio for every hour elapsing after the onset of the second stage.

When the operation can be performed at a fixed time, the patient should be prepared exactly as for an ordinary abdominal operation. On the night before, after she has received a full bath, the abdomen should be shaved, disinfected, and covered with a bichloride compress. The bowels should be evacuated by an appropriate cathartic, and an enema given a few hours before she is put upon the table.

Just before the beginning of the operation, the bladder is catheterized and the abdomen redisinfected in the usual manner with permanganate of potassium, oxalic acid, bichloride of mercury, alcohol, and ether. The woman is then placed in the dorsal or a slightly elevated Trendelenburg position, and the entire body, except the field of operation, is covered with sterile towels. If the patient is not seen until labour has set in, similar preparations should be made, except that the bath and the administration of a cathartic must, of course, be dispensed with.

In addition to the operator, four assistants are needed, one to give the anæsthetic, one to assist directly at the wound, and two to handle the instruments, ligatures, and sponges. With the exception of the anæsthetist, all should wear rubber gloves throughout the operation. A competent person should be charged with the reception and care of the child and receive careful instructions as to the best method of resuscitating it if necessary. The following instruments are required: 1 scalpel, 1 long blunt-pointed scissors, 2 dissecting forceps, 12 short and 6 long artery clamps, an abdominal retractor, a needle-holder and appropriate needles, as well as the usual sterile dressings, suture materials, and gauze sponges.

An incision from 16 to 18 centimetres long should be made in the linea alba with the umbilicus as its middle point. In this way injury to the bladder, which often extends one third or even one half of the distance between the symphysis and umbilicus, and also to the lower uterine segment, is avoided. The abdominal walls are usually very thin and bleed but little, rarely more than two or three clamps being required to check hæmorrhage.

The uterus will be found immediately beneath the incision. As soon as it is exposed, sterile gauze handkerchiefs should be tucked between it and the margins of the abdominal incision. If it lies obliquely, its long axis should be brought into coincidence with that of the wound, and the organ opened *in situ*, provided the patient is not infected. The escape of amniotic fluid into the peritoneal cavity can be prevented by having the assistant press the edges of the abdominal wound firmly against the uterus. If, however, there is any question as to the sterility of its contents, the uterus should be delivered through the abdominal incision and not cut into until it has been carefully packed off, so that all possibility of contaminating the abdominal cavity may be avoided.

The anterior surface of the uterus is opened longitudinally along its middle line. This is best accomplished by making an incision a few centimetres long with a scalpel, and then rapidly enlarging it with the scissors to 16 or 18 centimetres. The membranes are then ruptured, the child is seized by one foot and rapidly extracted. Two clamps are applied to the cord, which is cut between them, and the child handed to an assistant. This takes but a short time, and it is rare for more than ninety seconds to elapse between the beginning of the operation and the birth of the child. Many authorities recommend that an attempt be made to locate the position of the placenta beforehand, so that the incision may be made in such a way as to avoid it. This, however, is not necessary. If the placenta lies under the incision it should be rapidly cut through or pushed to one side and the child extracted. This is accompanied by a slight increase of hæmorrhage, but as the operation is necessarily bloody, and as the bleeding is only momentary, it is without significance. Immediately after the delivery of the child the uterus contracts down and hæmorrhage practically ceases. The contracted organ should then be delivered from the abdomen, and the edges of the abdominal incision above it brought together by an artery clamp and covered by a sterile towel, so as to prevent the uterus coming in contact with the skin surface. If the placenta and membranes have not become separated spontaneously they should be peeled off and removed with the hand, care being taken that no shreds of membranes are left behind. Disinfection of the uterine cavity is not necessary.

To prevent hæmorrhage, Litzmann recommended that an elastic ligature be applied about the cervix before opening the uterus. This is, however, an unnecessary precaution; nor is it devoid of danger, as the prolonged compression predisposes to uterine atony and hæmorrhage afterward. If, however, there is considerable loss of blood after the delivery of the child, the assistant should grasp the cervix firmly between his fingers and compress the uterine arteries. This effectually controls hæmorrhage and is preferable to the employment of a rubber ligature, as transient compression only is needed, and the fingers can be removed as soon as the object is accomplished.

Fritsch, in 1897, proposed opening into the uterus through a *transverse incision* over the fundus, instead of by the usual method, holding that, the course of blood-vessels in that location being parallel to the incision, the hæmorrhage would therefore be less. His proposal was at once tested by many operators. Trinks, Hübl, Hahn, and H. Schroeder have published tables of cases so operated upon, the latter having collected 94 cases. The results were excellent, but not better than those following the more usual incision.

There would appear to be no especial advantage in adopting Fritsch's suggestion, except in the small number of cases in which it is desired to sterilize the patient by excising the tubes. On the other hand, there are several objections to its employment. In the first place, it requires a longer abdominal incision and the evisceration of the uterus. Moreover, the intestines and omentum are more liable to become adherent to the uterine wound with the transverse than with the longitudinal incision. It is urged that the fundal wound is less likely to be followed by adhesions between the uterus and the anterior abdominal wall. This is no doubt correct, but at the same time, should infection of the uterine wound occur with the former incision, virulent material is more liable to gain access to the general peritoneal cavity; while, if it occurs with the latter, the abscess has more chance of opening through the abdominal wound.

No matter which incision has been employed, it is then closed by deep silk and superficial catgut sutures, or, if preferred, formol catgut may be used for both. The former are inserted at intervals of about 1 centimetre, and extend through the entire thickness of the muscularis, avoiding the decidua. They are then tied, and if accurate approximation is not secured, the gaping margins of the wound are brought together by superficial catgut sutures which extend through the peritonæum and the upper layers of the muscularis. Sänger recommended the formation of a small flap of peritonæum on either side of the wound, by excising a thin layer of muscularis from its margins and uniting the flaps by sero-serous sutures. This procedure, however, is not only unnecessary, but also considerably prolongs the operation. Any blood which may have escaped into the pelvic cavity is then carefully sponged out and the abdominal wound closed. This is best accomplished by suturing the peritonæum, muscles, fascia, and skin in separate layers.

(*b*) *Porro Cæsarean Section.*—Until after the delivery of the child, the operative steps are identical in the Porro and the conservative Cæsarean section. In the former, however, as the body of the uterus is to be amputated, it is unnecessary to remove the placenta. As soon as the child is delivered, an elastic ligature is tightly tied around the upper portion of the cervix. The infundibulo-pelvic ligaments are then ligated and cut through, after which the uterus is amputated a short distance above the rubber ligature. To prevent the stump from slipping backward, a long, straight needle is passed through it and allowed to rest upon the abdominal walls. The stump is then sewed into the lower angle of the abdominal wound, the remainder being closed in the usual manner. Within a short time the stump and elastic ligature slough off, leaving a depressed wound which heals by granulation. This operation is readily performed, but is rarely employed at present, because of the complicated healing necessary, and the in-drawn scar which results.

Instead of the typical Porro operation, when it is desirable to remove the body of the uterus, the stump is best treated as in an ordinary myomectomy. The infundibulo-pelvic and round ligaments on either side are ligated at their distal ends, clamped at their uterine ends and severed. With a single stroke of the scissors, the broad ligament on either side is cut through down to its base. An elliptical incision is then made through the peritonæum on the anterior surface of the uterus, just above the bladder, and a peritoneal flap rapidly peeled off by means of a piece of gauze applied around the end of the finger or the handle of a scalpel. The uterine arteries are then isolated, ligated, and severed, after which the body of the uterus is amputated. The peritoneal flap is stitched over the cervical stump, which is then dropped into the pelvic cavity. The openings in the broad ligaments are then closed by continuous catgut sutures, the pelvic cavity is sponged out, and the abdominal wound closed.

The operation is readily performed, and can be completed in less time than is required for an ordinary Cæsarean section; for, owing to the laxness of the pelvic floor and the abdominal walls, the upper portion of the cervix can be brought through the incision and the entire operation completed upon the surface of the abdomen instead of in the depths of the pelvis.

(*c*) *Total Hysterectomy.*—Bischoff was the first to remove the entire uterus after Cæsarean section, and at the present time, under thoroughly aseptic conditions, the operation gives satisfactory results. The technique is identical with that employed in supravaginal amputation of the uterus, except that after the ligation of the uterine arteries the vaginal vault is cut through and the entire uterus removed, after which the opening in the vagina is closed with catgut and the broad ligament wounds are sutured. Total hysterectomy is rarely indicated except in cancer of the uterus, or in the occasional cases of infection.

Choice of Operation.—In the vast majority of cases the conservative Cæsarean section is the operation of choice, as it is readily performed and gives most satisfactory results. On the other hand, when there is any possibility of infection, complete, or at least supravaginal, hysterectomy should be done. When the uterus is the seat of tumour formation, as well as in those cases in which osteomalacia is the cause of the pelvic deformity, or in which persistent hæmorrhage resulting from uterine atony complicates the conservative operation, supravaginal hysterectomy is the operation of choice.

In doing a Cæsarean section the question often arises as to the advisability of *sterilizing the patient* so as to avoid the possibility of future conception. This can be effected by supravaginal amputation of the uterus, by excising the tubes, or removing the ovaries.

It was formerly believed that sterilization could be effected by ligating the proximal end of either tube; but experience has shown that the ligatures eventually cut through or become absorbed, and that the lumen of the tube may subsequently become restored, and with it the possibility of future pregnancy. It was next suggested that the object might be accomplished by applying a double ligature to each tube and excising the portion between them; but the experiments of Fraenkel upon animals, and the experience of Zweifel upon the living woman, have shown that even these measures do not insure against conception, since the ligatures may be absorbed and the cut ends of the tube become united. In order, therefore, to render a woman permanently sterile by an operation upon the tubes, they must be excised by wedge-shaped incisions at the cornua of the uterus and the wounds closed by sutures. When this is to be done, the fundal incision is preferable, as it can readily be extended to the cornua of the uterus after the extraction of the child.

Sterilization should not be attempted by the removal of the ovaries, for the reason that the retracting uterus may exert such tension upon the pedicles that the sutures may slip and fatal hæmorrhage result. Of course the woman is effectually sterilized after supravaginal amputation or total hysterectomy, but in most cases it is better to excise the tubes and leave the uterus and ovaries, in order that the patient may escape the inconveniences attending a premature menopause.

The opinion of those authorities who consider that sterilization should form an integral part of every Cæsarean section is certainly open to question. If the patient is intelligent, the decision should be left to her or her family; whereas with the ignorant it is incumbent upon the physician to do what he thinks is best under the circumstances. Personally, I should be unwilling to sterilize the patient at the first operation, unless she comes from a district where proper operative help might not be available in a future pregnancy. On the other hand, if she is weak-minded or diseased and is liable to require repeated Cæsarean sections the operation is perfectly justifiable.

Prognosis.—When considering the history of Cæsarean section, reference was made to the mortality attending it in former times. Since the rehabilitation of the conservative operation by Sänger in 1882, and the constant advance in aseptic technique, there has been a corresponding steady improvement in the results: Caruso collected from the literature 135 cases which had been performed between the years 1882 and 1888, with a mortality of 25.56 per cent. Since then the death-rate has gradually fallen, so that at present on an average less than 10 per cent of the women are lost.

Indeed, in the hands of expert operators, still more favourable results are the rule. Thus, Zweifel has performed 76 Cæsarean sections with 1, and Reynolds 23 with no deaths. In 335 operations performed by Chrobak, Schauta, Leopold, Braun, Olshausen, Zweifel, Reynolds, Bar, Charles, and Cragin, there were only 23 deaths—a gross mortality of 6.87 per cent, which becomes reduced to 4.06 per cent on deducting the cases which were infected prior to the operation. In the 11 Cæsarean sections performed at the Johns Hopkins Hospital all the mothers were saved, and the only death in our clinic followed an operation performed upon a coloured woman at her own home, in a room so small as to make it necessary to remove the bed in order to find space for the operating table. Thus it will be seen that the mortality following the conservative Cæsarean section, when properly performed upon uninfected patients amid good surroundings, should hardly exceed that attending the removal of simple ovarian tumours. On the other hand, it should be remembered that when performed by inexperienced operators upon patients in poor condition and amid unhygienic surroundings, the results will be most disastrous.

The typical Porro operation and the supravaginal amputation of the uterus, with retroperitoneal treatment of the stump, have shown a similar improvement. Thus, 441 Porro operations performed up to the year 1891, and tabulated by Harris, give some idea of the rapid decrease in mortality. From 1876 to 1881 there were 95, from 1882 to 1886, 148, and from 1887 to 1891, 198 operations, with a mortality of 60 per cent, 45 per cent, and 22.8 per cent respectively. During the same period the mortality following retroperitoneal treatment of the stump was reduced from 85.7 per cent to 16.6 per cent. In 177 operations recently reported by Chrobak, Schauta, Leopold, and Braun, the gross mortality was 10.3 per cent, which became reduced to 2.5 per cent on deducting the cases which were infected prior to operation. On the other hand, when performed upon infected patients, no matter what method be employed, the results of the operation are still extremely unsatisfactory, Doktor, of Budapest, having collected 22 such cases, with a mortality of 23.5 per cent.

This marvellous diminution in the mortality is due to several factors. Primarily, of course, it must be attributed to the ever-increasing perfection of aseptic technique. At the same time, careful examination of the pelvis before labour and the determination to operate while the patient is in good condition, instead of only after the failure of other methods of delivery, have contributed markedly to the improvement. It should be remembered that the best results are obtained when the operation is resorted to at the end of pregnancy or at the onset of labour, and that they rapidly become worse the later in the second stage it is performed. In my experience convalescence in the former class of cases is uninterrupted, while in the latter it is usually more or less seriously interfered with.

Repeated Cæsarean Section.—The performance of conservative Cæsarean section does not interfere with future conception, as is shown by the fact that even in pre-antiseptic times not a few cases were reported in which the same woman had repeatedly been subjected to the operation. Leopold speaks of a patient upon whom he operated four times, while Ahlfeld and Birnbaum have reported cases of women who underwent five Cæsarean sections. The statistics of Abel, Bar, and Caruso show that 43 patients had been subjected to the procedure upon two or more occasions, without a death, thus apparently indicating that a subsequent operation is even better borne than the first.

The occurrence of pregnancy after a Cæsarean section, however, is not always devoid of danger, as Woyer and Targett have reported cases in which the uterine cicatrix ruptured in the latter part of the subsequent gestation. This, however, is a very unusual occurrence. It is also stated that the adhesions which sometimes form between the uterus and the anterior abdominal wall occasionally exert a deleterious influence in subsequent pregnancies. Aside, however, from the slight discomfort incident to their stretching, no serious consequences have been observed, and in not a few cases the subsequent operation has been done through the old adhesions without opening into the general peritoneal cavity.

Vaginal Cæsarean Section.—By this name Dührssen has described an operation by means of which the child is delivered by the vagina through an incision in the cervix and lower uterine segment. This, of course, is only practicable where the pelvis is approximately normal, and the indications are therefore quite different from those that hold good in the cases that have just been considered.

In this procedure the anterior and posterior *culs-de-sac* are opened and the bladder is separated from its connections, after which an incision is made through the cervix and lower uterine segment sufficiently large to permit the extraction of the child by version or forceps. After delivery the wounds are closed by sutures, or in other cases the entire organ is removed by vaginal hysterectomy. Dührssen, in 1900, collected 22 such operations with 5 deaths, the majority of them having been undertaken for carcinoma of the cervix, and several for eclampsia. The operation has a very limited field of usefulness, and should be reserved for cases complicated by carcinoma, in which it is desired to follow delivery by vaginal hysterectomy.

Laparo-elytrotomy.—This operation, which was recommended by Baudelocque in 1823, and rehabilitated by Gaillard Thomas in 1871, aims at delivering the child without opening the peritoneal cavity. For this purpose an oblique incision is made just above Poupart's ligament and the cervix reached extraperitoneally. After its exposure, an incision is made into it through which the child is extracted. This operation, while useful in pre-antiseptic times, is no longer employed, inasmuch as better and more certain results are obtained by the usual methods of procedure.

Post-mortem Cæsarean Section.—From the earliest times, when a patient died undelivered in the neighbourhood of full term, Cæsarean section was sometimes performed immediately after her death, in the hope of saving the life of the child. The number of children rescued by the procedure, however, has always been very small. In view of this fact, and the abhorrence in which it is more or less justly held by the laity, I do not consider that it should be recommended, more satisfactory results being obtainable from *accouchement forcé*, especially as the cervix just before or immediately after death is more readily dilatable than at other times.

Symphyseotomy.—By symphyseotomy is meant the division of the pubic joint in order to bring about an increase in the capacity of a contracted pelvis sufficient to permit the passage of a living child.

J. R. Sigault first performed the operation in 1777, and thereby successfully delivered a certain Madame Suchot, of Paris, who had a rhachitic pelvis with a conjugata vera of 6.5 centimetres and had previously given birth to four dead children. The procedure created a great sensation, though when the patient was exhibited before the Faculty of Medicine two months later she walked with considerable difficulty, and had a urinary fistula from which she never recovered.

The operation was taken up with great enthusiasm, and was performed upon 11 patients within the first year after Sigault's report. Opposition to it, however, soon developed, Baudelocque denouncing it as a "murderous and unphilosophical procedure"; and the discussion as to its merits waxed so bitter that the Parisian physicians became divided into two groups, Cæsareans and Symphyseans. As a result of poor technique and its employment in unsuitable cases, symphyseotomy soon fell into disrepute and was forgotten except in Italy, where it was performed sporadically until the year 1858.

The operation was rehabilitated in 1866 by Morisani, of Naples, who obtained very satisfactory results by its means, being able to report 50 operations with 40 recoveries to the International Medical Congress in

1881. It was reintroduced into France by Spinelli in 1891, who impressed its merits so strongly upon Pinard that he took it up and has since been its most enthusiastic advocate, being able to report in 1900 that 100 symphyseotomies had been performed in his clinic. The anatomical aspects of symphyseotomy were carefully studied by Farabeuf, who accurately demonstrated its theoretical possibilities. Dr. Robert P. Harris played a prominent part in directing attention to the operation in this country by a paper entitled The Remarkable Results of Antiseptic Symphyseotomy, read at the 1892 meeting of the American Gynæcological Society. Stimulated by this report, Jewett, a few years later, performed the first operation in America, and was soon followed by many others. Since then the question of symphyseotomy has been a burning one, and was the main theme of discussion at the German Gynæcological Congress in 1893, the International Medical Congress in 1897, and the Obstetrical Society of France in 1899.

Effect of Symphyseotomy upon the Size of the Pelvis.—As soon as the symphysis is cut through, the ends of the pubic bones gape from 3 to 6 centimetres. Owing to the structure of the sacro-iliac joints, the ossa innominata flare outward, while the tips of the pubic bones become depressed downward. As a result of these changes the capacity of the pelvic canal becomes considerably increased, particularly in its transverse and oblique, and less so in its antero-posterior diameters. It is usually stated that the conjugata vera becomes 2 millimetres longer for each centimetre of separation at the symphysis. As the latter may amount to 6 or 6.5 centimetres without imperilling the integrity of the sacro-iliac joints, the increase would aggregate 12 or 13 millimetres.

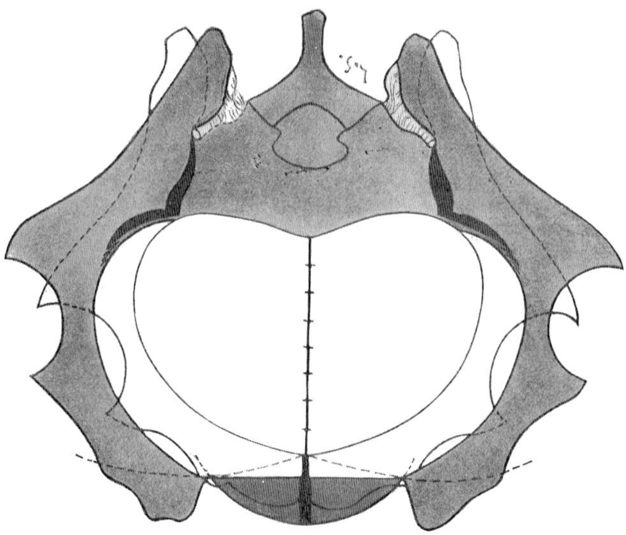

Fig. 402.—Diagram showing Effect of Symphyseotomy (Farabeuf).

According to Farabeuf this estimate is not strictly correct, as the increase varies with the size of the pelvis, being 13 millimetres when the true conjugate measures 6 centimetres, and 10 millimetres when it measures 9 centimetres. This, however, does not represent the actual enlargement of the superior strait from an obstetrical point of view; for, as Farabeuf has pointed out, one of the parietal bosses fits into the opening between the gaping pubic bones, thereby considerably increasing the space available for the passage of the head. Döderlein has calculated that when the pubic bones gape 6 to 7 centimetres the area of the superior strait is increased by one half.

Indications.—The field of usefulness of symphyseotomy is comparatively limited. It is available only when the conjugata vera exceeds 6.5 centimetres, since in smaller pelves the increase in the area of the superior strait will not be sufficient to permit the passage of the head. Accordingly, the operation cannot be considered as a substitute for Cæsarean section, except in a few cases at the upper limit of the old relative indication. Thus symphyseotomy must be regarded as a competitor of version, high forceps, and craniotomy, or with Cæsarean section for the broadened relative indication.

As the operation merely enlarges the pelvis, and must be followed by the extraction of the child by version or forceps, it is apparent that an error in the estimation of the size of the head or the pelvis may lead to very untoward results, cases having been reported in which Cæsarean section or craniotomy became necessary to effect delivery after an ill-chosen symphyseotomy. Moreover, the operation does not become available until the cervix is completely dilated, or is so softened as to be readily dilatable before delivery is attempted. On the other hand, its great advantage lies in the fact that it can be resorted to after some hours after second-stage pains, when Nature has shown herself unequal to the task of delivery—conditions under which Cæsarean section is usually contra-indicated.

Although Davis and Jewett have recommended the performance of the operation in face presentations when the chin is posterior, as well as in certain impacted posterior occiput presentations, I know of no cases in which it has been undertaken for such indications.

The operation is contra-indicated when one or both sacro-iliac joints are ankylosed, as under such circumstances the iliac bones cannot become flared outward; although Pinard, in a case of Naegele pelvis, performed a modified operation—*ischio-pubiotomy*—with success. Moreover, symphyseotomy is a questionable procedure when the patient is profoundly infected. I cannot agree with Jewett and others that it is permissible under such circumstances, as I consider that better results will be obtained from craniotomy; or, if the patient be extremely desirous of having a living child, from Cæsarean section followed by total hysterectomy.

Method of Operating.—The patient should lie upon her back with her buttocks at the edge of the table. After the external genitalia, Mons Veneris, and lower portion of the abdomen have been shaved and cleaned as carefully as for an abdominal operation, everything except the Mons Veneris and lowest portion of the abdomen should be covered with sterile towels. An incision is made in the middle line from a few centimetres above the upper margin of the symphysis almost to its lower margin, extending through the skin and subcutaneous fat down to the fascia upon its anterior surface. A finger is passed behind the symphysis and separates the underlying tissues until its lower margin is perfectly free. This step is frequently accompanied by profuse hæmorrhage from the antevesical plexus. The attachments of the clitoris to the lower margin of the symphysis are then separated by blunt dissection, after which a catheter is passed into the urethra and pushes it downward and to one side. The pubic cartilage is then cut through with a strong knife, either from its anterior or posterior surface. In the latter case, a blunt-pointed bistoury is passed behind the symphysis and the section made from below upward.

In many cases the pubic bones do not spring apart after the symphysis has been cut through, being held in position by the strong subpubic ligament, although as soon as this has been isolated and severed they will gape several centimetres. They should not be allowed to separate more than 6 centimetres, any tendency towards excessive gaping being counteracted by flexing the thighs upon the abdomen and having an assistant make firm pressure upon the trochanters. Following section of the symphysis, there is usually a profuse venous hæmorrhage, which is best controlled by packing the wound with sterile gauze, clamps and ligatures not being available.

After symphyseotomy, the child should be delivered by forceps or version, according to circumstances. During the extraction, firm pressure should be made upon the trochanters on either side to prevent too wide a separation of the symphysis and consequent injury to the sacro-iliac joints. Owing to the fact that the anterior vaginal wall, bladder, and clitoris have been deprived of their natural support, they are exposed to considerable tension and may be torn through if excessive force is employed. By adducting the thighs after delivery of the child, the ends of the pubic bones are brought together, so that the ligamentous structures upon their anterior surface can be united by mattress or figure-of-eight sutures, and the external wound closed in the usual manner.

Ayres recommends that the operation be performed subcutaneously by making a small incision immediately over the clitoris through which a blunt-pointed knife is introduced, the symphysis being divided from behind forward and from below upward. This, however, does not appear an advisable procedure, as it precludes the possibility of suturing the symphysis and of successfully checking hæmorrhage.

After the completion of the operation, the wound should be covered with sterile dressings and a broad strap of canvas applied over the trochanters and tightly buckled, the latter being well padded with cotton to avoid injurious pressure. The after-treatment is extremely complicated and onerous. Frequent catheterization is necessary, and the patient must lie on her back for three or four weeks after the operation. During this period it is well to re-enforce the action of the pelvic strap by placing the patient in a hammock bed, especially devised for the purpose, or by allowing the pelvis to rest upon two sand-bags.

Prognosis.—Contrary to the usual statements, my experience leads me to consider that symphyseotomy is a very serious operation, and one not to be lightly undertaken. In many cases the hæmorrhage is exceedingly profuse and is calculated to disconcert an inexperienced operator. Moreover, the vaginal tears frequently extend through to the retropubic wound, and are not easy to repair. Occasionally the bladder is injured by the sharp end of one of the pubic bones, while more frequently the clitoris is wounded and gives rise to alarming hæmorrhage. Such lesions should be repaired immediately, so as to avoid communication between the vagina and the pubic wound, or the formation of urinary fistulæ. If errors in technique have occurred during the operation, or the patient be already infected, the process may extend to the pubic wound and lead to destructive suppuration.

Considerable apprehension has been expressed as to the possibility of failure of union at the symphysis pubis, and several cases have been reported by Müllerheim which serve to show that the operation may permanently maim the patient. Fortunately, such accidents are extremely rare; although the recent investigations of Varnier by means of the Röntgen ray show that there is greater motility at the symphysis than before the operation, the pubic bones being united by a mass of fibrous tissue several centimetres wide. This does not necessarily lead to disturbances of locomotion, but the patients find that they tire more readily, and are less able to perform hard labour, than before the operation.

It appears that symphyseotomy is sometimes followed by a slight but permanent increase in the size of the pelvis, which is sometimes sufficient to permit spontaneous labour in subsequent pregnancies. A number of such instances have recently been collected by Madame Wulff.

The analysis by Neugebauer of 278 symphyseotomies indicated a maternal mortality of 11.1 per cent, while in the 100 cases operated upon in Pinard's clinic there were 12 maternal deaths; and even after deducting a number of instances in which he considered that the fatal termination was due to other causes, the mortality was as high as 5 per cent. Bar, basing his conclusions upon 140 operations performed by himself, Pinard, Zweifel, and Küstner, estimates the death-rate at 6.7 per cent. On the other hand, Zweifel has operated 31 times without a death. The fœtal mortality was 13 per cent in Pinard's, and 9.39 per cent in Bar's cases.

On comparing the results following symphyseotomy and Cæsarean section in the same class of cases, it would appear that little can be said in favour of the former. In the first place, the maternal mortality following it equals, if it does not exceed, that following Cæsarean section, while the fœtal mortality is considerably greater, being 9 or 10 per cent in the former and practically nothing in the latter operation. Moreover, if an error is made in estimating the relative size of the head and pelvis, the child is inevitably lost with symphyseotomy, while such an error is a matter of no consequence when Cæsarean section is done. Furthermore, there is no comparison as regards convalescence following the two operations. After the former the patient requires prolonged rest in bed in an uncomfortable position, whereas after the latter she recovers in a short time and with but slight inconvenience.

Abel has compared the results obtained in 25 symphyseotomies and 50

Cæsarean sections performed in Zweifel's clinic. There were no maternal deaths after either operation. He found that the convalescence was much more rapid and comfortable after the latter; and, what is more important, three to five weeks only were required before the patient was able to take up again her ordinary duties after it, as compared with thirteen weeks after symphyseotomy.

One of the chief advantages which is claimed for symphyseotomy is that it can be readily performed by the general practitioner in unfavourable surroundings, and even upon infected patients; while Cæsarean section requires considerable operative ability, the most rigid aseptic technique, and ideal surroundings. I cannot subscribe to such an opinion, as I believe that the same requirements must be fulfilled to insure success after either operation. Of the two I consider symphyseotomy the more difficult, and do not believe that either should be attempted upon infected patients. Bar, after a considerable experience with the two operations—22 symphyseotomies and 10 Cæsarean sections—has concluded that the latter is decidedly preferable, and that the field for the former is very limited. At the 1899 meeting of the Obstetrical Society of France similar views were expressed by Budin, Charles, and others. Personally, at the present time, I do not expect to perform symphyseotomy under any circumstances, and consider that the present enthusiasm for it will eventually disappear.

LITERATURE

Abel. Vergleich der Dauererfolge nach Symphyseotomie und Sectio Caesarea. Archiv f. Gyn., 1899, lviii, 294–367.

Ahlfeld. Lehrbuch der Geburtshülfe, II. Aufl., 1898, 547.

Ayres. Symphyseotomy, etc. N. Y. Polyclinic, 1896, vii, 129–139.

Bar. De l'opération Césarienne conservative, etc. L'Obstétrique, 1899, iv, 193–230.

La symphyséotomie. Ses résultats immédiates et éloignés, etc. L'Obstétrique, 1899, iv, 305–384.

Leçons de pathologie obstétricale. Paris, 1900.

Baudelocque, A. Nouveau procédé pour pratiquer l'opération Césarienne. Thèse de Paris, 1823.

Baudelocque, J. L. De la section du pubis. L'art des accouchements, nouv. éd., 1789, ii, 461–561.

Bauhin. ὑστεροτομοτοκια. Fr. Rousseti, etc. Basil, 1588.

Birnbaum. 5 Kaiserschnitte bei einer Person. Archiv f. Gyn., 1885, xxv, 422.

Bischoff. Die totale Exstirpation des schwangeren und carcinomatösen Uterus. Correspondenzbl. f. Schweizer Aerzte, 1880, Nr. 6.

Braun-Fernwald. Ueber den in den letzten 10 Jahren ausgeführten Sectiones Caesareae, Archiv f. Gyn., 1899, lix, 320–404.

Budin. Tarnier et Budin, Traité de l'art des accouchements, 1901, iv, 495.

Budin et Demelin. Symphyséotomie. Tarnier et Budin, Traité de l'art des accouchements, 1901, iv, 456–489.

Caruso. Die neuesten Ergebnisse des conservativen Kaiserschnittes mit Uterusnaht. Archiv f. Gyn., 1888, xxxiii, 211–269.

Charles. Parallèle entre les diverses opérations à pratiquer dans les vices du bassin. L'Obstétrique, 1899, iv, 280–286.

Chrobak. Quoted by Braun-Fernwald.

CRAGIN. Cæsarean Section. Medical Record, 1901, lix, 659–701 (May 4, 1901).

DAVIS. The Management of Face Presentation. Medical News, July 14, 1894.

DÖDERLEIN. Exp. anat. Untersuchungen über die Symphyseotomie. Verh. d. deutschen Gesell. f. Gyn., 1893, v, 27–34.

DOKTOR. Kaiserschnitt bei Sepsis. Archiv f. Gyn., 1899, lix, 200–216.

DÜHRSSEN. Der vaginale Kaiserschnitt. Berlin, 1896.

Ein neuer Fall von vaginalen Kaiserschnitt, etc. Archiv f. Gyn., 1900, lxi, 548–564.

FARABEUF. Sur la symphyséotomie. Annales de Gyn. et d'Obst., 1894, xli, 407–431.

FELKIN. Quoted by Ploss. Das Weib in der Natur- und Völkerkunde, IV. Aufl., 1895, ii, 297.

FRAENKEL, L. Experimente zur Herbeiführung der Unwegsamkeit der Eileiter. Archiv f. Gyn., 1899, lviii, 374–410.

FRITSCH. Ein neuer Schnitt bei der Sectio Caesarea. Centralbl. f. Gyn., 1897, 561–565.

HAHN. 11 konservative Kaiserschnitte mit querem Fundalschnitt. Centralbl. f. Gyn., 1899, 1457–1476.

HALBERTSMA. Eclampsia gravidarum. Eine neue Indikationsstellung für die Sectio Caesarea. Centralbl. f. Gyn., 1889, 901.

HARRIS. Remarks on the Cæsarean Operation. Amer. Jour. Obst., 1879, xi, 620–626.

Cattle-horn Lacerations of the Abdomen and Uterus in Pregnant Women. Amer. Jour. Obst., 1887, xx, 673–685, and 1033.

Results of the Porro Cæsarean Operation in all Countries. British Med. Jour., 1890, i, 68.

The Remarkable Results of Antiseptic Symphyseotomy. Trans. Amer. Gyn. Soc., 1892, xvii, 98–126.

The Porro Cæsarean Section tested by a Trial of Sixteen Years, etc. N. Y. Jour. of Gyn. and Obst., 1893, iii, 273–283.

HIRST. The Comparative Value of Cœliohysterotomy and Cœliohysterectomy in Cases requiring Cæsarean Section. Amer. Jour. Obst., 1898, xxxvii, 577–584.

HOLZAPFEL. Kaiserschnitt bei Mastdarmkrebs. Hegar's Beiträge zur Geb. u. Gyn., 1899, ii, 59–77.

HÜBL. Ueber dem queren Fundusschnitt nach Fritsch. Monatsschr. f. Geb. u. Gyn., 1899, 417–432.

JEWETT. A Case of Symphyseotomy. Brooklyn Med. Jour., 1892, vi, 790–792.

The Place of Symphyseotomy as contrasted with Cæsarean Section. Amer. Med., 1901, September 28, 488–489.

LEBAS. Jour. de Méd. et de Chirurgie, 1770, xxxiv (supplement).

LEOPOLD und HAAKE. Ueber 100 Sectiones Caesareae. Archiv f. Gyn., 1898, liv, 1–41.

LITZMANN. Kaiserschnitt mit temporärer Ligatur des Cervix. Centralbl. f. Gyn., 1879, 289–295.

MEYER. Sulla gastroisterotomia. Napoli, 1867.

MORISANI. De la symphyséotomie. Annales de Gyn. et d'Obst., 1881, xvi, 444–445.

MÜLLERHEIM. Die Symphyseotomie. Volkmann's Sammlung klin. Vorträge, 1894, Nr. 91, 1–54.

NEUGEBAUER. Ueber die Rehabilitation der Schamfugentrennung, etc. Leipzig, 1893.

OLSHAUSEN. Kaiserschnitt wegen Eklampsie. Zeitschr. f. Geb. u. Gyn., 1900, xlii, 348–351.

Ueber den Kaiserschnitt und seine Indikation bei Beckenverengerung. Zeitschr. f. Geb. u. Gyn., 1897, xxxvii, 533–541.

PINARD. De la symphyséotomie. Annales de Gyn. et d'Obst., 1892, xxxvii, 81–94.

Indication de l'opération césarienne considérée en rapport avec celle de la symphyséotomie, etc. Annales de Gyn. et d'Obst., 1899, lii, 81–117.

Du soi-disant fœticide thérapeutique. Annales de Gyn. et d'Obst., 1900, liii, 1–18.

PORRO. Della amputazione utero-ovarica, etc. Milan, 1876.

REYNOLDS. Circumstances which render the Elective Section Justifiable in the Interest of the Child Alone. Amer. Med., 1901, ii, 489–493, September 28.

ROUSSET. Traité nouveau de l'hystérotomotokie ou l'enfantement césarien. Paris, 1581.

SÄNGER. Der Kaiserschnitt bei Uterusmyomen, etc. Leipzig, 1882.

SCHAUTA. Quoted by Braun-Fernwald.

SCHROEDER, H. Zur Kaiserschnittsfrage. Monatsschr. f. Geb. u. Gyn., 1901, xiii, 22–39, und 206–230.

SIGAULT. Discours sur les avantages de la section de la symphyse dans les accouchements, etc. Paris, 1779.

SPINELLI. Les résultats de la symphyséotomie, etc. Annales de Gyn. et d'Obst., 1892, xxxvii, 2–15.

STORER. Extirpation of the Puerperal Uterus by Abdominal Section. Jour. Gyn. Soc. of Boston, 1861, i, 223.

TARGETT. Rupture of Uterus in Old Cæsarean Section Cicatrix. Trans. Lond. Obst. Soc., 1900, p. 242.

THOMAS. Gastro-elytrotomy: A Substitute for the Cæsarean Section. Amer. Jour. Obst., 1871, iii, 125–139.

TRAUTMANN. See Siebold, Versuch einer Geschicht der Geburtshülfe, 1845, ii, 108–111.

TRINKS. Neue Kaiserschnittfragen, Fundalschnitt, etc. Hegar's Beiträge zur Geb. u. Gyn., 1898, i, 449–469.

VARNIER. Étude anat. et radiographique de la symphyséotomie. Comptes rendus de la Soc. d'Obst., de Gyn., et de Péd. de Paris, 1899, i, 208–243.

WILLIAMS. Pelvic Indications for the Performance of Cæsarean Section. Amer. Med., 1901, September 28; Trans. Amer. Gyn. Soc., 1901, xxvi, 260–276.

WOYER. Ein Fall von Spontanruptur des schwangeren Uterus in der alten Kaiserschnittsnarbe. Monatsschr. f. Geb. u. Gyn., 1897, vi, 192–200.

ZWEIFEL. Ueber Symphyseotomie. Monatsschr. f. Geb. u. Gyn., 1897, vi, 227.

Referred to by Abel.

Quoted by Braun-Fernwald.

CHAPTER XXIII

DESTRUCTIVE OPERATIONS

Craniotomy.—Under this heading are included all operations which bring about a decrease in the size of the fœtal head, with a view to rendering its delivery easier.

Prior to the introduction of podalic version and forceps, artificial delivery could be effected only by means of craniotomy or embryotomy, one or other of which was resorted to in nearly every case of difficult labour. Accordingly, in former times, the perforator, sharp hook, and crotchet were the most important instruments in the obstetrician's armamentarium. Increased dexterity in the employment of forceps and version, however, brought about a rapid change, and craniotomy upon the living child became rarer and rarer.

Indications.—Craniotomy is positively contra-indicated when the conjugata vera measures less than 5.5 centimetres, since in such cases the extraction of the child, even after the skull has been crushed, is attended by a greater maternal mortality than Cæsarean section. On the other hand, in pelves above this limit, craniotomy may be indicated under any conditions that render the delivery of a mutilated child the most conservative procedure, so far as the safety of the mother is concerned.

The indications for its performance vary markedly. When the child is dead craniotomy is indicated whenever it will render delivery easier, and is preferable to forceps or version unless those operations can be undertaken without detriment to the mother. Æsthetic considerations should never deter the operator from resorting to it. On the other hand, if the child is alive, the operation is justifiable only in exceptional cases; indeed, Pinard and some others hold that, in view of the satisfactory results obtained from symphyseotomy and Cæsarean section, it should never be performed. This, however, must be looked upon as too radical a view and one demanding a certain amount of qualification; for, although it must ever be the duty of the obstetrician to do his best to save the life of both mother and child, it is nevertheless readily conceivable that conditions may arise under which craniotomy upon the living child may not only be perfectly justifiable, but even imperatively demanded.

Generally speaking, craniotomy should not be performed upon the living child if the mother is in good condition, amid suitable surroundings, and in the hands of a competent operator. Under such circumstances, if the obstacle to labour be due to a contracted pelvis or an excessively large child, Cæsarean section is preferable, inasmuch as the slightly increased risk to the mother is more than compensated for by the rescue of her offspring. On the other hand, if the woman is not seen until she has been in the second stage of labour for a considerable time, and has been subjected to repeated vaginal examinations and possibly presents signs of infection, Cæsarean section is not indicated, but the child should be sacrificed in the interests of the mother, inasmuch as the maternal mortality attending Cæsarean section under such circumstances is in the neighbourhood of 25 per cent. Again, if the child is not in good condition, as shown by a too rapid or too slow heart-beat, or by the passage of considerable quantities of meconium with a vertex presentation, its life is already in such peril that, against that of the mother, it is no longer entitled to serious consideration.

Moreover, in country districts, where the physician is unable to summon sufficient assistance, and is without the necessary appliances for an aseptic abdominal operation, Cæsarean section should not be undertaken and craniotomy becomes the operation of choice. But even under these adverse conditions the latter operation should be deferred as long as possible, and should not be resorted to until delivery becomes imperative in the interests of the mother, and then only after the failure of forceps.

Hydrocephalus affords a positive indication for craniotomy, which should be performed as soon as the cervix is completely dilated. In these cases spontaneous labour is out of the question, and even a successful Cæsarean section will only give us a child that is doomed to die shortly or remain an idiot.

When insuperable obstacles are encountered during the extraction of the after-coming head, craniotomy is a justifiable procedure, since the child is already dead, or dies within a few minutes after the nature of the obstacle has been recognised, and before preparations can be made for its delivery by symphyseotomy.

Craniotomy should not be performed until the external os has become completely dilated, as the imperfectly opened canal may offer a serious obstacle to the extraction of the child.

Method of Operating.—The patient should be brought to the edge of the bed or table, placed in the lithotomy position, and prepared as for an ordinary obstetrical operation. Craniotomy usually includes two steps: first, the perforation of the head and the evacuation of its contents; and, secondly, the extraction of the mutilated child.

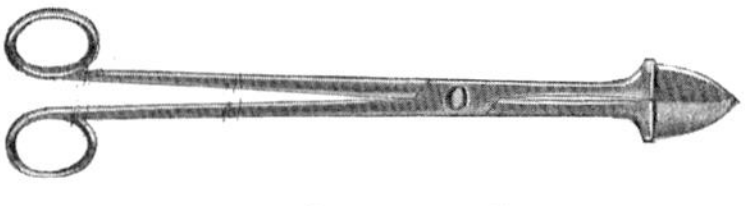

FIG. 403.—SMELLIE'S SCISSORS.

Numerous instruments have been devised for perforating the head, the most suitable of which are *Smellie's scissors* or Blot's perforator. Braun's trepan would serve the purpose admirably, but is not to be recommended on account of the difficulty with which it is kept clean.

If the head is engaged and firmly fixed, perforation is accomplished with but little difficulty. With two fingers the large or small fontanelle, as may be most convenient, is located, and the perforator plunged through it. The opening is then enlarged and the instrument briskly moved about within the skull, so as to disintegrate the brain to such an extent that it can be washed out with a douche of sterile water.

If, however, the head is movable above the superior strait, it must be firmly fixed by means of pressure exerted by an assistant through the abdominal walls. To avoid wounding the maternal soft parts, the perforation should be made through the portion of the head lying in the neighbourhood of the symphysis pubis; for, should the instrument slip from this position, it is less liable to inflict serious injury than if it were near the sacrum. In face presentations perforation should be effected through the brow.

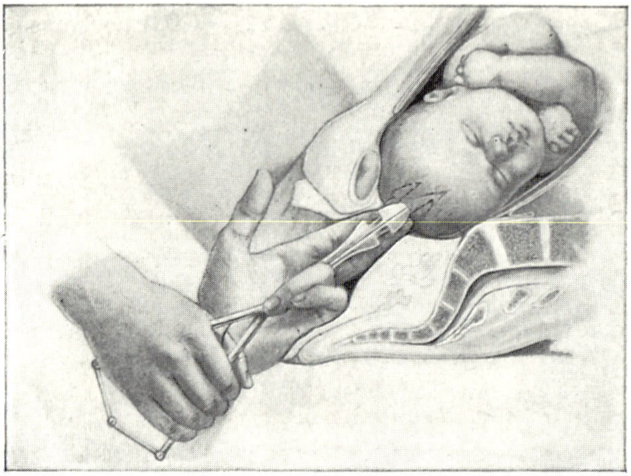

Fig. 404.—Method of Perforating Head (American Text-Book).

To pierce the after-coming head, the body of the child should be depressed and the instrument carried into the skull in the neighbourhood of the temporal suture. If, as occasionally happens, this point cannot be reached, the body of the child should be carried up over the abdomen of the mother, and perforation effected through the mouth and base of the skull. When a hydrocephalic child presents by the breech, and the head is arrested at the pelvic brim, the fluid contents of the skull may be evacuated by cutting through the arch of one of the cervical vertebræ, after which a metallic catheter is passed through the opening and carried along the vertebral canal into the skull.

After the brain has been washed out, although the vault of the cranium collapses and offers no further obstacle to labour, the base of the skull still remains unchanged, and as the bimastoid diameter measures between 7 and 7.5 centimetres, it is apparent that it cannot be delivered through a markedly contracted pelvis until it has been diminished in size.

When the conjugata vera exceeds 7.5 centimetres, the collapsed head may be expelled by the uterine contractions alone, or may be extracted by means of the forceps or a finger introduced through the perforation opening. But even in pelves of this size it is usually advisable to make use of a special instrument for grasping and crushing the base of the skull. The *cranioclast*, invented by Simpson and modified by Carl Braun, serves the purpose most satisfactorily. One blade is introduced

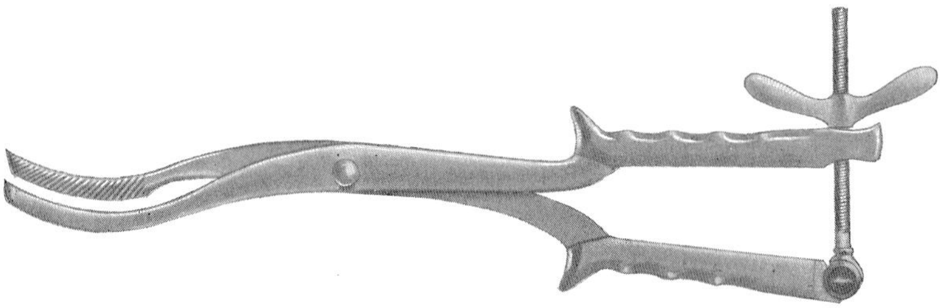

FIG. 405.—BRAUN'S CRANIOCLAST.

through the perforation until its free end impinges upon the base of the skull, while the fenestrated blade is applied over the face or lower portion of the occiput. The vise at the end of the instrument is then tightened, and as a result not only is the base of the skull more or less compressed, but at the same time a firm hold is obtained for the extraction that is to follow.

For crushing and extracting the head, Baudelocque the younger invented the *cephalotribe*. This is essentially a very heavy forceps, whose blades come closely together and forcibly compress the head when the vise at the ends of the handles is tightened. The instrument has been subjected to many modifications, one of the best being that of Tarnier (Fig. 407). At the same time it labours under the disadvantage that it aims to accomplish two purposes—i. e., crushing and extracting the head; and, unfortunately, whenever it is so constructed as to be an efficient crusher it is a poor tractor, and *vice versa*. For these reasons the cephalotribe, as such, is but little used.

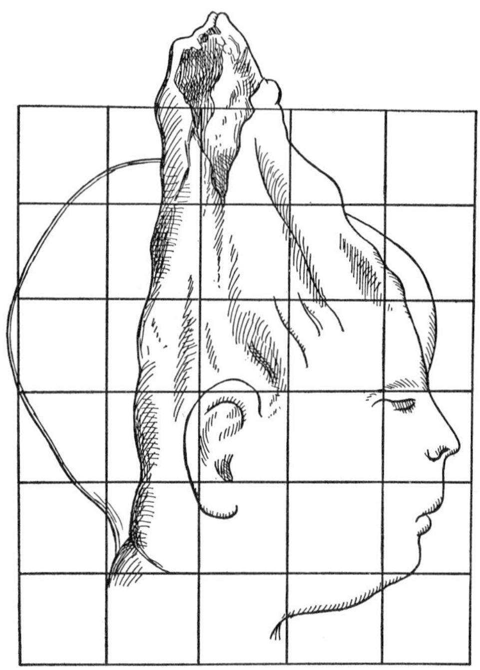

FIG. 406.—HEAD CRUSHED BY CRANIOCLAST (Simpson).

Tarnier, in 1883, invented the *basiotribe*, a three-bladed instrument which combines in one the advantages of the perforator, cranioclast, and cephalotribe. One blade is spear-pointed, and after serving as a perforator is forced into the base of the skull. The second blade is then introduced over the occiput and the third over the face of the child. All three are articulated, and the vise at the handles is screwed down, with the result that the base of the skull is fractured in many directions, and the head is compressed into

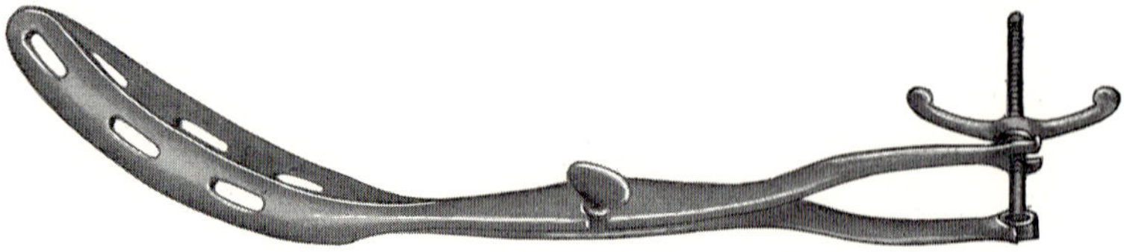

FIG. 407.—TARNIER'S CEPHALOTRIBE.

an elongated and shapeless mass. This is a most efficient instrument, and has been particularly recommended by Pinard and Bar.

J. R. Simpson, of Edinburgh, devised an instrument known as the *basilyst,* which likewise consists of three blades. The tips of two of them

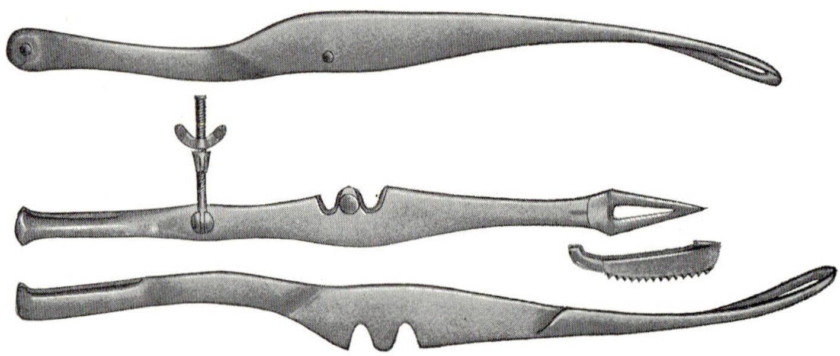

FIG. 408.—TARNIER'S BASIOTRIBE, DISARTICULATED.

come together and form a screw-like instrument. This first perforates the skull, and by a rotatory motion is then worked into the base, which is fractured in many directions by separating the two blades by pressure upon the handles. After this, the third blade is introduced over the face or

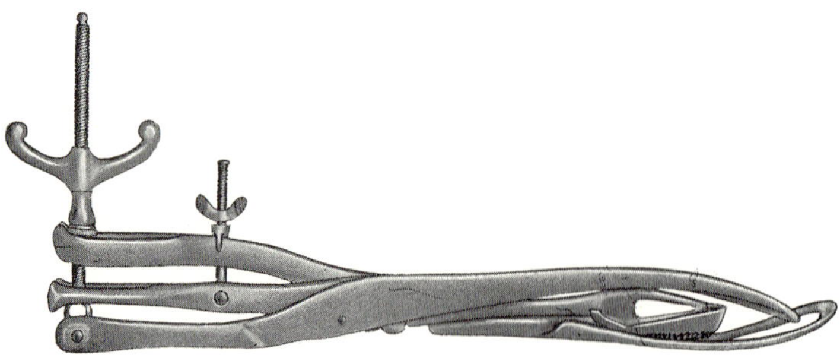

FIG. 409.—TARNIER'S BASIOTRIBE.

occiput and screwed tightly in place, thus converting the instrument into a typical cranioclast (Figs. 411 and 412). The basilyst gives very satisfactory results, and according to its inventor will compress the base of the skull into a mass 3.5 centimetres in diameter. Various other instruments have been invented for the same purpose, a full account of which is to be found in the work of Tarnier and Budin.

When perforating a hydrocephalic child, it is important to remember that the brain is spread out over the interior of the skull as a layer of tissue only a few millimetres thick. When this is perforated, the serum filling the dilated ventricles of the brain escapes and the skull collapses, after which delivery is readily effected. Occasionally perforation does not result in the death of the child, which promptly begins to cry after its birth. In order to guard against this most distressing occurrence, the obstetrician should not be content with merely perforating the skull at one point, but should carry the instrument back to the base of the brain and stir it around so as to effectually destroy the upper portion of the medulla. Especial care is necessary in this connection in order to avoid unpleasant complications, Pernice having recently reported the case of an infant who survived craniotomy and grew up an idiot. And a similar case has been known to occur in Baltimore.

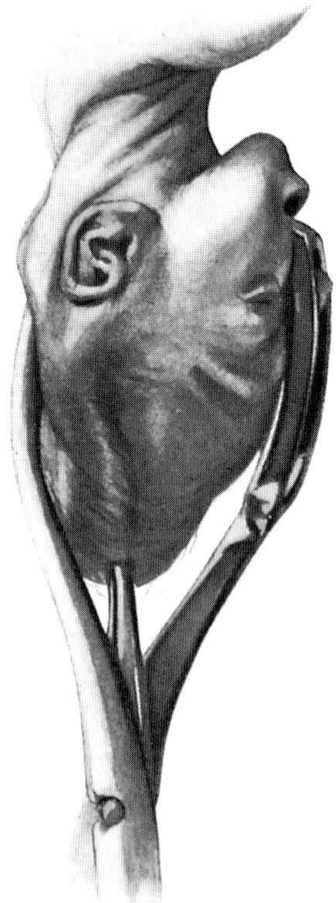

FIG. 410.—EFFECT OF BASIOTRIBE.

Prognosis.—In moderate degrees of pelvic contraction, craniotomy, if properly performed, is almost devoid of danger to the mother. On the other hand, when the conjugata vera measures 5.5 centimetres or less, the mortality exceeds that following Cæsarean section. It must be remembered, however, that favourable results are obtained only when the mother is in good condition; whereas, if the operation be deferred until infection has occurred, it is a most serious procedure, and is attended by a mortality of 10 to 15 per cent.

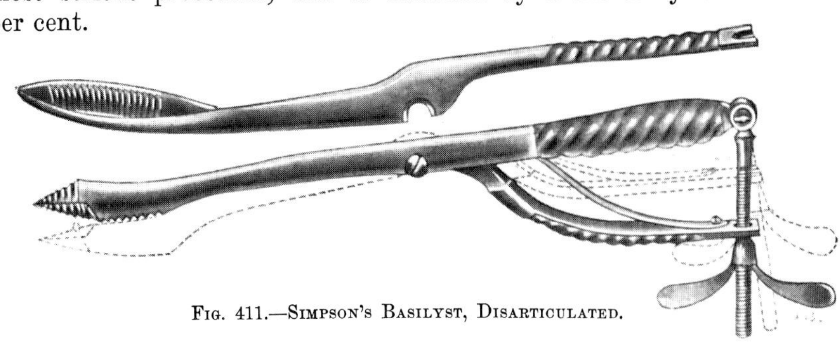

FIG. 411.—SIMPSON'S BASILYST, DISARTICULATED.

Embryotomy.—In embryotomy the viscera are removed through an opening in the thorax or abdomen of the child, or the head is severed from the body. The former operation is known as evisceration, the latter as decapitation.

At present *evisceration* is rarely employed, though it occasionally becomes necessary in order to effect the delivery of certain monstrosities or

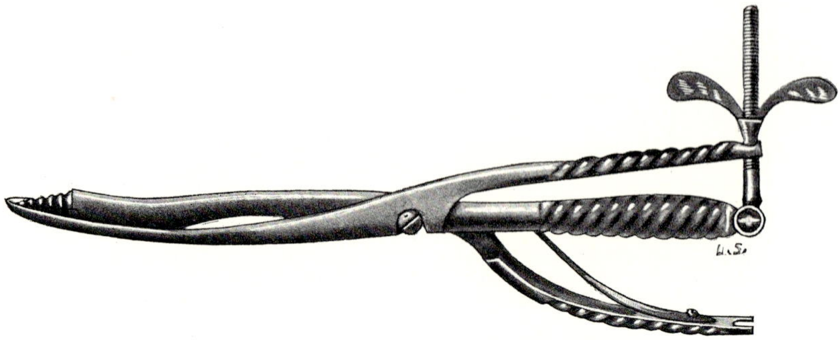

FIG. 412.—SIMPSON'S BASILYST, ARTICULATED.

children suffering from unusual enlargement of the thoracic or abdominal cavities, resulting from tumour formation or the accumulation of fluid. It may likewise become necessary in rare cases of transverse presentation, when the thorax or abdomen of the child lies over the superior strait and the neck is not accessible. Under such circumstances an opening is made by scissors through the thoracic or abdominal wall, as the case may be, sufficiently large to admit two fingers, with which the viscera are then torn loose from their attachments and slowly extracted.

Decapitation is much more frequently employed, and is indicated more particularly in *neglected transverse presentations*. As a rule, when seen early, such cases can be readily delivered by version and extraction; but exceptionally the condition is overlooked, and assistance is not called for until one shoulder has become firmly impacted in the pelvic canal, the lower uterine segment at the same time being so stretched as to make an attempt at version practically synonymous with rupture of the uterus. Under such circumstances the child can be delivered only by decapitation, which can readily be accomplished by means of Braun's blunt hook.

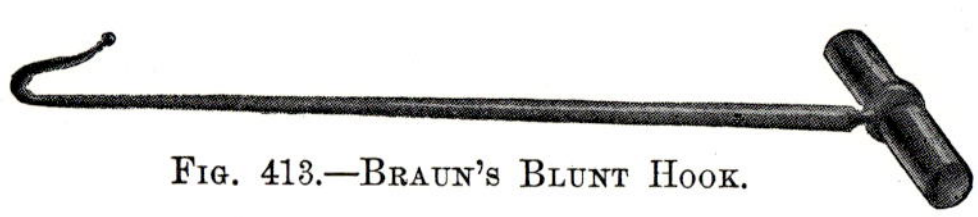

FIG. 413.—BRAUN'S BLUNT HOOK.

Fortunately, in neglected shoulder presentations, decapitation is often materially facilitated by the prolapse into the vagina of one arm. This having been seized and brought through the vulva, firm traction should be exerted upon it so as to put the neck on the stretch as much as possible. The index finger of one hand is then passed over the neck and used as a guide in applying Braun's hook as accurately as possible. When in position, the tip of the instrument is covered by the finger so as to avoid wounding the maternal soft parts. All being in readiness, strong traction is now made upon the handle of the instrument, which at the same time is given a rotary movement, by which the cervical vertebræ become disarticulated, and on continuation of the motion the neck is readily severed from the body. If any resistance is offered by the skin, it may be cut with scissors. After decapitation the body is extracted by traction upon the arm; or, if that be not available, by version. The head can frequently be expressed from the uterus by manœuvres similar to those employed for the delivery of the placenta, but if these prove unsuccessful, a finger is introduced into the uterus and inserted into the mouth of the child, after which, as a rule, extraction is readily effected by traction upon the lower jaw. If this is not effectual, delivery can be accomplished by means of a cephalotribe or after perforation.

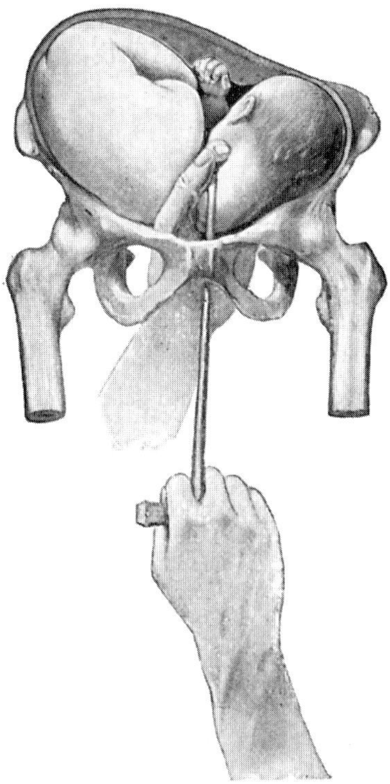

Fig. 414.—Decapitation with Braun's Blunt Hook (American Text-Book).

Zweifel believes that decapitation can be rendered easier by the use of the *trachelo rhekter,* which consists essentially of a double Braun's hook. So far as my own experience goes, I see no necessity for the new instrument, as I have always been able to effect decapitation by means of Braun's hook. Again, if the latter be not available, the operation can be readily performed by means of a pair of long curved scissors, similar to the embryotomy scissors of Hodge; while in cases of necessity the head may be severed from the trunk by passing a strong cord over the neck and using it as a saw. When this is employed, the vaginal walls must be protected by a speculum to prevent them from being cut through.

Occasionally, in head presentations, the excessive size of the shoulders

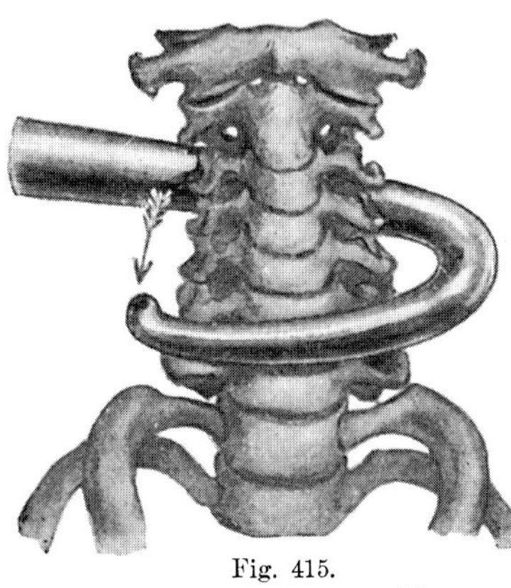

Fig. 415.

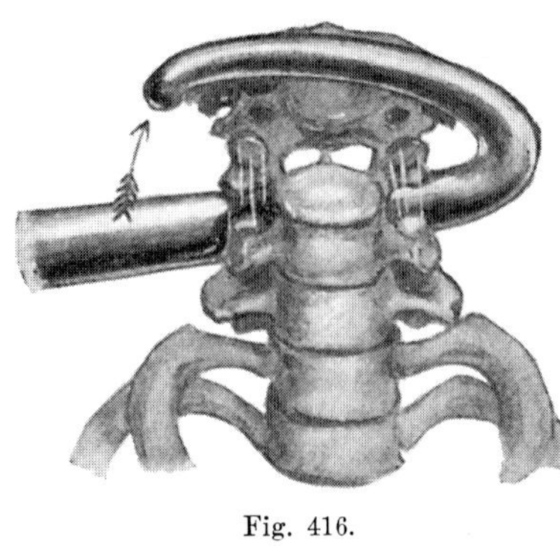

Fig. 416.

Figs. 415, 416.—Showing Mode of Action of Blunt Hook (American Text-Book).

may prove a serious obstacle to labour. In such cases *cleidotomy,* proposed by Von Herff and Strassmann, renders excellent service. In this operation a pair of long curved scissors are introduced under the guidance of the hand and cut through the clavicles on either side, after which the shoulder girdle collapses and delivery is readily effected.

LITERATURE

Bar. Embryotomie céphalique. Paris, 1889.

Baudelocque. Nouveau moyen pour délivrer les femmes contrefaites et en travail. Paris, 1829.

Braun. Ueber das technische Verfahren bei vernachlässigten Querlagen, etc. Wiener med. Wochenschr., 1861, No. 45.

Von Herff. Die Zertrümmerung des Schultergürtels (Kleideotomie). Archiv f. Gyn., 1895, liii, 542–546.

Pernice. Ueber einen günstig verlaufenen Fall von Perforation, etc. Centralbl. f. Gyn., 1900, 918–921.

Pinard. Le basiotribe Tarnier. Annales de Gyn. et d'Obst., 1884, xxii, 321–341 and 406–442.

Du soi-disant fœticide thérapeutique. Annales de Gyn. et d'Obst., 1900, liii, 1–18.

Simpson, A. R. Delivery by Basilysis. Scottish Med. and Surg. Jour., 1900 (May).

Simpson, J. Y. Cranioclast. Med. News and Gaz., 1860, vol. i.

Strassmann. Ueber die Geburt der Schultern und über den Schlüsselbeinschnitt (Cleidotomie). Archiv f. Gyn., 1897, liii, 135–143.

Tarnier. Le basiotribe. Acad. de méd. de Paris, 1883, December 11. Annales de Gyn. et d'Obst., 1884, xxi, 74–77.

Zweifel. Ueber die Dekapitation, etc. Centralbl. f. Gyn., 1895, 521–39.

CHAPTER XXIV

OPERATIVE PROCEDURES WHICH DO NOT AIM AT DELIVERY

In this chapter will be considered a number of procedures usually designated as minor operations, which may become necessary during pregnancy, labour, or the puerperium.

The Douche.—We distinguish between vaginal and uterine douches, according as a considerable quantity of fluid is injected into the vaginal canal alone or directly into the uterine cavity.

Vaginal Douche.—Following the introduction of antiseptic methods into surgery, the use of an antiseptic, *prophylactic vaginal douche* became a routine part of the conduct of labour, in the belief that by its means the countless pathogenic micro-organisms supposed to exist in the vaginal secretion of pregnant women could be destroyed, or at least rendered innocuous, and the risk of auto-infection minimized. Experimental work, however, has shown clearly that, with the exception of the gonococcus, the vaginal secretion during pregnancy rarely, if ever, harbours pyogenic bacteria, and that the prophylactic vaginal douche is unnecessary. Furthermore, clinical experience has demonstrated that it is not only useless but even directly harmful, as its routine employment is followed by a greater number of febrile cases during the puerperium than when it is omitted. This question will be dealt with more fully in the chapter upon puerperal infection.

Accordingly, at the present time the vaginal douche is employed only exceptionally during pregnancy and labour; as, for instance, when the pregnant woman presents a profuse vaginal discharge due to gonorrhœal infection. In such cases, four litres of a hot 1-to-10,000 bichloride solution may be injected into the vagina twice daily during the last few weeks of pregnancy, not so much in the hope of curing the disease as of avoiding infection of the child's eyes during labour. This is all that can reasonably be expected, inasmuch as the gonococci are rarely limited to the vaginal mucosa, but have usually invaded the glands of the cervical canal, where they are protected from the action of the antiseptic fluid.

Many authorities recommend the employment of a prophylactic vaginal douche if the patient has been subjected to repeated examinations during labour by persons who habitually neglect ordinary aseptic precautions, and particularly if signs of infection are present. Owing to the impossibility of thoroughly disinfecting the vagina at the time of labour, the value of such a procedure is questionable; but a douche consisting of several litres of hot sterile salt solution can do no harm in such cases.

After the first week of the puerperium, the vaginal douche is frequently employed when the lochia present an offensive odour. It need hardly be said, however, that it is of but little value as a disinfectant, but merely removes mechanically the secretion collected in the vagina, and thus adds materially to the comfort of the patient. Sterile salt solution or a $2\frac{1}{2}$-per-cent solution of carbolic acid, either alone or combined with boric acid and a little oil of peppermint, may be employed.

Occasionally, when a puerperal infection has become localized, and has given rise to induration at the base of the broad ligament or of Douglas's *cul-de-sac*, the application of heat by means of abundant douches of a hot fluid markedly alleviates suffering, hastens the maturation of the abscess, and prepares the way for its prompt evacuation.

Before giving a vaginal douche, the external genitalia should be carefully cleansed and the patient placed upon a douche-pan as she lies in bed, or brought to the edge of the bed and placed in the obstetrical position with a rubber pad beneath her. A fountain-syringe, containing four quarts and provided with an appropriately shaped glass nozzle, previously sterilized by boiling, is employed, and the fluid allowed to run in under moderate gravity pressure. For the first ten days of the puerperium rigid aseptic precautions should be observed in the use of the douche, and its administration should not be intrusted to the nurse, unless one is assured of her competency.

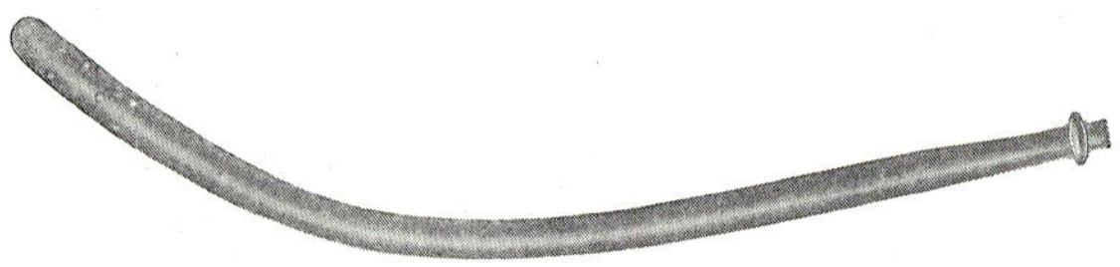

Fig. 417.—Glass Douche Tube.

Intra-uterine Douche.—The intra-uterine douche is not employed so long as the uterine cavity is occupied by the product of conception, but is frequently used immediately after labour and during the puerperium.

Formerly it was customary to give an intra-uterine douche after all obstetrical operations. Such a procedure, however, is indicated only when the patient has exhibited signs of infection during labour; but after delivery in these cases an intra-uterine douche of several litres of hot salt solution does no harm and occasionally is productive of good.

The most usual indication for its employment immediately after labour is afforded by *post-partum hæmorrhage* due to atony of the uterus. In such cases the administration of a douche of 4 or 5 litres of hot sterile salt solution will usually lead to efficient and permanent contraction, provided that fragments of the placenta are not retained *in utero.*

The intra-uterine douche is also frequently employed during the puerperium, especially in the presence of *infection.* It has, however, been greatly abused; for while it must be admitted that it is frequently a most valuable therapeutic agent, it is nevertheless true that it may be directly harmful. For these reasons great care should be taken in the selection of the cases in which it is employed. Generally speaking, it is contra-indicated in all cases of streptococcic infection, inasmuch as the necessary manipulations may give rise to an extension of the process. On the other hand, when the symptoms are due to infection by the so-called putrefactive organisms associated with retention of the lochial discharge, the introduction into the uterus of several litres of hot salt solution is frequently followed by an immediate fall of temperature and a permanent improvement in the condition of the patient. Usually a single douche brings about the desired result, though occasionally its daily repetition may be necessary.

Sterile salt solution should be employed for intra-uterine douching, instead of the antiseptic solutions which are usually recommended, since the latter, no matter how strong they may be made, can act only in a purely mechanical way, and cannot destroy the bacteria which have already invaded the endometrium. On the other hand, their use occasionally causes the death of the patient, particularly when bichloride of mercury is employed. On looking over the literature upon the subject several years ago, I collected over 40 cases in which death from mercurial poisoning followed the use of such solutions for intra-uterine injection.

Inasmuch as the administration of an intra-uterine douche must always be regarded as a serious matter, it should be given by the physician himself and not delegated to the nurse, no matter how competent she may be; since the most rigid aseptic precautions are necessary, and failure in this regard may result in infection of the patient. As a preliminary, the vagina should be douched out. Two fingers having then been employed to locate the external os, the douche-tube is passed through it until it impinges upon the fundus of the uterus. Four or five litres of fluid are then slowly injected, care being taken to insure a free return flow.

During the puerperium the cervical canal rapidly diminishes in calibre, and, owing to the marked anteflexion of the uterus which frequently occurs in this period, may become so bent as to offer a considerable obstacle to the introduction of the nozzle. To overcome this difficulty, traction is made upon the anterior lip of the cervix by means of a pair of bullet forceps, as a result of which the cervical canal becomes straightened out so that the nozzle can readily be introduced. Occasionally, the contraction ring offers an obstacle, and the nozzle is arrested in the collapsed lower uterine segment. By making traction upon the cervix, and cautiously moving the extremity of the douche-tube, it can usually be passed into the uterine cavity without further difficulty.

Curettage.—By this term is understood the removal of the lining membrane of the uterus by means of a curette. The operation may be indicated in three conditions: incomplete abortion, imperfect involution of the puerperal uterus, and certain cases of infection.

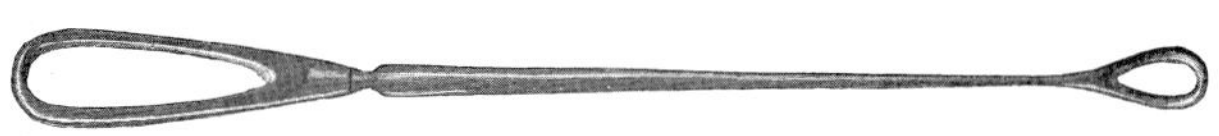

Fig. 418.—Curette.

When portions of the placenta and membranes are retained within the uterus after an *incomplete abortion*, many authorities recommend their removal by means of a dull curette. As a preliminary, the cervix, if not sufficiently pervious, must be dilated by a suitable instrument, preferably one modelled after that of Goodell (see Fig. 319). The curette is then introduced into the uterus and gently scrapes off the retained structures. The employment of an instrument, however, is rarely advisable, as it is far better to peel off the adherent placenta and membranes with one or two fingers, while the other hand controls their movements through the abdominal walls. After they are once loosened, the retained structures can be readily removed by means of the fingers or an ovum or placental forceps. The former procedure necessitates the introduction of the entire hand into the vagina, and can only be accomplished under anæsthesia.

After the uterus has been emptied in such cases, the fingers are again introduced and carefully palpate its cavity, in order to make sure that the offending structures have been entirely removed and all danger of subsequent hæmorrhage has been averted. If the curette is used, considerable portions of placenta may be left behind, which may later give rise to bleeding and necessitate another operation. On several occasions I have seen cases in consultation in which hæmorrhage had persisted after curettage, and on examination found that considerable portions of the placenta, or even the entire structure, had been left in the uterus, the physician having removed only a part of the decidua at the previous operation. Moreover, curettage always carries with it the possibility of perforating the uterus, the walls in many cases being so soft and friable that the accident may occur despite the exercise of the utmost caution. Fortunately, the injury in generally attended by but little danger, although, if the uterine contents be infected, it may give rise to fatal peritonitis; again, in rare cases, a loop of gut may prolapse through the rent in the uterus and necessitate a major operation.

Probably the most justifiable indication for curettage in obstetrical practice is the loss of blood during the latter part of the puerperium, resulting from *imperfect involution of the uterus*, which is frequently associated with the retention of portions of the placenta or membranes. Under such circumstances the operation gives excellent results, provided it be carried out in an aseptic manner.

Most authorities recommend curettage in *puerperal infection*, in the belief that by its means the focus of infection can be removed. The operation is undoubtedly beneficial in a certain number of cases, but should be instituted only in the presence of definite indications, as the routine employment of the curette is frequently more dangerous than the original infection, and has led to the death of many hundreds of women. Generally speaking, it is contra-indicated when the infection is due to the streptococcus, as under such circumstances the lesions attending its use simply offer new areas for infection. On the other hand, it is often followed by excellent results when the so-called putrefactive organisms are producing the mischief, and the uterine cavity contains necrotic tissue and occasionally larger or smaller portions of degenerated placenta. Nevertheless, in this class of cases it is generally far better to employ the fingers in emptying the uterus.

The Tampon or Pack.—The vaginal tampon is occasionally indicated in the following conditions: inevitable abortion, certain cases of placenta prævia, and to dilate the cervix in the early months of pregnancy. Profuse hæmorrhage occurring in the early months of pregnancy usually indicates that *abortion* is inevitable. In such cases, if the cervical canal is not sufficiently dilated to admit the finger, it is often advisable to pack it and the vagina tightly with sterile gauze and administer ergot. When the packing is removed twelve or twenty-four hours later, the product of conception is frequently found lying free in the vaginal vault, and when this does not occur the cervical canal will usually be sufficiently dilated to permit the introduction of the finger, by means of which the uterus can be emptied.

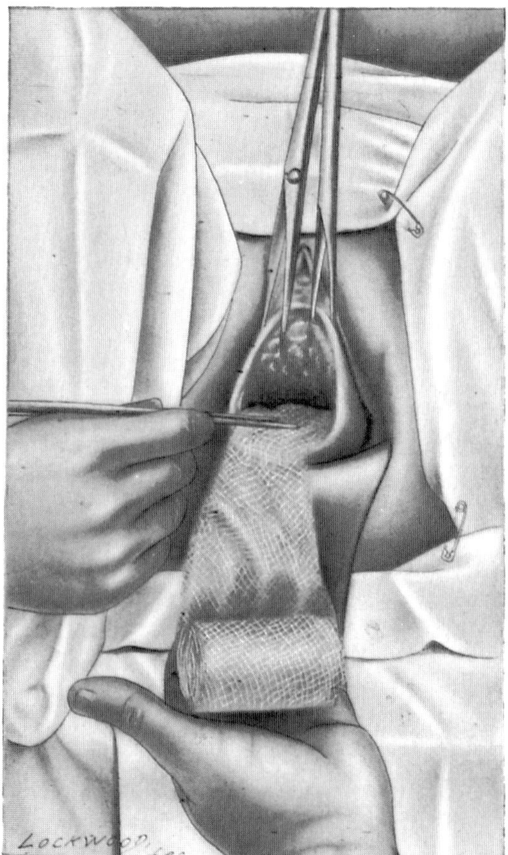

Fig. 419.—Packing the Uterus for Post-partum Hæmorrhage.

In *placenta prævia*, when the hæmorrhage is alarming and the cervical canal is not sufficiently dilated to admit a finger, excellent results occasionally follow the application of a tight tampon to the cervical canal and vagina. This effectually controls hæmorrhage, and on its removal a few hours later the cervix will usually be sufficiently dilated to admit two fingers, after which combined version by the Braxton Hicks method can be performed, or manual dilatation effected, followed by the immediate extraction of the child.

In the early months of pregnancy a tightly applied pack offers an excellent means of *dilating the cervix* in any condition which demands the evacuation of the uterine contents, and in many cases is preferable to rapid instrumental dilatation. This is particularly true in hydatidiform mole and in certain cases of so-called missed abortion.

The best material for a vaginal tampon is gauze, which is most conveniently handled in the shape of roller-gauze bandages, 3 or 4 inches wide, which have previously been carefully sterilized. For the introduction of the pack the patient should be brought to the edge of the bed and subjected to the usual preparations for an operation. A bivalve, or preferably a Simon speculum, is then introduced into the vagina and the cervix seized with a bullet forceps. Then with a long dressing forceps the bandage is carried up and tightly packed into the cervical canal, and afterward into the fornix, so that eventually the entire vagina is completely filled with it (see Fig. 323).

Intra-uterine Pack.—Dührssen, in 1887, advocated packing the uterus with iodoform gauze as a means of controlling hæmorrhage. Whenever there is persistent loss of blood following the third stage of labour, which does not yield to the ordinary methods of treatment, this procedure offers a most efficient method of controlling it, as the pack not only exerts pressure upon the bleeding vessels but mechanically stimulates the uterus to renewed contraction. Plain sterilized gauze may be substituted for that impregnated with iodoform or other antiseptics.

Before resorting to this procedure, however, it is essential that the hand be introduced into the uterus in order to ascertain that the hæmorrhage is not due to retention of portions of the placenta. If the uterus is empty, after the usual preparations for an operation have been carried out, the anterior lip of the cervix is seized with a bullet forceps and drawn down as near as possible to the vulva, after which sterilized bandages are rapidly packed into the uterine cavity by means of a long dressing forceps, the upper part of the vagina being also tamponed (Fig. 419). The pack should be allowed to remain in place for twenty-four hours, after which it can be removed by traction upon its free end.

Manual Removal of the Placenta.—When considering the treatment of the third stage of labour, it was pointed out that previous to the introduction of Credé's method of expressing the placenta its manual removal was frequently resorted to. With increasing knowledge as to the proper conduct at this time, however, the operation became less and less frequently demanded, so that at present competent obstetricians consider that it is indicated only about once in several hundred cases, and then only when abnormal adhesions exist between the placenta and the uterine wall, or when one has to do with a placenta membranacea or succenturiata.

Manual removal is indicated whenever there is alarming hæmorrhage and the placenta cannot be expressed by Credé's method, though such a condition is but rarely observed. On the other hand, if there is no hæmorrhage, the operation should not be resorted to merely to hasten the completion of the third stage of labour. Generally speaking, in such cases, repeated attempts at expression by Credé's manœuvre should be persisted in for at least an hour, under anæsthesia, if necessary, and manual removal resorted to only after prolonged effort has shown that more conservative methods are ineffectual. The procedure is attended by grave danger, and offers a greater opportunity for infection than any other obstetrical manipulation. In the ordinary operations, such as forceps and version, the hand, when introduced into the uterus, is within the amniotic cavity, and consequently micro-organisms which may have been introduced along with it, are cast off when the after-birth is expelled; whereas, in manual removal of the placenta the hand is inserted between the fœtal membranes and the uterine wall, and, in separating the placenta from its attachments, comes in direct contact with the gaping or thrombosed sinuses, so that if it be not absolutely sterile abundant facilities for infection are offered.

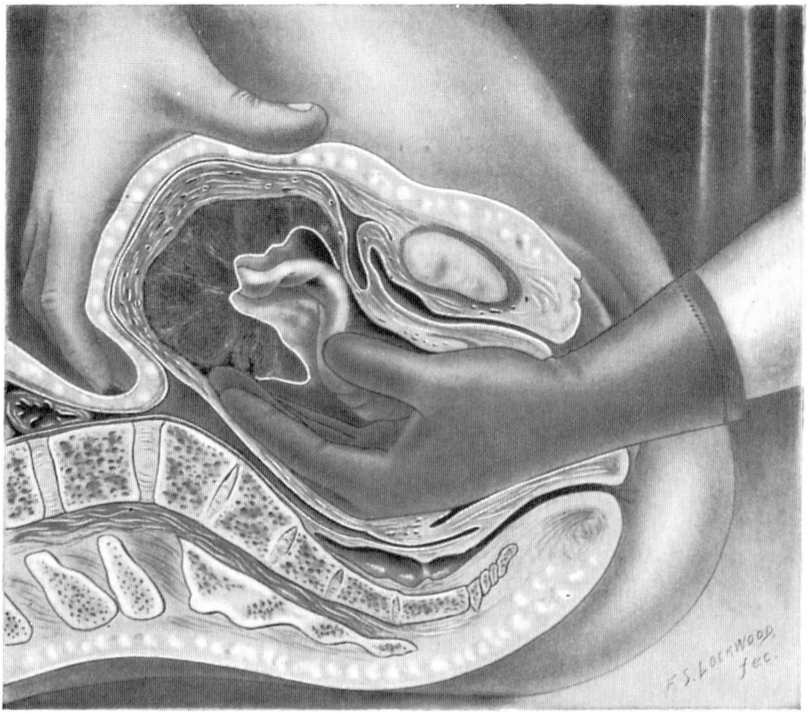

FIG. 420.—MANUAL REMOVAL OF PLACENTA.

When the operation becomes necessary, the strictest attention should be given to every aseptic detail. The external genitalia should be most rigorously cleansed, the hands and forearms of the operator carefully disinfected, and rubber gloves employed. After grasping the uterus through the abdominal wall with one hand, the other, lubricated with sterile vaseline, is introduced into the vagina and passed into the uterus, following the umbilical cord. As soon as the placenta is reached its margin should be sought for and the inner surface of the hand insinuated between it and the uterine wall. Then, with the back of the hand in contact with the latter, the placenta should be peeled off from its attachment by a motion similar to that employed in cutting the leaves of a book. After its complete separation, the placenta should be grasped in the entire hand, but not extracted immediately, the operator waiting until the uterus contracts down firmly over the hand, which should then gradually be withdrawn.

Once again the importance of a most rigid aseptic technique in carrying out this procedure must be emphasized. Naturally, when the obstetrician finds himself face to face with an alarming post-partum hæmorrhage, his only thought is likely to be as to the most rapid method of checking it, without regard to details. But even in such cases, the hand should be carefully redisinfected, or at least encased in a sterile rubber glove, for if it be introduced into the uterus without proper precautions, the patient, although saved from death from hæmorrhage, may succumb to a virulent infection a few days later.

PATHOLOGY OF PREGNANCY

CHAPTER XXV

ACCIDENTAL COMPLICATIONS OF PREGNANCY DUE TO DISEASE

Pregnancy may be associated with certain diseases which result from the condition itself, or by others which are to be regarded as accidental complications. The latter may have existed before the inception of pregnancy, or may have been acquired during its course.

As a rule, all diseases which subject the organism to a considerable strain are much more serious when occurring in the pregnant woman. Thus, a lung which is partially destroyed or thrown out of function may suffice for the respiration of an ordinary individual, but be unable to respond to the added demands of pregnancy, particularly in the latter months, when the enlarged uterus restricts the mobility of the diaphragm. Similarly, many a woman is unaware of the existence of a cardiac lesion, or at least leads a very comfortable existence, until the increased demands upon the activity of the heart incident to pregnancy bring about broken compensation with its attendant symptoms.

In general, it may be said that pregnancy exerts a deleterious influence upon all chronic organic maladies, while its effect is usually less marked in acute infectious processes. The latter, however, frequently lead to premature delivery, and the additional physical strain attending the latter may render the course of the disease much less favourable.

Pregnancy complicated by Acute Infectious Diseases.—*Small-pox.*—Small-pox complicating pregnancy carries with it a more serious prognosis than at other times. Thus Vinay reported a mortality of 36 per cent in 235 cases, as compared with 25 per cent in the non-pregnant condition. The hæmorrhagic form of the disease is particularly fatal in pregnant women, Mayer having recorded the loss of 13 consecutive cases.

Moreover, small-pox exerts a deleterious influence upon the product of conception, and frequently causes abortion or premature labour. This may be due to hæmorrhagic changes in the decidua, or to the direct transmission of the disease to the fœtus, with its subsequent death and expulsion. The occurrence of intra-uterine small-pox is well authenticated, as children are occasionally born in the eruptive stage of the disease or with distinct pock-marks. Mauriceau is said to have been infected in this manner, and the condition was well known to John Hunter and Smellie. Cordes reported a similar case in 1900.

Bollinger first suggested the possibility of the transmission from mother to fœtus of the protective influence of vaccinia, and stated that when the mothers are successfully vaccinated during pregnancy a certain number of the children fail to take when vaccinated soon after birth. Behm noted this insusceptibility once in 29 cases, and believed that it was due to the transmission of an immunizing substance through the placenta. Kolloch held similar views. On the other hand, most authorities are sceptical as to the possibility of such an occurrence, and consider that unsuccessful vaccination in young children indicates that they are refractory to its influence, or that the virus was of poor quality. In 46 cases reported by Wolff, Palm, and Gast there was not a single instance of successful intra-uterine transmission.

Scarlet Fever.—It is generally believed that the pregnant woman possesses a certain immunity to scarlet fever. Braxton Hicks and others considered that this was demonstrated by the fact that the disease occurs much less frequently during pregnancy than in the puerperium. Olshausen, who also held this view, was able to collect from the literature only 7 cases of scarlet fever occurring in the former, as compared with 134 in the latter period. It is quite possible, however, that many of the puerperal cases were not examples of true scarlet fever, confusion having arisen on account of the rash which sometimes occurs in puerperal infection. The correctness of this latter supposition is supported by the fact that many authors believe in the intercommunicability of the two diseases, a point that cannot be demonstrated until the *materies morbi* of scarlet fever has been discovered.

When occurring in the early months of pregnancy the disease frequently causes abortion. This accident is usually attributed to the high temperature of the mother, though in very rare instances it may be due to the direct transmission of the disease to the fœtus, Ballantyne having recorded a case in which the child presented a characteristic rash at birth. This view, however, has never met with any general acceptation.

Measles.—Measles is not a frequent complication of pregnancy, but when it occurs is very prone to cause premature delivery, which was observed by Klotz in 9 out of 11 cases. It is stated that intra-uterine transmission of the disease to the fœtus is now and again noted, Lomer, Fiori, and others having reported cases in which the child presented a characteristic eruption at birth.

Cholera.—Pregnant women do not appear to be attacked by cholera more frequently than others, although they succumb more readily to the disease. Schütz states that the mortality among them in the Hamburg epidemic of 1892 was 57 per cent.

The disease exerts a very deleterious effect upon pregnancy, 54 per cent of the cases, according to Schütz, ending in abortion or premature labour. This may be due to various causes. One third of the women suffering from cholera have more or less profuse uterine hæmorrhage, which when occurring during pregnancy gives rise to serious changes in the decidua, Slavjansky having described a peculiar form of hæmorrhagic endometritis in such cases. Moreover, in nearly every instance, the disease causes uterine contractions, which are supposed to result from the circulation of toxines in the blood.

Most authorities do not believe in the direct transmission of cholera bacilli to the child, Tizzoni and Cantani being the only investigators who have demonstrated it for human beings. On the other hand, Vitanza's experiments render it probable that such an occurrence is quite frequent in animals.

Typhoid Fever.—Typhoid fever is a serious, and often a dangerous complication of pregnancy. Moreover, it increases largely the fœtal mortality, abortion, or premature labour occurring in two thirds of the cases. Usually the death of the fœtus and its subsequent expulsion are due to the high temperature characterizing the disease, or to the transmission of toxines through the placenta. In a smaller number of cases, however, the bacilli themselves pass into the fœtal circulation. Thus, in my own clinic, F. W. Lynch was able to demonstrate them in the organs of a fœtus aborted by a woman suffering from typhoid fever at the Johns Hopkins Hospital, and similar cases have been reported by Lubarsch, Speier, and others.

Pneumonia.—The maternal mortality is materially augmented when pneumonia occurs during pregnancy, since the disease frequently leads to premature labour or abortion. This result is usually due to imperfect oxygenation of the fœtal blood, though in a small number of cases it is attributable to the direct transmission of bacteria to the fœtus, in whose organs pneumococci have been demonstrated by Levy, Netter, Carbonelli, Lubarsch, and others.

Premature labour is a very untoward complication in such cases, as the exertion incident to it subjects the already weakened maternal organism to so great an additional strain that death frequently results.

Influenza.—According to many authorities, influenza exerts a very pernicious influence upon pregnancy, Felkin and Müller having observed premature labour in 6 out of 7, and in 15 out of 21 cases respectively. In most of these cases the interruption of pregnancy was preceded by profuse metrorrhagia, which was supposed to be directly connected with the disease. On the other hand, Bar and Boullé, and Ahlfeld state that the disease is almost without influence upon gestation, the first-named observers having noted premature delivery only twice in 41 cases. It would appear, therefore, that the effects of influenza must vary with the severity of the epidemic, and more particularly with the frequency of pneumonic complications.

Erysipelas and Sepsis.—Erysipelas is a very serious disease at any time, but is particularly dangerous when occurring in pregnant women, in whom the possibility of a streptococcic puerperal infection is markedly increased. Occasionally, as noted by Lebedeff, the streptococci which have given rise to the erysipelas may be transmitted from mother to child, though this is unusual.

Furthermore, as a rule, any septic condition offers a worse prognosis in pregnancy than at other times. Krönig has reported several instances of transmission of the offending bacteria to the child. In one case he found that colon bacilli had been transmitted from a parametritic abscess to the fœtus, and could be demonstrated in its tissues. He made similar observations in an infectious process due to an anaerobic bacillus, as well as in several cases of streptococcic infection.

Gonorrhœa.—The occurrence of gonorrhœa in the pregnant woman should never be lightly regarded. In not a few instances the organisms invade the decidua and give rise to inflammatory conditions which lead to abortion. Gonococci have been demonstrated in decidual endometritis by Neumann, Maslovsky, myself, and others.

More important, however, are the consequences of gonorrhœal infection at the time of labour and during the puerperium, leaving out of consideration, for the present, the frequency of ophthalmia neonatorum, to which reference has already been made. After labour the gonococci, which have remained limited to the cervical canal during pregnancy, may gain access to the uterine cavity and give rise to febrile phenomena. The condition, although rarely fatal, is always serious, since it frequently leads to involvement of the uterine appendages, which may render the patient permanently sterile, or even necessitate operative measures at a later date. In rare instances the gonococcus may produce a general infection, Dabney and Harris having reported a case of gonorrhœal endocarditis which was observed in a woman delivered at the Johns Hopkins Hospital.

Tetanus.—Always a very dangerous disease, tetanus is fortunately a rare complication of pregnancy, nor does it appear to be more fatal than in non-pregnant women. Archambaud has recently reported a case which terminated favourably.

Anthrax.—Anthrax, or malignant pustule, is rarely observed in human beings under any circumstances, but is almost always fatal. Rostowzen met with three deaths in pregnant women, and was able in each case to demonstrate anthrax bacilli in the tissues of the child. A similar observation was made by Paltauf. Ahlfeld and Marchand have reported a case in which a child, born of a mother suffering from anthrax, died a few days after birth from the same disease. It remained doubtful, however, whether the case was one of intra-uterine transmission or of post-natal infection. In certain animals, on the other hand, the placental transmission of anthrax can frequently be demonstrated experimentally. The first observations of this character were made by Strauss and Chamberlent in 1882.

Pregnancy complicated by Chronic Infectious Diseases.—*Tuberculosis.*—Formerly it was believed that pregnancy exerted a beneficial effect upon tuberculosis, the mother improving markedly as long as she carried the child, though she frequently succumbed rapidly after its birth. At present, however, it is generally conceded that its effect is almost always harmful. Moreover, the strain incidental to labour and the extra drain upon the system, if the mother nurses the child, pull such patients down still further, so that the final result is usually hastened.

On the other hand, the disease does not appear to predispose to premature interruption of pregnancy, and it is not unusual for tuberculous patients to give birth to large and splendidly developed children at full term.

In very exceptional cases tuberculosis may be transmitted from mother to child. Hauser (1898) collected from the literature 18 cases in which the transmission of tubercle bacilli was definitely demonstrated. In 9 of these the children were distinctly tuberculous at birth, in 5 tubercle bacilli were found in the various organs, but specific foci were not present, while in 4 cases tuberculous lesions could be demonstrated in the fœtal portion of the placenta. Later Auché and Chamberlent discovered distinct evidences of tuberculosis in a child twenty-six days old, and considered that the disease was congenital. Full literature upon this subject is contained in the article of Dürck and Oberndorfer.

When one considers, however, the large number of tuberculous women who become pregnant, and the very small proportion of cases in which the transmission of the disease to the fœtus has been demonstrated, it is apparent that the latter must be a very exceptional occurrence. Presumptive evidence in favour of this view was supplied by a case occurring at the Johns Hopkins Hospital. The mother had died from a tuberculous peritonitis a short time after delivery, and at the autopsy the exterior of the uterus was found studded with tubercles, while the interior was covered with tuberculous ulcers and caseous material. The condition was suspected at the time of labour, and with a view of determining whether the placenta contained tubercle bacilli guinea-pigs were inoculated with portions of it, but with negative results. Cultures taken from the interior of the uterus during life revealed the presence of tubercle bacilli. The child, however, presented no signs of the disease, and was perfectly well some months later.

It would appear, therefore, that in the vast majority of cases the disease is not transmitted directly from the mother to the fœtus, and that Baumgärtner and Maffucci are correct in holding that the child is born with a tendency to the disease rather than with the disease itself. Hence it follows that the children of tuberculous mothers should be brought up under the best hygienic surroundings, and should not be nursed by their mothers. Various authorities have recommended the induction of premature labour in women suffering from advanced tuberculosis. This, however, is justifiable only in the interests of the child, in the rare cases in which the woman is so ill that it does not seem probable that she will live until the end of pregnancy.

Malaria.—Despite the somewhat widespread opinion to the contrary, it would appear that the ordinary forms of malaria have but little influence upon the course of pregnancy, although Goth has reported that 19 out of 46 cases ended in premature labour, and Edmonds states that this accident is very common in Africa.

I have observed 15 cases of malaria complicating pregnancy, the diagnosis being assured by the demonstration of the characteristic plasmodium. The character of the infection was as follows:

Tertian	1 case.
Double tertian	4 cases.
Triple tertian	1 case.
Æstivo-autumnal	6 cases.
Character of organism not recorded	3 cases.

None of these patients aborted, and in but two did pregnancy end prematurely, and then only a week or so before term. It is probable, however, that the pernicious forms of malaria may have a much more deleterious effect. There is a marked tendency towards recrudescence of the disease during pregnancy and the puerperium, just as is frequently observed after surgical operations.

It is generally stated that the disease is frequently transmitted to the fœtus, Runge believing that conclusive evidence of such an occurrence is afforded by the presence of characteristic pigmentation in its organs, while Kolloch says that it is not unusual for the new-born child to have characteristic malarial attacks. In a number of our cases the patients were suffering from malaria at the time of labour, but in no instance did the fœtus present signs of the disease, though in all such cases its blood was carefully and repeatedly examined for malarial parasites.

Quinine should be administered unhesitatingly to women suffering from malaria during pregnancy, as its oxytoxic properties are apparently in abeyance under such conditions, so that it can be used with impunity without fear of setting up uterine contractions.

Syphilis.—Syphilis is one of the most important complications of pregnancy, as it is one of the most frequent causes of abortion or premature labour. It should be suspected in all cases in which a perfectly satisfactory explanation for this accident cannot be adduced.

When infection occurs during pregnancy, owing to the vascularity of the parts, the initial sore assumes larger proportions than under ordinary circumstances, while the secondary lesions are often but slightly marked. The latter are practically limited to the genitalia, where they appear as large, elevated areas which occasionally undergo ulcerative changes, and sometimes lead to the destruction of superficial portions of the vulva.

The influence of syphilis upon pregnancy differs materially, and three classes of cases are distinguished, according as infection has taken place: (1) before pregnancy, (2) at the time of conception, and (3) during pregnancy.

When inoculation with the specific poison has occurred before conception, the disease nearly always gives rise to abortion or premature labour, more frequently the latter. Le Pileur obtained a striking illustration of the disastrous effects of syphilis from a study of the reproductive histories of 130 women before and after its inception, 3.8 per cent of the children being born dead before, as compared with 78 per cent after infection.

In premature labour due to syphilis, the child is usually dead when it comes into the world; less frequently it is born alive with definite manifestations of the disease; again, in a still smaller number of cases, it is born without signs of the disease, which, however, make their appearance later; while occasionally, particularly when the infection had occurred some years previously, the child may never manifest any signs of the disease.

When the mother is infected at the time of conception, the offspring is always syphilitic. Under such circumstances, however, it is a question whether the child owes the disease to paternal or maternal influences. On the other hand, when syphilis is contracted during pregnancy its effect upon the fœtus varies. If infection occurs within the first few months, the fœtus, as a rule, likewise manifests signs of the disease, but when it occurs later the child is not infected.

In the vast majority of cases fœtal syphilis is the result of paternal infection, and many a man suffering from the tertiary form has engendered a syphilitic child without infecting his wife. In such cases the child may present manifest signs of the disease, but the mother nevertheless may nurse it with impunity, whereas it would certainly infect another woman. This fact is well stated in the dictum known as Colles's law, the condition being explained by a previous transmission of immunity from the fœtus to the mother. Not a few syphilographers, however, believe that the mother is likewise infected, but without showing signs of the disease, or else suffers only from a very attenuated form—post-conceptional syphilis. That immunity is not always produced is evidenced by those rare instances in which the mother is infected by the child after birth.

The consideration of the syphilitic lesions of the child and the placenta will be taken up in the chapter upon Diseases of the Ovum.

Whenever we obtain a history of syphilis in the mother, no matter whether infection has occurred prior to or at the time of conception, radical specific treatment should at once be instituted, as by its means not only may the mother be cured, but at the same time fœtal transmission may be avoided.

In view of the general application of Colles's law, the syphilitic child should never be given to a wet nurse, but should be fed artificially in case its own mother is unable to nourish it.

Diseases of the Circulatory and Respiratory Systems.—*Valvular Lesions of the Heart.*—The occurrence of pregnancy in women suffering from valvular disease of the heart is generally believed to be a most serious complication. Guérard records a mortality of 28 per cent, and considers the condition more alarming than even eclampsia or placenta prævia. He states further that Schlayer, Leyden, Macdonald, and Lublinsky lost respectively 48, 54, 60, and 100 per cent of such patients. These figures, however, apply only to those cases in which compensation has long since failed and the condition is complicated by renal changes or the toxæmia of pregnancy. When all classes of cases are considered, of course, the mortality is much lower.

Routine examination shows that heart lesions are present in a considerable proportion of cases, being observed by Demelin in 1.23, by Vinay in 2, and by Fellner in 2.4 per cent of pregnant patients. In a series of 94 cases Fellner observed the following lesions:

Mitral insufficiency	37
Mitral stenosis	5
Combined mitral lesions	34
Aortic insufficiency	3
Aortic and mitral lesions	10
Uncertain lesions	5
Myocarditis	2

He also stated that only one seventh of the cases showed cardiac manifestations, whereas Demelin noted them in two thirds of his series.

Even when symptoms are present, it would appear that some authors have exaggerated the seriousness of the condition, inasmuch as the mortality noted by Fellner and Demelin, in 94 and 41 cases respectively, was only 6.3 and 5 per cent. From my own experience, I should say that one or two women in every 100 present heart lesions, the majority of which, however, do not give rise to symptoms. In a small proportion of cases, however, dyspnœa and œdema occur during the latter part of pregnancy, and occasionally some degree of collapse is noted shortly after labour. Out of more than 3,000 cases of labour I have seen only one in which the cardiac symptoms were alarming. The patient was a multipara suffering from uncompensated mitral disease, who collapsed in the last month of pregnancy, with signs of acute dilatation of the heart and intense pulmonary œdema. Death was averted by blood-letting and the induction of premature labour.

It is generally believed that the most untoward symptoms are observed in mitral stenosis. Lusk regarded this lesion as sufficiently serious to warrant the induction of abortion as soon as the diagnosis is made.

Generally speaking, the prognosis is good so long as compensation is retained. To this, however, there are certain exceptions, as Zweifel has recorded two cases in which collapse and death occurred in pregnant women who had previously been absolutely unaware of their condition. On the other hand, if compensation fails, and appropriate therapy does not bring about an amelioration of the symptoms, the prognosis becomes ominous; for even if the patient be saved from immediate death by the induction of premature labour, serious complications are usually in store for her in the future.

Grave heart lesions complicating pregnancy predispose to premature labour, as was noted in 20.2 per cent of Fellner's cases. This accident may result from uterine hæmorrhage directly attributable to the cardiac condition, from the death of the fœtus due to insufficient oxydation, or from changes in the placenta. In not a few cases there is more or less profuse hæmorrhage immediately following delivery; or again, at the time of labour, owing to the elevation of arterial pressure incident to the uterine contractions, compensation may fail and the woman's life may be in peril. Again, collapse may manifest itself immediately after the expulsion of the child as a result of the marked fall in the arterial pressure which occurs at that time.

If the lesion is fairly compensated the patient should be kept under close observation, rest being ordered and digitalis or some other heart tonic being employed as soon as symptoms appear. If this treatment fails to bring about the desired result, and the patient's life is threatened by œdema of the lungs, blood-letting occasionally gives excellent temporary results, and should be followed by prompt evacuation of the uterus.

The psychical disturbances incident to labour, and the elevation of arterial pressure brought about by the abdominal and uterine contractions, render it advisable to make use of an anæsthetic during the second stage. As soon as the cervix is completely dilated and the head well engaged in the pelvis, the termination of labour by forceps is indicated.

Some authorities recommend that women suffering from heart lesions should be dissuaded from marriage. This, however, appears to be an extreme view, though, of course, when the lesion is serious and the compensation faulty, the dangers of childbearing should be carefully explained.

Myocarditis.—Owing to the difficulty in making an exact diagnosis, myocarditis is rarely recognised during life. Nevertheless, it is a most serious complication of pregnancy, and is one of the frequent causes of sudden death during the second stage of labour and the first few hours of the puerperium.

Endocarditis.—Acute endocarditis may appear during pregnancy, just as at other times. It should always be regarded as a serious matter, but particularly at this time, as in a small number of cases the bacteria giving rise to it may be transmitted to the fœtus and cause its death, while at other times small portions of the vegetations upon the valves may be broken off and give rise to apoplexy or embolism.

Phlegmasia.—Thrombosis of the veins of the thigh, or phlegmasia, is a very rare complication of pregnancy. Brindeau has recently reported an instance and refers to two others in the literature. I have seen one case. It should be regarded as a very serious condition, particularly in view of the fact that incautious manipulations may lead to the detachment of small particles of a thrombus, which may then give rise to embolism of the pulmonary arteries. The symptoms and treatment are dealt with in Chapters XLIV and XLV.

Pulmonary Embolism.—Embolism of the pulmonary arteries is a very rare complication of pregnancy. Barnes reports one case which ended fatally within a few moments, while Sperling has reported a second which eventuated in recovery. The condition should always be borne in mind in cases of sudden death during pregnancy which cannot otherwise be explained.

Varices.—Owing to the pressure of the pregnant uterus upon the veins returning from the thighs, and the fact that they are but poorly supplied with valves, abnormalities in their circulation are frequently observed during pregnancy, and manifest themselves by the appearance of varicose veins. These may assume considerable proportions in the legs or about the vulva, and give rise to distressing symptoms. In rare cases, particularly when they are situated at the vulva, their rupture may lead to fatal hæmorrhage. When they occur in the legs, marked relief is often obtained by the use of neatly applied bandages or elastic stockings. Active treatment is useless in vulval varices, but the patient should be cautioned concerning the danger of their rupture.

Emphysema.—When pregnancy occurs in women suffering from advanced emphysema, the dyspnœa may become so intense as to demand its artificial interruption. In a certain number of cases abortion or premature labour occurs spontaneously, the untimely uterine contractions being attributed to insufficient aeration of the blood.

Asthma.—The symptoms of asthma are sometimes markedly aggravated during pregnancy. In some patients the disease makes its appearance only during pregnancy or at the time of labour, disappearing spontaneously after childbirth. If the usual methods of treatment fail, a radical change of air sometimes proves beneficial.

Dyspnœa.—Almost every woman in the last few weeks of pregnancy suffers more or less from shortness of breath resulting from interference with the motility of the diaphragm by the enlarged uterus. Dyspnœa occurring in the earlier months of pregnancy is usually due to cardiac or renal disease, and demands a thorough physical examination. Occasionally it follows excessive distention of the uterus, as in hydramnios.

Diseases of the Alimentary Tract and the Liver.—*Icterus.*—Pregnancy is comparatively seldom complicated by jaundice, which is usually due to catarrhal processes in the duodenum. The disease is generally without significance and undergoes spontaneous cure. In rare instances jaundice may appear in successive pregnancies, Ahlfeld having had a patient in whom it was noted upon four occasions.

Notwithstanding the fact that in most cases the jaundice disappears without treatment, too favourable a prognosis should not be ventured, for the reason that now and again the condition may represent the initial symptom of acute yellow atrophy of the liver.

Acute Yellow Atrophy of the Liver.—This is a very infrequent complication of pregnancy, though the latter appears to be a predisposing factor. Lomer noted that 30 out of 143 cases of acute yellow atrophy coming to autopsy were in pregnant women. The etiology is unknown, but the various hypotheses which have been advanced concerning it will be found in an article by Wendt.

Indigestion.—Pregnant women very frequently suffer from indigestion, and the symptoms arising from it are ofttimes very distressing. Such cases should be treated without reference to the existence of pregnancy.

Constipation.—Owing to distention by the growing uterus, the abdominal walls may become so impaired in tonicity that considerable difficulty is experienced in evacuating the bowels. Indeed, it may be said that the majority of pregnant women suffer from constipation. This condition should be carefully guarded against in order to avoid auto-intoxication and increased strain upon the kidneys. It is best overcome by appropriate diet, regularity in going to stool, and the occasional use of pills of aloin, belladonna, and strychnine, the fluid extract of cascara, or compound licorice powder. The stronger cathartics should be avoided on account of their tendency to cause abortion.

Enteroptosis.—The neurasthenoid symptoms which so frequently accompany enteroptosis, are often markedly ameliorated during pregnancy, inasmuch as the steadily enlarging uterus may tend to restore the displaced viscera to their normal positions. The comfort of the patient can be added to appreciably by the use of rational clothing, and especially by the application of a properly adjusted abdominal supporter. The condition, however, is prone to recur after childbirth unless the patient takes on considerable flesh. According to Maillart the improvement is sometimes permanent, especially if the relaxation of the abdominal walls be counteracted by the use of a snugly fitting binder during the puerperium and a suitable abdominal supporter afterward.

Diseases of the Kidneys and Urinary Tract.—*Chronic Nephritis.*—Pregnancy occurring in patients suffering from chronic nephritis is always a serious complication. The disease rarely eventuates in eclampsia, though the renal lesions may occasionally become so aggravated that uræmic poisoning results. More frequently, however, so great a portion of the placenta is thrown out of function by hæmorrhagic changes, that the fœtus dies and is expelled prematurely. Even when the placental changes are not sufficiently marked to interrupt pregnancy, the fœtus is often so poorly developed that it may weigh 2,000 grammes or less at birth.

Many cases which terminate favourably, so far as the pregnancy is concerned, persist after the birth of the child, and the fatal result is sometimes hastened. The treatment of chronic nephritis will be considered under albuminuria and the toxæmia of pregnancy.

Diabetes.—Formerly it was believed that diabetes was inconsistent with conception. This view was combated first in 1882 by Matthews Duncan, who was able to find in the literature 12 cases in which pregnancy was complicated by this disease. Later Partridge and Graefe each collected 26 cases in which the association was observed.

Diabetes may exist before the inception of pregnancy, or may not appear until labour. The prognosis is generally believed to be ominous for mother and child, but a review of the literature shows that less than 25 per cent of the mothers died from diabetic coma, while premature labour occurred in only one third of the cases, pregnancy going on to term in the other two thirds. The only patient in my practice presenting a marked glycosuria went on to full term, and the condition disappeared after labour.

It is interesting to note that 7 of the cases collected by Graefe were complicated by hydramnios, and that in 5 of these sugar could be demonstrated in the liquor amnii. These observations suggested the possibility of the fœtal origin of the glycosuria, which, however, was distinctly disproved in the cases of Rossa and Ludwig, the fœtal urine in both being free from sugar, although it was readily demonstrated in the liquor amnii.

According to Payer, sugar is found in the urine shortly before term in 4 per cent of pregnant women. Glucose is rarely demonstrated, whereas lactose or milk sugar is of comparatively frequent occurrence. The presence of lactose is simply a sign of mammary activity, and is without significance, while cane sugar is merely a manifestation of alimentary glycosuria. Payer has shown that women are less tolerant of sugar during pregnancy than at other times, as he was able to produce alimentary glycosuria in 80 per cent of his patients by increasing the amount of sugar ingested. Accordingly, whenever sugar is present in the urine, a prognosis should not be expressed until it has been determined whether one has to deal with glycosuria or lactosuria, as the former is a serious complication, whereas the latter is unattended by danger.

Hæmaturia.—The passage of bloody urine is rarely observed during pregnancy, and its occurrence should always lead one to suspect more or less serious lesions of the urinary tract. Nevertheless, Chiaventone has described an idiopathic hæmaturia due to pregnancy, and has collected 18 similar cases from the literature. He considers that the hæmorrhage is probably due to histological changes in the kidney which result from a hepato-toxæmia. He mentions, however, a case described by Albarran in which the bloody urine was probably due to the presence of varicose veins in the wall of the bladder.

Pyelo-nephritis.—According to Vinay, attention was first called to this complication of pregnancy by Reblaud in 1892. Since then numerous examples have been observed, Vinay being able to report 9 personal cases, while Brigand has collected 23 instances from the literature, which is well reviewed in a recent article by Reed.

The disease usually appears in the latter half of pregnancy, when the patient, who has previously been perfectly well, or has merely complained of slight vesical irritation, is suddenly seized with intense paroxysmal pains in one renal region. This is accompanied by a marked elevation of temperature and occasionally by chills, the temperature pursuing a hectic course. On palpation one kidney is found to be markedly enlarged. After a certain time a large amount of purulent urine is suddenly passed, when the pain disappears and the kidney becomes smaller, the symptoms reappearing as the kidney fills again. The condition results from compression of the ureter by the pregnant uterus, to which must be added an infectious process which usually makes its way upward from the bladder, though in a certain number of cases Vinay believes that the offending micro-organisms are derived from the intestines.

The disease may lead to death if not alleviated. The treatment consists of rest in bed and an abundant but bland diet. The patient should be encouraged to drink large quantities of lithia water, and the usual renal antiseptics should be administered. If improvement does not take place and the condition becomes alarming, premature labour should be induced without hesitation, as the emptying of the uterus removes the ureteral obstruction and allows of free drainage from the kidney into the bladder, the establishment of which, as a rule, is followed by complete recovery. In two cases of my own, the pain and fever disappeared immediately after the induction of labour, the patients made an uninterrupted recovery, nor did the symptoms recur.

Floating Kidney.—The symptoms arising from a movable or floating kidney are usually considerably alleviated during pregnancy, as the enlarged uterus tends to retain the kidney in its normal situation. In rare instances, however, the pedicle of the kidney may become twisted and give rise to intense pain, which may be mistaken for renal colic or appendicitis. Careful taxis will usually suffice for reduction, after which the symptoms at once disappear.

Owing to the increased laxity of the abdominal wall following childbirth, the symptoms are apt to become aggravated when the patient gets about, unless she has taken on considerable flesh, so that sufficient fat has formed about the kidney to hold it in place. A snugly applied bandage should be worn throughout the puerperium.

Dislocation of the Kidney.—Cragin has reported an instance in which one kidney occupied the pelvic cavity, and has collected 5 more or less similar cases from the literature. The condition is rarely diagnosed before the onset of labour, though in Cragin's case symptoms of incarceration led to vaginal examination and the diagnosis of the presence of a tumour, which was removed and found to be a kidney.

Cystitis.—Pregnancy is occasionally complicated by cystitis, which is usually due to gonorrhœal infection, though the colon bacillus may be the infective agent. In view of the possibility of an ascending ureteritis and a resulting pyelo-nephritis, the condition demands prompt treatment.

Diseases of the Nervous System.—*Paralysis.*—Paraplegia of spinal origin occasionally occurs during pregnancy, while in rare cases a patient suffering from paralysis may become pregnant. In either event the condition is without influence upon the course of pregnancy, and clinical experience teaches that labour in such cases is, as a rule, easy and comparatively painless.

Neuralgia.—Neuralgic pains are frequent concomitants of pregnancy. In rare instances they are very obstinate and resist all treatment, though they often disappear spontaneously after labour. During the later months of pregnancy the head of the child, after descending into the pelvis, may frequently compress one or other sciatic nerve and give rise to severe pain along its course, which is sometimes accompanied by intense muscular spasm. Owing to its mode of origin, this form of sciatica is not amenable to treatment.

Neuritis.—Winscheid has recently directed attention to an idiopathic neuritis which occurs during pregnancy. It usually disappears shortly after childbirth, and he considers that the condition is probably of toxæmic origin and not the result of pressure. The affection may be limited to a single nerve, or may appear as a multiple neuritis. It is characterized by paralysis of the affected region associated with muscular atrophy and the presence of the characteristic reaction of degeneration. There is marked sensitiveness along the course of the affected nerves, which is frequently associated with shooting pains. Sensibility of the parts is markedly impaired, and the patients frequently suffer from parasthesiæ. Occasionally the symptoms are so severe that the induction of premature labour may be justifiable.

Chorea.—Pregnancy occasionally occurs in choreic individuals, while in rare instances the disease does not appear until after conception. In the first class of cases it is comparatively unimportant, while in the latter the choreic movements are sometimes so intense as to interfere with sleeping or the taking of food. In these severe cases abortion frequently occurs, and death from exhaustion may follow.

Schrock has collected 154 cases of chorea complicating pregnancy, with a mortality of 22 per cent, and Buist 255, with a mortality of 17.5 per cent. In view of the serious prognosis attending the graver forms of the affection, Jolly recommends the induction of abortion or premature labour in aggravated cases, while Zweifel goes so far as to advocate its performance in all cases as soon as the diagnosis is made.

Epilepsy.—This disease appears to have no effect upon pregnancy, though at the time of labour it may be mistaken for eclampsia by inexperienced observers. If the attacks are frequent, the patient should be put upon large doses of potassium bromide and treated just as at other times. As a rule, it is not advisable to allow the mother to nurse her child, as lactation sometimes appears to aggravate the disease, while serious injury might possibly be done to the child during an attack.

Hysteria.—Hysteria is a not infrequent complication of pregnancy, but does not appear to exert a deleterious influence upon its course. Indeed, the physical condition often undergoes marked improvement at such times. Occasionally, however, the hysterical symptoms may become aggravated. Many authors have of late been inclined to attribute the nausea and vomiting of pregnancy to hysteria. This is no doubt true in many cases, but certainly cannot be regarded as the sole cause of the condition.

Tetany.—In rare instances tetany may occur during the course of pregnancy, Meinert, in 1898, being able to collect 20 cases from the literature. In some patients the disease appears only during pregnancy and is absent at other times. H. M. Thomas observed a case at the Johns Hopkins Hospital, in which the condition had appeared in 6 successive pregnancies. A full *résumé* of the literature is to be found in his article.

The ætiology of tetany is not clear, though Thomas thinks it probable that it is connected in some way with abnormalities in the function of the thyreoid gland. This was particularly manifest in one of Meinert's cases. The patient had had nine normal pregnancies; during the tenth she was operated upon for a goître which seriously interfered with respiration. The disease came on immediately afterward and persisted until after the birth of the child. It likewise reappeared in the eleventh pregnancy.

Apoplexy.—Apoplexy is rarely observed during pregnancy, though it is not an infrequent complication of eclampsia. When it occurs independently of the latter disease, it is usually the result of emboli due to endocarditis, or to phlebitis of the lower extremities.

Disturbances of Vision.—Disturbances of vision are rarely observed during pregnancy, but inquiries should always be made and the patient cautioned concerning their diagnostic significance if they appear. Amaurosis or total blindness occurring at this time is generally due to albuminuric retinitis, and the first indication of a serious renal affection is sometimes afforded by an ophthalmoscopic examination.

Diseases of the Blood.—*Pernicious Anæmia.*—According to Osler, this complication was first described by Channing in 1842. Since then a considerable literature has accumulated upon the subject, which is well reviewed in Davis's article. The disease occasionally appears during pregnancy, but most frequently not until after labour. It is characterized by marked pallor and anæmia, which is associated with weakness and shortness of breath, the extremities also becoming œdematous.

A positive diagnosis is made by the microscopical examination of the blood, when the number of red blood-cells is found to be markedly diminished. Many of the corpuscles are irregular in shape, while nucleated varieties are not infrequently observed. At the same time there is a relative increase in the amount of hæmoglobin, though its total amount is considerably below normal. As a rule, the disease ends in death if it be not properly treated, and marked fatty degeneration of the various organs is found at autopsy. Excellent results are obtained by the administration of Fowler's solution in increasing doses, beginning with 5 drops 3 times a day.

Leukæmia.—Leukæmia is a very rare complication of pregnancy, Herman and H. Schroeder being able to collect from the literature only 8 and 10 examples respectively. In 4 cases the disease had existed before the onset of pregnancy, while in the remainder it appeared after its inception. It exerts no direct effect upon gestation, though the association of the two conditions may seriously affect the mother. In several instances premature labour resulted, after which the symptoms underwent marked amelioration.

The diagnosis is rendered probable by the existence of marked anæmia associated with enlargement of the spleen, and is placed beyond doubt by a differential blood count. Examinations of the fœtal blood by Sänger, Cameron, and Laubenberg indicate that the characteristic leucocytes are not transmitted to the fœtus. In view of the good results which sometimes follow spontaneous premature labour, pregnancy should be terminated artificially in serious cases.

Hæmophilia.—Although the existence of a hæmophilic diathesis may be without effect upon gestation, in the third stage of labour it predisposes to obstinate post-partum hæmorrhages. In view of this danger, in the rare cases in which the conditions are associated, Kehrer recommended the induction of abortion, though it is probable that the bleeding would be as difficult to check after that operation as after full-term labour. In a case of extra-uterine pregnancy under my observation, hæmophilia proved a most serious complication at the time of operation.

Lead Poisoning.—C. Paul studied the histories of 141 pregnancies occurring in women suffering from chronic lead poisoning, and found that 86 ended in abortion or premature labour. Moreover, a large number of the children which were born alive perished at an early period, only 10 per cent remaining alive at the tenth year.

Diseases of the Skin.—*Impetigo Herpetiformis.*—According to Dühring, Hebra was the first to call attention to the serious nature of this disease. Impetigo herpetiformis occurs in pregnant women, and is characterized by superficial pustules, which are arranged in groups or clusters with inflammatory bases. New lesions appear on the borders of older and crusted confluent patches, while recovery takes place in their centres. The lesions occur on the trunk, thighs, and in the neighbourhood of the genitalia, but rarely upon the face. They are accompanied by itching and constitutional symptoms, chills and high fever. The recorded mortality is about 75 per cent, Debreuihl having collected 24 cases occurring in Austria and Germany with 18 deaths. The disease, as a rule, does not lead to abortion or premature labour, though many of the women affected with it died undelivered. The treatment is purely palliative.

Herpes Gestationis.—This disease, more frequently known as dermatitis herpetiformis, "is an inflammatory, superficially seated, multiform, herpetiform eruption, which is characterized by erythematous, vesicular, pustular, and bullous lesions." It occurs occasionally in pregnant women, and is accompanied by marked burning and itching. It pursues a chronic course, is often attended with fever, and sometimes ends in death.

Dühring believes that is probably toxæmic in origin, though similar lesions sometimes occur during the course of sepsis. In view of its depressing character, the patient should be placed upon tonic treatment, while the itching is best allayed by the use of ointments or lotions containing oil of cade, carbolic acid, or similar substances.

Pruritus.—Itching is often a distressing complication of pregnancy. It may extend over the greater part of the body or be limited to the genitalia. General pruritus should be regarded as a neurosis, which is probably toxæmic in origin. It often gives rise to intense suffering, the itching sometimes being so constant that the patient is unable to sleep. In some patients the loss of rest and the nervous strain attendant upon it exert a marked influence upon the general condition. Such cases are best controlled by the administration of nerve sedatives and general tonic treatment. A rigid milk diet is sometimes followed by excellent results. When the condition is not amenable to treatment and the patient shows marked signs of exhaustion, the termination of pregnancy may be justifiable.

Genital pruritus—*pruritus vulvæ*—may be due to several causes, among which are irritating vaginal discharges, parasites or glycosuria. When due to the first-named cause, the condition is best treated by the administration of astringent vaginal douches and the maintenance of absolute cleanliness. At the same time the itching may be allayed by the employment of ointments containing cocaine, menthol, or carbolic acid. Pruritus of diabetic origin is observed but rarely, but the possibility of its occurrence should always be borne in mind and the urine examined. If sugar is present, relief can be obtained only by placing the patient upon a rigid antidiabetic diet, while at the same time the appropriate ointments should be employed. Occasionally intense itching about the anus may be due to the presence of seat-worms, which are best destroyed by the use of rectal enemata of infusion of quassia. If local measures prove ineffectual, a dose of 5 grains of santonin at night, followed by Rochelle salts the next morning, will often bring about the desired result.

Abnormalities of Pigmentation.—During pregnancy abnormalities in pigmentation are not infrequently noted, which are particularly marked along the linea alba and about the breasts. In other cases unsightly yellowish splotches—*cloasma*—appear upon the face. They are not amenable to treatment, but usually disappear promptly after childbirth.

Accidents during Pregnancy.—The pregnant woman is exposed to the same possibility of injury as at other times, the prognosis not being materially altered except that abortion frequently occurs. Pregnancy itself may be complicated by accidents which are incident to that condition, the most important being rupture of an extra-uterine pregnancy, rupture of the uterus, and premature separation of the placenta—all very serious complications. Their mode of production and treatment will be considered in detail in the appropriate chapters.

Surgical Operations during Pregnancy.—Formerly it was believed that the performance of surgical operations during pregnancy would almost inevitably bring about abortion or premature labour, even the extraction of a tooth being considered a serious procedure. At present, however, thanks to anæsthesia and a perfected surgical technique, many operations can be performed at this time with but little additional risk. Accordingly, whenever a condition arises in the pregnant woman which imperatively demands surgical treatment, the necessary operation should be performed without hesitation. At the same time, if the indication is not pressing, it is advisable to defer interference until after labour, so as not to subject the patient to an added strain.

A review of the literature goes to show that amputations are not more dangerous than at other times. Several observers, notably Polk and Cragin, have removed the kidney without terminating pregnancy, and numerous cases are on record in which paranephritic or broad-ligament abscesses have been opened. Tumours of the generative tract can likewise be excised without great risk or markedly increasing the danger of premature labour. These conditions are considered in the chapter upon the Complication of Pregnancy by Diseases and Abnormalities of the Generative Tract.

Appendicitis.—Appendicitis is a very serious complication of pregnancy, as many women die if not operated upon, while surgical procedures for its relief are frequently followed by premature labour.

The diagnosis is more difficult than at other times, as the enlarged uterus renders it almost impossible to explore the right iliac region satisfactorily. At the same time, if a pregnant woman complains of pain in the appendix region, associated with muscular spasm and an elevation of temperature and pulse, there is usually but little doubt as to the condition, and surgical treatment should promptly be instituted. Mundé, in 1894, was the first to operate under such circumstances, and to demonstrate the justifiability of such a procedure. Since then his advice has been generally followed, and an extensive literature has developed upon the subject. The reader is referred more particularly to the articles of Abrahams, Gerster, and Pinard.

LITERATURE

ABRAHAMS. Appendicitis complicating Pregnancy. Amer. Jour. Obst., 1897, xxxv, 205–223.

AHLFELD. Pathologie der Schwangerschaft. Lehrbuch der Geburtshülfe, II. Aufl., 1898, 239–242.

AHLFELD und MARCHAND. Ahlfeld's Lehrbuch der Geburtshülfe, II. Aufl., 1898, 239.

ARCHAMBAUD. Le tétanos pendant la grossesse. La Revue Méd., 1896, 413.

AUCHÉ et CHAMBERLENT. Ein Fall von intrauteriner Uebertragung der Tuberculose. Ref. Centralbl. f. Gyn., 1898, 1102.

BALLANTYNE and MILLIGAN. A Case of Scarlet Fever in Pregnancy, with Infection of the Fœtus. Trans. Edinburgh Obst. Soc., 1893, xviii, 177.

BAR et BOULLÉ. Grippe et puerpéralité. L'Obstétrique, 1898, iii, 193–214.

BARNES. On the Thrombosis and Embolia of Lying-in Women. Trans. Lond. Obst. Soc., 1863, iv, 30–53.

BEHM. Ueber intrauterine Vaccination. Zeitschr. f. Geb. u. Gyn., 1882, viii, 1–21.

BOLLINGER. Ueber Menschen- und Thierpocken. Volkmann's Sammlung klin. Vorträge, 1877, Nr. 116.

BRIGAND. La pyélo-néphrite pendant la grossesse. Thèse de Paris, 1900.

BRINDEAU. Cas de phlegmasia alba dolens pendant la grossesse. L'Obstétrique, 1900, v, 417–420.

BUIST. Chorea Gravidarum. Trans. Edinburgh Obst. Soc., 1892, January 12.

CAMERON. The Influence of Leukæmia upon Pregnancy and Labor. Amer. Jour. Med. Sciences, 1888, N. S., xcv, 28–34.

CARBONELLI. Quoted by Lubarsch.

CHIAVENTONE. De l'hématurie de la grossesse. Annales de Gyn. et d'Obst., 1901, lvi, 196–219.

CORDES. Bulletin de la Soc. d'Obst. de Paris, Mars 15, 1900.

CRAGIN. Congenital Pelvic Kidney obstructing the Parturient Canal. Amer. Jour. Obst., 1898, xxxviii, 36–41.

DABNEY and HARRIS. Report of a Case of Gonorrhœal Endocarditis in a Patient dying in the Puerperium. Bulletin of the Johns Hopkins Hosp., 1901, xii, No. 120.

DAVIS. Puerperal Pernicious Anæmia. Trans. Amer. Gyn. Soc., 1891, xvi, 425–438.

DEBREUIHL. Impétigo herpetiformis. Besnier, Brocq et Jacouet, La Pratique dermatologique, 1901, ii, 915–920.

DEMELÍN. Contribution à l'étude des cardiopathies, etc. L'Obstétrique, 1896, i, 41–57.

DÜHRING. Impetigo Herpetiformis. Cutaneous Medicine, 1898, Part II., 436–439.

DUNCAN. On Puerperal Diabetes. Trans. Lond. Obst. Soc., 1882, xxiv, 256–285.

DÜRCK und OBERNDORFER. Die hereditäre u. kongenitale Tuberkulose. Lubarsch-Ostertag, Ergebnisse der allg. Path. u. path. Anat., 1901, vi, 300–310.

EDMONDS. Malaria and Pregnancy. Brit. Med. Jour., 1899, April 29.

FELKIN. The Influence of Influenza upon Women. Trans. Edinburgh Obst. Jour., 1892, xvii, 12.

FELLNER. Herz u. Schwangerschaft. Monatsschr. f. Geb. u. Gyn., 1901, xiv, 370–417 and 497–520.

FIORI. Un caso di transmissione di morbillo della madre al feto. Frommel's Jahresbericht, 1900, xiv, 722.

GAST. Experimentel. Beiträge zur Lehre von der Impfung. Schmidt's Jahrbücher, 1879, clxxxiii, 201.

GAULARD et BUÉ. Tuberculose pulmonaire. Accouchements et maladies des femmes en couches, 1901, 207–220.

GERSTER. The Surgical Treatment of Appendicitis occurring during Pregnancy. Phila. Monthly Med. Jour., 1899, i, 170–174.

GOTH. Ueber den Einfluss der Malariainfection auf Schwangerschaft, etc. Zeitschr. f. Geb. u. Gyn., 1881, vi, 17–34.

GRAEFE. Die Einwirkung des Diabetes mellitus, etc. Graefe's Sammlung zwangloser Abhandlungen, 1897, ii, Heft 5.

GUÉRARD. Herzfehler u. Schwangerschaft. Monatsschr. f. Geb. u. Gyn., 1900, xii, 571–577.

HAUSER. Zur Vererbung der Tuberkulose. Deutsche Archiv f. klin. Med., 1898, lxi, 221.

HERMAN. Leukæmia and Pregnancy. Lancet, 1901, October 12.

HICKS. A Contribution to our Knowledge of Puerperal Diseases, etc. Trans. London Obst. Soc., 1871, xii, 44–113.

JOLLY. Die Indikation des kunstlichen Abortus bei der Behandlung von Neurosen und Psychosen. Centralbl. f. Gyn., 1901, 1169–1170.

KEHRER. Die Haemophilie bei weiblichem Geschlechte. Archiv f. Gyn., 1876, x, 201–237.

KLOTZ. Beiträge zur Pathologie der Schwangerschaft. Archiv f. Gyn., 1887, xxix, 448–475.

KOLLOCH. The Protective Influence of Vaccination, etc. Amer. Jour. Obst., 1889, xxii, 1078.

KRÖNIG. Bakteriologie des Genitalkanales der schwangeren, kreissenden und puerperalen Frau, 1897, 180.

LAUBENBURG. Ueber Leukämie in der Schwangerschaft, 1891, xl, 419–438.

LEBEDEFF. Ueber die intrauterine Uebertragbarkeit des Erysipel. Zeitschr. f. Geb. u. Gyn., 1886, xii, 321–327.

LEPILEUR. Quoted by Ribemont-Dessaignes et Lepage. Précis d'Obstétrique, 1894, 642.

LEVY. Ueber intrauterine Infection mit Pneumonia crouposa. Archiv f. exp. Pathologie, xxvi.

LOMER. Ueber die Bedeutung des Icterus gravidarum, etc. Zeitschr. f. Geb. u. Gyn., 1886, xiii, 169–185.

Masern in der Schwangerschaft. Centralbl. f. Gyn., 1889, 826.

LUDWIG. Ein Beitrag zur Pathologie des Fruchtwassers. Centralbl. f. Gyn., 1895, 281–284.

LUSK. Mitral Stenosis in Pregnancy. Medical News, 1893, December 1.

LYNCH. Placental Transmission, with Report of a Case during Typhoid Fever. Johns Hopkins Hospital Reports, 1902, x, 283–322.

MAFFUCCI. Richerche sperimentale intorno al passaggio del veneno tubercolare dai genitori alla prole. Revista critica di clinica med., 1900, No. 12.

MAILLART. Ueber den gunstigen Einfluss der Schwangerschaft auf die Enteroptose. Centralbl. f. Gyn., 1900, 1342–1353.

MASLOVSKY. Endometritis decidualis gonorrhoica. Monatsschr. f. Geb. u. Gyn., 1896, iv, 212–218.

MEINERT. Fall von Tetanie in der Schwangerschaft, entstanden nach Kropfoperation. Archiv f. Gyn., 1898, lv, 446–453.

MÜLLER. Weitere Beobachtungen bezüglich des Einflusses der Influenza auf dem weibl. Sexualapparat. Münch. med. Wochenschr., 1895, Nr. 41, 952.

MUNDÉ. Appendicitis. N. Y. Med. Record, 1894, December 1.

NETTER. Transmission intrauterine de la pneumonie, etc. Comptes rendus de la Soc. de Biologie, 1889, Mai 15.

NEUMANN. Ueber puerperale Uterus-gonorrhöa. Monatsschr. f. Geb. u. Gyn., 1896, iv, 109–115.

OLSHAUSEN. Untersuchungen über die Complication des Puerperium mit Scharlach. Archiv f. Gyn., 1876, ix, 169–195.

OSLER. Puerperal Anæmia, etc. Boston Med. and Surg. Jour., 1888, xcix, 454–455.

PALM. Beitrag zur Vaccination schwangerer Wöchnerinnen u. Neugeborener. Archiv f. Gyn., 1901, lxii, 348–365.

PALTAUF. Zur Aetiologie der Hadernkrankheit. Wien. klin. Wochenschr., 1888, Nr. 18.

PARTRIDGE. Diabetes in Pregnancy. Medical Record, 1895, July 27.

PAUL. Considérations sur quelques maladies saturnines. Thèse de Paris, 1861.

PAYER. Ueber den Einfluss des Zuckers auf den Stoffwechsel der Schwangeren, etc. Monatsschr. f. Geb. u. Gyn., 1899, xi, 784–806.

PINARD. L'appendicité dans ses rapports avec la grossesse. Annales de Gyn. et d'Obst., 1900, liii, 357–368.

REED. Pyelo-nephritis of Pregnancy. Phila. Med. Jour., 1899, December 9.

ROSSA. Traubenzucker in Harn und Fruchtwasser. Centralbl. f. Gyn., 1896, 656–662.

ROSTOWZEN. Ueber die Uebergang von Milzbrandbacillen beim Menschen von die Mutter auf die Frucht bei Pustula maligna. Zeitschr. f. Geb. u. Gyn., 1897, xxxvii, 542–552.

RUNGE. Die acuten Infectionskrankheiten in ätiologischer Beziehung zur Schwangerschaftsunterbrechung. Volkmann's Sammlung klin. Vorträge, Nr. 174.

SÄNGER. Ueber Leukämie bei Schwangerschaft, etc. Archiv f. Gyn., 1888, xxxiii, 161–210.

SCHROCK. Ueber Chorea gravidarum. D. I., Königsberg, 1898.

SCHROEDER. Ueber wiederholte Schwangerschaft bei linealer Leukämie. Archiv f. Gyn., 1899, lvii, 26–35.

SCHÜTZ. Ueber der Einfluss der Cholera auf Menstruation, Schwangerschaft, Geburt u. Wochenbett. Centralbl. f. Gyn., 1894, 1138.

SPEIER. Zur Kasuistik des placentären Ueberganges der Typhusbacillen von der Mutter auf die Frucht. D. I., Breslau, 1897.

SPERLING. Zur Kasuistik der Embolie der Lugenarterie während der Schwangerschaft, etc. Zeitschr. f. Geb. u. Gyn., 1893, xxvii, 439-465.

STRAUSS et CHAMBERLENT. Comptes rendus de la Soc. de Biologie, 1882, novembre 11 et decembre 16.

THOMAS. Tetany in Pregnancy. Johns Hopkins Hosp. Bull., 1895, Nos. 50–51.

TIZZONI et CANTANI. Recherches sur le choléra asiatique. Ziegler's Beiträge zur path. Anat. u. zur allg. Path., 1888, iii, 189–237.

VINAY. Maladies valvulaires et grossesse. Archives de Tocologie, 1893, 805.

Vaccinia et variole au cours de la grossesse. Lyon Méd., 1900, mars 25.

VINAY et CADE. La pyélo-néphrite gravidique. L'Obstétrique, 1899, iv, 230–256.

VITANZA. Sulla transmissibilita dell' infezione colerica della madre al feto. Riforma medica, 1890, Nos. 48 and 49.

WENDT. Beitrag zur Lehre vom Icterus gravis in der Schwangerschaft. Archiv f. Gyn., 1898, lvi, 104–128.

WINDSCHEID. Neuritis gravidarum und Neuritis puerperalis. Graefe's Sammlung zwangloser Abhandlungen, 1898, ii, Heft 8.

WOLFF. Ueber Vererbung von Infectionskrankheiten. Virchow's Archiv, cxii, 177.

ZWEIFEL. Ueber plötzliche Todesfälle von Schwangeren u. Wöchnerinnen. Centralbl. f. Gyn., 1897, 1–16.

Kunstlicher Abortus bei Chorea gravidarum. Centralbl. f. Gyn., 1901, 1170.

CHAPTER XXVI

COMPLICATIONS RESULTING DIRECTLY FROM PREGNANCY

In the preceding chapter we considered the effect upon pregnancy of certain diseases which exist before its inception, as well as of others which may occur as accidental complications during its course. We shall now deal with certain disturbances which result directly from the pregnant condition itself, and are not due to extraneous causes.

Fortunately, in the vast majority of cases gestation pursues a perfectly physiological course, and is not attended by untoward symptoms. At the same time there is no other condition in which the border line between health and disease is less sharply marked, since a very slight irregularity often suffices to convert a physiological and normal into a pathological and abnormal state.

Toxæmia of Pregnancy and Albuminuria.—It is readily conceivable that the excretory functions are far more liable to various derangements when they are called upon to care for the elimination of the waste products of the fœtal, as well as of the maternal, metabolism. For this reason many women who are perfectly well at other times, suffer during pregnancy from the retention of certain excrementitious substances which may give rise to an auto-intoxication or toxæmia.

We know very little concerning the nature of the products of the fœtal regressive metabolism, but these, whatever they may be, gain access to the maternal organism through the placenta, being eventually carried to the liver, where they probably undergo further change, to be finally excreted through the kidneys along with the excrementitious materials of maternal origin. It is apparent, therefore, that abnormalities in the functioning of these organs, which under ordinary circumstances might be of but little importance, may be attended by serious consequences during pregnancy. Moreover, it is probable that heart lesions, particularly degenerative changes in the myocardium, as well as disturbances in the intestinal function, may predispose to such pathological conditions.

From the time of Bouchard, the French observers have insisted that all pregnant women suffer to a greater or lesser extent from auto-intoxication, the result of the retention of certain poisonous substances in the blood, holding that the correctness of such a view is clearly demonstrated by an increase in the toxicity of the blood serum and a decrease in that of the urine, as shown by their effect after injection into the circulation of rabbits. The force of this argument, however, has been greatly impaired by the recent investigations of Van der Bergh, Stewart, Schumacher, and others, who have shown that the results of such experiments are dependent upon so many factors as to make one sceptical in accepting conclusions based upon them.

Nevertheless, there can be no doubt that pregnant women frequently suffer from a toxæmia, which is accompanied by characteristic changes in the liver and kidneys. The hepatic lesions are analogous to, but less marked than those occurring in eclampsia, and consist of thrombotic processes which give rise to focal necroses, into which hæmorrhage frequently occurs, while the renal changes are degenerative in character. The former are so characteristic that many French obstetricians, notably Pinard and Bouffe de Saint Blaise, consider them the primary cause of the condition, which they designate as *hepato-toxæmia*. They believe that in such cases the hepatic metabolism is so interfered with that certain poisonous substances, ordinarily rendered innocuous in the liver, gain access to the blood.

The German observers, on the other hand, lay particular stress upon the renal changes. Leyden pointed out that degenerative changes in the epithelium of the uriniferous tubules were of such frequent occurrence as to justify one in describing the "*kidney of pregnancy*" as a pathological entity. This he believed was brought about by alterations in the arterial pressure and by the interference with the renal circulation incident to gestation. In a small proportion of cases an acute parenchymatous nephritis is observed.

It is generally believed that the frequency of renal involvement may be approximately determined by ascertaining the number of cases in which albumin can be demonstrated in the urine. Its presence was noted by Trantenroth and Saft in 50 and 5.41 per cent of their cases respectively, the former counting every case in which a trace of albumin could be detected, and the latter only those in which it was present in abundance.

H. M. Little has tabulated the results of the examination of the urine in 1,000 pregnant women at the Johns Hopkins Hospital. Traces of albumin were recorded in 50 per cent, and considerable quantities of albumin, together with tube-casts, in 7.3 per cent of the cases. As the urine was not obtained by catheterization, it is probable that in many cases the slight trace of albumin was due to contamination by vaginal or urethral discharge. On the other hand, it appears permissible to assume that renal lesions were present in the cases in which considerable quantities of albumin and tube-casts could be demonstrated. These conclusions are still further substantiated by the subsequent history of the patients. In the first group there were no serious disturbances, whereas nearly every patient in the second group presented symptoms of toxæmia, which in several instances eventuated in eclampsia in spite of appropriate treatment.

But even when renal lesions are present, it does not seem probable that they constitute the primary etiological factor in the condition. My own experience and reading have led me to the belief that these, as well as the hepatic changes, are due to the circulation in the blood of certain imperfectly oxidized metabolic products, with whose exact nature we are as yet unacquainted, and that the resulting disturbance of function causes still further retention of the offending substances, thus giving rise to a vicious circle.

The *symptoms* of the toxæmia of pregnancy may vary from a slight headache or nausea in one case to a fatal attack of eclampsia in another. Most frequently the patient complains of a certain amount of headache, lassitude, and a diminished urinary secretion, with which may be associated œdema of the face or lower extremities. In other cases the headache is more severe and persistent, and may be accompanied by disturbances of vision, which sometimes amount to total blindness; and now and again we meet with a patient suffering from hallucinations and bordering on the verge of insanity. Again, in very rare instances, the woman may pass into a somnolent condition, which gradually deepens into coma, usually followed by death. Schmorl has lately reported three such cases in which the autopsy revealed lesions identical with those observed in eclampsia. I have also met with a similar instance. Somewhat rarely the symptoms may be identical with those of an acute nephritis. When the toxæmia is pronounced, the child, as well as the mother, may suffer, and in not a few cases the death of the fœtus is to be attributed to the condition (Dienst).

The total amount of urine may be markedly diminished, and its examination usually shows the presence of a variable quantity of albumin and casts, associated with a diminished output of urea. Albumin and casts are not invariably present; occasionally a marked diminution in the amount of urea may be the only abnormality.

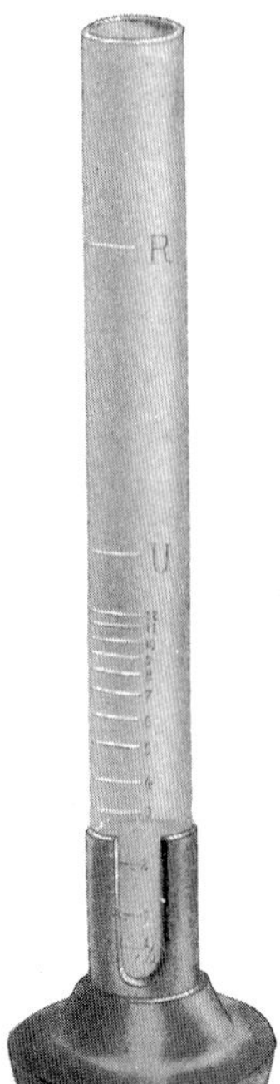

FIG. 421.—ESBACH'S ALBUMINOMETER.

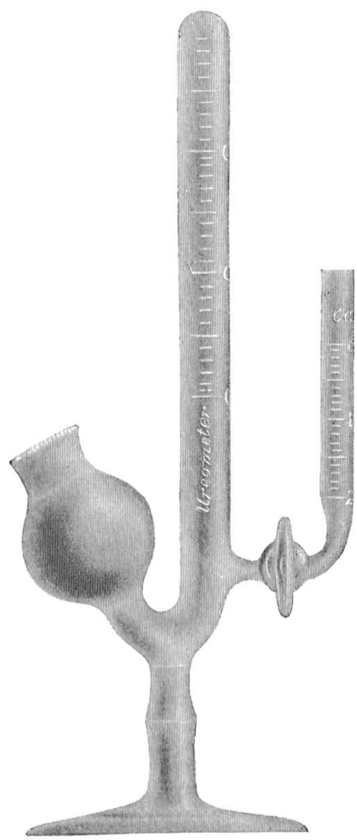

FIG. 422.—DOREMUS'S UREOMETER.

Treatment.—In the chapter upon The Management of Pregnancy, attention was directed to the necessity for the frequent and routine examination of the urine. Even in normal cases these examinations should be made once in four weeks during the first six months, and every two weeks during the last three months of pregnancy. The patient should also be cautioned to notify the physician whenever she suffers from headache, disturbance of vision, or œdema.

If the presence of albumin is detected, or the physician does not feel satisfied with the condition of the patient, the entire amount of urine passed in the twenty-four hours should be measured, and the total output of albumin and urea estimated. For practical purposes, approximate results may be obtained by the use of Esbach's albuminometer and Doremus's ureometer.

Esbach's albuminometer is a graduated test-tube provided with a stopper (Fig. 421). The reaction consists in the precipitation of the albuminous substances by a solution consisting of picric acid 10, citric acid 20, and distilled water 1,000 grammes. In order to estimate the amount of albumin, the tube is filled to the mark U with urine and afterward to R with the reagent. It is then corked and gently inverted ten or twelve times, after which it is allowed to stand for twenty-four hours, when the amount of

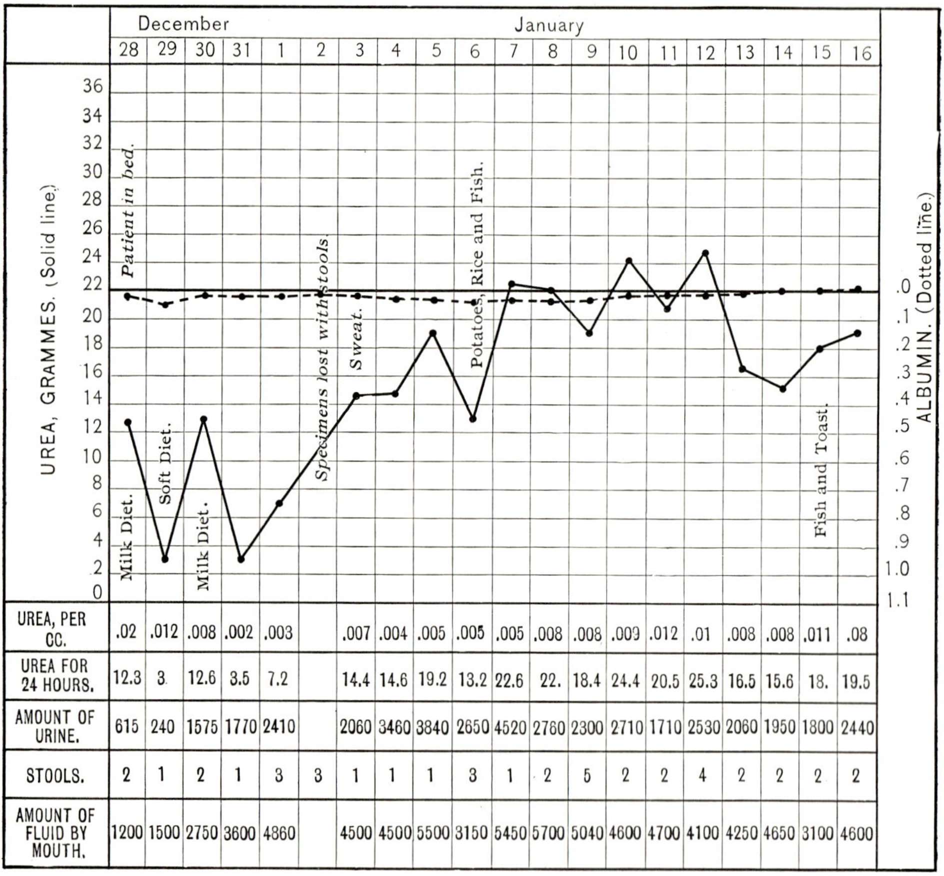

	28	29	30	31	1	2	3	4	5	6	7	8	9	10	11	12	13	14	15	16
UREA, PER CC.	.02	.012	.008	.002	.003		.007	.004	.005	.005	.005	.008	.008	.009	.012	.01	.008	.008	.011	.08
UREA FOR 24 HOURS.	12.3	3.	12.6	3.5	7.2		14.4	14.6	19.2	13.2	22.6	22.	18.4	24.4	20.5	25.3	16.5	15.6	18.	19.5
AMOUNT OF URINE.	615	240	1575	1770	2410		2060	3460	3840	2650	4520	2760	2300	2710	1710	2530	2060	1950	1800	2440
STOOLS.	2	1	2	1	3	3	1	1	1	3	1	2	5	2	2	4	2	2	2	2
AMOUNT OF FLUID BY MOUTH.	1200	1500	2750	3600	4860		4500	4500	5500	3150	5450	5700	5040	4600	4700	4100	4250	4650	3100	4600

FIG. 423.—UREA CHART.

Toxæmia of pregnancy; recovery under milk diet and rest in bed.

precipitate is read off on the scale, each division corresponding to 1 gramme of albumin to the litre.

Doremus's ureometer, which is represented in Fig. 422, enables one to estimate indirectly the amount of urea after decomposing it by means of sodium hypobromite, the reaction being shown by the following formula:

$$CON_2H_4 + 3NaOBr = 3NaBr + CO_2 + 2H_2O + N_2$$

The potassium bromide and carbon dioxide are dissolved, while the nitrogen gas rises to the top of the tube, where it can be measured.

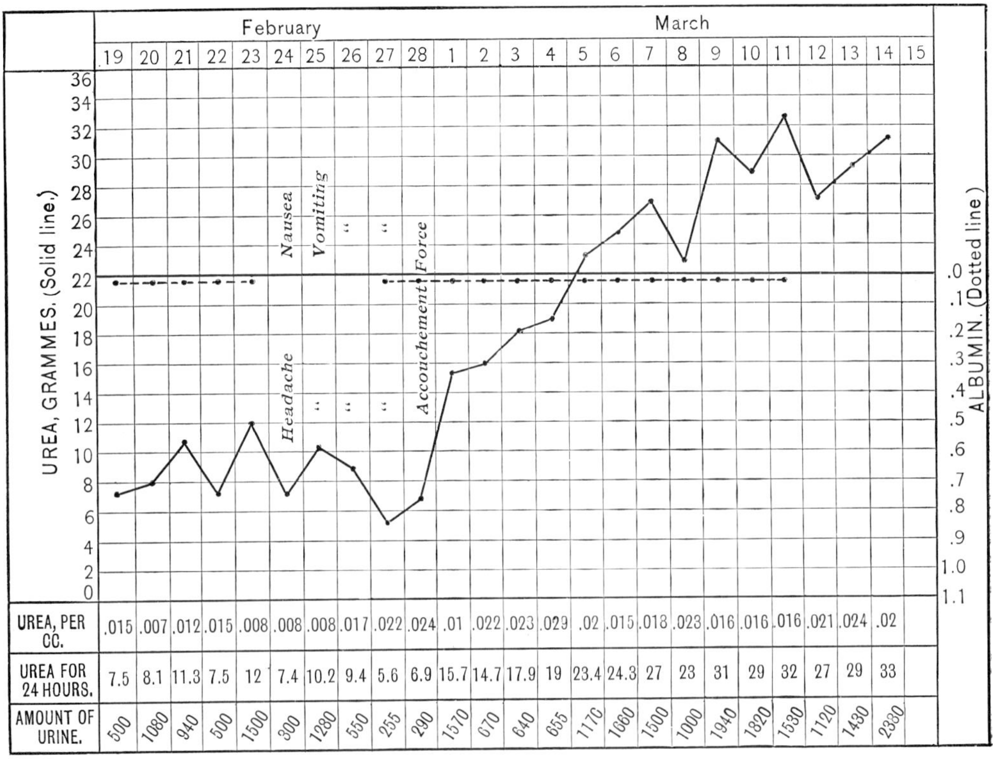

	Feb. 19	20	21	22	23	24	25	26	27	28	Mar. 1	2	3	4	5	6	7	8	9	10	11	12	13	14	15
UREA, PER CC.	.015	.007	.012	.015	.008	.008	.008	.017	.022	.024	.01	.022	.023	.029	.02	.015	.018	.023	.016	.016	.016	.021	.024	.02	
UREA FOR 24 HOURS.	7.5	8.1	11.3	7.5	12	7.4	10.2	9.4	5.6	6.9	15.7	14.7	17.9	19	23.4	24.3	27	23	31	29	32	27	29	33	
AMOUNT OF URINE.	500	1080	940	500	1500	300	1280	550	255	290	1570	670	640	655	1170	1660	1500	1000	1940	1820	1530	1120	1430	2330	

FIG. 424.—UREA CHART.

Toxæmia of pregnancy; treatment without effect; accouchement forcé followed by prompt recovery.

In employing this apparatus, the large branch is filled with a 40-per-cent solution of caustic soda, to which is added 1 cubic centimetre of bromine, the two together forming a fresh solution of sodium hypobromite. After the mixture has settled, the shorter branch is filled with urine, and by turning the stop-cock 1 cubic centimetre of it is allowed to enter the longer branch. Its admission is followed by an active formation of gas, which drives part of the fluid out of the tube into the adjoining bulb. When the process is completed, the amount of nitrogen formed is read off from the scale, each division indicating the presence of 0.001 gramme of urea to each cubic centimetre of urine. From this the total amount in the specimen is readily calculated.

Ordinarily, if the urea output is normal (20 to 24 grammes *per diem*), the presence of a slight amount of albumin may be regarded with indifference; whereas, if a considerable quantity is present and the urea at the same time falls considerably below normal, the patient should be regarded as in serious danger and should be kept under close supervision. During this time the twenty-four-hour specimen of urine should be examined daily, and the treatment based upon the relative amounts of albumin and urea present, as well as upon the subjective symptoms. (See Figs. 423 and 424.)

The patient should be put to bed, or at least confined to her room and placed upon a restricted diet, meats and the stronger vegetables being interdicted; or, better still, for a while she should depend solely upon milk, which is not only an excellent food, but also a most efficient diuretic. At least two quarts should be consumed in the twenty-four hours. To relieve the monotony, she may be allowed small quantities of lettuce salad, bread and butter, and occasionally a little herring roe as a relish. She should also be made to take considerable quantities of fluid in the shape of plain water, Buffalo lithia water, or cream of tartar lemonade (1 dram to the pint).

In most cases this treatment will be followed by a marked amelioration of the symptoms, an increased urinary secretion, a decrease in the amount of albumin, a rise in the amount of urea, and a prompt return to normal conditions (Fig. 423). If the desired result is not accomplished, a brisk purge of Rochelle or Epsom salts should be given daily, and the cutaneous functions stimulated by a daily hot pack or sweat bath. If under treatment the symptoms disappear, the albumin becomes less and the urea increased in amount, the outlook may be considered excellent. On the other hand, if the albumin steadily increases, and the urea decreases in amount, while the subjective condition of the patient remains unchanged, the prognosis becomes ominous, and the appearance of somnolence and coma or eclampsia can probably be avoided only by the induction of premature labour, no matter what be the period of pregnancy (Fig. 424).

In what has been said concerning the diagnostic value of the determination of the relative amounts of urea and albumin in the urine, we have not intended to convey the impression that the toxæmia results from the retention of urea. Nevertheless, the estimation of the latter affords a convenient clinical index as to the amount of waste material that is being excreted. In hospital practice a more accurate criterion is afforded by the total amount of nitrogen excreted during the twenty-four hours, and particularly the relation which it bears to the nitrogen contained in the urea.

Eclampsia.—When the symptoms of toxæmia do not disappear under the treatment just outlined, it is probable that eclampsia will shortly supervene. The consideration of this condition, however, will be taken up in Chapter XL.

Pernicious Vomiting of Pregnancy.—*Hyperemesis.*—Reference has already been made to the nausea and vomiting which so frequently accompanies pregnancy—the so-called *morning sickness.* This symptom is more or less marked in almost one half of the cases; it usually makes its appearance about the sixth week, disappearing spontaneously about the twelfth or fourteenth week of pregnancy. In other cases it persists for a longer period, and occasionally continues up to term. If the vomiting occurs only in the early morning, as is usually the case, and does not materially interfere with the ingestion of food, it must be regarded rather as an annoying than as a serious complication.

On the other hand, about once in 1,000 cases, according to Pick, the patient is constantly nauseated, and vomits whenever she attempts to take food. This pernicious vomiting of pregnancy, or *hyperemesis*, as it is termed, constitutes a most serious affection, and according to Merle terminates fatally in nearly 50 per cent of the cases which are subjected to purely medicinal treatment. At first the patient suffers merely from the discomfort incident to the condition, but in a short time, owing to the inability to retain nutriment, she begins to show signs of malnutrition and eventually those of actual starvation. Rapid emaciation occurs, the face assumes a drawn and haggard aspect, and the skin may become slightly jaundiced. The pulse increases in rapidity and the temperature becomes elevated, sometimes reaching 103° to 104° F. The fever is variously interpreted, but is probably indicative of the onset of a terminal infection. When this stage of the disease is reached the outlook becomes gloomy, as death will probably result, no matter what treatment may be instituted.

Ætiology.—That a vast literature has accumulated as to the causation and treatment of the affection goes to prove that it is not dependent upon a single ætiological factor. Kaltenbach, Klein, and many recent writers consider it a neurosis, which is more or less allied to hysteria, and base their belief upon the fact that its cure is frequently effected by suggestion or moral suasion. At the same time they advocate placing the patient at absolute rest and excluding all forms of excitement, while small amounts of nutritive and easily digestible food are administered at frequent intervals. In several cases under my observation, the neurotic nature of the condition was clearly demonstrated. One patient, who had vomited incessantly for several weeks, was promptly cured after I had drawn an alarming picture of the dangers incident to abortion, which I told her must inevitably be induced if she did not improve within the next twenty-four hours. Many similar cases are reported in which permanent cure followed simple methods, and was manifestly the result of suggestion.

Of late years there has been an increasing tendency to attribute certain cases of hyperemesis to the toxæmia of pregnancy. Lindemann, Dirmoser, Champetier de Ribes and Bouffe de Saint Blaise have reported fatal cases in which the autopsy showed lesions of the liver, kidneys, and other organs identical with those observed in eclampsia.

In many cases the condition is clearly the result of reflex irritation, which has its origin in certain abnormalities of the generative tract. Thus, it is sometimes associated with an incarcerated retroflexed uterus, the symptoms disappearing immediately after the organ is freed from its abnormal position. Again, a similar beneficial result has followed the closure of deep cervical tears. More frequently, the vomiting is attributable to the existence of endometritis, more or less recent inflammatory processes affecting the tubes and ovaries, especially when they are bound down by adhesions, extra-uterine pregnancy, hydramnios, or other complications.

Sometimes lesions of other organs are responsible, the condition being observed in women suffering from anæmia or gastric ulceration, and disappearing with the cure of the underlying affection. Davis reports a case which apparently resulted from cerebral metastases following a deciduoma malignum. Chronic pancreatitis appeared to have been the primary cause in a fatal case under my observation. Full literature upon the ætiology of the affection may be found in the exhaustive monograph of Pick.

Treatment.—The fact that a large proportion of the remedies in the pharmacopœia have been recommended for the treatment of the vomiting of pregnancy, is abundant evidence that drugs are often unavailing. Satisfactory results are sometimes obtained from one or other of the following: Capsules containing $\frac{1}{4}$ grain of nitrate of silver and 2 grains of pepsin, or 2 grains of menthol, dilute hydrocyanic acid, small doses of cocaine, drop doses of the tincture of iodine, subnitrate of bismuth, or oxalate of cerium, either in the form of 5-grain powders or the effervescent preparation. Occasionally the first remedy prescribed will lead to a marked amelioration of the symptoms, while in other cases the whole gamut may be prescribed in succession without appreciable result.

When the condition is serious the patient should be subjected to a careful physical examination, and if any abnormality is detected, whether in the generative tract or elsewhere, the treatment should be directed to its removal or correction. In a few cases the application of nitrate of silver or of the tincture of iodine to the cervical canal, or its moderate dilatation by means of a steel dilator or a small pack, seems to effect a cure, though the possibility of suggestion should always be borne in mind.

Excellent results are sometimes obtained by treating the condition as a pure neurosis, with rest in bed, avoidance of excitement, moral suasion, and particularly the administration of small quantities of easily digestible food at frequent intervals and, when nothing is retained by the stomach, the employment of nutritive rectal enemata. High injections of large quantities of normal salt solution, once or twice daily, are very valuable for allaying the thirst from which the patient so often suffers. Occasionally an examination of the urine will show that we have to deal with an auto-intoxication. In such cases the treatment previously outlined may give good results.

Unfortunately, the conscientious employment of the methods of treatment here suggested is sometimes of no avail, and the patient becomes progressively worse until she appears to be on the verge of death from starvation. Under such circumstances the only hope of saving her life lies in emptying the uterus, and abortion should be induced before her condition becomes desperate. Owing to the uncertain nature of the affection, and the fact that not a few cases recover spontaneously at the last moment, it is only natural that the physician should defer such a procedure as long as possible; but, unfortunately, this laudable desire has not infrequently resulted in postponing interference so long that the operation has been performed too late to prevent a fatal issue. I have seen several cases in consultation in which the death of the patient was undoubtedly due to this delay. Hence, although general therapeutic measures should be given a thorough trial, care should be taken to empty the uterus while the patient has still a chance of surviving the operation. Full literature concerning the induction of abortion under such circumstances will be found in Merle's article.

Salivation.—In exceptional instances the salivary secretion becomes markedly increased during pregnancy. As a rule, this is not a serious complication, but now and again the amount of saliva is so great as to cause the patient great annoyance, and sometimes even prevent her from sleeping. One of my own patients expectorated between 500 and 600 cubic centimetres of clear fluid every day for several weeks, while Lvoff has reported several cases in which the secretion in the twenty-four hours varied from 1,000 to 1,600 cubic centimetres.

The condition is usually attributed to a reflex neurosis incident to pregnancy, but sometimes it is a manifestation of auto-intoxication. In the first class of cases the treatment is very unsatisfactory, astringent mouth washes, and even comparatively large doses of atropine, being without effect. On the other hand, when the condition results from auto-intoxication, marked amelioration frequently results from placing the patient upon a rigorous milk diet.

Gingivitis.—Exceptionally, the gums of pregnant women become inflamed and spongy, and bleed upon the slightest touch. The condition is usually observed in run-down individuals, and is very refractory to treatment, although in many cases it disappears almost immediately after delivery. It is best met by the employment of astringent mouth washes, especially those containing tincture of myrrh, combined with general tonic treatment and an abundant diet.

Dental Caries—Toothache.—Many women suffer during pregnancy from dental caries, which is associated with more or less severe toothache. It is a popular belief that pregnancy predisposes to the condition, as is evidenced by the saying, "For every child a tooth." It is probable that the condition is somewhat allied to the minor degrees of osteomalacia which occur only during pregnancy. Such patients should be referred to a skilful dentist, and at the same time should be placed upon the sirup of the hypophosphites or the lactophosphate of lime.

Œdema.—Œdema is a very frequent complication of pregnancy. It may be general and involve any portion of the body, but is usually limited to the lower extremities. Occasionally the vulva becomes intensely œdematous. When limited to the extremities, the swelling probably results from pressure exerted by the enlarged uterus upon the veins returning from the legs. On the other hand, if it be generalized, it is likely to be a manifestation of toxæmia, or even of an acute nephritis, though occasionally it may be due to other causes. Similarly, œdema of the vulva may be purely mechanical or a manifestation of some systemic disturbance.

The patient should be cautioned as to the significance of œdema, and whenever it appears the urine should be carefully examined. If the kidneys are found to be doing their work properly, the swelling is probably of mechanical origin and usually is not amenable to treatment, though the condition may be markedly benefited by restricting the movements of the patient, or even confining her to her bed. If the urine be abnormal, the

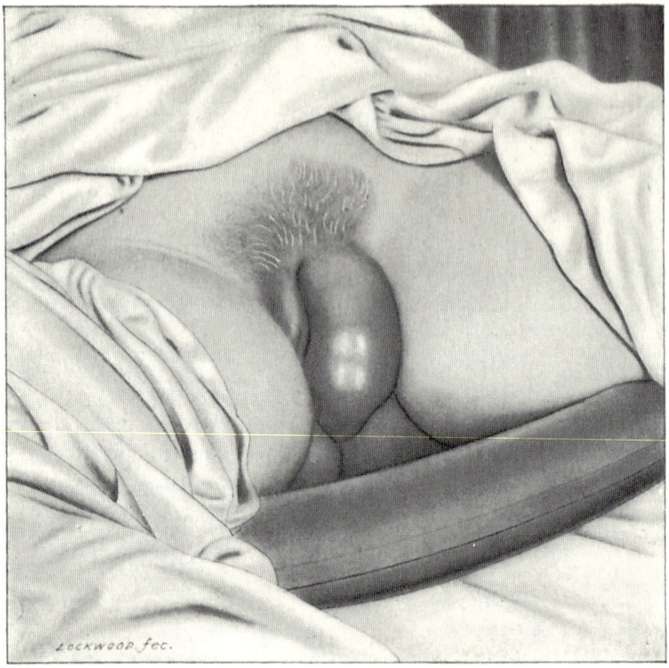

Fig. 425.—Œdema of Vulva.

condition is more serious, and the woman should be subjected to the treatment already outlined for the toxæmia of pregnancy.

When the marked swelling about the vulva is a source of discomfort and annoyance, and is not relieved by medicinal treatment, relief may be given by puncturing the most dependent portions of the swollen labia and allowing the serum to drain off. This slight operation should always be done under the strictest aseptic precautions, and the labia afterward covered with sterile dressings, inasmuch as infection can readily occur and may be followed by serious consequences.

Goître.—We have already referred to the slight enlargement which the thyroid frequently undergoes during pregnancy. Bignami has reported a case which, in his opinion, proved that pregnancy occasionally exerts a pathological influence upon this gland. During his patient's first pregnancy the thyroid underwent considerable hypertrophy, but returned to its normal size after delivery. The condition returned in the second pregnancy, the enlargement reaching such proportions that death resulted from suffocation.

In rare instances pregnancy appears to cause a rapid increase in the size of a thyroid tumour, which had been present before its inception.

Ahlfeld, Albers-Schönberg and Meinert have reported cases in which a goître, which had previously grown only slowly or had remained stationary in size, became so large during pregnancy as to render tracheotomy or the operative removal of the growth necessary in order to prevent death from suffocation.

Mental Derangements and Insanity.—Pregnancy is frequently accompanied by slight emotional or mental disturbances, many women becoming very irritable at such times. In rare instances the disturbances may become emphasized and the patients suffer from delusions, and occasionally from actual insanity. This is often a manifestation of auto-intoxication, which yields readily to appropriate treatment, although now and again the condition may eventuate in permanent insanity.

I recall one patient who during the later months of pregnancy suffered from delusions of persecution. At such times large amounts of albumin were present in the urine, while the urea output was greatly diminished. Sweat baths were repeatedly followed by an immediate improvement in the condition of the urine, after which the mental condition became normal, the delusions reappearing, however, within a few days, to again disappear under the same treatment. Complete recovery followed delivery.

Relaxation of the Pelvic Joints.—Owing to the great vascularity incident to pregnancy, the various pelvic joints always show a somewhat increased motility. In rare instances, however, the softening of the interarticular cartilage at the symphysis pubis admits of such abnormal motion in the joint as to interfere seriously with the comfort of the patient, who suffers from intense dragging pains in the pelvis and lower abdomen, while at the same time the gait may be so profoundly altered as to suggest the possible presence of cerebral or spinal trouble. In such cases the application of a tightly fitting bandage about the thighs is followed by marked improvement, though occasionally the symptoms are so pronounced that the patient is obliged to take to her bed. Occasionally the condition persists for a considerable time after childbirth. The whole subject has been studied in detail by Cantin (1899).

Hæmatoma of the Abdominal Walls.—Stoeckel has reported two cases of hæmatoma of the abdominal walls occurring during pregnancy. In one case the tumour was situated in the sheath of the right rectus muscle just above the symphysis, while in the other it appeared as a large mass in the right hypogastric region, which was mistaken for the head of the child. The condition resulted from rupture of the inferior and superior epigastric artery respectively.

LITERATURE

Ahlfeld. Schwangerschaft und Geburt complicirt durch Struma. Berichte u. Arbeiten, 1885, ii, 131.

Albers-Schönberg. Kompression der Trachea in Folge von Schilddrusenschwellung in der Gravidität, Tracheotomie. Centralbl. f. Gyn., 1895, 454–458.

Bignami. Tiroidismo e gravidanza. Ref. l'Obstétrique, 1896, i, 174.

Bouchard. Leçons sur l'autointoxication. Paris, 1887.

Bouffe de Saint Blaise. Les autointoxications gravidiques. Annales de Gyn. et d'Obst., 1898, l, 342–374 et 432–455.

Cantin. Relâchement des symphyses et arthralgies pelviennes d'origine gravidique. Thèse de Paris, 1899.

Champetier de Ribes et Bouffe de Saint Blaise. Note sur un cas de vomissements incoercibles avec autopsie. Comptes rendus de la Soc. de Gyn., d'Obst., et de Péd. de Paris, 1901, iii, 195–197.

Davis and Harris. Syncytioma Malignum and Ectopic Gestation causing Pernicious Nausea. Trans. Amer. Gyn. Soc., 1900, xxv, 364–389.

Dienst. Kritische Studien über die Pathogenese der Eklampsie, etc. Archiv f. Gyn., 1902, lxv, 369–464.

Dirmoser. Der Vomitus gravidarum perniciosus. Wien, 1901.

Kaltenbach. Ueber Hyperemesis gravidarum. Zeitschr. f. Geb. u. Gyn., 1891, xxi, 200–208.

Klein. Hyperemesis gravidarum. Zeitschr. f. Geb. u. Gyn., 1898, xxxix, 75–98.

Leyden. Einige Beobachtungen über Nierenaffectionen, welche mit Schwangerschaft im Zusammenhang stehen. Zeitschr. f. klin. Med., 1881, ii, 171–191.

Lindemann. Zur path. Anat. des unstillbaren Erbrechens der Schwangeren. Centralbl. f. allg. Path. u. path. Anat., 1893, Nr. 15.

Lvoff. Ptyalismus perniciosus gravidarum. Ref. Frommel's Jahresbericht, 1896, 595.

Meinert. Fall von Tetanie in der Schwangerschaft, entstanden nach Kropfoperation. Archiv f. Gyn., 1898, lv, 446–453.

Merle. De l'avortment forcé dans vomissements incoercibles graves. L'Obstétrique, 1900, v, 230–252.

Pick. Ueber Hyperemesis gravidarum. Volkmann's Sammlung klin. Vorträge, N. F., 1902, Nrs. 325–326.

Saft. Beitrag zur Lehre von der Albuminurie in der Schwangerschaft, etc., und von ihren Verhältniss zur Eklampsie. Archiv f. Gyn., 1896, li, 206–249.

Schmorl. Zur Lehre von der Eklampsie. Archiv f. Gyn., 1902, lxv, 504–529.

Schumacher. Exp. Beiträge zur Eklampsie-frage. Hegar's Beiträge zur Geb. u. Gyn., 1901, v, 257–309.

Stewart. Toxicity of Urine in Pregnancy. Amer. Jour. Obst., 1901, xliv, 506–575.

Stöckel. Zwei Fälle von Bauchdeckenhämatom in der Schwangerschaft. Centralbl. f. Gyn., 1901, 241–246.

Trantenroth. Studien über das Verhalten der Harnorgane, insbesondere der Nieren, in Schwangerschaft, etc. Zeitschr. f. Geb. u. Gyn., 1894, xxx, 98–175.

Van der Bergh. Ueber die Giftigkeit des Harns. Zeitschr. f. klin. Med., 1898. xxxv, 52–79.

CHAPTER XXVII

COMPLICATIONS DUE TO DISEASES AND ABNORMALITIES OF THE GENERATIVE TRACT

Diseases of the Vulva and Vagina.—*Varices.*—Varicose veins sometimes appear in the lower part of the vagina, but are more common around the vulva, where they may attain considerable proportions and give rise to a sensation of weight and discomfort. Treatment has practically no effect upon the local condition. In rare instances the varices may rupture during pregnancy, though this accident is more frequently observed at the time of labour, when profuse and sometimes fatal hæmorrhage may result if appropriate surgical treatment is not available.

Inflammation of Bartholin's Glands.—Infectious micro-organisms may gain access to Bartholin's glands and give rise to abscess formation. In such cases the labium majus on the side affected becomes swollen and painful, and on examination is found to inclose a large collection of pus. Most often the infection is gonorrhœal in origin, though other bacteria are sometimes associated with the gonococcus. Aside from the pain and discomfort, this complication is always a possible source of danger during labour and the puerperium, since it may be the starting-point of a puerperal infection. For these reasons, whenever a labial abscess develops during pregnancy it should be opened up and drained; or, better still, the entire pus sac should be excised.

Relaxation of the Vaginal Outlet.—In multiparous women the congestion incident to pregnancy not uncommonly causes the anterior or posterior vaginal wall to protrude through the relaxed or torn outlet as a distinct cystocele or rectocele. This condition is generally associated with dragging pains in the back and lower abdomen, and often interferes with locomotion. It is not amenable to treatment during pregnancy, though the symptoms may be temporarily relieved by rest in bed.

Vaginitis.—This complication has already been considered in Chapter XXV, under the heading of Gonorrhœa.

Colpo-hyperplasia cystica.—This rare condition, first described by Winckel, is characterized by the presence in the vaginal mucosa of numerous small cavities filled with clear fluid or gas and forming elevations upon its surface. Although not amenable to treatment during pregnancy, it usually disappears soon after childbirth. The recent researches of Lindenthal render it probable that the disease, in many cases at least, is due to infection with B. ærogenes capsulatus.

Diseases of the Cervix.—*Endocervicitis.*—Gonorrhœal infection of the cervical canal is frequently observed during pregnancy, the most prominent symptom being a profuse and persistent leucorrhœa. The treatment has already been considered.

Carcinoma.—About once in 2,000 cases, according to Sarwey, pregnancy is complicated by carcinoma of the cervix. It is most common in women between the thirtieth and fortieth years of life, two thirds of the cases collected by Sarwey having occurred within this decade, while the youngest patient was twenty-six years old.

In the majority of instances, the condition has existed before conception, but may make its appearance during pregnancy. A bloody, foul-smelling vaginal discharge is suggestive of malignant disease, but unfortunately the early stages are often unaccompanied by symptoms, and may escape detection unless a vaginal examination is made for some other reason, and an indurated and excavated ulceration of the cervix is discovered.

Pregnancy tends to bring about rapid growth and extension of a preexisting carcinoma. On the other hand, the malignant disease influences pregnancy very unfavourably, abortion being noted in 30 to 40 per cent of the cases. It likewise predisposes to the occurrence of placenta prævia, and at the time of labour markedly increases the risks of infection or spontaneous rupture of the uterus. In advanced cases, the cervix may be so indurated by carcinomatous infiltration that dilatation is either impossible, or may be accompanied by profuse hæmorrhage. In 603 cases collected by Sarwey, the mortality at the time of labour, or during the puerperium, was 43.3 per cent, 8 per cent of the patients dying undelivered.

The treatment of pregnancy complicated by carcinoma of the cervix differs according to the period at which the diagnosis is made and the extent to which the disease has progressed. If the condition is detected in the first half of pregnancy and the process has not extended beyond the cervix, immediate vaginal hysterectomy should be performed, Sarwey having reported 26 such operations without a death. On the other hand, if the case is inoperable, gestation should be allowed to continue in the interests of the child.

In the second half of pregnancy the choice of treatment is based upon similar indications, except that the large size of the uterus materially complicates vaginal hysterectomy. Hence, if a radical operation appears advisable, the uterus should be emptied and then removed through the vagina; or a laparotomy may be performed and the uterus removed unopened. In inoperable cases pregnancy should be allowed to go on to term, and then, if spontaneous delivery is out of the question, Cæsarean section should be performed in the interests of the child. For particulars concerning operative treatment, the reader is referred to the articles of Sarwey and Noble, the latter having collected the results obtained in 166 cases observed between the years 1886 and 1896.

Developmental Abnormalities of the Uterus.—Abnormalities in the development or fusion of one or both Müllerian ducts may result in malformations which sometimes possess an obstetrical significance. Various degrees of malformation—from an almost total absence of the uterus on the one hand to its duplication on the other (uterus didelphys)—are encountered. The accompanying diagrams (Figs. 426 to 431) give an idea of the nature of the more important varieties.

Pregnancy may be associated with any one of these malformations, provided an ovum be cast off from the ovaries and no serious obstacle be opposed to the upward passage of the spermatozoa and their subsequent union with it.

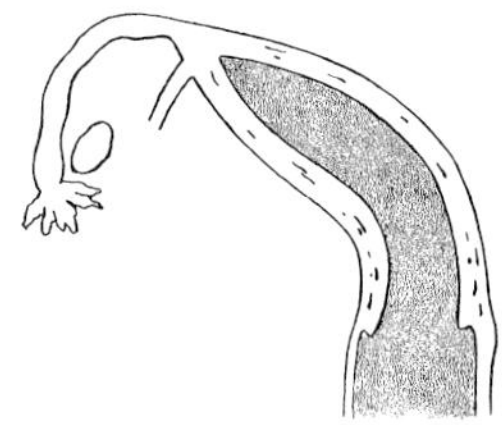

Fig. 426.—Diagram of Uterus Unicornis (Kehrer).

Pregnancy in the Rudimentary Horn of a Double Uterus.—In this condition the course of pregnancy is exposed to serious modifications. We owe to Mauriceau the first description of a case of this character, but since his time quite a number of examples have been reported.

In 78 per cent of the 84 cases collected from the literature by Kehrer in 1900, the proximal end of the rudimentary horn did not communicate

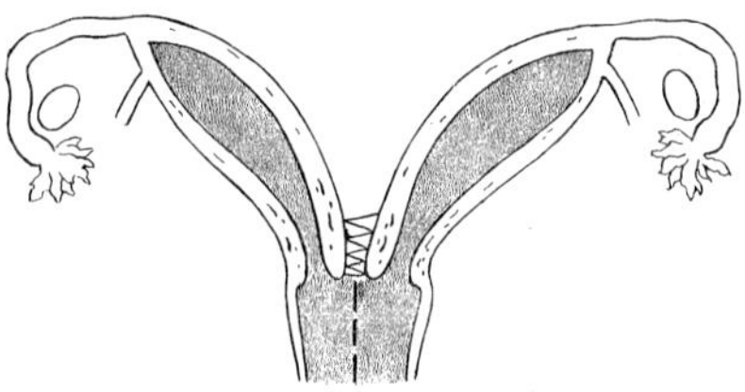

Fig. 427.—Uterus Pseudo-Didelphys (Kehrer).

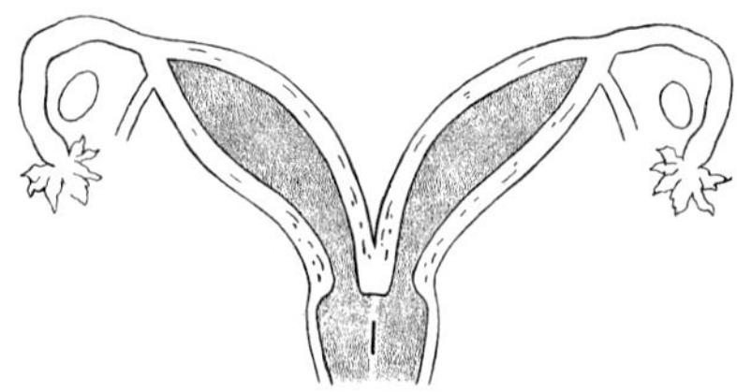

Fig. 428.—Uterus Bicornis Duplex (Kehrer).

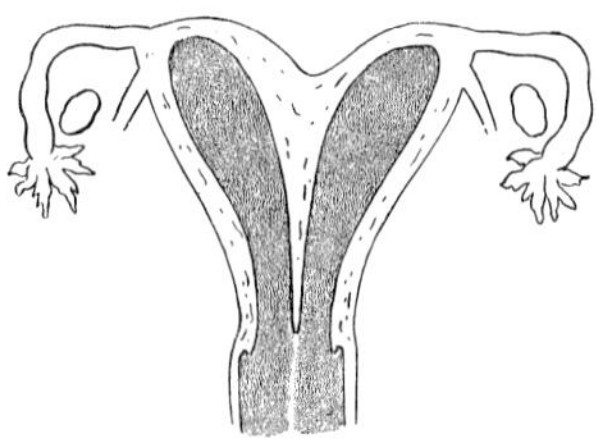

Fig. 429.—Uterus Bicornis Septus (Kehrer).

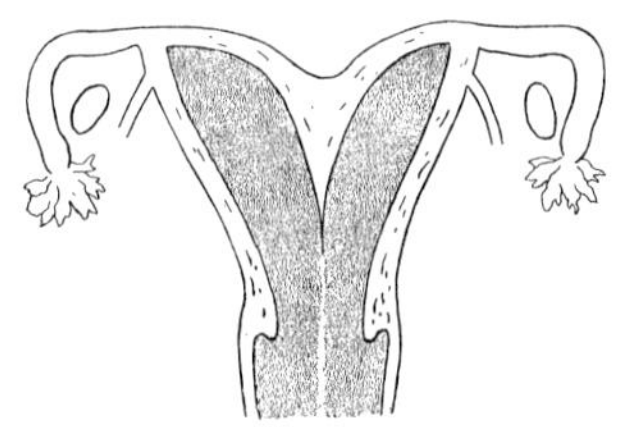

Fig. 430.—Uterus Bicornis Subseptus (Kehrer).

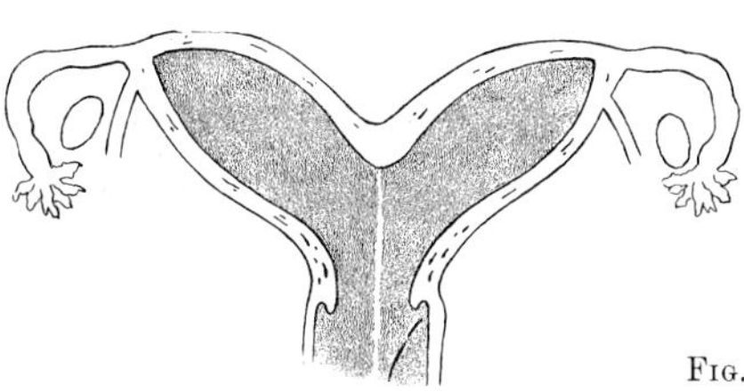

Uterus Bicornis Unicollis (Kehrer).

Fig. 431.

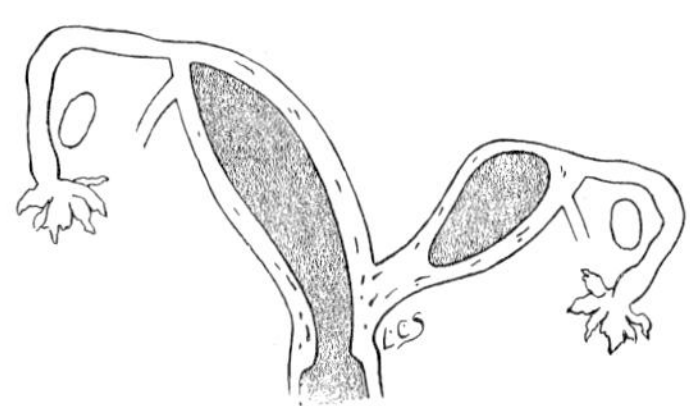

Uterus Bicornis Unicollis with Rudimentary Horn (Kehrer).

with the uterine cavity, so that in them pregnancy must have followed external migration of the spermatozoa or the ovum. In the former class of cases the spermatozoa pass up through the developed horn, gain access to the pelvic cavity, and then fertilize an ovum, either on the surface of the opposite ovary or within the tube of the rudimentary horn. In the latter an ovum is fertilized in the neighbourhood of the ovary of the normal side, and is then carried to the opposite tube, whence it gains access to the rudimentary horn, in which it undergoes development.

The occurrence of pregnancy in a rudimentary horn is accompanied by the development of a decidua in the non-pregnant horn, as well as by a marked increase in its size. Unless there is free communication between the two horns, which is but rarely the case, a pregnancy in this situation

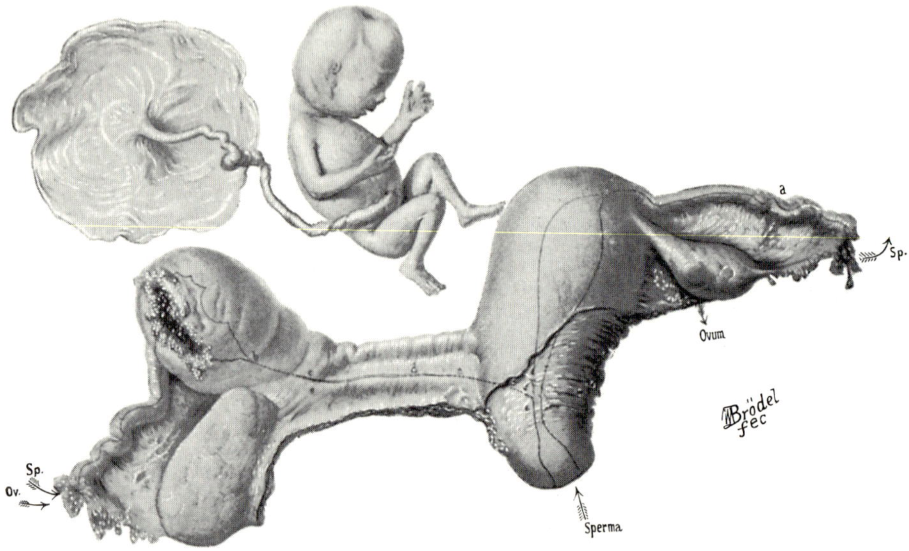

Fig. 432.—Pregnancy in a Rudimentary Left Uterine Horn. External Migration of Ovum (Kelly).

The specimen is viewed from behind. To the right is the well-developed uterus, which, after reaching the internal os, deviates to the right side. Attached to the cornu is the right tube, which is normal. The ovary is of the usual size, and at its inner and lower portion is the corpus luteum of pregnancy. Springing from the left side of the uterus at the internal os is a muscular band; on tracing this to the left it merges into the rudimentary uterine horn. On the posterior surface of this horn is a long slit representing the point of rupture. Protruding through the rent are placental remains. The left tube passes off from the outer side of the rudimentary horn. The left ovary is flattened. The lines on the well-developed uterus indicate the size of the uterine cavity. The line *b*, *c*, *d*, *e* indicates the course of the left Müller's duct. Between *c* and *d* it contains a lumen; where it is represented by dotted lines it consists of a solid muscular cord.

is a very serious occurrence, since it usually eventuates in rupture, which may lead to the death of the patient from intra-peritoneal hæmorrhage. This accident usually occurs within the first four months, and was noted in 87 and 47.6 per cent of the cases collected by Sänger and Kehrer respectively, in 1884 and 1900. The marked difference in the percentages is attributable to greater accuracy in diagnosis and more frequent recourse to operative interference, since the appearance of Sänger's work. In rare cases pregnancy may go on to term, the fœtus afterward being gradually eliminated by suppurative processes, or converted into a lithopædion.

Rupture is always attended by serious intra-peritoneal hæmorrhage, which usually ends fatally if operative procedures are not undertaken, 82 per cent of such patients in Kehrer's series having perished.

The existence of pregnancy in a rudimentary horn can occasionally be recognised during the early months, a positive diagnosis having been made in 20 per cent of Kehrer's cases. When a tumour corresponding in size to the duration of pregnancy can be detected alongside of what appears to be the slightly enlarged uterus, this condition should always be thought of. In differentiating it from a tubal pregnancy, it is important to remember that in the former the round ligament is felt coming off from the distal side of the tumour instead of from its proximal or uterine portion.

Treatment.—If the condition be diagnosticated, treatment consists in promptly opening the abdomen and amputating the pregnant horn. This operation was first performed by Sänger in 1884, and has since been repeated on 44 occasions, with a mortality of 13.3 per cent (Kehrer and Wells). Too frequently, however, the first suggestion of the existence of the abnormality is afforded by the symptoms of intra-peritoneal hæmorrhage, and an operation is usually undertaken in the expectation of finding a ruptured extra-uterine pregnancy.

Pregnancy in Uterus Unicornis.—Occasionally only one horn of the uterus is developed, the opposite tube and ovary being lacking or arising from the lower portion of the uterus. In such cases pregnancy usually pursues an uneventful course, and the condition is only accidentally recognised at the autopsy table.

Pregnancy in Uterus Bicornis.—When the two horns of the uterus are well developed, but no connection exists between them, as in uterus didelphys, or when they are partly fused, as in the various varieties of uterus bicornis, pregnancy may occur in either horn. In the very rare instances in which a twin pregnancy is observed, the two ova may occupy the same horn, although now and again an ovum has been found in each.

When pregnancy occurs in one horn of a bicornuate uterus, the other undergoes sympathetic hypertrophy and a distinct decidua is formed in its cavity. Ordinarily there is no interference with the course of pregnancy, and spontaneous labour may be looked for. Much more rarely the non-pregnant horn may partially fill up the pelvic cavity and give rise to serious dystocia similar to that produced by tumours of other origin. Nagel mentions three cases in which labour could not proceed until this structure had been pushed out of the pelvic canal. In two other instances—one reported by Löhlein and one observed in the Out-Patient Department of the Johns Hopkins Hospital and reported by Bettman—the non-pregnant horn obstructed the pelvic cavity and gave rise to rupture of the uterus. In the latter case, the condition was not recognised at the time of labour; the child presented by the breech and was extracted with considerable difficulty. The woman died thirty-six hours later from a subperitoneal hæmatoma following an incomplete rupture of the uterus, which was clearly due to impaction of the non-pregnant horn in the pelvis. Werth has reported a case in which the non-pregnant horn became retroflexed.

The diagnosis is usually not made, as in the majority of cases spontaneous labour occurs at term. Our own patient had given birth to 8 children without any suspicion of the existence of the deformity having arisen. Sometimes the existence of a double vagina or a double cervix puts one on the alert. The former may occur with a normal uterus, whereas the latter condition almost invariably indicates the existence of a double, or at least a bicornuate, uterus. When there is only a single cervix, as in uterus bicornis unicollis, the condition always escapes observation, unless the patient is subjected to examination at an early period of pregnancy, and the depression noted between the two halves of the uterus gives a clew to the true state of affairs.

Displacements of the Uterus.—*Anteflexion.*—Slight degrees of anteflexion are frequently observed in the early months of pregnancy, but are usually without significance. In the later months, particularly when the pelvis is markedly contracted or the abdominal walls are very lax, the uterus may fall forward, the sagging being occasionally so marked that the fundus lies considerably below the lower margin of the symphysis pubis. Even in less marked instances of the so-called *pendulous abdomen,* the patient may complain of various annoyances, more especially of exhaustion on exertion and dragging pains in the back and lower abdomen. Marked amelioration frequently follows the wearing of a properly fitting abdominal supporter.

Anteversion of the pregnant uterus is occasionally observed in patients who have previously been subjected to operative procedures for the relief of symptoms incident to retroflexion of the uterus, particularly after vaginal fixation, less frequently after an improperly performed ventrofixation, and now and again after shortening of the round ligaments. The condition is accompanied by marked discomfort during pregnancy, and at the time of labour may give rise to serious dystocia, which will be considered in Chapter XXXII.

Retrodisplacement of the Pregnant Uterus.—Retroflexion and retroversion of the uterus are frequently observed in non-pregnant women, and usually cause more or less inconvenience, though occasionally the condition may exist for years without any abnormal manifestation. In women who have never borne children, inflammatory or other changes in the endometrium, resulting from circulatory disturbances incident to the displacement, offer a serious obstacle to the occurrence of pregnancy. In parous women, on the other hand, this influence is less pronounced, but pregnancy, when it occurs, is prone to early interruption, retroflexion being one of the most frequent causes of spontaneous abortion.

In the vast majority of cases of pregnancy complicated by retrodisplacements, the uterus was already out of place before conception; although, as has been pointed out by Keitler and others, the abnormality may arise during gestation.

Pregnancy is more frequently complicated by retroflexion than by retroversion, though the latter usually gives rise to more serious symptoms. In these cases several eventualities are possible: the displacement may undergo spontaneous reduction without any interruption to pregnancy; abortion may occur; or, if neither takes place, the uterus may become incarcerated in the pelvic cavity and serious consequences follow.

If the displaced uterus is not adherent, spontaneous reduction usually occurs during the second or third month. This is rendered possible by an eccentric hypertrophy of the organ, owing to which the anterior wall becomes more rapidly distended than the posterior, and emerging above the superior strait eventually draws up the rest of the uterus. After the fundus has once passed the promontory of the sacrum there is no fear of a recurrence of the condition. Moreover, spontaneous reduction is not wholly out of the question, even when adhesions exist, since they often become stretched and occasionally disappear without any treatment. Retroflexion offers better prospects than retroversion; indeed, as Dührssen and Keitler have pointed out, when the latter condition is marked spontaneous restitution is almost impossible, for the reason that the cervix rises above the symphysis pubis, while the fundus is held back by the promontory of the sacrum.

In a certain number of cases, especially when the fundus is firmly adherent, pregnancy may remain uninterrupted for a long while. This prolongation is rendered possible by the marked upward growth of the anterior wall of the uterus, while the posterior wall retains its original situation and forms a cavity in which one pole of the fœtus is retained. This so-called *sacculation of the uterus* has been described in detail by Oldham, Dührssen, and others. Owing to the abnormal position of the cervix and the fact that the presenting part lies far below it, serious difficulties are to be expected at the time of labour, which will be considered in Chapter XXXII.

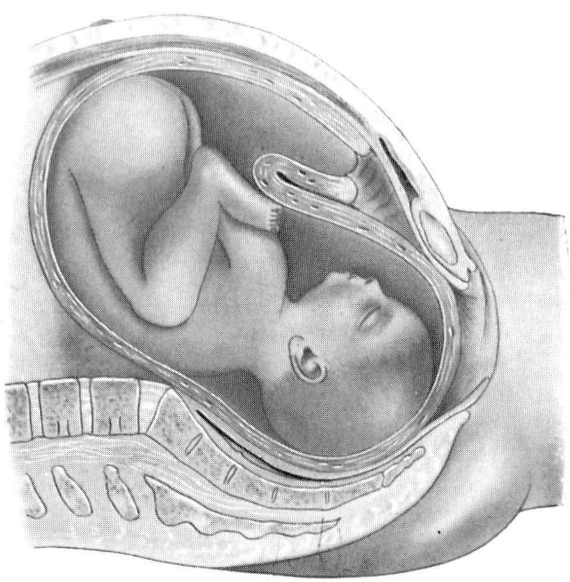

Fig. 433.—Sacculation of Retroflexed Pregnant Uterus (Oldham).

Abortion is common in pregnancies complicated by retrodisplacements. It usually occurs in the course of the third month, when the growing uterus pretty well fills the pelvic cavity and, becoming irritated by the pressure to which it is subjected, begins to contract, and thus brings about the expulsion of the ovum.

In other cases the abortion results from an endometritis which may have existed before the onset of pregnancy, or have been produced by circulatory disturbances incident to the displacement. This termination is particularly likely to occur when the sacrum possesses a marked vertical concavity, since the projecting promontory opposes a serious obstacle to spontaneous restitution.

If pregnancy continues and the displacement is not reduced in the natural course of events, or as the result of manipulations on the part of the physician, the uterus will continue to increase in size until it completely fills the pelvic cavity and, being unable to free itself, becomes impacted, and we have what is known as *incarceration.* Untoward effects, due to pressure, come on sooner in retroversion than in retroflexion, for the reason that in the former the cervix compresses the lower portion of the bladder at an earlier period. Incarceration is accompanied by characteristic symptoms, the woman complaining of pain in the lower portion of the abdomen and back, and disturbances in the functions of the urethra, bladder, and rectum. As the pelvis becomes more and more filled by the growing uterus, the pressure upon the neck of the bladder and urethra becomes so intense as to cause retention of the urine with consequent overdistention. When the latter has reached a certain limit, the overstretched viscus squeezes out a small amount of urine at frequent intervals, but never empties itself—*paradoxical incontinence.* If the condition is not soon relieved, the symptoms become more intense, cystitis develops, the urine becomes bloody, and eventually gangrene of the bladder may result, necrotic portions of its lining membrane being cast off and finally expelled through the urethra with intense cramp-like pains. In other cases the weakened walls of the bladder are unable to withstand the distention and rupture occurs, followed by a fatal peritonitis.

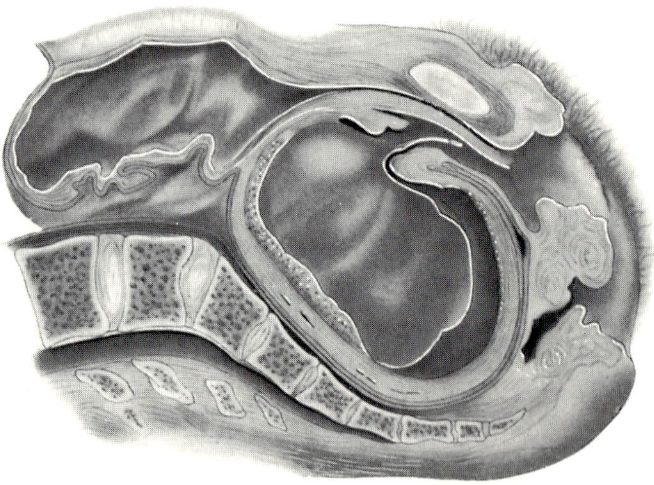

Fig. 434.—Incarceration of Retroflexed Pregnant Uterus (Swytzer).

Occasionally the uterus may undergo inflammatory changes as the result of the pressure to which it is subjected, and become densely adherent to the surrounding parts, while now and again the organ may be forced down and out of the pelvic cavity and emerge through the vulva or anus. In some cases the rectum is compressed to such an extent that defecation becomes impossible and gangrene results. Ileus, however, has not been observed.

Gottschalk found that the following were the most frequent causes of death in 67 cases reported in the literature up to 1894:

Peritonitis of vesical origin	17
Uræmia	16
Rupture of the bladder	11
Septicæmia of vesical origin	4
Gangrene of the bladder	3

A retrodisplacement of the pregnant uterus should always be suspected when a woman in the early months of pregnancy complains of long-continued, frequent, and painful micturition, especially if there is a history of antecedent uterine trouble. Incontinence of urine during pregnancy is a most suggestive sign, and always calls for a thorough vaginal examination. With the bimanual method, the soft body of the uterus will be found occupying the pelvic cavity, while the cervix is forced up against the symphysis or lies above it, according as one has to deal with a retroflexion or retroversion. It should be remembered that a pregnant tube lying behind the uterus may give somewhat similar signs, and this possibility should not be ruled out until careful examination has shown that the slightly enlarged uterus does not lie in front of the soft mass.

Treatment.—If the condition be detected in the first three months of pregnancy, bimanual reposition of the uterus should be attempted, aided by traction upon the cervix by means of a tenaculum or bullet forceps. After reposition has been effected, a properly fitting Smith-Hodge pessary should be introduced. On the other hand, if these simple manœuvres fail, the patient should be left alone until well on into the third month, in the hope that spontaneous reduction will still occur. If this has not taken place by that time, a more determined effort at replacement should be made, with the patient in the knee-chest position. If this proves unsuccessful, reduction can usually be effected by bimanual manipulations under anæsthesia.

When dense adhesions are present, various procedures have been recommended—the forcible breaking up of the adhesions under anæsthesia, attempts to loosen them by means of a succession of vaginal packs, the colpeurynter, or the "watch-spring" pessary, from the use of which Sinclair has reported excellent results.

Generally speaking, these methods are not to be recommended, and if the uterus cannot be replaced under anæsthesia, laparotomy should be performed and the adhesions separated under the guidance of the eye, as recommended by Mann and Fry. In one of my cases this course was pursued with most satisfactory results.

On the other hand, if symptoms of incarceration supervene, prompt treatment is imperative. The bladder should be immediately emptied. This cannot always be accomplished with the ordinary catheter on account of the elongation of the urethra and neck of the bladder resulting from the displacement (Fig. 434), so that in many cases the male instrument must be employed. Its introduction may often be facilitated by making traction upon the cervix with a tenaculum. After the bladder has been emptied, attempts should be made to replace the uterus—under anæsthesia, if necessary. But if this cannot be effected, most authors advise emptying it immediately, either by dilating the cervical canal or by puncturing the corpus through the vaginal vault. At present, however, I believe that better results will be obtained in such cases by laparotomy. This operation, however, should never be attempted if symptoms of infection or gangrene are present, since the weakened and necrotic bladder may be injured, or dense adhesions may be encountered which have formed over the uterus, practically shutting it off from the abdominal cavity and rendering the freeing of it almost impossible. Under these circumstances the obstetrician should content himself with emptying the uterus in the most conservative manner and then rely upon palliative treatment.

Lateral Displacements of the Pregnant Uterus.—Slight degrees of lateral displacement of the uterus during pregnancy are relatively frequent, but usually have no effect upon its course and do not give rise to symptoms. In two cases reported by Löhlein and Gottschalk the uterus had undergone a considerable degree of torsion, its left margin showing marked rotation towards the right, which in the second case was associated with retroflexion.

Prolapse of the Pregnant Uterus.—Impregnation in a totally prolapsed uterus is very rare on account of the difficulties attending a successful coitus, but if the prolapse is only partial it is comparatively frequent. In such cases the cervix, and occasionally a portion of the corpus, may protrude to a greater or lesser extent from the vulva during the early months, but as pregnancy progresses the uterus gradually rises up in the pelvis, and, as soon as it has passed beyond the superior strait, prolapse is no longer possible. On the other hand, if it retains its abnormal position, symptoms of incarceration appear during the third or fourth month, and abortion is the inevitable result, there being no cases on record in which pregnancy has progressed to term with the uterus outside of the body.

If there is a tendency towards prolapse during pregnancy, the uterus should be replaced and held in position by a suitable pessary. If, however, the pelvic floor be too relaxed to permit its retention, the patient should be kept in a recumbent position as far as possible until after the fourth month. When the cervix reaches to or slightly protrudes from the vulva, the greatest cleanliness is necessary, as several cases of fatal infection have been reported as occurring even without any internal examination. If the uterus lies outside of the vulva and cannot be replaced, it should be promptly emptied of its contents.

When the vaginal outlet is markedly relaxed, the congested anterior or posterior vaginal walls not infrequently prolapse during pregnancy, although the uterus may still retain its normal position. This condition may give rise to considerable discomfort and interfere with locomotion. It is not amenable to treatment until after delivery. At the time of labour these structures may be forced down in front of the presenting part and interfere with its descent. When this occurs they should be carefully cleansed and pushed back over it.

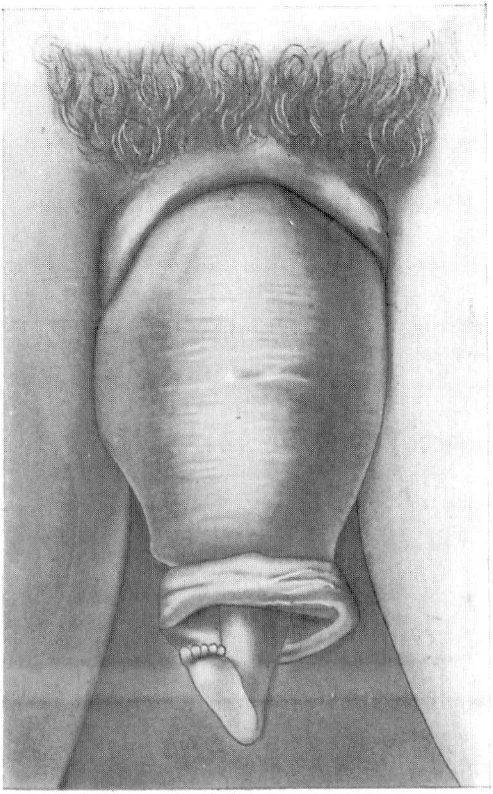

Fig. 435.—Prolapsed Pregnant Uterus (Wagner).

In rare instances a hernial protrusion may occur through the vagina, the anterior or posterior wall forming part of the sac. Such a *vaginal enterocele* may form a tumour of considerable size filled with intestines. Hirst has collected 27 instances from the literature. If the condition occurs during pregnancy, the protrusion should be replaced and the patient kept in the recumbent position. At the time of labour it may seriously interfere with the advance of the head. In such cases the mass should be pushed up if possible, and when this cannot be done it should be held out of the way as well as may be, and the head delivered past it.

Hypertrophic Elongation of the Cervix.—An abnormally elongated cervix seriously interferes with the occurrence of conception, but, as a rule, does not complicate the course of pregnancy or labour. The canal usually becomes shorter and more dilatable as term is approached. In the case of a patient whom I saw recently, the vaginal portion of the cervix in the early months was 5 centimetres in length and the external os protruded from the vulva, whereas later it had undergone marked softening and become reduced to normal dimensions, so that labour occurred spontaneously.

Acute Œdema of the Cervix.—In very rare instances, and usually without apparent cause, the cervix, particularly its anterior lip, may become acutely œdematous and attain such proportions as to protrude from the vulva. This condition has been exhaustively considered by Geyl in a recent publication.

Hernia.—Pregnancy occurring in women suffering from *inguinal hernia* is not influenced by the condition, although, owing to the increased intra-abdominal pressure, the previous defect may become aggravated. Generally speaking, the hernia should be treated palliatively by rest and the use of a truss, operative treatment being deferred until after delivery.

Very exceptionally, the uterus may form part of the contents of an inguinal hernia, and, indeed, several cases are on record in which conception has occurred under such circumstances. Full literature upon the subject will be found in the articles of Adams and Eisenhart, the latter having reported a case in which one horn of a five-months' pregnant bicornuate uterus occupied the right inguinal canal.

Umbilical herniæ are frequently noted during pregnancy, but are usually without effect upon the condition. During the early months the uterus is not in the neighbourhood of the hernial opening, while later, when the fundus reaches its level, it is usually too large to gain access to it. In exceptional cases, however, when the abdomen is markedly pendulous, such an occurrence is not beyond the range of possibility, and several such instances are on record. Much more common are the cases in which the cicatrix of an abdominal incision yields to the increased intra-abdominal pressure incident to pregnancy, and along the linea alba is formed a hernia into which the pregnant uterus often makes its way, being then covered merely by a thin layer of skin, fascia, and peritonæum.

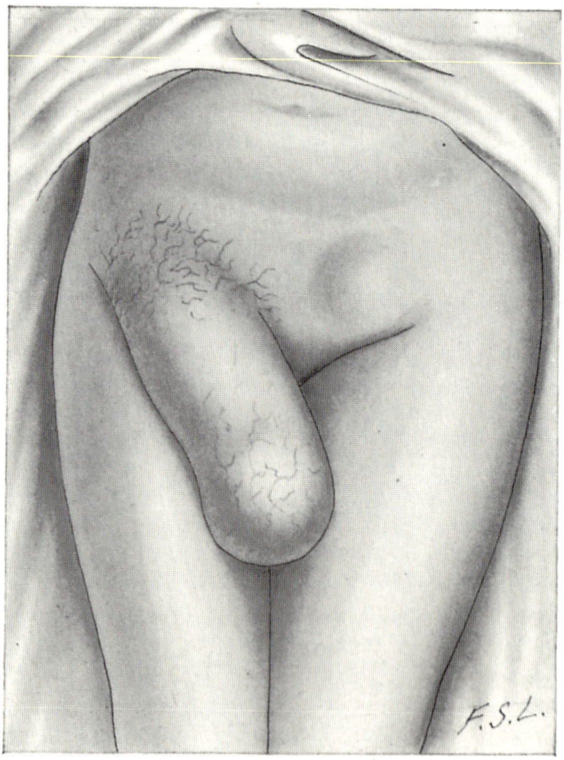

Fig. 436.—Pregnancy in Horn of Uterus contained in Inguinal Canal (Eisenhart).

A similar condition is occasionally observed in women suffering from marked *diastasis of the recti muscles*. Fig. 437 represents a patient in whom a hernia of this kind occurred suddenly during labour. Ordinarily, such herniæ have no effect upon pregnancy, although they may add markedly to the discomfort of the patient. Temporary relief is frequently obtained by holding the uterus in its normal position by a properly fitting bandage. At the time of labour, owing to the loss of muscular tone in the abdominal walls, the second stage is liable to be prolonged, and the employment of forceps is often called for.

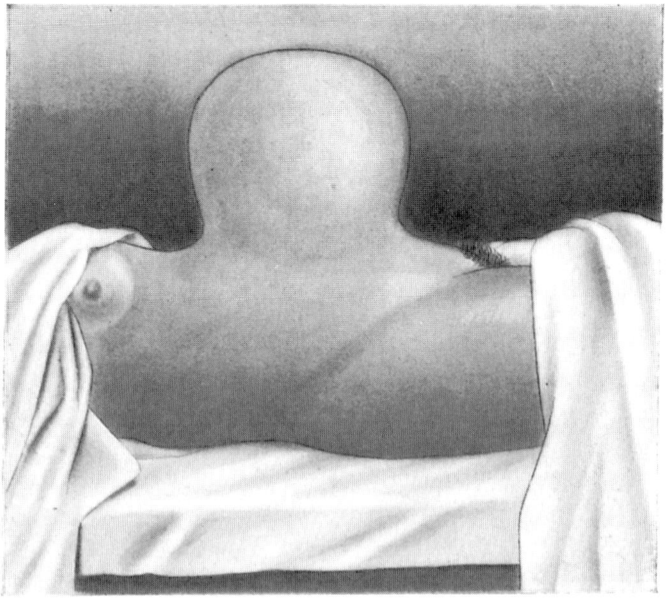

FIG. 437.—HERNIA OF PREGNANT UTERUS (Adams).

Diseases of the Decidua.—In non-pregnant women the endometrium is frequently the seat of lesions which are grouped together clinically under the general heading of *endometritis*. Careful histological examination shows, however, that the term is usually a misnomer, as the changes are generally trophic rather than inflammatory in character. The most important varieties are:

Hyperplastic endometritis—general hyperplasia, localized hyperplasia, polypoid growths.

Glandular endometritis—glandular hyperplasia.

Interstitial endometritis—general hypoplasia.

Acute and subacute endometritis—inflammatory changes.

These conditions are prototypes of more or less similar lesions occurring in the decidua, except, of course, that the latter are modified by the histological characteristics incident to pregnancy.

In the vast majority of cases, as was first pointed out by Veit, the decidual affection represents the extension of a lesion already existing at the time of pregnancy, conception occurring in a uterus affected by one of the various forms of so-called endometritis. In rare cases, however, it may be primary.

It is generally believed that endometritis is almost necessarily associated with sterility, the abnormal secretion of the uterine glands interfering with impregnation, and, even if conception occurs, the diseased mucosa does not offer a favourable nidus for the implantation of the ovum. Certainly this belief is justified in any marked grade of the affection, and every physician can recall instances in which the patient remained sterile until appropriate treatment had restored the endometrium to its normal condition. On the other hand, slight degrees of endometritis do not, as a rule, interfere with conception.

Diffuse Thickening of the Decidua.—Hegar, Kaltenbach, Kaschewarowa, and others have described a general hyperplasia of the decidua, in which the membrane, instead of becoming thinner, as is generally the case after the first few months, assumes unusual proportions. The condition frequently results in abortion, as a large part of the nutritive material intended for the fœtus is diverted to nourishing the decidua. After abortion or labour, a thickened decidua may cause abnormalities in the separation of the placenta.

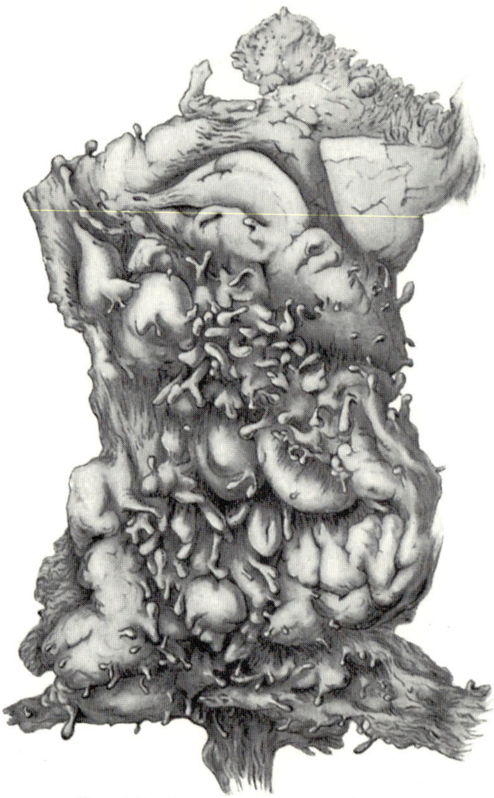

FIG. 438.—DECIDUA POLYPOSA (Bulius).

Localized Thickening of the Decidua (Decidua polyposa).—In this affection the entire decidua is somewhat thickened, but its characteristic feature consists in the projection of irregularly shaped, knob-like masses from the inner surface. Virchow first described this condition as decidua tuberosa or polyposa, and considered it to be syphilitic in origin, which, however, is not always the case. Ahlfeld states that it is frequently observed, whereas Bulius holds that it occurs but rarely. Personally I have never met with an instance.

Glandular Hyperplasia of the Decidua (Endometritis decidua glandularis).—Occasionally marked hyperplasia of the glandular structures of the decidua is present, and is usually associated with persistence of the glandular ducts. This affection commonly manifests itself by a profuse secretion of clear fluid, which may dribble away as rapidly as it is produced, or be retained in the uterus to be suddenly discharged in large quantities at variable intervals—*hydrorrhœa gravidarum.* The amount of fluid expelled varies considerably, though Ahlfeld has reported a case in which it exceeded 500 cubic centimetres on several occasions. This condition precludes the fusion of the decidua vera and reflexa, and theoretically the secretion should cease during the third or fourth month. In the occasional instances, however, in which it continues throughout pregnancy, it must be assumed that fusion of these structures has failed to occur.

During the last few years considerable discussion has arisen concerning the nature of hydrorrhœa gravidarum. Stoeckel, Reifferscheid, and others believe that it does not result from changes in the decidua, but is simply due to premature rupture of the membranes and the escape of the liquor amnii, which is not followed by the immediate termination of pregnancy. Van der Hoeven inclines to the older view, and bases his belief upon the analysis of specimens of the fluid expelled, which differs from the liquor amnii in having a lower specific gravity and in not containing albuminous materials or urinary constituents.

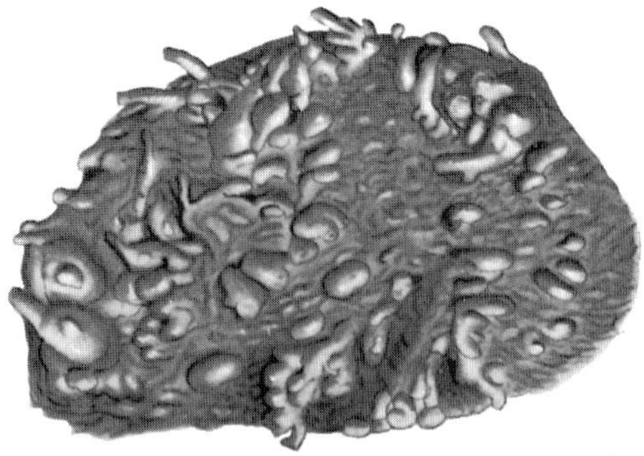

FIG. 439.—ENDOMETRITIS DECIDUA CYSTICA (Breus).

In rare cases the openings of the uterine glands may become occluded, small retention cysts being formed which project from the surface of the decidua, giving it a nodulated appearance. The affection has been described by Hegar and Breus as *endometritis cystica.*

Atrophic Endometritis decidua.—Under this heading Hegar, Ahlfeld, and others have described a disease in which large portions of the decidua vera and serotina undergo atrophic changes similar to those which occur normally in the portions corresponding to the lateral margins of the uterus. They offer no suggestion as to its ætiology, but consider that it interferes with the nutrition of the ovum and is a frequent cause of abortion.

Acute Endometritis decidua.—Acute inflammatory lesions of the decidua not infrequently follow attempts at criminal abortion, though now and again they may occur without such a history, cases having been reported by Donat, Emanuel and Wittkowsky, and others. Reference has already been made to the lesions of the endometrium which are sometimes associated with the acute infectious diseases.

In one of Emanuel's two cases bacilli were obtained in pure culture and were likewise present in the sections, while in the other cultures were not made, but cocci were demonstrated in the tissues. In one instance I was able to demonstrate the presence of cocci in sections, but unfortunately failed to make cultures before placing the specimens in the hardening fluid. These observations prove beyond doubt the bacterial origin of the lesions, and it is probable that future investigations will show that such conditions are not uncommon.

I have also observed several cases in which the decidua presented the characteristic features of acute inflammation, the vera and serotina being thickened and their external surface covered with a yellowish purulent exudate. Under the microscope the tissue was found to be infiltrated with leucocytes, and presented the typical picture of acute inflammation, with here and there areas of necrosis. More commonly, however, the changes are less marked, and only a few leucocytes are seen lying between the decidual cells.

Maslowsky and Neumann have been able to demonstrate the presence of gonococci in several cases of acute inflammation of the decidua; it is

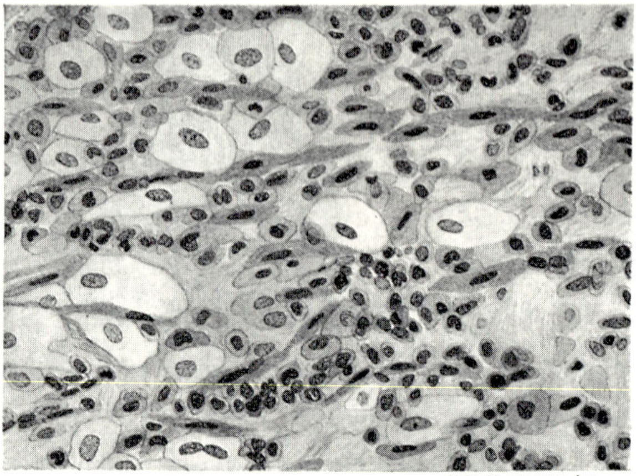

K. M. Montague, fec.

FIG. 440.—DECIDUAL ENDOMETRITIS. × 280.

probable that such conditions are not uncommon, and would serve to explain the origin of not a few cases of abortion.

The various forms of endometritis decidua complicating pregnancy are the most important factors in the causation of spontaneous abortion, and the existence of some one of them should be suspected whenever the patient complains of a sensation of weight in the lower abdomen associated with a slightly blood-stained or dirty brownish discharge, particularly when there is a history of gonorrhœal infection or repeated abortions.

It is permissible to assume that such conditions, particularly the hyperplastic forms, sometimes seriously interfere with the mechanism of the third stage of labour, owing to the abnormal consistency of the decidua and the consequent difficulty experienced in its separation.

Endometritis is not amenable to treatment during pregnancy. Should the patient present the slightest sign of its existence after abortion or childbirth, appropriate measures should at once be instituted, since the condition frequently persists to a slight degree, and may become seriously aggravated in a subsequent pregnancy.

Metritis.—Unless it results from infection, metritis is a very rare complication of pregnancy, and when it exists was usually present before conception. It predisposes to abortion and is not amenable to treatment during pregnancy.

Peri-uterine Inflammation.—When pregnancy occurs in women suffering from peri-uterine inflammation, considerable discomfort may result from the stretching of old adhesions. Not uncommonly abortion results.

Now and again the inflammatory changes undergo exacerbation during pregnancy, and may eventuate in abscess formation, which is accompanied by the usual symptoms of pelvic peritonitis. Very exceptionally rupture may occur and give rise to acute peritonitis, which usually ends fatally unless appropriate operative measures are promptly undertaken.

Pregnancy complicated by Tumours.—Pregnancy is occasionally complicated by the presence of ovarian or uterine tumours. Although, as a rule, they do not materially affect its course, they frequently offer a marked obstacle to labour, and will therefore be considered in detail in Chapter XXXII.

LITERATURE

ADAMS. Hernia of the Pregnant Uterus. Amer. Jour. Obst., 1889, xxii, 225–246.

AHLFELD. Ueber Endometritis decidualis tuberoso-polyposa. Archiv f. Gyn., 1876, x, 168–176.

Hydrorrhoea gravidarum. Endometritis atrophicans. Lehrbuch der Geb., II. Aufl., 1898, 253.

BETTMAN. A Case of Labour in a Bicornuate Uterus. Johns Hopkins Hosp. Bulletin, 1902, xiii, 57.

BREUS. Ueber cystöse Degeneration der Decidua vera. Archiv f. Gyn., 1882, xix, 483–489.

BULIUS. Ueber Endometritis decidua polyposa et tuberosa. Münchener med. Wochenschr., 1896, Nr. 28.

DONAT. Endometritis purulenta in der Schwangerschaft. Archiv f. Gyn., 1884, xxiv, 481–486.

DÜHRSSEN. Aussackungen, etc., der schwangeren Gebärmutter. Archiv f. Gyn., 1899, lvii, 70–223.

EISENHART. Fall von Hernia inguinalis cornu dextri uteri gravidi. Archiv f. Gyn., 1885, xxvi, 439–459.

EMANUEL. Zur Lehre von der Endometritis in der Schwangerschaft. Zeitschr. f. Geb. u. Gyn., 1895, xxxi, 187–198.

EMANUEL und WITTKOWSKY. Ueber Endometritis in der Gravidität. Zeitschr. f. Geb. u. Gyn., 1895, xxxii, 98–111.

FRY. Cœliotomy in the Treatment of the Incarcerated Pregnant Uterus when Irreducible. Amer. Gyn. and Obst. Jour., 1899, xiv, 25–27.

GEYL. Zum Œdema acutum cervicis uteri gravidi, etc. Volkmann's Sammlung klin. Vorträge, N. F., 1895, Nr. 128.

GOTTSCHALK. Zur Lehre von der Retroversio uteri gravidi. Archiv f. Gyn., 1894, xlvi, 358–383.

HEGAR. Kysten-bildung in der Decidua. Monatsschr. f. Geburtsk., 1863, xxi, Supplement-Heft, 11.

Die Drüsen der Decidua und die Hydrorrhoea gravidarum. Monatsschr. f. Geburtsk., 1863, xxii, 429–451.

HEGAR und MAIER. Beiträge zur Pathologie des Eies. Virchow's Archiv, 1871, lii, 161–192.

HIRST. Vaginal Enterocele in Pregnancy and Labour. Trans. Amer. Gyn. Soc., 1893, xviii, 351–357.

KALTENBACH. Diffuse Hyperplasie der Decidua am Ende der Gravidität. Zeitschr. f. Geb. u. Gyn., 1878, ii, 225–231.

KASCHEWAROWA. Ueber die Endometritis decidualis chronica. Virchow's Archiv, 1868, xliv, 103–113.

KEHRER. Das Nebenhorn des doppelten Uterus. Heidelberg, 1900.

KEITLER. Ein Beitrag zur Retroflexion und Retroversion der schwangeren Gebärmutter. Monatsschr. f. Geb. u. Gyn., 1901, xiii, 285–305.

LINDENTHAL. Aetiologie der Kolpohyperplasia cystica. Wiener med. Wochenschr., 1897, Nrs. 1–2.

LÖHLEIN. Ueber Achsendrehung des Uterus, besonders des graviden Uterus. Deutsche med. Wochenschr., 1897, Nr. 14.

MANN. The Surgical Treatment of Irreducible Retroflexion of the Gravid Uterus. Trans. Amer. Gyn. Soc., 1898, xxiii, 135–140.

MASLOWSKY. See Chapter XXV.

MAURICEAU. Histoire d'une femme, etc. Traité des maladies des femmes grosses, 6me éd., 1721, T. I., 86–91.

NAGEL. Entwickelungsfehler des Uterus und der Scheide. Veit's Handbuch der Gyn., 1897, i, 563–604.

NEUMANN. See Chapter XXV.

NOBLE. One Hundred and Sixty-six Cases of Cancer of the Pregnant Uterus, etc. Amer. Jour. Obst., 1896, xxxiii, 873–882.

OLDHAM. Case of Retroflexion of the Gravid Uterus, etc. Trans. London Obst. Soc., 1860, i, 317–322.

REIFFERSCHEID. Beitrag zur Lehre von der Hydrorrhoea uteri gravidi. Centralbl. f. Gyn., 1901, 1143–1145.

SÄNGER. Ueber Schwangerschaft im rudimentären Nebenhorn bei Uterus duplex. Centralbl. f. Gyn., 1883, 324.

SARWEY. Carcinom u. Schwangerschaft. Veit's Handbuch der Gyn., 1899, iii, 2te Hälfte, 1ste Abth., 489–532.

SINCLAIR. A Contribution to the Diagnosis and Treatment of Retro-flexio-versio Uteri Gravidi. Trans. London Obst. Soc., 1900, xlii, 338–355.

STOECKEL. Beitrag zur Lehre von der Hydrorrhoea uteri gravidi. Centralbl. f. Gyn., 1899, 1353–1361.

VAN DER HOEVEN. Hydrorrhoea gravidarum. Monatsschr. f. Geb. u. Gyn., 1899, x, 329–337.

VEIT. Ueber Endometritis decidua. Volkmann's Sammlung klin. Vorträge, 1885, Nr. 254.

Allgemeines über die Aetiologie der Endometritis in der Gravidität. Zeitschr. f. Geb. u. Gyn., 1895, xxxii, 111–116.

VIRCHOW. Endometritis decidua tuberosa. Die krankhafte Geschwülste, 1864, ii, 478–481.

WELLS. The Clinical Significance of Developmental Duplications of the Uterus and Vagina. Amer. Jour. Obst., 1900, xli, 317–365.

WERTH. Retention einer Ausgetragenen Frucht in dem unvollkommen entwickelten Horne eines Uterus bicornis. Archiv f. Gyn., 1881, xvii, 281–297.

WINCKEL. Ueber die Cysten der Scheide, etc. Archiv f. Gyn., 1871, ii, 383–413.

CHAPTER XXVIII

DISEASES AND ABNORMALITIES OF THE OVUM

ANY portion of the ovum—chorion, amnion, placenta, or fœtus—may be the seat of disease, or may present abnormalities. In many instances the morbid process is limited to a single portion, while in others a large part, or even the ovum as a whole, may be implicated. Accordingly, we shall take up successively those lesions or abnormalities which are limited to the chorion, amnion, or placenta; next, those in which the entire ovum, and finally those in which the fœtus alone is affected.

Diseases of the Chorion.—*Hydatidiform Mole.*—In this condition, also known as vesicular mole, cystic degeneration of the chorion, or myxoma chorii, the terminal extremities of the chorionic villi are converted into transparent vesicles with clear, viscid contents. These vary in size from minute bodies a few millimetres in diameter to cystic structures the size of hazel-nuts, and hang in clusters from the villous stems, to which they are connected by thin pedicles, giving to the external surface of the chorion a grape-like appearance. The formation may involve the entire periphery of the membrane, but more frequently is limited to portions of it.

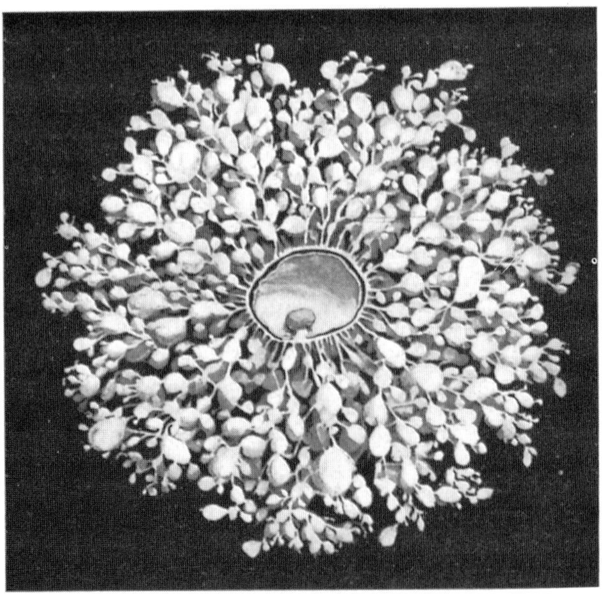

FIG. 441.—HYDATIDIFORM MOLE (Bumm).

It is generally stated that the condition was first described by Schenck von Grafenberg in 1565, but Kossmann has pointed out that Ætius, of

Amida, in the early part of the sixth century, wrote intelligently about an hydatidiform mole, although he had no clear idea of its nature.

Owing to its peculiar appearance and the fact that it frequently contained no trace of a fœtus, the hydatidiform mole was a source of not a little speculation to the early writers upon medicine, and all sorts of theories were advanced concerning its origin. As the name implies, the condition was long considered to be analogous to the hydatid cysts observed in other parts of the body, Goeze, Percy, and others believing that the vesicles contained worm-like structures. De Graaf held that the vesicles were mature ova, while some authors thought that each represented an early pregnancy. It

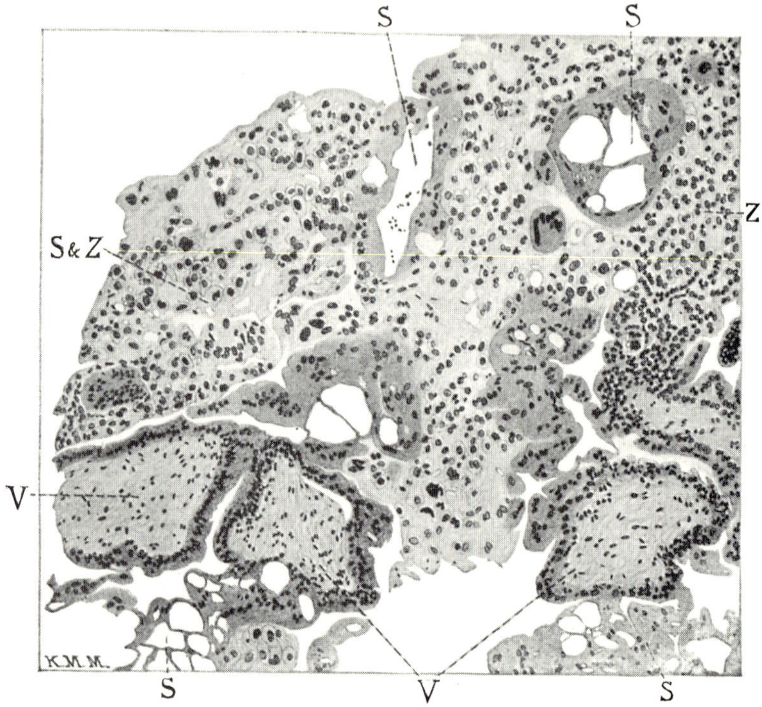

FIG. 442.—SECTION OF HYDATIDIFORM MOLE, SHOWING PROLIFERATION OF SYNCYTIUM AND LANGHANS'S CELLS. ×75.

S., syncytium ; *V.*, normal chorionic villi ; *Z.*, Langhans's cells.

is probable that many of the extraordinary cases of multiple gestation recorded in the early literature, such as that of the Countess Hagenau, who was believed to have given birth to 365 embryos at a single labour, were really instances of hydatidiform mole.

The true nature of the affection was first recognised by Velpeau and Madame Boivin in 1827, and since then it has been universally admitted to be a disease of the chorion. Numerous theories were advanced as to the nature of the lesion, until Virchow in 1853 stated that the process was essentially a myxomatous degeneration of the connective tissue of the chorionic villi, and designated it as *myxoma chorii*. This view obtained immediate acceptance and held its ground until 1895, when Marchand demonstrated that the essential feature of the affection was to be found not so much in the stroma as in the epithelial covering of the villi. He showed that both the syncytium and Langhans's layer of cells underwent profuse and irregular proliferation, penetrating Nitabuch's fibrin layer and making their way into the depths of the decidua, and not infrequently into the uterine musculature as well. At the same time the blood-vessels of the terminal villi disappeared and the stroma degenerated, so that in advanced cases its nuclei failed to take up the usual histological stains and the cells presented a necrotic appearance. Moreover, inasmuch as the fluid contents of the vesicles failed to give the characteristic reaction for mucin, Marchand felt justified in attributing them to œdema.

This work obtained almost immediate acceptance, and was promptly confirmed by many investigators, among whom Neumann, Fraenkel, Pick, Ouvry, Schwab, and Van der Hoeven may be mentioned. Fig. 442 represents a section through the most recent one of the four specimens which I have examined, all of which abundantly confirm Marchand's view.

With the discovery that the so-called *deciduoma malignum* resulted from a malignant proliferation of the epithelial elements of the chorion, and particularly that it was preceded in from one third to one half of the recorded cases by the expulsion of an hydatidiform mole, great interest arose as to the nature of the latter condition and the relation which it bore to the production of the former. The similarity in the microscopic structure of the two pathological processes made it apparent that there must be a genetic relationship between them, and the question arose whether it existed in all cases.

Neumann, in 1897, held that it was possible to differentiate between two forms of hydatidiform mole—malignant and benign—one of which was and the other was not followed by the development of a deciduoma malignum. He considered that in the former the proliferating epithelium invaded the stroma, while in the latter it was limited to the periphery of the villus. Pick likewise believes that there are two forms of mole which are very difficult to separate, inasmuch as he thinks that in the early stages, at least, the difference is biological rather than histological. On the other hand, Van der Hoeven believes that all moles are essentially malignant, and that the development of a deciduoma depends upon the completeness with which the original growth has been expelled from the uterus.

Causation.—Virchow and Veit agree that the development of the condition is dependent upon endometritic changes. Marchand and most recent writers, however, hold that such changes are secondary. At the 1901 meeting of the German Gynæcological Congress, Aichel stated that he had been able to produce the condition experimentally in dogs by destroying the vessels going to the decidua, and thereby interfering with the nutrition of the chorionic villi. His experiments were very briefly reported, and until satisfactory and conclusive evidence of their correctness is adduced they should be received with caution. On the other hand, it is not unlikely that in many cases, at least, the process originates primarily in the ovum, plausibility being lent to such a view by the fact that in rare cases of twin pregnancy one ovum may be perfectly normal, while the other presents the lesion in question. It is hardly probable, if the endometrium were the primary cause, that the changes would be limited to one ovum. A characteristic case of this kind has been reported by Kahn-Benzinger.

Clinical History.—Hydatidiform mole is a rare disease, occurring, according to Madame Boivin, once in 20,000 cases. On the other hand, the recent statistics of Williamson would indicate that it may be found about once in 2,400 cases. It may occur at any period of reproductive life, but is particularly frequent in the third decade, having been noted between the twentieth and thirtieth years in 41 and 38 per cent of the cases collected by Dorland and Kehrer respectively. It likewise appears with comparative frequency after the fortieth year—in 16 and 22 per cent of the cases, according to the same author.

The process usually comes on early in pregnancy, rarely making its appearance after the third month. When it develops comparatively late it does not implicate the entire chorion; but whenever a considerable portion of the membrane is involved, atrophic changes affecting the fœtus are constantly found, and the development of the latter is materially influenced even when the disease is relatively mild in character. In the former class of cases the fœtus dies at an early period, and often undergoes complete dissolution, all trace of it disappearing except the maternal end of the umbilical cord. As the chorionic villi are nourished by the maternal blood, the condition may persist after the death of the fœtus, and the growth attain considerable proportions, though spontaneous expulsion usually occurs before the sixth month.

The clinical history is very characteristic. The uterus enlarges much more rapidly than usual, so that the fundus is often found at the level of or above the umbilicus in a woman who gives a history of being only three or four months pregnant. After a longer or shorter period more or less profuse hæmorrhage occurs, which persists until the mole is cast off spontaneously or removed by the physician.

In a small number of cases, the hypertrophic villi invade the uterine wall, following the course of venous channels. This happens in what is known as the destructive mole, characteristic examples of which have been reported by Krieger, Volkmann, Jarotsky, and Waldeyer. Now and again the growth reaches the peritoneal surface of the uterus and gives rise to perforation, followed by fatal intra-peritoneal hæmorrhage. This complication was observed by Wilton, Madame Boivin, Ouvry, and others.

In rare instances, at varying periods after the expulsion of the mole, small purplish or reddish tumours appear in the vagina or about the vulva. On microscopic examination, after excision, these are found to consist for the most part of blood, through which are scattered dropsical villi showing the characteristic epithelial changes. In a number of cases recorded the uterus was perfectly normal, and complete excision of the nodule was followed by permanent recovery. The question has accordingly arisen whether such tumours represent metastases from a deciduoma malignum or a malignant hydatidiform mole, or whether they are merely due to the accidental transportation of particles of a benign growth. Neumann and

Schmidt take the former, while Pick and Schlagenhauser incline to the latter view. The observations of Veit, Poten, and myself, concerning the transportation of villi in normal pregnancy, lend a certain probability to the latter theory, although the question must remain to be settled by future investigations (see Fig. 610).

Aside from the possibility of the development of a deciduoma malignum, the hydatidiform mole is a serious affection, since Dorland noted an immediate mortality in 10 per cent of the 100 instances which he collected from the literature, death being due to hæmorrhage at the time of operation in 3 per cent, to perforation of the uterus in 2 per cent, and to infection in 5 per cent of the cases.

Diagnosis.—Hydatidiform mole should always be suspected when hæmorrhage occurs in a patient whose uterus is considerably larger than it should be for the duration of pregnancy, though in not a few cases similar symptoms are noted in hydramnios. A positive diagnosis may be made when one finds one or more vesicles in the uterine discharges, or when the finger introduced through the cervical canal is able to palpate the characteristic grape-like masses.

Treatment.—Owing to its inherent danger, but especially to the possible subsequent development of a deciduoma malignum, the uterus should be emptied as soon as a positive diagnosis is made. By means of a gauze pack or a steel dilator, the cervix should be dilated sufficiently to admit two fingers, with which the growth is peeled off from the uterine wall and then removed. Care should be taken that the manipulations are made as gently as possible in order to avoid a possible perforation of the uterus, whose walls are likely to have been weakened by the invasion of the growth. After removal of the mole, the uterine cavity should once more be explored to make sure that it is thoroughly empty.

Every woman who has suffered from a hydatidiform mole should be carefully watched for the next few months, and if hæmorrhage makes its appearance the interior of the uterus should be palpated. Whenever a small nodular growth is present it should be removed and subjected to microscopic examination; and if the characteristic lesions of deciduoma are found to be present immediate hysterectomy is imperative, in the hope of avoiding metastases. On the other hand, as has already been pointed out, vaginal or vulval metastases occasionally occur without any apparent involvement of the uterus. Under such circumstances they should be excised, but the uterus left in place, as the history of similar cases shows that the majority of the patients recover permanently.

Deciduoma Malignum, Chorionic Epithelioma.—The term deciduoma malignum was applied by Sänger to a very malignant variety of uterine tumour which develops after a full-term labour, abortion, or hydatidiform mole, and in rare instances before the last is expelled from the uterus. Strictly speaking, this subject should be considered in the section upon the pathology of the puerperium, but owing to the frequent genetic relationship of this tumour to the hydatidiform mole, it is best considered in this place.

The nature of the growth has given rise to a great deal of discussion, and various appellations have been suggested for it, the most important being sarcoma deciduo-cellulare, chorio-epithelioma, syncytioma malignum, and carcinoma syncytiale.

Sänger read his first paper upon the subject before the German Gynæcological Society in 1892, and based his report upon the following case: A woman, twenty-three years of age, aborted in the eighth week and died seven months later. At autopsy four large, soft, reddish, spongy tumours were found in the uterine wall, with metastases exhibiting similar characteristics in the lungs, diaphragm, tenth rib, and right iliac fossa. Microscopic examination showed that the tumour was made up in great part of blood spaces bounded by large cells, which Sänger identified as decidual cells. The metastases presented a similar appearance and had resulted from the transportation of tumour masses through the venous channels. As Sänger believed that the tumour was derived from decidual cells and was therefore of connective-tissue origin, he designated it *decidual sarcoma* or *sarcoma uteri deciduo-cellulare.* The appearance of his monograph in 1893, in which was collected all that was then known upon the subject, created profound interest, and was soon followed by the publication of many similar cases.

In 1895 I published a monograph upon the subject, in which I reported a case and collected 24 others from the literature. My patient was a coloured woman who had a spontaneous full-term labour. A week later she noticed a small painful nodule upon the right labium majus, which rapidly increased in size, so that two weeks later it had attained the size of a hen's egg and resembled a hæmatoma in appearance. Shortly afterward it underwent necrotic changes, which were accompanied by a profuse, foul-smelling discharge. The patient gradually grew worse, eventually developed a cough and bloody expectoration, and finally died six months after delivery. The nature of the vulval tumour was not suspected during life, but at autopsy the lungs were found to be studded with large numbers of metastases of varying size, which resembled placental tissue in appearance. Similar but smaller growths were present in the kidneys, spleen, and ovary, while a small nodule about 1 centimetre in diameter was found in the uterus.

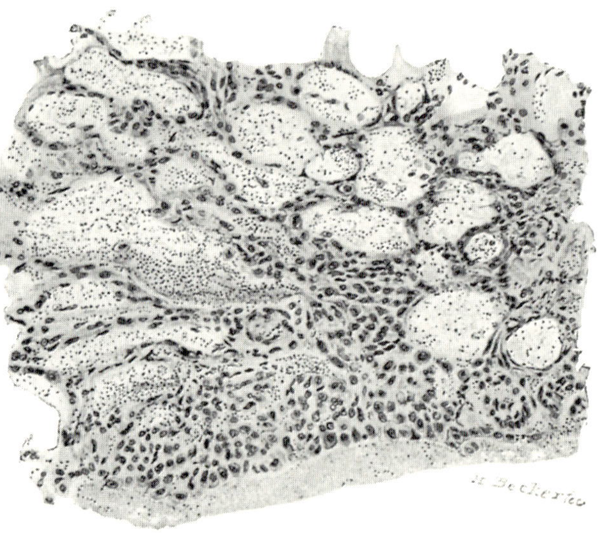

Fig. 443.—Deciduoma Malignum, showing Alveolar Arrangement of Primary Tumour. × 60.

Microscopic examination showed that the uterine growth and the metastases were made up in great part of blood spaces, whose walls were formed by large clear cells with definite vesicular nuclei. At the margins of the primary growth, invading the adjacent musculature, were large masses of vacuolated protoplasm which was not divided into individual cells. The

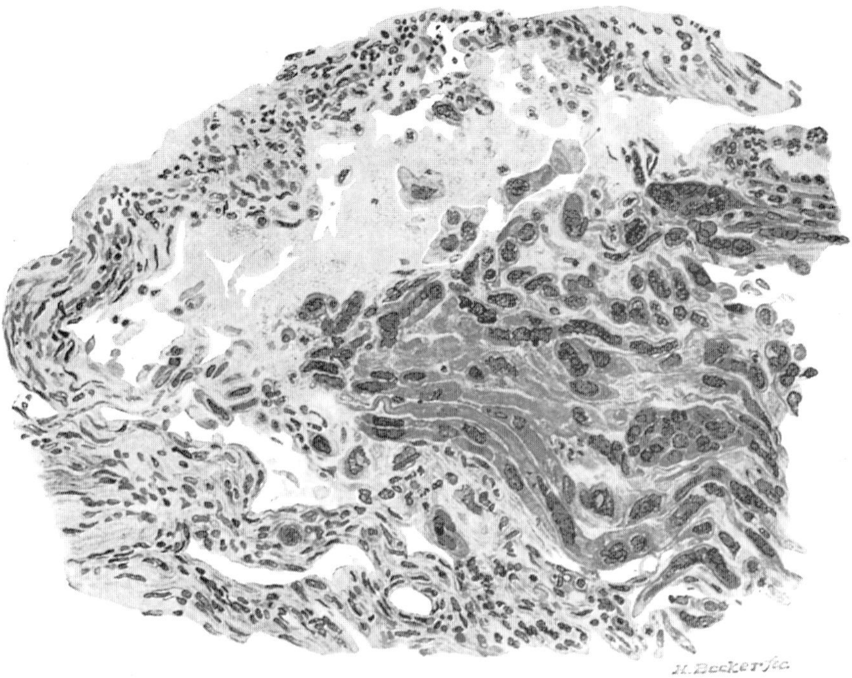

FIG. 444.—DECIDUOMA MALIGNUM, SHOWING SYNCYTIAL MASSES INVADING A VENOUS CHANNEL.

nuclei were irregular in shape and stained intensely. Closer examination showed that these protoplasmic masses were similar to and identical in structure with the syncytial layer of the chorionic epithelium; the nature of the individual cells was not so clear, although I was inclined to consider them due to transverse and oblique sections through the syncytial masses.

The same year, Marchand wrote a most important monograph upon the subject. He identified the protoplasmic masses with the syncytium, and the individual cells with those of Langhans's layer. At that time it was generally believed that the former was of maternal and the latter of fœtal origin, so that according to this view the tumour would be composed partly of maternal and partly of fœtal tissue. Later investigations indicated that the syncytium was also of fœtal origin, and this was demonstrated beyond peradventure by the findings in Peters's ovum. Hence it follows that the tumours in question are entirely fœtal in origin, and arise from the malignant proliferation of the two layers of chorionic epithelium. This being the case, they cannot correctly be described as deciduomata or decidual sarcomata, and Marchand, in his second article (1898), proposed the term *chorio-epithelioma.* In view, however, of the multiplicity of designations, and especially the fact that the growth was so described by Sänger, it appears advisable to retain the term deciduoma malignum for clinical purposes.

Marchand's conclusions have received abundant confirmation at the hands of all who have studied the subject, with the exception of Veit and certain English authorities. Veit holds that the tumour is simply a sarcoma whose cells have undergone changes in appearance under the influence of pregnancy. Eden, Kanthack, and other English observers stated before the London Obstetrical Society in 1896 that it did not differ materially from other sarcomata, and they therefore saw no reason to place it in a class by itself.

The monographs of Sänger and Marchand were merely the beginning of an extensive literature upon the subject, which rapidly increased in volume every year. Thus, Dorland, in 1897, was able to collect 52 cases, while Marchand, in 1898, described 2 new cases and mentioned 59 others, in addition to those recorded in his first monograph. In 1902 Ladinski was able to collect 132 cases.

The deciduoma malignum consists, as a rule, of a small primary growth which gives rise to abundant metastases, particularly in the lungs, vagina, and brain. Thus, in the 52 cases collected by Dorland, metastases were observed in the lungs of 78.38 per cent, in the vagina of 54 per cent, and in the kidney, spleen, and ovary of 13.5 per cent; of the liver, broad ligament, and pelvis respectively 10.8 per cent, and in the brain 5.4 per cent.

The vaginal metastases are of particular significance, and in several instances growths have been observed in the vagina without the discovery of a primary focus in the uterus. Schmorl has even reported a case in which generalized metastases developed while the uterus remained perfectly free. Under such circumstances it must be assumed that the primary growth originated during pregnancy and was limited to the placenta, particles of which became broken off and were carried into the circulation, giving rise to metastases at the points at which they were arrested, while the primary tumour itself was cast off with the after-birth. Poten and Vassmer have recently reported a case in which vaginal metastases appeared while an hydatidiform mole was still in the uterus.

Clinical History.—Deciduoma malignum may occur at any age during the childbearing period, and always follows a pregnancy, whether the latter terminates in full-term labour, abortion, or hydatidiform mole, the last condition being noted in nearly 50 per cent of the cases. In several instances it originated from an extra-uterine pregnancy.

Ordinarily there is no suspicion of the existence of the growth during pregnancy, or even during the first few weeks after delivery. In a small number of cases hæmorrhage in the latter part of the puerperium may be the first indication of its existence, though this symptom is usually lacking. In more than one half of the cases the first indication is the appearance of vaginal or vulval metastases. These are usually not noted until some weeks or months after the puerperium, though in Poten and Vassmer's case they appeared before the extrusion of the mole, and in my case one week after a full-term labour. The development of metastases in the lungs is usually associated with pulmonary symptoms, cough, and bloody expectoration, though these are frequently lacking. Unless diagnosed and removed by operative procedures, the tumour rapidly causes death, the majority of patients succumbing within the first year. Indeed, it may be said that this is the most rapidly fatal malignant growth with which we are acquainted.

Diagnosis.—In a considerable number of cases, the diagnosis is not made until uterine hæmorrhage, occurring at a varying period after the puerperium, necessitates curettage, when the microscopic examination of the scrapings reveals characteristic changes. In other instances, as has already been said, the occurrence of vaginal metastases is the first indication of the existence of the growth.

The possibility of its development should always be borne in mind whenever a woman has expelled a hydatidiform mole, and the appearance of hæmorrhage or of other more obscure symptoms should be an imperative indication for curettage and the microscopic examination of the scrapings.

Treatment.—If curettage reveals the existence of characteristic lesions, immediate hysterectomy is imperative. On the other hand, when vaginal metastases are present, the indications for this operation are not so clearly marked, as we know that in many such cases the uterus contains no growth, and that the excision of the vaginal tumours is frequently followed by complete recovery. If a tumour in the uterus is diagnosed, hysterectomy as well as excision of the metastases is indicated, though the chances for ultimate recovery are very slight. Full literature upon the subject will be found in the articles of Sänger, Marchand, Williams, Veit, Pierce, Münzer, and Ladinski.

Diffuse Myxoma of the Chorion.—Breslau and Eberth have called attention to a rare affection of the chorionic membrane, in which its connective tissue layer undergoes myxomatous degeneration and becomes converted into a jelly-like substance analogous to the Whartonian jelly of the cord. This layer may attain a thickness of 4 to 5 millimetres, but does not appear to exert any special influence upon pregnancy.

Myxoma Fibrosum of the Chorion.—Virchow called attention to the fact that a greater or lesser number of the chorionic villi, which enter into the formation of the placenta, may lose their original structure and take part in the formation of a tumour made up of dense connective tissue with larger or smaller areas of myxomatous tissue scattered through it. As the change is limited to the placenta, its consideration will be deferred until the tumours of that structure are studied.

Diseases of the Amnion.—*Hydramnios.*—By hydramnios is understood the presence of an excessive quantity of liquor amnii. Exactly when the proper limit is passed cannot be stated with accuracy, for the reason that the authorities do not agree as to the amount to be considered normal, Fehling placing it at 680 and Gassner at 1,877 cubic centimetres, though, generally speaking, a quantity greater than 2 litres may certainly be considered excessive.

Minor degrees of hydramnios—2 to 3 litres—are common, but the more marked grades are of infrequent occurrence. In rare cases the uterus may contain an almost incredible amount of liquor amnii, Küstner having observed 15 litres, and Schneider 30 litres at the fifth and sixth month of pregnancy respectively. In most cases the increase in the amount of amniotic fluid is quite gradual, but exceptionally it takes place very suddenly, so that the uterus may become immensely distended within a few days—*acute hydramnios.*

The fluid in a case of hydramnios is usually identical in appearance and composition with that which is normally found in the amniotic cavity, although Prochownick states that the former occasionally contains a slightly increased amount of urea.

Ætiology.—In view of the fact that there is still considerable discussion as to the source of the liquor amnii in normal pregnancy, it is manifestly impossible in many cases to give a satisfactory explanation for its excessive production. As was said when the physiology of the fœtus was dealt with, it must be assumed that the amniotic fluid is derived in great part from the mother, since the experiments of Schaller appear to demonstrate that the fœtal kidneys function only to a very slight extent, if at all, during intra-uterine life. At the same time it is not *a priori* impossible that fœtal urine should be passed into the amniotic cavity under certain pathological conditions.

Generally speaking, writers upon hydramnios state that the excess of amniotic fluid may be derived from several sources—from the fœtus, from the mother, from both fœtus and mother, and in rare cases from the amnion itself.

In something less than one half of the cases, careful examination of the fœtus after death reveals the presence of some abnormality which may or may not bear a causal relation to the disease. Thus, hydramnios is sometimes, although not always, noted when the fœtus presents some abnormality or deformity, particularly hemicephalus or spina bifida. Under such circumstances many authors believe that the superabundant fluid is the result of an excessive urinary secretion, which is brought about by the stimulation of cerebral or spinal centres which have been deprived of their usual coverings, just as happens in the *piqûre* experiments of the physiologists. Hydramnios is also found associated with other deformities, such as hare-lip, the various varieties of club-foot, ectopia of the bladder, etc., as well as certain tumours of the kidneys.

More frequently, however, the abnormality which is supposed to give rise to hydramnios is to be found in lesions which cause obstruction to the circulation either in the cord or within the fœtus. In other instances the condition is attributed to renal changes or to abnormalities in the cutaneous functions.

Sallinger has shown that an obstruction to the circulation in the umbilical vein is accompanied by an exudation of fluid from the external surface of the umbilical cord and from the fœtal surface of the placenta. This he attributed to the persistence of the so-called vasa propria of Jungbluth, which, springing from the fœtal end of the cord, lie between the chorion and amnion and usually become obliterated in the second half of pregnancy. Analogous observations have been made by Levison. According to Franqué, obliterative changes in coats of the arteries of the chorionic villi may lead to similar results. Leopold and Bar have shown that the obstruction may be due to stenosis or thrombosis of the umbilical vein, while Fehling has attributed it to torsion of the cord.

More frequently the obstruction lies within the fœtus. Thus Opitz observed cirrhotic changes in the liver in all of his cases. Others have attributed it to syphilitic changes, though my experience leads me to believe that lues is an unimportant factor, as hydramnios does not appear to occur much more frequently in syphilitic than in normal children. In a considerable proportion of cases the obstruction to circulation is due to cardiac abnormalities. Thus Woerz found the right auricle almost entirely occluded by a rhabdomyoma. Bar observed tricuspid insufficiency and stenotic changes about the pulmonary arteries; Lebedeff, aortic stenosis, and Nieberding a narrowing of the ductus Botalli.

Many authorities believe that hydramnios is due to an excessive urinary secretion resulting from renal or cardiac lesions. As has already been pointed out, this mode of origin cannot be accepted without reservation, since it now appears fairly certain that the kidneys normally play little if any part in the production of the liquor amnii. The correctness of such a view is now and again forcibly demonstrated by the presence of certain abnormalities in the urinary tract of the fœtus. Rissmann, for example, has reported a case in which a fœtus showing complete absence of both kidneys was born alive just before term, thus proving that the renal function is not necessary to intra-uterine life, and that, in some cases at least, the urine plays no part in the production of the amniotic fluid.

Opitz thought he had demonstrated that the liquor amnii in hydramnios contained a lymphagogue substance, which is normally absent. He considered that its presence in the tissues of the fœtus resulted in the extraction from the intervillous spaces of the placenta of a greater amount of fluid than usual. This necessitated increased exertion on the part of the heart, which eventually resulted in its hypertrophy. As a consequence a larger amount of fluid circulated through the kidneys, giving rise to an increased urinary secretion.

It is generally believed that the ætiological importance of increased renal activity is strikingly illustrated in hydramnios occurring in single-ovum twins. Wilson (1899) analyzed the histories of 101 cases of hydramnios, 51 of which occurred in single and the remainder in multiple pregnancies—46 twins and 4 triplets. Twenty-two of the twins were uni-oval in origin, and when one considers that these are much less frequently observed than double-ovum twins, it is apparent that something connected with the former must exert an appreciable influence in the production of the disease. In such cases, as a rule, the excess of liquor amnii is limited to a single amnion, while the other contains a normal or diminished amount of fluid. At autopsy the heart and kidneys of the fœtus suffering from hydramnios are found to be both relatively and actually larger than those of the normal twin. Wilson attributed this difference to the presence in the single placenta of an area of circulation common to both twins, and believed that one, for some reason, received a larger amount of blood than the other, this excess giving rise to cardiac hypertrophy which still further accentuated the condition, and in turn was followed by renal hypertrophy with increased secretion. He considered that the primary cause for the difference in the amount of fluid received by the two twins was to be found in abnormalities of the umbilical cord, by which the flow of blood to one child was rendered more difficult, as in the cases which he analyzed the affected twin always presented some abnormality of that structure—velamentous insertion, excessive length, or marked narrowing.

The mode of production of hydramnios in such cases has been considered in detail by Schatz, Werth, and Küstner. The last-named authority believes that the cardiac hypertrophy comes about in the manner already mentioned, and leads to a still further increase in the amount of circulating fluid. Eventually the heart becomes unequal to its task and insufficiency results, which is followed by signs of obstruction, particularly in the liver, thereby completing a vicious circle.

Some authors consider that the skin plays a not unimportant part in the excessive formation of liquor amnii. Budin in one case was inclined to attribute it to a large nævus, through which he believed excessive exudation occurred. Furthermore, Wilson and others consider that excessive cutaneous activity is ofttimes associated with cardiac hypertrophy.

In a small number of cases inflammatory conditions of the amnion itself are believed to play a part in the production of the condition, leading to increased exudation through that membrane.

Occasionally diseases of the mother which are attended by circulatory disturbances, particularly cardiac and renal affections and visceral syphilis, lead to œdema of the placenta, with increased transudation into the amniotic cavity. One or other of the conditions just mentioned may account for the excessive production of amniotic fluid in a considerable proportion of the cases; but at the same time they do not always afford a satisfactory explanation, inasmuch as in many instances careful search fails to reveal the presence of any lesion which can be supposed to play a part in the production of the anomaly.

Symptoms.—The symptoms accompanying hydramnios arise from purely mechanical causes, and are due to the pressure exerted by the overdistended uterus upon adjacent organs. The effects are particularly marked in the respiratory functions, and when the distention is excessive the patient may suffer from severe dyspnœa and cyanosis, and in extreme cases be able to breathe only in an upright position. Œdema often occurs, especially in the lower extremities and about the vulva.

It is surprising what great degrees of abdominal distention can sometimes be borne by the patient with comparatively little discomfort, although this is the case only when the accumulation of fluid has taken place gradually. On the other hand, in acute hydramnios, a much slighter degree of distention may lead to disturbances sufficiently serious to threaten the life of the patient.

Diagnosis.—In moderate degrees of hydramnios, palpation and percussion enable one to feel confident that the fluctuant tumour is the distended uterus, in which a readily ballottable fœtus can be felt, although the heart sounds are heard with difficulty.

The excessive enlargement of the abdomen due to multiple pregnancy occasionally renders the differentiation from hydramnios almost impossible; and, moreover, the latter is a frequent complication of the former condition. Thus it appears that the hydramnios is usually detected, whereas a multiple pregnancy associated with it often passes unnoticed. On the other hand, in a multiple pregnancy not complicated by hydramnios, the diagnosis is comparatively easy, inasmuch as the uterus offers a firm consistence to the touch, and careful palpation will reveal the presence of several fœtal poles and an unusual number of small parts, as contrasted with a marked fluctuation and the difficulty of mapping out the fœtus in hydramnios.

When the uterine distention is excessive, the diagnosis of hydramnios becomes even more difficult, and many cases are recorded in which the condition was mistaken for a large ovarian cystoma, with the result that the contents of the amniotic cavity were evacuated by means of a trocar, or laparotomy was performed. Inquiry as to the possibility of pregnancy, and careful examination will generally serve to prevent such an error.

Excessive abdominal enlargement due to ascites can usually be differentiated by the characteristic changes in percussion. In rare instances pregnancy, complicated by a large ovarian cystoma, may be mistaken for hydramnios. In some cases, the detection of two tumours—one corresponding to the uterus and the other to the cyst—will permit a correct diagnosis, but in others the condition may escape detection until after childbirth.

Treatment.—Minor grades of hydramnios rarely require active treatment. On the other hand, when the abdomen is immensely distended and respiration is seriously hampered, the termination of pregnancy is urgently indicated no matter to what period it may have advanced. In such cases interference is the more justifiable since experience teaches that spontaneous premature labour frequently occurs if the patient is left alone, and the children are frequently so poorly developed or so deformed that their chances of living are minimal.

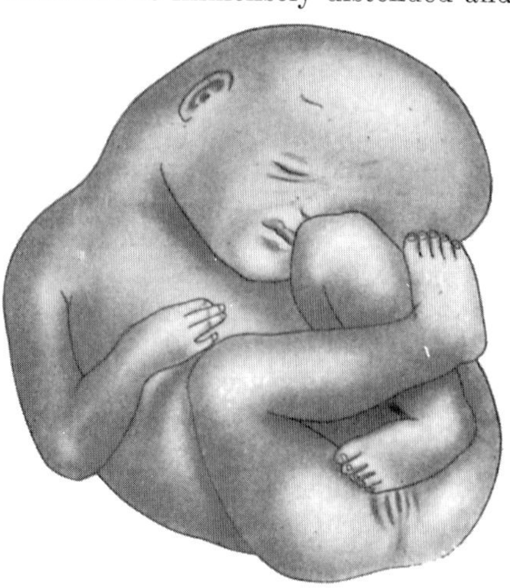

Fig. 445.—Compression of Fœtus in Oligohydramnios (Ahlfeld).

In such cases, the symptoms can be promptly relieved by perforating the membranes through the cervix, after which the amniotic fluid drains off and labour pains set in. When the abdomen has been enormously distended, and the course of labour particularly rapid, there is an increased risk of atonic hæmorrhage during and just after the completion of the third stage. For this reason the uterus should be carefully watched and appropriate treatment instituted at the slightest sign of danger.

Oligo-hydramnios.—In rare instances the amount of amniotic fluid may fall far below the normal limits, and occasionally be represented by only a few cubic centimetres of clear, viscid fluid.

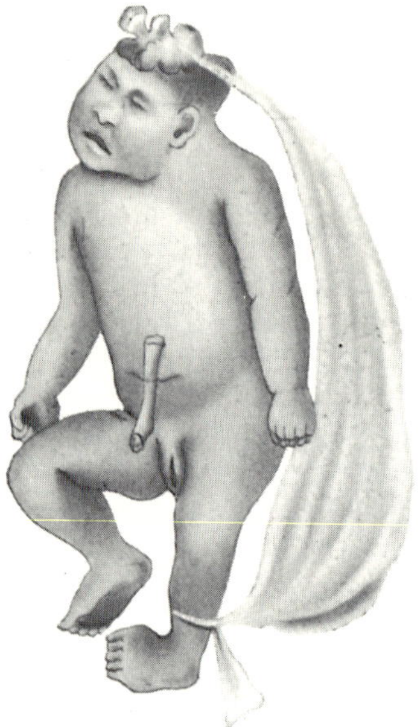

Fig. 446.—Encephalocele resulting from Amniotic Adhesions (Ahlfeld).

The ætiology is even less well understood than that of hydramnios. Jaggard, in 1894, reported a case in which the fœtus presented an imperforate urethra with absence of one and cystic degeneration of the other kidney, and he therefore concluded that the lack of amniotic fluid was the result of non-secretion of urine. He likewise collected several instances from the literature, in which the anomaly was associated with complete absence of both kidneys.

When oligo-hydramnios occurs early in pregnancy it is attended by serious consequences to the fœtus, as adhesions may be formed between its external surface and the amnion and give rise to serious deformities. When occurring later, its effect upon the fœtus, though less marked, is quite characteristic. Under such circumstances the latter is subjected to pressure from all sides and takes on a peculiar appearance, and many minor deformities, such as club-foot, are frequently observed (Fig. 445).

In some cases of oligo-hydramnios, the skin of the fœtus is markedly thickened, and presents a dry, leathery appearance. Most authorities attribute this to the lack of amniotic fluid, but Ahlfeld is inclined to believe that it is the cause and not the result of the condition, since the skin lesion may be so marked as to interfere with the normal cutaneous functions and thus do away with one of the sources of the liquor amnii.

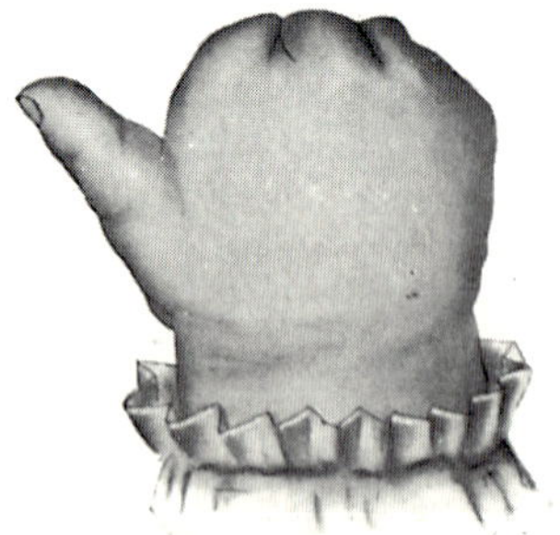

Fig. 447.—Amputation of Fingers by Amniotic Adhesions (Küstner).

Amniotic Adhesions.—In oligo-hydramnios, and occasionally even when the liquor amnii is present in normal amounts, adhesions may form between the amnion and the surface of the fœtus. According to Simonart, Chaussier, in 1812, was the first to direct attention to this condition, and its consequences were further studied by Montgomery, G. Braun, Küstner, Ahlfeld, and others.

The effects of amniotic adhesions are variable and depend in great measure upon their location. As a rule, when they develop early in pregnancy they give rise to serious deformities of the fœtus. The following abnormalities have been directly traced to the condition: Encephalocele or hemicephalus; fissure of the face, jaw, or lips; fissure of the thorax with ectopia cordis, and eventration with hernia of the umbilical cord.

In other instances, amniotic bands may encircle an extremity of the fœtus and so compress it as to lead to strangulation and subsequent spontaneous amputation. Fig. 447 represents intra-uterine amputation of the fingers, and Fig. 448 amputation of the arms, produced in this way. Braun has reported two cases in which the death of the fœtus was attributable to strangulation of the umbilical cord by such bands.

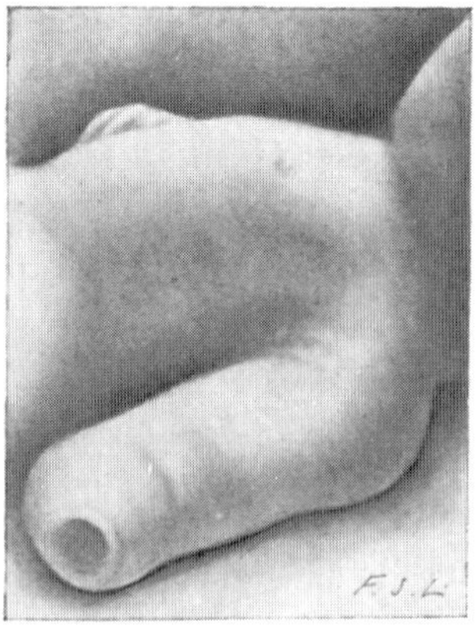

FIG. 448.—AMPUTATION OF ARM BY AMNIOTIC ADHESIONS.

Inflammation of the Amnion.—In rare cases inflammatory processes implicate the amnion. These are usually associated with similar changes in the chorion and decidua, and result from attempts at criminal abortion or from the extension of an infection that has originated in the decidua.

Cysts of the Amnion.—Now and again small cystic structures, lined by typical epithelium, may be formed in the amnion. They generally result from the fusion of amniotic folds with subsequent retention of fluid. Special attention has been devoted to this subject by Ahlfeld. The same observer has also described a dermoid cyst of the amnion, which does not, however, bear critical examination, inasmuch as the small particles found in it were probably mere concretions.

Abnormalities and Diseases of the Placenta.—*Abnormalities in Size, Shape, and Weight.*—The normal placenta is a flattened, roundish, or discoid organ, which averages from 15 to 20 centimetres in diameter, and from 1.5 to 3 centimetres in thickness. It is relatively larger in the earlier than in the later months of pregnancy, and varies considerably in size at term, though, generally speaking, the thickness is in inverse proportion to its area. The placenta, as a rule, presents more or less rounded outlines, but now and again when inserted in the neighbourhood of the internal os it may take on a horseshoe-like appearance, its two branches running partially around the orifice. In very rare instances, as in one reported by Taurin, it may be a broad annular organ which encircles the uterine cavity just as in carnivorous animals.

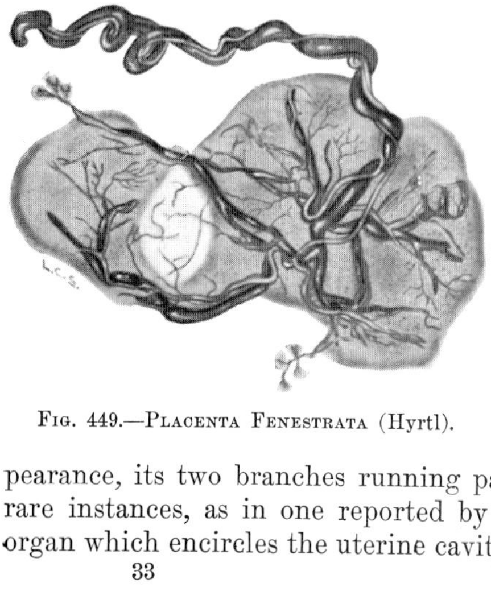

FIG. 449.—PLACENTA FENESTRATA (Hyrtl).

The normal full-term placenta on an average weighs about one sixth as much as the child—i. e., somewhere in the neighbourhood of 500 grammes. Exceptionally it may be considerably heavier, Levy having reported a number of cases in which it exceeded 1,000 grammes in weight. In diseased conditions, on the other hand, this proportion no longer holds good, and in syphilis the placenta may weigh one fourth, one third, or even one half as much as the fœtus. In albuminuria it also undergoes a relative increase in weight, due almost entirely to the imperfect development of the fœtus which characterizes such conditions. The largest placentæ with which we are familiar are observed in cases of general dropsy of the fœtus and placenta. In a case of this character under my observation the weights of the fœtus and of the placenta were 1,140 and 1,200 grammes respectively, and Cohen has reported a case in which the latter weighed 2,900 grammes.

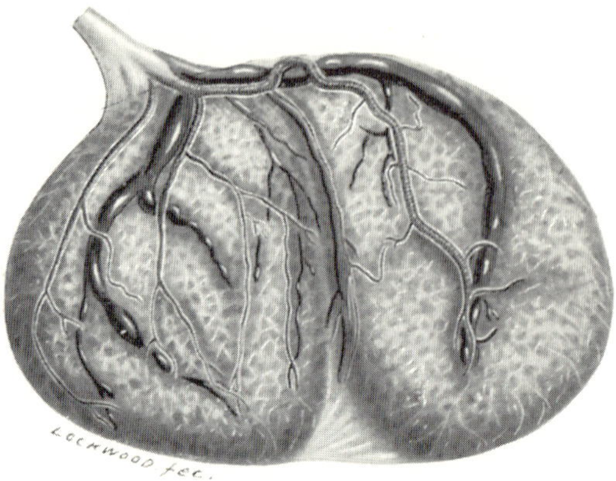

Fig. 450.—Placenta Bipartita.

Multiple Placenta in Single Pregnancies.—Occasionally in a single pregnancy the placenta is divided into several parts, which may be absolutely distinct or more or less closely united. Such abnormalities have been studied more particularly by Hyrtl and Ribemont-Dessaignes, the latter stating that they occur about once in 352 cases.

In rare cases the placenta may be oblong in shape with an aperture of varying size somewhere in the neighbourhood of its centre. To this abnormality Hyrtl applied the term *placenta fenestrata.* More frequently the organ is more or less completely divided into two lobes. When the division is incomplete, and the vessels extend from one lobe to the other before uniting to form the umbilical cord, we speak of a *placenta dimidiata* or *bipartita.* According to Ahlfeld, this anomaly is noted about once in 600 cases. Again, the placenta may consist of two separate lobes, the vessels

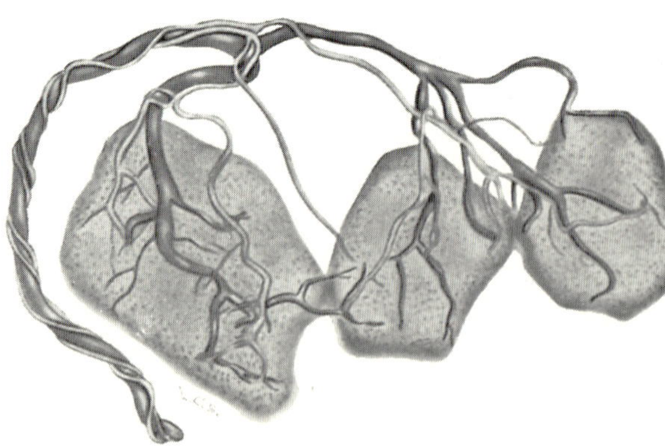

Fig. 451.—Placenta Tripartita (Hyrtl).

of which are perfectly distinct and do not unite until just before entering the cord—*placenta duplex* (see Fig. 454). Occasionally the organ may be made up of three distinct lobes—*placenta triplex*; while in very rare instances it may consist of a number of small lobes, Hyrtl having described as many as seven—*placenta septuplex*.

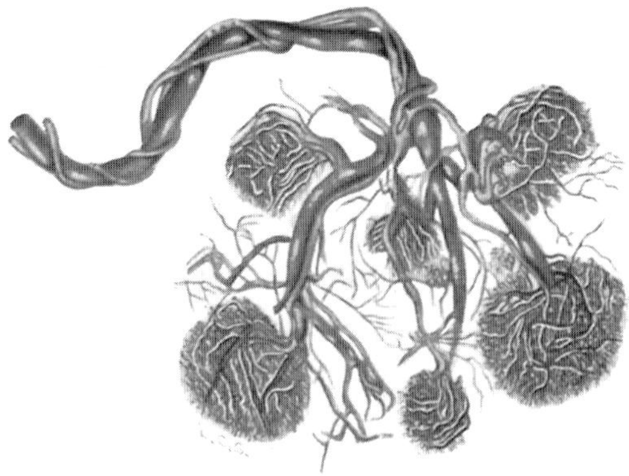

FIG. 452.—CORROSION PREPARATION OF PLACENTA SEPTUPLEX (Hyrtl).

All of these conditions result from abnormalities in the blood supply of the decidua. Generally speaking, the portion of the ovum which is to become converted into the chorion frondosum, and later into the fœtal portion of the placenta, is that which is in contact with the most highly vascularized portion of the decidua. If the vascularization, instead of being practically limited to a single area, develops in several separate portions of the decidua, some such anomaly is bound to occur. Küstner believes that certain cases of placenta bipartita or duplex owe their origin to extensive infarct formation by which the intervening tissue is destroyed. Occasionally this is undoubtedly true, but such an explanation cannot be accepted when the various lobes or lobules are separated from one another by apparently normal membranes.

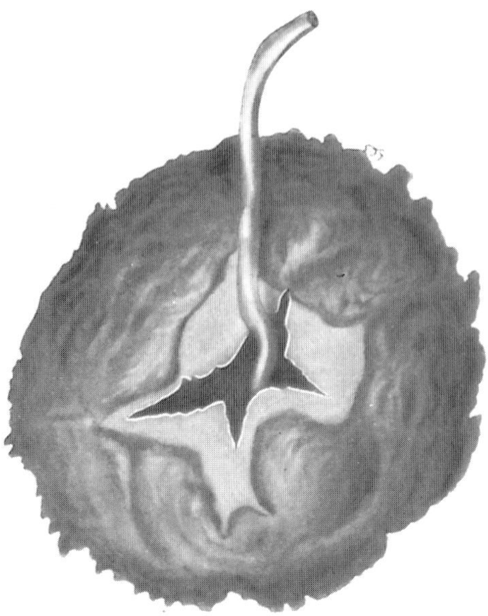

FIG. 453.—PLACENTA MEMBRANACEA (von Weiss).

In rare instances the decidua reflexa is so abundantly supplied with blood that the chorion læve in contact with it fails to undergo atrophy. Under such circumstances, the entire periphery of the ovum is covered by functioning villi, so that the placenta, instead of being a discoid organ limited to the decidua serotina, corresponds to the entire chorion — *placenta membranacea*. This abnormality does not interfere with the nutrition of the ovum, but occasionally gives rise to serious complications during the third stage of labour, since the thinned-out placenta is not readily separated from its area of attachment and is retained, manual removal becoming necessary.

An important and not infrequent anomaly is the so-called *placenta succenturiata,* in which one or more small accessory lobules are developed in the membranes at some distance from the periphery of the main placenta. Ordinarily they are united to the latter by vascular connections. Occasionally, however, these are lacking, and as a result we have what are known as *placentæ spuriæ.*

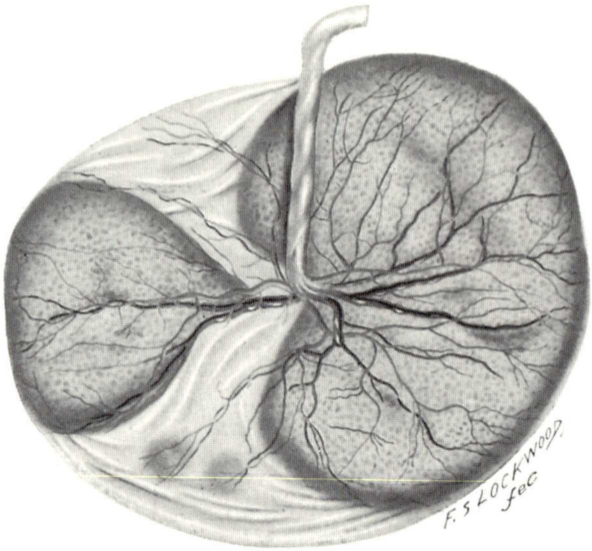

Fig. 454.—Placenta Duplex, with Two Succenturiate Lobules. ×½.

The placenta succenturiata is of considerable clinical importance, because the accessory lobules are sometimes retained in the uterus after the expulsion of the main placenta, and may give rise to serious hæmorrhage. For this reason one should always bear in mind the possibility of their existence, and the examination of the after-birth should not be limited merely to the inspection of the placenta, but should extend to the membranes as well. Should small, roundish defects be present in the latter a short distance from the placental margin, the retention of a succenturiate lobe should be suspected. If, in such cases, the slightest signs of hæmorrhage occur, the hand should be introduced into the uterus for the purpose of locating and removing the offending structure.

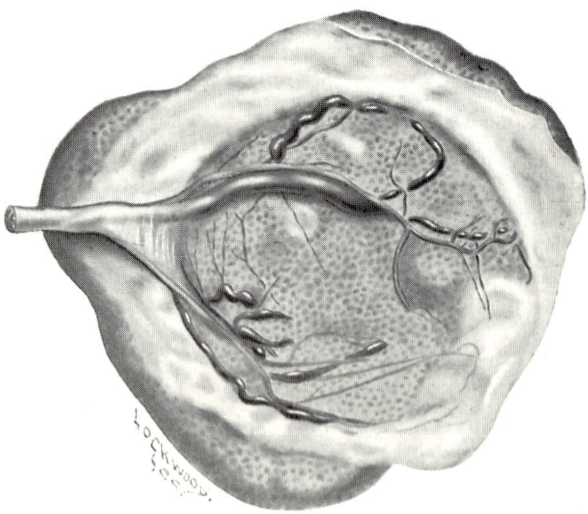

Fig. 455.—Placenta Marginata. ×½.

Placenta marginata will be considered when we come to speak of infarcts of the placenta.

In exceptional instances the fœtal surface of the placenta may present a central depression surrounded by an elevated portion, the amnion extending from the edges of the former. This condition is designated as *placenta circumvallata*, and is due to a proliferation of the villi at the margin of the placenta after the definite attachment of the amnion has occurred.

Once in several hundred cases the placenta, instead of being inserted upon the lateral walls or the fundus of the uterus, is implanted upon the lower uterine segment in such a manner as more or less completely to overlap the internal os—*placenta prævia.* As this condition is unavoidably associated with hæmorrhage during the first stage of labour, and is a most serious complication, it will be dealt with in a separate chapter.

Diseases of the Placenta.—*Infarct Formation.*—The most frequent abnormality of the placenta consists in the development of certain degenerative changes, which have been variously designated as schirrus, atrophy, placentitis, hepatization, apoplexy, phthisis, fatty and fibro-fatty degeneration of the placenta, etc., but which are most appropriately described as *placental infarcts.*

These structures vary materially in size, shape, and appearance, and are best described under the following headings:

1. Small, whitish or yellowish fibrous formations occurring upon either the fœtal or maternal surface of the placenta, and varying in size from areas hardly visible to the naked eye to those having a diameter of several centimetres. These rarely attain a thickness of more than a few millimetres, and are sharply differentiated from the surrounding placental tissue.

2. On section through the placenta one frequently sees wedge-shaped or irregularly round areas, which are usually dull white in colour and exhibit a striated, fibrous appearance. They present a striking contrast to the surrounding tissue, which appears to be perfectly normal.

3. Less commonly, considerable portions of the placenta are implicated in the process, and one occasionally finds one or more cotyledons converted into a pale white, dense, more or less fibrous area, in which the usual spongy structure of the placenta is lacking. In other instances a large portion of the organ may be involved in the change, one half and sometimes nearly its entire substance being implicated.

4. Not infrequently a broad rim of whitish or yellowish-white material is observed extending for a varying distance around the margin of the fœtal surface of the placenta, taking in a larger or smaller portion of its periphery, and occasionally forming a complete ring around it. These bands vary from a few millimetres to 3 or 4 centimetres in breadth. They lie beneath the amnion and rarely attain a thickness of more than a few millimetres, except at the extreme margin of the placenta, where it merges into the membranes. This condition is known as *placenta marginata.* In a certain number of cases the band, instead of being situated at the margin of the placenta, lies somewhere between it and the centre of the organ, thus forming a broad zone more or less parallel to the periphery, but sepa-

rated from it by apparently normal placental tissue. To this condition the term *margo placentæ* is sometimes applied.

5. In rarer instances a larger or smaller portion of the placenta is occupied by a pinkish or brickdust-coloured, irregularly shaped, more or less solid mass, which is sharply marked off from the surrounding tissue. Such masses are usually most prominent on the maternal surface of the placenta, but not infrequently extend through its entire thickness; they are sometimes termed *red infarcts.*

Still more rarely, scattered through the substance of the placenta, are seen roundish areas varying from bright red to almost black in colour, and measuring from one to three centimetres in diameter. They are apparently composed almost entirely of blood, and are sharply differentiated from the surrounding tissue by a capsule which presents a more or less fibrous appearance. They may occur singly or in considerable numbers, so that occasionally the entire placenta is studded with them and presents a nodular surface, and on section an appearance which Pinard has aptly described as *placenta truffé.*

These structures are also designated as red infarcts, though many authors prefer to speak of apoplexy or hæmatoma of the placenta. They differ markedly in structure and appearance from the other form of so-called red infarcts, and probably have nothing in common with them.

Frequency.—Minute white infarcts are to be found in every placenta, while similar areas, measuring 1 centimetre or more in diameter, were observed in 63 per cent of 500 consecutive placentæ which I examined. If not present in excessive numbers, they possess no clinical significance, and according to the researches of Eden and myself are to be regarded as signs of senility of the organ. On the other hand, when they are of large size and abundant, they may mechanically throw out of function so great a portion of the placenta as seriously to interfere with the nutrition of the fœtus, and sometimes cause its death.

Mode of Formation.—According to the researches of Ackermann, Orth, Eden, Kermauner, and myself, infarct formation is the ultimate result of obliterating endarteritis in the vessels of the chorionic villi, and is brought about in the following manner: As soon as the circulation through the arteries of the chorionic villi is interfered with by the endarteritic process, necrotic changes begin to appear at their periphery (Plate XIV, Fig. 2). Owing to the fact that the syncytium is in direct contact with the maternal blood, the changes occur first in the layer of tissue just beneath it, and manifest themselves as coagulation necrosis of Langhans's layer of cells or the tissue which has replaced it. As the process becomes more marked this is gradually converted into the so-called canalized fibrin. A little later the syncytium becomes implicated and undergoes a similar change, the fibrin then coming in direct contact with the maternal blood in the intervillous spaces. As a consequence, the blood immediately adjoining the necrotic tissue coagulates with eventual fibrin formation.

When necrotic changes occur simultaneously in several adjacent villi, the maternal blood lying between them undergoes coagulation, so that eventually a number of villi become fused together by fibrin. Still further

PLATE XIV.

Fig. 1.

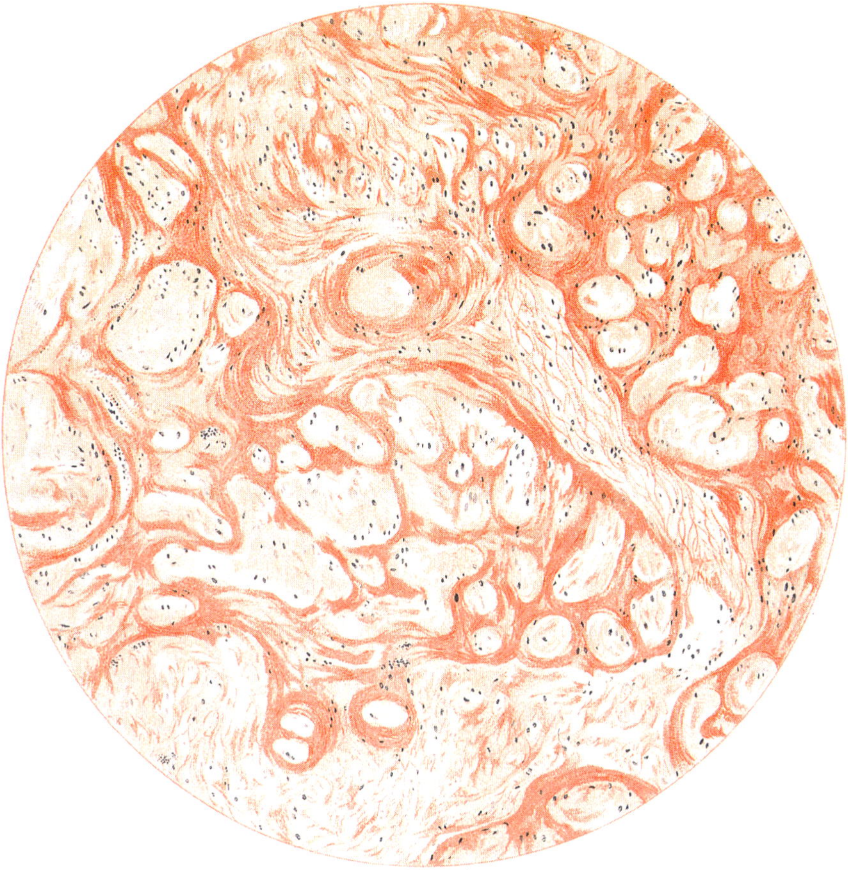

Fig. 2.

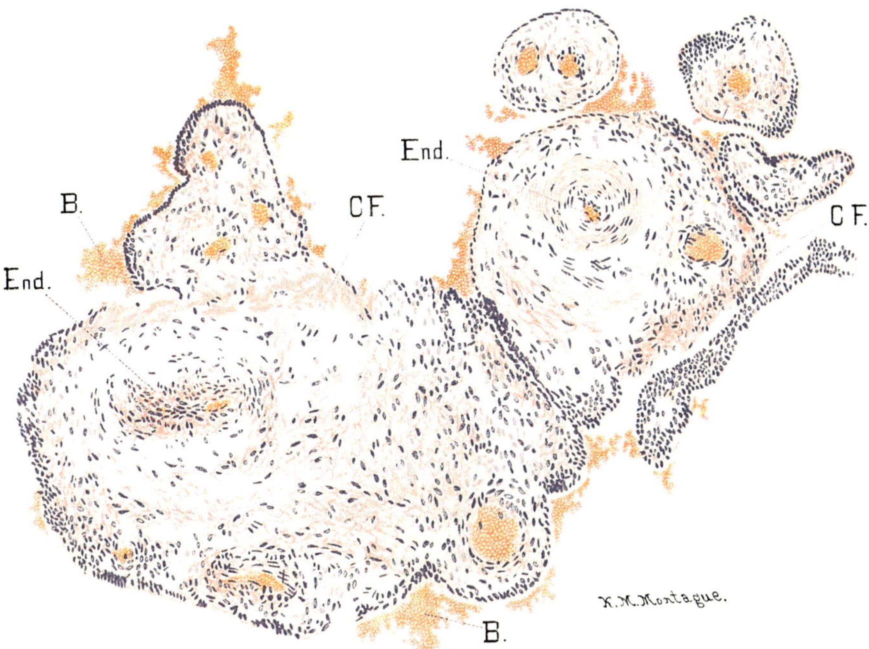

INFARCT FORMATION. × 60.

FIG. 1.—Fully developed infarct.

FIG. 2.—Chorionic villi, showing endarteritis and formation of canalized fibrin. *B*, blood in intervillous spaces; *C. F.*, canalized fibrin; *End.*, arteries showing obliterating endarteritis.

changes then occur in the stroma of the incarcerated villi, the cells undergo coagulation necrosis, and finally the conversion into fibrin becomes so extensive that large areas are produced in which only the shadows of degenerated villi can be distinguished (Plate XIV, Fig. 1). Ultimately the outlines of the villi disappear, and the entire mass takes on a homogeneous fibrinous appearance, in which it is impossible to distinguish the component parts. For full particulars concerning the process the reader is referred to my monograph upon the subject.

Steffeck and many recent writers are inclined to attribute the starting-point of the process to inflammatory and degenerative changes in the decidua. It would seem, however, that there are no grounds for such a belief, and that their conclusions were based upon faulty premises, in that these authors considered that the cells making up the so-called decidual septa were of maternal instead of fœtal origin, as has been rendered probable by recent investigations.

Red infarcts of the placenta are less frequently observed. In some cases they are associated with albuminuria on the part of the mother, which was present in 33, 60, and 67 per cent of the cases collected by Cagny, Rossier, and Martin respectively. Unlike white infarcts, they possess a considerable clinical significance and, whenever well marked, are associated with imperfect development of the fœtus, and sometimes cause its death. Unfortunately, we are not in a position to explain satisfactorily their mode of formation, and must be content with pointing out the relation which they bear to albuminuria on the one hand and to imperfect development of the child on the other.

Red infarcts are not, as a rule, observed in the placentæ of eclamptic women, being noted only in those cases in which the onset of the disease has been preceded by distinct and continued nephritic disturbances.

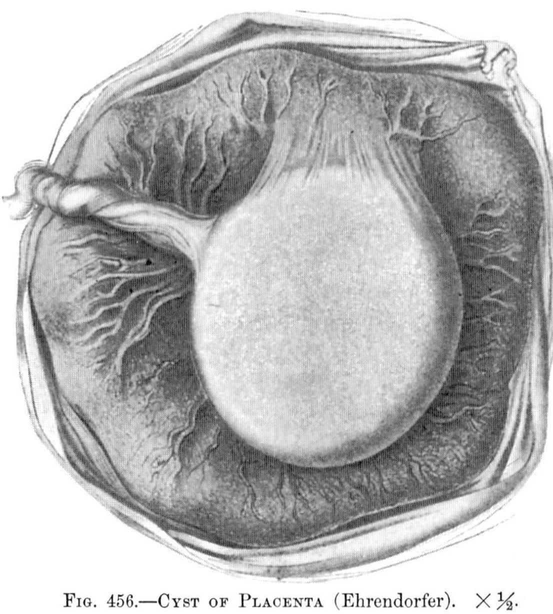

FIG. 456.—CYST OF PLACENTA (Ehrendorfer). × ½.

Cysts of the Placenta.—Cystic structures are frequently observed upon the fœtal surface and occasionally in the depths of the placenta. Small cysts a few millimetres in diameter were noted in 56 per cent of the cases collected by Kermauner. Larger ones, occasionally attaining the size of a lemon, are observed but rarely.

Cysts projecting from the fœtal surface of the placenta are derived from the chorion, as is shown by the fact that the amnion can be readily stripped off from them. Their contents are usually clear and transparent, but are sometimes bloody or grumous in character. The walls, especially the portions adjacent to the intervillous spaces, are lined in great part by a dull whitish membrane, while occasionally a portion is occupied by a white infarct.

On microscopic examination, the lining membrane is found to be made up mainly of one or more layers of tolerably large epithelial cells with round vesicular nuclei which frequently present various degrees of degeneration. Here and there, corresponding to the situation of a white infarct, the cells are absent and the wall consists of fibrin. The researches of Ehrendorfer, Peiser, De Jong, and Vassmer have clearly shown that the cells in question correspond to those of Langhans's layer, and are derived from the trophoblastic tissue which forms the epithelial covering of the chorionic membrane, and that the cysts result from their degeneration.

The cysts occurring in the depths of the placenta rarely exceed 1 centimetre in diameter. They frequently occupy the centre of an infarct, are filled with grumous contents, and were mistaken by the older writers for abscesses. In other cases the contents are clear. Such structures may be derived in one of two ways: either by the softening and breaking down of an infarct, the cyst-wall then consisting of fibrin, or from the degeneration of the trophoblastic cells which make up most of the so-called decidual septa. In the latter case, the walls are composed of cells identical with those observed in the cysts occurring upon the fœtal surface of the placenta.

So far as present experience goes, cystic formations, whether occurring upon the fœtal surface or in the depths of the placenta, are of interest purely from a pathological point of view, and exert little or no influence upon the course of pregnancy or labour.

Tumours of the Placenta.—John Clarke, in 1798, described a solid tumour about the size of a man's fist, which made up a large part of the placenta. Since then a number of similar tumours have been described, something less than 50 being recorded. Niebergall and Albert, in 1897 and 1898, respectively, were able to collect 30 and 36 cases from the literature. Since then Guéniot, Osterloh, and Bode and Schmorl have described additional instances.

All tumours of the placenta which have thus far been studied are of connective-tissue origin. The most frequent variety is the *myxoma fibrosum* of Virchow, which is a tumour of varying size, composed in great part of fibrous tissue having abundant oval nuclei, with typical myxomatous areas scattered through it.

The 36 tumours collected by Albert can be classified as follows:

Myxoma fibrosum	14
Fibroma	10
Angioma	9
Sarcoma	2
Hyperplasia of chorionic villi	1

The two cases of sarcoma were described by Hyrtl as "*placenta in placenta.*" Their nature, however, is open to considerable doubt, but in all probability they were fibromata.

We are absolutely ignorant as to the ætiology of placental tumours, but it is interesting to note that several have originated in a succenturiate placenta, while the main organ remained intact.

According to Albert they exert a deleterious influence upon the course of pregnancy and labour. In the 36 cases collected by him, only one third of the children were born alive or were normal in size. Premature labour was noted in 13, and hydramnios in 4 instances. The tumour formation appeared to interfere with the separation of the placenta, as its manual removal was necessary in 3 cases, while hæmorrhage during or immediately after the third stage of labour occurred 5 times.

Inflammation of the Placenta.—Under the term *placentitis* many of the older writers described changes which we now recognise as infarct formation. Moreover, as has already been said, small placental cysts filled with grumous contents were formerly thought to be abscesses. Hence it follows that most of the statements in the abundant early literature upon inflammatory lesions of the placenta must be received with the greatest caution. At the same time acute inflammation of the placenta is occasionally met with. It is not a primary condition, but is due to the extension of a similar process from the decidua, the latter resulting from an exacerbation of a pre-existing chronic gonorrhœa or from an acute infection due to the gonococcus or other pyogenic bacteria.

In several instances, upon examining sections of placental tissue under the microscope, I found the decidua serotina infiltrated with leucocytes and presenting the characteristic picture of an acute inflammation, while the adjacent intervillous spaces were crowded with leucocytes. Franqué observed similar conditions, but is inclined to believe that in most instances the implication of the placenta is secondary to the death of the fœtus.

Tuberculosis of the Placenta.—Tubercle formation in the fœtal portion of the placenta is extremely infrequent. For particulars concerning the cases which have thus far been reported, the reader is referred to the chapters upon the Physiology of the Fœtus and the Infectious Diseases complicating Pregnancy.

Calcification of the Placenta.—Small calcareous nodules, sometimes occurring in the form of flat plaques, are frequently observed upon the maternal surface of the placenta, and are occasionally so abundant as to cause it to resemble a piece of coarse sand-paper. Fränkel showed that the chalky material was usually deposited in the necrotic tissue surrounding the ends of the "fastening" villi, as well as in the superficial layers of the decidua serotina.

When the almost universal occurrence of degenerative changes in the placenta is remembered, it should be a matter of surprise, not that calcification is occasionally met with, but rather that it is not noted in almost every placenta, inasmuch as apparently ideal conditions for its formation are constantly present in the later months of pregnancy.

Abnormal Adherence of the Placenta.—In the vast majority of cases the term *adherent* placenta is a misnomer, since the interference with its expulsion is usually due to abnormalities in the uterine contractions rather than to abnormal adhesions between it and the uterine wall. In rare instances, on the other hand, the adhesions may be so firm and extensive that spontaneous separation becomes impossible, and occasionally cannot be effected even at autopsy except by tearing either the placenta or the uterine wall.

Neumann and Hense have recently examined two uteri in which this condition obtained. Microscopic examination in each case showed that the decidua serotina was almost entirely absent, and that the chorionic villi were in direct contact with the uterine muscle and the connective tissue separating its fibres. Under such circumstances the absence of the spongy layer of the decidua readily explains the clinical phenomena.

Abnormalities of the Umbilical Cord.—*Variations in Insertion.*—The umbilical cord is usually inserted eccentrically upon the fœtal surface of the placenta, somewhere between its centre and periphery. A central insertion is less common, while in a still smaller number of cases the junction has taken place near the margin, giving rise to a condition known as *battledore placenta.*

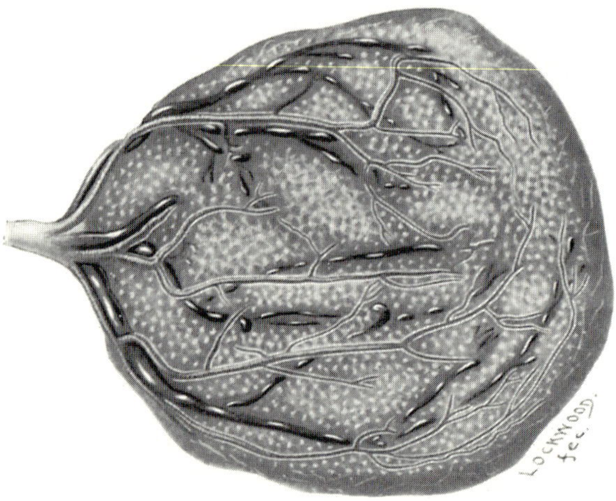

Fig. 457.—Marginal Insertion of the Cord. Battledore Placenta.

In 2,000 placentæ examined at the Johns Hopkins Hospital the insertion was eccentric in 73.25 per cent, central in 18.25 per cent, and marginal in 7.25 per cent. These variations possess no clinical significance.

On the other hand the so-called *velamentous insertion of the cord*—insertio velamentosa—is of considerable practical importance. In this condition the vessels of the cord separate some distance from the placental margin and make their way to the latter in a fold of amnion (Fig. 309). This mode of insertion was noted in 0.84 per cent of 15,894 placentæ examined by Lefèvre, and in 1.25 per cent of our cases. According to Mironoff it occurs nine times more frequently in twin than in single pregnancies, being noted in 5 and 0.57 per cent of the cases respectively.

Its mode of production has given rise to a great deal of speculation. So long as the old views were in vogue concerning the part played by the allantois and the amnion in the formation of the umbilical cord, Schultze's explanation obtained almost universal acceptance. According to this, the anomaly was the result of abnormal adhesions between the umbilical vesicle and the chorionic membrane, whereby the amnion was prevented from applying itself in the usual manner to the cord. At present, however, the allantois is known to play an insignificant part in the formation of the cord in human beings, since the researches of His have clearly shown that the abdominal pedicle—the forerunner of the cord—is present from the earliest periods, and represents an extension of the caudal end of the embryo, in which the allantois is represented by a mere epithelial ductlet. Moreover, the cord is not provided with a sheath of amnion, and therefore abnormal adhesions of the umbilical vesicle can have no effect upon its covering.

Franqué, in 1900, advanced the following theory as to the mode of origin of the velamentous insertion. In the vast majority of cases, the abdominal pedicle extends from that portion of the chorion which is in contact with the most richly vascularized portion of the decidua—ordinarily the decidua serotina—so that the cord becomes inserted upon the placenta. Occasionally, however, during the first few days of pregnancy, the area of greatest vascularization may be in the decidua reflexa, and the abdominal pedicle then takes its origin from the portion of chorion in contact with it. With the advance of pregnancy, however, the area of vascularization shifts to the decidua serotina—the site of the future placenta—while the abdominal pedicle retains its original position, and from its maternal end the vessels extend to the placental margin. Peters, while recognising the fallacy of Schultze's explanation, is not prepared to accept that proposed by Franqué.

As has already been pointed out, the velamentous insertion is noted comparatively often in twin pregnancy, and in single-ovum twins is supposed to play a part in the production of hydramnios. According to Lefèvre, the condition not very uncommonly predisposes to premature labour.

When the placenta is inserted low down in the uterus, the velamentous vessels may extend partially across the internal os—vasa prævia—and as dilatation progresses be pressed upon the presenting part, the interference with the circulation causing asphyxia of the fœtus. In rare cases such vessels are torn through when the membranes rupture, and the fœtus bleeds to death. The full literature upon this subject up to 1898 has been collected by Peiser, while Knapp has reported a case in which the accident led to the death of both twins developed from a single ovum.

Variations in Length of Cord.—Normally, the umbilical cord averages about 55 centimetres in length, though it may present marked variations—3.5 to 198 centimetres (Dyhrenfurth and Hyrtl). In rare instances it may be so short that the abdomen of the fœtus is almost in contact with the placenta, but under such circumstances a congenital umbilical hernia is always present.

According to Kaltenbach the cord must be of a certain length in order to permit of delivery of the child—that is, it must be sufficiently long to reach from its placental insertion to the vulva, 35 centimetres when the placenta is inserted high up, and 20 centimetres when low down. As a matter of fact it rarely measures less than 25 centimetres.

On the other hand, it not infrequently happens that cords which actually exceed the normal in length may be so twisted about the child as to become practically too short. Accordingly, one distinguishes between absolute and accidental or relative shortness of the cord. Either of these conditions may give rise to serious dystocia. Brickner, who has carefully studied the subject, states that delivery cannot occur under such circumstances unless one of the following accidents occur: separation of the placenta, inversion of the uterus, umbilical hernia of the fœtus, or rupture of the cord, the last two being of infrequent occurrence.

Rupture of the cord may result from absolute or accidental shortness, being due to the former in Dyhrenfurth's, and to the latter in Ahlfeld's case, in which the cord measured 44 centimetres in length, but was tightly twisted about the fœtus. Ordinarily an excessively long cord exerts no deleterious influence, although it predisposes to the formation of loops during pregnancy and to prolapse at the time of labour.

Knots of the Cord.—It is customary to distinguish between false and true knots, the former being due to developmental abnormalities in the cord, while the latter result from the active movements of the child. True knots occur very frequently, and occasionally are of the most complicated character. Ordinarily they are of no clinical importance, but occasionally they may be pulled so taut as to compress the vessels and lead to asphyxia of the fœtus.

Loops of the Cord.—The cord frequently becomes wrapped around portions of the fœtus, and in every third or fourth case of labour the child's neck will be found loosely encircled by one or more loops. In rare instances these may produce strangulation. In most of these cases, however, the accident is not due to any drawing taut of the loop, but rather to the fact that it does not become looser in proportion as the neck of the child increases in size. In other cases, loops of the cord may so tightly encircle the body or one of the extremities of the child as to give rise to deep depressions, which in extreme cases may eventuate in the strangulation or gangrene of the affected part.

In single-ovum twins in which the amniotic partition wall has been broken through, it not infrequently happens that the cord of one fœtus may become wrapped around some portion of the other so tightly as to cause its death. A number of cases of this character have been collected by Hermann.

Torsion of the Cord.—As the result of movements on the part of the fœtus, the cord may become more or less twisted. Occasionally the torsion is so marked as to interfere seriously with the circulation. The most extreme degrees are observed only after the death of the fœtus, Schauta having reported a case in which 380 twists were noted. In rare instances separation of the cord is produced, though this is possible only after the death of the fœtus in the early months of pregnancy.

Inflammation of the Cord.—As long as the child is alive inflammatory conditions are rarely noted, but after its death the Whartonian jelly is found to be infiltrated with leucocytes. Not uncommonly obliterative changes occur in the vessels, the lumina becoming almost completely occluded. This is especially liable to occur in syphilis, although it is observed in other conditions, and, as has already been pointed out, is believed to be an occasional factor in the production of hydramnios.

In rare instances *varices of the cord* may be subjected to undue pressure as the result of such changes. Meier has reported a case in which the death of the fœtus was attributable to the rupture of such a structure.

Tumours of the Cord.—Tumour formations implicating the cord are rarely seen. Hæmatomata occasionally result from the rupture of a varix with subsequent effusion of blood into the cord. In one instance I observed such a tumour, 5 centimetres in diameter, at the fœtal end of the cord. Myxomata and myxosarcomata have also been described. Winckel has reported two cases of sarcoma of the cord, while Budin has described an apparently typical dermoid.

Cystic structures occasionally occur in the course of the cord. As a rule they are only apparent, and result from the liquefaction of the myxomatous tissue of the cord. In other cases, as reported by Kleinwächter, they may develop from the duct of the umbilical vesicle, which is included in the cord.

Œdema of the Cord.—This condition is rarely noted by itself, but not infrequently complicates œdematous conditions of the fœtus. It is very common in dead and macerated children. In one of my cases, in which the child was born alive at full term, the cord was 3 centimetres in diameter and resembled an eel in appearance. Microscopic examination showed that the condition was simply due to an increase in the amount of Whartonian jelly.

Fœtal Syphilis.—Syphilis is the most frequent cause of fœtal death in the later months of pregnancy, and, as was said in Chapter XXV, may be maternal or paternal in origin. The mother may be suffering from the disease at the time of conception, or may contract it during the course of pregnancy. In the one case, it is believed that transmission to the fœtus occurs through the ovum, whereas in the other it takes place through the placenta. As a rule, the latter mode of infection is possible only when the mother is inoculated during the early months of pregnancy, though exceptions are occasionally noted. So far as my own experience goes, I am inclined to believe that in most instances the disease is paternal in origin, and is transmitted by the spermatozoa. In such cases the mother will or will not contract the disease, according as the father does or does not present infectious lesions at the time of coitus. Since these are usually absent, the fœtus ordinarily becomes inoculated, while the mother escapes —*Colles's law.*

It has long been known that a syphilitic infection exerts a most deleterious influence upon the product of conception. It frequently is responsible for the death of the fœtus and its premature expulsion from the uterus. Less commonly the child is born alive showing distinct manifestations of the disease, while in other cases they do not appear until a later period.

It is of the greatest importance that the practitioner should become thoroughly familiar with the characteristic lesions of fœtal and placental syphilis, as upon their recognition the future treatment of the patient often depends. This is a point especially worthy of emphasis, inasmuch as, in consequence of ignorance or design on the part of one or both parents, the first intimation that the physician has of the existence of the disease is often afforded by the birth of a dead child or the appearance of syphilitic stigmata in a living one.

Syphilis not only gives rise to characteristic lesions in the skin and internal organs of the fœtus, but also affects the placenta, so that frequently a diagnosis can be made from an examination of the latter organ. This fact is of special importance in those cases in which the fœtus is born alive, or when an autopsy is not permitted upon a dead child. The appearance of the syphilitic fœtus varies materially according as it is born alive or dead. In either instance it is markedly undersized, and the subcutaneous fat is poorly developed or entirely lacking. In the living child the skin presents a dry, drawn appearance, and has a peculiar grayish hue. It is very brittle,

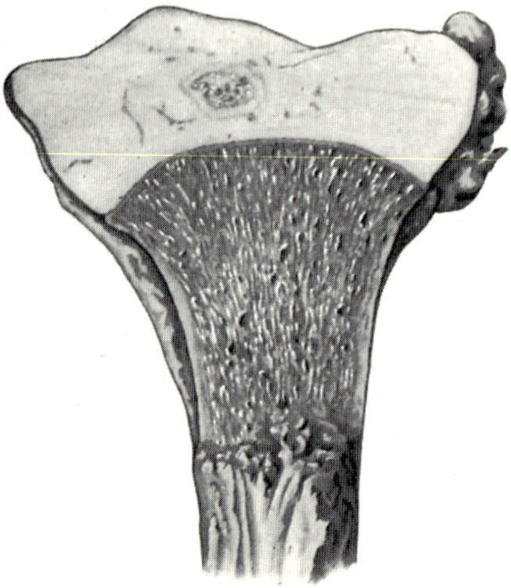

Fig. 458.

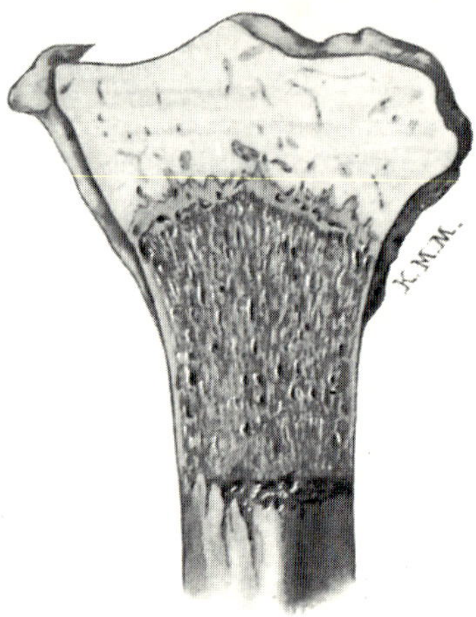

Fig. 459.

Figs. 458, 459.—Normal and Syphilitic Fœtal Epiphysis. ×2.

especially at the flexor surfaces of the joints, where abrasions readily occur and expose the underlying corium. The skin covering the soles of the feet and palms of the hands is often thickened and glistening, and suggests the condition observed in the hands of washerwomen. In other cases, characteristic cutaneous lesions are noted, particularly the appearance of pemphigoid vesicles upon the palms of the hands and soles of the feet.

If intra-uterine death has occurred, the fœtus rapidly undergoes maceration, the skin peeling off upon the slightest touch and exposing the underlying discoloured corium. Inexperienced persons have regarded this condition in itself as due to syphilis, but it is by no means pathognomonic, since it occurs in all macerated children, no matter what the cause of death. At the same time it must be remembered that this defect may entirely obliterate or at least obscure the specific skin lesions.

The lesions in the internal organs consist essentially in interstitial changes in the lungs, liver, spleen, and pancreas, and osteochondritis in the long bones.

It is generally stated that the lungs frequently contain gummatous nodules. These, however, were lacking in the specimens which I have examined. In many cases the lungs are enlarged, pale, and scarcely float when thrown into water. On microscopic examination the alveoli are found filled with cast-off epithelial cells — catarrhal pneumonia, the *pneumonia alba* of Virchow. In other cases the lesion consists in an increase in the interstitial tissue between the alvéoli, by which the latter are compressed, but do not become quite impervious to air. These changes have been exhaustively studied by Heller.

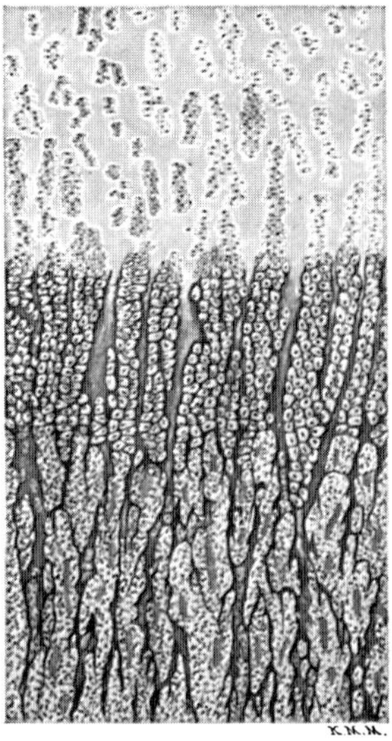

Fig. 460.—Normal Fœtal Epiphysis. × 60.

As the result of hypertrophic cirrhosis, the liver undergoes a marked increase in size, and according to Ruge its weight may equal one tenth or even one eighth of that of the whole body, instead of one thirtieth as usual. Under the microscope there is a marked increase in the connective tissue surrounding the individual lobules and acini, with here and there small areas of round-cell infiltration.

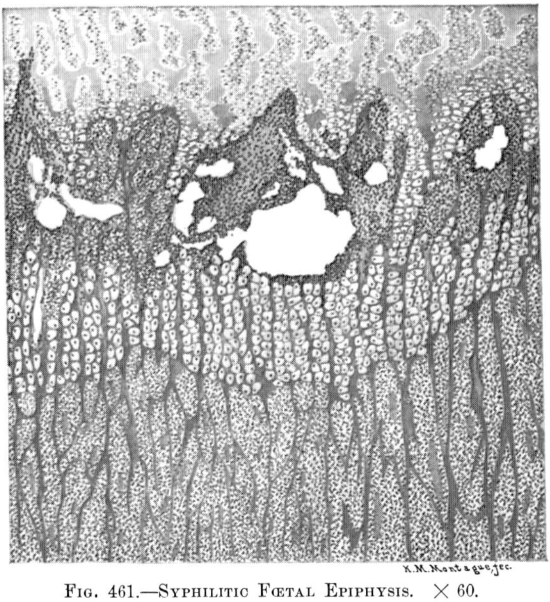

Fig. 461.—Syphilitic Fœtal Epiphysis. × 60.

The spleen likewise undergoes interstitial changes and increases markedly in size, so that it frequently weighs two or three times as much as usual, which, roughly speaking, is one three-hundredths of the body weight. The pancreas also presents interstitial changes, and is slightly larger than normal.

The recognition of these lesions requires some little pathological experience, though if the liver and spleen are found markedly increased in size and weight the diagnosis of syphilis is permissible.

A much more characteristic sign, and one which is readily detected, is afforded by changes occurring at the junction of the epiphysis with the diaphysis in the long bones—Wegner's bone disease. Normally the two are separated by a narrow, whitish, slightly curved line, 0.5 to 1 millimetre in diameter—Guérin's line—representing the area of preliminary calcification, which constitutes the scaffolding upon which the new bone is developed. In syphilis, on the other hand, this undergoes characteristic changes, becoming converted into an irregular, jagged, yellowish line 2, 3, or more millimetres in thickness. In advanced cases this alteration is associated with considerable softening and the formation of a soft pultaceous material, which occasionally leads to complete separation of the epiphysis (Figs. 458 and 459).

Upon microscopical examination of the normal epiphysis, as shown in Fig. 460, the cartilage cells are found to be arranged in parallel rows at

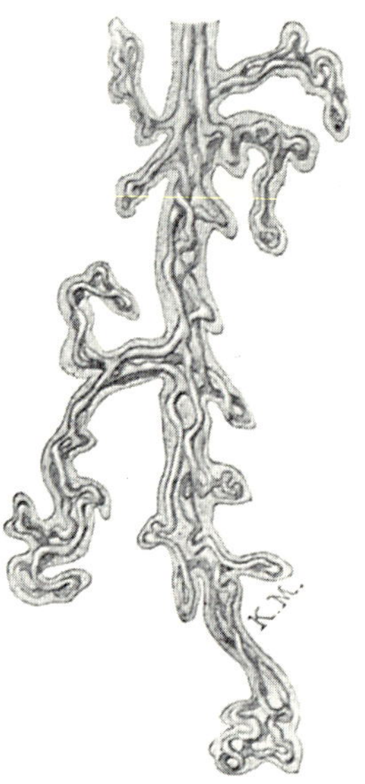

Fig. 462.

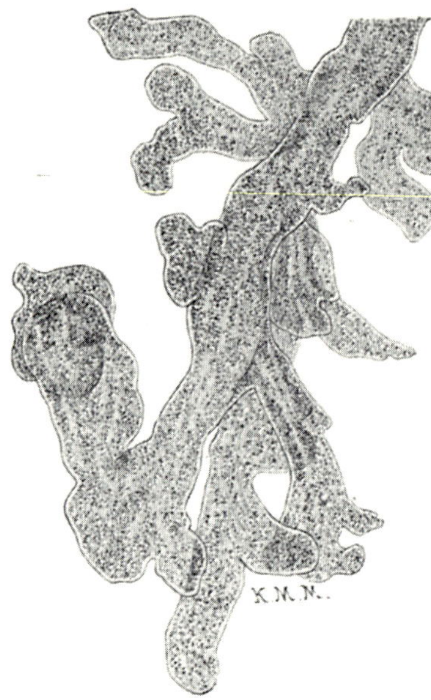

Fig. 463.

Figs. 462, 463.—Normal and Syphilitic Chorionic Villi teased out in Salt Solution, Slightly Magnified.

right angles to Guérin's line, while below it is the typical bony structure of the diaphysis with its marrow cavities. The line itself is formed by a deposit of lime salts between the median ends of the rows of cartilage cells, and is gradually invaded by the newly formed bone.

In syphilis, as is illustrated in Fig. 461, the changes are due to *osteochondritis,* as the result of which there is no longer a sharply marked zone of preliminary calcification between the cartilage and the growing bone; but areas of bone formation and calcification are found scattered irregularly through the lower portions of the epiphysis, giving an irregular appearance to this region.

These changes have been carefully studied by Wegner and R. Müller, and are most readily recognisable at the lower end of the femur, and fairly well at the lower ends of the tibia and radius. They are less clearly defined at the upper ends of the tibia, fibula, and femur, and only in rare instances can they be made out at the ends of the ribs. They are extremely characteristic, and their detection justifies one in making a positive diagnosis and placing the patient under specific treatment.

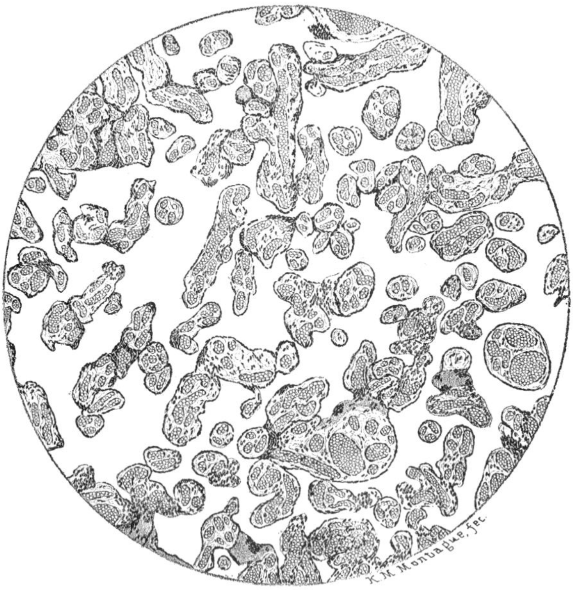

FIG. 464.—NORMAL FULL-TERM PLACENTA. ×50.

Placental Syphilis.—Under the influence of syphilitic infection the placenta undergoes very characteristic changes. It becomes larger and paler in colour, and if the fœtus is dead often presents a dull, greasy appearance. Its increase in size is very marked, and according to the researches of Correa-Dias and Schwab, which I have been able to confirm, instead of one sixth it may represent as much as one fourth or even a larger fraction of the entire body weight of the fœtus.

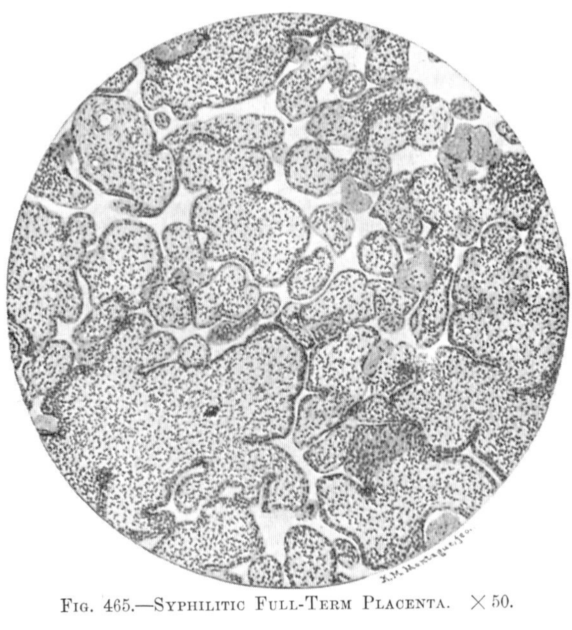

FIG. 465.—SYPHILITIC FULL-TERM PLACENTA. ×50.

Still more characteristic, however, are the changes in the chorionic villi, to which Fränkel called attention in 1873. In syphilis the villi, when teased out in salt solution, are seen to have lost their characteristic arborescent appearance and to have become thicker and more club-shaped (Figs.

462 and 463). At the same time there is a marked decrease in the number of blood-vessels, which disappear almost entirely in advanced cases. This results partly from endarteritic changes, but principally from a proliferation of the stroma cells, which lose their normal stellate appearance, becoming round or oval in shape, and closely packed together.

Similar changes are observed in sections made from hardened specimens. As will be seen on comparing Figs. 464 and 465, the individual villi are markedly increased in size and almost devoid of blood-vessels, while their stroma is made up of closely packed, round, or oval cells. This appearance is so characteristic as to enable one with a little practice to make a probable, if not a positive diagnosis, and at the same time affords a satisfactory explanation for the poor development of the fœtus.

It is generally stated that distinct syphilitic lesions, varying from a marked thickening of the membrane to distinct gumma formation, are frequently noted in the decidua. I am inclined to believe, however, that many of the conditions which have been described as such have no connection with lues, but are analogous to the various hyperplastic conditions of the decidua, which were formerly attributed to the same cause.

Zilles, and many of the earlier writers, described gummata occurring in the fœtal portion of the placenta. I have never met with such lesions, and am of the opinion that careful histological study will show that the majority of the so-called placental gummata are merely infarcts in various stages of development or degeneration.

General Dropsy of the Fœtus.—In this rare condition, 65 instances of which have been collected by Ballantyne, the fœtus and placenta are markedly œdematous. As the result of infiltration with serum the former may attain immense proportions and the latter be increased to three or four times its normal size. In a case recently under my observation the fœtus, at the seventh month of pregnancy, weighed 1,140 and the placenta 1,200 grammes. Cohn has described a placenta weighing 2,900 grammes.

Although a good deal has been written upon the subject, no satisfactory explanation of the anomaly has as yet been arrived at. Formerly it was supposed to result from œdematous conditions of the mother, but the researches of Ballantyne have shown that this view does not always hold good, and that in the majority of the cases submitted to a thorough study lesions were noted in the organs of the fœtus sufficient to explain the production of the condition. It is interesting to note that in several cases collected by Seifert it was attributed to fœtal leukæmia.

The disease always leads to the death of the fœtus, which in no instance survived its birth for more than a few hours. In the majority of cases on record labour was spontaneous, though occasionally the increased size of the fœtus and the placenta may give rise to dystocia.

Diseases of the Fœtus.—In most text-books upon obstetrics, numerous morbid conditions of the fœtus are described under this heading. The majority of them, however, are of interest mainly from a pathological point of view, and have no obstetrical significance, except in those cases in which they lead to an increase in the bulk of the fœtus, which in turn may give rise to difficult labour. Accordingly, they will not be considered in this place, though certain of them will be referred to in the chapter upon Fœtal Dystocia.

LITERATURE

ACKERMANN. Der weisse Infarct der Placenta. Archiv f. path. Anat., 1884, xcvi, 439–452.

Zur normalen u. path. Anat. der menschlichen Placenta. Virchow's Festschrift, Berlin, 1891, 585–616.

AHLFELD. Multiple Dermoidcysten des Amnion. Berichte u. Arbeiten, 1885, ii, 200–202.

Die Verwachsungen des Amnion mit der Oberfläche der Frucht. Berichte u. Arbeiten, 1887, iii, 158–165.

Zerreissung der Nabelschnur eines reifen Kindes während der Geburt. Zeitschr. f. Geb. u. Gyn., 1897, xxxvi, 467–472.

Mangel des Fruchtwassers. Lehrbuch der Geb., 1898, II. Aufl., 271.

AICHEL. Ueber die Blasenmole eine experimentelle Studie. Habilitationsschrift, Erlangen, 1901.

ALBERT. Ueber Angiome der Placenta. Archiv f. Gyn., 1898, lvi, 144–159.

BALLANTYNE. General Dropsy of the Fœtus. The Diseases of the Fœtus, Edinburgh, 1892, i, 102–164.

BAR. Recherches pour servir à l'histoire de l'hydramnios. Thèse de Paris, 1881.

BODE und SCHMORL. Ueber Tumoren der Placenta. Archiv f. Gyn., 1898, lvi, 73–83.

BOIVIN, Madame. Nouvelles recherches sur la nature, l'origine et le traitement de la mole vésiculaire. Paris, 1827.

BRAUN, G. Ligatur der Nabelschnur durch Amnionstränge. Zeitschr. f. Ges. d. Aerzte zu Wien, 1854, ii, 192.

BRESLAU und EBERTH. Diffuses Myxom der Eihäute. Virchow's Archiv, 1867, xxxix, 191–192.

BRICKNER. A New Symptom in the Diagnosis of Dystocia due to a Short Umbilical Cord. Amer. Jour. Obst., 1902, xlv, 512–521.

BUDIN. Note sur une tumeur du cordon ombilical. Femmes en couches et nouveau-nés, 1897, 179–184.

Tarnier et Budin, Traité des l'art des accouchements, 1886, ii, 276.

CAGNY. Hémorrhagies placentaires de l'albuminurie. Thèse de Paris, 1891.

CLARKE. Account of a Tumour found in the Substance of the Human Placenta. Philosophical Transactions, London, 1798.

COHN. Ueber das Absterben des Foetus bei Nephritis der Mutter. Zeitschr. f. Geb. u. Gyn., 1888, xiv, 596.

CORREA-DIAS. De l'hypertrophie placentaire dans les cas de syphilis. Thèse de Paris, 1891.

DORLAND and GERSON. Cystic Disease of the Chorion. University Medical Magazine, May, 1896, 565–590.

DYHRENFURTH. Inversio uteri bedingt durch zu kurzen Nabelstrang. Centralbl. f. Gyn., 1885, 801–804.

EDEN. Deciduoma Malignum: A Criticism. Trans. Lond. Obstet. Soc., 1896, xxxviii, 149–162.

A Study of the Human Placenta. Jour. Path. and Bacteriology, 1897, v, 265–282.

EHRENDORFER. Cysten und cystoide Bildungen der menschlichen Placenta. Wien, 1893.

FEHLING. Ueber die physiologische Bedeutung des Fruchtwassers. Archiv f. Gyn., 1879, xiv, 221–244.

FRÄNKEL. Ueber Verkalkungen der Placenta. Archiv f. Gyn., 1871, ii, 373–382.

Ueber Placentarsyphilis. Archiv f. Gyn., 1873, v, 1–54.

FRAENKEL. Die Histologie der Blasenmole, etc. Archiv f. Gyn., 1895, xlix, 481–507.

Franqué. Anat. und klin. Beobachtungen über Placentarerkrankungen. Zeitschr. f. Geb. u. Gyn., 1894, xxviii, 293–348.

Ueber histologische Veränderungen in der Placenta und ihre Beziehungen zum Tode der Frucht. Zeitschr. f. Geb. u. Gyn., 1897, xxxvii, 277–298.

Die Entstehung der velamentosen Insertion der Nabelschnur. Zeitschr. f. Geb. u. Gyn., 1900, xliii, 463–488.

Gassner. Menge des Fruchtwassers. Monatsschr. f. Geburtsk., 1862, xix, 30–33.

Goeze. Quoted by Kossmann.

von Grafenberg. Observationes medicae rariores. Frankfurt, 1565.

Guéniot. Tumeur du placenta observée chez une primipara. L'Obstétrique, 1897, ii, 275–276.

Heller. Die Lungenerkrankungen bei angeborener Syphilis. Deutsches Archiv f. klin. Med., xliii, 159.

Hense. Adhärenz der Placenta. Zeitschr. f. Geb. u. Gyn., 1901, xlv, 272–279.

Hermann. Ueber Verschlingungen der Nabelschnüre bei Zwillingen. Archiv f. Gyn., 1891, xl, 253–260.

Hyrtl. Die Blutgefässe der menschlichen Nachgeburt. Wien, 1870.

Jaggard. Note on Oligohydramnion. Amer. Jour. Obst., 1894, xxix, 432–446.

Jarotsky und Waldeyer. Traubenmole in Verbindung mit dem Uterus, etc. Virchow's Archiv, 1867, xli, 528–534.

De Jong. Ueber das Entstehung von Cysten in der Placenta. Monatsschr. f. Geb. u. Gyn., 1900, xi, 1072–1092.

Jungbluth. Zur Lehre vom Fruchtwasser, etc. Archiv f. Gyn., 1872, iv, 554–557.

Kahn-Bensinger. Myxoma chorii bei einem Zwillingsei. D. I., Giessen, 1887.

Kaltenbach. Zu kurze Nabelschnur. Lehrbuch der Geb., 1893, 316.

Kanthack. Discussion on Deciduoma Malignum. Trans. Lond. Obst. Soc., 1896, xxxviii, 171–184.

Kehrer. Ueber Traubenmolen. Archiv f. Gyn., 1894, xlv, 478–505.

Kermauner. Zur Lehre von der Entwickelung der Cysten u. des Infarctes in der menschlichen Placenta. Zeitschr. f. Heilkunde, 1900, xxi, 1–36.

Kleinwächter. Ein Beitrag zur Anatomie des Ductus omphalo-mesentericus. Archiv f. Gyn., 1876, x, 238–247.

Knapp. Eineiige Zwillingsplacenta: velamentöse Insertion; Verblutung beider Früchte unter der Geburt. Archiv f. Gyn., 1896, li, 586–594.

Kossmann. Zur Geschichte der Traubenmole. Archiv f. Gyn., 1900, lxii, 153–169.

Krieger. Fall von interstitiellen Molenbildung. Berliner Beiträge zur Geb. u. Gyn., 1872, i, 10–15.

Küstner. Hydramnios. Müller's Handbuch der Geburtsh., 1889, ii, 557–579.

Mehrfache Placenta, etc. Müller's Handbuch der Geburtsh., 1889, ii, 624–625.

Ueber eine noch nicht bekannte Entstehungsursache amputirender amniotischer Fäden u. Stränge. Zeitschr. f. Geb. u. Gyn., xx, 445–458.

Ladinski. Deciduoma Malignum. Amer. Jour. Obst., 1902, xlv, 465–509.

Lebedeff. Quelques données sur la fonction physiologique de l'amnios. Annales de gyn. et d'obst., 1878, ix, 241–251.

Lefèvre. De l'insertion vélamenteuse du cordon. Thèse de Paris, 1896.

Levison. Fruchtwasser und Hydramnios. Archiv f. Gyn., 1876, ix, 517–519.

Levy. Rapports existant entre le poids du fœtus et celui du placenta. Thèse de Paris, 1900.

Marchand. Ueber die sogenannten "decidualen" Geschwülste, etc. Monatsschr. f. Geb. u. Gyn., 1895, i, 419–438; 513–560.

Ueber den Bau der Blasenmole. Zeitschr. f. Geb. u. Gyn., 1895, xxxii, 405–472.

Die Blasenmole. Zeitschr. f. Geb. u. Gyn., 1898, xxxix, 206–216.

Ueber das maligne Chorionepitheliom, nebst Mittheilung 2 neuen Fälle. Zeitschr. f. Geb. u. Gyn., 1898, xxxix, 173–258.

MARTIN. De l'influence des altérations du placenta sur la development du fœtus. Thèse de Paris, 1896.
MONTGOMERY. On the Spontaneous Amputation of the Fœtal Limbs in Utero. An Exposition of the Signs and Symptoms of Pregnancy. 1863, 2d ed. (reprinted), 625–695.
MÜLLER, R. Beitrag zur path. Anatomie der Syphilis hereditaria. Virchow's Archiv, 1883, xcii, 523–556.
MÜNZER. Chorioepithelioma malignum. Centralbl. f. allg. Path. u. path. Anatomie, 1902, xiii, 197–265.
NEUMANN. Beitrag zur Lehre von der Anwachsung der Placenta. Monatsschr. f. Geb. u. Gyn., 1896, iv, 307–318.
Beitrag zur Kenntniss der Blasenmole, etc. Monatsschr. f. Geb. u. Gyn., 1897, vi, 17–36; 157–177.
NIEBERDING. Zur Genese des Hydramnios. Archiv f. Gyn., 1882, xx, 310–316.
NIEBERGALL. Ueber Placentargeschwülste. Monatsschr. f. Geb. u. Gyn., 1897, vi, H. 5.
OPITZ. Beiträge zur Aetiologie des Hydramnios. Centralbl. f. Gyn., 1898, 553–560.
ORTH. Infarct der Placenta. Lehrbuch der spec. path. Anat., 1893, ii, 603–607.
OSTERLOH. Kapillarangiom der Placenta. Centralbl. f. Gyn., 1899, 1232.
OUVRY. Étude de la mole hydatidiforme. Thèse de Paris, 1897.
PEISER. Verblutungstod der Frucht in folge Ruptur einer Umbilicalarterie bei Insertio velamentosa. Monatsschr. f. Geb. u. Gyn., 1898, viii, 619–624.
Beitrag zur Pathologie der Placenta. Monatsschr. f. Geb. u. Gyn., 1899, x, 613–626.
PERCY. Mémoire sur les hydatides utérines, etc. Jour. de méd. chir. et pharm., Paris, 1811, p. 171.
PETERS. Beitrag zur Casuistik der Vasa prævia, etc. Monatsschr. f. Geb. u. Gyn., 1901, xiii, 1–21.
PICK. Von der gut- und bös-artig metastasirenden Blasenmole. Berliner klin. Wochenschr., 1897, 1069–1073; 1097–1102.
PIERCE. Chorio-epithelioma malignum. Amer. Jour. Obst., 1902, xlv, 321–351.
POTEN. Die Verschleppung der Chorionzotten. Archiv f. Gyn., 1902, lxvi, 590–617.
POTEN und VASSMER. Beginnendes Syncytiom mit Metastasen, beobachtet bei Blasenmolenschwangerschaft. Archiv f. Gyn., 1900, lxi, 205–276.
RIBEMONT-DESSAIGNES. Des placentas multiples dans les grossesses simples. Annales de Gyn. et d'Obst., 1887, xxvii, 12–52.
ROSSIER. Klin. und histolog. Untersuchungen über die Infarcte der Placenta. Archiv f. Gyn., 1888, xxxiii, 400–412.
RUGE. Ueber den Foetus sanguinolentus. Zeitschr. f. Geb. u. Gyn., 1877, i, 57–119.
SALLINGER. Ueber Hydramnios, etc. D. I., Zürich, 1875.
SÄNGER. Deciduoma malignum. Verh. d. deutschen Gesellsch. f. Gyn., 1892, iv, 333.
Sarcoma uteri deciduo-cellulare, etc. Archiv f. Gyn., 1893, xlix, 89–149.
SCHALLER. Ueber Phloridzin-diabetes Schwangerer, etc. Archiv f. Gyn., 1899, lvii, 566–596.
SCHATZ. Eine besondere Art von einseitiger Polyhydramnie, etc. Archiv f. Gyn., 1882, xix, 329–369.
SCHAUTA. Zur Lehre von der Torsion der Nabelschnur. Archiv f. Gyn., 1881, xvii, 19–23.
SCHLAGENHAUFER. Zwei Fälle von Tumoren des Chorionepithels. Wiener klin. Wochenschr., 1899, Nr. 18.
SCHMIDT. Zur Kasuistik der chorio-epithelialen Scheidentumoren. Centralbl. f. Gyn., 1900, 1257–1265.
Ein neuer Fall von primären Chorio-epitheliom der Scheide. Centralbl. f. Gyn., 1901, 1350.
SCHMORL. Demonstration eines syncytialen Scheidentumors. Centralbl. f. Gyn., 1897, 1217.
SCHNEIDER. Quoted by Küstner.

SCHULTZE. Die genetische Bedeutung der velamentalen Insertion des Nabelstranges. Jenaische Zeitschr. f. Med. u. Naturwiss., 1867, iii, 198.

Ueber velementale u. placentale Insertion der Nabelschnur. Archiv f. Gyn., 1887, xxx, 47–56.

SCHWAB. De la syphilis du placenta. Thèse de Paris, 1896.

De la mole hydatidiforme. L'Obstétrique, 1898, iii, 405–427.

SIMONART. Note sur les amputations spontanées. Archiv de médecine Belge, 1845, T. 18, 112–119.

STEFFECK. Der weisse Infarct der Placenta. Hofmeier, "Die Placenta," Wiesbaden, 1890, 91–116.

VAN DER HOEVEN. Ueber die Aetiologie der Mola hydatidosa, etc. Archiv f. Gyn., 1901, lxii, 316–347.

VASSMER. Zur Aetiologie der Placentarcysten. Archiv f. Gyn., 1902, lxvi, 49–69.

VEIT. Das Deciduome malignum. Veit's Handbuch der Gyn., 1899, iii, 2te Hälfte, erste Abth., 535–596.

Ueber Deportation vom Chorionzotten. Zeitschr. f. Geb. u. Gyn., 1901, xliv, 466–504.

VELPEAU. Quoted by Virchow.

VIRCHOW. Myxom der Placenta. Die krankhaften Geschwülste, 1863, i, 405–414.

Myxom fibrosum placentæ. Die krankhaften Geschwülste, 1863, i, 415.

VOLKMANN. Ein Fall von interstitieller Molenbildung. Virchow's Archiv, 1867, xli, 528–534.

WEGNER. Ueber hereditäre Knochensyphilis bei jungen Kindern. Virchow's Archiv, 1870, l, 305–323.

WERTH. Einseitiges Hydramnion mit Oligohydramnie der zweiten Frucht. Archiv f. Gyn., 1882, xx, 353–377.

WILLIAMS, J. WHITRIDGE. Deciduoma malignum. Johns Hopkins Hosp. Reports, 1895, iv, No. 9.

The Frequency and Significance of Infarcts of the Placenta. Amer. Jour. Obst., 1900, xli, 775–801.

WILLIAMSON. The Pathology and Symptoms of Hydatidiform Degeneration of the Chorion. Trans. London Obst. Soc., 1900, xli, 303–338.

WILSON. Hydramnion in Cases of Uni-oval or Homologous Twins. Trans. Lond. Obst. Soc., 1899, xli, 235–272.

WILTON. Hydatids, terminating Fatally by Hæmorrhage. Lancet, 1840, i, 691–693.

WINCKEL. Teleangiektatisches Myxosarkom der Nabelschnur. Centralbl. f. Gyn., 1894, 397.

WOERZ. Ein Fall von Hydramnios. Centralbl. f. Gyn., 1895, 580–581.

ZILLES. Studien über Erkrankungen der Placenta bedingt durch Syphilis. Tübingen, 1885.

CHAPTER XXIX

ABORTION, MISCARRIAGE, AND PREMATURE LABOUR

SPONTANEOUS expulsion of the ovum may occur at any period of pregnancy, and is variously designated according to the degree of development which the product of conception has attained. Thus, it is customary to speak of abortion, of miscarriage, or of premature labour, respectively, according as pregnancy has terminated before the sixteenth week, between the sixteenth and twenty-eighth week, or at a later period.

Prior to the sixteenth week, owing to the imperfect development of the placenta, the entire ovum often comes away intact. From that time on, however, the placenta forms a definite organ and the expulsion of an intact ovum is exceptional, the fœtus, as a rule, being extruded first, and followed after a longer or shorter period by the placenta and membranes. After the twenty-eighth week the course of labour differs but little from that observed at full term, and the child, if properly cared for, may survive, its chances of so doing increasing in almost geometrical proportion with every additional week.

As the term abortion is somewhat suggestive of a criminal procedure, it is rarely employed in popular parlance, all cases terminating prior to the period of viability being designated as miscarriages. Among medical men, on the other hand, the latter term is but little used, and it is customary to speak of all cases ending before the twenty-eighth week as abortions.

Frequency.—It is difficult to arrive at accurate conclusions concerning the frequency with which abortion occurs. Inasmuch as a comparatively small proportion of such cases are treated in the lying-in hospitals, the statistics based upon their records would give too low an estimate. On the other hand, sufficiently large series from private practice are not available. Franz states that abortion occurred in 15.4 per cent of the cases admitted to the lying-in hospital at Halle, the accident being more than twice as frequent in multiparæ as in primiparæ. A conservative estimate would indicate that about every fifth or sixth pregnancy in private practice ends in abortion, and the percentage would be increased considerably were the very early cases taken into account, in which there is profuse loss of blood following the retardation of the menstrual period for a few weeks.

Ætiology.—In the early months of pregnancy spontaneous expulsion of the ovum is nearly always preceded by the death of the fœtus. For this reason the consideration of the ætiology of abortion practically resolves itself into determining the cause of fœtal death. In the later months, on the other hand, the fœtus is frequently born alive, and other factors must be looked for to explain its expulsion. Fœtal death may be due to abnormalities occurring in the ovum itself or due to some disease on the part of the mother, and now and again of the father.

(*a*) The death of the fœtus is frequently due to abnormalities in the development of the embryo which are inconsistent with fœtal life. More often, however, it results from changes in the fœtal appendages, which interfere with its nutrition, such as excessive torsion of the cord, hydramnios, hydatidiform mole, or syphilis. In the last two affections the nutritive material conveyed by the maternal vessels to the intervillous spaces merely suffices to nourish the hypertrophic chorionic villi, little or none remaining to be transmitted to the child.

Again, other diseases and abnormalities of the placenta may lead to the same result. Thus Merttens and Franqué have described an obliterating endarteritis in the vessels of the chorionic villi, independent of syphilis, which interferes with the fœtal circulation to such an extent as to be incompatible with life. In other cases, the abundant formation of red and white infarcts may throw so large a portion of the placenta out of function that the remainder is not sufficient to supply the needs of the fœtus. Abnormalities in development, such as placenta prævia or velamentous insertion of the cord, as well as premature separation of the placenta, may likewise bring about circulatory conditions inconsistent with fœtal life.

(*b*) As was pointed out in the chapter upon the Accidental Complications of Pregnancy, all acute infectious diseases have a tendency to bring about the death of the child and its subsequent expulsion from the uterus. The fatal result is usually due to the transmission of toxines, and occasionally of the specific micro-organisms from the mother to the child. Poisoning with phosphorus, lead, illuminating gas, and other substances may lead to similar results.

Diseases of the heart and kidneys may likewise play a prominent part in the causation of fœtal death. In the former it is attributed to imperfect aeration of the blood; in the latter it may result directly from the accumulation of excrementitious substances in the maternal blood and their subsequent transmission to the fœtus; or indirectly, from the fact that large portions of the placenta are thrown out of function by extensive infarct formation. Less commonly diseases of the liver or lungs of the mother may be indirectly responsible.

Fœtal death is sometimes attributable to malnutrition on the part of the mother, although this is very exceptional. On the other hand, it is not unusual for women suffering from wasting diseases to give birth to fully developed children.

Abnormalities in the generative tract likewise play an important part in the ætiology of abortion. Thus, developmental anomalies of the uterus, or imperfect development of the normally formed organ, may be responsible for conditions which are unfavourable for the implantation of the ovum and later for the development of the placental circulation. Chronic metritis is also supposed to act in the same way. Dense adhesions about the tubes and ovaries, resulting from inflammatory processes, only rarely interfere with the expansion of the uterus sufficiently to give rise to abortion, since in most cases the bands of adhesions gradually stretch and become elongated.

Displacements of the uterus, more particularly retroflexion and prolapse, are justly considered as most important factors in the causation of abortion. As a rule, the interruption of pregnancy is due less to the abnormal position of the uterus than to changes in its endometrium incident to the displacement. In the rare cases of incarceration, however, the accident must be attributed to the persistent abnormal position of the organ.

The most important factor in the production of abortion is afforded by diseases and abnormalities of the decidua. In the hypertrophic forms of decidual endometritis—decidua polyposa—the bulk of the maternal blood brought to the placental site goes to nourish the hyperplastic decidua, while in the atrophic forms the conditions are unfavourable for the normal implantation of the ovum and the development of the placenta. More important still is the part played by chronic glandular endometritis and acute inflammation of the decidua. The former is usually accompanied by hæmorrhagic changes, and is the most frequent cause of abortion in the early months. The presence of myomata in the walls of the uterus must be looked upon as an occasional factor, abortion resulting less from the mechanical effect of the tumour itself than from the changes in the decidua incident to it.

In a few cases the cause of abortion is to be sought for in reflex influences which take their origin from lesions of the generative tract or from irritative conditions about the breasts. In very rare instances the accident is attributable to intense mental emotions—anger, fright, or grief.

It is customary to distinguish between *predisposing* and *exciting causes* of abortion. The various factors to which allusion has just been made, predispose to abortion, while the exciting cause is often of a mechanical nature, such as a slight fall, jar, or overexertion. The statements of the patient concerning the latter, however, must be received with caution, as in many cases they are merely incidental and have no connection with the interruption of pregnancy. At the same time it must be admitted that the apparently healthy uterus in certain women possesses an abnormal degree of irritability, and will react to stimuli which in others would be without effect. In such patients the slightest violence, such as coitus, a misstep, tripping over a carpet, or a ride over a rough road may bring on an abortion; while in others the most violent exercise and the rudest manipulations may be borne with impunity. Occasionally a simple bimanual examination may be followed by an abortion; while, on the other hand, every physician can recall cases in which a sound has been introduced into the pregnant uterus without ill effects, and in rare instances, in the later months, the repeated introduction of a large bougie, or even of a Champetier de Ribes balloon, will fail to bring about satisfactory uterine contractions.

(*c*) Practically the only paternal cause of abortion is syphilis, which, as has already been said, frequently leads to changes in the placenta and the organs of the fœtus, which bring about its death and its premature expulsion from the uterus.

To sum up, the most important ætiological factors in the interruption of pregnancy in the first four months are endometritis and uterine displacements, while after this period syphilis and Bright's disease play a similar *rôle*. Thus, Sentex, in 485 cases of intra-uterine death occurring in the later months of pregnancy in Pinard's clinic, found the underlying cause to be syphilis in 42.7, albuminuria in 19.8, and diseases and abnormalities of the fœtus in 11.1 per cent.

It is not unusual to meet with women who give a history of repeated abortion or premature labour occurring at about the same time in a number of successive pregnancies. Careful examination of such patients will usually demonstrate the existence of an endometritis or a uterine displacement, if the interruption has occurred in the first half of pregnancy; and it is only after the cure of the underlying condition that subsequent pregnancies can be expected to progress to full term. When repeated premature labour has occurred in the second half of gestation, signs of albuminuria, Bright's disease, or syphilis will usually be discovered. This subject has recently been considered in detail by Lomer.

Pathology.—In the first half of pregnancy, the immediate cause of the expulsion of the ovum is to be found in hæmorrhagic changes in the decidua. Concerning their mode of production we must confess a profound ignorance, although when endometritis is the underlying cause their origin is readily understood. These changes, which are most marked in the decidua serotina, are followed by degeneration of the affected tissues, as the result of which the attachment of the ovum to the uterine wall becomes more or less loosened, and the product of conception comes to act as a foreign body and gives rise to uterine contractions, which, after a longer or shorter period, lead to its expulsion.

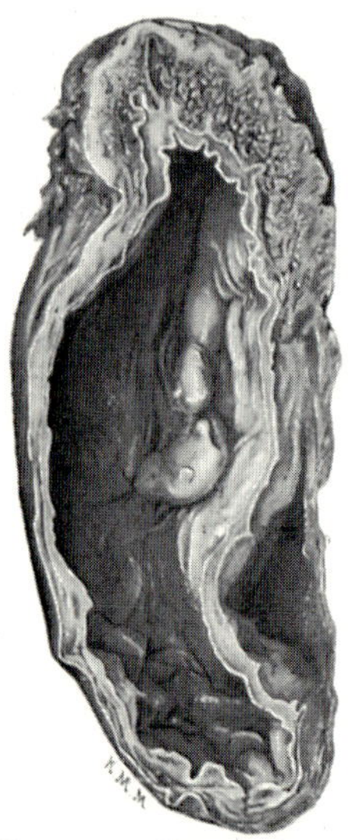

Fig. 466.—Early Abortion, showing Decidua Reflexa and Serotina with Degenerate Embryo. × 1.

Sometimes, especially in the early months, the entire ovum may be expelled after a few premonitory symptoms, and not infrequently the entire decidual lining of the uterine cavity is cast off at the same time. In such cases a triangular sac comes away which represents the decidua vera and is made up of blood-stained tissue several millimetres in thickness. It contains in its interior the rounded vesicular ovum, covered by the decidua reflexa. More frequently, however, the decidua vera remains *in utero*, while the ovum, surrounded by the decidua reflexa, is expelled. Occasionally the reflexa is torn through, and a shaggy, more or less spherical structure is cast off—the ovum surrounded by the chorionic villi.

As pregnancy advances, the expulsion of the entire ovum is observed less frequently, so that after the fourth month it is the rule for the membranes to rupture and the fœtus to be expelled by itself, followed by the placenta and membranes. Occasionally the intact ovum may be expelled even at a later period, and I have seen several cases in which this occurred as late as the seventh or eighth month. This, however, is very unusual, the course of premature labour being identical with that observed at full term.

In many instances the process of abortion occurs very slowly, so that the blood poured out between the periphery of the ovum and the decidua has an opportunity to coagulate. Under such conditions, the ovum on

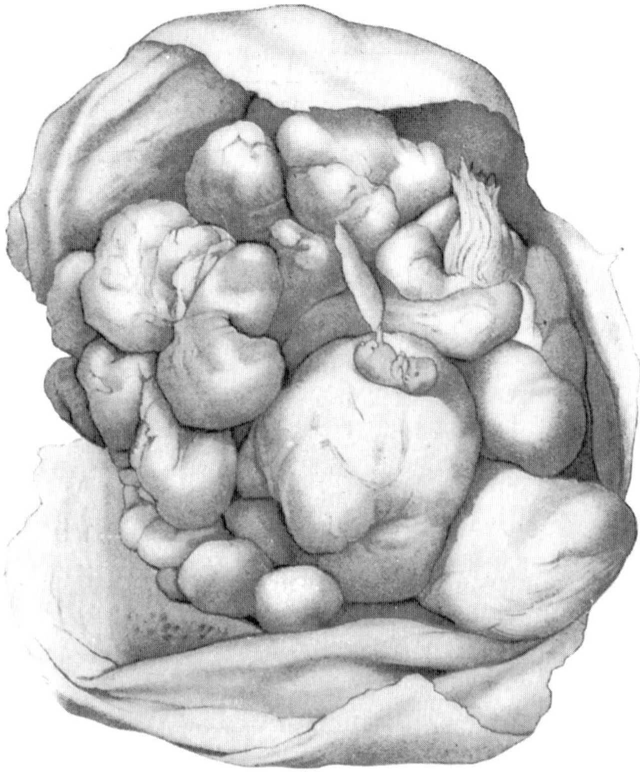

FIG. 467.—TUBEROUS SUBCHORIAL HÆMATOMA (Breus). × 1.

its expulsion is surrounded by a capsule of clotted blood of varying thickness with degenerated chorionic villi scattered through it. In its interior is a small cavity filled with clear fluid and lined by a thin, glistening membrane (the amnion) from one point of which hangs the umbilical cord and the partially degenerated fœtus. Such structures are classified as *blood or carneous moles*, according to their appearance. In the former the capsule of coagulated blood is red in colour, while in the latter it presents a paler appearance, the result of fibrin formation (Fig. 468).

Now and then, the interior of such structures, instead of being lined by the smooth amnion, may present an irregular nodular appearance, which is due to the formation of hæmatomata of varying size beneath the amnion and chorion. This condition, to which Granville applied the term *ovum tuberculosum*, has been more particularly studied by Breus, who designated it as *tuberous subchorial hæmatoma* of the decidua (Fig. 467). He believed that the tuberous appearance was the result of hæmorrhage into collapsed folds of the amnion, while Gottschalk, Walther, and others considered that the hæmorrhage was the primary factor. Davidsohn, in a recent article, takes the view that the disproportion between the size of the fœtus and the ovum is the result of hydramnios, and after the death of the former the amniotic fluid is gradually absorbed, when the redundant amnion becomes folded upon itself, the blood being effused into its folds.

In all uterine moles the fœtus is relatively smaller in size than would naturally correspond with the menstrual history. This fact indicates that the process is of gradual formation, and that a considerable period elapses between the death of the fœtus and the expulsion of the ovum. Not uncommonly, indeed, the fœtus may undergo complete dissolution, or be represented merely by a stub of umbilical cord hanging from the interior of the ovum; while in rare instances all trace of it may disappear, and, after resorption of the amniotic fluid, the ovum may be represented by a solid mass of varying size, composed of chorionic villi embedded in coagulated blood.

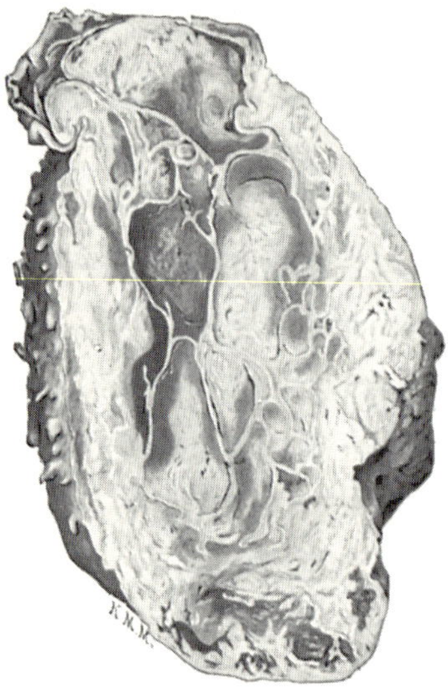

FIG. 468.—SECTION THROUGH BLOOD MOLE. × 1.

Dissolution of the dead fœtus is possible only in the early weeks of pregnancy, and cannot occur after it has attained any considerable proportions. In the latter class of cases the retained fœtus may undergo *maceration*. Under such circumstances the brain degenerates, the bones of the skull collapse, the abdomen becomes distended with a blood-stained fluid, and the entire fœtus takes on a dull reddish colour due to staining with blood pigment. At the same time the skin softens and peels off at the slightest touch, leaving behind the bright-red corium. The internal organs become soft and friable, and lose their capacity for taking up the usual histological stains. In rarer instances the fœtus becomes compressed and takes on a dry, parchment-like appearance—*mummification*. This is rarely observed in ordinary abortion, but is noted with comparative frequency in twin pregnancies, when one fœtus has died at an early period while the other has gone on to full development—fœtus papyraceus.

In very exceptional instances the fœtus may be retained *in utero* for a long period, until the deposition of lime salts upon it converts it into what is known as a *lithopædion*. This phenomenon, though extremely rare in uterine pregnancy in human beings, is relatively common in the lower animals. In extra-uterine gestation, on the other hand, such a condition is not of unusual occurrence.

Clinical History.—From a clinical standpoint it is a matter of considerable importance to distinguish the period at which the pregnancy is terminated. When it occurs in the first half it is not unusual for the ovum to be expelled as a whole, while in the second half of pregnancy the course of events is similar to that observed at a full-term labour.

The onset of abortion is usually preceded by certain premonitory symptoms, the most important of which are hæmorrhage and pain in the back and lower abdomen. Loss of blood, no matter how slight, in the early months of pregnancy, should always be regarded with suspicion, for if it be not a premonitory symptom of abortion it usually indicates the existence of a hyperplastic endometritis or an abnormal implantation of the placenta. When due to the former the discharge is usually not very profuse, and is of a dirty brown or brownish-red colour, while when due to the latter it is apt to be more profuse and distinctly bloody in character. The premonitory bleeding may persist for weeks or be promptly followed by the expulsion of the ovum. Indeed, in some cases the latter event may occur so rapidly as to surprise the patient.

When a patient in the first few weeks of pregnancy begins to lose blood, and the flow is associated with pain in the lower abdomen and back, an abortion is *threatened.* It, however, does not become *imminent* unless the hæmorrhage be profuse or the cervix considerably dilated; even in the latter case it is not impossible for the disturbance to subside, and for pregnancy to go on without interruption. On the other hand, rupture of the membranes and escape of the liquor amnii indicate that abortion is *inevitable.*

When abortion becomes imminent, the hæmorrhage is usually quite profuse, though as a rule not sufficient to endanger the life of the woman. At the same time she experiences severe cramp-like pains in the abdomen due to the uterine contractions, which later become distinctly bearing-down in character. After the cervix has become sufficiently dilated the detached ovum may be expelled intact from the uterus, and when not retained in the vagina comes away satisfactorily. This is known as *complete abortion.*

Not uncommonly, on the other hand, after rupture of the membranes and the escape of the amniotic fluid, the fœtus alone is expelled, while the placenta and membranes remain in the uterus—*incomplete abortion.* In such cases the hæmorrhage usually persists until the retained structures are extruded spontaneously or are removed artificially, though the pains usually cease with the expulsion of the fœtus. After the uterus has rid itself of the product of conception, the hæmorrhage and pain cease, and a process of involution begins, identical with that observed after full-term labour.

Treatment.—Prophylactic treatment is most important, although, as a rule, it is not available in women aborting for the first time. If, however, the patient presents a history of repeated abortion or premature labour, precautionary measures should be instituted before conception has again taken place.

The general and local condition should be carefully investigated and any abnormality subjected to appropriate treatment. If the patient has a retroflexed uterus, the organ should be replaced and held in position by a properly fitting pessary. If the desired results are not obtained in this way, ventrosuspension or some other suitable operation should be performed. If endometritis be present, the patient should be curetted and warned against becoming pregnant until sufficient time has elapsed to allow the uterus to recover from the morbid condition. If the symptoms reappear, the operation should be repeated. If there is no abnormality in the generative tract, the possibility of syphilis in either parent should be borne in mind, and appropriate treatment instituted in suspicious cases. The urine should always be carefully examined with a view to determining the presence or absence of renal lesions.

If past experience has shown that the patient has an irritable uterus and is predisposed to abort upon the slightest provocation, coitus should be interdicted during pregnancy, and the patient be cautioned against overexertion and encouraged to lead a careful, well-ordered existence. Moreover, she should be instructed to take to her bed immediately upon the appearance of any untoward symptom.

Treatment of Threatened Abortion.—Whenever symptoms of threatened abortion appear, the patient should be placed in bed and kept in a recumbent position. If pains occur, a hypodermic injection of $\frac{1}{4}$ grain of morphine should be administered at once, to be followed by 1-grain rectal suppositories of extract of opium, repeated at intervals of every four or six hours. Better results are occasionally obtained by combining the opium with the extracts of hyoscyamus and viburnum prunifolium. The following suppository, administered every four or six hours, according to circumstances, often gives most satisfactory results:

℞.	Codiæ sulphat.	gr. ss.
	Ext. hyoscyami	gr. j.
	Ext. viburni prunifolii	gr. v.
	Ol. theobromæ	q. s.

In many instances the symptoms rapidly subside under such treatment, but the patient should be kept in bed for at least a week after their disappearance, in the hope of avoiding any repetition.

In other cases, the pain yields to the administration of sedatives, but the hæmorrhage persists, and we then have to decide how long we are justified in permitting the bloody uterine discharge to continue, and whether there is any probability that an interruption of pregnancy will not occur.

So long as the loss of blood does not exceed that usually observed at the menstrual period, the flow is not necessarily incompatible with the continuance of pregnancy, and may be permitted to go on for some time. On the other hand, if it becomes so profuse that the patient begins to show signs of anæmia, the uterus should be emptied by the methods to be described later. In many instances, notwithstanding appropriate treatment and rest in bed, slight hæmorrhage may persist for several weeks, and it then becomes necessary to ascertain whether there is any possibility of the pregnancy continuing. Unfortunately, this problem usually requires several weeks for its solution. Thus, if bimanual examination shows at the end of two weeks that the uterus has remained stationary in size, one is justified in concluding that the fœtus has perished; while, on the other hand, an increase probably indicates that the fœtus is still alive, but does not necessarily mean that pregnancy will go on to a happy termination. As soon as we are convinced that the fœtus is dead, the uterus should be promptly emptied. In such cases nothing can be gained by delay, as abortion will inevitably occur sooner or later, whereas temporizing treatment sometimes exposes the patient to serious danger.

Treatment of Inevitable Abortion.—When convinced that abortion is inevitable, particularly in those cases in which the hæmorrhage is profuse, the uterus should be emptied in the most conservative manner, the choice of procedure depending upon the degree of dilatation of the cervix. If it be sufficiently patulous to admit one or two fingers, the patient should be anæsthetized, brought to the edge of the bed, and prepared for operation. The carefully sterilized hand, anointed with sterile vaseline, having been introduced into the vagina, one or preferably two fingers are carried up into the uterine cavity, and under the guidance of the other hand applied over the abdomen, peel off the ovum from the uterine wall and slowly extract it. If this cannot be effected the ovum should be broken up by the finger and the fragments extracted by means of a placental or ovum forceps, under the guidance of a finger within the uterus.

But if, as often happens, the cervix is not sufficiently dilated to permit the introduction of a finger, the cervical canal and vagina should be packed tightly with a sterile gauze bandage, as described in Chapter XXIV, and 30 drops of the fluid extract of ergot administered every four hours. When removed at the end of twenty-four hours, the pack frequently brings with it the intact ovum; but, even if this does not occur, the cervix will generally be sufficiently dilated to permit the introduction of the finger, when the ovum can be removed as recommended above.

This method of procedure is preferable to the rapid dilatation of the cervix with a Goodell or some similar dilator, followed by the immediate removal of the ovum by means of a curette or polypus forceps. Moreover, the cervix is sometimes so resistant that it is impossible to dilate it sufficiently by means of metallic dilators to permit the introduction of the finger, the employment of which, in my opinion, is essential for the proper evacuation of the uterus and a careful exploration of its cavity after removal of the ovum, in order to make sure that it is perfectly empty, and that there is consequently no danger of subsequent hæmorrhage.

No doubt the uterus can be satisfactorily evacuated in most cases by means of the curette and polypus forceps, but no instrument has ever been invented which will prove an efficient substitute for the carefully trained sense of touch when it becomes necessary to satisfy one's self that no remnants of the ovum are still retained in the uterus. On several occasions I have seen patients suffering from profuse hæmorrhage following the supposed thorough removal of the product of conception by curetting, and, on introducing the finger into the uterus, I have found that it still contained the bulk of the ovum. Experiences of this kind have therefore led me to do away with the use of instruments except in very rare cases. Moreover, in addition to the fact that they fulfil their object only imperfectly, they are not devoid of danger. Every gynæcologist is familiar with cases in which the softened uterus has been perforated by the curette, and knows of rare instances in which a loop of gut has prolapsed through the opening so made.

When the ovum has been expelled intact, as in complete abortion, there is no necessity for further interference; and, as a rule, if the decidua vera is not cast off, it is not advisable to attempt its removal by means of the curette, for it is usually expelled spontaneously within a few days. At the same time the physician should always satisfy himself by careful inspection that the entire ovum has come away, and that portions of it are not retained. In incomplete abortion, on the other hand, the retained placenta and membranes should be removed manually by the methods already described. As soon as the uterus is emptied it contracts and the danger of hæmorrhage has passed.

It often happens that the physician does not see the patient until some days after the expulsion of the fœtus, when the cervix has retracted to such a degree that it will not admit the finger. Under these circumstances it can readily be sufficiently dilated by means of a Goodell dilator, after which the remnants of the ovum are removed by the finger. In other cases infection has resulted, and the uterine discharge may be very foul-smelling. In such cases the cervix should be dilated and the uterus, after being emptied, should be washed out with an abundance of sterile salt solution. If the symptoms still persist after this procedure, the uterine wall has been invaded by the offending micro-organisms, and we have to deal with a case of puerperal infection, the treatment of which is considered in the appropriate chapter.

The treatment of abortion in the second half of pregnancy and of premature labour is identical with that already described for full-term labour, and does not require further mention.

Missed Abortion.—This term was applied by Oldham to the rare cases in which the fœtus is retained in the uterine cavity for months or even years after its death. Retention may exist for a long period without giving rise to symptoms, and this possibility should always be borne in mind in the case of an abortion occurring in a woman who has been for some time separated from her husband, inasmuch as an error in this regard occasionally results in irreparable damage to her character. In other cases the patient may believe herself to be in the seventh or eighth month, and yet on examination the uterus will be found to correspond in size to that of a three-months' pregnancy. Seventy instances of this kind have been collected by Graefe, 11 of the cases having been seen by him, and the rest having been recorded in the literature. In quite a number the fœtus had been retained for more than a year, and in one instance for twenty-eight years.

According to Veit and Graefe, the retention is to be attributed to a lack of irritability on the part of the uterus, which does not contract as usual under the stimulation excited by the dead ovum acting as a foreign body. Not uncommonly the condition, after persisting for some time without symptoms, may exert an appreciable effect upon the patient, who may suddenly begin to lose flesh, suffer from a foul taste in her mouth, perhaps present a slight elevation of temperature, and occasionally manifest symptoms of mental derangement.

Whenever the diagnosis is established beyond doubt, the cervix should be dilated by means of a vaginal and cervical pack, and the uterus emptied of its contents. In several instances under my observation the cervix was so resistant that its dilatation by means of steel instruments was out of the question.

LITERATURE

BREUS. Das tuberöse subchoriale Haematom der Decidua. Leipzig u. Wien, 1892.

DAVIDSOHN. Zur Lehre von der Mola haematomatosa. Archiv f. Gyn., 1902, lxv, 181–216.

FRANQUÉ. Ueber histologische Veränderungen in der Placenta und ihre Beziehungen zum Tode der Frucht. Zeitschr. f. Geb. u. Gyn., 1897, xxxvii, 277–298.

FRANZ. Zur Lehre des Aborts. Hegar's Beiträge, 1898, i, 493–514.

GOTTSCHALK. Zur Lehre von den Hämatommolen, etc. Archiv f. Gyn., 1899, xviii, 134–169.

GRAEFE. Ueber Retention des menschlichen Eies im Uterus nach dem Fruchttod. Festschrift zu Carl Ruge, Berlin, 1896, 38–79.

GRANVILLE. Graphic Illustrations of Abortion, etc. London, 1834.

LOMER. Zur Therapie wiederholter Aborte und der Frühgeburt todter Kinder. Zeitschr. f. Geb. u. Gyn., 1901, xlvi. 282–306.

MERTTENS. Beiträge zur normalen und path. Anatomie der menschlichen Placenta. Zeitschr. f. Geb. u. Gyn., 1894, xxx, 1–97.

OLDHAM. Missed Labour. Guy's Hosp. Reports, 1847, 105–112.

SENTEX. Des causes de la mort du produit de la conception pendant la grossesse. Thèse de Paris, 1901.

VEIT. Vorzeitige Unterbrechung der Schwangerschaft. Müller's Handbuch der Geburtshülfe, 1889, ii, 23–57.

WALTHER. Ein Fall von tuberösem, subchorialem Hämatom der Decidua. Centralbl. f. Gyn., 1892, 707–710.

CHAPTER XXX

EXTRA-UTERINE PREGNANCY

In *extra-uterine pregnancy* the fertilized ovum is arrested at some point between the ovary and the uterus, and there undergoes more or less complete development. *Ectopic gestation,* which is sometimes used as a synonymous term, has a broader meaning, inasmuch as it includes not only the usual forms of extra-uterine pregnancy, but also those in which the ovum is implanted in the rudimentary horn of a bicornuate uterus. Reference has already been made to this class of cases in Chapter XXVII.

For a long time extra-uterine pregnancy was of interest chiefly from a pathological point of view, but since 1883, when Tait first operated upon a case of ruptured tubal pregnancy, the subject has attained a markedly practical interest, as is manifested by the immense literature of recent years. The history of its development is treated in detail in the monographs of Campbell, Hecker, Parry, Tait, Werth, and Webster.

Prior to 1876, extra-uterine pregnancy was considered so rare an affection that Hennig stated that even the directors of large obstetrical institutions might never encounter a case, and Parry was able to collect only 500 instances from the entire literature. It was only with the gradual development of abdominal surgery that its relative frequency became recognised. Thus Schrenck, in 1892, collected 610 cases which had been reported in the preceding five years, and recently many operators have placed on record large series, Küstner having operated upon 105 cases in the course of five years, while Noble encountered extra-uterine pregnancy in from 3 to 4 per cent of all his laparotomies.

Ætiology.—Unfortunately, concise and definite statements cannot be made concerning the ætiology of the condition, although quite a number of explanations, of greater or less plausibility, have been advanced. Broadly speaking, these may be divided into three main groups: (1) Conditions which interfere mechanically with the downward passage of the ovum; (2) Those resulting from inflammatory diseases of the tubes, ovaries, and pelvic peritonæum; (3) Physical and developmental abnormalities which favour decidual formation in the tubes.

I. *Conditions which Interfere Mechanically with the Downward Passage of the Ovum.*—(*a*) Fritze, in 1779, first directed attention to the fact that peritoneal adhesions, by compressing the lumen of the tube or by interfering with its peristalsis, might cause the arrest of the ovum.

(*b*) Leopold, Breslau, Beck, Wyder, and others have reported cases in which they believed that polypi projecting into the lumen of the tube had interfered with the descent of the ovum. It is quite possible, however, that such structures were merely decidual outgrowths, and appeared only after conception.

(*c*) Some observers believe that myomata or other tumours, situated in the wall of the tube or in adjacent organs, may so compress the tubal lumen as to interfere with the passage of the ovum.

(*d*) Schroeder, in 1887, but more particularly Tait, a few years later, advanced the theory that the most frequent cause of tubal pregnancy was an endosalpingitis, whence had resulted the destruction of the cilia, and the consequent cessation of the downward current which was thought to prevent the entry of spermatozoa into the tube.

This view presupposed that fertilization occurred in the uterine cavity, and was based upon the belief that the ciliary current was directed downward in the tubes and from below upward in the uterus, the entry of spermatozoa into the uterine cavity being thereby facilitated, while their access to the tubes was rendered very difficult. The recent work of Hofmeier and Mandl has demonstrated the fallacy of these suppositions. Moreover, animal experiments and a few observations upon human beings make it reasonably certain that fertilization occurs normally in the tubes, every pregnancy being therefore primarily tubal. Accordingly, the problem to be solved in a case of extra-uterine pregnancy is not how the spermatozoa may have gained access to the tubes, but why the fertilized ovum failed to make its way to the uterus.

Tait's theory found many adherents, but careful study of specimens obtained at operation go to show that in most cases it is without foundation.

I have been able to demonstrate the presence of cilia in nearly every pregnant tube which I have examined, while Zedel saw them in motion in three out of four specimens which he examined in the fresh condition.

(*e*) Abel, Kreisch, and others believe that the fœtal convolutions of the tube occasionally persist in later life, and hinder the downward passage of the fertilized ovum either by constricting the lumen or by interfering with peristalsis.

(*f*) In 1891 Landau and Rheinstein and the writer demonstrated the presence of *diverticula* from the lumen of the tube, and suggested that a fertilized ovum entering such a structure would eventually be arrested at its blind end, and there might undergo further development (Fig. 469). For a number of years I believed that a considerable number of my cases had originated in this way. In such specimens the fœtal sac lay entirely outside of the lumen of the tube, being separated from it by a layer of tissue of varying thickness (see Fig. 482). After further examination of my specimens, while not wishing to deny such a possibility, I am of the opinion that these conditions can be more satisfactorily explained by supposing that the fertilized ovum had burrowed beneath the mucosa of the tube, just as it does into the decidua in uterine pregnancy.

Now and again, in serial sections through the pregnant tube, it is possible to demonstrate the presence of accessory lumina—long processes which extend from the main lumen and continue parallel to it for a considerable distance, and then rejoin it or end blindly. I have noted such a condition in several instances, and see no reason why a fertilized ovum arrested in such a structure should not go on to further development.

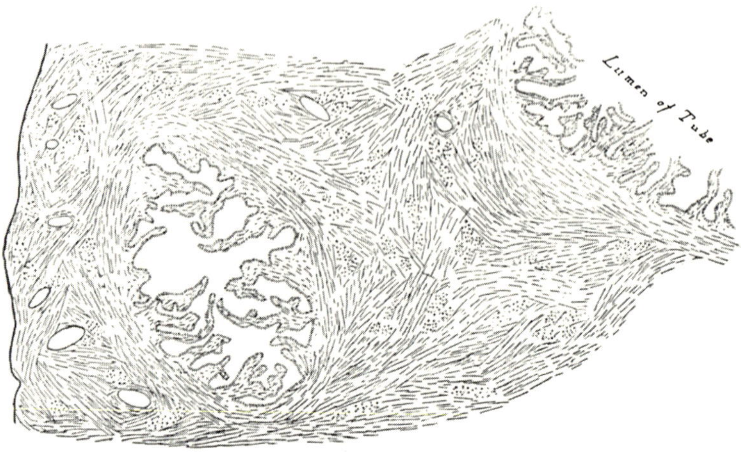

Fig. 469.—Diverticulum from the Lumen of Tube.

Sometimes accessory tubal ostia, instead of communicating with the lumen of the tube, represent mere *culs-de-sac*. That the fertilized ovum may be arrested in such a structure and go on to further development was conclusively demonstrated by Henrotin and Herzog (Fig. 470).

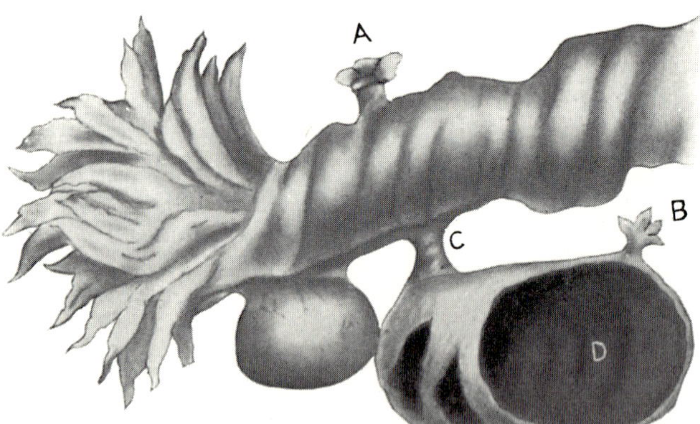

Fig. 470.—Pregnancy in Accessory Tubal Ostium (Henrotin and Herzog).
A, small accessory ostium; *B*, opening of pregnant ostium; *C*, blind end of same; *D*, blood-clot containing remnants of ovum.

(*g*) Dührssen believes that in occasional instances the arrest of the ovum may be due to puerperal atrophy of the tube, whereby its normal peristalsis is markedly impaired.

(*h*) In a considerable number of the cases which I have examined, the corpus luteum was situated not in the ovary corresponding to the pregnant tube, but in the opposite one, indicating that *external migration* had occurred, and that the fertilized ovum had made the transit of the pelvic cavity. Sippel believes that such a phenomenon may favour the production of extra-uterine pregnancy, since the fertilized ovum may attain such proportions during its migration as to prevent its passage through the tube.

II. *Conditions resulting from Inflammatory Conditions of the Tubes, Ovaries, and Pelvic Peritonæum.*—As has already been said, Schroeder and Tait pointed out that such conditions may result in the production of tubal pregnancy. This view is supported by the fact that many cases of extra-uterine pregnancy have been preceded by pelvic inflammatory trouble. Thus Dührssen, Mandl and Schmidt, Küstner, and others were able to elicit a history of gonorrhœal salpingitis or inflammatory conditions of the appendages in more than two thirds of their cases. Martin was formerly an enthusiastic advocate of this view, but has recently abandoned it, and now considers that extra-uterine pregnancy is nearly always the result of mechanical interference with the downward passage of the ovum.

III. *Physical and Developmental Conditions which Favour Decidual Formation in the Tubes.*—Webster believes that the explanation for the comparatively infrequent occurrence of extra-uterine pregnancy is to be found in the fact that the decidual reaction, which he considers essential to the proper implantation of the fertilized ovum, readily occurs in the uterus, but is usually lacking in the tubes. He holds that tubal pregnancy can come about only when the tubes are capable of this reaction. Furthermore, he considers that such an occurrence probably represents a reversion to an earlier type, and may therefore be looked upon as a sign of degeneracy. This view was soon indorsed by Pantellani, Mandl and Schmidt, Wormser, Moericke, and others, but their belief was based upon theoretical considerations rather than upon anatomical facts.

That Webster's theory is not entirely without foundation is rendered probable by the experimental work of Tainturier and Mandl and Schmidt, in which an artificial obstruction was produced in the generative tract of rabbits by applying ligatures to one or both sides at a certain period of time after copulation. When these were placed about the middle of the cornua, ova were arrested above them and went on to development; but when the uterine ends of the tubes themselves were ligated extra-uterine pregnancy never occurred, notwithstanding the fact that in rare instances degenerated ova could be demonstrated above the ligatures. In a control series of experiments, in which the uterine end of only one tube was ligated, pregnancy occurred in the non-ligated, but not in the ligated uterine horn, thus showing that the experiment had been performed at the proper time. These observers, therefore, concluded that something more than a mere mechanical obstruction was necessary, and believed that a decidual reaction was the essential pre-requisite for the production of tubal pregnancy.

In the presence of an abundance of theories concerning the ætiology of extra-uterine pregnancy, it still remains uncertain which of them is correct. Theoretically, it would appear that many mechanical conditions must occasionally play a part in the production of the abnormality; but whereas, certain of the former are noted with considerable frequency, extra-uterine pregnancy is nevertheless comparatively rare.

That extra-uterine pregnancy is dependent upon a pre-existing inflammatory disease of the generative tract cannot be demonstrated in the majority of cases, since in many instances, as in the 43 cases reported by Taylor, no history of previous inflammatory disease could be elicited. Moreover, even when such lesions are noted, it still remains doubtful whether they existed before the occurrence of pregnancy or were secondary to it. Sutton inclines to the latter view, and believes that the occlusion of the fimbriated end of the tube, which is so often noted, is the result of the pregnancy itself.

Nor is Webster's decidual reaction theory entirely satisfactory, since recent histological work has shown that the decidua does not play nearly so important a part in tubal pregnancy as was formerly supposed, many recent authorities going so far as to deny its formation.

The idea that the abnormality is a sign of degeneracy and reversion, while extremely interesting and to a certain extent borne out by facts, cannot be accepted as universally true, for an extra-uterine pregnancy sometimes occurs in perfectly healthy women, living amid the very best surroundings. Moreover, its relative infrequency in the lower animals speaks against such a view.

Accordingly, it is apparent that the ætiology of extra-uterine pregnancy is not a simple matter, and that there is no universal cause. As a rule, the history of the patient and a careful study of the specimen will afford a satisfactory explanation for its occurrence, but in not a few instances the underlying cause will remain as great a problem to us as to our predecessors.

Classification.—The fertilized ovum may be arrested at any point on its way from the Graafian follicle to the uterine cavity, and may undergo development in the ovary or in any portion of the tube, giving rise to ovarian or tubal pregnancy respectively. It is extremely doubtful whether the ovum can become implanted upon the peritonæum and a primary abdominal pregnancy follow.

Ovarian Pregnancy was first described in the seventeenth century, by Mercerus and St. Meurice, after which it was generally recognised until 1835, when Velpeau stated that none of the cases which had been described up to that time afforded conclusive evidence of ovarian origin. Similar views were expressed by Mayer in 1847, and were indorsed by Pouchet, Allan Thompson, and others. This scepticism was probably quite justifiable at the time, since most of the early cases collected by Campbell and Gurgui were simply dermoid cysts of the ovary.

With the exception of Mayer, the possibility of ovarian pregnancy has always been admitted by the German writers, but was strenuously denied until 1901 by the English authorities, particularly by Tait, Webster, and Bland Sutton.

So far as I can ascertain, only 6 cases of so-called ovarian pregnancy have been reported in England during the past hundred years—2 by Granville in 1834, and 1 each by Oliver, Croft, Gilford, and Anning and

Littlewood. Of the instances reported in this country up to 1902, Thompson's case only will stand a rigid scrutiny.

The earlier unsatisfactory condition of affairs was largely due to the fact that proper criteria were lacking, and as a consequence many specimens were described as ovarian pregnancy which had little or no claim to that title. In 1878, however, Spiegelberg formulated certain conditions which must be fulfilled in order to justify such a diagnosis. He demanded that (1) the tube on the affected side must be intact; (2) the fœtal sac must occupy the position of the ovary; (3) it must be connected with the uterus by the ovarian ligament; and (4) definite ovarian tissue must be found in the sac wall. The last criterion should be still further modified, and it must be shown that ovarian tissue is present in several portions of the sac wall at some distance from one another before the evidence becomes convincing. This requirement is necessary, for the reason that in certain cases of tubal or broad-ligament pregnancy the ovary may become flattened out, and to a certain extent become incorporated in the sac wall.

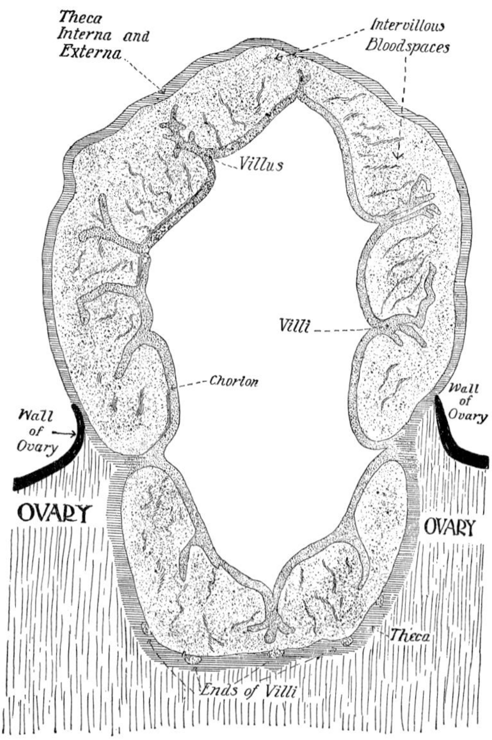

FIG. 471.—DIAGRAM ILLUSTRATING THOMPSON'S SPECIMEN OF OVARIAN PREGNANCY (Amer. Gyn.).

After a fairly thorough search through the literature upon ovarian pregnancy for the past hundred years, I have collected a number of cases, which I have classified as positive, highly probable, fairly probable, doubtful and negative, according to the extent to which they fulfil the above-mentioned criteria.

In only 5 cases has the primary ovarian character of the pregnancy been conclusively demonstrated—those of Gottschalk, Kouwer and Tussenbroeck, Anning and Littlewood, Franz, and Thompson. In none of these was there any doubt concerning the anatomical conditions. Gottschalk's case was the most advanced, the ovary being converted into a mass the size of a small orange in which was a distinct fœtus. In the others the product of conception was smaller. Anning and Littlewood exhibited a specimen before the London Obstetrical Society in 1901, which was so convincing as to silence the objections of even so persistent a sceptic as Bland Sutton.

Among the highly probable cases I have included 13—those reported by Granville, Hein, Uhde, Franck, Schrenck, Walther, Spiegelberg, Herzfeld, Larsen, Leopold, Martin, Gottschalk, and Ludwig. The first 5 had not progressed beyond the third month, while the others had reached full

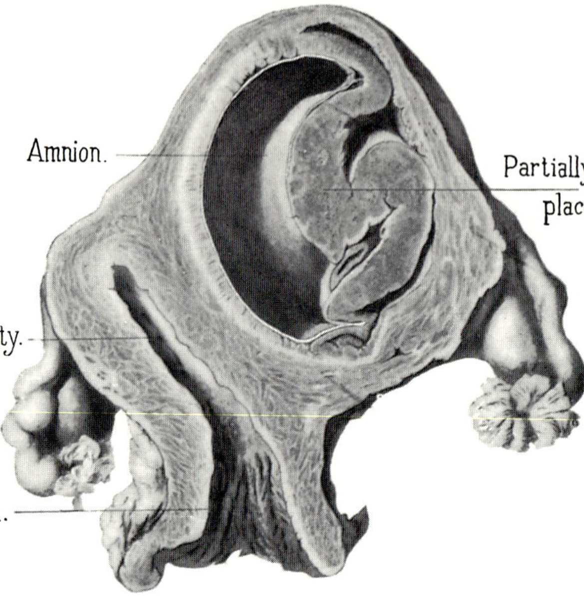

FIG. 472.—INTERSTITIAL PREGNANCY (Bumm).

term. In the cases of Leopold, Gottschalk, and Martin the product of conception had been retained in the abdomen for a number of years.

Among the fairly probable cases I have included those of Peuch, Patenko, Geuer, Küstner, Toth, Croft, and Gilford, making a total of 25 cases in which a positive or more or less probable diagnosis is justifiable.

One of the interesting points in connection with the cases thus far recorded is that 10 of the 25 reached full term. This would go to show that the ovary can accommodate itself more readily than the tube to the growing pregnancy. At the same time, it should be remembered that 4 of the 5 positive cases ruptured at an early period.

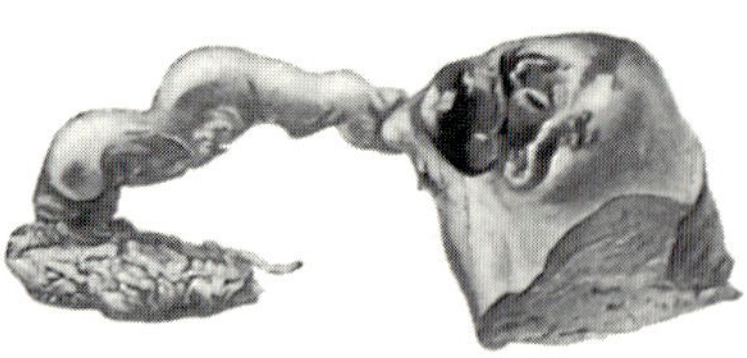

FIG. 473.—ISTHMIC PREGNANCY. RUPTURE TEN DAYS AFTER LAST MENSTRUAL PERIOD. × 1.

Ovarian pregnancy results from the fertilization of the ovum before it escapes from the Graafian follicle, the spermatozoa entering the follicle immediately after its rupture. Leopold believes that in a certain number of cases a deep-lying follicle may rupture into a more superficial one, the ovum contained in the former remaining *in situ* and being fertilized by spermatozoa gaining access to it through an opening in the more superficial follicle.

Tubal Pregnancy.—In this, by far the most frequent variety of extra-uterine pregnancy, the ovum may develop in any one of the three portions of the tube, giving rise to an *interstitial*, *isthmic*, or *ampullar pregnancy* respectively. In rare instances it may be implanted upon the fimbriated extremity, and occasionally even upon the fimbria ovarica. From these primary types certain secondary forms—tubo-abdominal, tubo-ovarian, and broad-ligament pregnancy—occasionally develop.

According to Rosenthal, the interstitial is the rarest variety, having occurred in only 3 per cent of the 1,324 cases of tubal pregnancy which he collected from the literature. Of 57 cases analyzed by Martin and Orthman, 48 were ampullar, 8 isthmic, and only 1 was interstitial. More recent writers, as Lindenthal, state that the isthmic variety is the commonest, and this has also been my experience.

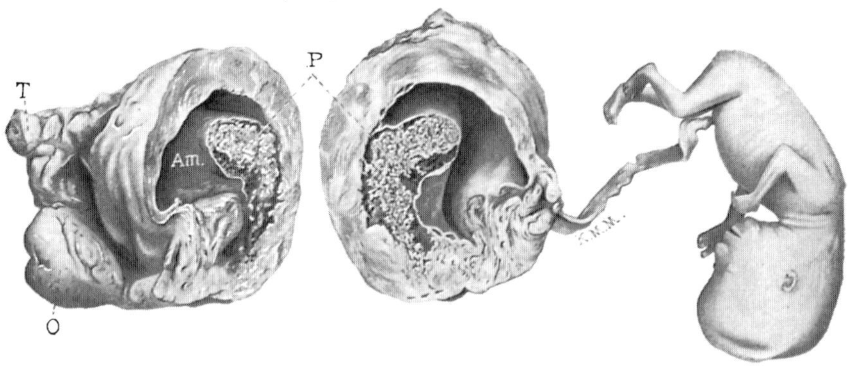

FIG. 474.—RUPTURED AMPULLAR PREGNANCY. × 1.
Am., amnion; *O.*, ovary; *P.*, placenta; *T.*, uterine end of tube.

According to Tait, rupture occurring not later than the twelfth week is the universal termination of tubal pregnancy. More careful study, however, has shown that only one fourth of the cases end in this way, the other three fourths terminating by abortion at an early period. Very exceptionally, the pregnancy may go on to full term without rupture, as in the cases reported by Saxtorph, Spiegelberg, Chiari, Gutzwiller, Emanuel, and others. My own collection also contains a specimen of a similar case.

Tubal Abortion.—After Werth, in 1887, had directed attention to the possibility of tubal abortion, it has gradually been demonstrated that this is the most frequent outcome of tubal pregnancy. The marked change of opinion upon this point which has taken place being clearly indicated by the following figures: Thus, whereas in 1892 Schrenck found only 6 cases of abortion in 610 cases of tubal pregnancy collected from the literature, the recently published reports of Martin, Wormser, Mandl and Schmidt, Fehling and Glitsch, comprising 289 cases, show that 78 per cent ended by abortion and only 22 per cent by rupture. According to Martin, "this termination is the general rule, spontaneous rupture occurring only in those cases in which occlusion of the abdominal end of the tube precludes the possibility of an abortion, or in which the ovum, being inserted in a hernia of mucosa, burrows directly through the tube wall."

In abortion, the connection between the ovum and the tube wall is loosened, the former becoming completely or partially separated from its site of implantation as the result of hæmorrhage due to the sudden opening up of maternal vessels by the growing trophoblast and chorionic villi. If the separation is complete, the effused blood gradually forces the ovum towards the fimbriated end of the tube, through which it is extruded into the peritoneal cavity, whereupon the hæmorrhage usually ceases. On the other hand, if the separation is only partial, the ovum remains *in situ*, and the hæmorrhage continues. Accordingly, we distinguish between *complete* and *incomplete abortions*, the latter occurring far more frequently than the former—10 to 1, according to Wormser.

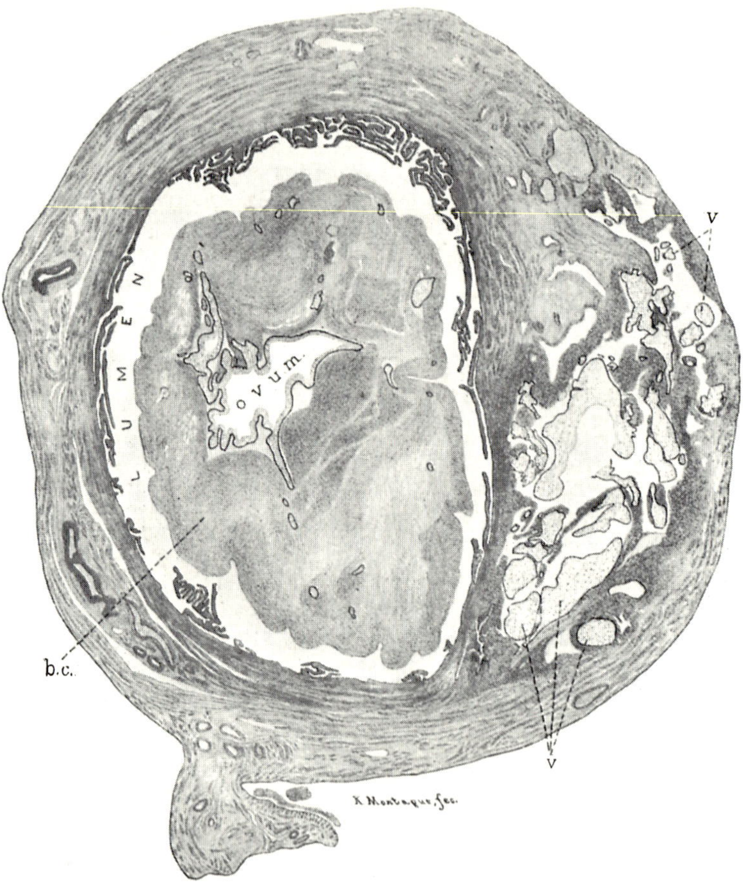

FIG. 475.—EARLY TUBAL PREGNANCY, WITH ABORTION OF OVUM INTO LUMEN OF TUBE. × 6. *b.c.*, blood-clot ; *v.*, chorionic villi.

In a small number of cases the ovum may be observed in the act of abortion (Fig. 476). Thus, among my own specimens are two which show the fœtus surrounded by its membranes, protruding from the dilated fimbriated extremity of the tube.

When the hæmorrhage is moderate in amount and the ovum remains *in situ,* it may become infiltrated with blood and increase markedly in

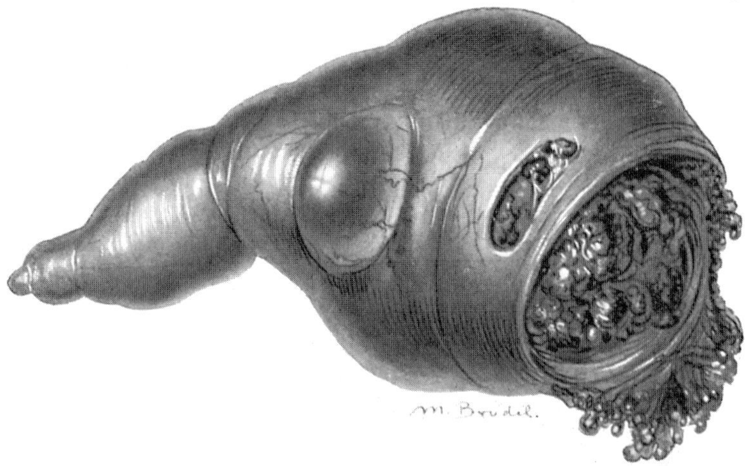

FIG. 476.—TUBAL ABORTION, OVUM BEING EXTRUDED THROUGH FIMBRIATED EXTREMITY (Kelly). × 1.

size, being converted into a structure analogous to the blood or fleshy mole observed in uterine abortions (Fig. 477). The hæmorrhage usually persists as long as the mole remains in the tube, and the blood slowly trickles from the fimbriated extremity into the peritoneal cavity, where it becomes encapsulated, giving rise to an *hæmatocele.* If the fimbriated extremity is occluded, the tube may gradually become distended by blood—*hæmatosalpinx.*

After incomplete abortion small particles of the chorion may remain attached to the tube wall, and, becoming surrounded by fibrin, give rise to a placental polypus, just as is often noted after an incomplete uterine abortion.

Rupture into the Peritoneal Cavity.—About one fourth of the cases of tubal pregnancy end within the first twelve weeks by rupture, which usually occurs spontaneously, but occasionally is the result of violence. Generally speaking, when rupture occurs in the first few weeks, the pregnancy is situated in the proximal end of the tube, a short distance from the cornu of the uterus (see Fig. 473). On the other hand, when the ovum is implanted in the interstitial portion of the tube, rupture occurs later than in the other varieties—as a rule, not until after the fourth month, sometimes considerably later. This difference is due to the fact that the interstitial portion of the tube is surrounded by uterine musculature, which reacts promptly to the stimulation of pregnancy, and by its hypertrophy allows the ovum to attain a considerable size before rupture occurs.

The underlying causes of rupture are perforation of the tube wall by the growing villi, or acute overdistention as a result of hæmorrhage into a tube whose fimbriated end is occluded. The mechanism will be more clearly understood when the anatomical relations of the ovum to the tube wall are studied. Rupture, as a rule, occurs in the neighbourhood of the placental site, and may take place either into the peritoneal cavity or between the folds of the broad ligament. In the former case the entire ovum may be extruded or remain within the tube. In either event the accident is usually accompanied by a profuse and often fatal hæmorrhage. If the patient recovers, the effect of the rupture upon the course of pregnancy varies according to circumstances. If the ovum be expelled entire the fœtus must inevitably die, and the product of conception will be rapidly absorbed, unless the pregnancy has advanced beyond the third month. This fact was proved by Leopold's experimental work upon animals, although some authors still believe that under such circumstances the placenta may become attached to any portion of the peritonæum and there establish vascular connections, thus rendering further development of the ovum possible. That these could be developed soon enough and before the ovum became irreparably damaged seems very unlikely.

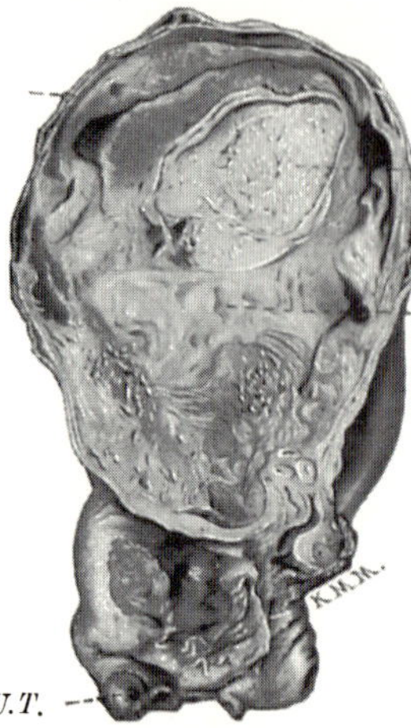

Fig. 477.—Section through Tubal Mole. × 1.

B.C., blood-clot; *Ov.*, ovum; *T.W.*, tube wall; *U.T.*, uterine end of tube.

If the fœtus only escapes, while the placenta remains within the tube, the effect will vary according to the amount of injury sustained by the placenta. If the latter be much damaged, the termination of pregnancy is inevitable. On the other hand, if it is intact and remains attached to the tube wall, further development is possible, and gestation may go on to full term as a so-called *abdominal pregnancy.* In such cases, after the escape of the fœtus, the tube often closes down upon the placenta and forms a sac in which the latter remains during the rest of pregnancy. Less frequently the placenta remains attached to the tube wall, but as it increases in size its peripheral portions extend beyond the latter, so that the organ eventually becomes implanted partly upon the tube and partly upon the uterus, pelvic floor, rectum, or even the intestines. The placenta does not become attached directly to organs outside of the pelvic cavity—for example, to the stomach or the diaphragm. When such a condition is noted, it is probable that one has to deal with a broad-ligament pregnancy, in which the placenta is situated in the upper portion of the gestation sac, and that the latter has become adherent to the organ in question.

When the fœtus escapes into the peritoneal cavity, according to the general belief, further growth is impossible unless it is surrounded by the amnion. Both has, however, reported an exceptional case in which a fully developed fœtus lay perfectly free in the abdominal cavity, all that was left of its membranes being found in the tubal sac.

Rupture into the Broad Ligament.—In a small number of cases rupture may occur at the portion of the tube uncovered by peritonæum, so that the contents of the gestation sac are extruded into a space formed by the separation of the folds of the broad ligament. Generally speaking, this is the most favourable variety of rupture, and may terminate either by the death of the ovum and the formation of a *broad-ligament hæmatoma*, or by the further development of the pregnancy between the folds of the broad ligament. The outcome depends largely upon the degree of completeness with which the placenta has been separated from its tubal attachment.

If the placenta remains attached to the tube on the side opposite the point of rupture, it generally becomes displaced upward as pregnancy advances, and comes to lie above the fœtus; but when it is situated near the point of rupture it gradually extends down between the folds of the broad ligament, being implanted partly upon the tube and partly upon the pelvic connective tissue. In either event, the fœtal sac lies entirely outside of the peritoneal cavity, and as it increases in size the peritonæum is gradually

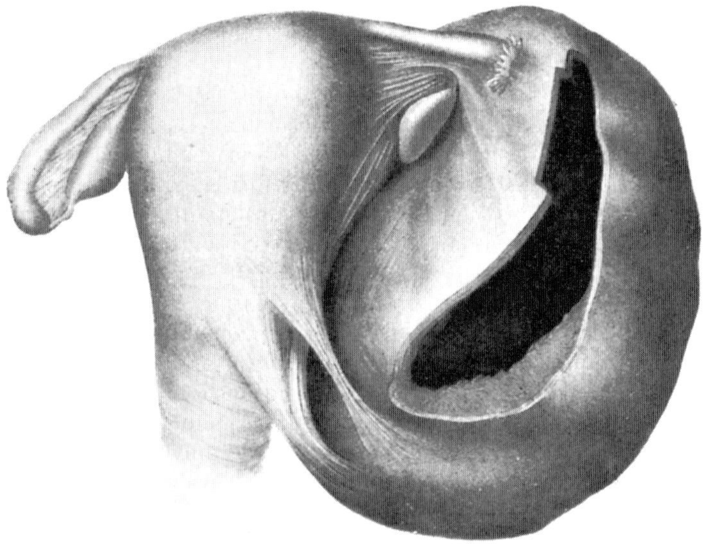

FIG. 478.—BROAD-LIGAMENT PREGNANCY (Zweifel).

dissected up from the pelvic walls. This condition is designated as *extra-peritoneal* or *broad-ligament pregnancy*, and was carefully studied by Dezeimeris in 1836. Occasionally the broad-ligament sac may rupture at a later period, and the child be extruded into the peritoneal cavity, while the placenta retains its original position—*secondary abdominal pregnancy.*

The importance of rupture into the broad ligament was particularly emphasized by Tait, who believed that it was only under such circumstances that extra-uterine pregnancy could go on to full term. But since tubal pregnancy does not necessarily end in rupture, it is evident that his statements were based upon imperfect information. The frequency of this mode of rupture seems to have been considerably overestimated. It was noted in only 4 out of 276 cases collected from the articles of Mandl and Schmidt, Küstner, and Fehling, and only once in 50 specimens of extra-uterine pregnancy examined by the writer.

The so-called *tubo-uterine pregnancy* results from the gradual extension into the uterine cavity of an ovum which was originally implanted in the interstitial portion of the tube. *Tubo-abdominal pregnancy*, on the other hand, is derived from a tubal pregnancy in which the ovum has been inserted in the neighbourhood of the fimbriated extremity, and gradually extended into the peritoneal cavity. Under such circumstances the portion of the fœtal sac projecting into the peritoneal cavity forms adhesions with the surrounding organs, which often seriously complicate its removal at operation. Neither of these conditions are very common, nor do they deserve to be classified separately; in reality, they are merely tubal pregnancies developed at unusual portions of the tubes.

The term *tubo-ovarian pregnancy* is employed when the fœtal sac is composed partly of tubal and partly of ovarian tissue. Such cases owe their origin to the development of an ovum in a tubo-ovarian cyst, or in a tube whose fimbriated extremity was adherent to the ovary at the time of fertilization. They are therefore primarily either tubal or ovarian in origin.

Abdominal Pregnancy.—Until comparatively recently it was generally believed that the ovum could be implanted upon any portion of the peritonæum and give rise to a primary abdominal pregnancy. Thus, in Hecker's statistics abdominal was recorded twice as frequently as tubal pregnancy. Later, however, when the specimens were more carefully studied, it became apparent that the great majority of abdominal pregnancies were secondary in character, having resulted from ruptured tubal pregnancy.

Gradually doubt began to be cast upon the existence of primary abdominal pregnancy, so that at present most authors, while admitting its theoretical possibility, are extremely sceptical as to its actual occurrence. Occasionally, as was shown by Zweifel, Martin, Voigt, and Leopold, the fertilized ovum may become implanted upon the fimbria ovarica. Such cases closely resemble primary abdominal pregnancy, inasmuch as the surface to which the ovum is primarily attached is so small that as pregnancy advances the margins of the placenta soon extend beyond the primary seat of implantation and become attached to the surrounding organs, thus giving the impression that it was primarily implanted upon the peritonæum. A careful microscopical examination, however, will enable one to differentiate between the two conditions.

Fate of Extra-uterine Fœtus.—As has already been pointed out, absorption is the universal fate of small embryos which are extruded into the peritoneal cavity, unless the placenta retains its attachment to the tube wall and still offers conditions suitable for the continuance of the circulation. Moreover, the young fœtus is frequently absorbed while still within the tube, as is shown by the fact that upon opening early gestation sacs it is sometimes represented by an amphorous mass of tissue attached to the umbilical cord. At times the only indication of its previous existence is found in a small portion of the cord hanging free in the amniotic cavity. On the other hand, when the fœtus has attained a certain size before death it cannot be absorbed in this manner, and must undergo suppuration, mummification, lithopædion, or adipocere formation.

Pyogenic bacteria often gain access to a gestation sac which is adherent to the intestines, and give rise to *suppuration* of its contents. Eventually the abscess perforates at the point of least resistance, and if the patient does not die from septicæmia, portions of the fœtus may be extruded through the abdominal wall or into the intestines or bladder, according to the situation of the perforation. This outcome is particularly frequent in broad-ligament pregnancies, on account of their proximity to the rectum and the liability to infection by intestinal bacteria.

Mummification and *lithopædion formation* have already been referred to in the chapter on Abortion, and are dealt with fully in Küchenmeister's article. The latter is generally regarded as the most favourable of the possible eventualities in cases of advanced extra-uterine pregnancy, as in many instances the calcified product of conception may be carried for years as a harmless foreign body and do no harm, unless it gives rise to serious dystocia in a subsequent pregnancy. In several instances a lithopædion has been known to remain in the abdomen for fifty years or more, and the literature contains more than 30 cases in which a period of twenty to thirty years elapsed before its removal at operation or autopsy.

Much more rarely the fœtus may become converted into a yellowish greasy mass to which the term *adipocere* is applied. The fatty material is supposed to be an ammoniacal soap, but a satisfactory explanation of its formation has not as yet been advanced.

Anatomical Considerations.—*Structure of the Fœtal Sac.*—In extra-uterine pregnancy there is a marked increase in the vascularity of the affected tube, the larger arteries and veins being much hypertrophied, while the smaller vessels, especially in the neighbourhood of the placental site, are markedly engorged.

Microscopical sections through the sac in the early months show a slight hypertrophy of the muscle cells, but no apparent increase in their number. Except at the placental site, the tube wall is considerably thickened and its cells are spread apart by œdema. At a still more advanced period, the muscular constituents of the gestation sac appear to diminish in number, so that at full term almost its entire thickness is made up of a connective tissue poor in cells, with only here and there a muscle fibre. This indicates that the muscularis of the tube does not possess the same tendency to hypertrophy as the uterus, though occasionally it is quite marked, Pinard having reported a case in which the fœtal sac contracted so strongly that he mistook it for a pregnant uterus.

In most cases the exterior of the tube gives evidence of peritonitic involvement, and a considerable portion of the thickness of the fœtal sac is often due to peritoneal adhesions.

In order for complete tubal abortion to occur, the fimbriated extremity must remain patent, but in other cases its condition varies, being sometimes closed, sometimes open. As a rule the lumen of the tube communicates directly with either end of the fœtal sac. Less commonly, however, this communication is noted only at one end, while still more rarely the fœtal sac is completely shut off from the main lumen. A satisfactory explanation of these differences has not as yet been adduced.

Uterine Decidua.—Under the influence of extra-uterine gestation, the endometrium becomes converted into a decidua similar to that observed in uterine pregnancy, and differing from it only in a less marked development of the spongy layer and a greater abundance of blood spaces just beneath its free surface. Soon after the death of the fœtus the decidua is thrown off in small pieces, and occasionally as a triangular cast of the uterine cavity. Its discharge is usually considered of marked diagnostic significance: so much so that in doubtful cases many observers recommend curetting the uterus, and base their diagnosis upon the presence or absence of decidual tissue.

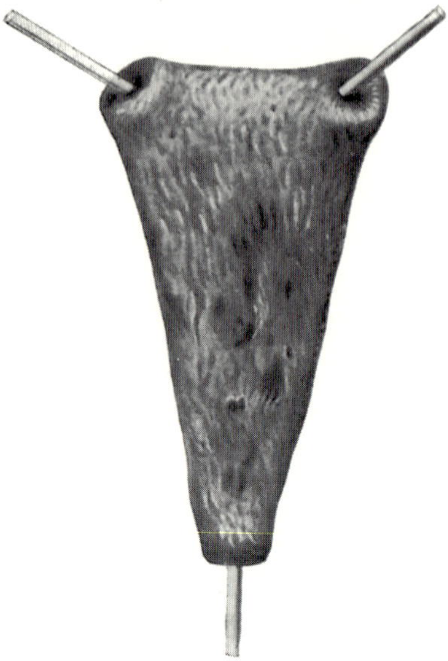

Fig. 479.—Uterine Decidua from a Case of Extra-Uterine Pregnancy (Zweifel).

Decidua Vera and Serotina.—All the early observers stated that the interior of the pregnant tube was lined by a distinct decidual membrane analogous to the decidua vera in uterine pregnancy. This view was accepted without question until 1891, when Bland Sutton denied the existence of such a structure. Later, other investigators, notably Griffiths, Kühne, Aschoff, and Kreisch, stated that decidual cells were not developed in the pregnant tube, and that the structures which had been considered as such were fœtal in origin and represented the proliferated trophoblast or fœtal ectoderm.

While there is no doubt that a great part of the so-called decidual cells are really fœtal in origin, I am, nevertheless, confident that a decidual formation occurs, though to a far less marked degree than was believed by the early observers. At the same time it must be admitted that the authors just mentioned were correct in denying the existence of a continuous membrane of considerable thickness, analogous to the decidua vera of the uterus, as the decidual formation is limited and *occurs only in discrete patches.*

That the tubes are capable of a decidual reaction has been conclusively proved by the observations of Mandl, Lange, and others, who demonstrated its occurrence in rare cases of intra-uterine pregnancy. In a number of specimens of tubal pregnancy which I have examined, there was a distinct decidual formation not only at the site of implantation of the ovum, but also in folds of the mucosa some distance from it—a condition also noted by Webster, Voigt, Both, and Dobbert. In one case, as is shown in Fig. 480, I was able to demonstrate the formation of decidual cells not only in the pregnant, but also in the non-pregnant tube. A similar observation was also made by Webster. These observations would appear to place the question beyond all doubt, as in such cases there could be no possibility of confusing fœtal with maternal cells.

What has been said concerning the decidua vera in tubal pregnancy applies equally well to the decidual serotina. This likewise never occurs as a continuous membrane, but at most consists of a few patches of decidual cells, which can be distinguished from the more abundant fœtal cells only by the most careful examination (see Fig. 481). As will be pointed out later, it is to this scanty development of decidual tissue that the characteristic course of extra-uterine pregnancy is to be attributed.

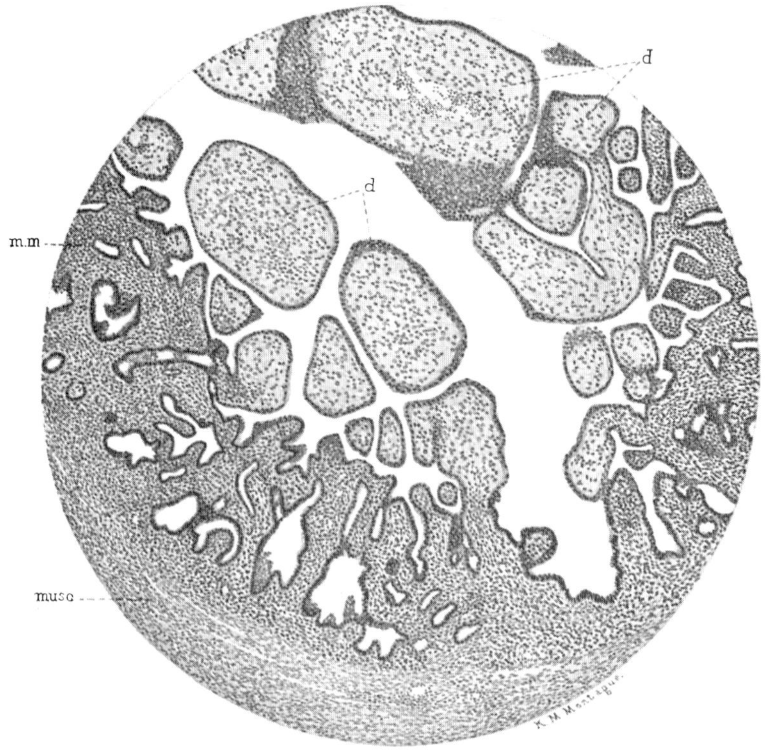

FIG. 480.—SECTION SHOWING FORMATION OF DECIDUAL CELLS IN RIGHT TUBE, WHILE THE PREGNANCY WAS IN THE OPPOSITE TUBE; CONCLUSIVELY DEMONSTRATING THAT THEY COULD NOT BE OF FŒTAL ORIGIN.

m.m., tubal mucosa; *musc.*, muscularis; *d.*, decidua.

Decidua Reflexa.—As to the mode of implantation of the ovum, and whether or not a decidua reflexa is developed in the tube, there has been not a little discussion. So far as can be gathered from the literature, none of the more recent writers describe a decidua reflexa analogous to that observed in uterine pregnancy, but most of them agree that, in the early stages, at least, the ovum is separated from the main lumen of the tube by a thicker or thinner layer of tissue, which practically represents the decidua reflexa—the *pseudo-reflexa* (see Fig. 482). This, no doubt, contains isolated decidual cells at an early period, but its inner surface soon becomes invaded by fœtal ectoderm and undergoes fibrinous or hyalin changes. Such a structure was present in all the early tubal pregnancies which I have examined, and the recent work of Couvelaire, Heinsius, Füth, Petersen, and others confirms my experience.

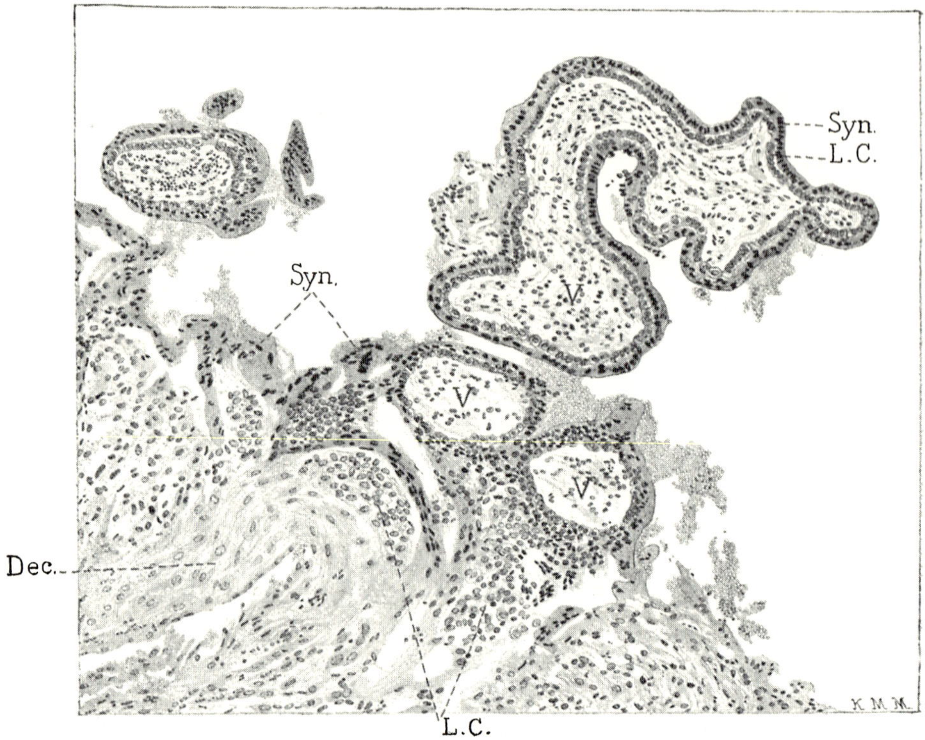

FIG. 481.—SECTION SHOWING ATTACHMENT OF CHORION TO TUBE WALL. × 90.
Dec., decidual cells ; *L.C.*, Langhans's cells ; *Syn.*, syncytium ; *V.*, villi.

Mode of Attachment of the Ovum.—The ovum becomes attached to the tube wall just as it does to the endometrium—that is, it penetrates the surface epithelium and burrows down into the tissue beneath it. As was said before, several specimens, which I had previously taken as indicating the development of the ovum in a diverticulum from the lumen of the tube, are to be interpreted in this manner (see Figs. 475 and 482).

Owing to the relative paucity of decidual cells, the changes following the implantation of the ovum differ considerably from those occurring in normal uterine pregnancy. As there is no distinct decidual membrane to separate the growing ovum from the underlying muscular and connective tissue, the rapidly proliferating trophoblast comes at once in contact with the tube wall, and promptly leads to its necrosis and ultimate conversion into fibrin. Since this tissue opposes but slight resistance to the growing fœtal elements, the chorionic villi within a short time extend through the entire thickness of the tube wall and come to lie just beneath its peritoneal covering, so that perforation becomes imminent. For the same reason, the maternal vessels are opened up much more rapidly than in uterine pregnancy, with the result that in many cases sudden hæmorrhage occurs beneath the ovum, thereby separating it from its attachments and causing an abortion. Again, if any obstacle is opposed to the escape of the blood from the fimbriated extremity, the thinned-out wall yields to the sudden increase in pressure and rupture occurs.

The formation of the placenta is analogous to that observed in uterine pregnancy, the only difference being that the maternal portion is made up of a tissue containing very few decidual cells, instead of the thick membrane observed in the uterus. As has already been pointed out, it is to the absence of a characteristic decidua that the early occurrence of abortion or rupture is to be attributed.

Diseases of Extra-uterine Ovum.—If an extra-uterine pregnancy goes on without interruption beyond the first few months, the ovum is exposed to all the diseases which may occur in the ordinary uterine form. Thus, hydatidiform mole has been observed by Otto, Recklinghausen, and Wenzel; hydramnios by Teuffel, Webster, and others; and deciduoma malignum by Ahlfeld and Marchand.

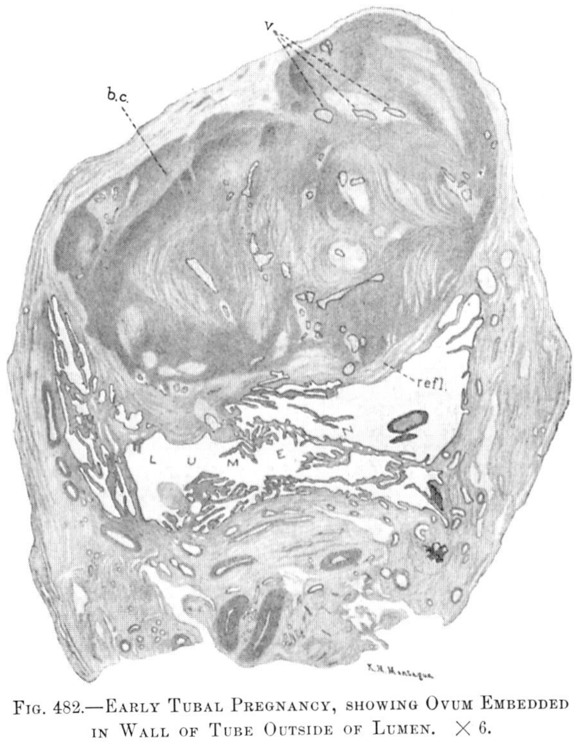

FIG. 482.—EARLY TUBAL PREGNANCY, SHOWING OVUM EMBEDDED IN WALL OF TUBE OUTSIDE OF LUMEN. × 6.
b.c., blood-clot; *v.*, chorionic villi; *refl.*, decidua reflexa.

Symptoms.—Unfortunately, the manifestations belonging to an uninterrupted extra-uterine pregnancy are not characteristic, and the patient and her physician are usually entirely unaware of the existence of any abnormality until rupture or tubal abortion occurs. Ordinarily the patient considers herself pregnant, presents the usual subjective symptoms, and possibly suffers from slight pains in one or other ovarian region, which she regards as the usual concomitants of her condition. In rare instances, indeed, she may have no idea that she is pregnant, and rupture may occur and perhaps prove fatal, even before she has missed a single menstrual period.

Suppression of the menses is not associated so regularly with this condition as with normal pregnancy, being noted in only 43 per cent of the cases observed by Martin and Orth, Mandl, Bouilly, and Wormser. These statements, however, do not carry as much weight as would appear at first sight, for frequently the hæmorrhage does not represent a genuine menstrual flow, but is due to endometritis, or to the fact that the dilated vessels in the uterine decidua are not covered by a layer of fœtal tissue. Moreover, the death of the extra-uterine fœtus at an early period, if not accompanied by rupture or abortion, is usually associated with more or less uterine hæmorrhage, which is frequently mistaken for the menstrual flow or for an early abortion, the latter belief being still further confirmed by the discharge of decidua.

In many cases the first manifestation of the abnormal pregnancy is the sudden occurrence of intense, lancinating pain in one or other ovarian region, which is soon followed by faintness, the patient rapidly passing into a condition of collapse. This indicates the occurrence of abortion or rupture. In the former case the patient usually rallies promptly, whereas, if rupture has occurred, the collapse deepens, the face becomes extremely pallid, and the patient complains of intense pain in the lower abdomen. The temperature is persistently subnormal, and an examination of the blood shows a marked diminution in the number of red corpuscles and in the amount of hæmoglobin. Death may occur within a few hours unless the hæmorrhage is checked by operative means. On the other hand, in most cases of abortion the general condition is not so alarming, and the patient gradually recovers. Vaginal examination a few days later frequently reveals the presence of a large fluctuant mass which fills a greater or lesser portion of the pelvic cavity—*pelvic hæmatocele.*

In the earlier text-books on gynæcology, hæmatocele was considered as a distinct disease, and it was mainly owing to Veit's observations that its connection with extra-uterine pregnancy was established. It is described as *diffuse* or *solitary,* according as the collection of blood occupies a considerable portion of the pelvic cavity or is confined to the neighbourhood of the fimbriated end of the tube. The diffuse variety usually occurs when pre-existing adhesions about the pelvic organs facilitate the coagulation of blood and aid in the formation of an organized membrane over it, thus shutting it off from the peritoneal cavity. According to Sänger, the solitary hæmatocele, on the other hand, does not require the presence of adhesions for its formation, but results from the gradual trickling of blood from the fimbriated end of the tube, the outer portions gradually coagulating and becoming organized, thus forming a capsule about the more fluid portions.

Hæmatocele formation, for the most part, promises a very favourable termination, for if left alone the mass gradually undergoes absorption and complete recovery occurs. Thorn has reported 157 cases with two fatalities, and Fehling 91 cases without a single death. Occasionally, however, if the hæmorrhage persists, the hæmatocele becomes larger and larger until it finally ruptures and its contents are poured out into the peritoneal cavity. Such an accident is speedily followed by collapse. Again, bacteria sometimes make their way into the mass from the intestines and cause suppuration.

If the patient survives the rupture of a tubal pregnancy, a *secondary abdominal pregnancy* may result, provided the placenta has not been separated to too great an extent. Under such circumstances the usual symptoms of pregnancy persist, except that the woman suffers more pain and feels the fœtal movements more acutely than usual. The pain is due partly to stretching and possibly to contractions of the fœtal sac, but principally to the pulling apart of adhesions which have formed between the sac and the various abdominal organs.

In a small number of cases of broad-ligament pregnancy, *secondary rupture* into the peritoneal cavity may occur at a later period, and the patient may bleed to death, or else a secondary abdominal pregnancy may result. In such cases the fœtus lies within the peritoneal cavity, while the placenta remains partly within the tube and partly between the folds of the broad ligament.

If a secondary abdominal pregnancy or, as now and again occurs, an unruptured tubal pregnancy goes on to term, *false labour* sets in, associated with distinct pains similar to those occurring in the early stages of labour in normal pregnancy. They are due to uterine contractions, since the fœtal sac contains so few muscular fibres that it cannot contract, and of course cannot lead to the birth of the extra-uterine child. False labour may last for a few hours or several days, and is soon followed by the death of the child, although in a small number of cases the fœtal movements have been known to persist for a considerable time after the cessation of the pains.

After the death of the fœtus, the placental circulation gradually becomes abolished, the amniotic fluid is absorbed, and the fœtal sac retracts, so that it occupies a much smaller space than formerly. The abdomen consequently becomes smaller, and its change in size is soon noticed by the patient. After its initial shrinking, the tumour may remain stationary in size for a number of years, the child becoming mummified or converted into a lithopædion; while in rare instances suppurative changes may lead to its gradual discharge or to the death of the patient from peritonitis.

Combined and Multiple Pregnancies.—Parry stated in his monograph that 22 out of the 500 cases of tubal pregnancy collected by him were complicated by a coexisting intra-uterine pregnancy. He designated the condition as *combined pregnancy*. The subject has since been investigated by Browne, Pantellani, Gutzwiller, Strauss, Zincke, and others, Strauss having collected 32 cases which had been reported up to 1898, not including a number of Parry's cases. Zincke, in 1902, collected 88 cases.

In rare instances twin tubal pregnancy has been observed, the embryos being sometimes found in the same tube, while in other cases there was a fœtus in each tube, both showing the same development. Sänger and Krusen have reported cases of triplet tubal pregnancy.

Repeated Tubal Pregnancy.—Parry collected 8 cases in which tubal pregnancy had occurred a second time in the same patient, and stated that Primrose, in 1594, was the first to describe such a condition. With the increased employment of abdominal surgery, the abnormality has been recognised quite frequently, the first series of cases was reported by Abel in 1893, and soon followed by those of Dorland, Weil, Varnier, and Pestalozza, the last author having collected 111 cases. In several instances only a few months had elapsed between the two pregnancies, while in others they were separated by an interval of several years.

Effects of Extra-uterine Pregnancy upon Subsequent Childbearing.—The presence of the products of an old extra-uterine pregnancy occasionally gives rise to dystocia and necessitates the performance of a major obstetrical operation. Thus, in the cases reported by Hugenberger, Schauta, and Sänger, Cæsarean section was performed; while in another, reported by Ott, the same operation would have been necessary had miscarriage not occurred at the sixth month. Hennigsen, Dibot, and Brossi induced premature labour, and Stein and Cheston resorted to craniotomy under similar circumstances.

As a rule, however, dystocia is not encountered, Funck-Brentano having collected 92 cases in which spontaneous labour occurred in patients still carrying the remains of a previous extra-uterine pregnancy.

Diagnosis.—Unfortunately, the symptoms to which uninterrupted extra-uterine pregnancy gives rise are usually so slight that the woman does not consult a physician, and as a result the diagnosis is rarely made before rupture or abortion occurs. If, however, a patient presenting the usual subjective and some of the objective symptoms of pregnancy be examined for any reason, and a unilateral tubal tumour be found, the diagnosis is fairly certain, especially if she has been sterile for a number of years or a long interval has elapsed since her last pregnancy. In such cases the uterus is somewhat enlarged and softened, while the tubal tumour is soft and doughy, and corresponds roughly in size to the supposed duration of pregnancy. The first positive diagnosis of unruptured tubal pregnancy was made by Veit in 1883, and in this country by Janvrin in 1886.

As a matter of fact, however, it very often happens that when laparotomy is performed for a supposed unruptured tubal pregnancy a tumour of some other origin is found. On the other hand, the unruptured pregnant tube may prolapse into Douglas's *cul-de-sac* and be mistaken for the body of a retroflexed pregnant uterus, so that an attempt at its reposition not infrequently leads to rupture and occasionally to death.

When the fœtus has died before the occurrence of rupture or abortion, errors in diagnosis are common, and many cases are mistaken for incomplete uterine abortions or for tubal tumours associated with uterine hæmorrhage. For this reason no attempt should ever be made to empty the uterus in a case of suspected incomplete abortion unless the tubes and ovaries have been previously palpated. If a careful examination shows that a tumour is present on either side, the possibility of tubal pregnancy should be seriously considered.

It is generally taught that the discharge of a distinct decidual cast from the uterus, without evidence of a fœtus, is a characteristic sign of tubal pregnancy. But that now and again such a structure may be discharged without the existence of pregnancy of any kind was demonstrated by Griffiths and Dakin. Ott and Ayers believe that the presence of decidual tissue in the uterus, in the absence of a fœtus, affords conclusive evidence of the existence of tubal pregnancy, especially if a tumour mass can be detected on one side. In doubtful cases they recommend curettage for diagnostic purposes. My own experience has taught me that the presence of decidua under such circumstances usually affords strong presumptive evidence, but that its absence is not an equally convincing negative proof, for occasionally the decidua may have been cast off at an early period and been replaced by normal endometrium by the time the patient is examined.

The diagnosis of tubal abortion or rupture, on the other hand, usually offers no difficulty, and should be made without hesitation whenever a patient who is believed to be pregnant has complained of pain in the lower part of the abdomen, and suddenly becomes faint, deathly pale, and sinks into a state of collapse. If the collapse becomes more profound and the temperature is subnormal, rupture has probably occurred. On the other hand, if rapid recovery ensues, the probabilities are that one has to deal with an abortion, and the subsequent formation of an hæmatocele settles the question.

As has already been pointed out, rupture may occur at a very early period, even before the patient believes herself pregnant. In view of such a possibility, therefore, one should regard sudden collapse associated with symptoms of abdominal hæmorrhage in a woman during the childbearing period, as *primâ facie* evidence of a ruptured tubal pregnancy. By so doing, and operating promptly in suitable cases, a number of lives will be saved which otherwise would inevitably be lost.

Very often the patient comes into the hands of the physician some time after she has recovered from the primary shock due to abortion or rupture. Under such circumstances vaginal examination will show a mass on one side of the uterus which is usually mistaken for pelvic inflammatory trouble. In a small number of cases, a fluctuant tumour can be felt posterior and lateral to the uterus, and when exploratory puncture through the vagina reveals the presence of a dark bloody fluid, the diagnosis of a pelvic hæmatocele or a broad-ligament hæmatoma is assured.

The diagnosis of secondary abdominal pregnancy is rarely made until false labour supervenes, unless the physician's attention is particularly directed to the previous history of the case. If, however, a careful physical examination is made, the uterus will be found much smaller than it should be for the duration of the pregnancy, and more or less displaced by the fœtal sac, which makes up the greater part of the abdominal enlargement. Moreover, the child can be palpated much more readily than usual, and its movements are often very painful to the mother. In doubtful cases the introduction of a sound into the uterus is permissible.

The diagnosis of broad-ligament pregnancy can be made by finding the uterus pushed to one side by a tumour intimately connected with it, which at the same time depresses the vaginal vault instead of being high up in the abdominal cavity.

The diagnosis of combined intra-uterine and extra-uterine pregnancy is rarely made until rupture of the extra-uterine pregnancy, or the persistence of symptoms after the expulsion of the uterine fœtus, leads to a very careful examination. The condition has never been diagnosed in the later months of pregnancy, although in several instances the presence of twins was recognised.

After extra-uterine pregnancy has reached full term the diagnosis is usually easy, and is based upon the history of pregnancy followed by a false labour and a gradual decrease in the size of the abdomen. Examination shows the uterus to be practically normal in size, and displaced to a varying extent by a large tumour more or less intimately connected with it, in which the outlines of the child can occasionally be distinguished.

To recapitulate, a positive diagnosis is occasionally made before rupture, but in the vast majority of cases the condition escapes recognition until symptoms of collapse point to the probability of rupture or abortion. In advanced cases careful examination will usually disclose the real condition of affairs, and when full term has been passed the history is so characteristic that mistakes should hardly occur.

Treatment.—As soon as an unruptured extra-uterine pregnancy is positively diagnosed, its immediate removal by laparotomy is urgently indicated, since rupture may occur at any time and the patient die from hæmorrhage before operative aid can be obtained. The importance of immediate operation cannot be too strongly emphasized, and all methods of treatment which aim at destroying the fœtus and thus terminating pregnancy without operation are absolutely unjustifiable. This applies not only to the use of electricity, but also to the injection of various poisonous substances into the gestation sac. Even when such procedures are successful, the danger to the mother is by no means at an end, since rupture sometimes takes place after the death of the fœtus; and, even if this accident does not occur, the retention of the product of conception renders the tube a useless organ.

Tait, in 1883, performed the first laparotomy for the purpose of checking hæmorrhage from a ruptured tubal pregnancy. After he had demonstrated the ease with which the procedure could be performed and the surprisingly good results obtained thereby, the operation came into general use. Its beneficent results were clearly demonstrated by Schauta, who, after a careful study of the literature, found that 123 cases operated upon and 121 cases treated without operation presented a mortality of 5.7 and 86.9 per cent respectively.

For these reasons, whenever we see a possibly pregnant woman in a state of profound collapse, and presenting a deathly pallor of the face, a subnormal temperature, and other symptoms of intra-abdominal hæmorrhage, immediate operation is demanded, unless, indeed, her condition is so desperate that death is imminent.

The abdomen should be opened rapidly, under cocaine anæsthesia if necessary. In many cases blood spurts from the abdomen as soon as the peritonæum is incised, and completely obscures the field of operation. Under these circumstances the hand passed down alongside of the uterus seizes the tubal mass, which is then clamped on either side by long forceps. The hæmorrhage having been controlled in this way, the blood-clots are removed and the field of operation is cleaned up, after which the operator will be able to remove the mass and replace the clamps by ligatures, under the guidance of the eye, at comparative leisure. After the fœtal sac has been taken away, it is not advisable to attempt to remove all the blood from the peritoneal cavity unless the patient's condition is fairly satisfactory.

Not infrequently the appendages on the opposite side may be the seat of chronic inflammatory lesions. Some discretion should be exercised as to their removal at this time, it being far better to allow them to remain than to prolong the operation if the patient is in a very bad condition. In desperate cases it is advisable to begin the subcutaneous or intravenous infusion of sterile salt solution while the necessary preparations for the operation are being made. In less severe cases good results follow the introduction of several litres of it into the abdomen just before the wound is closed.

In certain cases of tubal abortion, Prochownick, Martin, and others advocate attempting to save the tube, if possible, by opening it and removing the product of conception, after which it is closed by sutures. Such a procedure may occasionally be advisable if the patient is in good condition, but proof is still lacking that a tube so treated regains its normal functions.

A freshly ruptured tubal pregnancy should not be attacked through the vagina, for the reason that the procedure is often more difficult than a laparotomy, and affords but a limited view of the field of operation, while there is always a possibility that it cannot be completed by the vaginal route, and that an eventual resort to laparotomy will become necessary.

If the patient is not seen until the acute symptoms have subsided and the effused blood has become encapsulated as an hæmatocele, she should be put to bed and carefully watched, operative procedures being instituted only when the hæmatocele steadily increases in size or presents symptoms indicative of suppuration. This condition, however, rarely presents itself, and Thorn operated upon only 6 out of 157 such cases. When, however, the occasion demands it, excellent results are obtained by evacuating the hæmatocele through an incision in the vaginal fornix and packing the cavity with sterile gauze, as has been recommended by Kelly, Segond, and others. Broad-ligament hæmatomata should be treated in a similar manner.

In the later months, the treatment of extra-uterine pregnancy differs markedly according as the fœtus is alive or dead. In very rare cases a living fœtus may be inclosed in an unruptured tubal or ovarian sac, or lie between the layers of the unfolded broad ligament. More frequently, however, one has to deal with a secondary abdominal pregnancy, with the child lying in the peritoneal cavity and inclosed in a sac composed of the fœtal membranes and newly formed adhesions, the placenta being within the tube or broadly implanted upon the floor of the pelvis. Whatever the anatomical conditions, the mother is constantly exposed to the possibility of sudden and acute hæmorrhage so long as pregnancy continues, and accordingly prompt laparotomy is the only conservative method of treatment.

When the child has nearly attained the period of viability, certain authorities urge the propriety of deferring the operation for a few weeks in its interests. Such a course may be permissible in exceptional cases, provided the increased dangers of waiting are carefully explained to the patient and her family and accepted by them.

In a small number of cases the operation is comparatively easy and the fœtal sac can be removed as readily as a large ovarian cyst. More frequently, however, the fœtal sac is markedly adherent to surrounding organs, or the placental attachment is spread over a broad area, thereby markedly increasing the difficulty of the operation.

Now and again, in broad-ligament pregnancies it will be found that the portion of the broad ligament immediately adjoining the uterus has not been spread apart by the growing ovum, and under such circumstances the entire sac may be removed without great difficulty by ligating the vessels at the pelvic brim and at the uterine cornu before attempting its enucleation.

As a rule, however, the complete removal of the gestation sac is by no means easy, and can only be effected by removing the uterus as well. When, as occasionally happens, it is apparent that the operation cannot be completed without markedly endangering the life of the patient, the sac should be incised, the placenta being avoided, if possible, and the fœtus extracted. The margins of the sac are then stitched to the abdominal incision, the umbilical cord is cut off short, and the cavity packed with sterile gauze, the placenta being left *in situ* and afterward allowed to come away piecemeal. This method necessarily entails a prolonged convalescence, but is much safer than any attempt at removal of the placenta. Occasionally, however, partial separation of the placenta gives rise to such profuse hæmorrhage that its removal must be effected at any cost in the hope of preventing immediate death.

The results following laparotomy in advanced cases of extra-uterine pregnancy with a living child have improved markedly since the introduction of aseptic methods. This fact was clearly shown by Harris, who collected 27 such cases in 1887 and 145 additional cases ten years later, with a mortality of 93 and 31 per cent respectively. Nevertheless, the operation is still one of the most dangerous which the gynæcologist is called upon to perform.

When the fœtus is dead the conditions are much more favourable, as the dangers incident to bleeding from the placental site are markedly diminished. For this reason the operation should be deferred for six or eight weeks after fœtal death in order to permit the obliteration of the maternal blood spaces in the placenta, and thus render possible its removal without hæmorrhage. In such cases, however, should dangerous symptoms supervene, immediate interference is indicated. On the other hand, the operation should not be deferred too long, as there is always a possibility that the fœtal sac may become infected from the intestinal tract, when a fatal peritonitis may result. Lusk, in 1886, made an earnest plea for prompt operation in such cases, and supported his contention by a long array of statistics.

In a small number of cases of advanced extra-uterine pregnancy, operation through the vagina has been recommended. This method of procedure, however, has a very limited field, and Herman is right in saying that it should be performed only when the fœtus is firmly impacted in the pelvis and depresses the vaginal vault to such an extent as to make it probable that it can be extracted without difficulty. In all other cases laparotomy is the operation of choice.

LITERATURE

ABEL. Zur Anatomie der Eileiterschwangerschaft nebst Bemerkungen zur Entwickelung der menschlichen Placenta. Archiv f. Gyn., 1891, xxxix, 393–436.

Ueber wiederholte Tubengravidität bei derselben Frau. Archiv f. Gyn., 1893, xlv, 55–89.

AHLFELD. Ein Fall von Sarcoma uteri deciduo-cellulare bei Tubenschwangerschaft. Monatsschr. f. Geb. u. Gyn., 1895, i, 209–213.

ANNING and LITTLEWOOD. A Case of Primary Ovarian Pregnancy, etc. Trans. London Obst. Soc., 1901, xliii; Lancet, 1901, i, 100.

ASCHOFF. Anatomie der Extrauterinschwangerschaft. Ziegler's Beiträge, 1899, xxv, H. 2.

Die Beziehungen der tubaren Placenta zum Tubenabort und zur Tubenruptur. Archiv f. Gyn., 1900, lx, 523–533.

Neuere Arbeiten über die Anat. u. Aetiologie der Tubenschwangerschaften. Centralbl. f. allg. Path. u. path. Anat., 1901, Nr. 11 u. 12.

AYERS. Decidua in the Diagnosis of Extra-uterine Pregnancy. Amer. Jour. Obst., 1892, xxvi, 289–306.

BECK. Ectopic Pregnancy Twice in the Same Patient, the Second Time complicated by Intestinal Obstruction. Amer. Jour. Obst., 1893, xxvii, 570–576.

VON BOTH. Rechtsseitige Tubarschwangerschaft. Ruptur im 5ten Monat. Entbindung des frei in der Bauchhöhle lebenden Kindes durch Laparotomie im 8ten Monat. Monatsschr. f. Geb. u. Gyn., 1899, 782–794.

BOUILLY. Notes sur la grossesse extra-utérine tirées de l'analyse de cinquante observations personelles. La Gynécologie, 1898, iii, 1–16.

BRESLAU. Zur Aetiologie und path. Anatomie der Extrauterinschwangerschaft. Monatsschr. f. Geb. u. Gyn., 1863, xxi, Supplement Heft, 119–124.

BROSSI. Quoted by Sänger.

BROWNE. A Contribution to the History of Combined Intra-uterine and Extra-uterine Twin Pregnancy. Trans. Amer. Gyn. Soc., 1882, vi, 444–462.

CAMPBELL. Abhandlung über die Schwangerschaft ausserhalb der Gebärmutter. Translated from the English by Dr. Ecker, Karlsruhe and Freiburg, 1841.

CHESTON. Quoted by Funck-Brentano.

CHIARI. Beiträge zur Lehre von der Graviditas tubaria. Zeitschr. f. Heilkunde, 1887, viii.

COUVELAIRE. Note sur l'anatomie de la réfléchie dans la grossesse tubaire. Comptes rendus Soc. d'obst. de gyn. et de pæd. de Paris, 1900, ii, 50–61.

Quelques points de l'anatomie des grossesses tubaires en évolution, etc. Revue de gyn., 1902, vi, 51–84.

CROFT. An Anomalous Case of Ectopic Pregnancy, probably Ovarian. Trans. London Obst. Soc., 1900, xlii, 316–323.

DAKIN. Cast from the Uterus having all the Characters of the Decidual Membrane Found in Connection with Ectopic Gestation, etc. Trans. Lond. Obst. Soc., 1897, xxxviii, 385–388.

DEZEIMERIS. Grossesses extra-utérines. Jour. des conn. méd.-chir., Paris, Dec., 1836.

DIBOT. Quoted by Sänger. Monatsschr. f. Geb. u. Gyn., 1895, i, 21–28.

DOBBERT. Sechzig Fälle in frühen Entwickelungsstadien unterbrochener Tubenschwangerschaften. Archiv f. Gyn., 1902, lxvi, 70–123.

DORLAND. Repeated Extra-uterine Pregnancy. Amer. Jour. Obst., 1898, xxxvii, 478–491.

Dührssen. Ueber operative Behandlung, insbesondere die vaginale Coeliotomie bei Tubarschwangerschaft, nebst Bemerkungen zur Aetiologie der Tubarschwangerschaft und Beschreibung eines Tubenpolypen. Archiv f. Gyn., 1897, liv, 207–323.

Emanuel. Eine zwanzigjahre getragene Extrauterinschwangerschaft. Centralbl. f. Gyn., 1894, 1306.

Fehling. Die Bedeutung der Tubenruptur und des Tubaraborts für Verlauf, Prognose und Therapie der Tubarschwangerschaft. Zeitschr. f. Geb. u. Gyn., 1898, xxxviii, 67–100.

Franck. Ueber Extrauterinschwangerschaft mit besonderer Berücksichtigung der Ovarialgravidität. Centralbl. f. Gyn., 1895, 545.

Franz. Ueber Einbettung u. Wachstum des Eies im Eierstock. Hegar's Beiträge zur Geb. u. Gyn., 1902, vi, 70–81.

Funck-Brentano. Des grossesses utérines survenant après la grossesse extra-utérine. Thèse de Paris, 1898.

Füth. Ueber die Einbettung des Eies in der Tube. Archiv f. Gyn., 1901, lxiii, 97–158.

Geuer. Ovarialschwangerschaft. Centralbl. f. Gyn., 1894, 391.

Gilford. Ovarian Pregnancy. British Med. Jour., 1901, ii, 963–964.

Glitsch. Zur Aetiologie der Tubenschwangerschaft. Archiv f. Gyn., 1900, lx, 385–425.

Gottschalk. Ein Präparat von Ovarialschwangerschaft aus der 3.–4. Woche der Gravidität. Centralbl. f. Gyn., 1886, 727.

Ein Lithokelyphopädion, das gleichzeitig als Fall von reiner Eierstocksschwangerschaft sehr bemerkenswerth ist. Verhandlungen der deutschen Ges. f. Gyn., 1893, 304–305.

Granville. Graphic Illustrations of Abortion and Diseases of Menstruation. London, 1834.

Griffiths. Note on the Importance of a Decidual Cast as Evidence of Extra-uterine Gestation. Trans. London Obst. Soc., 1894, xxxvi, 335–340.

Gestation in the Fallopian Tube, and the Structural Changes that take Place in its Walls. Jour. of Pathology and Bacteriology, 1898, v, 443–459.

Gurgui. Die Ovarialschwangerschaft vom path. anat. Standpunkte. Stuttgart, 1880, 150.

Gutzwiller. Ein Fall von gleichzeitiger Extra- und Intrauteringravidität. Zusammenstellung und Betrachtung derartiger Fälle. Archiv f. Gyn., 1893, xliii, 223–251.

Harris. Operation of Primary Laparotomy in Cases of Extra-uterine Pregnancy, with a Tabular Record showing the Results in 27 Women under 26 Operators. Amer. Jour. Obst., 1887, xx, 1154–1167.

Weitere Fortschritte der Entbindung ektopischer lebensfähiger Früchte durch Koeliotomie. Monatsschr. f. Geb. u. Gyn., 1897, vi, 137–156.

Hecker. Beiträge zur Lehre von der Schwangerschaft ausserhalb der Gebärmutterhöhle. Monatsschr. f. Geburtsk., 1859, xiii, 81–123.

Hein. Eierstockschwangerschaft. Archiv f. path. Anat. u. Physiol., 1847, i. 513–537.

Heinsius. Beiträge zur Lehre von der Tubengravidität, etc. Zeitschr. f. Geb. u. Gyn., 1901, xlvi, 385–434.

Ueber tubare Einbettung des menschlichen Eies. Monatsschr. f. Geb. u. Gyn., 1902, xv, 315–322.

Hennig. Die Krankheiten der Eileiter und die Tubenschwangerschaft. Stuttgart, 1876.

Hennigsen. Abdominalschwangerschaft bei einer Sechstgebärenden. Archiv f. Gyn., 1870, i, 335–340.

Henrotin et Herzog. Anomalies du canal de Müller comme cause des grossesses ectopiques. Revue de gyn., 1898, 633–649.

Herman. On Delivery by the Vagina in Extra-uterine Gestation. Trans. London Obst. Soc., 1887, xxix, 429–455.

Herzfeld. Ueber einen Fall von Ovarialgravidität, uterine Schwangerschaft. Laparotomie. Heilung. Wiener klin. Wochenschr., 1891, Nr. 43, 802–804.

HOFMEIER. Zur Kenntniss dem normalen Uterusschleimhaut. Centralbl. f. Gyn., 1893, Nr. 33, 764–766.

HUGENBERGER. Bericht aus dem Hebammen-Institut in Moskau. St. Petersburg, 1863, 122.

JANVRIN. A Case of Tubal Pregnancy of Unusual Interest. Trans. Amer. Gyn. Soc., 1886, xi, 471–484.

KELLY. The Treatment of Extra-uterine Pregnancy ruptured in the Early Months by Vaginal Puncture and Drainage. Trans. Amer. Gyn. Soc., 1896, xxi, 190–209.

KOUWER. Fall von Schwangerschaft im Graaf'schen Follikel. Centralbl. f. Gyn., 1897, 1426.

KREISCH. Beitrag zur Anatomie und Pathologie der Tubargravidität. Monatsschr. f. Geb. u. Gyn., 1899, ix, 794–812.

KÜCHENMEISTER. Ueber Lithopädion. Archiv f. Gyn., 1881, xvii, 153–359.

KÜHNE. Beitrag zur Anatomie der Tubenschwangerschaft. Marburg, 1899.

KÜSTNER. Der Fick'sche Fall von Abdominalschwangerschaft—eine Eierstocksschwangerschaft. Verh. der deutschen Ges. f. Gyn., 1890, 213–334.

Ueber Extrauterinschwangerschaft. Volkmann's Sammlung klin. Vorträge, N. F., 1899, Nr. 244–245.

LANDAU und RHEINSTEIN. Beiträge zur pathologischen Anatomie der Tube. Archiv f. Gyn., 1891, xxxix, 273–290.

LANGE. Beiträge zur Frage der Deciduabildung in der Tube, etc. Monatsschr. f. Geb. u. Gyn., 1902, xv, 48–71.

LARSEN. See Tainturier.

LEOPOLD. Zur Lehre von der Graviditas interstitialis. Archiv f. Gyn., 1878, xiii, 355–365.

Ovarialschwangerschaft mit Lithopädionbildung von 35-jähriger Dauer. Archiv f. Gyn., 1882, xix, 210–218.

Beiträge zur Graviditas extrauterina. 1. Graviditas interstitialis. 2. Graviditas auf der Fimbria ovarica bez. Plica infundibulo-ovarica. 3. Graviditas ovarialis. Archiv f. Gyn., 1899, lviii, 526–565.

Beitrag zur Graviditas extra-uterina. 4. Die Graviditas tubo-ovarialis. Archiv f. Gyn., 1899, lix, 557–594.

LUDWIG. Eierstocksschwangerschaft neben normaler uteriner Schwangerschaft, etc. Wiener klin. Wochenschr., 1896, Nr. 27, 600–604.

LUSK. The Desirability of the Early Performance of Laparotomy in Cases of Abdominal Pregnancy. British Med. Jour., 1886, ii, 1083–1090.

MANDL. Ueber den feineren Bau der Eileiter während und ausserhalb der Schwangerschaft. Monatsschr. f. Geb. u. Gyn., 1897, V. Ergänzungsheft, 130–139.

Ueber die Richtung der Flimmerbewegung im menschlichen Uterus. Centralbl. f. Gyn., 1898, Nr. 13, 323–328.

MANDL und SCHMIDT. Beiträge zur Aetiologie und path. Anatomie der Eileiterschwangerschaften. Archiv f. Gyn., 1898, lvi, 401–487.

MARTIN. Ein Fall von Ovarialschwangerschaft mit Carcinoma colli uteri. Zeitschr. f. Geb. u. Gyn., 1892, xxiii, 179.

Zur Kenntniss der Tubarschwangerschaft. Monatsschr. f. Geb. u. Gyn., 1897, v, 1–7 and 244–246.

MARTIN und ORTHMANN. Eileiterschwangerschaft. Die Krankheiten der Eileiter von A. Martin, Berlin u. Leipzig, 1895, 303–399.

MAYER. Kritik der Extrauterinschwangerschaft, etc. Giessen, 1845.

MOERICKE. Zur Aetiologie der Tuben-gravidität. Sammlung zwangloser Abhandlungen aus dem Gebiete der Frauenheilkunde u. Geb., 1900, Bd. iii, H. 4 u. 5.

NOBLE. Remarks on Ectopic Pregnancy. Amer. Gyn. and Obst. Jour., 1895, vi, 167–171.

OLIVER. Ovarian Pregnancy. Lancet, 1896, ii, 241.

OTT. Beiträge zur Kenntniss der ektopischen Formen der Schwangerschaft. Leipzig, 1898.

OTTO. Ueber Tubenschwangerschaft, mit Berücksichtigung eines Falles von Graviditas tubaria molaris hydatidosa. D. I., Greifswald, 1871.

PANTELLANI. Die mehrfache Schwangerschaft, die Extrauteringravidität, etc. Zeitschr. f. Geb. u. Gyn., 1896, xxv, 373–413.

PARRY. Extra-uterine Pregnancy. London, 1876.

PATENKO. Zur Lehre von der Extrauterinschwangerschaft (Graviditas ovarialis). Archiv f. Gyn., 1879, xiv, 156–164.

PESTALOZZA. Sulla gravidanza tubarica recidivante. Annali di ost. e gin., 1901, No. 1.

PETERS. Ueber die Einbettung des menschlichen Eies. Wien, 1899.

PETERSEN. Beiträge zur path. Anatomie der graviden Tube. Berlin, 1902.

PINARD. Nouveaux documents pour servir a l'histoire de la grossesse extra-utérine. Annales de Gyn., 1892, xxxviii, 1–11; 99–118; 181–188.

PROCHOWNICK. Ein Beitrag zur Mekanik des Tubenaborts. Festschrift der Ges. f. Geb. u. Gyn. in Berlin, Wien, 1894, 266–295.

Zur Mekanik des Tubenaborts. Archiv f. Gyn., 1895, xlix, 177–241.

ROSENTHAL. Ein Fall intramuraler Schwangerschaft. Centralbl. f. Gyn., 1896, 1297–1305.

SÄNGER. Ueber einen Fall von ektopischer Drillingsschwangerschaft. Centralbl. f. Gyn., 1893, 148.

Ueber solitäre Hämatocele und deren Organisation. Verhand. der deutschen Ges. f. Gyn., 1893, 281–302.

Conception durch ein accessorisches Tubenostium. Kaiserschnitt bedingt durch frühere ektopische Schwangerschaft. Monatsschr. f. Geb. u. Gyn., 1895, i, 21–28.

SAXTORPH. Quoted by Spiegelberg.

SCHAUTA. Beiträge zur Casuistik, Prognose und Therapie der extrauterinen Schwangerschaft. Prag, 1891.

VON SCHRENCK. Ueber ektopischer Gravidität. D. I., Dorpat, 1893.

SEGOND. Traitement des grossesses extra-utérines. Annales de Gyn., October, 1898, l, 241–316.

SIPPEL. Ueber äussere Ueberwanderung des Eies. Centralbl. f. Gyn., 1901, 289–296.

SPIEGELBERG. Eine ausgetragene Tubenschwangerschaft. Archiv f. Gyn., 1870, i, 406–414.

Zur Casuistik der Ovarialschwangerschaft. Archiv f. Gyn., 1878, xiii, 73–79.

STEIN. Quoted by Funck-Brentano.

STRAUSS. Tubargravidität bei gleichzeitiger intrauteriner Schwangerschaft. Zeitschr. f. Geb. u. Gyn., 1900, xliv, 26–38.

SUTTON, BLAND. Tubal Pregnancy. Surgical Diseases of the Ovaries and Fallopian Tubes. Philadelphia, 1891, 313–326.

TAINTURIER. Etiologie de la grossesse ectopique. Thèse de Paris, 1895.

TAIT. Lectures on Ectopic Pregnancy and Pelvic Hæmatocele. Birmingham, 1888, 107.

TAYLOR. Extra-uterine Pregnancy. A Clinical and Operative Study. London, 1899, 205.

THOMPSON. Ovarian Pregnancy, with Report of a Case. American Gynecology, 1902, i, 1–15.

THORN. Ueber Beckenhämatome. Volkmann's Sammlung klin. Vorträge, N. F., Nr. 119 u. 120.

TOTH. Beiträge zur Frage der ektopischen Schwangerschaft. Archiv f. Gyn., 1896, li, 410–482.

TEUFFEL. Hydramnion bei Extrauterinschwangerschaft. Archiv f. Gyn., 1884, xxii, 57–64.

TUSSENBROEK. Un cas de grossesse ovarienne (Grossesse dans un Follicule de Graaf). Annales de Gyn., 1899, lii, 537–573.

UHDE. Graviditas ovarii. Monatsschr. f. Geburtsk., 1857, x, 339–342.

VARNIER. Recidive de grossesse ectopique. Comptes rendus Soc. d'obst. de gyn., et de pæd. de Paris, 1900, ii, 296–301.

VEIT. Die Eileiterschwangerschaft. Stuttgart, 1884.

VELPEAU. Traité complet de l'art des accouchements. Paris, 1835, t. i, 214.

VOIGT. Schwangerschaft auf der Fimbria ovarica. Monatsschr. f. Geb. u. Gyn., 1898, viii, 222–232.

WALTER. Einige Beobachtungen über Schwangerschaft ausserhalb der Gebärmutter. Monatsschr. f. Geburtsk., 1861, xvii.

WEBSTER. Ectopic Pregnancy. Edinburgh and London, 1895.

WEIL. Ueber wiederholte Eileiterschwangerschaft. Prager med. Wochenschr., 1899, Nrs. 1, 2, 3.

WENZEL. Blasenmole im Eileiter. Alte Erfahrungen im Lichte der neuen Zeit, Wiesbaden, 1893, 85–89.

WERTH. Beiträge zur Anatomie und zur operativen Behandlung der Extrauterinschwangerschaft. Stuttgart, 1887.

WILLIAMS. Contribution to the Normal and Pathological Histology of the Fallopian Tubes. Amer. Jour. Med. Sciences, October, 1891.

WORMSER. Beiträge zur Kenntniss der Extrauteringravidität. Hegar's Beiträge f. Geb. u. Gyn., 1899, 289-321.

WYDER. Beiträge zur Lehre von der Extrauterinschwangerschaft und dem Orte des Zusammentreffens von Ovulum und Spermatozoen. Archiv f. Gyn., 1886, xxviii, 325–407.

ZEDEL. Zur Anatomie der schwangeren Tube mit besonderer Berücksichtigung des Baues der tubaren Placenta. Zeitschr. f. Geb. u. Gyn., 1893, xxvi, 78–143.

ZINCKE. A Case of Extra- and Intra-uterine Pregnancy. Amer. Jour. Obst., 1902, xlv, 623–646.

ZWEIFEL. Ueber Extrauteringravidität und retro-uterine Hämatome. Archiv f. Gynäkologie, 1891, xli, 1–61.

PATHOLOGY OF LABOUR

CHAPTER XXXI

DYSTOCIA DUE TO ANOMALIES OF THE EXPULSIVE FORCES

Dystocia or *difficult labour* may be due to various ætiological factors, and is most commonly encountered in the following groups of cases: (1) Those in which the expulsive forces are subnormal and are not sufficiently strong to overcome the natural resistance offered to the birth of the child by the bony canal and the maternal soft parts. (2) Those in which, although the expulsive forces may be of normal strength, abnormalities in the structure or character of the birth canal offer an insuperable mechanical obstacle to the descent of the presenting part. (3) Those in which the fœtus, on account of faulty presentation or excessive development, cannot be extruded by the *vis a tergo*. (4) Those cases in which accidental complications, such as eclampsia, hæmorrhage, or rupture of the uterus, lead to various irregularities which interfere with the normal progress of labour.

Dystocia due to Anomalies of the Expulsive Forces.—The expulsion of the fœtus is brought about by the contractions of the uterus, re-enforced towards the latter half of the second stage of labour by the action of the muscles of the abdominal wall. Either of these factors may be lacking in force or intensity, while occasionally they may be abnormally strong.

Unfortunately, there is no absolute standard by which the character of the labour pains can be gauged. Thus, in many multiparous women a rapid and happy termination of labour not uncommonly follows a few relatively slight pains, which in primiparæ would prove quite inadequate to bring about the desired result. Clinically the efficiency of the uterine contractions may be measured by their effect upon the course and duration of labour, provided there is no serious mechanical obstacle to be overcome, so that, other things being equal, prolonged or precipitate labour occurs as a result of abnormalities in their frequency and intensity.

Prolonged Labour.—Normally, in the early stages of labour, the uterine contractions occur at infrequent intervals, and gradually increase in frequency, intensity, and duration as its termination is approached. Moreover, a proper alternation between the contraction and relaxation of the uterus is a very important requisite for the successful accomplishment of delivery.

Anomalies are often noted in the first stage of labour, the contractions recurring in some patients at frequent intervals and being cramp-like in character and very painful, but exerting very little influence upon the dilatation of the cervix and the expulsion of the child. As a result, obliteration of the cervical canal is brought about very slowly, and the external os undergoes but little change. As a rule, such conditions do not give rise to serious complications, since under appropriate treatment the pains assume a more normal character, after which the termination of labour is speedily accomplished.

More frequently, however, the first-stage pains recur at long intervals and are feeble in character, so that labour, instead of being terminated within the usual period, may drag on for days. If the membranes are unruptured and the patient is in good condition, the delay may be regarded with equanimity, since in the great majority of instances the pains eventually become stronger and more frequent, when the birth of the child is effected without interference. For this reason, the obstetrician should not interfere too hastily, but should encourage the patient to bear her suffering patiently by a plain statement of the facts of the case, and the assurance that a favourable outcome may be expected not only for her but also for the child.

Again, labour sometimes begins in a perfectly typical manner and gives every promise of an ordinarily speedy termination, and yet after a certain lapse of time, without any appreciable cause, the pains become less frequent and less intense, although giving rise to quite as much or even more suffering than previously. At the same time, the cervix, which was becoming obliterated and dilated in a satisfactory manner, ceases to make further progress, and labour apparently comes to a standstill. Such a condition is frequently due to what is termed *inertia uteri.*

In all of these cases, the prolongation of labour is commonly attributed to the imperfect dilatation of the cervix, which is supposed to be due to an abnormal rigidity of its tissues. Ordinarily, however, the converse is true, and the condition is the direct result of faulty uterine contractions. That this latter view is correct, is shown by the fact that the appearance of satisfactory contractions is promptly followed by rapid dilatation of the cervix and a happy termination of labour. On the other hand, however, especially in primiparæ of thirty years of age or over, excessive rigidity of the cervix and its consequent tardy and imperfect dilatation may be the essential factor in the production of the dystocia, especially when a further complication has been introduced by the premature rupture of the membranes.

This accident occurs occasionally in primiparæ, and not infrequently in multiparous women before the onset of uterine contractions, and gives rise to what is designated as "*dry labour,*" which is usually unduly prolonged and very painful. The delay is due in great part to the absence of the hydrostatic action of the bag of waters, in consequence of which the changes in the cervix must be brought about almost entirely by the direct pressure of the presenting part, which acts as a dilating wedge of imperfect shape and consistency.

This complication is usually not so serious in multiparous as in primiparous women, since in the former labour, as a rule, sets in within a short time after the discharge of the liquor amnii. Occasionally, however, hours, days, and in rare instances even weeks may elapse before it occurs.

Not uncommonly obliteration of the cervical canal takes place without difficulty, while the external os alone appears to offer the obstacle to dilatation. In such cases its margins are often extremely thin and sharp, and during a contraction may not exceed a sheet of paper in thickness. On the other hand, especially when labour is unduly prolonged, they may become thick and œdematous.

In the absence of any mechanical obstacle, prolongation of the second stage of labour is rarely due to abnormalities in the uterine contractions, but rather to deficient action of the abdominal muscles. In primiparous women, especially, the tardy labour is often ascribed to the resistance offered by a rigid perinæum and a small vaginal outlet, but in the majority of cases this is only apparent, the delay being really due to an insufficient *vis a tergo.*

Ætiology.—Uterine insufficiency is usually attributed to one of three causes: faulty development or diseased conditions of the uterine musculature, anomalies in its innervation, or mechanical interference with its contraction. The first factor is the one most frequently concerned in the causation of tardy labour, and is especially likely to be associated with imperfect general development, being frequently observed in patients presenting varieties of the justo-minor pelvis, but only rarely in sufferers from rhachitic deformities. On the other hand, faulty development of the musculature is occasionally noted in apparently normal women, and is relatively common in large, pale, and corpulent individuals.

Sometimes the faulty action of the uterine muscle is attributable to a loss of tonicity incident to excessive distention, and is therefore frequently met with in women who have passed through a number of pregnancies in rapid succession, or in whom the uterus has been subjected to acute distention, as in certain cases of multiple pregnancy and hydramnios. Much less commonly the defect is due to general weakness following exhausting diseases, but that this is rarely responsible is shown by the common observation that the pains are usually very efficient even in patients suffering from advanced stages of tuberculosis.

Although direct proof of the existence of abnormalities in the innervation of the uterine musculature cannot be adduced, clinical observation affords strong presumptive evidence in favour of this view, or at least indicates clearly the possibility that extraneous causes can interfere reflexly with the activity of the uterus. Thus, it is a matter of common experience that the entrance of the obstetrician into the lying-in chamber is frequently followed by a cessation of the labour pains, which is generally transient, but sometimes persists for quite a long while. Moreover, extreme nervousness, profound mental emotions, or excruciating pain may have a similar effect. In such cases the severe pain is often due to the irregular action of the uterus, and in turn, by acting reflexly, interferes still further with its function, thus giving rise to a vicious circle. That reflex nervous influences are responsible is shown by the fact that the administration of a sedative is frequently followed by a return of satisfactory contractions.

That the action of the uterus is occasionally influenced by mechanical conditions is shown by the cases in which tumour formations in its wall, especially myomata, have been found to be responsible for faulty labour pains. Much the same effect is exerted by uterine displacements, especially when the organ sags markedly forward in a pendulous abdomen. Old adhesions about the uterus and appendages, and fresh inflammatory areas in the same location may act in a similar manner.

Defective abdominal contractions may be due to a number of causes. Sometimes the insufficiency results from faulty development of the abdominal muscles, but more frequently is due to a loss of muscular tone following excessive distention, so that it is much more common in multiparous than in primiparous women. Not infrequently the insufficiency is only apparent, and is due to the fact that for fear of increased pain the patient is unwilling to bring her abdominal muscles into full play, and makes efforts to restrain them. For this reason the obstetrician is often obliged to terminate labour by means of low forceps, although he feels sure that a few minutes' effective use of the abdominal muscles would lead to spontaneous delivery. In many such cases the administration of chloroform is attended by most happy results, since it dulls the sensation of pain sufficiently to enable the patient to bring her abdominal muscles into action.

Treatment of Prolonged Labour.—Active treatment is rarely demanded when the tardy labour is the result of infrequent pains of slight intensity, as in the majority of such cases they gradually become more severe and eventually bring about a spontaneous delivery. If the condition lasts for several days it is important that the patient should sleep well at night, and the administration of hypnotics, or even of morphine hypodermically, is indicated.

On the other hand, when the pains are inefficient, cramp-like, and follow one another in rapid succession without exerting any appreciable effect upon the course of labour, excellent results often follow the administration of a hypodermic injection of morphine (grain $\frac{1}{4}$), combined with the sulphate of atropine (grain $\frac{1}{150}$); or a rectal injection containing 30 grains of chloral hydrate in 4 ounces of warm milk may be given, and repeated, if necessary, in one hour.

When the dystocia is due to secondary uterine inertia the problem is more difficult; though, as a rule, if the patient can obtain several hours of sound sleep, more satisfactory pains will appear when she wakens. For this reason the use of a hypnotic is often indicated. Some authors recommend the administration of quinine in this class of cases. It would appear, however, that the oxytocic properties of the drug have been a good deal exaggerated, since in many cases large doses produce no visible effect. Occasionally, however, 5 grains of the sulphate given in a freshly prepared pill or in solution, and repeated in one hour, may prove of great benefit. A third dose is not necessary, for, if the uterus has not responded to the amount already given, the further administration of the drug may be regarded as useless.

Ergot was formerly used with a free hand in this condition, but this practice cannot be too strongly reprehended. It is true that its administration is often followed by an increase in the intensity of the uterine contractions, but experience has shown that they soon lose their normal characteristics and become tetanic. As a result the uterus is liable to remain firmly contracted upon its contents, and no longer alternating between contraction and relaxation, loses its expulsive power, so that the final action of the drug is to defeat the very purpose for which it was given. Moreover, if the existence of a mechanical obstacle has been overlooked, the use of ergot may lead to so pronounced an overstretching of the lower uterine segment that rupture occurs. From the very first the young physician should make up his mind never to employ ergot for its oxytocic properties, and to use it only as a prophylactic for uterine hæmorrhage after the expulsion of the placenta.

As has already been pointed out, abnormalities in the contraction of the uterus are usually associated with imperfect dilatation of the cervix, and in elderly primiparæ, and occasionally in younger women who have suffered from inflammatory conditions about the cervix, rigidity of the tissues can sometimes be invoked as its underlying cause. In many cases the administration of a sedative is followed by satisfactory results. The use of an anæsthetic, although it frequently leads to satisfactory dilatation of the cervix, is generally inadvisable, inasmuch as the patient, having once experienced its soothing effect, refuses to dispense with it, so that the obstetrician will often be obliged to continue its use throughout the entire second stage, thereby so prolonging labour that the application of forceps becomes necessary. Occasionally a copious vaginal douche of hot sterile salt solution or a hot full bath is attended by satisfactory results.

In other cases, if interference becomes imperative, the introduction of a bougie into the uterus, or the employment of a small Champetier de Ribes rubber bag acts as an efficient uterine irritant, and brings about complete dilatation. As a rule, however, if the condition of the mother or the child demands the prompt termination of labour, rapid dilatation of the cervix is best effected manually by Harris's method, provided the internal os and cervical canal are already obliterated.

When labour is complicated by premature rupture of the membranes, the patient should be informed concerning its probable effect, and should be encouraged to bear her sufferings as patiently as possible. At the same time she should be most carefully watched, and care should be taken that the child's head is not subjected for too long a time to injurious pressure. Moreover, the premature opening up of the amnion greatly increases the danger of intrapartum infection. Accordingly, if symptoms of exhaustion appear, and an objective examination shows that the mother or child will suffer from further delay, interference is indicated, particularly if the temperature becomes elevated, or changes in the fœtal pulse-rate, the passage of meconium or a markedly œdematous condition of the cervix be noted. Under such circumstances dilatation may be effected either by means of the rubber bag or manually, after which delivery should be brought about as soon as possible by the most conservative method available. Forceps, however, should never be applied until the cervix is completely dilated, nor while the head is freely movable above the superior strait.

Tardy labour, due to the prolongation of the second stage, is usually best treated by the application of forceps, except in those cases in which there is some mechanical obstacle, or when the patient refuses to use her abdominal muscles. In the latter case the necessity for instrumental delivery may often be obviated by the judicious administration of chloroform.

Precipitate Labour.—Precipitate labour may result from an abnormally slight degree of resistance offered by the soft parts, as in certain multiparous women, or from abnormally strong uterine and abdominal contractions.

Generally speaking, precipitate labour is not attended by serious consequences, although the child is sometimes extruded so rapidly that the patient is unable to secure proper attention. Under such circumstances deep tears of the perinæum are common. Cases are on record in which the woman has been suddenly overtaken by intense labour pains and has given birth to the child before she could reach her bed. Under such circumstances the child has sometimes fallen to the ground and sustained severe or even fatal injuries. Occasionally the cord is torn through and the child may bleed to death before aid is obtainable.

If tempestuous pains come on while the patient is under the observation of a physician, they should be controlled by the administration of chloroform, in order that the head may be held back and prevented from being born too brusquely. The effects of precipitate labour have been studied particularly by Winckel.

Tetanic Contraction of the Uterus.—Occasionally in the first, and more frequently in the second stage of labour, the uterus may cease to relax at regular intervals, and remain in a condition of continued or tetanic contraction. This condition is usually encountered in prolonged labours, in which a mechanical obstacle is opposed to the passage of the child. In such cases the danger of rupture of the uterus becomes imminent, although now and again this accident occurs when everything seems to be going on normally.

So long as the tetanic condition persists the extrusion of the contents of the uterus is out of the question, while at the same time the patient suffers intense pain, and the child is exposed to considerable danger, owing to interference with the placental circulation. If the condition is not due to an obstruction it can be temporarily controlled by the administration of sedatives or an anæsthetic, after which delivery should be effected as soon as practicable.

Closely related to this form of dystocia is that which is sometimes attributed to a stricture resulting from tonic *contraction of Bandl's ring.* Considerable attention has been directed to this complication within the last few years, and numerous cases have been described by Budin, Demelin, Cheron, Rossa, and others. The French observers believe that while the portions of the uterus above and below it remain flaccid, Bandl's ring can undergo isolated contraction, and thereby so strongly compress the neck or some other portion of the child as to interfere seriously with its delivery. Cheron has reported instances of transverse presentation in which this kind of stricture developed and confined the child to the upper portion of the uterus, at the same time offering an almost insuperable obstacle to the introduction of the hand for the performance of version.

Veit is probably correct in denying the existence of such conditions, and in believing that the reports are due to faulty observation. That the contraction should be confined to Bandl's ring would appear highly improbable, and it is much more likely that the entire active portion of the uterus may pass into a condition of tetanic rigidity, and that under such circumstances its lower margin would be felt as a contracted ring. In ssch cases the lower uterine segment would be flabby, while the upper portion of the uterus would be tightly contracted, thereby opposing a serious obstacle to the expulsion of the child and to the introduction of the hand or instruments into the uterus. In cases of this character the administration of an anæsthetic relaxes the spasmodic contractions, and delivery can then be accomplished by the most appropriate procedure.

It is likewise probable that, in a certain number of cases in which the dystocia has been attributed to the contraction of Bandl's ring, the condition was really due to more or less rigidity of the internal os, while the cervical canal below it had undergone satisfactory dilatation.

As the result of the misuse of ergot or of extensive adherence of the placenta, the uterus sometimes undergoes such an extreme degree of retraction during the third stage that the latter becomes imprisoned in its cavity. In such cases the greater part of the upper segment of the uterus is tightly contracted over the retained placenta, while its lower portion undergoes still further retraction, and is felt by the examining finger as a tightly contracted ring below the placenta. The lower uterine segment and the cervix, not having recovered from the distention to which they have been subjected, are flabby in character, and widen from above downward to the vaginal insertion. From the shape thus imparted to the uterus the condition is generally designated as an "*hour-glass contraction.*" Its occurrence usually necessitates the manual removal of the placenta, which can sometimes be accomplished only under anæsthesia.

LITERATURE

Budin. De la dystocie causée par l'anneau de Bandl L'Obstétrique, 1898, iii, 289–310.

Cheron. Des difficultés de la version causées par la retraction de l'anneau de Bandl. Thèse de Paris, 1899.

Demelin. De la retraction utérine avant la rupture des membranes. L'Obstétrique, 1898, iii, 49–59.

Rossa. Der Contractionsring in seinen Beziehungen zur Mechanik der Geburt. Monatsschr. f. Geb. u. Gyn., 1900, xii, 457–480.

Veit. Ueber die Dystocie durch den Contractionsring. Monatsschr. f. Geb. u. Gyn., 1900, xi, 493–501.

Winckel. Ueber die Bedeutung präcipitioter Geburten für die Aetiologie des Puerperalfiebers. München, 1884.

CHAPTER XXXII

DYSTOCIA DUE TO ABNORMALITIES OF THE GENERATIVE TRACT

Vulva.—Complete atresia of the vulva or the lower portion of the vagina is usually congenital, and unless corrected by operative measures would oppose an insuperable obstacle to conception. Von Meer has reported an exceptional case in which the lower two thirds of the vagina were lacking, while the upper third communicated with the bladder. Coitus was accomplished *per urethram*, through which a three-months' fœtus was subsequently expelled.

More frequently vulval atresia is incomplete, and is due to adhesions and cicatricial changes resulting from injury or inflammatory processes. The defect may offer a considerable obstacle to labour, but the resistance is usually overcome by the continued pressure exerted by the head, though frequently only at the expense of deep perineal tears.

Cases are on record in which an almost imperforate hymen has remained intact until the time of labour, and only ruptured when distended by the child's head. In rare instances, as was pointed out by Coester, a thick septate hymen may form a bridge of tissue opposing the advance of the presenting part, and may require to be cut through before delivery can be completed.

In some women, especially in elderly primiparæ, the vulval outlet is very small, rigid, and altogether lacking in elasticity. Again, as the result of pressure or renal lesions, the vulva may become so œdematous that its orifice is almost occluded. The latter condition does not necessarily give rise to dystocia, but in both the brittleness of the soft parts predisposes to perineal laceration. Moreover, when the œdema has been excessive, and has persisted for some time, the tone of the tissues may be so lowered that they even become gangrenous as a result of the strain incident to labour.

The formation of thrombi or hæmatomata about the vulva, although more common during the puerperium, occasionally occurs during the latter part of pregnancy, and gives rise to a slight retardation of labour. Inflammatory lesions about the vulva, as well as malignant new growths, may have a similar effect.

Vagina.—Complete vaginal *atresia* is nearly always congenital in origin, and is an effectual bar to pregnancy. Incomplete forms, on the other hand, are sometimes manifestations of faulty development, but more frequently result from accidental complications.

Somewhat rarely the vagina is divided into two halves by a longitudinal septum extending from the vulva to the cervix; more often the structure is incomplete, being limited to either the upper or lower portion of the canal. Such conditions are frequently associated with abnormalities in the development of the generative tract, and their detection should always lead to further careful examination, with a view to determining whether the uterus and appendages are normal.

A complete longitudinal septum rarely gives rise to dystocia, as the half of the vagina through which the child descends gradually undergoes satisfactory dilatation. On the other hand, an incomplete septum occasionally interferes with the descent of the head, becoming stretched over it as a fleshy band of varying thickness. Such structures are usually torn through spontaneously, but occasionally are so resistant that they must be severed by the obstetrician.

Occasionally the vagina may be obstructed by ring-like strictures or bands of congenital origin. These, however, rarely offer a serious obstacle to labour, as they usually yield before the oncoming head, though in extreme cases incision may be necessary.

Sometimes the upper portion of the vagina is separated from the remainder of the canal by a diaphragm-like structure with a small central opening. Such a condition is occasionally mistaken by inexperienced observers for the vaginal fornix, and at the time of labour for the undilated external os. A careful examination, however, should reveal the presence of the opening, through which a finger can be passed, the cervix then being distinguished above it. After the external os is completely dilated, the head impinges upon the abnormal structure and causes it to bulge downward. If it does not yield, slight pressure upon its opening will usually lead to further dilatation; but if this is not effectual crucial incisions may be necessary in order to allow of delivery.

Accidental atresia is always secondary in origin, and results from the formation of adhesions following injuries or inflammatory processes. It not infrequently follows severe puerperal infections, during the course of which the entire lining of the vagina may have sloughed off, so that as healing occurs its lumen has become almost entirely obliterated. A similar result is sometimes noted after diphtheria, small-pox, cholera, and syphilis; while in rare instances, as in a case reported by Schenk, it may be due to the action of corrosive fluids injected into the vagina in the hope of inducing abortion. That the most frequent cause of atresia is injury or inflammatory conditions following labour is shown by the fact that 209 of the 1,000 cases collected by Neugebauer presented such a history.

The effects of such conditions vary greatly. In the majority of cases, owing to the softening of the tissues incident to pregnancy, the obstruction is gradually overcome by the pressure exerted by the presenting part; less often manual or hydrostatic dilatation or incisions may become necessary; while in very rare cases extreme dystocia may demand Cæsarean section. Full literature concerning this complication is to be found in the articles of Ward and Brindeau.

Among the rare causes of serious dystocia, *vaginal neoplasms* are worthy of mention, Güder, in 1893, having collected 60 cases from the literature. The obstruction was due to the presence of cystic structures, fibromata, carcinomata, sarcomata, or hæmatomata, arising from the vaginal walls or the surrounding tissues. When the tumour is accessible it is best treated by excision, no matter what its origin. If this is not practicable, and the growth is cystic, tapping becomes the operation of choice. The presence of a solid tumour may occasionally afford an indication for Cæsarean section.

Exceptionally *tetanic contraction of the levator ani muscle* may seriously interfere with the descent of the head. In this condition, which is analogous to the vaginismus of non-pregnant women, a thick, ring-like structure completely encircles and markedly constricts the vagina several centimetres above the vulva. In a recent thesis Davet has collected a number of such cases.

Ordinarily the condition yields to the administration of sedatives or anæsthetics, though in one of my patients the obstruction persisted in spite of profound anæsthesia, and it was only after steady pressure had been exerted upon it for ten minutes or more that it relaxed sufficiently to permit the passage of the hand folded in the shape of a cone.

Cervix.—Inasmuch as complete atresia of the cervix is incompatible with conception, it must be assumed, whenever such a condition is met with in a pregnant woman, that conception had occurred before its formation. In the majority of cases, however, the atresia is only apparent, and is simulated by a very minute external os.

A good illustration is afforded by the so-called *conglutinatio orificii externi*. In this condition the cervical canal undergoes complete obliteration at the time of labour, while the os remains extremely small with very thin margins, the presenting part being separated from the vagina only by a very thin layer of tissue. Formerly, this appearance was attributed to the existence of adhesions between the lips of the external os, but Schroeder was probably right in stating that it is simply due to a very small and resistant os. Ordinarily, complete dilatation promptly follows firm pressure with a finger tip, though in rare instances manual dilatation or crucial incisions may become necessary.

Cicatricial stenosis of the cervix frequently follows difficult labour associated with considerable destruction of tissue. Less frequently it is due to syphilitic ulceration and induration, several instances of which have been reported by Le Bigot. Now and again it results from the employment of corrosive substances for the purpose of producing abortion.

Ordinarily, owing to the softening and succulence of the tissues incident to pregnancy, the stenosis, whatever its cause, gradually yields to the natural forces; but in other cases dilatation has to be accomplished by manual methods or by the employment of rubber bags. In rare instances, however, the resistance may be too great to be overcome, and as labour progresses the lower uterine segment may become stretched to such a degree that rupture becomes imminent, an accident which can be averted only by the performance of Cæsarean section.

Rigidity of Cervix.—Reference has already been made to the unyielding cervix of elderly primiparæ. Occasionally still greater rigidity is encountered in patients who have suffered from inflammatory lesions, though such conditions rarely give rise to serious dystocia. On the other hand, in certain extreme cases of hypertrophic elongation of the cervix, considerable difficulty is experienced in effecting dilatation, although, as a rule, one is surprised to see how completely the abnormality may be effaced during the course of pregnancy.

Dystocia due to malformations of the uterus has already been considered in Chapter XXVII.

Uterine Displacements.—*Anteflexion.*—Marked anteflexion of the uterus is usually associated with a pendulous abdomen. In primiparæ the condition is usually indicative of disproportion between the size of the head and the pelvis; whereas in multiparæ it is more often the result of extreme flaccidity of the abdominal walls incident to repeated childbearing. In the latter class of cases the abnormal position of the uterus prevents the force of its contractions from being properly transmitted to the cervix, hence the dilatation of the latter is interfered with. Marked improvement in this respect frequently follows the application of a properly fitting abdominal bandage, by means of which the uterus is maintained in an approximately normal position.

Retroflexion.—As was said in Chapter XXVII, retroflexion of the pregnant uterus is usually incompatible with advanced pregnancy, since, if spontaneous or artificial reposition does not occur, the patient either aborts or presents symptoms of incarceration before the end of the fourth month. In the very exceptional instances in which pregnancy goes on to term, the fundus remains attached to the floor of the pelvis, while the anterior wall hypertrophies to such an extent as to afford room for the product of conception. In this condition, which is known as *sacculation*, the head of the child occupies the fundus, while the cervix is sharply bent and so drawn up that the external os lies above the upper margin of the symphysis pubis. At the time of labour the contractions tend to force the child through the most dependent portion of the uterus, while the cervix dilates only partially, so that spontaneous labour is out of the question. As a rule, the cervix can be dilated manually under anæsthesia, and the child delivered by version; but in rare instances the cervix is so inaccessible that Cæsarean section will afford the most conservative method of delivery.

Dystocia Due to Operations for the Relief of Retroflexion of the Uterus.—Unfortunately, several of the operations which have been suggested for the relief of retroflexion of the non-pregnant uterus, while rectifying the condition, occasionally give rise to serious dystocia. Thus, in rare instances, after a *ventrofixation*, when the fundus has become firmly adherent to the lower portion of the abdominal parietes, the anterior wall of the uterus is unable to expand, and the enlargement of the organ is effected solely at the expense of its posterior wall, the anterior wall forming a thick layer of muscle which extends backward from the point of attachment to the cervix. Under such circumstances the latter is gradually drawn upward from its usual position, until the external os lies on a level with the promontory of the sacrum, and sometimes considerably above it. When labour sets in, dilatation of the cervix is effected very imperfectly, since the bag of waters and the presenting part, instead of impinging upon it, are forced down upon the thickened anterior wall of the uterus. Accordingly, the uterine contractions, no matter how strong they may be, are unable to effect the completion of labour, and unless suitable operative procedures are undertaken, rupture of the uterus will occur, as in one of Dickinson's cases.

Noble, in 1896, collected the histories of 177 cases of labour occurring in women who had been subjected to ventrofixation, and found that dystocia was frequently noted, Cæsarean section having been necessary four times, not to speak of numerous versions and other operations. Dickinson, in 1901, reported a case of Cæsarean section for the same cause, and collected 9 others from the literature.

I have delivered some 20 women after the performance of ventrofixation or suspension of the uterus, but in only one was there any serious dystocia. In this case the patient was a multipara, who had had several spontaneous labours before the operation and conceived soon afterward. During pregnancy she complained of a great deal of pain at the lower end of the abdominal incision, which was distinctly drawn inward. Internal examination showed that the cervix pointed backward, the external os being on a level with the promontory of the sacrum. After some sixteen hours of strong labour pains the cervical canal was not obliterated and the os measured only 2 centimetres in diameter, while the head was jammed down upon the anterior wall of the uterus. The propriety of performing Cæsarean section was considered, but it was believed that the cervix could be dilated manually; this was accomplished after considerable difficulty, when version was performed and a living child extracted. The patient made an uneventful recovery, except that she continued to complain of intense pain in the lower abdomen. For this reason the abdomen was opened a few weeks later, and the fundus was found to be firmly adherent, having been attached to the fascia and muscles of the abdominal wall by several silkworm-gut sutures. Permanent relief followed the freeing of the uterus.

In view of such experiences, the question arises whether the performance of ventrofixation in women during the childbearing period is a justifiable procedure. My experience leads me to believe that *suspension* of the uterus is devoid of danger from an obstetrical point of view, as in this operation the uterus is attached merely to the peritonæum, so that it is eventually held in place by pressure exerted by the abdominal contents assisted by two newly formed peritoneal ligaments. If, however, it be firmly sutured to the fascia—a real *ventrofixation*—serious consequences may result in the next pregnancy, and for this reason the latter operation should be employed only in women past the menopause.

The *vaginofixation*, suggested by Dührssen and Mackenrodt, in which the fundus is firmly stitched to the anterior vaginal wall, has been followed by such serious dystocia that it has been practically abandoned during the childbearing period. Rühl has collected 9 cases of Cæsarean section following this operation, and Rieck has suggested a modified vaginal Cæsarean section for the relief of the resulting dystocia.

Prolapse.—Pregnancy cannot go on to full term when the uterus is completely prolapsed, although the size of the uterine tumour which occasionally projects from the vulva may give rise to a belief in its possibility. In such cases, however, careful examination will show that the fundus occupies its usual level, while the protrusion from the vulva is made possible by elongation of the lower uterine segment and hypertrophic elongation of the cervix. As a rule, the cervix becomes retracted when labour sets in, though in rare cases it may continue to protrude from the vulva and becomes markedly œdematous and so swollen as to give rise to serious dystocia. Under such circumstances multiple incisions of the cervix may be necessary in order to effect delivery.

Dystocia Due to Tumours of the Generative Tract and Pelvis.—*Carcinoma of the Cervix.*—The effect of this condition upon pregnancy and labour and its appropriate treatment has been considered in Chapter XXVII.

Fibro-myomata of the Uterus.—Myomata were observed by Pinard in 84 out of 13,915 consecutive cases of labour—0.6 per cent. It is a matter of general observation that women suffering from this disease are relatively sterile. Thus, 49 of Pinard's patients were over thirty years of age when pregnancy first occurred.

The obstacle to conception is most marked when the tumour is of the submucous or interstitial variety, and much less so when it is subserous in origin. Moreover, when pregnancy occurs, owing to the hæmorrhagic changes in the endometrium which are frequently associated with the presence of submucous myomata, there is an increased tendency towards premature expulsion of the ovum. On the other hand, pregnancy is not without influence upon the tumours themselves, which frequently increase rapidly in size, more as a result of œdema than of actual hypertrophy. Moreover, owing to the pressure to which they are subjected by the growing ovum, the softened tumours undergo changes in shape and become markedly flattened. At the same time the pedicles may become twisted and gangrene and peritonitis may ensue; while a submucous tumour may sometimes become loosened from its bed and hang down into the uterine cavity or cervix as a polypus.

The diagnosis of the association of pregnancy and myomata is not always easy, as hæmorrhage may occur at intervals as the result of changes in the endometrium, and be mistaken by the patient herself for the menstrual flow, so that the idea of pregnancy may never suggest itself. On the other hand, a sudden increase in the rapidity of the growth of the uterine tumour should direct attention to the possibility of pregnancy, and the diagnosis becomes assured when careful palpation shows the presence of soft areas interspersed between the firmer myomatous nodules. Subperitoneal myomata occasionally escape observation, being mistaken for small parts, or sometimes for the head of the fœtus, so that a diagnosis of multiple pregnancy may be made.

At the time of labour the effect exerted by the myomata depends entirely upon their size and situation. Generally speaking, subserous tumours are without great significance, except when their large size leads to pressure symptoms. On the other hand, a pedunculated tumour occasionally prolapses into the pelvic cavity and gives rise to serious dystocia. As a rule, however, interstitial myomata, developed in the cervix or lower uterine segment, offer serious obstacles to labour and may so obstruct the pelvic cavity that normal delivery will be impossible. As a result of the uterine contractions, submucous myomata may become partially separated from their bed and protrude from the cervix as a polypoid mass. Under such circumstances, since they effectively prevent the descent of the head, they must be removed by cutting through the pedicle.

Even when the tumour does not interfere with the course of labour by its size and situation, it frequently exerts a deleterious influence upon the position of the child. Thus Olshausen, in tabulating the cases reported in the literature, found only 53 per cent of vertex presentations, as compared with 24 and 19 per cent of breech and transverse presentations respectively. Moreover, the mere presence of the tumour may so interfere with the character of the uterine contractions as to cause dystocia. In not a few cases the condition appears to predispose towards placenta prævia, as well as to favour the occurrence of post-partum hæmorrhage. The latter is due partly to the fact that the myomatous nodules interfere with the normal contraction and retraction of the uterus, and partly because they offer mechanical obstacles to the separation and expulsion of the placenta.

In the puerperium, myomata not infrequently undergo degenerative changes, and if they have been subjected to prolonged pressure may become gangrenous. On the other hand, in not a few cases the effect of pregnancy is beneficent, as the tumours become smaller after the birth of the child, and occasionally disappear entirely.

Prognosis.—In preantiseptic times the outlook in labours complicated by the presence of myomatous tumours was most serious. Thus, the maternal and fœtal mortality was respectively 25 and 79 per cent in 307 cases collected from the literature by Lefour in 1880. At present, thanks to early diagnosis and prompt recourse to operative procedures in suitable cases, the prognosis is much more favourable, though at the same time the condition is sometimes one of the most serious with which the obstetrician has to cope. Pinard reported that labour was spontaneous in 54, and required operative aid in 30 of his cases, while the maternal mortality was only 3.6 per cent.

Treatment.—When extreme distention, serious hæmorrhage, or symptoms of impaction occur before the child has attained the period of viability, laparotomy is indicated; but whether removal of the tumour can be best effected by excision, enucleation, supravaginal or total hysterectomy will vary according to circumstances and the predilections of the individual operator. Generally speaking, isolated subserous myomata are best treated by excision, and those of the interstitial variety by enucleation; whereas, if numerous tumours are present, supravaginal hysterectomy is indicated without reference to the existence of pregnancy.

Myomectomy and enucleation are frequently followed by abortion or miscarriage, but do not necessarily destroy all chance of saving the life of the child. Notwithstanding this, however, my own inclination is towards supravaginal amputation, whenever operation is imperatively demanded, as being a less dangerous procedure as far as the mother is concerned. Thumin has collected 62 myomectomies, 40 enucleations, and 98 supravaginal hysterectomies performed between the years 1885 and 1901, with a mortality of 10, 5, and 11.23 per cent respectively.

If serious symptoms do not supervene during pregnancy, the patient should be examined thoroughly under anæsthesia shortly before the expected date of confinement. If the tumour is found to be firmly impacted in the pelvis, Cæsarean section should be performed before labour sets in, followed by supravaginal amputation or complete hysterectomy, according to the judgment of the operator. On the other hand, if there is apparently no danger of impaction, and spontaneous delivery is probable, the patient may be allowed to go into labour. But if symptoms of obstruction occur, Cæsarean section should be promptly performed in preference to attempts at delivery by the more usual obstetrical procedures.

Ovarian Tumours.—The presence of an ovarian tumour is one of the most serious complications of pregnancy, as it markedly increases the

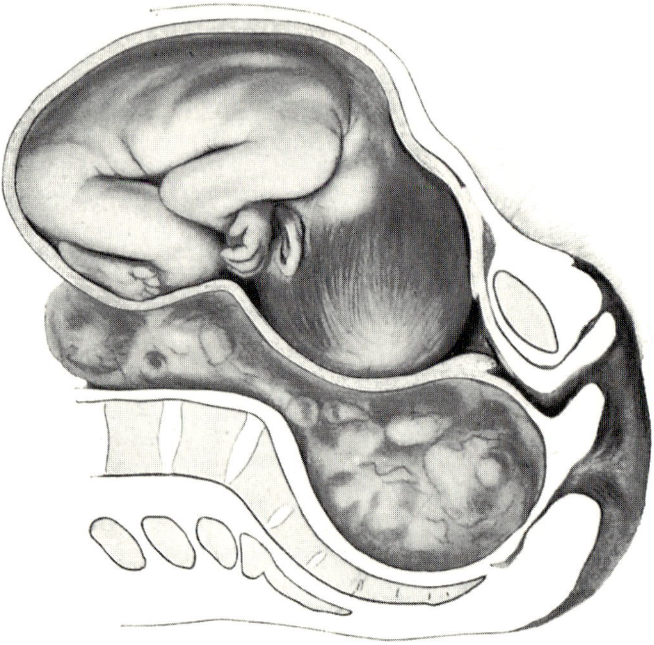

Fig. 483.—Dystocia Due to Ovarian Cyst (Bumm).

probability of abortion and frequently offers an insuperable obstacle to delivery at the time of labour. Moreover, even after a spontaneous labour, its presence occasionally gives rise to disturbances during the puerperium.

While any variety of ovarian tumour may complicate pregnancy and labour, dermoid cysts have been described comparatively frequently in this connection. Thus, in 107 cases collected by McKerron, in which the nature of the tumour was stated, there were 47 cystomata, 46 dermoid cysts, 9 malignant tumours, 5 fibromata, and 2 colloid cysts. Swan, in 1898, was able to collect 14 cases of solid ovarian tumours.

Of the 321 pregnancies complicated by ovarian tumours collected by Remy, spontaneous abortion or premature labour occurred in 17 per cent.

If the tumour occupies the pelvic cavity it may give rise to most serious dystocia. Thus, McKerron, in 183 cases collected from the literature, noted a maternal mortality of 30.5 per cent, while more than half of the children were lost. The majority of these cases, however, were reported prior to the introduction of more radical surgical methods, very few laparotomies having been performed, and interference for the most part being limited to puncture or incision of cysts through the vagina. Moreover, the danger to the patient does not end with the birth of the child, as in not a few cases peritonitis follows gangrene of the tumour resulting from excessive pressure, while in others torsion of the pedicle may lead to a fatal termination.

Again, the cyst may rupture and extrude its contents into the peritoneal cavity during a spontaneous labour or as the result of operative interference. This event is a matter of indifference with the ordinary cystomata, but in the case of a dermoid cyst is frequently followed by fatal peritonitis. In other instances rupture of the uterus occurs, or the tumour is forced into the vagina and occasionally even into the rectum.

Diagnosis.—Unfortunately, the presence of an ovarian tumour complicating pregnancy often remains unrecognised, the condition having escaped observation in all but 18 of McKerron's cases. Nevertheless, more careful observation would certainly eliminate a large proportion of these errors. Any excessive enlargement of the abdomen or the appearance of pressure symptoms should always lead one to make a careful examination, and in not a few cases a tumour will be found occupying the pelvic cavity. Again, failure of the presenting part to engage, when the pelvis is known to be normal, suggests an obstructing mass. On the other hand, if the tumour does not occupy the pelvic cavity, the diagnosis is extremely difficult, and the abdominal enlargement is frequently attributed to the presence of twin pregnancy or hydramnios, and the true condition is not recognised until after labour.

Treatment.—If the tumour is detected prior to the last month of pregnancy, it should be removed at once by laparotomy. Orgler has collected 142 such operations, with a maternal mortality of 2.77 per cent.

It has been objected that such a procedure increases the chances of premature delivery, which occurred in 22.5 per cent of Orgler's cases. It should, however, be remembered that a similar accident may take place even if the patient is not interfered with, being noted in 17 per cent of Remy's cases. This difference is so slight that the chances for the child are little, if at all, impaired by operation, while those of the mother are markedly improved.

On the other hand, when the diagnosis is not made until the last month of pregnancy, it is usually advisable to postpone the operation until term, for the reason that the fresh abdominal cicatrix is not well adapted to the strain of parturition. At the time of labour, if the tumour is impacted in the pelvis, unanimous opinion favours its immediate removal by laparotomy. Bland Sutton and most authorities advise that the abdomen should then be closed and the birth of the child left to Nature, or at most assisted by forceps. On the other hand, Hirst is strongly of the opinion that a supplementary Cæsarean section should immediately follow, believing that the woman should not be submitted to the strain of labour immediately after a severe operation, and, when all things are considered, the latter appears to me to be the wiser course.

Formerly it was advised to attempt the reposition of the mass under anæsthesia. This practice, however, is not to be recommended, for the reason that the tumour is very liable to give rise to trouble during the puerperium. Moreover, since operative interference will be necessary sooner or later, it would seem far better to institute radical measures without delay. Puncture through the vagina, although strongly advocated at one time, must be considered as a dangerous and extremely reprehensible practice, inasmuch as we possess no means of preventing the tumour contents from contaminating the peritoneal cavity.

If spontaneous labour has occurred, the patient should be carefully watched during the puerperium for the appearance of untoward symptoms. Should they arise, prompt operation is imperatively demanded. In any event, a woman suffering from an ovarian tumour should not be discharged from treatment until the tumour has been removed, or at least until the importance of operative procedures have been strongly urged upon her.

Tumours of Other Origin.—Labour is occasionally obstructed by tumours of various origin, which encroach upon the cavity of the pelvis to such an extent as to render delivery difficult or even impossible. In Chapter XXXVIII reference will be made to dystocia due to tumours arising from the pelvic walls.

In rare instances a normal sized or *enlarged kidney* or *spleen* may prolapse into the pelvic cavity and offer an obstacle to labour. Bland-Sutton has added an additional case of displaced kidney complicating pregnancy to those collected by Cragin; he has also reported the removal of a prolapsed spleen in the second month of pregnancy, which would have given rise to serious dystocia at the time of labour had it remained *in situ.*

Echinococcus cysts are occasionally implanted in the pelvic cavity. Franta, in 1902, collected 22 cases noted during pregnancy and discussed their effect upon the course of labour.

In Chapter XXX reference was made to those cases in which an old extra-uterine gestation sac so obstructed the pelvic canal as to interfere with the delivery of a subsequent intra-uterine pregnancy.

Enterocele or hernia through the vaginal walls occasionally gives rise to dystocia, though in the majority of cases the prolapsed intestine can be replaced and the obstacle temporarily overcome. Where this is not possible, Cæsarean section is indicated as a more conservative procedure than forcibly dragging the child over a large irreducible hernia.

In occasional instances *tumours of the bladder* or large *vesical calculi* may likewise offer an impediment to the passage of the child, though it is rarely so serious as to demand operative interference. On the other hand, cases have been reported in which it has been necessary to remove a large calculus from the bladder before delivery could be effected.

A large *rectocele* or *cystocele*, though occasionally offering an obstacle to labour, can generally be replaced while delivery is being effected.

Tumours arising from the lower part of the rectum or pelvic connective tissue may likewise give rise to serious dystocia, Holzapfel having collected the cases in which *carcinoma of the rectum* rendered Cæsarean section necessary.

LITERATURE

Bland-Sutton. The Surgery of Pregnancy and Labour complicated with Tumours. Lancet, 1901, i, 382–386; 452–456; 529–532.

Brindeau. De l'atrésie acquise du vagin au point de vue obstétricale. L'Obstétrique, 1901, vi, 97–122.

Coester. Ueber Geburtshindernisse durch hymenale Balken, etc. D. I., Marburg, 1900.

Cragin. Congenital Pelvic Kidney obstructing the Parturient Canal. Amer. Jour. Obst., 1898, xxxviii, 36–41.

Davet. De la dystocie due à la contracture du muscle reléveur de l'anus. Thèse de Paris, 1900.

Dickinson. Pregnancy following Ventrofixation. Amer. Jour. Obst., 1901, xliv, 34–45.

Franta. Les kystes hydatiques du bassin et de l'abdomen au point de vue de la dystocie. Annales de gyn. et d'obst., 1902, lvii, 165–197; 296–308.

Güder. Ueber Geschwülste der Vagina als Schwangerschaft und Geburtskomplikationen. D. I., Bern, 1889.

Hirst. Ovarian Cysts. A Text-Book of Obstetrics. Third edition, 1901, 515–517.

Holzapfel. Kaiserschnitt bei Mastdarmkrebs. Hegar's Beiträge zur Geb. u. Gyn., 1899, ii, 59–77.

Le Bigot. De l'influences du chancre syphilitique de col de l'utérus sur l'accouchement. Thèse de Paris, 1899.

Lefour. Quoted by Olshausen.

McKerron. The Obstruction of Labour by Ovarian Tumours in the Pelvis. Trans. Lond. Obst. Soc., 1897, xxxix, 334–382.

von Meer. Conception und Abort durch den Ausführungsgang der Blase bei angeborener Defect der Vagina. Hegar's Beiträge zur Geb. u. Gyn., 1900, iii, 409–424.

Neugebauer. Zur Lehre von den angeborenen und erworbenen Verwachsungen und Verengerungen der Scheide. Berlin, 1895.

Noble. Suspensio Uteri with Reference to its Influence upon Pregnancy and Labour. Trans. Amer. Gyn. Soc., 1896, xxi, 247–268.

Oldham. Sacculation of the Uterus. A Case of Retroflexion of the Gravid Uterus. Trans. Lond. Obst. Soc., 1860, i, 317–322.

Olshausen. Myom und Schwangerschaft. Veit's Handbuch der Gyn., 1897, ii, 765–814.

Orgler. Zur Prognose und Indikation der Ovariotomie während der Schwangerschaft. Arch. f. Gyn., 1901, lxv, 126–160.

Pinard. Fibromes et grossesse. Annales de gyn. et d'obst., 1901, lv, 165–167.

Remy. De la grossesse compliquée de kyste ovarique. Paris, 1886.

Rieck. Vaginifixur und Geburt. Monatsschr. f. Geb. u. Gyn., 1901, xiv, 237–254.

Rühl. Kritische Bemerkungen uber Geburtsstörungen nach Vaginalfixatio-uteri. Monatsschr. f. Geb. u. Gyn., 1901, xiv, 477–911.

Schenk. Hochgradige frische Aetzstenose der Cervix und des Fornix in der Schwangerschaft. Centralbl. f. Gyn., 1900, 161–170.

Schroeder. Conglutinatio orificii externi. Lehrbuch der Geburtsh., XIII. Aufl., 1899, 590–592.

Swan. The Management of Solid Tumours of the Ovaries complicating Pregnancy, with Report of a Successful Case. Bull. Johns Hopkins Hosp., 1898, ix, 56–61.

Thumin. Chirurgische Eingriffe bei Myomen der Gebärmutter in Schwangerschaft und Geburt. Archiv f. Gyn., 1901, lxiv, 457–525.

Ward. Atresia Vaginæ complicating Labour. Obstetrics, 1899, i, 623–625.

CHAPTER XXXIII

CONTRACTED PELVIS—HISTORY, FREQUENCY, METHODS OF DIAGNOSIS, AND CLASSIFICATION

We consider a pelvis contracted when it is shortened to such an extent in one or more of its diameters as to affect materially the mechanism of labour, but without necessarily retarding the birth of the child. According to Litzmann this is the case when the conjugata vera measures 9.5 centimetres or less in flat, and 10 centimetres or less in generally contracted pelves.

History.—Inasmuch as Vesalius was the first to describe the normal pelvis correctly, it is clear that the conception of contracted pelves could not have existed before his time. His pupil, J. C. Arantius (1530–'89), gave the first anatomical description of an abnormal pelvis, but his discovery exerted no appreciable effect upon the obstetrical art of the period, for the reason that Ambroise Paré still held to the old view of the separation of the pubic bones during labour, and promulgated it in his writings.

During the next century knowledge of the subject advanced but slowly, and we find Mauriceau (1637–1709) stating that in his very large experience he had observed only two instances of contracted pelvis. In one of these Chamberlen was permitted to apply the forceps invented by his uncle, but failed to effect a delivery.

We are indebted to Heinrich van Deventer for our first knowledge of contracted pelves from an obstetrical standpoint. In his New Light for Midwives, which appeared in 1701, he described the two most usual varieties of contracted pelvis—the generally contracted and the flat—and discussed the influence which they exerted upon labour. From that time on mention of the subject is to be found in all the text-books, De la Motte, Puzos, and Dionis being the obstetricians of the first half of the eighteenth century who devoted most attention to it. The last-named observer was the first to point out the causal relation which rhachitis bears to many cases of pelvic deformity.

Most important contributions to the subject were made by Smellie. In his treatise on The Theory and Practice of Midwifery, published in 1752, is to be found an excellent description of the normal pelvis, as well as of the most usual varieties of deformity to which it is subject. He also laid down practical rules for the estimation of the degree of contraction, carefully described the mechanism of labour in such cases, and gave excellent pictures showing the influence exerted by the contracted pelvis upon the fœtal head.

Baudelocque (1746–1810) contributed largely towards the development of our knowledge of the subject, as he devoted particular attention to the diagnosis of the condition in the living woman, and showed that it could be detected by measuring the distance between certain external bony parts of the pelvis by means of a pair of calipers. He was the first to describe the external conjugate, which is now generally known by his name, and taught that the length of the conjugata vera could be readily and accurately estimated by deducting 3 inches from it.

At the same time G. W. Stein, in Germany, did good work upon somewhat similar lines and devised a pelvimeter for the direct mensuration of the conjugata vera.

The real foundation, however, for the modern doctrine concerning contracted pelves was laid by Michealis and Litzmann. The former was Professor of Obstetrics in the University of Kiel from 1843 to 1850, and during that time carefully measured the pelvis in 1,000 consecutive cases of labour. He designated as contracted all pelves in which the conjugata vera measured 8.75 centimetres or less, and found 72 such cases in his series, a percentage of 7.2. After his death he was succeeded by Litzmann, who continued the work, and soon reported accurate measurements based upon a second series of 1,000 cases. He advanced the definition which was given at the beginning of the present chapter, and considered as contracted all pelves having a conjugata vera of 10 or 9.5 centimetres or less, according as they were generally contracted or flat, respectively. Judged by these criteria he found that 14.9 per cent of his pelves were abnormal, and estimated that had Michealis employed the same standard his percentage would have been 13.1.

Litzmann's definition and criteria have been adopted throughout the world, and since the appearance of his work scientific obstetricians have devoted a considerable amount of attention to the subject. To mention all who have added materially to our knowledge would be equivalent to writing the history of obstetrics for the past fifty years; but Naegele, Kilian, Schauta, and Breus and Kolisko may be cited as among the most important contributors.

Frequency.—In this country and in England very few statistics are available upon which to base accurate statements as to the frequency of contracted pelves, but in Germany and France many of the large lying-in hospitals supply valuable data. The frequency of pelvic deformity varies considerably in different countries, and even in various parts of the same country. Thus, as is shown by the following table, a frequency ranging from 8 to 24 per cent is reported from the various German clinics.

Goenner (Basel)	observed	7.9	per cent	in 2,433	cases.
Glaser (Würzburg)	"	8.4	"	" 1,812	"
Heinsius (Breslau)	"	8.5	"	" 1,641	"
Pfund (Munich)	"	9.5	"	" 1,199	"
Fuchs (Erlangen)	"	11.43	"	" 1,766	"
Michealis (Kiel)	"	13.1	"	" 1,000	"
Köttgen (Bonn)	"	13.45	"	" 2,000	"
Litzmann (Kiel)	"	14.9	"	" 1,000	"
Müller (Berne)	"	16	"	" 1,177	"
Weidenmüller (Marburg)	"	18.7	"	" 3,224	"
Leopold (Dresden)	"	24.3	"	" 2,415	"

Winckel states that contracted pelves are observed in from 10 to 15 per cent of all German women, while Schauta estimates that the condition is met with in one woman out of seven. The statistics from the Austrian Empire seem to indicate a lesser frequency than in Germany, as is shown by the following table:

Knapp (Prague)...........	observed	2.44	per cent	in	4,289	cases.
Ludwig and Savor (Vienna)..	"	3.84	"	"	50,621	"
Pawlik (Prague)...........	"	7.8	"	"	29,615	"

Large series of statistics are not available for France. The yearly reports from Pinard's clinic, however, indicate a frequency of about 5 per cent, while Budin gives 8 per cent in 7,687 cases, and Tarnier 16 per cent in 715 cases.

Fancourt Barnes, in 1897, reported that only 0.5 per cent of contracted pelves were observed in 38,065 cases of labour in London. In view of the fact, however, that every year a considerable number of Cæsarean sections are performed in that city for this indication, it would appear probable that his figures in no way represent the true condition.

It has been a matter of general belief that in this country contracted pelves are very rare, and Dewees stated in 1824 that he had observed only three cases in his large experience. Lusk held a similar opinion, and said that rhachitis is rarely, and osteomalacia never, observed among native American women. Hirst, on the other hand, states that these diseases are not of infrequent occurrence, and that no one who practises obstetrics can fail to meet with occasional examples.

We owe to Reynolds the first statistical statement upon the subject in this country. In 1890 he reported that he had observed 1.34 per cent of contracted pelves in 2,227 women delivered in Boston. His statements, however, must be accepted with reserve and as underestimating the frequency of the condition, since he measured the pelvis only in those cases which required operative interference, and left out of consideration those in which labour terminated spontaneously. Had he taken these into account he would, in all probability, have reported a frequency of 6.8 per cent. Flint observed 1.42 per cent of contracted pelves in 10,233 consecutive cases delivered in New York; but his figures cannot be considered to represent the frequency of the condition in this country, as his material was composed almost entirely of Polish and Russian Jewesses, only 9 per cent of his patients being native-born Americans.

Crossen, of St. Louis, reports a frequency of 8 per cent, and Davis states that there were 25 per cent of contracted pelves in 1,224 cases delivered under his supervision in Philadelphia. The latter's estimates, however, were based almost entirely upon external pelvic mensuration, which, as will be pointed out later, gives an exaggerated idea of the frequency of the condition.

Since the opening of the lying-in department of the Johns Hopkins Hospital, it has been our rule to measure both externally and internally the pelvis of every pregnant woman who comes into our hands. In 1899 I reported that we had met with 131 contracted pelves in the first 1,000 women delivered. In June, 1901, I gave the results obtained in 1,123 additional cases, which showed exactly the same percentage as in the previous report. Thus, a total of 2,133 cases gave a percentage of 13.1.

One reason for the marked frequency of contracted pelves in Baltimore is probably due to the fact that more than half of our patients are coloured, 941 in the entire series being white and 1,182 black women. In the former we found 6.9 and in the latter 18.82 per cent of contracted pelves. In other words, about every fourteenth white and every fifth coloured woman of the poorer classes in Baltimore has an abnormal pelvis. From the statistics of Reynolds, Crossen, and my own—derived from Boston, St. Louis, and Baltimore respectively—it would appear that contracted pelves occur in from 7 to 8 per cent of the white women of this country. Hence, it will be evident that no one can practise obstetrics without encountering a certain number of such cases.

Methods of Diagnosis.—It is essential that the obstetrician be able to diagnose the existence and extent of the condition before the onset of labour, in order that he may, as far as possible, decide in advance upon the proper line of treatment to be instituted in each case. With this object in view accurate pelvic mensuration should constitute an integral part of the preliminary examination of pregnant women, and, in the present state of our knowledge, a physician who practices obstetrics without pelvimetry must be regarded as no better than one who treats diseases of the heart and lungs without the aid of auscultation and percussion.

At the *preliminary examination*, which should be made four to six weeks before the expected time of confinement, the physician should neglect no means of obtaining all possible data bearing upon the case. Generally speaking, large, well-built women are likely to have normal, and undersized women contracted pelves; but this rule by no means always holds good, and it is not unusual for examination to disclose some abnormality in the former and perfectly normal pelves in the latter.

The gait of the patient should be carefully noted, since the existence of a limp or some peculiar way in which the feet are placed upon the floor may serve to direct attention to the possibility of a pelvic deformity. Marked abnormalities of the spinal column—kyphosis or lordosis—are also suggestive, and even slight degrees of spinal curvature should not be overlooked, as they are not infrequently of rhachitic origin. The more usual signs of rhachitis—deformities of the extremities, the characteristically shaped head, and the rhachitic rosary—should also be looked for. Inquiry should always be made as to the age at which the patient first learned to walk, and if she is found to have been backward in this respect the possibility of a rhachitic pelvis should be borne in mind, even though the usual external manifestations of the disease may be lacking.

If the patient has already borne children she should be questioned as to the course of previous labours, and the history of any serious difficulty should always suggest the possibility of an abnormal pelvis. On the other hand, a negative history is by no means so valuable, as it is a well-known fact that in moderate degrees of pelvic contraction the first labour may be relatively easy, while each successive one becomes more difficult.

In primiparous women a markedly pendulous abdomen should always be regarded as evidence of the existence of a marked disproportion between the child's head and the pelvis until careful examination shows that such is not the case.

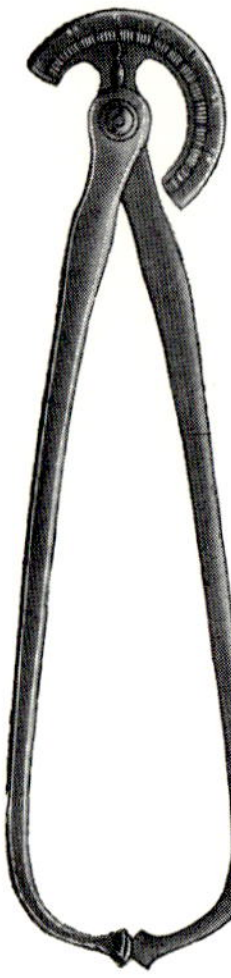

FIG. 484.—BUDIN'S PELVIMETER.

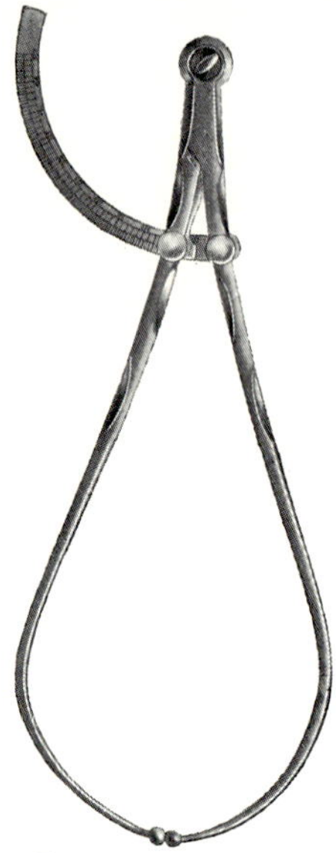

FIG. 485.—MARTIN'S PELVIMETER.

Pelvimetry.—While the abovementioned conditions are of value in suggesting the possibility of pelvic deformity, accurate information as to its existence and extent can be obtained only by measuring the pelvis.

For this purpose external or internal pelvimetry may be employed, according as the measurements are taken from the surface of the body or through the vagina. As has already been said, Baudelocque was the first to insist upon the importance and value of the former, and invented the first pelvimeter, which consisted of a pair of calipers or compasses provided with a scale to indicate the extent to which they are opened. Innumerable instruments of this kind have since been devised, but, although most of them give satisfactory results, before buying one it is always well to see that the blades are sufficiently curved to allow them to span the thighs of stout patients. Thus, Budin's pelvimeter (Fig. 484), which can readily be carried in the pocket, gives satisfactory results in the vast majority of cases; but it cannot be used to measure the external conjugate in stout women, owing to the slight curvature of its blades. Personally, I usually employ the instrument devised by E. Martin (Fig. 485).

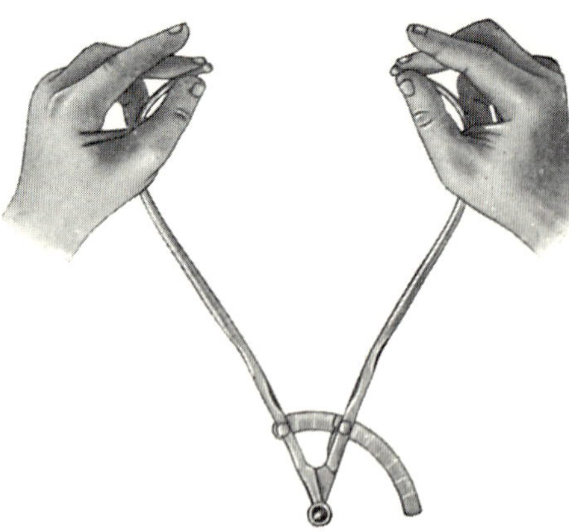

FIG. 486.—METHOD OF HOLDING PELVIMETER.

In *external pelvimetry* the ordinary measurements are four in number. Thus we ascertain accurately the distance between the anterior superior spines of the ilium, between the external edges of the crests of the ilium, between the heads of the trochanters, and between the spinous process of the last lumbar vertebra and the anterior surface of the symphysis pubis. Normally these measure 26, 29, 32, and 21 centimetres respectively. Naegele suggested certain other measurements, which as a rule, however, are not employed unless one suspects the existence of an obliquely contracted pelvis.

When the pelvis is to be measured externally, the patient should lie upon a bed or table with her abdomen and hips either bared or covered only by a thin chemise. The legs and upper portions of the body should not be exposed. The physician, sitting on the side of the bed facing the patient, grasps the tips of the pelvimeter between the thumb and second finger of each hand, the index fingers being left free. With the latter he locates the outer edges of the *anterior superior spines*, and with the other

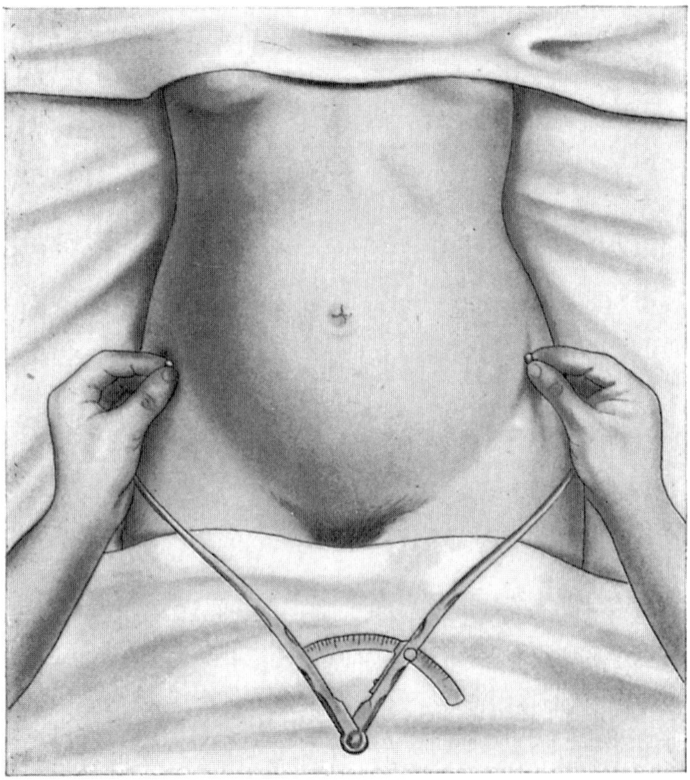

FIG. 487.—MEASURING THE DISTANCE BETWEEN THE ANTERIOR SUPERIOR SPINES.

fingers presses the tips of the pelvimeter upon them as closely as possible, the distance between them being indicated on the scale of the instrument.

In measuring the distance between the *iliac crests*, the most widely separated portions are located, and the tips of the pelvimeter applied to their outer edges. In taking these measurements, it should be borne in mind that the iliac spines and crests present an outer and inner lip and an intermediate ridge, and that the distance between the outer lips of the spines and crests is 1.5 to 2.5 centimetres greater than that between the inner lips.

In determining the distance between the *trochanters,* the patient's legs having been brought into close apposition, the examiner carefully palpates the upper portion of the thighs until the most prominent points of the trochanters are felt on either side. The tips of the pelvimeter are then

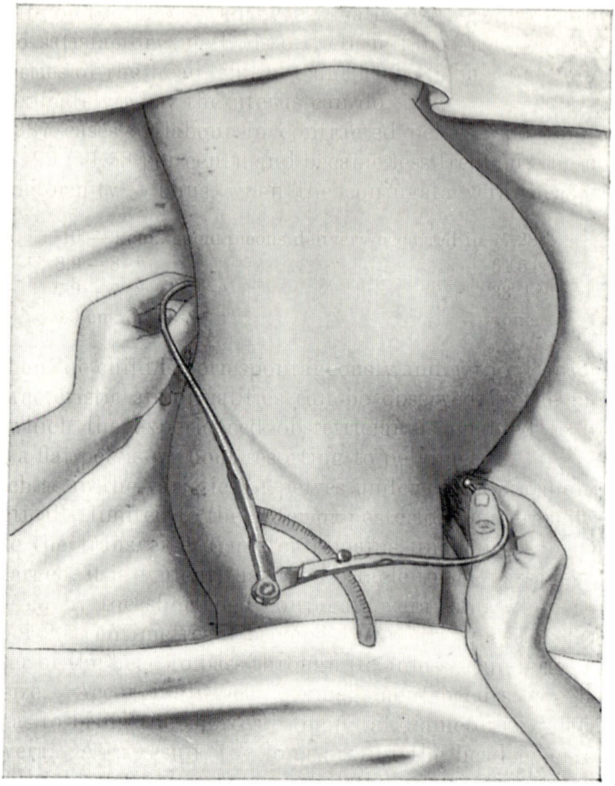

Fig. 488.—Measuring the External Conjugate.

firmly pressed against them, so that they come into closest possible contact with the bones, after which the measurement is read off on the scale.

The external conjugate, or *Baudelocque's diameter,* extends from a depression just beneath the spine of the last lumbar vertebra to the anterior and upper margin of the symphysis pubis. For this measurement, the woman should lie on her side with her back towards the physician. As a rule the spine of the last lumbar vertebra is readily found by palpating the spinous processes from above downward, the last and most prominent being usually that of the last lumbar vertebra. Immediately beneath it is a slight depression, which forms the posterior extremity of the diameter to be measured. Into this one tip of the pelvimeter should be inserted and held firmly in place, while the other hand seeks the upper margin of the symphysis pubis, and firmly applies the other tip of the pelvimeter to it. The distance separating them is then read off on the scale.

In stout women considerable difficulty may be experienced in locating the posterior extremity of the diameter, owing to the fact that the spinous process of the last lumbar vertebra cannot be identified. This difficulty can usually be obviated in the following manner: A line is drawn between the depressions marking the attachment of the fascia to the superior posterior spines of the ilium, and which are usually clearly visible. A point 2.5 centimetres above the middle of this line will usually correspond to the point required, and will lie at the apex of a rhomboidal figure—Michealis's rhomboid—whose upper and lower margins are formed by the transverse and sacro-spinalis and gluteus muscles respectively.

The Value of External Pelvimetry.—As was said above, the external conjugate was first described by Baudelocque, who stated that by deducting 3 inches from it the length of the true conjugate could be accurately estimated. He based his opinion upon the fact that he had rarely observed a difference of more than 1 or 2 lines between the estimated and the actual conjugata vera in 30 to 35 cases which he had measured during life and at autopsy. Later experience, however, has shown that Baudelocque's conclusions were erroneous, and that the length of the external conjugate gives a very imperfect idea of that of the conjugata vera, since several modifying factors may exist. Thus, the amount to be deducted varies with the thickness of the sacrum and the symphysis pubis, and also depends, to a great extent, upon the elevation of the promontory of the sacrum and the length of the spinous process of the last lumbar vertebra. Unfortunately, these factors cannot be accurately estimated in the living woman, and Skutsch has shown that in 100 pelves examined by him the difference between the length of the external and of the true conjugate varied from 5.5 to 10 centimetres. Baisset has recently arrived at similar conclusions after studying 120 dried pelves; and at the present time I have in my possession two specimens whose true conjugates are of equal length, but whose external conjugates show a difference of 5 centimetres.

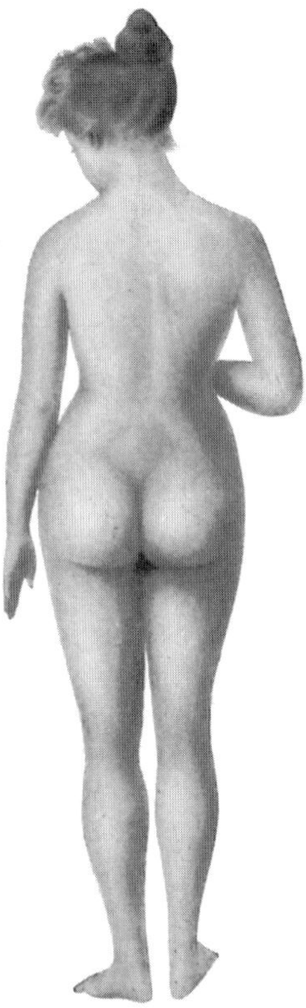

Fig. 489.—Michealis's Rhomboid (Stratz).

But although the measurement of the external conjugate does not give us accurate information concerning the length of the conjugata vera, it nevertheless enables us to draw certain important conclusions. Thus, generally speaking, when the former measures between 20 and 21 centimetres, the conjugata vera will rarely be found to be shortened; when, however, it measures between 18 and 19 centimetres, the conjugata vera is shortened in about one half of the cases; and when it is below 17 centimetres pelvic contraction is almost uniformly present.

It was formerly believed that one could form a fairly accurate estimate of the length of the transverse diameter of the superior strait by making certain deductions from the distances between the anterior superior spines and between the crests of the ilium. The incorrectness of this conclusion, however, was first demonstrated by Scheffer, who showed that the transverse diameter of the superior strait may be of the same length in two pelves, while at the same time the distances between the iliac crests vary by as much as 3.3 centimetres. This source of error depends in great part upon the angle which the iliac fossa forms with the rest of the innominate bone, and the extent to which its anterior portion is flared out.

The distance between the trochanters is the least valuable of all the external pelvic measurements, as its length depends, to a great extent, upon

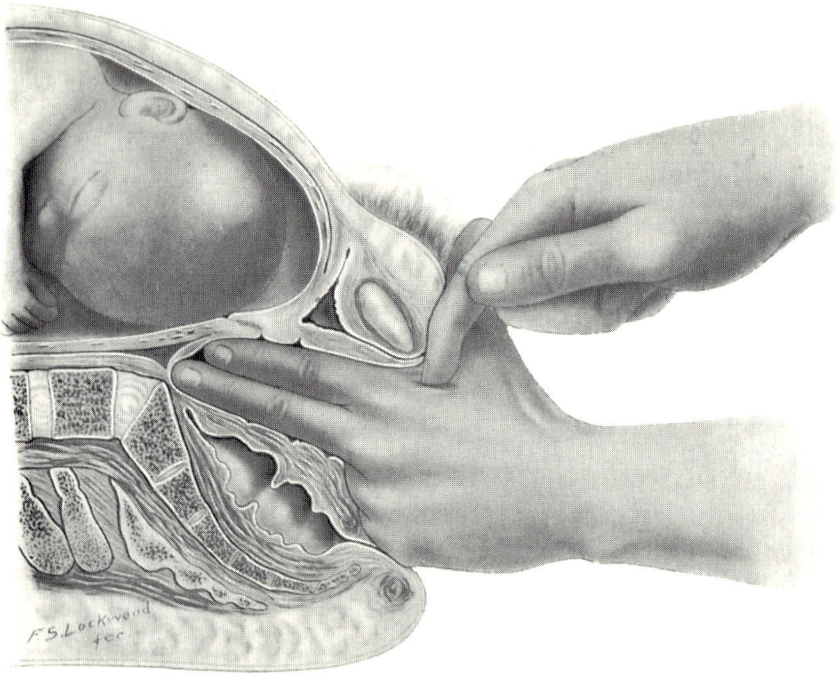

Fig. 490.—Measuring Diagonal Conjugate.

the angle which the neck of the femur forms with its shaft; and as a consequence its shortening, unless very marked, does not indicate a corresponding decrease in the transverse diameters of the pelvic cavity.

Nevertheless, despite many possible inaccuracies, the external measurements are of considerable value, in that they serve to indicate with tolerable certainty the variety of pelvis with which one has to deal. Normally the distance between the spines is 2.5 to 3 centimetres less than that between the crests; but in the rhachitic pelvis, owing to the flaring of the iliac bones, this proportion becomes deranged, and the two diameters approximate one another in length, the former frequently being equal to, and occasionally exceeding the latter. If, however, both measurements are considerably below the normal, but preserve their usual relation to one another, and at the same time the external conjugate is also shortened proportionately, it is permissible to conclude that the entire pelvis measures below normal in all its diameters, or, in other words, is generally contracted.

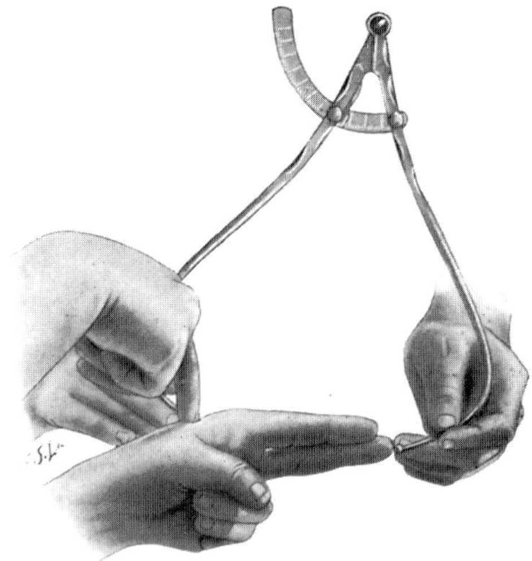

FIG. 491.—MEASURING THE LENGTH OF DIAGONAL CONJUGATE UPON THE FINGERS.

Goenner, in 1901, demonstrated the fallacy of attempting to diagnose the existence of a contracted pelvis by external pelvimetry alone. After measuring the external diameters in 100 cadavers, he compared them with those of the pelvic cavity as revealed at autopsy, and found that whereas the former would seem to indicate that nearly all of the pelves were contracted, the latter proved that such was the case in only 22 instances. My own observations bear out Goenner's conclusions, particularly in coloured women, in whom, had we estimated the frequency of contracted pelves from external measurements alone, our figures would

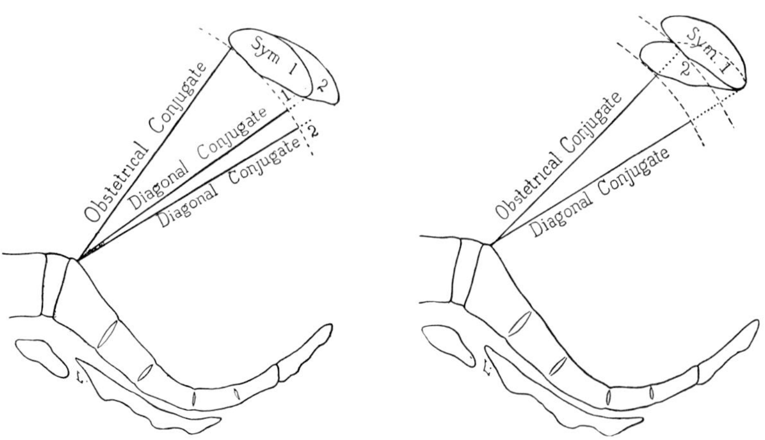

Fig. 492. Fig. 493.

FIGS. 492, 493.—DIAGRAMS SHOWING VARIATIONS IN LENGTH OF DIAGONAL CONJUGATE DEPENDENT UPON THE HEIGHT AND INCLINATION OF THE SYMPHYSIS PUBIS.

have shown a frequency of about 75 per cent, whereas internal pelvimetry showed that in reality it was only 18.8 per cent.

Notwithstanding all these possible fallacies, external pelvimetry is of considerable value to the obstetrician and should not be neglected. In private practice it is my rule to employ it at the preliminary examination four to six weeks before the expected date of confinement. If the measurements are approximately normal, the patient being a primipara and the child's head fixed in the pelvic cavity, internal mensuration is not practised. But if they are abnormal, and especially if the diagonal conjugate measures 18 centimetres or less, internal pelvic measurements should be resorted to no matter what the position of the head may be or how many children the patient may have borne previously.

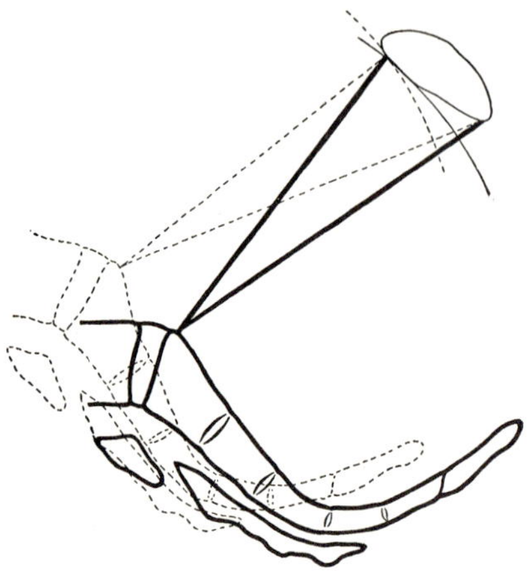

Fig. 494.—Diagram showing Effect of Position of Promontory of Sacrum upon the Length of the Diagonal Conjugate.

Internal Pelvimetry.—In the vast majority of abnormal pelves the most marked deformity affects the antero-posterior diameter of the superior strait, and as a consequence we are especially anxious to arrive at the length of the conjugata vera. Unfortunately, this cannot be measured directly in the living woman, and in practice it is estimated by measuring the diagonal conjugate—the distance from the promontory of the sacrum to the lower margin of the symphysis pubis—and making a certain deduction from it. This method was introduced by Smellie and still further elaborated by Baudelocque.

Measuring the Diagonal Conjugate.—For this purpose the patient should be placed upon an examining table with her knees drawn up. If this cannot be conveniently arranged, she should be brought to the edge of the bed and a firm pillow placed beneath her buttocks. Two carefully disinfected fingers are introduced into the vagina, and the anterior surface of the sacrum

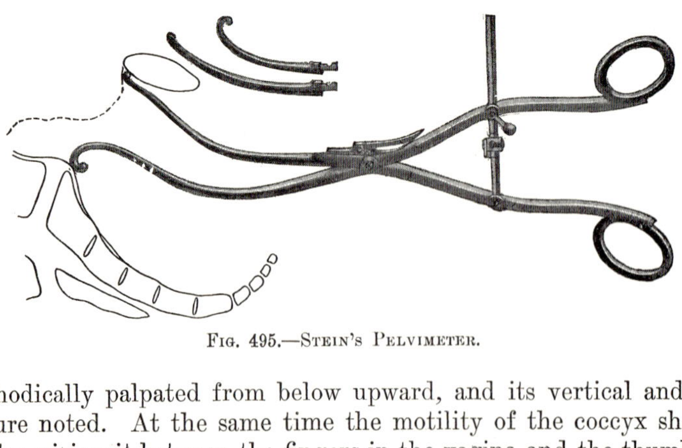

Fig. 495.—Stein's Pelvimeter.

is methodically palpated from below upward, and its vertical and lateral curvature noted. At the same time the motility of the coccyx should be tested by seizing it between the fingers in the vagina and the thumb externally. In normal pelves only the last three sacral vertebræ can be felt without pushing up the perinæum, whereas in markedly contracted varieties the entire anterior surface of the sacrum is readily accessible.

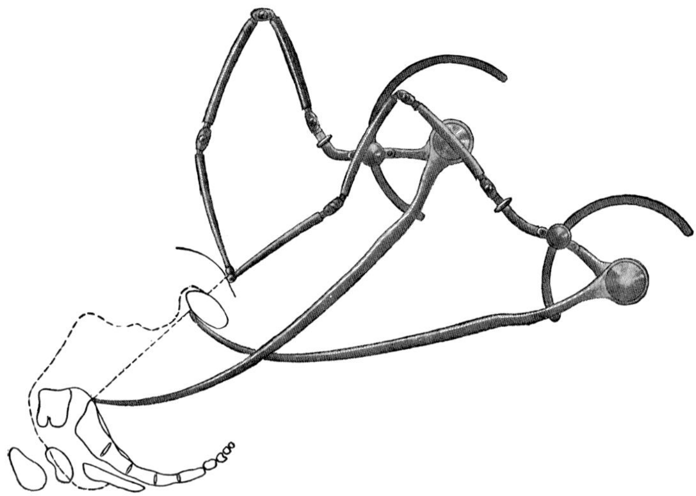

FIG. 496.—MEASURING CONJUGATA VERA WITH SKUTSCH'S PELVIMETER.

In ordinary cases, in order to measure the diagonal conjugate the elbow is depressed and the perinæum forcibly pushed upward by the knuckles of the third and fourth fingers, while the index and second fingers are held firmly together and directed upward in the direction of the umbilicus. The promontory of the sacrum is soon felt by the tip of the second finger as a projecting bony margin at the base of the sacrum. With the finger

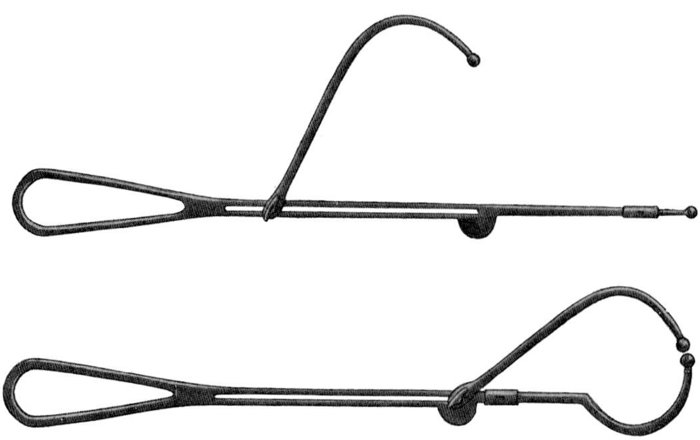

FIG. 497.—HIRST'S PELVIMETER.

closely applied to its most prominent portion, the hand is elevated until the radial surface of the index finger is brought into close contact with the pubic arch. This point is then marked by the index finger of the other hand, after which the fingers are withdrawn from the vagina and the distance between it and the tip of the second finger is measured (Figs. 490 and 491). This measurement gives the diagonal conjugate, from which the true conjugate is estimated by deducting 1.5 to 2 centimetres, according to the height and inclination of the symphysis pubis.

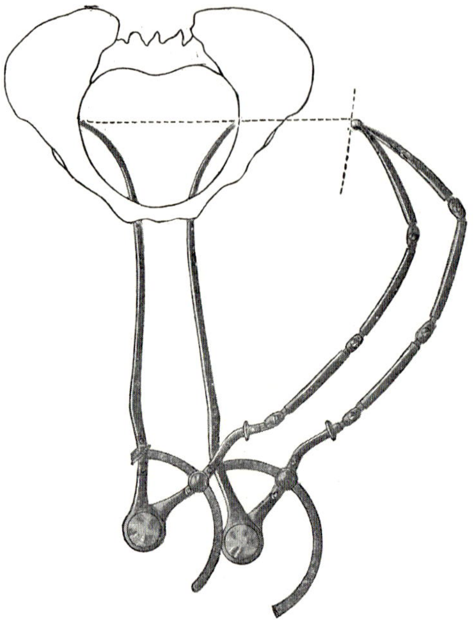

Fig. 498.—Measuring Transverse Diameter of Superior Strait with Skutsch's Pelvimeter.

In this method the problem consists in estimating the length of one side of a triangle, the conjugata vera; the other two—the diagonal conjugate and the height of the symphysis pubis—being known. Were we able to measure satisfactorily the angle formed between the symphysis and conjugata diagonalis, the exact length of the true conjugate could readily be ascertained by the ordinary rules of trigonometry; but unfortunately this cannot be done in the living woman, and for practical purposes it suffices to estimate the length of the diagonal conjugate as just described, deducting 1.5 centimetre from it if the pubis is low and slightly inclined, and 2 centimetres if it is high and has a marked inclination. The rationale of this is clearly shown in Figs. 492 and 493. The length of the diagonal conjugate also varies according to the position of the promontory, being longer when it is elevated, and *vice versa* (Fig. 494).

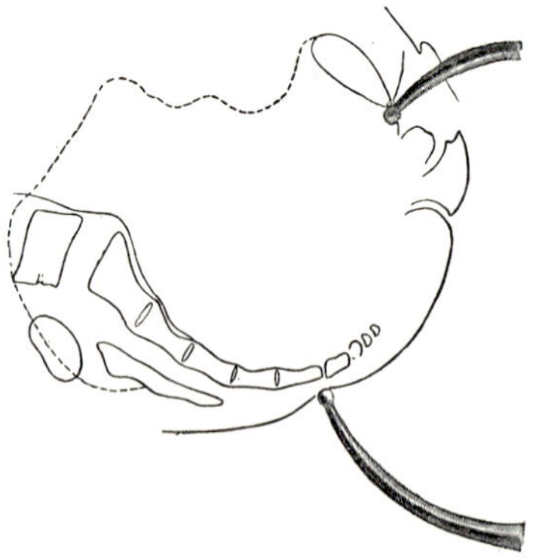

Fig. 499.—Breisky's Method of Measuring Antero-Posterior Diameter of Pelvic Outlet.

Since the time of G. W. Stein (1772), numerous instruments have been devised by means of which the conjugata vera could be directly measured; but unfortunately the majority of them, while theoretically correct, are practically useless on account of the difficulty of their application. Descriptions and illustrations of many of these instruments are to be found in Skutsch's excellent monograph.

Skutsch, in 1886, devised a pelvimeter by which the conjugata vera could be indirectly though accurately measured (Fig. 496). Hirst has more recently described a simple device for the same purpose. Both of these instruments give satisfactory results when properly used, but their employment is usually so painful to the patient as to require the administration of an anæsthetic. Naturally, therefore, they are employed only in those rare cases in which accurate information concerning the length of the conjugata vera is urgently called for.

Neumann and Ehrenfest, in 1900, described a complicated instrument —the *pelvigraph*—by means of which the contour of the anterior and posterior walls of the pelvis can be graphically outlined, and whence the exact length of the various antero-posterior diameters can be readily ascertained. This instrument gives excellent results, but is too complicated for use outside of a well-regulated hospital.

Measuring the Transverse Diameter of the Superior Strait.—This diameter cannot be measured directly in the living woman, and as a rule for

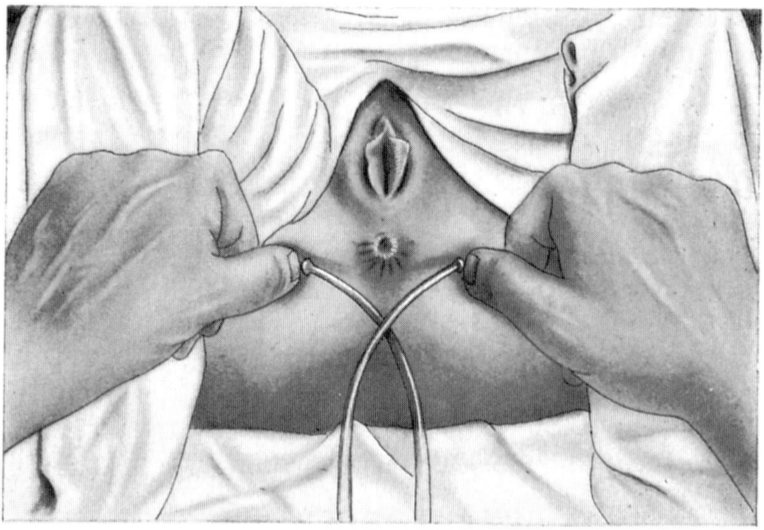

Fig. 500.—Measuring the Distance between the Tubera Ischii.

all practical purposes it is necessary only to palpate the linea terminalis with the examining fingers, and in this way roughly estimate the outlines of the superior strait. If, however, we wish to learn its exact length, it can be ascertained indirectly by the employment of Skutsch's instrument.

Measuring the Diameters of the Pelvic Outlet.—Occasionally it is desirable to measure the diameters of the pelvic outlet—the distances between the lower margin of the symphysis pubis and the tip of the sacrum, and between the tubera ischii respectively. Breisky described a practical method of measuring the former. For this purpose the woman having been placed on her side, one end of the pelvimeter is introduced into the vagina and applied to the lower margin of the symphysis pubis, the other end being applied over the tip of the sacrum externally. A deduction of 1.5 centimetre from this measurement will give a tolerably accurate idea of the antero-posterior diameter of the inferior strait.

The distance between the tubera ischii can be approximately estimated by Schroeder's method or by a modification of it. In the former the tubera ischii are carefully palpated through the skin and marks made with a dermatographic pencil on the external surface at points apparently corresponding to their inner margins. The distance between these is then measured with a tape-measure. It is often convenient to palpate the inner margins of the ischial tuberosities with the thumbs, so that the nails are directly over the points to be measured, when an assistant ascertains the distance between them with Budin's pelvimeter. If precise information is desired, it is advisable to use the pelvimeter described by Klien. By the routine employment of this instrument, its inventor claims that contraction of the inferior strait will be found to be of comparatively frequent occurrence.

Use of X Rays.—After the discovery of the Roentgen ray and the demonstration of the various uses to which it might be put, it was thought possible that it might also afford a valuable method of investigating the shape and size of the pelvis. Budin and Varnier, in 1897, reported their experience with it, and showed that, while it often gave an excellent idea of its shape, the ideas as to size obtained by it were erroneous.

Varnier continued to experiment with the method, but although he reported in 1899 that he had discovered a method by which it could be employed for estimating the actual size of the pelvis, no details have as yet been published.

A comprehensive review of the literature upon the subject was given by Müllerheim in 1898. Bouchacourt, in 1900, devised a method for which he claimed excellent results. Up to that time all radiographs of the pelvis gave distorted ideas in regard to its dimensions, owing to the fact that the sacrum lay much nearer the sensitive plate than the symphysis, and consequently the anterior portion of the pelvis was enlarged out of all proportion to the posterior. This defect rendered out of the question any attempt to utilize the radiograph for purposes of mensuration. Bouchacourt suggested that it might be obviated by placing a rectangular metal frame about the woman's hips, more or less corresponding to the plane of the superior strait, each side of the frame being marked by dentations 1 centimetre apart. When the picture was taken these would also be reproduced, and on connecting the corresponding points upon the four sides of the picture a definite idea could be obtained as to the dimensions of the superior strait. The method, however, is quite complicated, and has not come into general use.

Classification of Contracted Pelves.—For the first classification of abnormal pelves we are indebted to Deventer, who distinguished three groups: too large, too small, and too flat pelves.

Most recent attempts at classification have been based upon the shape of the pelvis, without taking into consideration the ætiological factors which lead to its production. This method was adopted by Michealis, and reached its greatest perfection in Litzmann's hands. The former thoroughly realized its inherent defects and regretted that other methods of classification could not be employed. Kilian, Busch, and Siebold had previously recognised the necessity of taking into account the ætiological factors which are concerned in the production of pelvic abnormalities, but their knowledge was too meagre to permit of such a course.

It was not until 1889 that Schauta was able to suggest a fairly satisfactory ætiological classification, which soon obtained general acceptance, although it is still far from ideal. Tarnier and Budin, in their treatise issued in 1898, followed somewhat similar lines. Breus and Kolisko do not consider that either are perfectly satisfactory, and have suggested a substitute for them.

Owing to the fact that our knowledge of the fundamental factors underlying the production of many forms of abnormal pelves is still very meagre, and occasionally entirely lacking, it is apparent that at the present time no ætiological classification can be perfectly satisfactory, though from a practical point of view the one employed by Tarnier and Budin would seem to approach more nearly to it.

For convenience of reference we shall give the classifications of Tarnier and Budin and of Schauta in parallel columns; but although we shall generally follow the former in describing the several varieties, we shall not necessarily adhere to the order in which the different groups are arranged.

TARNIER AND BUDIN'S CLASSIFICATION

I. *Pelvic Anomalies due to Excess of Malleability of Pelvic Bones:*

(*a*) Rhachitic pelvis.
(*b*) Flat, non-rhachitic pelvis.
(*c*) Osteomalacic pelvis.

II. *Anomalies due to Abnormal Transmission of the Body Weight to Pelvis:*

(*a*) Lordosis.
(*b*) Scoliosis.
(*c*) Kyphosis.

III. *Anomalies resulting from Abnormal Articulation of the Vertebral Column with the Sacrum:*

(*a*) Spondylolisthesis.
(*b*) Spondylizème.

IV. *Anomalies resulting from the Abnormal Direction of the Upward and Inward Force exerted by the Femora:*

(*a*) Unilateral lameness.
(*b*) Bilateral lameness.

SCHAUTA'S CLASSIFICATION

II. *Pelvic Anomalies resulting from Diseases of the Pelvic Bones:*

(*a*) Rhachitic pelvis.
(*b*) Osteomalacic pelvis.
(*c*) New growths.
(*d*) Fracture.
(*e*) Atrophy, caries, and necrosis.

IV. *Anomalies resulting from Diseases of the Superimposed Skeleton:*

(*a*) Spondylolisthesis.
(*b*) Kyphosis.
(*c*) Scoliosis.
(*d*) Kyphoscoliosis.
(*e*) Lordosis.
(*f*) Anomalies resulting from the fusion of the last lumbar with the first sacral vertebra, as well as of the first sacral vertebra with the iliac bones (assimilation pelvis).

V. *Anomalies resulting from Abnormalities of the Subjacent Skeleton:*

(*a*) Coxitis.
(*b*) Luxation of the head of the femur.
(*c*) Luxation of the heads of both femora.
(*d*) Unilateral or bilateral club-foot.
(*e*) Absence or deformity of one or both lower extremities.

Tarnier and Budin's Classification	Schauta's Classification
V. *Anomalies resulting from Primary Defects in the Development of the Pelvic Bones:*	I. *Anomalies resulting from Faulty Development:*
(*a*) Generalized and symmetrical: 1. Excess of general development (justo major pelvis). 2. Lack of general development (generally contracted pelvis). (*b*) Localized and asymmetrical: 1. Obliquely contracted (Naegele) pelvis. (*c*) Localized and symmetrical: 1. Double oblique (Robert) pelvis. 2. Split pelvis. 3. Ossification of sacro-iliac joints. 4. Arrest of development of the body of the sacrum.	(*a*) Generally contracted pelvis. (*b*) Simple flat, non-rhachitic pelvis. (*c*) Generally contracted flat pelvis. (*d*) Narrow, funnel-shaped fœtal or undeveloped pelvis. (*e*) Imperfect development of one sacral ala (Naegele pelvis). (*f*) Imperfect development of both sacral alæ—Robert pelvis. (*g*) Generally, equally enlarged (justo major pelvis).
VI. *Atypical Deformities:* Tumours and fractures of the pelvic bones.	III. *Anomalies in the Articulation of the Pelvic Bones:* (*a*) Abnormally firm union (synostosis): 1. Of the symphysis. 2. Of one or both sacro-iliac synchondroses. 3. Of the sacrum with the coccyx.

LITERATURE

Arantius. See Chapter I.

Baisset. De la mensuration externe du bassin. Thèse de Lyon, 1901.

Barnes. Internat. Gynæcolog. Congress, Geneva, 1896. Centralbl. f. Gyn., 1896, 1089.

Baudelocque. L'art des accouchements. Nouvelle éd., 1789, t. I, 76–90.

Bouchacourt. De la radiographie du bassin de la femme adulte. L'Obstétrique, 1900, v, 320–351.

Breisky. Beiträge zur geburtshülflichen Beurtheilung der Verengerungen des Beckenausganges. Wien. med. Jahrb., 1870, xix.

Breus und Kolisko. Die pathologischen Beckenformen. Wien, 1900, Theil I.

Budin. Statistiques de la Maternité de Paris. L'Obstétrique, 1896, iii, 134.

Photographie par les rayons x d'un bassin de Naegele. L'Obstétrique, 1897, ii, 490.

Busch. Geburtskunde, Berlin, 1849.

Crossen. Partial Report of Eight Hundred Cases of Labour. Amer. Gyn. and Obst. Jour., 1898, xiii, 53.

Davis. Frequency and Mortality of Contracted Pelves. Amer. Jour. Obst., 1901, xli, 11–15.

Deventer. Operationes chirurgicæ novum lumen exhibentes obstetricantibus, 1701.

Dewees. A Compendious System of Midwifery. Philadelphia, 1824.

Dionis. Traité général des accouchements, etc. Paris, 1718.

Flint. Deformed Pelves. Rep. of Soc. of the Lying-in Hosp., New York, 1897, 258–271.

Fuchs. Statistik der in den letzten 10 Jahren in der Erlanger Universitäts-Frauenklinik vorgekommenen engen Becken. D. I., Würzburg, 1899.

Glaser. Ueber spontane Geburten bei engen Becken. D. I., München, 1898.

Goenner. Zur statistik des engen Beckens. Zeitschr. f. Geb. u. Gyn., 1882, vii, 314.

Ein hundert Messungen weiblicher Becken an der Leiche. Zeitschr. f. Geb. u. Gyn., 1901, xliv, 308–325.

HEINSIUS. Die Geburten bei engen Becken in den Jahren, 1894–'97. D. I., Breslau, 1898.
HIRST. American Text-Book of Obstetrics, 1897, 498–510.
KILIAN. Die Geburtslehre von Seiten der Wissenschaft und Kunst dargestellt. Frankfurt, 1840.
KLIEN. Die geburtshülfliche Bedeutung der Verengerungen des Beckenausgangs. Volkmann's Sammlung klin. Vorträge, N. F., Nr. 169.
KNAPP. Bericht über 105 Geburten bei engen Becken aus den Jahren 1881–'95. Archiv f. Gyn., 1886, xl, 489–586.
KÖTTGEN. Zur Statistik des engen Beckens. D. I., Bonn, 1895.
LEOPOLD (Franke). Enges Becken und spontane Geburt. Arbeiten aus d. königl. Frauenklinik in Dresden, 1895, ii, 29–48.
LITZMANN. Die Formen des Beckens. Leipzig, 1861.
Die Geburt bei engen Becken. Leipzig, 1884.
LUDWIG und SAVOR. Klin. Bericht über die Geburten bei engen Becken in den Zeitraum 1878–'92. Bericht aus der II. geb. gyn. Klinik in Wien, R. Chrobak, 1897, 120–394.
LUSK. The Science and Art of Midwifery. Fourth ed., 1895.
MAURICEAU. Observations sur la grossesse et l'accouchement des femmes. Nouv. éd., 1738.
MICHEALIS. Das enge Becken. Leipzig, 1851.
DE LA MOTTE. Traité complet des accouchements naturels, etc. Nouv. éd., Leiden, 1729.
MÜLLER. Zur Frequenz und Aetiologie des allgemeinen verengten Beckens. Archiv f. Gyn., 1880, xvi, 155.
MÜLLERHEIM. Verwerthung der Röntgen Strahlen in der Geburtshülfe. Deutsche med. Wochenschr., 1898, Nr. 39.
NAEGELE. Das weibliche Becken, etc. Carlsruhe, 1839.
Das schräg verengte Becken, etc. Mainz, 1839.
NEUMANN und EHRENFEST. Eine neue Methode der inneren Beckenmessung an der lebenden Frau. Monatsschr. f. Geb. u. Gyn., 1900, xi, 237–253.
PARÉ. See Chapter I.
PAWLIK. Internat. Gyn. Congress, Geneva, 1896. Centralbl. f. Gyn., 1896, 1090.
PFUND. Aerztl. Intelligenzblatt, 1895, xxxii, 247.
PINARD. Fonctionment de la Maison d'accouchement Baudelocque. For various years.
PUZOS. Traité des accouchements, etc. Paris, 1749.
REYNOLDS. The Frequency of Contracted Pelves. Tr. Am. Gyn. Soc., 1890, xv, 367–377.
SCHAUTA. Die Beckenanomalien. Müller's Handbuch der Geb., Bd. II, 1889.
SCHEFFER. Ueber das Verhältniss des Abstandes der Spinae und Cristae ilium an dem des Querdurchmesser des Beckeneinganges. Monatsschr. f. Geb., 1868, xxxi, 299–309.
SKUTSCH. Die Beckenmessung. Jena, 1886.
Die praktische Verwerthung der Beckenmessung. Deutsche med. Woch., 1891, Nr. 21.
SIEBOLD. Lehrbuch der Geburtshülfe, 1854.
SMELLIE. Treatise on the Theory and Practice of Midwifery, with Collection of Cases. Eighth ed., London, 1774.
STEIN, G. W. Beschreibung des kleinen und einfachen Beckenmesser, etc. Klein Werke zur prak. Geburtsh., Marburg, 1798, 135.
VARNIER. Étude anat. et radiographique de la symphyse pubienne apres le symphyséotomie. Comptes rendus de la Soc. d'obst., de gyn. et de paed. de Paris, 1899, i, 208.
WIEDENMÜLLER. Zur Statistik des engen Beckens. D. I., Marburg, 1895.
WILLIAMS, J. WHITRIDGE. Pelvimetry for the General Practitioner. Medical News, March 21, 1891.
Frequency of Contracted Pelves in Baltimore. Johns Hopkins Hosp. Bulletin, Aug., 1896.
Frequency of Contracted Pelves in the first One Thousand Women delivered in the Obstetrical Department of the Johns Hopkins Hospital. Obstetrics, 1899, i, Nos. 5 and 6.
Pelvic Indications for the Performance of Cæsarean Section. Amer. Medicine, 1901, ii, 483–488.

CHAPTER XXXIV

ANOMALIES DUE TO ABNORMAL MALLEABILITY OF THE PELVIC BONES

Flat Non-Rhachitic Pelvis.—This is the most frequent variety of pelvic deformity occurring in white women, but it is comparatively rare in the black race. It was noted in 43 per cent of the 72 contracted pelves described by Michealis. Litzmann stated that its frequency, as compared with that of the rhachitic pelvis, was as 7 to 5. In our material at the Johns Hopkins Hospital it constituted 49.33 per cent of the contracted pelves occurring in white women, as compared with 9.86 of those in coloured women.

Most German authors confirm the statements of Michealis and Litzmann as to its frequency. On the other hand, Ahlfeld dissents from this view, holding that many of the pelves which have been designated as of the simple flat variety are really of rhachitic origin, and Tarnier and Budin state that only one sixteenth of the abnormal pelves with which they met could be attributed to other causes than rhachitis.

This variety is frequently described as the pelvis plana Deventeri, or *simple flat pelvis,* although it is doubtful whether Deventer differentiated between it and the rhachitic form. It was accurately described by Betschler in 1832, but Michealis and Litzmann were the first to insist upon its importance and frequent occurrence.

The characteristic feature of the flat non-rhachitic pelvis consists in a shortening of all the antero-posterior diameters of the pelvic cavity, while the transverse measurements remain practically normal.* This condition is due to the fact that the entire sacrum approaches more nearly than

* The illustrations in the chapters on Contracted Pelves have been prepared with the greatest care and accuracy. The half-tone illustrations are exactly one third natural size. Those from specimens in our possession were drawn from photographs which were taken with the pelvis as nearly as possible in the same position—that is, with the tip of the coccyx and upper margin of the symphysis pubis on the same horizontal level. Accordingly, the various illustrations can be accurately compared.

The diagrams of the superior strait and the sagittal sections through the pelvic cavity are one sixth natural size, and are accurate to within one millimetre. The former were made by means of the camera with the pelvis held so that the plane of its superior strait was at a right angle to the horizon. The latter were made from tracings of casts of the pelvic cavity obtained by means of dental wax, which were then reduced by the pantograph.

normal to the symphysis pubis. At the same time it undergoes a slight rotation about its transverse axis, since the contraction is always more marked in the antero-posterior diameter of the superior than in that of the

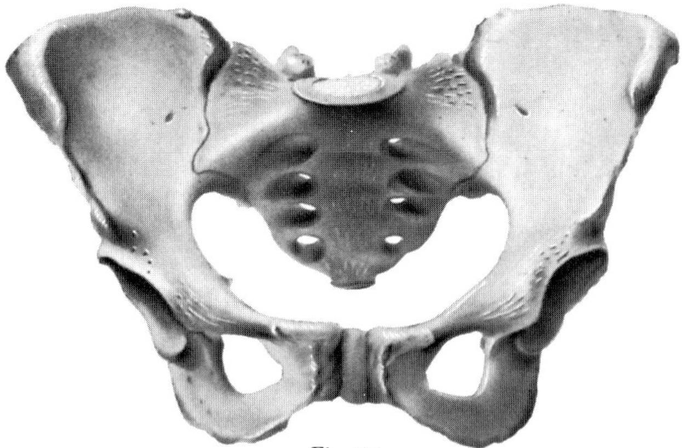

Fig. 501.

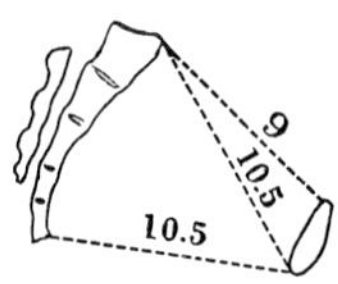

Fig. 502.

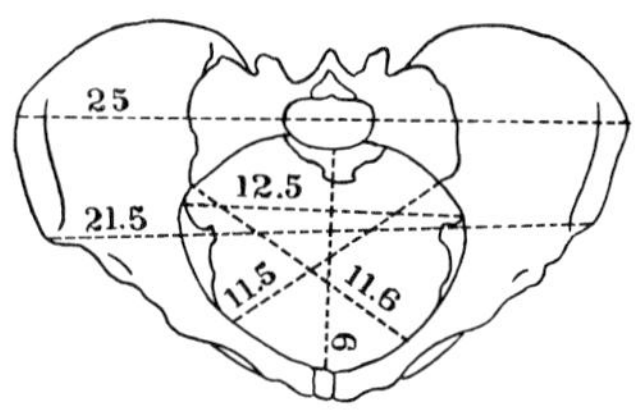

Fig. 503.

FIGS. 501–503.—FLAT NON-RHACHITIC PELVIS.

inferior strait. The degree of contraction is usually not very pronounced, and it is rare to find the conjugata vera measuring less than 8 centimetres. In fact, whenever this limit is passed the probability that one has to deal with a flat rhachitic pelvis should always be borne in mind.

The sacrum does not present the characteristic features of rhachitis, and preserves its normal vertical and side to side concavity. Occasionally it may appear somewhat more delicately shaped than usual, and be narrower transversely. Under such circumstances the transverse diameters of the pelvic cavity are slightly decreased.

In not a few pelves of this character the line of ossification between the first and second sacral vertebræ is more marked than usual, thus giving rise to a so-called second or accessory promontory.

Ætiology.—Unfortunately we are not able to make positive statements as to the cause of this deformity. By many it is believed that the approach of the sacrum to the symphysis results from the carrying of heavy burdens upon the back or head during early life, though such an explanation cannot apply to all cases, especially in this country, where it is unusual for girls to carry heavy loads. In other cases the condition is attributed to the fact that the child was allowed to sit up at too early an age and for too long periods.

Ahlfeld, Tarnier, and others think that a part in the production of the deformity is played by rhachitis, which, they hold, may be present in a larval form without giving rise to its usual and characteristic manifestations. It is quite possible that this may be true in many cases, but in others no history even suggestive of rhachitis in childhood can be elicited.

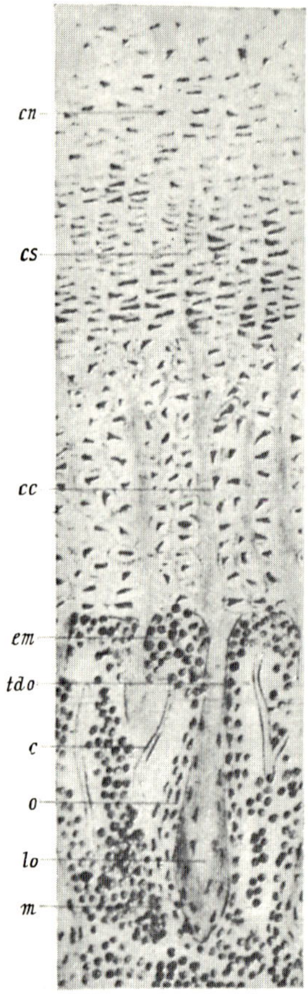

Fig. 504. — Section through Normal Epiphysis of Child (Spillmann).

cn., normal cartilage; *cs.*, cartilage cells arranged in parallel rows; *cc.*, area of preliminary calcification; *em.*, medullary spaces; *o.*, osteoblasts; *lo.*, osseous lamellæ; *m.*, marrow.

Fehling and Schliephake consider that this variety of pelvic anomaly is congenital in a certain number of instances, as they have shown that the pelves of newly born children may occasionally present a flattened appearance. In several cases studied by them the relation between the conjugata vera and the transverse diameter of the superior strait was as 100 to 145, 100 to 160, or 100 to 177, instead of 100 to 122, as is usually the case. Under such circumstances the mechanical factors above alluded to could certainly not have come into play.

Diagnosis.—The presence of a simple flat pelvis, as a rule, is readily diagnosed. By external pelvimetry the distances between the spines and crests of the ilium and that between the trochanters are found to be approximately normal, whereas Baudelocque's diameter is more or less shortened. On internal examination the diagonal conjugate is found to be shortened, and the entire anterior surface of the sacrum appears to be nearer the symphysis than usual, but presents its normal curvatures. There is no widening of the transverse diameter of the pelvic outlet, as in the rhachitic form.

The consideration of the effect of the flat pelvis upon the course of labour, and the treatment of such cases, will be deferred until the flat rhachitic pelvis is studied, as there is no essential difference in the mechanism of the two varieties.

Rhachitic Pelves.—In many parts of Europe the most prominent factor in the production of contracted pelves is an abnormal softening of the bones in early life resulting from rhachitis. In this country the disease is observed comparatively rarely in white children, occasionally in coloured children inhabiting the country districts, and very frequently in those living in large cities.

In not a few cases the disease undergoes spontaneous cure, so that no trace of its existence can be discovered in later life; while in many instances permanent skeletal deformities result which are not infrequently localized in the pelvis. Again, it is also not unusual to meet with women who to all appearances are quite normally formed, but whose pelves upon examination present rhachitic deformities. Six and fifteen hundredths per cent of the abnormal pelves occurring in the white, and 22.54 per cent in the coloured women delivered at the Johns Hopkins Hospital were rhachitic in origin, thus showing that even in this country the disease is of not a little importance from an obstetrical standpoint.

Nature and Pathology of Rhachitis.—Before describing the various changes in the pelvis which may result from rhachitis, it will be well to consider briefly the nature and pathology of the disease.

According to Kassowitz, Spillmann, and others, rhachitis is to be looked upon as an osteitis associated with an excessive formation of osteoid tissue at the epiphyses and beneath the periosteum of the long bones, as well as in the flat bones of the skull and pelvis. This proliferation is accompanied by defective calcification of the newly formed tissue, Zweifel stating that only 18 to 24 per cent of inorganic salts are present in rhachitic, as against 63 to 65 per cent in normal bone.

It is customary to distinguish three stages in the disease: that of congestion, that of softening, and that of progressive deformity or cure, as the case may be. In the stage of congestion there is a great increase in vascularity, which is most marked at the union of the articular cartilages with the diaphyses of the long bones and also beneath the periosteum.

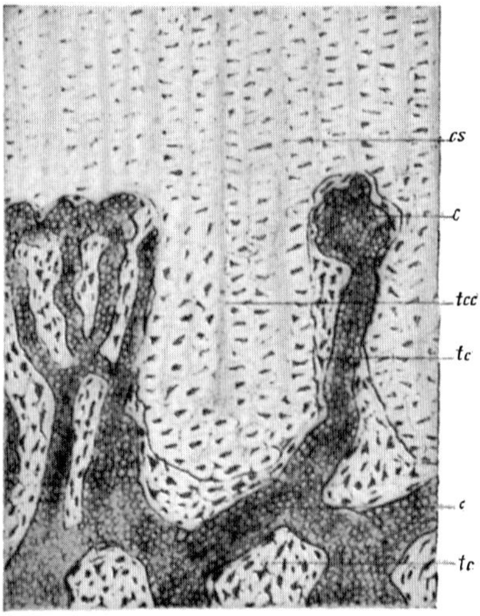

FIG. 505.—SECTION THROUGH EPIPHYSIS IN EARLY STAGES OF RHACHITIS (Spillmann).
cs., cartilage cells arranged in parallel rows; *tcc.*, area of preliminary calcification; *c.*, capillary; *tc.*, unossified connective tissue.

In studying the epiphysis of a long bone at this period, we find that the zone of preliminary calcification—Guérin's line—is slightly thickened, and its lower portion adjacent to the newly formed spongy bone is perforated by numerous vascular loops. A similar condition may also be observed beneath the periosteum covering the long and the flat bones (Fig. 505).

In the second stage, while Guérin's line has become markedly thickened and very irregular, the vascular proliferation has advanced to a marked degree. Under the microscope, the former is seen to be broken up in all directions by the rapidly growing vascular loops which subdivide it into large numbers of small, irregularly shaped calcific areas. At the same time the formation of osseous tissue just beneath it proceeds in an irregular manner, ossification either failing to occur or taking place imperfectly. The newly formed tissue is penetrated in all directions by vascular loops which break it up into small masses, between which and the marrow cavities is a considerable formation of connective tissue, with spindle- and star-shaped cells, which does not become ossified at all.

To summarize these changes briefly, one may say that the growing end of the bone, instead of undergoing normal ossification, consists in great part of dilated capillaries which separate irregularly shaped masses of calcified cartilage from areas of connective tissue and imperfectly formed bone

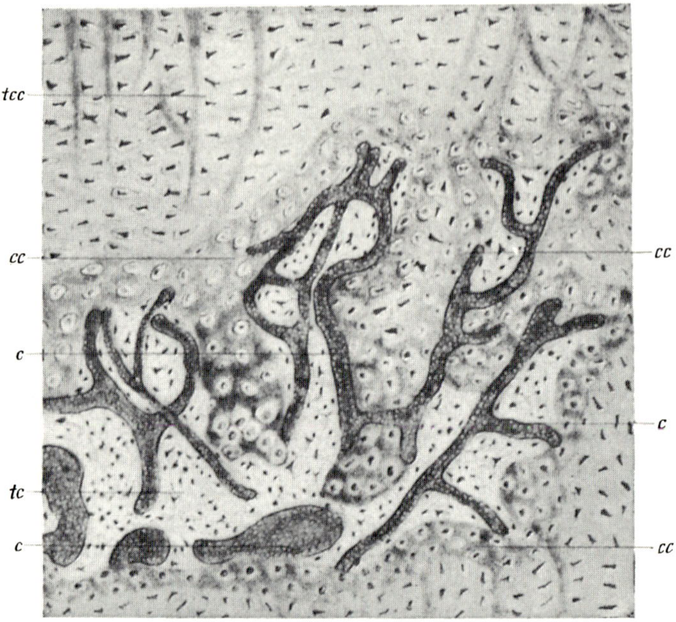

Fig. 506.—Section through Epiphysis in Advanced Stages of Rhachitis (Spillmann). *tcc.*, area of preliminary calcification; *cc.*, calcified cartilage; *c.*, capillaries; *tc.*, connective tissue.

(Fig. 506). More or less similar changes take place under the periosteum of the long and flat bones, so that the shaft of the bone soon becomes converted into a spongy tissue corresponding closely to that observed at the epiphyses.

In the third period these changes continue until death occurs; or, if recovery ensues—the usual outcome—there is a progressive decrease in vascularity, and the normal process of ossification is resumed, so that after a time the only trace of the disease is to be found in a thickening of the bone, not infrequently associated with an increased porosity. It is therefore apparent that the bones become abnormally soft and yielding in the acute stages of the disease, so that if the child uses its extremities at the time, more or less marked deformities of the various bones must result, depending upon the mechanical conditions which are liable to modify the evolution of the infantile pelvis.

Forms of Rhachitic Pelves.—As has already been said, the rhachitic type is one of the most frequently observed varieties of contracted pelvis, and in extreme cases presents the most marked deformities with which we are familiar, with the exception of those resulting from osteomalacia. Fortunately, however, the degree of contraction is usually not very pronounced,

Tarnier having stated that the conjugata vera measured less than 8.5 centimetres in only 14.4 per cent of the 1,020 rhachitic pelves studied by him.

With the exception of the cases which are complicated by abnormalities of the vertebral column, or by deformities giving rise to a marked difference in the length of the limbs, rhachitic pelves are usually classified as follows:

1. Flat rhachitic pelvis.
2. Generally contracted, flat rhachitic pelvis.
3. Generally and equally contracted rhachitic pelvis.
4. Pseudo-osteomalacic pelvis.

1. *Flat Rhachitic Pelvis.*—This variety corresponds with the flat, nonrhachitic pelvis, in so far that the greatest contraction occurs in the antero-posterior diameter of the superior strait, while the transverse diameter is seldom affected, or may even be slightly longer than usual. At the same time it differs materially from it in several particulars.

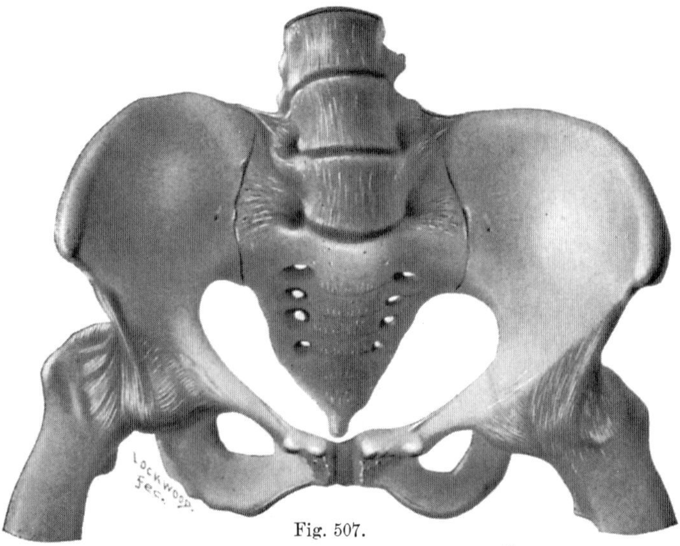

Fig. 507.

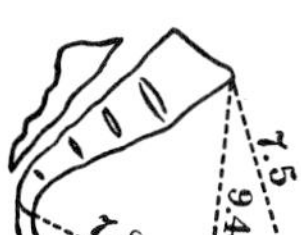

Fig. 508.

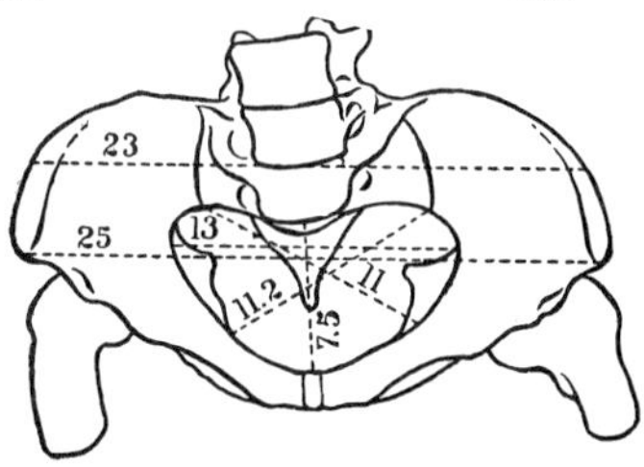

Fig. 509.

Figs. 507–509.—Flat Rhachitic Pelvis.

Generally speaking, the bones are less dense in texture than usual, and not infrequently are delicate in form, though occasionally they may appear clumsy and swollen. Owing to the marked lordosis which not infrequently results from rhachitis, the pelvic inclination, as a rule, is considerably increased.

The most important changes, however, are to be noted in the sacrum and in the relation which it bears to the rest of the pelvis, the whole bone

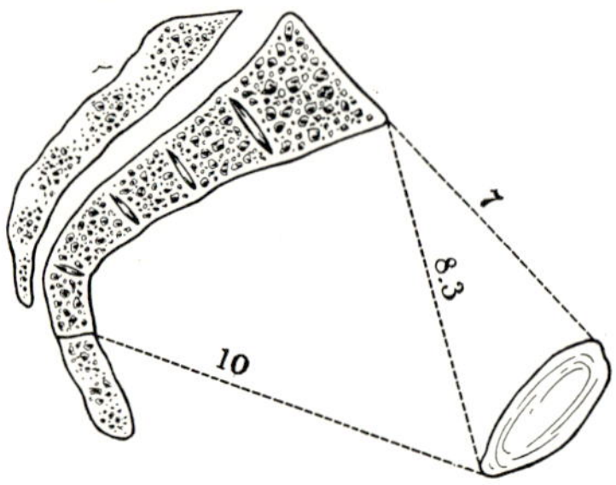

Fig. 510.—Accentuation of Vertical Concavity of Sacrum in Rhachitis.

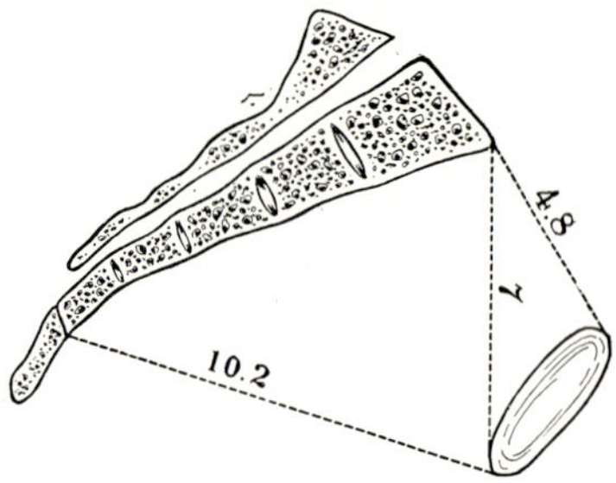

Fig. 511.—Showing Obliteration of Vertical Concavity of Sacrum in Rhachitis.

being rotated forward in such a manner that its promontory lies at a lower level than usual and encroaches markedly upon the area of the superior strait. Moreover, the entire bone is usually sharply bent upon itself in the neighbourhood of its third vertebra, its vertical concavity becoming markedly accentuated. In extreme cases the upper portion of its anterior surface extends almost horizontally, while the lower portion looks upward and forward. At the same time the bodies of the individual vertebræ are pushed out beyond the level of their alæ, the lateral concavity of the sacrum being thereby diminished, and not infrequently becomes converted into a convexity. Occasionally the lower extremity of the sacrum and the coccyx are not bowed inward, and in such cases the former bone, instead of presenting an increased vertical concavity, may be straight or even convex from above downward.

It is not unusual for the body of the first sacral vertebra to be more markedly displaced forward than those below it, so that its lower margin projects beyond the general surface, when it can be felt as a *false promontory.* Under such circumstances the distance between it and the symphysis pubis is frequently the shortest antero-posterior diameter of the pelvis.

As the upper part of the sacrum becomes displaced downward and inward, its posterior surface recedes from the superior posterior spines of the ilium, which approach one another more closely than in the normal condition.

The iliac bones, in addition to being more delicately shaped than usual, are directed almost horizontally, and, what is more important, flare outward to a marked degree, so that the distance between their anterior superior spines approaches that between their crests, and occasionally even exceeds it in length. Not infrequently the iliac bones bend just in front of the sacro-iliac synchondrosis, so that the ilio-pectineal line, instead of following a gentle curve, forms a sharp angle at that point, thus adding materially to the narrowing of the superior strait. At the same time the acetabula are displaced forward and come to lie upon the anterior, instead of upon the lateral portion of the pelvic ring. The pubic arch is somewhat wider than usual, and the tubera ischii are everted, so that the transverse diameter of the pelvic outlet appears to be exaggerated, and occasionally measures more than in the normal pelvis.

These changes exert a decided influence upon the shape of the pelvic cavity, the effect being most marked in the superior strait, which may become oval, reniform, or even heart-shaped in outline, according to the degree of displacement of the promontory of the sacrum. The conjugata vera is always shortened, while the transverse diameter seems to be enlarged, although this may be only apparent unless the pelvis be of large size.

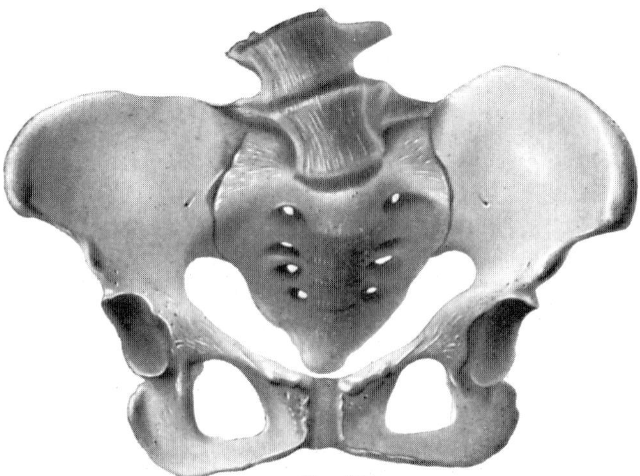

Fig. 512.

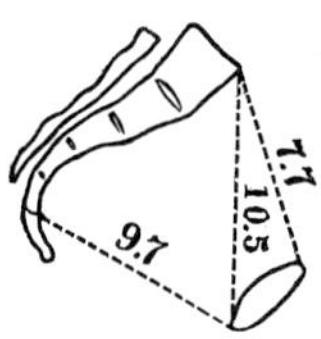

Fig. 513.

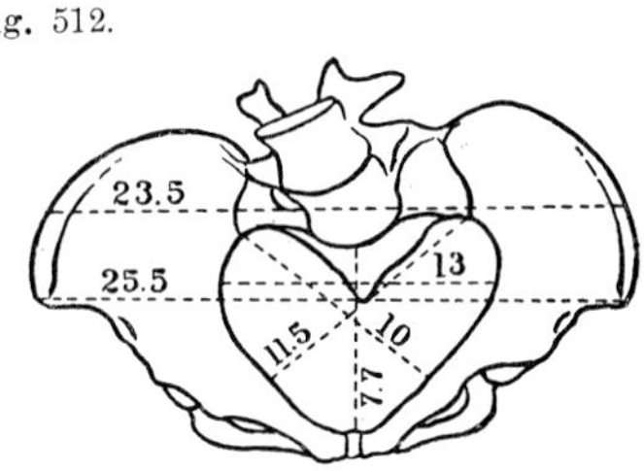

Fig. 514.

Figs. 512–514.—Flat Rhachitic Pelvis, showing Double Promontory.

Owing to the approach of the anterior and posterior walls of the pelvis, the oblique diameters of the superior strait are always shortened, as are also the sacro-cotyloid diameters. As a result of the upward and backward displacement of the lower portion of the sacrum, the pelvic cavity below the superior strait undergoes a relative increase in size, which is more particularly marked in the various antero-posterior diameters.

In occasional cases sharp exostoses may make their appearance upon the pubic crests, the ilio-pectineal eminences, and in front of the sacro-iliac synchondroses—*pelvis spinosa.* When such structures are not well covered by soft parts, they may lead to serious injuries of the uterus at the time of labour.

2. *Generally Contracted, Flat Rhachitic Pelvis.*—It is in this variety of pelvis that marked degrees of contraction are often encountered, thé conjugata vera sometimes being reduced to 3 or 4 centimetres. This pelvis corresponds closely to the ordinary flat rhachitic type, except that the shortening applies to all its diameters instead of being limited to the conjugata vera.

The decrease in size is particularly marked in the sacrum, which may present a considerable diminution in its transverse measurements. The small size of the pelvis in such cases may be due either to atrophic changes in the bones resulting from the rhachitis itself or to a primarily small pelvis that has become affected with the disease.

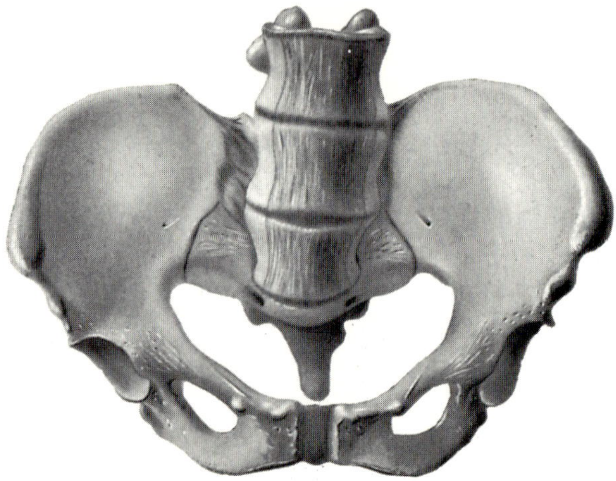

Fig. 515.

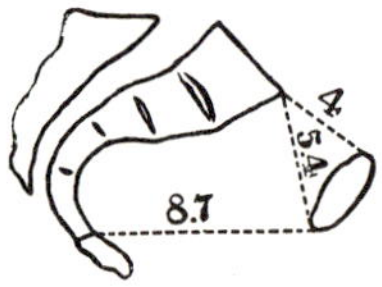

Fig. 516.

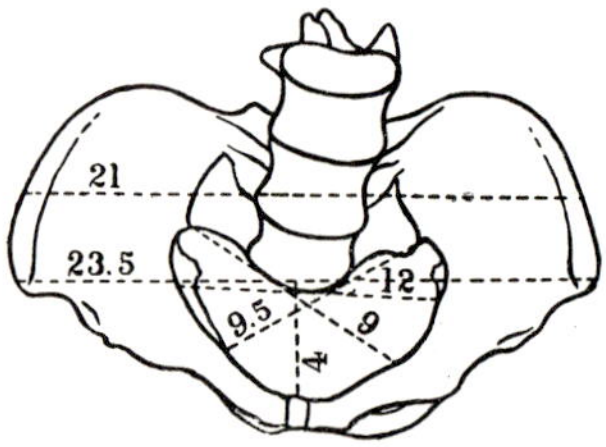

Fig. 517.

Figs. 515–517.—Generally Contracted, Flat Rhachitic Pelvis.

3. *Generally Equally Contracted Rhachitic Pelvis.*—This variety was first described by Michealis, and according to most authors is observed but rarely. Müller, however, considers that not a few cases which were previously described as instances of simple, generally contracted (justo-minor) pelvis, belong under this category, and my own experience, particularly in the negro race, has tended to confirm his observations.

According to Litzmann, this type differs from the justo-minor pelvis in its ungainly and angular appearance, and in the marked prominence of the pubic crests. The superior strait appears to be equally shortened in all its diameters instead of merely flattened, while the rest of the pelvis presents indisputable signs of a past rhachitis, which is more particularly marked in the sacrum and in the eversion of the tubera ischii.

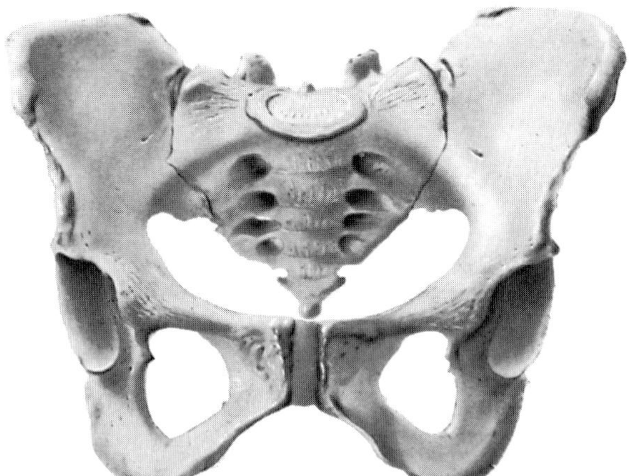

Fig. 518.

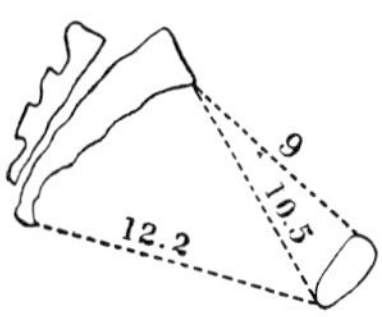

Fig. 519.

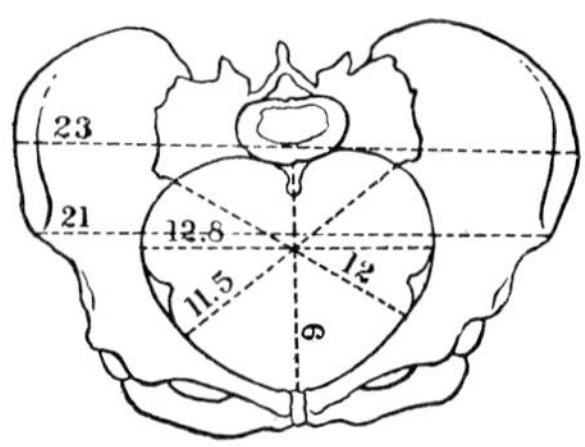

Fig. 520.

FIGS. 518–520.—GENERALLY EQUALLY CONTRACTED RHACHITIC PELVIS.

4. *Pseudo-osteomalacic Rhachitic Pelvis.*—This variety is a manifestation of the severest forms of rhachitis, and affords examples of the most marked

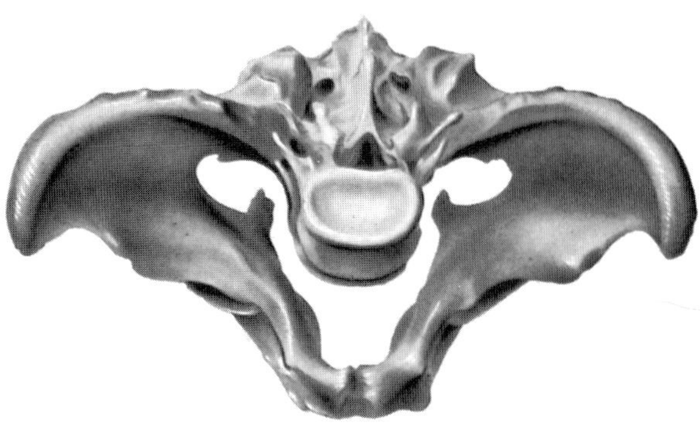

FIG. 521.—PSEUDO-OSTEOMALACIC PELVIS (Naegele).

degrees of contraction. In such cases, as the name implies, the pelvis resembles one deformed by osteomalacia, the sacrum and lateral walls approaching one another so as to give rise to a very small triangular superior strait, the contraction also extending to other portions of the pelvic cavity.

This form of pelvis was first described by Smellie, who gave an illustration of it in his anatomical plates. More particular attention was directed to it by Stein, and especially by Naegele. It is not of frequent occurrence, though Fasbender in 1878 was able to collect 40 cases from the literature, not a few of which occurred in young children.

Mode of Production of Deformity in Rhachitic Pelves.—We have already considered the part played in the transformation of the fœtal into the adult pelvis by the action of the body weight and the upward and inward force exerted by the femora. Abnormalities and variations in the mode of action of these forces also serve to explain the way in which most of the characteristic rhachitic deformities are produced.

These views were developed in great part by Litzmann, and have obtained almost general acceptance, although Fehling, Freund, Kehrer, and others take exception to them.

In the acute stages of rhachitis the young child is unable to walk, and spends its time in a sitting or reclining position, in which the upward and

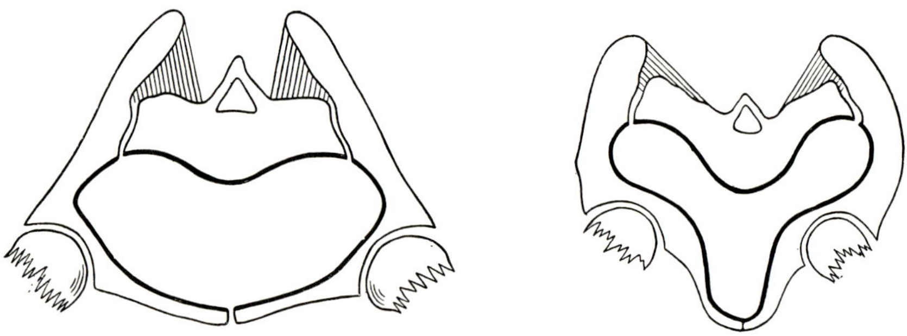

Fig. 522. Fig. 523.

FIGS. 522, 523.—DIAGRAMS SHOWING CHANGES IN SHAPE IN RHACHITIC AND OSTEOMALACIC PELVES (Schroeder).

inward force exerted by the femora is in abeyance. Consequently, when it sits up, the body weight is the only force which comes into play, and on being transmitted from the vertebral column to the sacrum, it is resolved into two forces—one directed downward and the other forward. As a result, the sacrum rotates about its transverse axis, the promontory being pressed forward and downward, while the remainder of the bone moves in the opposite direction and tends to assume a more or less horizontal position. The extreme upward dislocation of its lower end is resisted by the traction exerted upon it and the coccyx by the strong sacro-sciatic ligaments, and consequently the softened bone becomes sharply flexed at its lower portion, whereby its vertical concavity is accentuated. At the same time, owing to the softened condition of the sacrum and the imperfect union between the bodies and alæ of its vertebræ, the former are pushed out beyond the latter, thus converting its normal lateral concavity into a convexity.

As the promontory is displaced forward and downward under the influence of the body weight, the posterior surface of the sacrum recedes from the superior posterior spines of the ilium, thus subjecting the strong iliosacral ligaments to marked tension. As a result the spines are drawn nearer to the middle line, while at the same time the anterior portions of the iliac bones flare out, thus accounting for the changed position of the anterior superior spines. This movement is resisted by the cohesive force exerted by the anterior pelvic wall, and as a consequence the softened bones bend just in front of the sacro-iliac synchondrosis, so that the iliopectineal line on either side, instead of following a gentle curve, becomes sharply bent at that point.

Coincident with these changes, the positions of the acetabula become altered, being situated upon the anterior, instead of upon the lateral walls of the pelvis. As a result, when the child begins to walk the forces exerted by the femora also add to the flattening of the superior strait. On the other hand, owing to the previous non-use of the lower extremities, these last forces have not been called into play early enough to counteract the widening of the pelvis as a result of prolonged sitting, and consequently the ischial tuberosities become flared out.

The same factors are concerned in the production of the generally contracted rhachitic pelvis, its small size being due either to atrophy following the rhachitis, or to the effect of the disease upon a pelvis already abnormally small.

The pseudo-osteomalacic form results when the rhachitic softening of the bones is very marked and the child persists in walking. Under such circumstances not only are the characteristic changes in the sacrum and iliac crests produced, but at the same time the anterior and lateral portions of the pelvis are pushed in towards the sacrum, the pelvic cavity becoming almost obliterated.

As has already been said, these views have not been universally accepted, Fehling believing that the characteristic form of the pelvis may result *in utero*, before these factors can come into play. In not a few cases of fœtal pelvic deformity the embryo has suffered from so-called fœtal rhachitis, which has been designated as *achondroplasia* and *chondrodystrophia fœtalis* by Porak and Kaufmann respectively, both of whom, however, have shown that it differs radically from rhachitis. They agree, therefore, that deformities resulting from this process cannot be compared with those resulting from true rhachitis (Fig. 544).

Freund has attempted to show that in view of the peculiar nature of the sacro-iliac joints the sacrum cannot rotate about its transverse axis. His description of these structures, however, appears to have been based in great part upon conditions observed in adult life, and he seems to have lost sight of the fact that articular surfaces in early life are almost entirely cartilaginous, and thus readily permit of motion in any direction.

Kehrer believes that the action of certain groups of muscles plays a most important part in the production of abnormal pelves. No doubt this is true to a certain extent, but it is hardly probable that it is the only factor concerned.

Diagnosis of Rhachitic Pelves.—Important information as to the presence of rhachitis may be elicited by the inspection and examination of the patient when characteristic deformities may be noted about the head, vertebral column, and lower extremities. In not a few cases, the thickened epiphyses at the costal margins—the so-called rhachitic rosary—may also serve to call attention to the existence of the disease.

A decidedly pendulous abdomen in primiparous women is always suggestive of marked disproportion between the size of the head and the pelvis, and should always suggest a search for rhachitic changes.

The age at which the patient first learned to walk is also of considerable importance, as it is well known that children suffering from rhachitis are usually backward in this respect. Again, when the disease appears after the first year of life, the child usually ceases to walk during its acute stages, and has to learn again at a later period.

Accurate information concerning the pelvis, however, can be obtained only by pelvimetry. On external mensuration the distances between the spines and crests of the ilium no longer show their normal relations, the former approaching and not infrequently exceeding the latter in length. Normally, there is a difference of 2.5 to 3 centimetres between the two, and whenever this becomes reduced to 1 centimetre or less, rhachitis should be suspected. The distance between the trochanters will be normal or not, according as one has to deal with a flat or generally contracted rhachitic pelvis. Baudelocque's diameter is always considerably shortened. At the same time Michealis's rhomboid loses its regular outlines, and in marked cases, owing to the sinking downward and forward of the sacrum, becomes converted into a triangular area.

Still more definite information may be gained by internal pelvimetry. The diagonal conjugate is always shortened. The anterior surface of the sacrum is much more readily accessible to the examining fingers, and on careful palpation its upper portion is found to be flatter than usual, while its lower portion is sharply bent forward. Moreover, owing to the prominence of the vertebral bodies, the sacrum is found to be convex from side to side, instead of concave, as normally. At the same time the pelvic outlet appears to be widened.

The flat rhachitic pelvis is ordinarily diagnosed when the transverse external measurements show but slight diminution, whereas in the generally contracted variety they measure considerably less than normal. The generally and equally contracted variety is rarely diagnosed during life, while the characteristic deformity of the pseudo-osteomalacic form will be recognised on internal examination, and the decision as to whether it is due to rhachitis or osteomalacia will be determined by the history of the patient.

Osteomalacic Pelves.—Inasmuch as osteomalacia gives rise to the most marked pelvic deformities with which we are familiar, it was only natural that the attention of obstetricians should have been directed to it at an early date. Cooper performed Cæsarean section for this condition in 1768, but for the main pioneer work we are indebted to Stein, Kilian, and Litzmann.

Nature and Clinical History of Osteomalacia.—Osteomalacia, halisteresis, mollities ossium or malacosteon disease, is a chronic inflammatory disease of the bones, which become soft, yielding, and occasionally brittle, and consequently undergo marked changes in shape as the result of the action of the various mechanical forces to which they are subjected.

The disease is one of adult life, and is very rarely met with in children. It occurs far more frequently in women than in men, especially during pregnancy or the puerperium. Litzmann, in 1861, collected 131 cases from the literature, 85 of which were in pregnant or puerperal women, 35 in non-pregnant women, and 11 in men. Since that time the number of cases in women has markedly increased, whereas in 1900 Hahn was able to add only 31 additional instances in males.

The disease may occur in any part of the world, but is especially frequent, and may even be said to be endemic, in certain localities, notably in the Rhine Valley, the Ergolz Valley in Switzerland, the Olona Valley and Calabria in Italy, and in the city of Vienna. It is very rarely observed in this country, England, or France, Dock having been able to collect only 10 cases in America up to 1896. Tarnier, in his large experience, encountered only 3 cases in Paris, Hirst saw 3 in Philadelphia, and up to the present time 3 have come under my observation in Baltimore.

As yet no satisfactory explanation for its endemic occurrence has been adduced, but it seems to be intimately connected with unsanitary surroundings and inferior food. This was strikingly illustrated by the experience of Winckel, Sr., in Gummersbach in Germany, and of Hoebecke in Sottegem in Holland. The former performed 13 and the latter 14 Cæsarean sections upon osteomalacic patients prior to 1840. Since that time improvement in the hygienic conditions of both villages, together with more healthy occupation for their inhabitants, has led to an almost total disappearance of the disease.

Osteomalacia may affect any portion of the skeleton, but seems to select more particularly the pelvis, vertebræ, and ribs. The fresh bones are yellowish or yellowish-brown in appearance, and very soft and brittle. In advanced cases their consistence is that of leather or wax, so that they can readily be cut with a knife. In the later stages of the disease the spongy bones present a markedly areolated appearance on section, and in some instances are so rarefied that only the outer layers remain intact. At the same time they become much lighter, the specific gravity being frequently reduced by one half.

Under the microscope the marrow spaces are found to be greatly enlarged, and there is a marked increase in vascularity. The most important change, however, consists in the substitution of osteoid tissue in place of the true bone surrounding the Haversian canals.

All of the earlier writers upon the subject considered that the changes in the bone resulted from decalcification, which was due to the presence of lactic or a related acid in the circulating blood. But after the correctness of this view had been denied by Virchow in 1852, the writers upon the subject have been divided into two camps: the one claiming that the essential feature of the disease is decalcification, and the other, a disturbance in the relation between resorption and deposition, by which osteoid instead of osseous tissue is formed. Full details of this discussion are to be found in the writings of Gelpke, Ribbert, Winckel, and Laufer, in which the entire subject is carefully considered.

One of the most important contributions to the subject was made by Fehling in 1888, who advanced the theory that the disease was a tropho-

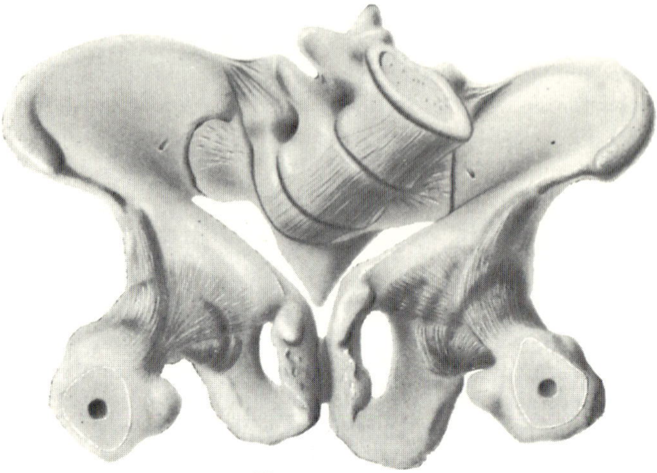

Fig. 524.

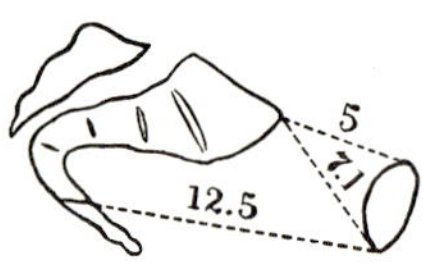

Fig. 525.

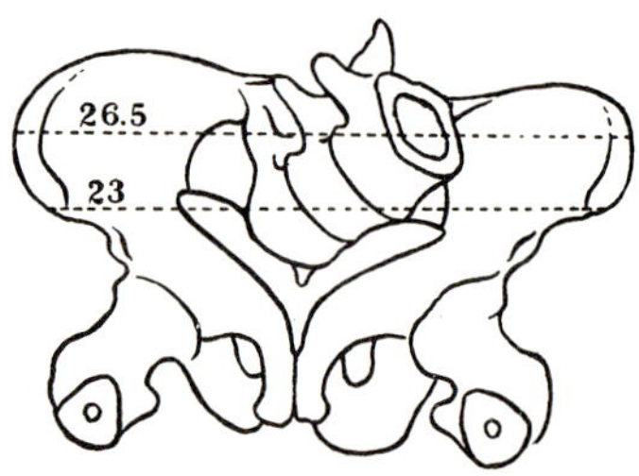

Fig. 526.

FIGS. 524–526.—OSTEOMALACIC PELVIS.

neurosis of ovarian origin. He believed that characteristic changes could be made out in the ovaries, and that these gave rise to reflex stimulation of the vasodilators supplying the bones. Although this theory serves to explain the brilliant results following castration in this disease, the various authorities are not yet agreed concerning the changes in the ovaries, and Bulius, in 1898, stated that they were not characteristic.

More important, from a practical standpoint, is the clinical history of the affection. In its earliest stages it is characterized by peculiar muscular palsies, which more especially affect the ilio-psoas, and which are often accompanied by contractures of the abductor muscles of the thigh and increased patellar reflexes. A little later rheumatoid pains make their appearance in various portions of the body, and at the same time the pelvis, ribs, and vertebral column become very sensitive upon pressure. As the disease advances still further and the bones become softer, various deformities appear, which are particularly marked in the vertebral column and pelvis.

The history of osteomalacic patients is usually of this character: The woman has had one or more normal labours. During the next pregnancy she complains of muscular symptoms and rheumatoid pains, and greater difficulty is experienced at the time of labour. The same symptoms recur with added intensity in the succeeding pregnancy, and the labour is still more difficult, probably requiring craniotomy. In the succeeding pregnancy the rheumatoid pains become so intense and locomotion is interfered with to such an extent that for the last months the patient is obliged to take to her bed. This labour also generally requires craniotomy or Cæsarean section. After its termination the pains disappear, and when the patient is able to get about again she notices that she has become some inches shorter than previously, the diminution in stature being sometimes associated with kyphotic changes in the vertebral column.

To sum up, a history of rheumatoid pains and difficult locomotion requiring rest in bed during pregnancy, associated with a decrease in height, is almost pathognomonic of osteomalacia.

Changes in the Shape of the Pelvis.—The extent of the deformity resulting from osteomalacia depends entirely upon the degree of softening which the various pelvic bones have undergone. According to Kehrer, in the early stages of the disease the pelvis is simply flattened as the result of the forcing downward and forward of the promontory of the sacrum. At the same time the bodies of the vertebræ are pushed out and beyond the alæ, and its lower extremity becomes markedly curved inward, the changes being usually much more pronounced than in the rhachitic pelvis.

In the later stages of the disease, when the bones have become very soft, the pelvis takes on a characteristic compressed appearance. The body weight presses the promontory still further downward and forward, while the upward and inward forces exerted by the femora push the lateral walls

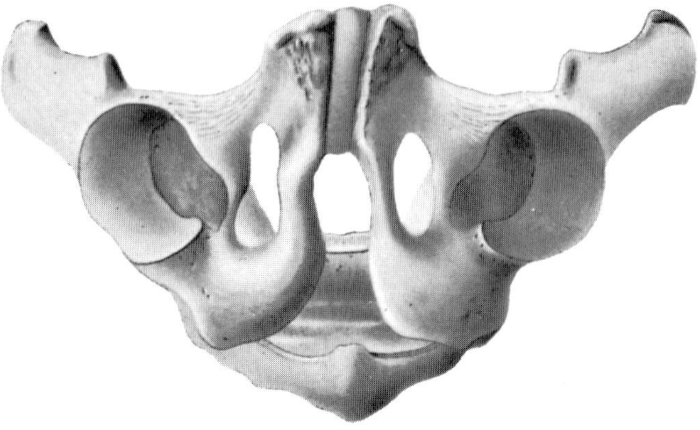

FIG. 527.—OSTEOMALACIC PELVIS, INFERIOR STRAIT.

of the pelvis inward, until in very marked cases the superior strait becomes almost entirely obliterated. At the same time the ischio-pubic rami are approximated, and the pubic arch is converted into a narrow slit into which it is sometimes impossible to insinuate the fingers. The pubic rami are pushed markedly forward, giving rise to a beak-like protuberance upon the anterior wall of the pelvis. Coincident with these changes, there is a marked diminution in the size of the pelvic cavity and of the inferior strait, though in not a few cases, owing to constant sitting upon the softened bones, the tubera ischii are considerably flared out. In advanced cases the pelvis is very much deformed, and may present any one of an almost infinite variety of bizarre shapes.

Diagnosis.—The diagnosis is readily made, as careful inquiry will usually elicit the characteristic clinical history of the disease; while examination of the pelvis will show that it is markedly compressed in all directions, and the pathognomonic changes in the pubic arch can hardly escape detection. Indeed, the only form of pelvis with which it might be confounded is the very rare transversely contracted Robert pelvis, but the absence of the characteristic clinical history and the lack of antero-posterior shortening in the latter will usually enable one to differentiate between them.

LITERATURE

Ahlfeld. Die Diagnose des einfach platten Beckens an der Lebenden. Zeitschr. f. Geb. u. Gyn., 1895, xxxii, 356–367.

Betschler. Annalen der klin. Anstalten, Breslau, 1832, i, 24–60, ii, 31.

Bulius. Osteomalacie u. Eierstock. Hegar's Beiträge, 1898, i, 138.

Deventer. Neues Hebammenlicht, III. Aufl., Jena, 1728, 199.

Dock. Osteomalacia, with a New Case. Amer. Jour. Med. Sciences, 1895, cix, 499–516.

Fasbender. Ueber das pseudo- und das rachitisch-osteomalacische Becken. Zeitschr. f. Geb. u. Gyn., 1878, ii, 332–345.

Fehling. Die Entstehung der rachitischen Beckenform. Archiv f. Gyn., 1877, xi, 173–183.

Ueber Kastration bei Osteomalacie. Verh. d. deutschen Gesellsch. f. Gyn., 1888, ii, 311–318.

Freund. Ueber das sogenannte kyphotische Becken. Gyn. Klinik, 1885, 1–134.

Gelpke. Die Osteomalacie im Ergolzthale. Basel, 1891.

Hahn. Ueber Osteomalacie beim Manne. Zusammenfassendes Referat: Centralbl. f. die Grenzgebiete der Med. u. Chir., 1900, iii.

Hirst. A Text-Book of Obstetrics. Third edition, 465. Philadelphia, 1901.

Kassowitz. Die normale Ossification und die Erkrankungen bei Rachitis und hereditärer Syphilis. Wien, 1882.

Kaufmann. Untersuchungen über die sogenannte fötale Rachitis. Berlin, 1892.

Kehrer. Zur Entwickelungsgeschichte des rachitischen Beckens. Archiv f. Gyn., 1873, i, 55–99.

Pelvis plana osteomalacica. Centralbl. f. Gyn., 1901, 986–990.

Kilian. Beiträge zu einer genauen Kenntniss der allgemeinen Knochenerweichung der Frauen. Bonn, 1829.

Das halisteretische Becken. Bonn, 1857.

Latzo. Beiträge zur Diagnose und Therapie der Osteomalacie. Monatsschr. f. Geb. u. Gyn., 1897, vi, 571–608.

Laufer. Zur Path. u. Therapie der Osteomalacie des Weibes. Centralbl. f. die Grenzgebiete der Med. u. Chir., 1900, iii, Nr. 1.

Litzmann. Die Formen des Beckens, nebst einem Anhange über Osteomalacie. Berlin, 1861.

Die Geburt bei engem Becken. Leipzig, 1884, 36.

MICHEALIS. Das enge Becken, Leipzig, 1851.
MÜLLER. Zur Frequenz und Aetiologie des allgemein verengten Beckens. Archiv f. Gyn., 1880, xvi, 155–174.
NAEGELE. Das schräg verengte Becken. Mainz, 1839.
PORAK. De l'achondroplasie. Nouvelles Archives d'Obst. et de Gyn., December, 1889.
RIBBERT. Die Osteomalacie. Bibliotheca Medica.
SCHLIEPHAKE. Ueber path. Beckenformen beim Fötus. Archiv f. Gyn., 1882, xx, 435–454.
SMELLIE. Anatomical Tables, etc. Plate III, new edition, Edinburgh, 1787.
SPILLMANN. Le Rachitisme. Thèse de Nancy, 1900.
STEIN. Kleine Werke zur prakt. Geburtshülfe, 1798, 283–340, dazu, Taf. X.
Die Lehranstalt der Geburtshülfe zu Bonn, I. Heft, Elberfeld, 1823.
TARNIER et BUDIN. Traité de l'art des accouchements, 1898, iii.
VIRCHOW. Archiv f. path. Anat. u. Physiol., 1852, iv.
WILLIAMS, J. WHITRIDGE. Pelvic Indications for the Performance of Cæsarean Section. American Medicine, 1901, ii, 483.
WINCKEL. Behandlung der Osteomalacie. Pentzoldt u. Stintzing. Handbuch der spec. Therapie, 1896, Bd. v, Abth. vii, 214–242.
ZWEIFEL. Aetiologie, Prophylaxis und Therapie der Rachitis. Leipzig, 1900.

CHAPTER XXXV

PELVIC ANOMALIES DUE TO ABNORMAL MALLEABILITY OF THE PELVIC BONES (*Continued*)

EFFECT UPON THE COURSE OF PREGNANCY AND THE MECHANISM OF LABOUR—TREATMENT

MARKED degrees of pelvic deformity exert a pronounced influence upon the course of pregnancy as well as upon the mechanism of labour. Indeed, to be unaccompanied by more or less untoward effects the contraction must be minimal.

Effect of Contracted Pelves upon the Course of Pregnancy.—*The Position of the Uterus.*—In the early months of pregnancy a minor grade of pelvic malformation may exert little or no influence upon the position of the uterus, but when present in any marked degree it may interfere with the normal rising up of that organ, particularly if the promontory of the sacrum projects so far into the superior strait as markedly to overhang the pelvic cavity. In such cases the fundus impinges upon the anterior surface of the sacrum, and as the uterus increases in size it assumes a position of more or less pronounced retroflexion, which later may give rise to characteristic symptoms of incarceration.

When the deformity is sufficient to interfere with the descent of the presenting part into the pelvis, marked abnormalities in the position of the uterus are observed in the later months of pregnancy. Under such circumstances, particularly in primiparæ, the fundus occupies a higher position than usual, and serious respiratory and circulatory disturbances often result. At the same time, owing to the fact that the lower portion of the uterus is not fixed by the engaged head, the entire organ is much more freely movable than usual.

More important, however, is the sharply anteflexed position which the uterus assumes as a consequence of serious disproportion in size between the head and the pelvis. This is emphasized more particularly in small women suffering from marked lumbar lordosis, in whom the capacity of the abdomen is so greatly diminished that the growing uterus seeks to gain room by pushing forward the anterior abdominal walls. The presence of a *pendulous abdomen* is a sign of considerable importance in primiparous women, and should always cause one to suspect the existence of marked pelvic deformity. The converse, however, by no means always holds good, and its absence does not necessarily indicate that no disproportion exists. Moreover, a pendulous abdomen is often observed in multiparous women, and may have no great significance, being generally due to a loss of tonicity of the uterine and abdominal walls as a result of previous pregnancies.

Position and Presentation of Fœtus.—A contracted pelvis plays an important part in the production of abnormal presentations. In primiparous women, when the pelvis is normal, the presenting part, as a rule, descends into the pelvic cavity during the last six weeks of pregnancy; but when the superior strait is considerably contracted this does not occur until after the onset of labour, and sometimes not at all. Vertex presentations still predominate; but since the head floats freely above the superior strait, or rests upon one of the iliac fossæ, very slight influences may cause the fœtus to assume other positions. According to Michealis, vertex presentations are rarer by 10 per cent in contracted than in normal pelves; while face, breech, and transverse presentations occur 2 or 3 times, and prolapse of the cord and the extremities 4 to 6 times more frequently.

Abnormal presentations increase in frequency with the degree of contraction, as is shown by the following figures of Michealis, Litzmann, and Schwartz:

Conjugata vera 9.5 – 8.5 cm., 93.1% vertex presentations.
" " 8.4 – 7.5 " 83.8% " "
" " 7.4 cm. or less, 64.7% " "

Tarnier, in 1,030 cases of labour complicated by contracted pelves, observed 882 vertex (85.13 per cent instead of 96 per cent), 72 breech (7 per cent instead of 3 per cent), 32 face (3 per cent instead of 0.6 per cent), and 44 transverse presentations (4.2 per cent instead of 0.5 per cent).

As has been seen, abnormal presentations occur more frequently in multiparous than in primiparous women even under favourable conditions, and, as might be expected, they become still more common when the pelvis is contracted. Thus, Schauta estimated that they are 3 times more frequent in the fifth than in the first pregnancy.

Face and transverse presentations possess a peculiar significance in primiparous women, and their occurrence is nearly always associated with marked disproportion between the size of the head and the pelvis, so that whenever either variety is encountered one can feel certain that the head is abnormally large or the pelvis abnormally small.

Size of Fœtus.—La Torre, Pinard, and others have stated that the children of women with abnormal pelves usually attain a larger size than usual. Pinard attributes this to the fact that in such cases the head does not become engaged during the last few weeks of pregnancy, and therefore cannot press upon the lower uterine segment, thus doing away with one of the factors predisposing to the premature termination of pregnancy. Wilcke, after careful study, has concluded that such is not the case, and that the children, under such circumstances, are generally slightly smaller than usual. This is particularly the case when the pelvis is generally contracted, as such women are usually under-sized and would naturally give birth to smaller children than would larger and better formed individuals.

Mechanism of Labour in Simple Flat and Flat Rhachitic Pelves.—The possibility of the occurrence of spontaneous labour in flat pelves depends primarily upon the degree of contraction, and, when this is not excessive, upon the following additional factors: the size, compressibility, and malleability of the fœtal head, and the character of the expulsive forces. The measurements of the pelvis can be estimated with tolerable accuracy, but there are no satisfactory methods of determining in advance the size and other properties of the head, and not until labour has come on can one tell at all approximately what the uterus can do.

In our 287 cases of labour in contracted pelves, spontaneous delivery occurred in 199 (71.58 per cent), and became less frequent the more maıked the pelvic deformity. Thus, when the conjugata vera measured

10 — 9 cm., spontaneous delivery occurred in				77.28%.
8.9 — 8 "	"	"	"	61.54%.
7.9 — 7 "	"	"	"	33-⅓%.
6.9 cm. or less,	"	"	"	none.

Even when the child is born spontaneously and without any undue delay, certain characteristic abnormalities can be observed in the mechanism of labour by which the experienced obstetrician is enabled to diagnose the presence of a flat pelvis without resorting to pelvimetry.

Inasmuch as in the varieties of pelves under consideration, the contraction is practically limited to the anterior posterior diameter of the superior strait, while the transverse diameter remains unchanged, or may even be slightly enlarged, it is evident that the obstacle to the passage of the child's head is offered by the shortened conjugata vera; and when this measures less than 9 or 9.5 centimetres it becomes out of the question for the biparietal diameter of the head to pass through it, unless it undergoes some diminution in size. Accordingly, when engagement occurs, the head slips to one side so as to bring the shorter bitemporal diameter in relation with the conjugata vera. As a result, the long arm of the head lever becomes displaced to the side of the occiput, so that the anterior portion of the head descends under the influence of the uterine contractions, while the occipital portion rises up. Under these conditions the large fontanelle is found to be readily accessible to the examining finger on one side of the pelvis, while the small fontanelle is reached with some difficulty on the other. At the same time, owing to the fact that the transverse diameter of the superior strait is not shortened, the head tends to accommodate itself to it, so that its long axis, as indicated by the sagittal suture, comes to lie transversely.

More characteristic still is the abnormal attitude which the head assumes when the disproportion between it and the pelvis is at all marked, so that we have what is known as an *anterior parietal presentation*. In this the presenting part, which is the anterior parietal bone, occupies the superior strait in such a manner that the sagittal suture lies just in front of the promontory. Under such circumstances the anterior shoulder is readily distinguished upon external palpation. According to the explanation generally accepted, this condition is brought about by the abnormal relation borne by the axis of the anteflexed uterus to the plane of the superior strait, as the result of which the posterior portion of the head is pressed against the promontory of the sacrum, where it becomes arrested, while its anterior portion is forced into the pelvis.

This presentation is simply an exaggeration of the so-called Naegele's obliquity, and the mechanism of descent is readily understood when we compare the passage of the head through the abnormal superior strait to the manœuvre necessary to pass a stick of a certain length through a ring of a somewhat shorter diameter. To do so, one must depress one end of the stick so as to allow it to enter the ring obliquely, and after it has nearly passed through its other end must likewise be lowered.

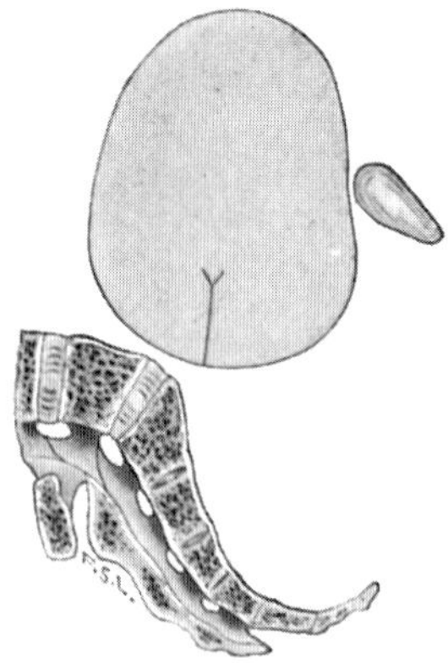

FIG. 528.—SHOWING ANTERIOR PARIETAL PRESENTATION.

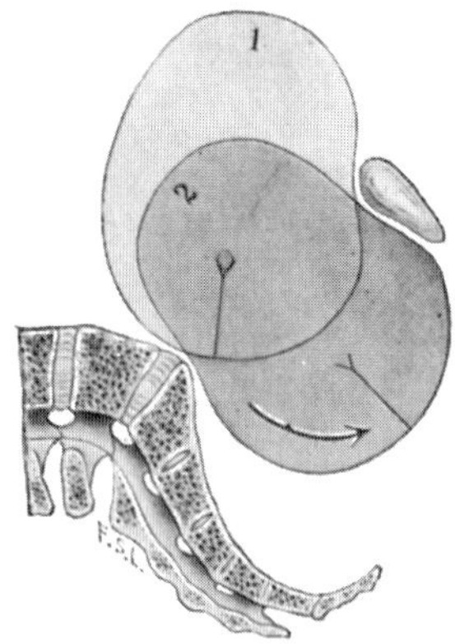

FIG. 529.—SHOWING THE PASSAGE OF AN ANTERIOR PARIETAL PRESENTATION THROUGH THE SUPERIOR STRAIT.

In order for descent of the head to occur, the posterior parietal bone is firmly pressed against the promontory of the sacrum, while under the influence of the uterine contractions the anterior portion of the head is slowly forced down into the pelvis along the posterior surface of the symphysis pubis; after this is accomplished the posterior portion passes over the promontory and enters the pelvis, the sagittal suture at the same time moving forward. Under such circumstances, when the contraction is marked, considerable pressure must be exerted upon the posterior portion of the head. Evidence of this is usually afforded after birth by a more or less well-defined curved depression, just behind the coronal suture, upon the side of the head which was in contact with the promontory. After the posterior parietal bone has passed the superior strait, all resistance has been overcome, and, owing to the fact that the lower portion of the pelvis is often larger than usual, the rest of the labour is promptly accomplished.

In a small number—according to Litzmann about one fourth of the cases—the reverse condition—the *posterior parietal presentation*—is observed. The sagittal suture now lies almost in contact with the symphysis pubis, while the posterior parietal bone occupies the superior strait, and in marked cases the posterior ear of the child can be felt just above the promontory, so that the condition is sometimes spoken of as an *ear presentation.* The long axis of the child's body forms an obtuse angle with its head, and upon palpation the anterior portion of the latter can be felt as a prominent tumour lying above the symphysis.

In order for the head to enter the pelvis, its posterior portion must be pushed down past the promontory of the sacrum, after which its anterior

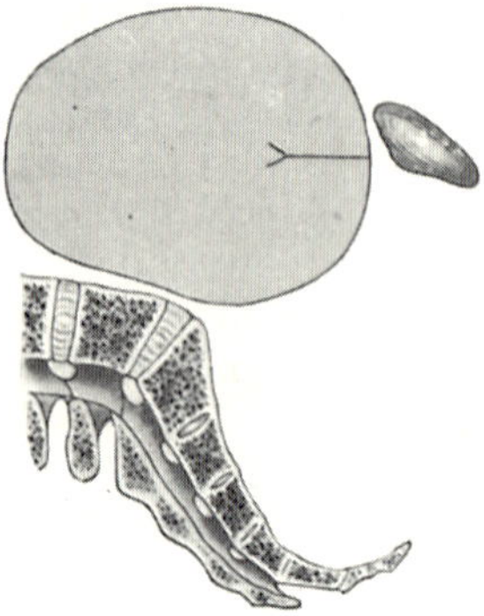

Fig. 530.—Showing Posterior Parietal Presentation.

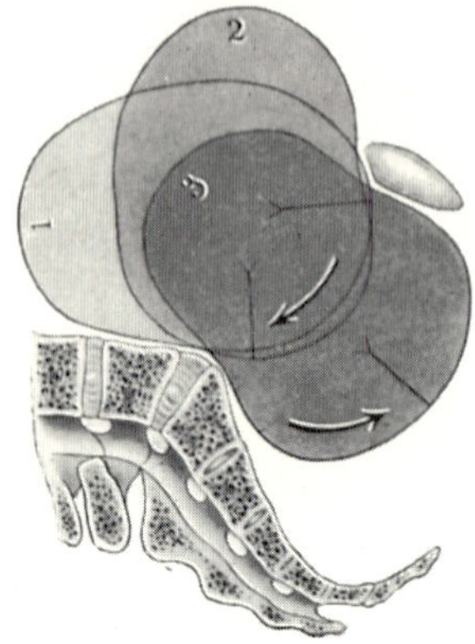

Fig. 531.—Showing the Passage of a Posterior Parietal Presentation through Superior Strait.

portion descends along the symphysis pubis, while at the same time the sagittal suture approaches the middle line of the pelvis. After this has occurred labour takes place in the usual manner.

The mode of production of this abnormality is not definitely understood, although it is observed most frequently when the grade of contraction is marked, the pelvic inclination considerably increased, and the abdomen not pendulous. The presentation is generally considered as very unfavourable by the Germans, as the line along which the uterine contractions are transmitted is given another direction at the neck and is much less advantageous than when the spinal column and head form a continuous axis. Tarnier and Varnier, on the other hand, hold that it occurs much more frequently than the anterior parietal presentation, and is without ominous prognostic significance. Indeed, they believe that it is merely an exaggeration of the process observed in the normal mechanism of labour. In my experience, however, it has occurred far less frequently than the anterior parietal presentation, although in many cases it has not been associated with a particularly difficult labour.

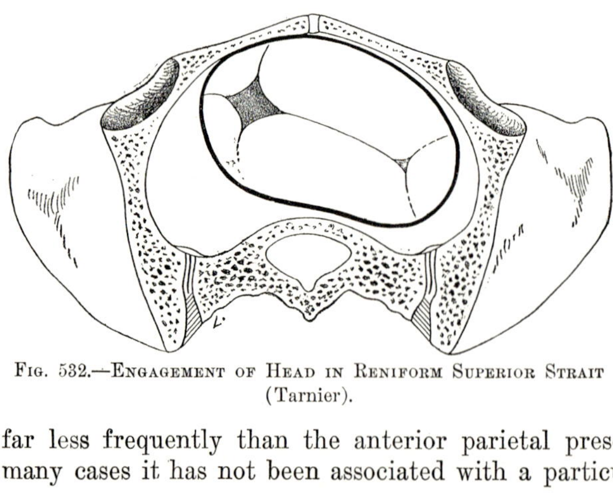

Fig. 532.—Engagement of Head in Reniform Superior Strait (Tarnier).

When the promontory of the sacrum protrudes into the superior strait in such a way as to render it reniform in outline, it is impossible for the head to assume its usual transverse position, and the sagittal suture must occupy an oblique diameter (Fig. 532).

In rare instances the promontory may project so far forward as to make the superior strait resemble the figure 8. Under such circumstances only one side of it is available for the passage of the head, and Breisky has designated the condition as *extra-median engagement*. It is, however, of very rare occurrence, and need not be considered further.

When the pelvic contraction is complicated by the existence of a face presentation, the prognosis becomes more dubious, as it is more difficult for the face than for the vertex to pass the contracted superior strait, and accordingly the course of labour is unduly prolonged.

Breech presentations likewise complicate matters to some extent, as they are very frequently accompanied by prolapse of the cord or of one or more of the extremities, owing to the imperfect adaptation of the breech to the superior strait. Under such circumstances, although the prognosis for the mother remains favourable, the child's life is endangered. This is especially true when the contraction is marked, as considerable difficulty may be experienced in extracting the after-coming head, and if this be not promptly accomplished the child will inevitably perish.

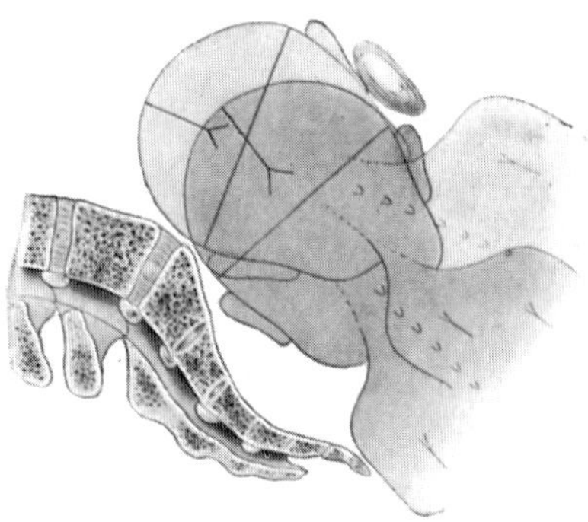

Fig. 533.—Showing Passage of After-coming Head through Superior Strait; Darker Child Last.

The after-coming head, in passing through the contracted superior strait, follows a mechanism analogous to that observed in anterior parietal presentations. In other words, its posterior portion is arrested at the promontory, while its anterior portion passes down behind the symphysis, after which its posterior portion descends.

Mechanism of Labour in Generally Contracted Flat and Generally Equally Contracted Rhachitic Pelves.—The mechanism of labour in generally contracted flat pelves varies according to the extent of the deformity and the shape of the pelvis—that is, according as it approaches more closely to the flat or to the generally contracted type. In the former case, provided the contraction be not too marked, the mechanism of labour will be identical with that just described for flat pelves, whereas in the latter the head will become sharply flexed and be born by the mechanism which we shall consider in detail when we study the generally contracted or justo-minor pelvis.

In the generally and equally contracted rhachitic pelvis the mechanism corresponds to that observed in the justo-minor pelvis.

In the pseudo-osteomalacic forms the contraction is usually so marked as to preclude the possibility of the head entering the superior strait, and the child cannot be born *per vias naturales*.

Course of Labour in Contracted Pelves.—When the pelvic deformity is sufficiently marked to prevent the head from entering the superior strait during the last few weeks of pregnancy or at the onset of uterine contractions, the course of labour is usually unduly prolonged. In the first stage this is due to imperfect dilatation of the cervix, and in the second to the time required to so mould and configure the head as to render possible its entrance into the pelvic cavity.

Abnormalities in Dilatation of Cervix.—Normally, dilatation of the cervix is brought about by the unruptured membranes acting as a hydrostatic wedge, and after their rupture by the direct action of the presenting part. In contracted pelves, on the other hand, when the head is arrested at the superior strait, the entire force exerted by the uterus acts directly upon the portion of membranes in contact with the internal os, and consequently, as its force is not broken by the intervening head, as in normal labour, *premature rupture* frequently results, occurring, according to Litzmann, in 26 per cent of the cases.

After rupture of the membranes, further dilatation cannot take place until the presenting part is able to exert a direct pressure upon the cervix, and this is out of the question until a long succession of strong pains have moulded the head sufficiently to permit its descent. In not a few instances, however, a *caput succedaneum* forms upon the most dependent portion of the presenting part, and aids materially in the dilatation of the cervix.

Even after the cervix is completely dilated considerable delay may occur, and it sometimes requires hours to mould the head to the pelvis; but in flat pelves the labour is promptly terminated as soon as the contracted superior strait is passed. In the generally contracted varieties, however, this is not the case, inasmuch as the hindrance persists throughout the entire pelvic canal.

Abnormalities in Uterine Contractions.—Not infrequently the course of labour is still further prolonged owing to faulty uterine contractions. This is rarely the case in rhachitic primiparæ, in whom the pains are usually very efficient; but in multiparæ, in whom previous difficult labours have weakened the uterine musculature, secondary uterine inertia not infrequently occurs as the result of exhaustion.

In a small number of cases the uterus, instead of presenting signs of secondary inertia, may become *tetanically contracted.* This is an extremely serious condition, as it cannot lead to the termination of labour, and at the same time markedly increases the danger of uterine rupture. If this complication does not yield promptly to the administration of sedatives, it affords an imperative indication for the termination of labour by one means or another.

Danger of Uterine Rupture.—Abnormal conditions in the lower uterine segment not infrequently constitute a very serious danger, especially when the disproportion between the head and the pelvis is pronounced.

Under such circumstances, after a prolonged second stage, with the head still at the superior strait, the lower uterine segment becomes markedly stretched, so that the danger of rupture becomes imminent. In such cases, the contraction ring can be felt as a transverse or oblique ridge extending across the uterus a short distance below the umbilicus and occasionally at its level, while in not a few instances its position is clearly visible. Thinning of the lower uterine segment is particularly liable to occur in the generally contracted variety of rhachitic pelves, since the lower end of the cervix may be caught between the child's head and the pelvic brim, and thus be prevented from retracting, thereby facilitating the stretching of the lower uterine segment. Whenever this condition is noted prompt delivery is urgently indicated; but at the same time great caution is necessary on the part of the physician lest his manœuvres give rise to traumatic rupture.

Production of Fistulæ.—When the presenting part is firmly wedged into the superior strait, but makes no advance for a long time, portions of the generative tract lying between it and the pelvic wall may be subjected to undue pressure for a considerable length of time. As a result the circulation is interfered with and necrosis follows, which may manifest itself a few days after labour by the appearance of vesico-vaginal, vesico-cervical, or recto-vaginal fistulæ, depending upon the part subjected to pressure. These conditions are not to be feared so long as the membranes remain intact, but are liable to follow a very prolonged second stage.

Intra-partum Infection.—Infection is another serious danger to which the patient is exposed in prolonged labours complicated by contracted pelves, particularly when she is examined repeatedly by a physician who does not observe the most stringent aseptic technique. The amniotic fluid may become infected and give rise to febrile symptoms during labour, while in not a few cases the micro-organisms may pass through the fœtal membranes and invade the uterine walls, giving rise to the characteristic manifestations of infection during the puerperium.

In other instances, gas-producing bacteria may be introduced into the uterus, which soon becomes distended with gas as a result of their activity —*tympanites uteri* or *physometra.* This condition usually follows infection with bacillus aerogenes capsulatus, particularly when the child is dead. It was formerly attributed to the entrance of air into the uterus, but at present such an explanation must be regarded with scepticism. For further details, the reader is referred to the chapter upon Puerperal Infection.

Rupture of the Pelvic Joints.—In rare instances, particularly when the pelvis is contracted in its lower portion, spontaneous rupture of the symphysis pubis or of one or both sacro-iliac joints has been observed. Such cases have been reported by Ahlfeld, Schauta, Braun-Fernwald, Rudaux, De Lee, and others, though in the majority the injury is produced by injudicious methods of delivery.

Effect of Labour upon the Child.—So long as the membranes remain intact the child suffers but little from the prolonged labour; but after their rupture frequent and prolonged uterine contractions exert a deleterious influence upon it. This is due in great part to interference with the placental circulation, owing to which the child receives imperfectly aerated blood, which sooner or later leads to manifestations of asphyxiation. Now and again premature separation of the placenta occurs, causing certain death to the child.

After the membranes have ruptured, and particularly during the second stage of labour, prolonged pressure exerted upon the head is not without influence upon the child, in some cases leading to vagus stimulation with its resulting slow pulse and consequent gradual asphyxiation.

Prolapse of the Cord.—A much more serious and frequent complication for the child is prolapse of the cord, the occurrence of which is facilitated by imperfect adaptation between the presenting part and the pelvic inlet. The condition exerts no influence upon the course of labour, but in the majority of cases death of the child results from compression of the cord between the presenting part and the pelvic wall, unless prompt delivery can be accomplished. This must be regarded as one of the most frequent causes of fœtal death in spontaneous labour in contracted pelves.

Changes in Scalp and Skull.—As has already been stated, a marked caput is frequently developed upon the most dependent part of the head in prolonged labour, and allusion has been made to the part which it sometimes plays in the dilatation of the cervix. In many instances it may assume very considerable proportions, but is without significance so far as the life of the child is concerned, usually disappearing within a few days after birth. When it is well marked it may lead to serious diagnostic errors, as it may project well down into the pelvic cavity while the head is still above the brim, so that an inexperienced physician may mistake it for the head and thus be tempted to resort to ill-timed operative measures.

When the disproportion between the size of the head and the pelvis is considerable, it is apparent that the former can only pass through after a process of moulding and accommodation, which is usually spoken of as *configuration.* In very exceptional cases the head may descend at a comparatively early period into the pelvic cavity, and as it cannot readily escape it undergoes further development in the pelvic cavity, and in consequence presents characteristic deformities at birth, the part within the pelvis being markedly flattened, while that above it is unusually large, as shown in Fig. 534.

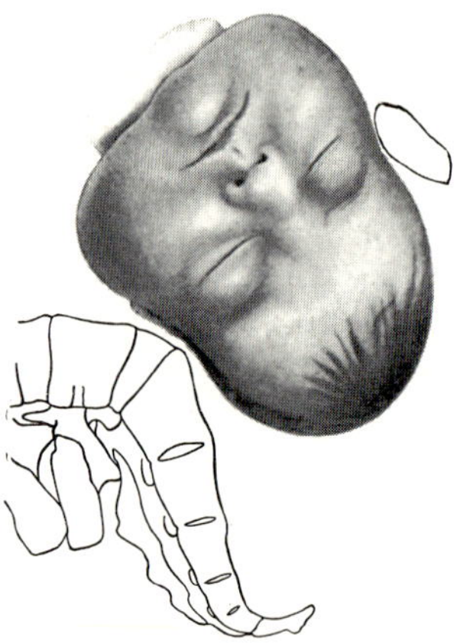

Fig. 534.—Showing Moulding of Head in a Generally Contracted Rhachitic Pelvis.

Under the influence of the strong uterine contractions, the various bones comprising the skull come to overlap one another at the various sutures. As a rule the median margin of the parietal bone, which is in contact with the promontory, becomes overlapped by that of its fellow, and the same occurs with the frontal bones. The occipital bone, on the other hand, becomes shoved under the parietal bones, so that the posterior margins of the latter frequently overlap it. These changes are usually accomplished without detriment to the child, though when the distortion is marked they occasionally lead to rupture of the longitudinal sinus, followed by fatal hæmorrhage.

At the same time the head also becomes moulded, and the parietal bone, which was in contact with the promontory, usually shows signs of having been subjected to marked pressure, sometimes becoming very much flattened. This process is more readily accomplished when the bones of the head are imperfectly ossified, in rare instances the skull being so soft that it yields to pressure as readily as the shell of a soft crab. This property is of marked importance, and serves to explain the difference in the course of

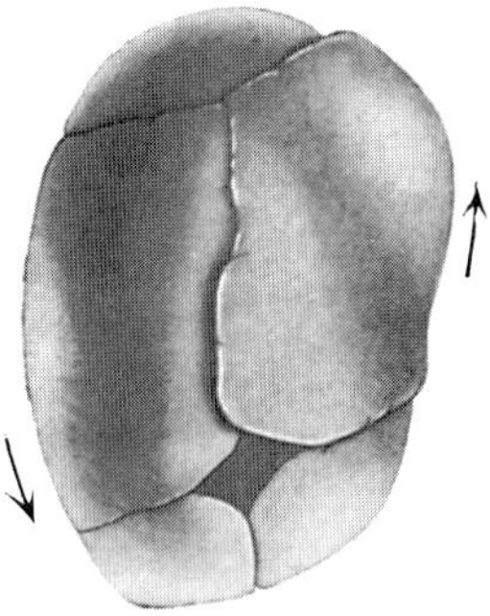

FIG. 535.—OVERLAPPING OF BONES OF SKULL (Tarnier).

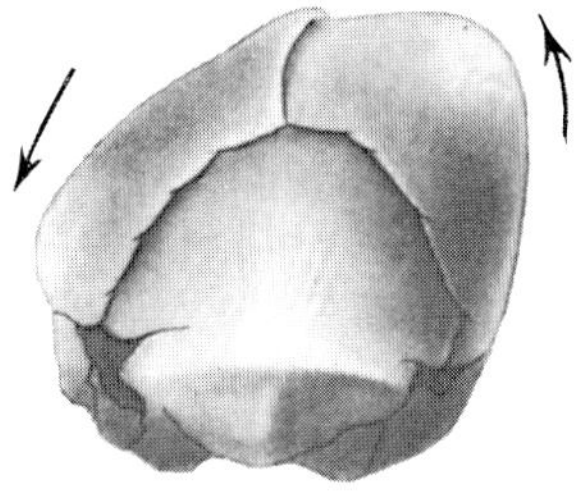

FIG. 536.—OVERLAPPING OF BONES OF SKULL (Tarnier).

labour in two apparently similar cases in which the pelvis and the head present identical measurements. In the one the head is soft and readily moulded, so that spontaneous labour can result; in the other the more resistant head retains its original shape, and a severe operative procedure becomes necessary for its delivery.

We have already referred to the *pressure marks* upon the scalp covering the portion of the head which passes over the promontory of the sacrum. These are frequently very characteristic in appearance, and from their course enable one to determine the movements which the head has undergone in passing through the superior strait. Much more rarely similar marks appear on the portion of the head which has been in contact with the symphysis pubis. These marks have no influence upon the well-being of the child, and usually disappear a few days after birth, although in exceptional instances the scalp may have been subjected to such severe pressure as to lead to necrosis and sloughing.

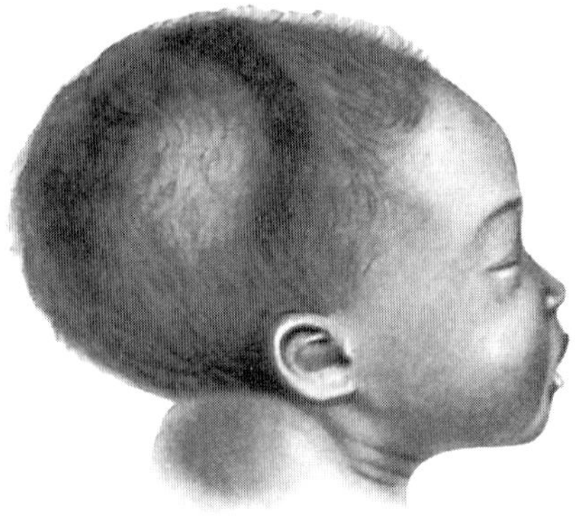

FIG. 537.—CHILD BORN SPONTANEOUSLY THROUGH GENERALLY CONTRACTED RHACHITIC PELVIS, CONJUGATA VERA 7.25 CENTIMETRES, SHOWING CAPUT SUCCEDANEUM AND DEPRESSION OF SKULL.

In a small number of cases *fractures of the skull* are met with. This accident usually follows violent attempts at delivery, though occasionally it may occur spontaneously. These fractures are of two varieties, appearing either as a shallow, gutter-like groove or as a spoon-shaped depression just posterior to the coronal suture. The former is relatively common, and as it involves only the external plate of the bone is not very dangerous; whereas the latter, according to Schroeder, leads to the death of the child in about 50 per cent of

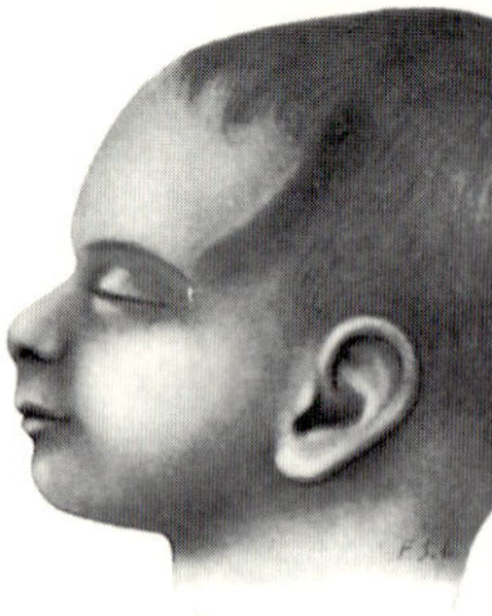

FIG. 538.—PRESSURE MARKS FROM PROMONTORY.

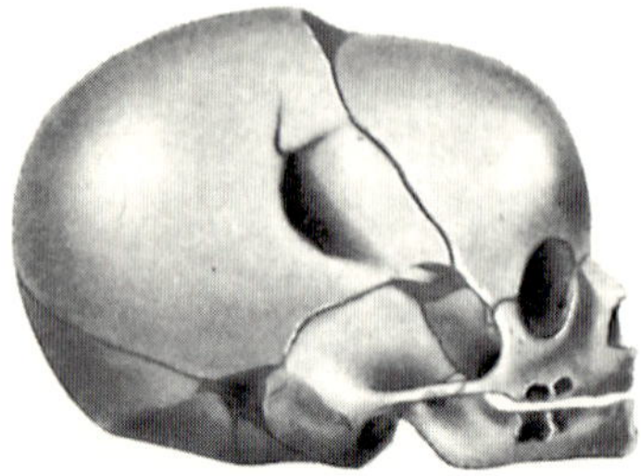

FIG. 539.—SPOON-SHAPED FRACTURE OF SKULL (Tarnier).

the cases, since it extends through the entire thickness of the skull and gives rise to projections upon its interior, which exert an injurious pressure upon the brain.

Prognosis for the Mother.—The prognosis as to the outcome of labours complicated by contracted pelves depends not only upon the degree of contraction but also upon the other factors to which we have already alluded. It may be said, however, that spontaneous delivery of a fully developed child rarely occurs when the conjugata vera measures 7 centimetres or less. Above this limit it will occur in a varying proportion of cases, and becomes more frequent the less marked the pelvic distortion.

In our 278 cases, 71.58 per cent of the children were delivered spontaneously, as compared with 68.6 per cent reported by Glaser, 69 per cent by Valency, 76.5 per cent by Bar, and 78.48 per cent by Krönig. The probability of spontaneous labour decreases with the degree of pelvic contraction. Thus, in our material a spontaneous termination occurred in 77.28 per cent of the cases when the conjugata vera measured between 10 and 9 centimetres; in 61.54 per cent between 8.9 and 8 centimetres; in 33⅓ per cent between 7.9 and 7 centimetres, and in not one with a measurement below 7 centimetres. The experience of Ludwig and Savor is shown by the following table:

Conjugata	vera	9.5 c. m.,	75.6%	spontaneous	labours.
"	"	9 "	58.7%	"	"
"	"	8.5 "	49.7%	"	"
"	"	8 "	25%	"	"
"	"	7.5 "	15%	"	"
"	"	7 "	no	"	"

Generally speaking, the probability of spontaneous labour is less in generally contracted than in flat pelves presenting the same conjugata vera, it being customary to calculate that half a centimetre must be added to the conjugata vera of the former to reduce it to terms of the latter.

The danger to the mother depends upon the course of labour, the perfection with which aseptic technique is observed, and the treatment pursued in operative cases. Speaking broadly, the maternal mortality after spontaneous labour should be hardly greater than that observed with normal pelves, if the case is conducted properly and the patient is among good surroundings. On the other hand, if spontaneous labour does not occur, and the patient is left to herself, she will almost always die undelivered, either from hæmorrhage resulting from uterine rupture or from infection. In operative cases the prognosis depends entirely upon the choice of the operation, the surroundings of the patient, and the degree of perfection of the technique.

In our 278 cases of labour complicated by contracted pelves, there were 8 maternal deaths (2.88 per cent). It should be said, however, that 6 of these patients were profoundly infected when first seen, as the result of attempts at delivery outside of the hospital, and cultures taken from the uterine cavity immediately after the expulsion of the placenta demonstrated the presence of the micro-organisms which caused the fatal infection, leaving only two cases whose death can be fairly attributed to us—a mortality of 0.72 per cent.

Bar, in 166 cases, had one maternal death—a mortality of 0.59 per cent—and Ludwig and Savor reported a maternal mortality of 0.8 per cent in 706 cases of spontaneous labour complicated by contracted pelves, as compared with 5.2 per cent in 591 operative cases. All these results, however, were obtained within the last few years—after the perfection of aseptic technique. Previously, such results were impossible, as Michealis and Litzmann reported a mortality of 10 per cent and 7.3 per cent respectively.

A very instructive comparison between the conditions existing then and now was furnished by Tarnier, who stated that the maternal mortality was 22 per cent in 334 cases occurring in the Maternité in Paris between the years 1860 and 1869, as compared with 1.91 per cent in 1,036 cases occurring between 1884 and 1892. In the latter series 764 labours were spontaneous, with a mortality of 0.78 per cent, and there were 272 operative cases with a mortality of 5.15 per cent.

Prognosis for the Child.—The prognosis for the fœtus is always more serious in contracted than in normal pelves, even though labour occurs spontaneously. It likewise depends to a great extent upon the methods chosen for delivery; and, broadly speaking, it may be said that the fœtal mortality increases with the degree of pelvic contraction, unless Cæsarean section is frequently performed. This is clearly shown by the following table of Michealis, Litzmann, and Schwartz:

Conjugata	vera	9.25 — 8.5	cm.,	fœtal	mortality	5%.
"	"	8.4 — 7.5	"	"	"	16.9%.
"	"	7.4 — 7	"	"	"	52.9%.

According to Ludwig and Savor the mortality was 9.4 per cent in 706 spontaneous labours as compared with 46.3 per cent in 591 operative cases. Bar reports a mortality in 11 per cent in 127 spontaneous, and 23 per cent in 39 operative labours. The difference between the results obtained by the latter and by Ludwig and Savor is due to the fact that Bar performed

Cæsarean section frequently, while Ludwig and Savor resorted to craniotomy in the difficult cases.

In our 278 cases 36 children were born dead, a mortality of 12.96 per cent. One half of these, however, died from causes not connected with the condition of the pelvis, being macerated or having died from eclampsia. The other half—6.5 per cent—however, died directly from the effects of the pelvic deformity or from operations performed for its relief. Of these children, however, 7 were dead when first seen, having succumbed to a too prolonged labour or to operative measures undertaken outside of the hospital; leaving 11, or 4 per cent, who died in our hands.

Treatment of Labour complicated by Contracted Pelves.—The treatment of labour complicated by contracted pelves varies according to the degree of contraction and the possibility of the occurrence of spontaneous labour. Generally speaking, a normally developed full-term child cannot be born spontaneously when the conjugata vera measures less than 7 centimetres in flat, and 7.5 centimetres in generally contracted pelves; above these limits its possibility steadily increases as the contraction becomes less marked.

We have therefore to consider in the first place the treatment of two great groups of pelvic deformities—those below and those above the limits just mentioned. In the first group the problem is comparatively simple, whereas in the latter it is ofttimes extremely complex and requires the utmost nicety of judgment for its proper solution.

Conjugata Vera less than 7 Centimetres in Flat, or 7.5 Centimetres in Generally Contracted Pelves.—When the pelvic contraction falls within these limits the treatment will vary according as the child is alive or dead, and also depends upon the physical condition of the mother and her surroundings.

If the deformity be diagnosed during pregnancy, the patient should be sent to a well-regulated hospital for the performance of Cæsarean section within a few days of the expected date of confinement or at the onset of labour pains, as the operator deems best. Such a procedure will give almost ideal results, and all of the children and nearly all of the mothers should be saved, inasmuch as the maternal mortality following Cæsarean section, when performed by competent operators upon healthy women, need not exceed that following the removal of ovarian cystomata.

On the other hand, if the condition of the pelvis is not diagnosed until the woman has fallen into labour, the treatment to be pursued will vary with circumstances. If the patient is uninfected, has not been examined repeatedly by the vagina, and is among suitable surroundings, Cæsarean section will offer every prospect for saving both mother and child, provided the latter is in good condition and a competent operator is procurable. But if the patient is infected or the child is dead or dying, the line of treatment to be pursued will be determined by the degree of pelvic contraction. If the conjugata vera be above 5 centimetres, craniotomy should be performed; but with a measurement below this limit we have to deal with the *absolute indication* for Cæsarean section, no matter what the condition of the child or the mother, as under such circumstances the delivery of a mutilated child through the natural passages will be impossible, or at least more dangerous to the mother than the performance of Cæsarean section, even under satisfactory conditions. If the patient is infected, the delivery of the child should be followed by a total hysterectomy, whereas the classical conservative operation should be chosen if she is in good condition. Symphyseotomy should not be thought of here, as its field of usefulness is limited to those cases in which the conjugata vera measures at least 7 centimetres.

Conjugata Vera above 7 Centimetres in Flat, and 7.5 Centimetres in Generally Contracted Pelves.—Here the question as to the proper treatment cannot be so readily disposed of, since definite rules cannot be laid down for the entire group, and each case must be considered upon its own merits.

We know in general that spontaneous labour will occur in many of these cases, and that its frequency increases with a lessening degree of pelvic contraction. But at the same time it is very difficult to predict what will occur in an individual case, as we have to reckon not only with the degree of pelvic deformity, but also with the size of the child's head, the extent to which it may become moulded and compressed, and the character of the labour pains. Moreover, although we can determine the size of the pelvis with tolerable accuracy, unfortunately we can form only a very imperfect estimate concerning the other factors; and until some method is devised by which this becomes possible, the treatment of labour complicated by moderate degrees of contraction will remain a very difficult problem.

Methods of Determining the Size of Head.—Despite the existence of numerous methods devised for accurately determining the size of the head, we are still without one that is thoroughly satisfactory.

In multiparous women, important information can occasionally be gained from the character of the heads of previous children of the same mother; and if they were large and firmly ossified, it is extremely probable that the child in question will possess a head showing similar characteristics, and that it may even be somewhat larger, as it is well known that the size is liable to increase with successive pregnancies.

Again, in some instances, *Müller's method of impression* may afford material aid. In making use of this procedure, the patient having been anæsthetized, the obstetrician seizes the brow and occiput of the child with his fingers through the abdominal wall and makes firm pressure downward in the axis of the superior strait, the effect of which may be controlled by the fingers of an assistant in the vagina. If there be no disproportion, the head will readily enter the pelvis and spontaneous labour may be predicted. On the other hand, the fact that the head cannot be forced into the superior strait does not necessarily indicate that spontaneous labour is out of the question, as we have no means of foretelling the extent to which moulding and configuration will occur at the time of labour.

A somewhat similar method is employed by Pinard—*le palper mensurateur.* In this procedure, the brow and occiput having been grasped by the two hands, the head is moved from side to side, so as to bring it into close contact with the pelvic brim. When this is accomplished, one hand is placed upon the child's neck and the head pushed strongly downward and backward so as to bring its posterior portion in close contact with the promontory. An attempt is then made to insinuate the fingers of the other hand between the anterior surface of the head and the symphysis. If this can be done it indicates that there is no disproportion; but if it is impossible, and the anterior portion of the head forms a prominent tumour over the symphysis pubis, the probabilities are that engagement will not occur.

Ahlfeld showed that the biparietal diameter of the head bears a definite relation to the length of the child, and suggested attempting to measure the latter *in utero*. To do this, one blade of the pelvimeter is placed upon the abdomen over the breech of the child, while the other is introduced into the vagina and applied to the vertex. The measurement thus obtained is taken to represent one half the length of the child, and from this the size of the head is calculated, as shown by the following table:

For a child	50	cm. long,	biparietal	diameter	9.06	cm.
" "	49	"	"	"	8.72	"
" "	48	"	"	"	8.56	"
" "	47	"	"	"	8.44	"
" "	46	"	"	"	8.34	"

These figures, however, represent only the average obtained from the measurements of a number of children, but do not necessarily hold good for any given case.

All of these methods may be employed during pregnancy or at the time of labour, and not infrequently give us valuable information. But at the same time they afford no indication as to the consistency or the extent to which the head may become moulded. Accurate information as to this point can be gained only by watching the course of labour during the second stage. In not a few cases a fairly correct estimate may be arrived at by anæsthetizing the patient soon after complete dilatation has taken place, and carefully examining the head with the entire hand in the vagina, aided, if necessary, by pressure from above.

Full details concerning this subject are to be found in the recent articles of Denys and Dardel.

For convenience in considering the treatment in this class of pelvic deformities, it is advisable to subdivide them into two groups. In the first the conjugata vera varies from 10 to 9 centimetres in generally contracted, and from 9.5 to 8.5 centimetres in flat pelves; while in the second group it varies from 8.9 to 7.5 centimetres, and from 8.4 to 7 centimetres respectively.

Conjugata Vera from 10 to 9 and 9.5 to 8.5 Centimetres.—Spontaneous labour is the rule in pelves belonging in this category, unless the head is unusually large or the expulsive forces are very deficient, since a moderate-sized head will become moulded sufficiently to pass through the contracted superior strait. Accordingly, in pelves of this character the course of labour should be left to Nature as long as possible, and interference resorted to only when absolutely necessary. In most cases the head becomes engaged and generally descends into the pelvis after a few hours of second-stage pains, or at least becomes sufficiently moulded to permit the safe application of high or mid forceps.

On the other hand, if engagement fails to occur after complete dilatation of the cervix, the patient should be placed in Walcher's position for as long a time as she will bear it. In many cases this procedure will bring about a lengthening of the anterior posterior diameter of the superior strait sufficient to permit engagement. As soon as the head has descended into the pelvis the patient should be placed upon her back, as the hanging position tends to contract the pelvic outlet and thus retards delivery.

If the child should die during the course of labour, craniotomy should be resorted to without hesitation, as it is far safer for the mother than the application of forceps, unless the greatest diameter of the head has already passed the contracted portion of the pelvis.

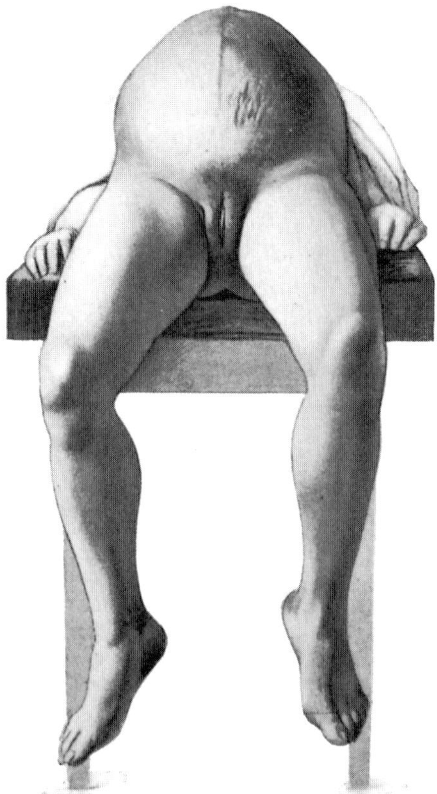

Fig. 540.—Walcher's Hanging Position (Bumm).

Conjugata Vera 8.9 to 7.5 and 8.4 to 7 Centimetres.—It is in pelves contracted within these limits that the greatest difficulty is experienced in predicting the course of labour and in laying down rules for treatment. About one half of the patients will be delivered spontaneously, the number decreasing as the lower limit is approached; but at the same time it is impossible to foretell what will occur in a given case. Accordingly, the labour should be left to Nature as far as possible, in the hope that spontaneous delivery will result, unless the history of previous labours or the excessive size of the child's head renders it almost certain that such a termination is out of the question. The most rigorous aseptic technique should be employed, and the course of labour followed by external palpation, internal examination being restricted as far as possible. If the condition of the pelvis has been ascertained before labour, a vaginal examination should not be made until after rupture of the membranes, as there is no possibility of the head descending before its occurrence. The fœtal heart, of course, should be auscultated at frequent intervals.

In a large number of cases spontaneous delivery will occur after a longer or shorter second stage; but if the head shows no tendency to descend after several hours of efficient second-stage pains, a spontaneous termination can scarcely be hoped for, and it then remains to determine what will be the most desirable method of delivery.

If the patient is in a well-regulated hospital, or can be surrounded by every convenience in her own home, the second stage of labour should be allowed to go on for one or two hours before the internal examination is made. If at that time the head is found to be well moulded but still above the superior strait, and shows no sign of advance, the pains having been efficient, Cæsarean section or symphyseotomy should be considered, according to the preference of the operator. The necessary preparations for the operation should then be made and the patient anæsthetized. But before proceeding to operate a thorough vaginal examination should be made with the entire hand, and the size and character of the head estimated. If there seems to be no likelihood of engagement occurring, the operation should be performed at once, but in other cases it should be deferred.

On the other hand, if the patient be in a tenement house and refuses to enter a hospital, or is in the country where the physician cannot command the necessary assistance and appliances for an aseptic operation, the second stage should be allowed to continue until the appearance of signs of danger on the part of the mother or child. Occasionally spontaneous labour will occur contrary to all expectation. Failing such a fortunate outcome, forceps should be applied obliquely to the head and a few tractions made. If the head shows a tendency to advance, they should be persisted in, but if not, the instrument should be removed and craniotomy performed at once. In such cases forceps should be employed only *tentatively,* it being understood that prolonged traction and brutal methods of extraction are positively contra-indicated, as by their means the child is almost as surely lost as by craniotomy, while the life of the mother is unnecessarily endangered.

Of course if the patient is a devout Catholic, the well-known views of that Church concerning craniotomy must be recognised, and the physician may feel called upon to perform Cæsarean section when, from a purely professional point of view, its justifiability might be open to criticism.

In all grades of moderately contracted pelves, craniotomy should always be performed if the child has died during the course of labour, as any other operation subjects the mother to increased danger for the purely sentimental consideration of not mutilating the child.

Likewise, if the patient has not been seen until far advanced in labour, and has been repeatedly examined by persons not skilled in aseptic technique, or if she presents symptoms indicative of a beginning infection, Cæsarean section is contra-indicated on account of its very high mortality under such circumstances. Tentative attempts at delivery with forceps should be made, and if these fail craniotomy should be performed unless the patient is very anxious for a living child and is willing to undergo the markedly increased risks of Cæsarean section after these have been clearly set before her and her family. In such cases the entire uterus should be removed. Not a few authorities advise symphyseotomy under these conditions, but in my opinion the results obtained are by no means commensurate with the added risk to which the patient is subjected.

If the line of treatment which we have outlined for hospital practice be rigorously carried out, I feel sure that the fœtal mortality will hardly exceed that occurring in normal labour, while the maternal mortality will be reduced to a minimum. On the other hand, when the forceps is employed tentatively and followed by craniotomy in unsuccessful cases, the fœtal mortality will approach 50 per cent, but the danger to the mother will be only slightly increased.

Breech and Face Presentations in Contracted Pelves.—The existence of a breech presentation in moderate degrees of pelvic deformity should be regarded as a complication especially unfavourable for the child, inasmuch as in the early stages of labour prolapse of the cord is facilitated and in the later stages serious delay may be encountered in the delivery of the after-coming head, which is followed by almost uniformly fatal results. On the other hand, so far as the mother is concerned it is rather favourable, for the soft breech does not subject her soft parts to such injurious pressure as the hard head; and if delivery becomes imperative, extraction can usually be accomplished without great difficulty, unless the pelvic contraction is very marked. In most of these cases, however, the child is sacrificed.

In frank breech presentations, when there is reason to believe that operative interference will become necessary and the pelvis is but slightly contracted, it is advisable, as a prophylactic measure, to bring down one foot soon after rupture of the membranes, so that prompt delivery can be effected when indicated.

Face and brow presentations should be regarded as much more serious complications, as their existence usually indicates a marked degree of disproportion and an increased probability of the necessity for operative interference. If the pelvic contraction is at all serious, too much should not be expected from Nature, and radical measures should be promptly employed. On the other hand, when one feels fairly satisfied that the disproportion is not excessive and can be overcome, an attempt should be made to convert the presentation into a vertex by one of the recognised procedures.

Use of Forceps in Contracted Pelves.—Generally speaking, the employment of forceps is contra-indicated in contracted pelves, especially when the head is freely movable above the superior strait. The persistence of the condition after several hours of efficient second-stage pains generally indicates that the disproportion between the head and pelvis is too great to be overcome. In such cases forcible attempts to drag the head through the pelvis will lead to fatal injury of the child, and not infrequently to the death of the mother or to serious lesions on her part. Too many cases in hospital and consultation practice abundantly bear out the truth of this assertion. On the other hand, the tentative application of forceps, after the head has become well moulded and is fixed at the pelvic brim, is a justifiable procedure, provided brutal traction is not made.

When the greatest circumference of the head has passed the superior strait, the employment of forceps is governed by the same rules as in normal pelves, for in such cases the operation is not performed on account of the contracted pelvis, but for one of the usual indications.

Version in Contracted Pelves.—Version is frequently recommended as a satisfactory method in delivery in contracted pelves, and many authorities compare its advantages with those obtained with the forceps.

Sir James Y. Simpson pointed out that the after-coming head offered more favourable conditions than the vertex for passing through the contracted superior strait, as smaller diameters are the first to encounter and overcome the resistance offered by the pelvis. But although version undoubtedly presents some advantages so far as the mother is concerned, these are more than counterbalanced by the dangers to which it exposes the child. Thus Rosenthal states that the fœtal mortality attending this operation in Leopold's clinic was 35 per cent. Moreover, the advantages of version are markedly diminished by the fact that it must be performed soon after rupture of the membranes if satisfactory maternal results are to be obtained. This limits considerably its range of usefulness, as one is compelled to operate before the uterine contractions have had an opportunity to exert their full effect in moulding the head, and consequently version is done in many cases, which if let alone would have terminated spontaneously.

Formerly many of the German authorities recommended the performance of so-called *prophylactic version*—turning at the onset of the second stage—in all cases of moderate disproportion. This practice, however, would not appear justifiable for several reasons. In the first place, it does away with the possibility of spontaneous labour and converts all into operative cases; and, on the other hand, when the operation is performed at the proper time, the head has had no chance of becoming moulded, and accordingly must be dragged through the pelvis with only such diminution in size as results from a few minutes' traction. Moreover, the death of the child is inevitable if any serious obstacle to extraction is experienced, as only a few minutes can elapse between the birth of the umbilicus and the delivery of the head, and sufficient time is not available to permit of any other operation being performed in the hope of saving the child. For these reasons a mistake in the estimation of the degree of disproportion always results in fœtal death.

Induction of Premature Labour.—In moderate degrees of pelvic deformity, many authorities recommend the induction of premature labour at the thirty-fourth or thirty-sixth week of pregnancy, in the hope that the smaller and softer head will be born more readily than at term. This is undoubtedly the case, and the operation, if properly performed, is practically without danger for the mother. Personally, I have never induced labour for this indication and do not recommend the procedure. It is applicable only to very moderate degrees of contraction, and the children not infrequently succumb to the operation, or, when born alive, are in so imperfect a state of development that even with the most careful attention hardly more than 50 per cent survive the first few months.

Schoedel, in 1901, reported a mortality of 36.6 per cent from Leopold's clinic, and gives a table showing the results of other operators. These results, to my mind, are not so good as those following the expectant treatment at full term, and are far inferior to those following the more general performance of Cæsarean section in the class of cases under discussion. Indeed, the fœtal mortality, direct and indirect, attending the induction of premature labour is so great that it appears to be merely a question of degree between its employment and bringing about artificial abortion in the early months of pregnancy.

In conclusion, it cannot be too forcibly impressed upon the general practitioner and the student that the repeated delivery of dead children in cases of contracted pelves is absolutely unjustifiable. The loss of a child is frequently perfectly excusable in a single pregnancy, but its repeated occurrence indicates a neglect of human life which should not be tolerated, and physicians should learn that it is their duty, if they do not feel competent to cope successfully with such cases, to send them to a well-regulated hospital or to confide them to the care of a competent specialist for appropriate treatment.

Treatment of Labour complicated by Osteomalacic Pelves.—The course of labour in osteomalacic pelves varies according to the stage of the disease and the degree of contraction. When the deformity is slight its influence upon the labour is minimal, but when marked it not infrequently gives the absolute indication for Cæsarean section.

Some idea of the obstacles offered to labour by this class of pelves may be gained from the figures of Litzmann, who in 1861 collected from the literature and tabulated 79 cases. He found that the following operations had been performed: 40 Cæsarean sections, 16 perforations, 1 symphyseotomy, 2 inductions of premature labour; while 7 women had succumbed to rupture of the uterus, and 4 others had died undelivered.

Latzo, in 1897, considered the effect of osteomalacia upon the course of labour in 85 patients who came under his observation. The women in question had 459 labours, 290 of which occurred before and 169 after the appearance of the disease. In the first group, operative interference was necessary once in every 48 cases, and in the second once in every 4.9 cases, thus showing that labour had become about 10 times more difficult.

If the patient is seen during the early months of pregnancy and is suffering from the disease in its acute stage, she should be at once removed to a hospital where she can live under the best hygienic surroundings and be supplied with an abundance of suitable food. Phosphorus in doses of 2.4 to 4 milligrammes per day in pill form or combined with cod-liver oil or almond oil should be given, as Latzo, Winckel, and others claim that many cases can be permanently cured by its administration.

On the other hand, if the patient is not seen until the end of pregnancy or the time of labour, the treatment to be pursued depends altogether upon the degree of pelvic contraction. In such cases attention should be paid not only to the length of the conjugata vera, but more particularly to the dimensions of the inferior strait, as the pelvic outlet is usually very markedly contracted.

In florid cases the bones may be so soft as to resemble leather in consistency, and the pelvis readily assumes various forms. This affords an explanation for the fact that one is occasionally surprised to see delivery accomplished through a pelvis which at first glance appears to offer no possibility of such an occurrence. Quite a number of such cases are referred to in Schroeder's text-book, but such an outcome should be regarded as very exceptional, and should not lead us to expect too much of Nature.

If the pelvis is markedly contracted, Cæsarean section should be performed without hesitation, followed by the removal of the uterus and ovaries or by castration alone. Fehling has shown that either of these operations leads to the permanent cure of the disease in about 80 per cent of the cases, and his results have been confirmed by Löhlein, Schauta, Latzo, and many other observers. On the other hand, if delivery occurs spontaneously, or has been effected by forceps or version, castration should be performed soon after the puerperium in the hope of checking the disease.

Exactly why this operation should have such a marked effect has not as yet been definitely determined. As was said in the preceding chapter, Fehling considers the disease as a trophoneurosis of ovarian origin, and believes that the removal of the ovaries does away with the reflex stimulation of the vaso-dilators, which he considers plays so important a part in the production of the bone changes.

Caratulo and Tarulli made careful studies of the metabolism occurring in dogs before and after castration, and showed that the excretion of lime salts and phosphoric acids was markedly diminished after it. Hence they argue that the presence of the ovaries in some way either favours decalcification or prevents calcification of the newly formed osteoid tissue. Their conclusions, however, have lately been denied by Falk, and cannot be accepted without reserve until further confirmation is supplied by the work of other observers.

LITERATURE

Ahlfeld. Ueber die Zerreissung der Schamfuge während der Geburt. D. I., Leipzig, 1868.
Bestimmungen der Grösse und des Alters der Frucht vor der Geburt. Archiv f. Gyn., 1871, ii, 353–372.

Bar. Leçons de pathologie obstétricale. Paris, 1900.

Braun von Fernwald. Ueber Symphysenlockerung und Symphysenruptur. Archiv f. Gyn., 1894, xlvii, 104–129.

Breisky. Extramediane Einstellung des Kindeskopfes, etc. Archiv f. Gyn., 1870, i, 173–174.

Caratulo et Tarulli. Comment la castration guérit l'osteomalacie. Annales de gyn. et d'obst., 1897, xlvii, 239–250.

Dardel. Sur l'évaluation du diamètre bi-pariétal du fœtus, etc. Thèse de Paris, 1898.

De Lee. Two Cases of Rupture of the Symphysis Pubis during Labour. Amer. Jour. Obst., 1893, xxxviii, 483–499 (full literature); also 1901, xliii, 630–633.

Denys. Mensuration de la tête fœtale pendant la vie intra-utérine. Thèse de Paris, 1897.

Falk. Ein Beitrag zur Kenntniss des Stoffwechsels nach Entfernung der Ovarien. Archiv f. Gyn., 1899, lviii, 565–579.

FEHLING. Ueber Wesen und Behandlung der puerperalen Osteomalacie. Archiv f. Gyn., 1891, xxxix, 171–196.

Ueber Osteomalacie. Zeitschr. f. Geb. u. Gyn., 1894, xxx, 471–476.

Weitere Beiträge zur Lehre von der Osteomalacie. Archiv f. Gyn., 1895, xlviii, 472–498.

GLASER. Ueber spontane Geburten bei engen Becken. D. I., München, 1898.

KRÖNIG. Die Therapie bei engen Becken. Leipzig, 1901.

LA TORRE. Die developpement du fœtus chez les femmes à bassin vicié. Paris, 1887.

LATZO. Beiträge zur Diagnose und Therapie der Osteomalacie. Monatsschr. f. Geb. u. Gyn., 1897, vi, 571–608.

LITZMANN. Die Formen des Beckens nebst einem Anhange über die Osteomalacie. Berlin, 1861.

Ueber die hintere Scheitelbeineinstellung. Archiv f. Gyn., 1871, ii, 433–440.

Die Geburt bei engem Becken. Leipzig, 1884.

LÖHLEIN. Erfahrungen über den Werth der Castration bei Osteomalacie. Zeitschr. f. Geb. u. Gyn., 1894, xxix, 18–47.

LUDWIG und SAVOR. Klin. Bericht über die Geburten beim engen Becken, Bericht aus der II geb.-gyn. Klinik in Wien. Wien, 1897, 120–353.

MICHEALIS. Das enge Becken. Leipzig, 1851.

MÜLLER. Ueber die Prognose der Geburt bei engem Becken. Archiv f. Gyn., 1896, xxvii, 311.

PINARD. Du palper mensurateur. Traité de palper abdominale, 2me éd., Paris, 1889, 202–222.

Note pour servir à l'histoire de la puériculture pendant la grossesse. Annales de gyn. et d'obst., 1898, l, 80–89.

ROSENTHAL. Die Wendung und Extraktion bei engem Becken. Arbeiten aus der königl. Frauenklinik in Dresden, 1893, 125–226.

RUDAUX. De la rupture de la symphyse pubienne au cours de l'accouchement. Thèse de Paris, 1898.

SCHAUTA. Allg. Pathologie der Beckenanomalien. Müller's Handbuch der Geb., 1889, ii, 265–284 (full literature).

Die Castration bei Osteomalacie. Wiener med. Wochenschr., 1900.

SCHOEDEL. Erfahrungen über künstliche Frühgeburt, etc. Archiv f. Gyn., 1901, lxiv, 151–164.

SCHROEDER-OLSHAUSEN-VEIT. Lehrbuch der Geburtshülfe, 1899, XIII. Aufl., 659.

SCHWARTZ. Ueber die Häufigkeit des engen Beckens. Monatsschr. f. Geburtsk., 1865, xxvi, 437–442.

SIMPSON. Memoir on Turning, as an Alternative for Craniotomy and High Forceps, etc., 1850.

Selected Obstetrical and Gynæcological Works, Edinburgh, 1871, i, 393.

TARNIER et BUDIN. Traité de l'art des accouchements. 1898, t. iii, 70–135 (full literature).

VALENCY. De l'accouchement spontané dans les bassins rétrécis rachitiques. Thèse de Paris, 1900.

VARNIER. Accommodation de la fête fœtale au bassin maternal. L'obstétrique journalière, Paris, 1900, 131–149.

WILCKE. Das Geburtsgewicht der Kinder bei engem Becken. Beiträge zur Geb. u. Gyn., 1901, iv, 291–302.

WILLIAMS, J. W. Pelvic Indications for the Performance of Cæsarean Section. American Medicine, September 28, 1901.

WINCKEL. Behandlung der Osteomalacie. Penzoldt u. Stintzing's Handbuch der spec. Therapie, v. Abth., 1896, vii, 214–242 (full literature).

Ueber die Erfolge der Kastration bei der Osteomalacie. Volkmann's Sammlung klin. Vorträge, N. F., Nr. 28.

CHAPTER XXXVI

ABNORMAL PELVES RESULTING FROM PRIMARY ANOMALIES IN DEVELOPMENT

THREE separate groups of cases are differentiated according as the abnormalities are: (*a*) Generalized and symmetrical; (*b*) localized and asymmetrical; (*c*) localized and symmetrical.

I. Generalized and Symmetrical Anomalies in Development.—Abnormal development may manifest itself in an excess or in a lack of the general growth of the pelvis. In the former case we have to do with the generally enlarged or justo-major pelvis, and in the latter with one of several varieties—the generally contracted (justo-minor) pelvis, the infantile, the masculine, or the dwarf type.

The Generally Enlarged (justo-major) Pelvis.—This variety of pelvis is symmetrically enlarged in all its parts, and differs from the normal only by its increased size. It is usually observed in giantesses, and occasionally in women of normal stature; indeed, if the external measurements alone are taken as a criterion, it is of quite frequent occurrence in the latter.

According to Schauta, the various diameters in this type rarely exceed the normal by more than 2 centimetres, though he refers to De la Tourette's case, in which the antero-posterior and transverse diameters of the superior and inferior straits measured 14.9, 17, and 14.9, 14.9 centimetres respectively. In not a few cases the greatest increase is in the antero-posterior diameter, while the others remain practically normal. Occasionally the enlargement may be limited to the superior strait, while the lower portions of the pelvic canal retain their usual proportions, thus producing a funnel-shaped pelvis. In rare instances excessive transverse external measurements may be due to the fact that the fossæ join the main body of the iliac bones at a less obtuse angle than usual.

This variety of pelvis has no effect upon the course of labour, except that its excessive size now and again obviates the necessity for the usual mechanism, and the head may be born so rapidly and suddenly that serious perineal tears result.

The Generally Contracted (justo-minor) Pelvis.—This type was first described by Deventer as the *pelvis nimis parva,* while Stein later applied to it the designation *justo-minor.* All of its measurements are more or less proportionately shortened, so that at first glance the pelvis appears perfectly normal, the narrowing being discovered only after careful mensuration.

As a rule, the generally contracted pelvis is lighter in texture, and its component parts are more delicately formed than usual. The sacrum is smaller, and the alæ proportionately shorter than the bodies of its vertebræ. At the same time its vertical concavity is not infrequently increased. On careful examination it is found that the decrease in size is not uniform,

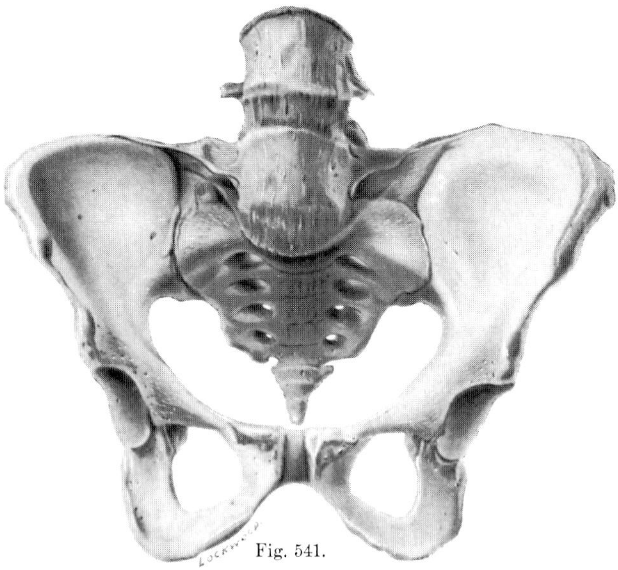

Fig. 541.

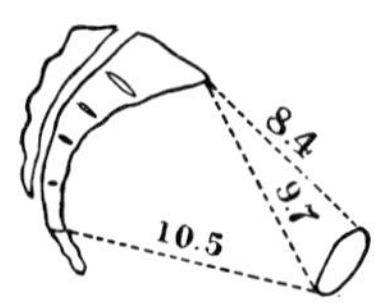

Fig. 542.

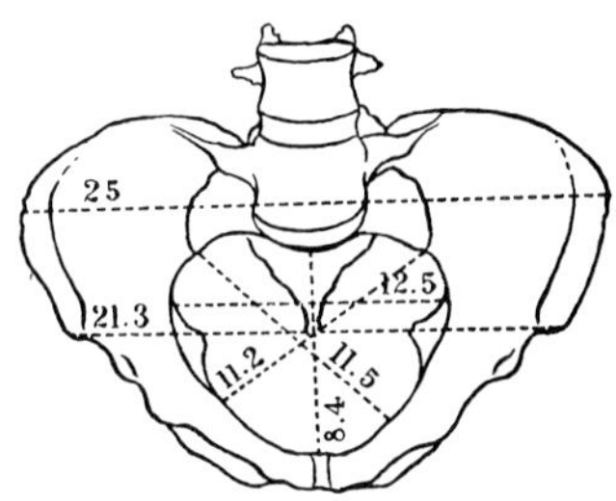

Fig. 543.

Figs. 541–543.—Generally Contracted Pelvis.

as occasionally the conjugata vera is relatively shorter than the transverse diameter of the superior strait, and exceptionally the inferior is relatively smaller than the superior strait, so that we have a type approaching the simple flat or funnel-shaped pelvis respectively. Michealis considered that the antero-posterior shortening in this class of pelves rarely exceeds 1.5 centimetre; and, although this appears to be be too conservative a figure, it may be said that whenever the conjugata vera measures less than 8 centimetres, rhachitic changes should be suspected.

This pelvis is usually met with in small women, although one is occasionally surprised to find it in those of large stature. It has generally been said to occur but rarely in Germany and France, although it was observed in 37 and 28 per cent of the contracted pelves reported by Müller and

Gönner respectively; and Richelet states that it is much more common in France than has generally been believed. Our own observations show that it is by no means unusual in Baltimore, as it was noted in one third of the contracted pelves occurring in white, and in two thirds of those occurring in black women. In the latter it is undoubtedly a sign of degeneration, and is a manifestation of the imperfect physical development which characterizes negroes living in large cities.

Müller considered that its frequency in Berne was probably due to the prevalence of cretinism in that locality, but the fact that Gönner observed it almost as frequently in Basel, where the latter disease occurs but rarely, militates against such a view. It is quite possible that not a few so-called justo-minor pelves are really of rhachitic origin, especially in negroes, and that in such cases the other more characteristic changes are lacking.

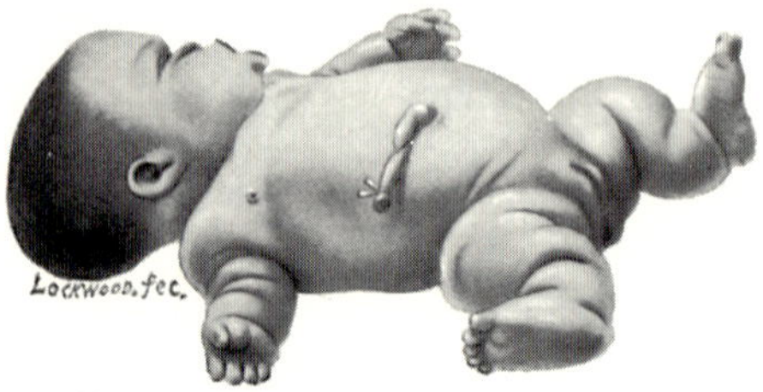

FIG. 544.—CHONDRODYSTROPHIA FŒTALIS.

The *diagnosis* is readily made. The existence of a generally contracted pelvis should always be suspected in small women, and especially in poorly developed working women, although it should not be forgotten that it may occur in large and apparently well-formed individuals. Accurate information can be obtained by means of pelvimetry. All of the external measurements are considerably and uniformly shortened. Internal examination shows a shortened conjugata vera with general smallness of the pelvic cavity, typical rhachitic changes being absent.

The effect of the generally contracted pelvis upon labour is very characteristic. Owing to the fact that all the diameters of the superior strait are shortened instead of only the conjugata vera, as in flat pelves, the head encounters more or less equal resistance from all sides of the pelvic inlet, and consequently enters it in a sharply flexed position, so that on vaginal examination the small fontanelle is readily felt, whereas the large fontanelle is almost or quite out of reach. Moreover, as the cantraction involves all portions of the pelvic canal, labour is not rapidly completed after the head has passed the superior strait, and as a rule is considerably prolonged. This is due partly to the resistance offered by the pelvis, and partly to the faulty character of the uterine contractions incident to the imperfect development of the uterus, which frequently characterizes such cases.

As has already been said, a generally contracted pelvis with a conjugata vera of a given length offers a greater obstacle to labour than a flat pelvis offering a similar measurement, and for practical purposes half a centimetre must be added to the latter to reduce it to terms of the former.

The Masculine Pelvis.—Michealis directed attention to the fact that generally contracted pelves are occasionally encountered in which the bones are thicker and clumsier than usual and approach the male type. Pelves of this class are not of infrequent occurrence, and have the same effect upon labour as the ordinary generally contracted variety, though in exceptional instances the relative contraction of the inferior strait may give rise to serious dystocia.

The Infantile Pelvis.—In rare instances, as the result of disease, which has caused the individual to spend her entire life in bed without attempting to sit up or walk, the pelvis retains the characteristic infantile form to which reference was made in Chapter I. Examples of this abnormality have been described by Naegele, Leisinger, Büttner, and Gurlt, but naturally it possesses no obstetrical significance.

The Dwarf Pelvis.—According to Breus and Kolisko, several varieties of dwarfs must be distinguished—i. e., the chondrodystrophic, the "true," the cretin, the rhachitic, and the hypoplastic dwarf.

In the first-mentioned variety the deformity results from chondrodystrophia fœtalis (Kaufmann), achondroplasia (Parrot and Porak), or fœtal rhachitis, as the disease has been variously designated. The affection is not allied to rhachitis, but is characterized by well-marked changes in the epiphyseal cartilages which lead to imperfect development of the shafts of the long bones.

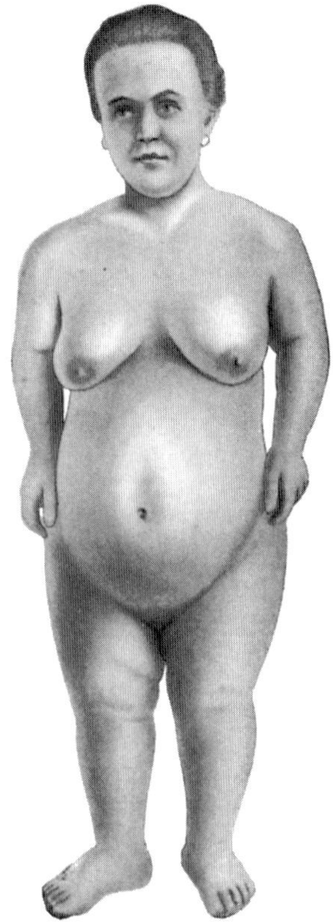

FIG. 545.—CHONDRODYSTROPHIC DWARF (Breus and Kolisko).

In the "true" dwarf there is a proportionate lack of general development, which is particularly characterized by the fact that the various epiphyses do not undergo ossification, but remain cartilaginous until an advanced age.

In the *cretin dwarf* the lack of development is general. The bony changes are allied to those observed in the true dwarf, but are less marked.

The term *rhachitic dwarf* should not be applied to individuals whose short stature is due to skeletal deformities, but should be restricted to those who would fall far below the normal height even if the deformities were straightened out and compensated for.

In the *hypoplastic dwarf* the changes are quantitative instead of qualitative, so that the individual differs from the normal only in its miniature appearance.

Each of these varieties of dwarfs has a characteristically shaped pelvis, which is more or less generally contracted.

The Chondrodystrophic Dwarf Pelvis.—Fig. 544 represents a chondrodystrophic infant, and Fig. 545 a chondrodystrophic dwarf, whose pelvis is reproduced in Fig. 546. This specimen was described by Breus and Kolisko, and was obtained from a woman twenty-seven years old and 123 centimetres tall, who died after a Cæsarean section.

This variety of pelvis is characterized by a marked antero-posterior flattening, so that on first glance one might believe that one had to deal with a rhachitic pelvis. On closer examination, however, it is seen that the flattening is due to the imperfect development of the portion of the iliac bone entering into the formation of the ilio-pectineal line, owing to which the sacral articulation is brought much nearer the pubic bone than usual. In 6 pelves of this character described by Breus and Kolisko, the conjugata vera varied from 4 to 7 centimetres, while the transverse diameter of the superior strait was but slightly shortened, varying from 11 to 12 centimetres.

The True Dwarf Pelvis (*Pelvis Nana*).—This variety of pelvis is extremely rare, only 4 well-marked specimens being in existence—those

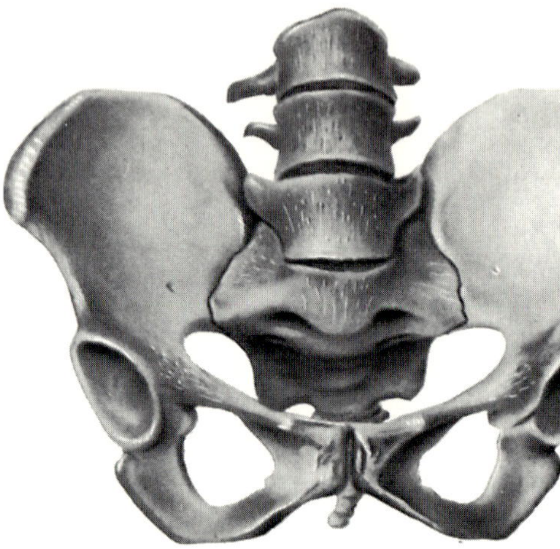

Fig. 546.

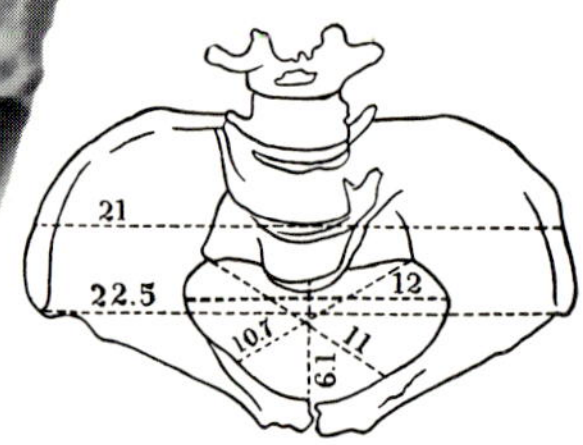

Fig. 547.

Figs. 546, 547.—Chondrodystrophic Pelvis (Breus and Kolisko).

described by Naegele and Boeckh, Schauta, Paltauf, and Breus and Kolisko, two of which were in females. The pelvis is generally contracted and tends towards the infantile type, but its most characteristic feature is the persistence of cartilage at all the epiphyses. Thus, in Boeckh's pelves, which belonged to a thirty-one-year-old woman, 108 centimetres tall, the Y-shaped cartilage at the acetabulum was clearly marked and the sacral vertebræ were not fused together (Fig. 548).

The Cretin Dwarf Pelvis.—This is a generally contracted pelvis with poorly developed and imperfectly formed bones. Unlike that of the true dwarf, it does not present infantile characteristics, but shows signs of a steady though imperfect growth throughout early life. Unossified cartilage may be present here and there in young subjects, but it disappears with advancing age and is never found in all the epiphyses as in the true dwarf pelvis.

The Rhachitic Dwarf Pelvis.—True rhachitic dwarfs are rare, and possess generally contracted, flat rhachitic pelves, which do not differ from those described in the previous chapter except by their extremely small size.

The Hypoplastic Dwarf Pelvis.—According to Breus and Kolisko this variety of pelvis is observed in very small individuals, and is simply a normal pelvis in miniature. It differs materially from that of the true dwarf in that it is completely ossified.

II. **Localized and Asymmetrical Anomalies in Development**—*The Obliquely Contracted or Naegele Pelvis.*—Naegele, in 1803, was the first to recognise the significance of this variety of pelvis, and in 1839 published a monograph upon the subject based upon the study of 35 specimens, one of which had been obtained from an Egyptian mummy.

The Naegele pelvis presents the following characteristics: The alæ of the sacral vertebræ are either lacking or imperfectly developed upon one side, while the corresponding sacral foramina are smaller than those on the normal side. In the great majority of cases the sacrum and the innominate bone are firmly synostosed on the affected side. At the same time the latter is pushed upward and backward as well as inward from the region of the acetabulum, and its crest is at a higher level than that of its fellow. The ilio-pectineal line is less curved than normally, being almost straight when the deformity is marked, while upon the opposite side its curvature is accentuated, particularly in the anterior portion. Corresponding with the change in position of the innominate bone, the ischial tuberosity and

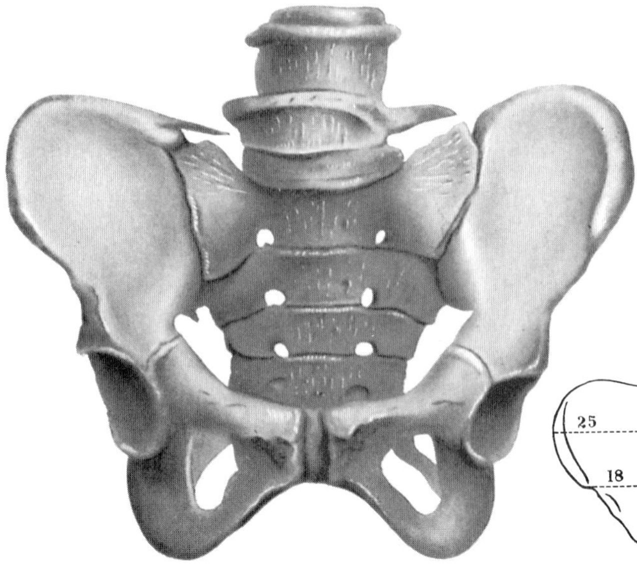

Fig. 548.

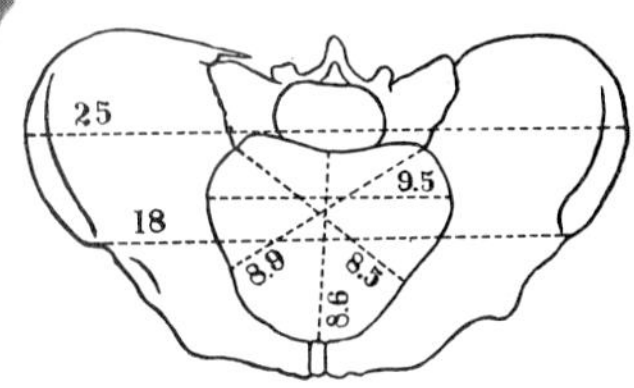

Fig. 549.

FIGS. 548, 549.—TRUE DWARF PELVIS (Boeckh).

spine are displaced inward, upward, and backward, thereby approaching the outer margin of the sacrum and narrowing the sacro-sciatic notch. The symphysis pubis is displaced towards the well side, while the pubic arch instead of looking directly forward is directed towards the abnormal side of the sacrum. The sacrum itself is displaced towards the ankylosed side, while its anterior surface is directed more or less obliquely towards it.

As a result of these changes the pelvis becomes obliquely contracted, the superior strait being ovate in shape, with its small pole directed towards the abnormal sacro-iliac joint and its larger end towards the horizontal ramus of the pubis on the well side. Its oblique diameters are of unequal length, the shorter extending from the sacro-iliac synchondrosis of the well side to the ilio-pectineal eminence on the diseased side, while the conjugata vera is usually somewhat lengthened and is directed obliquely.

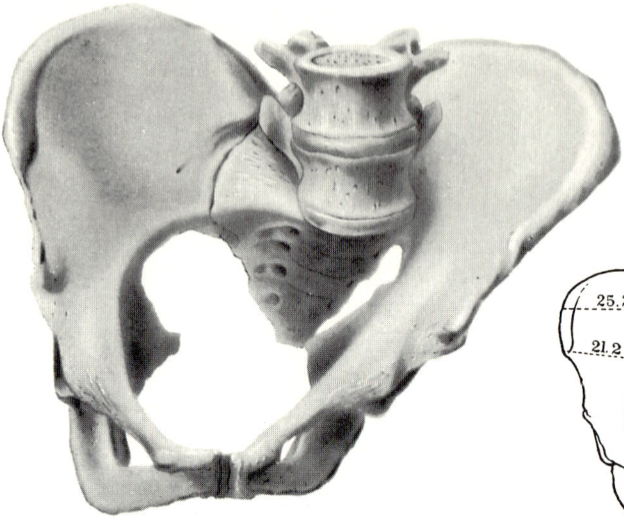

Fig. 550.

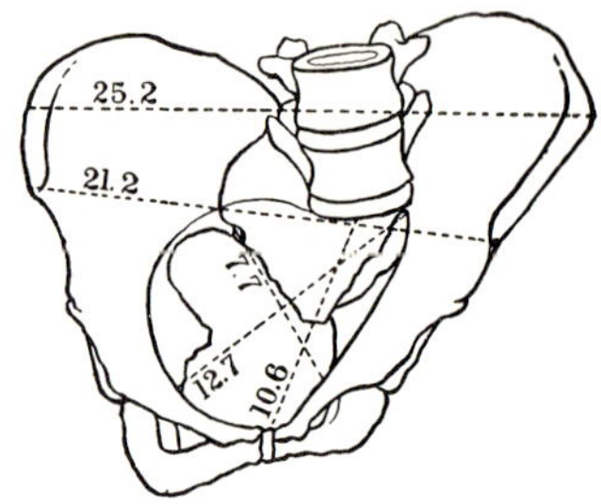

Fig. 551.

Figs. 550, 551.—Anterior View of Obliquely Contracted Pelvis (Naegele).

The distances from the promontory of the sacrum to the acetabulum and from the tip of the sacrum to the ischial spine are markedly diminished on the diseased side. At the same time the distance between the tuber ischii of the diseased side and the opposite posterior superior spine is less than that between the tuber ischii of the well and the corresponding spine of the diseased side. Moreover, the tip of the spinous process of the last lumbar vertebra is nearer the anterior superior spine of the ilium on the diseased than on the well side, while the distance from the lower margin of the symphysis to the posterior superior spine is less upon the well side.

The walls of the pelvis converge below, so that the contraction involves the entire pelvic cavity but is relatively greater in the plane of least pelvic dimensions and the inferior strait than at the superior strait. The acetabulum on the diseased side is directed more anteriorly, while that on the well side looks almost directly outward.

Mode of Production.—The genesis of this variety of pelvic deformity has given rise to a great deal of discussion, some writers claiming that the defect in the sacrum is primary and the synostosis secondary; others, that the synostosis results primarily from changes which bring about more or less destruction of the sacral alæ. The former view was advocated particularly by Unna, Hohl, Litzmann, Olshausen, and Schauta, and the latter by Betschler, E. Martin, Thomas, and others.

It is now generally admitted that the first-mentioned view is correct, Hohl and others having shown that the entire sacral alæ might be lacking without a sign of synostosis. Moreover, Thomas and Kundrat, among other observers, have demonstrated that the alæ of one or more sacral vertebræ may be absent or imperfectly developed while the others are normal. Accordingly, while the synostosis usually occurs at the affected sacro-iliac synchondrosis, it is not a necessary characteristic of this variety of pelvis.

The mechanism by which the deformity is produced is as follows: Owing to the asymmetry of the sacrum there is compensatory scoliosis of the lumbar portion of the vertebral column with its convexity on the diseased side. This causes the pelvis to assume an angle with the horizon, thereby bringing about a lowering of the acetabulum on the diseased side. As a consequence greater pressure is exerted by the femur on that side, which gradually brings about an upward, backward, and inward displacement of the corresponding innominate bone. Owing to the increased pressure, the synovial membrane at the sacro-iliac synchondrosis gradually undergoes pressure necrosis, and synostosis eventually results.

Frequency.—Thomas, in 1861, was able to collect from the literature a description of 50 pelves of this character. Since then several additional cases have been described, but at present the entire number does not exceed 100.

Diagnosis.—Generally speaking, the condition is readily recognisable, provided that one's attention is directed to the possible existence of such a

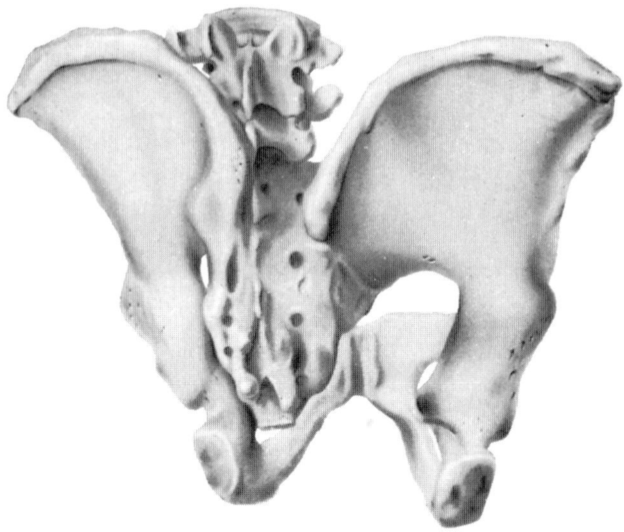

Fig. 552.—Posterior View of Obliquely Contracted Pelvis (Naegele).

deformity. Unfortunately, since the customary external measurements give no clew to its presence, the diagnosis is usually not made until labour is far advanced, when the evident dystocia forces one to look for the cause. The patients do not limp, and as a rule give no history suggestive of trouble at the sacro-iliac joint. On the other hand, the existence of scoliosis, a variation in the height of the hips, or a difference in the distance between the spine of the last lumbar vertebra and the posterior superior spines, should cause one to suspect its possibility.

Naegele suggested five measurements which should be made in such cases: (1) From the tuber ischii of one side to the opposite posterior superior spine; (2) from the anterior superior spine of one side to the opposite posterior superior spine; (3) from the spine of the last lumbar vertebra to the anterior superior spine on either side; (4) from the trochanter to the opposite posterior superior spine; (5) from the lower margin of the symphysis pubis to the posterior superior spines on either side. Normally, these various measurements should be the same on both sides, but differ considerably in obliquely contracted pelves.

Owing to the difficulty of definitely locating their end points, the first, fourth, and fifth measurements are rarely employed; but the information obtained from the second and third is of very considerable value. A difference of more than 1 centimetre between these measurements on the two sides indicates an obliquely contracted pelvis, but is not sufficient to enable one to differentiate between the Naegele and the other varieties. On internal examination the conjugata vera is not shortened, but on measuring the diagonal conjugate it is found that the symphysis pubis, instead of being situated directly in front of the promontory, lies considerably to

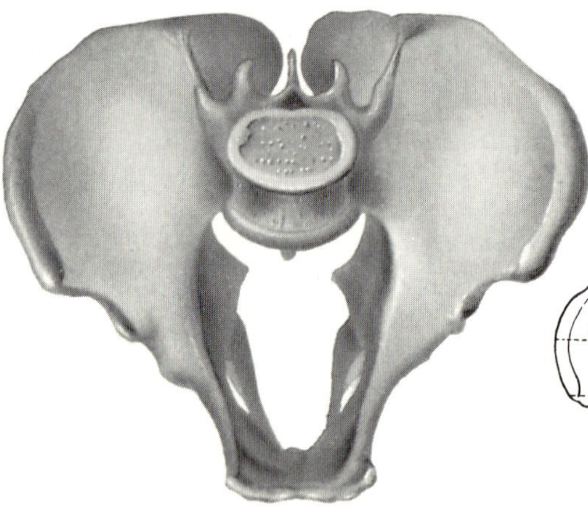

Fig. 553.

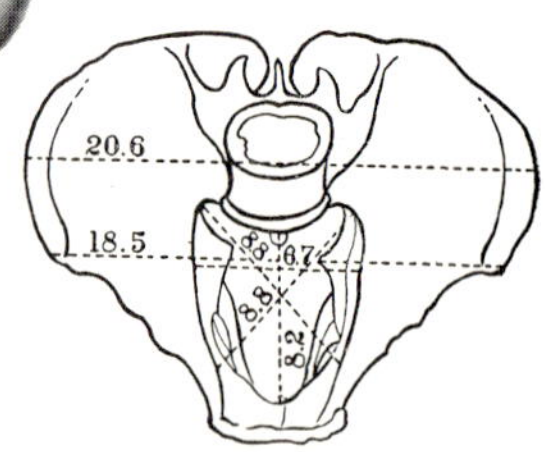

Fig. 554.

Figs. 553, 554.—Transversely Contracted Robert Pelvis (Robert).

one side of it. On palpation it is found that the lateral wall of the pelvis, as well as the ischial spine and tuberosity, approaches the sacrum much more closely on the diseased than on the opposite side, while the ilio-pectineal line is markedly flattened. At the same time the distance between the tubera ischii is markedly diminished.

Effect upon Labour.—When the deformity is at all pronounced, the side of the pelvis corresponding to the small end of the oval is so contracted as to be of no practical value for the passage of the child, so that engagement, if it is to occur at all, must take place on the opposite side. In effect, the pelvic inlet becomes converted into one of the generally contracted variety, and an idea of its available space is gained by measuring not the conjugata vera, but the distance between the symphysis pubis and the sacro-iliac synchondrosis on the normal side. If engagement is possible, labour will progress more favourably when the occiput is directed towards the ilio-pectineal eminence of the diseased than towards that of the well side, for the rea-

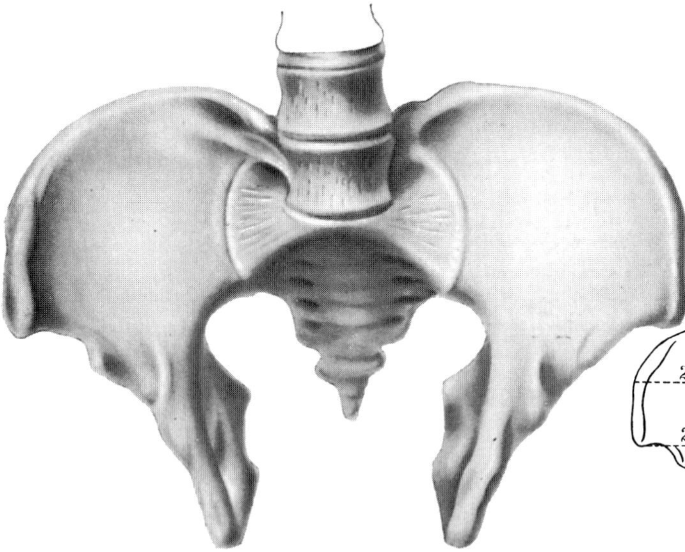

Fig. 555.

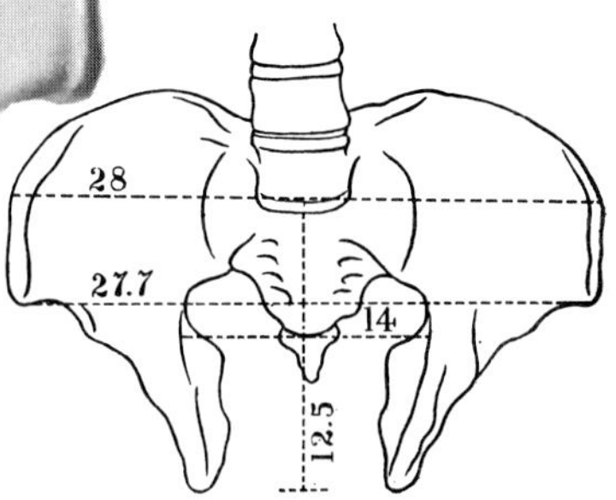

Fig. 556.

FIGS. 555, 556.—SPLIT PELVIS (Breus and Kolisko).

son that in the first instance the biparietal diameter lies in the long oblique instead of in the short oblique diameter of the superior strait.

Owing to the steady increase of the contraction in the lower portion of the pelvis, marked difficulty is experienced when the head attempts to pass between the ischial spines and tuberosities, and the possibility of delivery depends upon the distance between these points.

Prognosis.—If the deformity is marked the prognosis is bad, unless Cæsarean section be performed. Litzmann states that 22 out of 28 mothers died in the first labour, and that only 6 labours ended spontaneously out of the 41 making up his entire series.

Generally speaking, spontaneous labour is out of the question unless the short oblique diameter measures 8.5 centimetres. When this limit is reached, Cæsarean section is the only rational method of treatment if the child is alive and the patient in good condition. Pinard in 1 case performed a modified symphyseotomy, which he designated as *ischio-pubiotomy*, and thereby gained sufficient room for the delivery of the child. He sawed through the horizontal ramus of the pubis and the ascending ramus of the ischium on the diseased side instead of cutting through the symphysis. The operation is strongly condemned by Budin, and its performance is certainly not to be recommended.

III. **Localized and Symmetrical Anomalies in Development.**—These may be of several characters: (*a*) Imperfect development of both sacral alæ; (*b*) lack of union at the symphysis pubis; (*c*) lack of development of the vertebral bodies of the sacrum; (*d*) assimilation of the last lumbar

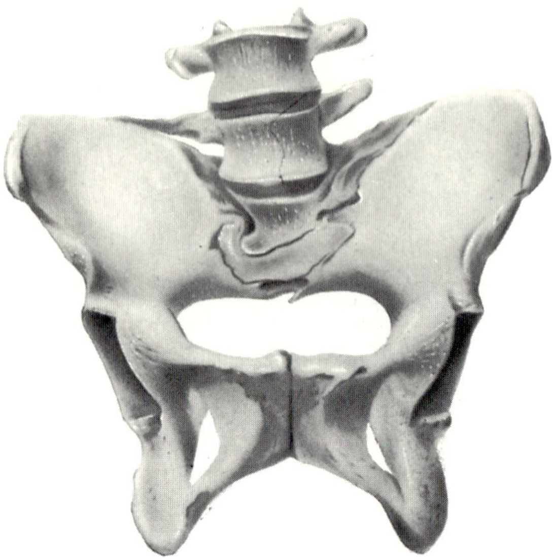

FIG. 557.—CONTRACTED PELVIS DUE TO ABSENCE OF BODIES OF SACRAL VERTEBRÆ (Litzmann).

vertebra with the sacrum, or of the first sacral vertebra with the lumbar column.

The Transversely Contracted or Robert Pelvis.—Imperfect development of the sacral alæ on both sides produces a pelvis which is markedly contracted transversely, and is sometimes described as the *double Naegele pelvis.* This variety is extremely rare, Tarnier stating that only 10 cases had been described up to 1898 (Fig. 553).

In the pelvis described by Robert the alæ on both sides of the sacrum were lacking, and the innominate bones firmly synostosed with the rudimentary sacrum. The anterior surface of the latter was convex in both directions. Owing to the imperfect development of the sacrum, the pelvis was markedly contracted transversely, and only slightly antero-posteriorly, the antero-posterior and transverse diameters of the superior and inferior straits measuring 9.7 and 7, and 10.6 and 5.1 centimetres respectively.

Just as in the Naegele pelvis, bony union between the sacrum and innominate bones is not an essential characteristic, and is occasionally lacking, sometimes on one, much more rarely on both sides. Where there is a difference in the development of the alæ on the two sides it can readily be understood how an asymmetrically transversely contracted pelvis may result.

The diagnosis is readily made, all of the transverse external measurements being markedly shortened while the external conjugate remains practically normal. Internal examination shows the conjugata vera to be only slightly changed, while it is hardly possible for the marked approach of the ischial spines and tuberosities to one another to escape recognition. In all cases thus far reported the transverse narrowing of the pelvis was so great as absolutely to preclude the possibility of the birth of a living child, and accordingly Cæsarean section is the only rational method of treatment.

Split Pelvis.—In rare instances union between the pubic bones at the symphysis does not occur, and the anterior portions of the pelvis gape widely (Fig. 555). This condition is usually associated with ectopia of the bladder

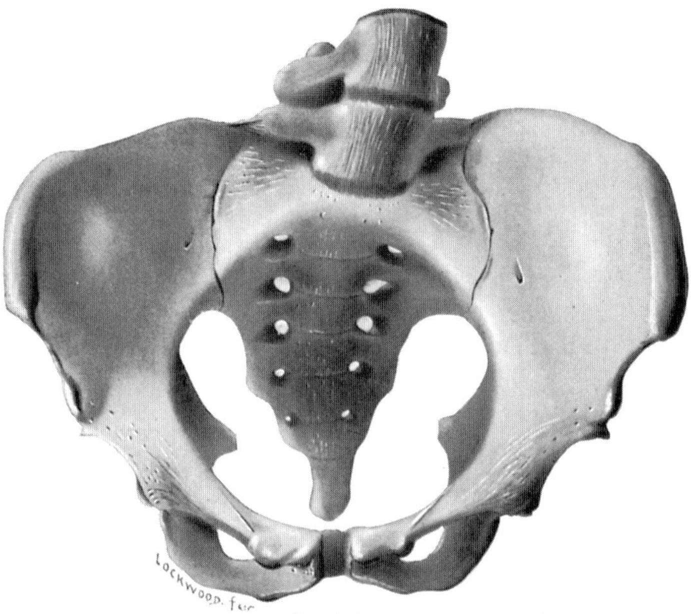

Fig. 558.

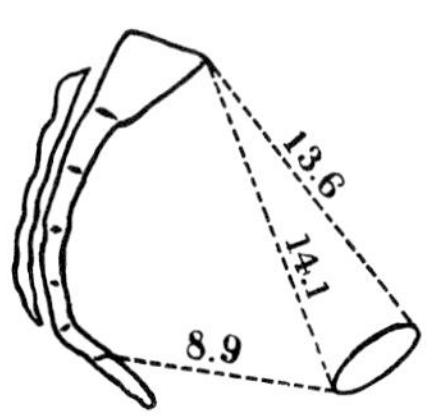

Fig. 559.

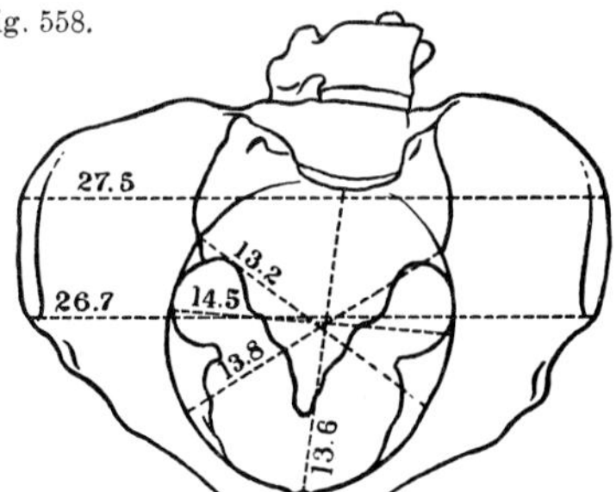

Fig. 560.

FIGS. 558–560.—HIGH ASSIMILATION PELVIS.

and imperfect development of the lower portion of the anterior abdominal wall. It has been observed in adults, but naturally is more common in young children. We are indebted to Litzmann for the first accurate description of a pelvis of this character from an obstetrical point of view.

In the split pelvis, owing to descent of the promontory of the sacrum and the absence of union at the symphysis, there is marked transverse

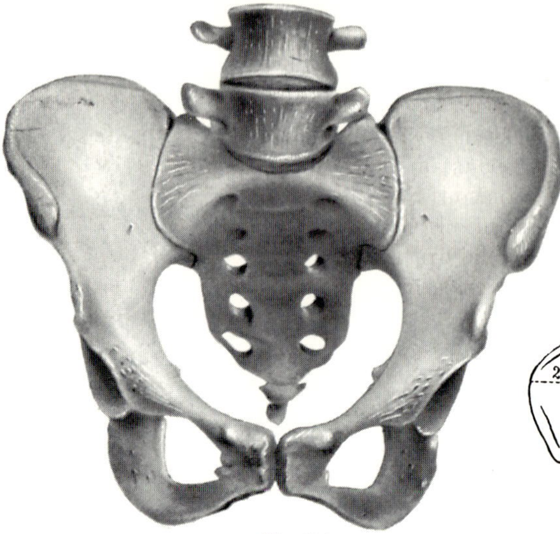

Fig. 561.

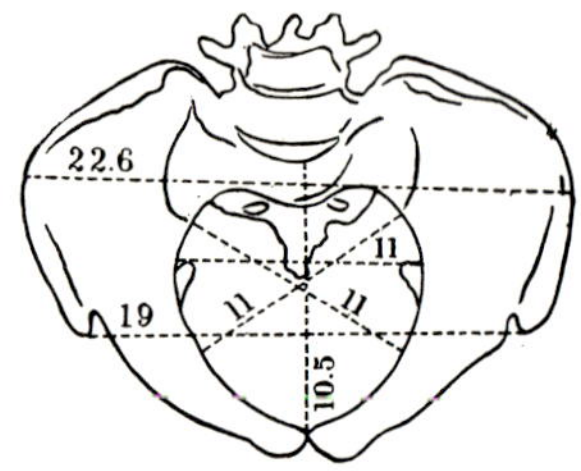

Fig. 562.

FIGS. 561, 562.—TRANSVERSELY CONTRACTED ASSIMILATION PELVIS (Breus and Kolisko).

widening of the posterior portion of the pelvis, while its anterior portions are more or less parallel. External examination in such cases shows a marked flaring of the anterior superior spines of the ilium, and were the defective condition of the anterior portion of the pelvis not clearly evident a rhachitic pelvis might be suspected.

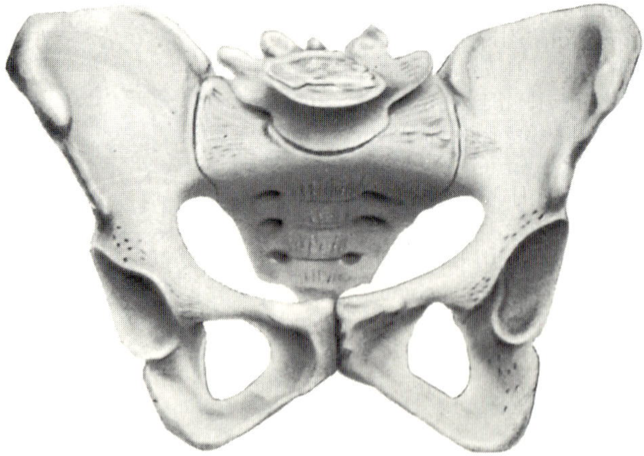

FIG. 563.—LOW ASSIMILATION PELVIS (Breus and Kolisko).

The distance between the extremities of the pubic bones varies considerably, and occasionally is as great as 14 centimetres. This space is usually filled by a fibrinous band. Schickele has lately reported a case of labour in a pelvis of this character, and states that 8 others are to be found in the literature. In only 2 of them was labour perfectly spontaneous, but in none of them was great difficulty experienced, as for practical purposes the pelvis may be considered as generally enlarged, the dystocia being due to abnormalities of mechanism resulting from the absence of a resistant anterior pelvic wall. Breus and Kolisko give an excellent description of several hitherto undescribed cases, and discuss fully the mechanical factors concerned in their production.

Imperfect Development of the Vertebral Bodies of the Sacrum.—Litzmann has described a remarkable pelvis, in which almost the entire sacrum was lacking. This defect was associated with considerable transverse contraction, which increased as the inferior strait was approached, the transverse diameter of the superior strait measuring 10.5 centimetres, while the dis-

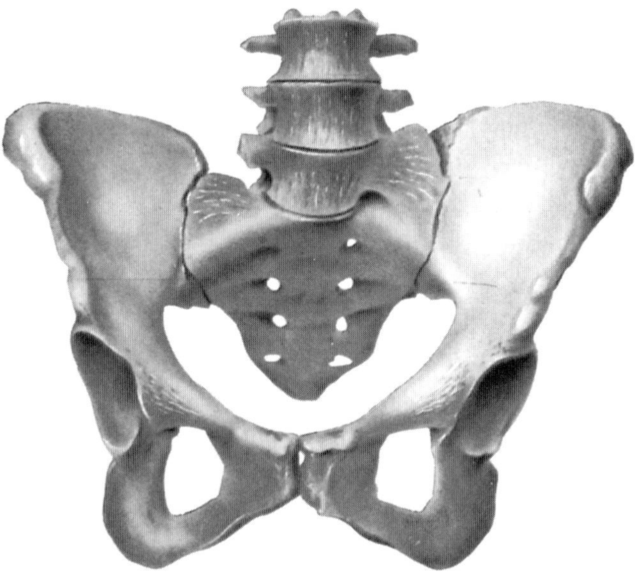

FIG. 564.—ASYMMETRICAL ASSIMILATION PELVIS (Breus and Kolisko).

tance between the ischial spines and ischial tuberosities was 6.5 and 8.5 centimetres respectively (Fig. 557).

Assimilation Pelvis.—Occasionally the transverse processes of the last lumbar vertebra may be transformed into structures similar to the lateral masses of the sacral vertebræ. Hence the former assumes the functions of the first sacral vertebra, the sacrum being now composed of 6 instead of 5 pieces. In other instances the first sacral vertebra may take on the characteristics of a lumbar vertebra and be assimilated with the lumbar column, so that there are 6 lumbar and only 4 sacral vertebræ. Occasionally the first coccygeal vertebra may become assimilated with the sacrum, but this has no effect upon the character of the pelvis. With the exception, then, of the last, these conditions give rise to marked changes in the shape of the pelvis.

When the last lumbar is assimilated with the first sacral vertebra, so that the sacrum consists of 6 pieces, important changes in the shape of the pelvis result, which depend in great part upon the manner in which the sacrum and innominate bones articulate, as well as upon the width of the former. In some cases the condition gives rise to a pelvis which is very high in its posterior portion, and whose superior strait is almost round, the walls in its inferior portion converging, thus producing a funnel-shaped pelvis (see Fig. 558). In other cases the condition gives rise to a somewhat transversely contracted pelvis (see Fig. 561).

On the other hand, when the first sacral vertebra is assimilated with the lumbar column, a pelvis results which is very shallow in its posterior portion, but which offers no particular obstacle to labour (see Fig. 563).

Occasionally the assimilated vertebra may undergo only a partial change, one side of it retaining the characteristics of a lumbar or sacral vertebra, as the case may be, while the other side undergoes considerable modification. Under such circumstances asymmetrical pelves result which are not infrequently obliquely contracted (see Fig. 564).

LITERATURE

Betschler. Neue Zeitschr. f. Geb., 1840, ix, 121.

Boeckh. Ueber Zwergbecken. Archiv f. Gyn., 1893, xliii, 347–472.

Breus und Kolisko. Die path. Beckenformen, 1900, i. Spaltbecken, 107–139. Assimilationsbecken, 169–256. Zwergbecken, 259–366.

Budin. Recherches expérimentales à propos de l'ischio-pubiotomie. Femmes en couches et nouveau-nés, 1897, 468–482.

Büttner. Beschreibung des inneren Wasserkopfs und des ganzen Beinkörpers einer von ihrer Geburt an bis im 31. Jahr krank gewesenen Person weiblichen Geschlechts. Königsberg, 1873.

Deventer. Neues Hebammenlicht. II. Aufl., 1728, 196.

Gönner. Zur Statistik der engen Becken. Zeitschr. f. Geb. u. Gyn., 1882, vii, 314–331.

Gurlt. Ueber einige Missgestaltungen des weiblichen Beckens. Berlin, 1854.

Hohl. Das schräg verengte Becken. Leipzig, 1852.

Kaufmann. Untersuchungen über die sogenannte fötale Rachitis. Berlin, 1892.

Kundrat. Quoted in full by Breus and Kolisko. Die path. Beckenformen, 1900, i, 147–153.

Leisinger. Anat. Beschreibung eines kindlichen Beckens. D. I., Tübingen, 1847.

Litzmann. Das schrägovale Becken. Kiel, 1853.

Das gespaltene Becken. Archiv f. Gyn., 1872, iv, 266–284.

Ein durch mangelhafte Entwickelung des Kreuzbeines querverengtes Becken. Archiv f. Gyn., 1885, xxv, 31–39.

Martin, E. De pelvi oblique ovate. June, 1841.

Müller. Zur Frequenz u. Aetiologie des allg. verengten Beckens. Archiv f. Gyn., 1880, xvi, 155–173.

Naegele. Das schräg verengte Becken. Mainz, 1839.

Olshausen. Schrägverengtes Becken, etc. Monatsschr. f. Geburtsk., 1862, xix, 161–185.

Paltauf. Quoted in full by Breus and Kolisko.

Pinard. De l'ischio-pubiotomie ou opération de Farabeuf. Annales de gyn. et d'obst., 1893, xxxix, 139–143.

PORAK. De l'achondroplasie. Nouv. archives d'obst. et de gyn., décembre, 1889.
RICHELET. Du bassin généralement rétréci, etc. Thèse de Paris, 1896.
ROBERT. Beschreibung eines im höchsten Grade querverengten Beckens, etc. Karlsruhe u. Freiburg, 1842.
SCHAUTA. Die Beckenanomalien. Müller's Handbuch der Geb., 1889, ii, 220–496.
Das durch mangelhafte Entwickelung eines Kreuzbeinflügels schrägverengten Becken. Müller's Handbuch der Geb., 1889, ii, 319–331.
Die Beckenformen bei symmetrischen und asymmetrischen Assimilation. Müller's Handbuch der Geb., 1889, ii, 447–458.
SCHICKELE. Beitrag zur Lehre des normalen und gespaltenen Beckens. Beiträge zur Geb. u. Gyn., 1901, iv, 243–272.
STEIN. Lehre der Geburtshülfe, etc., 1825, i, 78.
TARNIER et BUDIN. Traité de l'art des accouchements, 1898, iii, 314–318.
THOMAS, S. Das schrägverengte Becken, etc. Leipzig, 1861.
UNNA. Zur Genese des schrägverengten Beckens. Hamburger Zeitschr. f. die ges. Med., 1843, xxiii, 281.

CHAPTER XXXVII

PELVIC ANOMALIES DUE TO DISEASE OF THE VERTEBRAL COLUMN

Kyphotic Pelvis.—Kyphosis or humpback, the result of spinal caries, plays an important part in the production of pelvic abnormalities, for when situated in the lower portion of the vertebral column it is nearly always associated with a characteristically funnel-shaped pelvis.

We are indebted to Rokitansky for the first accurate work upon the subject, although as early as 1759 Madame Boursier de Coudray reported a Cæsarean section performed upon a patient having a pelvis of this character.

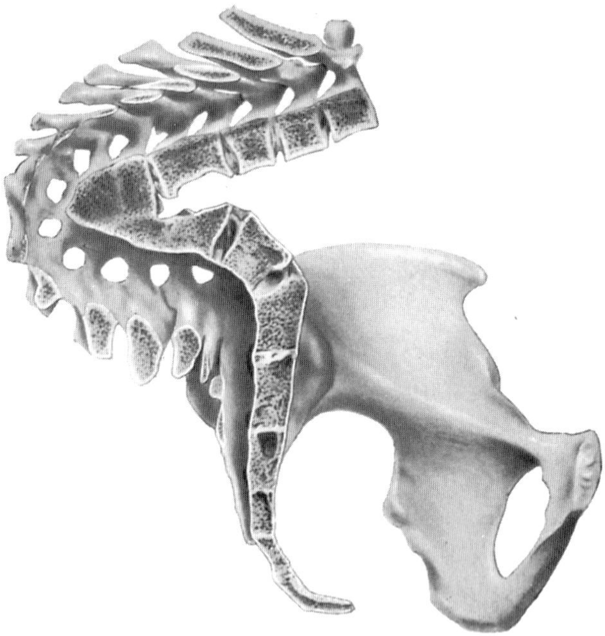

Fig. 565.—Longitudinal Section through Pelvis and Spinal Column in Dorso-lumbar Kyphosis (Breus and Kolisko).

The most important contribution to our knowledge concerning the kyphotic changes was made by Breisky (1865), who clearly set forth the mechanical factors by which the alteration in shape was brought about. Later Chantreuil, Champneys, Barbour, Treub, and particularly Breus and Kolisko, added materially to our knowledge of the subject.

The effect exerted upon the pelvis by kyphosis differs according to its location. When the gibbus or hump is situated in the dorsal region it is usually compensated for by marked lordosis beneath it, so that the pelvis itself is but little changed. On the other hand, when situated at the junction of the dorsal and lumbar portions of the vertebral column its effect upon the pelvis becomes manifest, and is still further accentuated when the kyphosis is lower down, being most marked when it is at the lumbo-sacral junction.

Klien analyzed 85 cases reported in the literature, and found that the kyphosis was dorso-lumbar in 24, lumbar in 17, and lumbo-sacral in 37

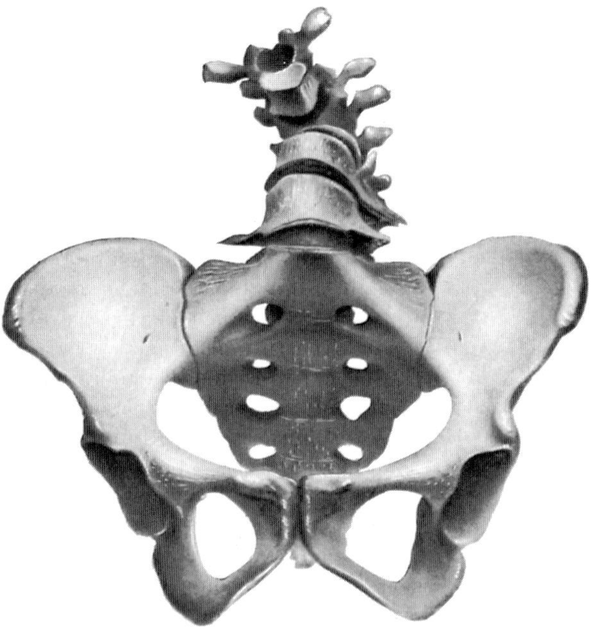

FIG. 566.—KYPHOTIC PELVIS, SHOWING ELONGATION OF CONJUGATA VERA.

cases, while in 7 other cases the vertebral column so overhung the superior strait as to produce a "*pelvis obtecta*" (Fig. 567).

The characteristic feature of the kyphotic pelvis is a retropulsion and rotation of the sacrum, by which the promontory becomes displaced backward and the tip forward. At the same time the entire bone becomes elongated vertically, and narrowed from side to side. These changes are associated with a rotation of each innominate bone about an axis, which extends through the symphysis pubis and the sacro-iliac articulation, so that the iliac fossæ become flared outward while the lower portions of the ischial bones are turned toward the middle line.

When the kyphosis is in the dorso-lumbar region, marked lordosis below it indicates an attempt at compensation, but as this is imperfect, the body weight is transmitted to the sacrum in such a manner that the latter becomes markedly retroposed and lengthened, its promontory being farther backward and at a higher level than usual. At the same time its normal vertical concavity is replaced by a straight or even convex surface, while its lateral concavity becomes obliterated by the projection of the vertebral bodies beyond their alæ. The bodies themselves are considerably narrower than usual, and the alæ of the first sacral vertebra appear to be drawn out and to extend obliquely upward to the promontory.

Owing to its backward displacement, the posterior surface of the sacrum approaches the superior posterior spines, thereby relaxing the ilio-sacral ligaments. At the same time the posterior extremities of the innominate bones are pushed apart, and as a consequence their upper portions tend to rotate outward and the lower portions inward, so that the crests are flared out and are situated at a lower level than usual, while the ischial spines and tuberosities approach the middle line. This movement of rotation is still further accentuated by the increased tension exerted by the ilio-femoral ligaments resulting from a diminution of the pelvic inclination. The acetabula also are shifted slightly and look more to the front than usual. Coincident with the displacement of the sacrum, the ilio-pectineal line becomes longer, particularly in its iliac portion.

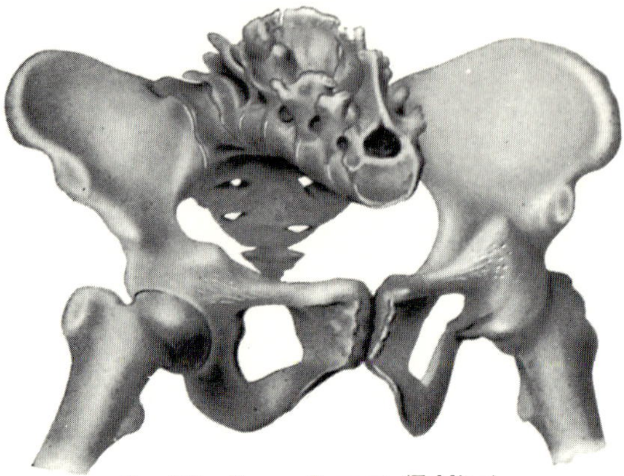

FIG. 567.—PELVIS OBTECTA (Fehling).

These changes give rise to a funnel-shaped pelvis, in which, as the result of the marked increase in the length of the conjugata vera, the superior strait becomes round or oval in shape, with the long diameter running antero-posteriorly, while the transverse diameter remains unchanged or may even be somewhat shorter than usual. There is also a gradual diminution of all the antero-posterior diameters of the pelvis below the superior strait, but the most characteristic change is the shortening of the various transverse diameters, especially between the ischial spines, and to a somewhat less extent between the ischial tuberosities. The pelvic inclination is usually decreased, though in some cases it is only slightly altered.

In 18 kyphotic pelves described by Breus and Kolisko, the conjugata vera varied from 10.7 to 16.5 centimetres in length, the distance between the spines from 5.2 to 8.2 centimetres, and that between the ischial tuberosities from 6 to 12.1 centimetres. At the same time it should be remembered that in not a few cases the entire cavity is smaller than usual, Klien having pointed out that 30 per cent of all the kyphotic pelves described were also generally contracted, so that a conjugata vera which at first glance appears normal may in reality be relatively increased in length.

When the kyphosis is situated at the junction between the last lumbar and the first sacral vertebræ, the pelvic changes are generally more marked than those just described, as the promontory of the sacrum is usually cari-

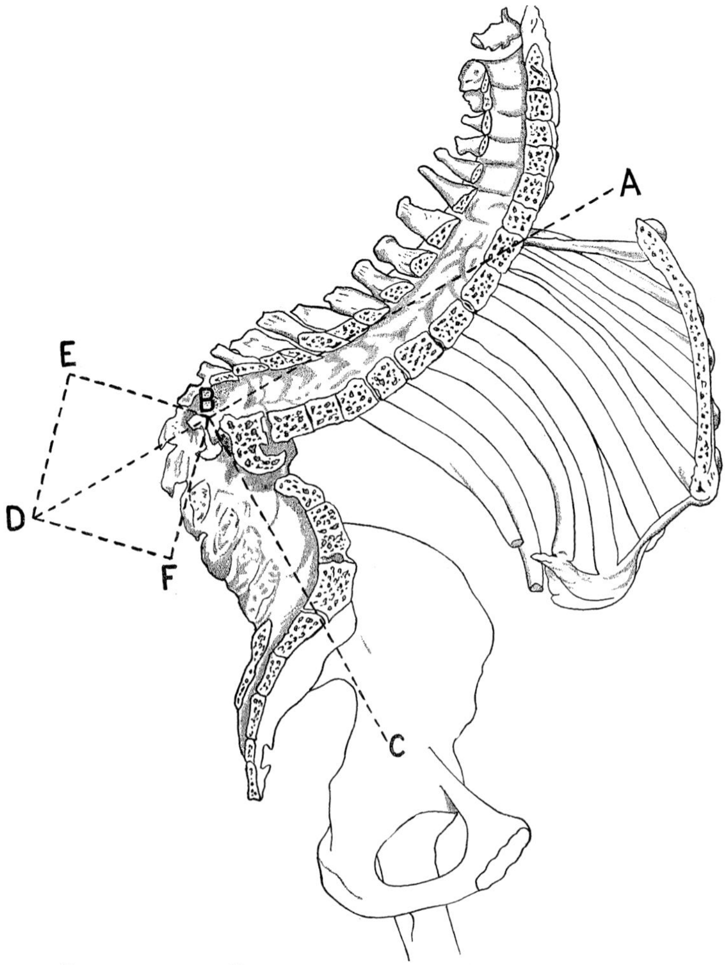

FIG. 568.—DIAGRAM SHOWING FORCES CONCERNED IN THE PRODUCTION OF KYPHOTIC PELVIS (Tarnier).

ous and takes part in the formation of the gibbus. In such cases there can be no attempt at compensation, as the body weight is transmitted directly to the anterior surface of the sacrum, so that its upper part is pushed far backward. It is not lengthened, and its alæ are usually very small. In such cases the transverse contraction becomes still more marked, so that the distance between the ischial spines may be reduced to 3 or 4 centimetres, as in the cases described by Schroeder and Doktor. The pelvic inclination is always diminished, and in some cases is entirely obliterated.

When the kyphosis is very marked, the lumbar vertebræ may so overhang the superior strait as effectively to prevent the child's head from entering it. This condition was described by Fehling as *pelvis obtecta.* In his specimen the distance between the symphysis pubis and the nearest point on the vertebral column was 3.8 centimetres. The pelvis obtecta was noted in 8 per cent of the cases analyzed by Klien. A similar condition was described by Herrgott as *spondylizème.*

Mode of Production.—A kyphosis in the dorsal region is usually compensated for by a marked lordosis below it, so that the body weight is transmitted to the sacrum in the usual manner. On the other hand, as Breisky pointed out, when the hump is situated lower down the body weight is transmitted through its upper limb, and on reaching the gibbus becomes resolved into two components, one of which is directed downward and the other backward. This latter force draws the promontory of the sacrum backward and upward, thus leading to rotation of the entire bone (Fig. 568).

Breus and Kolisko have shown that, owing to the necrosis of one or more of the vertebral bodies forming the gibbus, the body weight is not transmitted directly through the vertebral bodies below it, but through their arches and spinous processes. As a result the latter come into close contact, while the anterior portions of the vertebræ become widely separated, thus leading to marked lordosis beneath the gibbus. This causes an upward drag upon the bodies of the sacral vertebræ, which become stretched and elongated. Coincident with these changes the innominate bones likewise undergo rotation, which brings about a narrowing of the lower portion of the pelvis, and is due partly to the backward displacement of the sacrum and partly to increased tension exerted by the iliofemoral ligaments.

Frequency.—According to Klien's statistical study a kyphotic pelvis is met with once in every 6,016 labours, although he himself believes that this estimate was too low, in view of the fact that humpbacked women are relatively numerous. On the whole, it is probable that any one who has much obstetric practice is liable to meet with one or more cases complicated by this abnormality.

Diagnosis.—The diagnosis is usually easy, as the external deformity is readily detected and at once suggests the possible existence of a funnel-shaped pelvis.

External pelvimetry is of great value, as it shows that the distance between the iliac crests is equal to or exceeds that between the trochanters, whereas normally the reverse is true. In a patient suffering from this deformity, lines drawn through the iliac crests and trochanters will meet somewhere in the neighbourhood of the feet, instead of near the head as is generally the case.

On internal examination the transverse narrowing of the pelvic outlet should be noted, as well as the antero-posterior lengthening of the conjugata vera. In the lumbo-sacral variety the promontory no longer exists, and the bodies of the lower lumbar vertebra overhang the superior strait. Accordingly, particular attention should be devoted to estimating the length of the "pseudo-conjugate"—the distance from the upper margin of the symphysis pubis to the nearest portion of the vertebral column. Occasionally the condition may be confounded with spondylolisthesis, and the differential diagnosis will be considered under the latter heading.

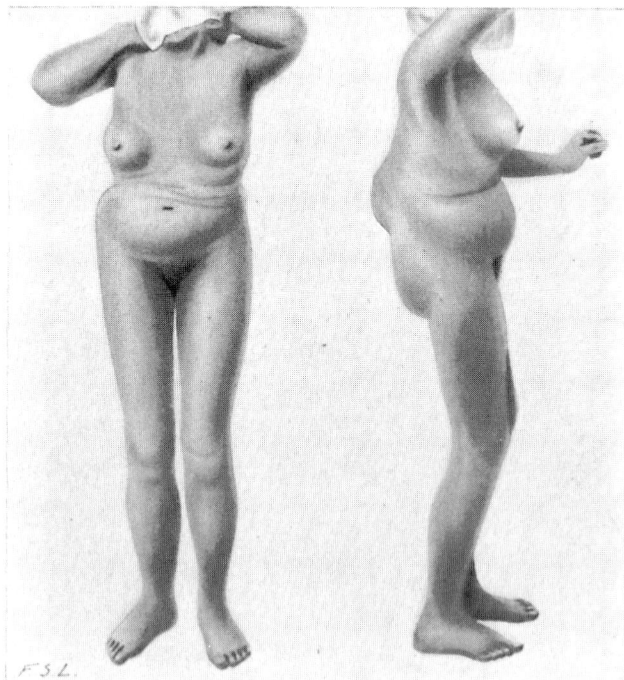

FIG. 569.—FRONT AND SIDE VIEW OF PATIENT WITH LUMBO-SACRAL KYPHOSIS (Hirst).

Effect upon Labour.—Owing to the collapse of the vertebral column the ribs approach the pelvic brim and markedly lessen the capacity of the abdomen, which in consequence becomes markedly pendulous at an early period of pregnancy, these mechanical conditions favouring the occurrence of certain abnormal positions of the fœtus. Thus Klien, in 103 cases, found 100 longitudinal and 3 oblique presentations. Of the former 90 were vertex, 4 face, and 6 breech presentations.

It is interesting to note that left occipito-iliac anterior presentations occurred much less frequently than usual, being noted in only one third of the cases, while the remainder were equally divided between right anterior and posterior presentations. It is difficult to give a satisfactory explanation for the unusual frequency of the R. O. I. A. position, but the production of posterior positions is readily seen to be due to the pendulous abdomen, as under such circumstances the concave anterior surface of the child tends to apply itself to the convex anterior surface of the uterus.

At the time of labour the presenting part experiences no difficulty in entering the superior strait, and no obstacle is met with until it reaches the lower part of the pelvis, particularly between the ischial spines. If the transverse contraction be not too marked to prevent the passage of the head, further difficulty is encountered when the latter attempts to pass beneath the pubic arch, which, owing to the approach of the tubera ischii, has become more angular than usual, so that the head is prevented from coming in contact with the lower margin of the symphysis pubis and must descend lower than usual in order to be born. This fact readily explains the deep perineal tears so frequently observed.

Generally speaking, it may be said that when the distance between the ischial spines is less than 8.5 centimetres, labour becomes difficult or impossible, according to the degree of contraction. Owing to the narrowing of the pubic arch, occipito-anterior are less favourable than occipito-posterior presentations, as in the former the wide biparietal diameter has to accommodate itself to the narrow pubic arch, whereas in the latter its place is taken by the brow. According to Klien, face presentations are still more favourable for the same reason.

Prognosis.—If the contraction is at all marked, the prognosis is bad unless Cæsarean section is resorted to. Klien has analyzed the histories of 175 labours occurring in 95 women, and found that 40 per cent of the children died. The maternal mortality varied according to the degree of contraction; when the disproportion between the biparietal diameter of the child's head and the distance between the spines was slight it was 6.2 per cent, as compared with 17 per cent in marked cases.

Neugebauer has likewise analyzed the histories of 199 labours occurring in 118 women, and found that only 44 ended spontaneously. The maternal mortality was 24.3 per cent, and 49 per cent of the fœtuses died.

Treatment.—When the distances between the spines and tuberosities of the ischium do not fall below 8 centimetres, spontaneous labour, or at least a probable delivery with forceps, can be looked for, but when the measurements fall below this limit, operative interference becomes necessary. If the case be seen in the later weeks of pregnancy, the propriety of the induction of premature labour may be considered. As a rule, however, Cæsarean section at term is far preferable unless the child is very small. Symphyseotomy is urged by many as an appropriate operation in this class of deformity, and will certainly give a sufficient increase in the size of the pelvic outlet to permit the passage of the head, provided the distance between the spines does not fall below 6 centimetres. If the child is already dead, craniotomy is the operation of election.

Kypho-Rhachitic Pelvis.—Kyphosis is nearly always of carious origin, but when due to rhachitis it is usually associated with a greater or lesser degree of scoliosis. In the rare cases of pure rhachitic kyphosis, however, the pelvic changes are slight, as the effect of the kyphosis is counterbalanced to a great extent by those of the rhachitis, the former leading to an elongation and the latter to a shortening of the conjugata vera, while tending respectively to narrow and widen the inferior strait. Thus it may happen that a woman presenting a markedly deformed vertebral column of this character may still have a practically normal pelvis. The two processes, however, do not always counteract one another, and, as a rule, when the kyphosis is high up the pelvic changes are predominantly rhachitic.

Scoliotic Pelvis.—Pronounced scoliosis, or lateral curvature of the spine, is usually of rhachitic origin; but, on the other hand, minor degrees of the deformity are often observed which have no connection with rickets. When the scoliosis involves the upper portion of the vertebral column it is usually compensated for by a corresponding curvature in the opposite direction lower down, thus giving rise to a double or S-shaped curve. In such cases the body weight is transmitted to the sacrum in the usual manner. But when the scoliosis is lower down and involves the lumbar region, the sacrum takes part in the compensatory process and accordingly assumes an abnormal position which leads to slight asymmetry of the pelvis.

Breus and Kolisko have devoted particular attention to the pelvic anomalies resulting from non-rhachitic scoliosis, but the changes in shape are usually so slight as to have little or no effect upon the course of labour.

When due to rhachitis, the scoliosis may be very pronounced, and give rise to marked pelvic deformity, in which the characteristic changes

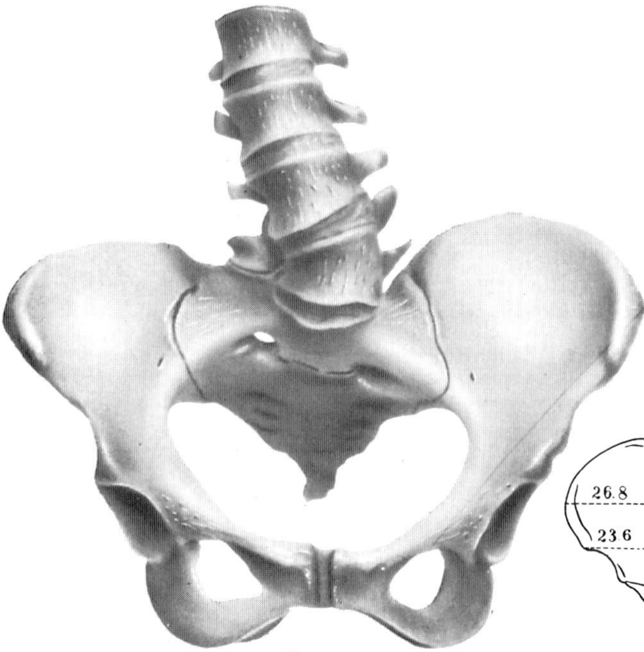

Fig. 570.

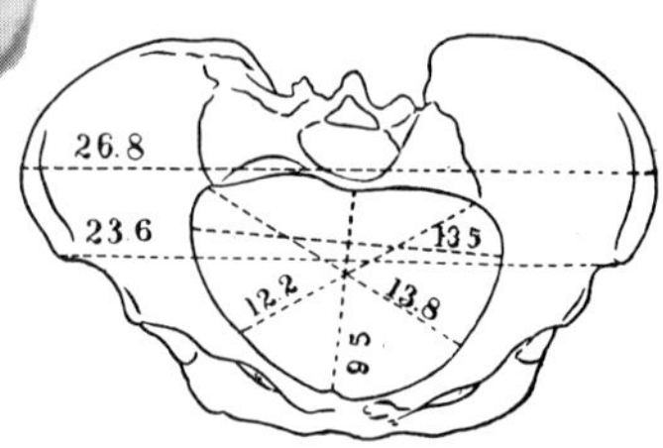

Fig. 571.

FIGS. 570, 571.—OBLIQUELY CONTRACTED PELVIS, DUE TO NON-RHACHITIC SCOLIOSIS (Breus and Kolisko).

due to the anomaly of the vertebral column are superadded to those resulting from rhachitis. In such cases the scoliotic convexity is usually directed to the right side, as was noted in 7 out of the 9 cases described by Leopold.

Under such circumstances the sacrum takes part in the compensatory scoliosis, one side being compressed and the other elongated, so that its long axis becomes directed obliquely towards one side. At the same time it undergoes a partial rotation about its vertical axis, the spinous processes being directed towards the compressed side, a result which indicates the abnormal direction along which the body weight is transmitted to the iliac bone, and thence to the femur. Owing to the abnormal pressure exerted upon one side, the pelvis becomes obliquely contracted, usually upon the side corresponding to the lumbar convexity; but, owing to the coexistence of rhachitic changes, the contraction is in great part limited to the superior strait.

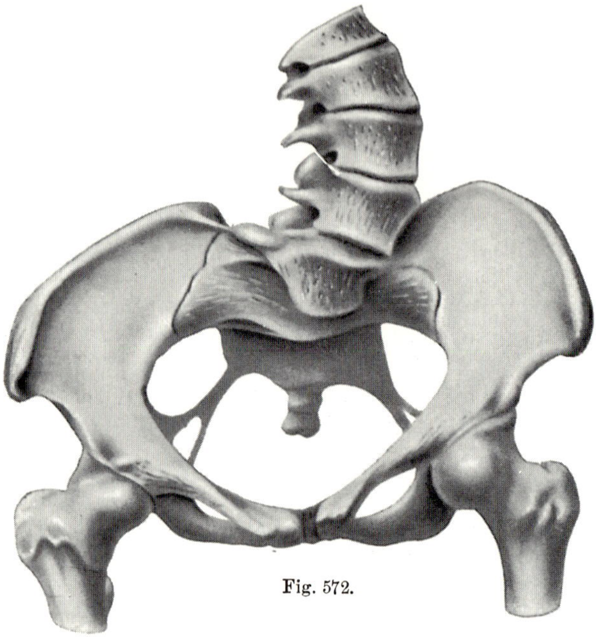

Fig. 572.

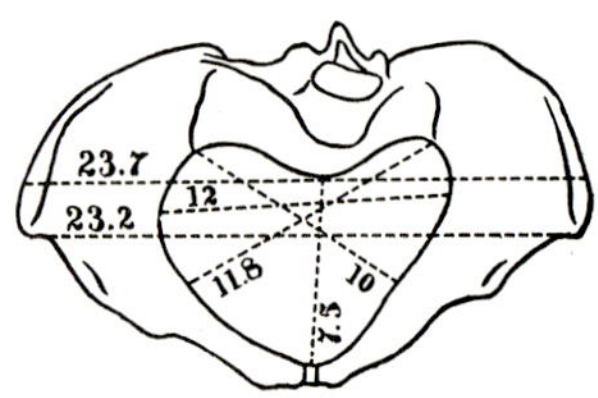

Fig. 573.

Figs. 572, 573.—Scolio-rhachitic Pelvis (Tarnier).

Owing to the pressure exerted upon the compressed side of the sacrum, ankylosis at the sacro-iliac articulations often occurs. At the same time the innominate bone on the affected side is displaced upward, inward, and backward, while its acetabulum looks more forward than usual. The symphysis pubis is brought somewhat nearer to the opposite side, and owing to the rhachitic changes the pubic arch is widened, while the tubera ischii are directed outward instead of inward as in the Naegele pelvis. In marked cases the superior strait assumes an obliquely ovate appearance, and occasionally the acetabulum on the affected side may come almost in contact with the promontory.

The location of the contraction can be determined by external examination, as it always lies upon the side towards which the convexity of the scoliosis is directed. The contracted side is valueless from an obstetrical standpoint, and for practical purposes the superior strait becomes generally narrowed. If, however, the head manages to pass through it, no further difficulty is experienced in its downward course, owing to the rhachitic widening of the lower portion of the pelvis.

Kypho-Scoliotic Pelvis.—The distortion of the pelvis will vary according as the kyphosis or the scoliosis is the predominant factor in the deformity of the spinal column. When the former is more pronounced, the pelvis will partake of the kyphotic character, and *vice versa*. When the two deformities are approximately equal, however, the kyphotic changes in the pelvis predominate, although the influence of the scoliosis tends to counteract, to a certain extent, the transverse narrowing of the inferior strait.

Kypho-Scolio-Rhachitic Pelvis.—This variety of pelvic deformity has been studied more particularly by Leopold and Barbour. As has already been pointed out, a kyphosis due to rhachitis is nearly always complicated by a scoliosis, and the latter nearly always predominates in the production of pelvic deformity, for the reason that the kyphosis and the rhachitis tend mutually to counteract one another in their effect upon the pelvis. Accordingly, the resulting pelvis does not differ materially from that observed in scolio-rhachitis, except that the tendency to antero-posterior flattening is partially counteracted by the action of the kyphotic vertebral column. Nevertheless, owing to the presence of the scoliosis, the oblique deformity of

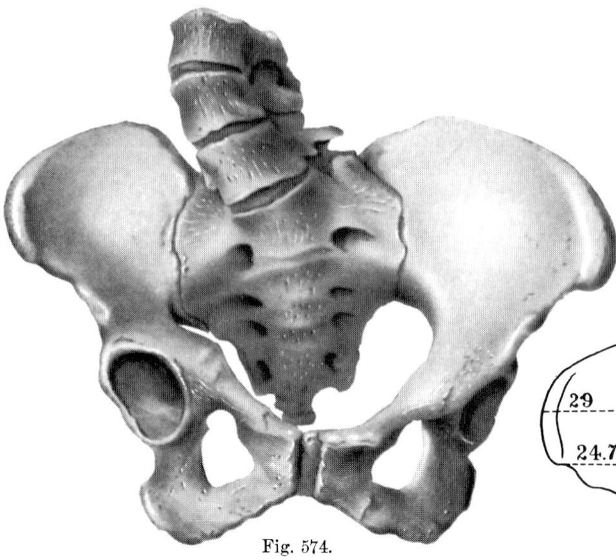

Fig. 574.

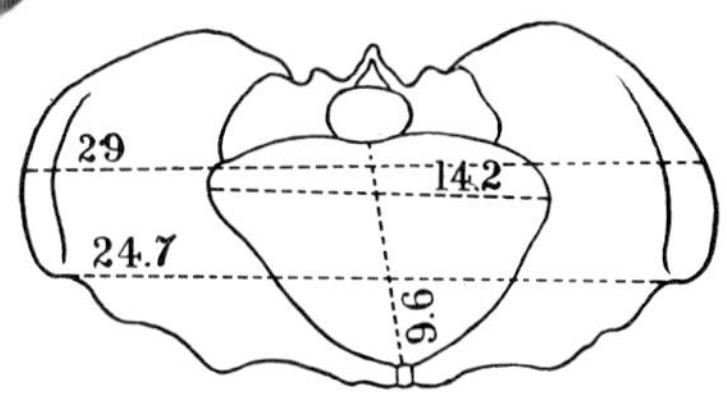

Fig. 575.

Figs. 574, 575.—Kypho-Scoliotic-Rhachitic Pelvis (Leopold).

the superior strait is usually quite marked. Generally speaking, however, this class of pelvis is more favourable from an obstetrical standpoint than that due to scolio-rhachitis alone.

Spondylolisthetic Pelvis.—The term spondylolisthesis (from σπόνδυλος, vertebra, and ὀλισθησις, slipping or sliding) was introduced by Kilian in 1853, in describing a pelvis in which the last lumbar vertebra had become displaced downward over the anterior surface of the sacrum.

The degree of displacement may vary greatly. When the deformity is slight the anterior inferior margin of the last lumbar vertebra merely projects a short distance beyond the anterior margin of the promontory of the sacrum, while in pronounced cases the entire body of the vertebra is displaced downward and forward into the pelvic cavity, so that its inferior surface comes in contact with and more or less completely covers the body of the first, and occasionally that of the second sacral vertebra. As a consequence, a greater or lesser portion of the lumbar column comes to occupy the upper portion of the pelvic cavity, the superior strait assuming a reniform shape.

The lower lumbar vertebræ may overhang the pelvic inlet to such an extent that the obstetrical or pseudo-conjugate will be represented by a line drawn from the upper margin of the symphysis to the lower margin of the fourth, third, or even second lumbar vertebra, as the case may be. In the specimen described by me in 1899 the pseudo-conjugate extended to the lower margin of the third lumbar vertebra and measured 6.5 centimetres, as compared with a distance of 7.6 centimetres to the lower margin of the fourth lumbar.

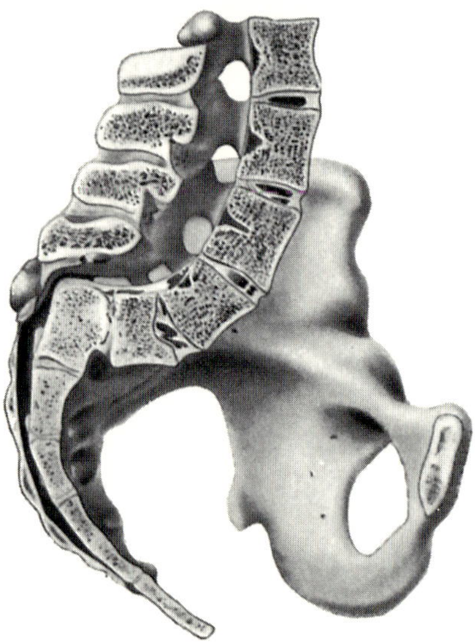

Fig. 576.—Vertical Section through Spondylolisthetic Pelvis (Kilian).

The displacement of the last lumbar vertebra is due not to luxation, but to the lengthening and bending of its interarticular portions. Its inferior articular processes still retain their normal relation to the superior articular processes of the first sacral vertebra, whereas its body and its superior articular processes, together with the rest of the vertebral column, become displaced forward and eventually downward. As a result of the new position assumed by the body of the last lumbar vertebra, the superior and anterior surfaces of the promontory become more or less worn away by friction, the defect being not infrequently followed by ankylosis which definitely checks further displacement. In advanced cases the inferior articular processes of the last lumbar and the superior articular processes of the first sacral vertebra are usually firmly synostosed together, as are also the inferior articular processes of the fourth and the superior articular processes of the fifth lumbar vertebra.

Owing to the collapse of the vertebral column into the pelvic cavity, the centre of gravity falls in front of instead of just behind the acetabula, and consequently the pelvis must be tilted backward in order that the individual may retain an upright position. In other words, the pelvic inclination must be diminished, and when the deformity is marked the plane of the superior strait becomes parallel to the horizon. This is rendered possible by changes in the ilio-femoral ligaments, which are manifested on the one hand by a marked roughening of the portions of the

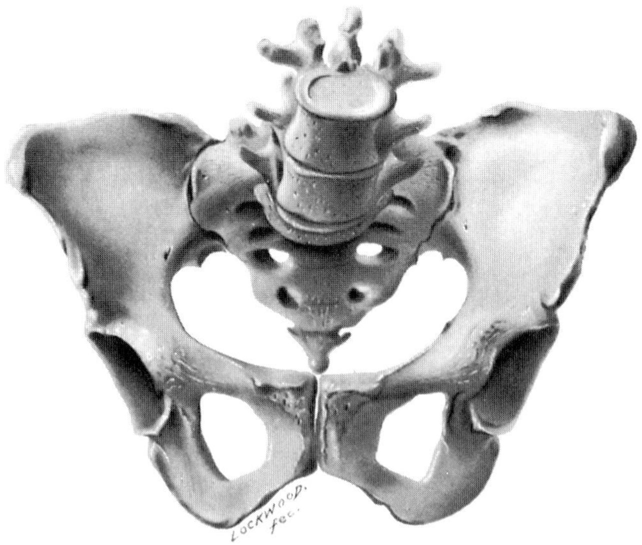

Fig. 577.

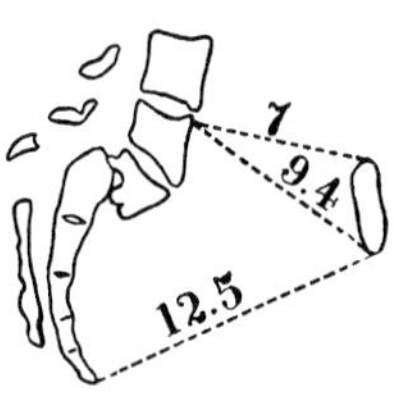

Fig. 578.

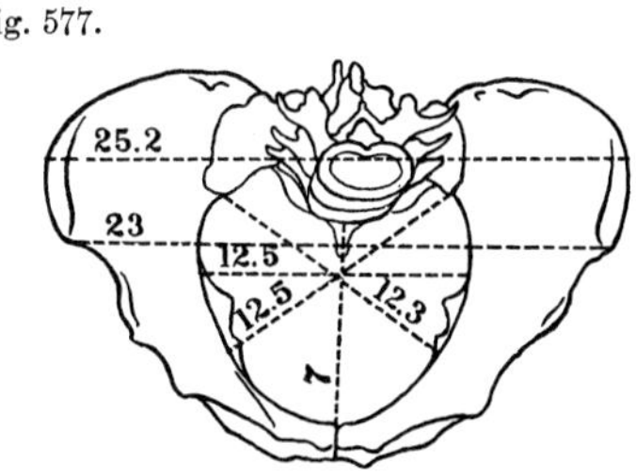

Fig. 579.

FIGS. 577–579.—SPONDYLOLISTHETIC PELVIS.

pelvis to which they are attached, and on the other by characteristic changes in gait of the patient. In my own case the pelvic inclination was obliterated; but, had it remained normal, the vertebral column would have formed a right angle with the legs, necessitating the patient's going upon all-fours, whereas, as a matter of fact, she was able to walk erect.

As the inferior surface of the last lumbar vertebra is in contact with the anterior instead of the superior surface of the first sacral vertebra, the action of the body weight tends to force the promontory of the sacrum backward, thereby causing it to rotate about its transverse axis, while its tip approaches the anterior pelvic wall. The retropulsion and rotation of the sacrum, together with the increased traction exerted by the ilio-femoral ligaments, causes each innominate bone to rotate about an axis extending from the symphysis to the sacro-iliac joint, and tends to give the pelvis a funnel shape, just as in kyphosis, the inferior strait becoming considerably contracted transversely and the pubic arch narrowed.

Ætiology.—Kilian considered that the displacement of the last lumbar vertebra was rendered possible by inflammatory softening of the intervertebral disk. Later, various hypotheses were advanced as to its mode of production. Robert, Lambl, and Königstein showed that the displacement could not take place so long as the inferior articular processes of the last lumbar were normal and in contact with the superior articular processes of the first sacral vertebra, unless the entire vertebra became lengthened.

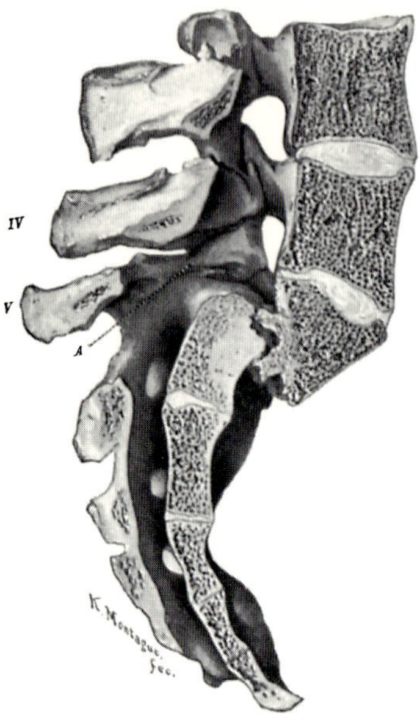

Fig. 580.—Spondylolisthesis; Vertical Section through Last Three Lumbar Vertebræ and Sacrum. × ½.

Neugebauer devoted thirteen years (1882–'95) to the study of this subject, and during that period published 15 journal articles and 3 monographs upon it, covering nearly 900 pages, not to mention the discussions and demonstrations in which he took part. He showed conclusively that in the vast majority of cases the deformity was rendered possible by a lengthening and thinning out of the interarticular portions of the last lumbar vertebra, by which its superior and inferior articular processes become separated by a long, thin lamina of bone instead of being almost in the same vertical line (Fig. 581).

This condition he attributed to imperfect development of the interarticular portion (spondylolysis) or to its fracture, with subsequent stretching of the callus. He considered that the former was the more frequent cause, as he was able to demonstrate it in many vertebræ which presented no signs of spondylolisthesis. When the displacement is marked the interarticular portion is not only lengthened and thinned out, but also becomes bent over the promontory of the sacrum, thus forming a *dolicho-kyrto-platy-spondylus.*

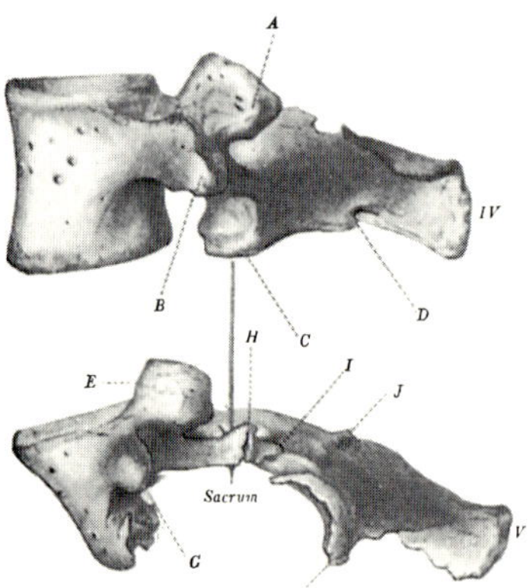

Fig. 581.—Fourth and Fifth Lumbar Vertebræ from my Case of Spondylolisthesis. × ½.

A, superior articular process; *B*, transverse process; *C*, inferior articular process; *D*, lamina of fourth lumbar vertebra; *E*, superior articular process; *F*, inferior articular process; *G*, transverse process; *H*, *I*, *J*, fissures in interarticular portion of last lumbar vertebra.

In opposition to Neugebauer's statement that the deformity always results from changes in the interarticular portion, Chiari definitely showed, in one case at least, that it can follow fracture of the articular processes without the characteristic changes in the vertebra.

Arbuthnot Lane stated that the disease is more common than is generally supposed, as he observed several examples of it in coal-heavers. He considers that in such cases, at least, the changes in the interarticular portion are due not to abnormalities in development but to excessive pressure, which results from carrying heavy burdens. Complete literature upon the subject will be found in my own article and in that of Breus and Kolisko.

Frequency.—Neugebauer, in 1893, was able to collect 115 cases of spondylolisthesis, most of which were clinical observations. In 1899 the author collected 123 cases, 6.5 per cent of which occurred in males. According to Breus and Kolisko only 20 indisputable anatomical specimens of this condition are in existence, 2 of which they described for the first time.

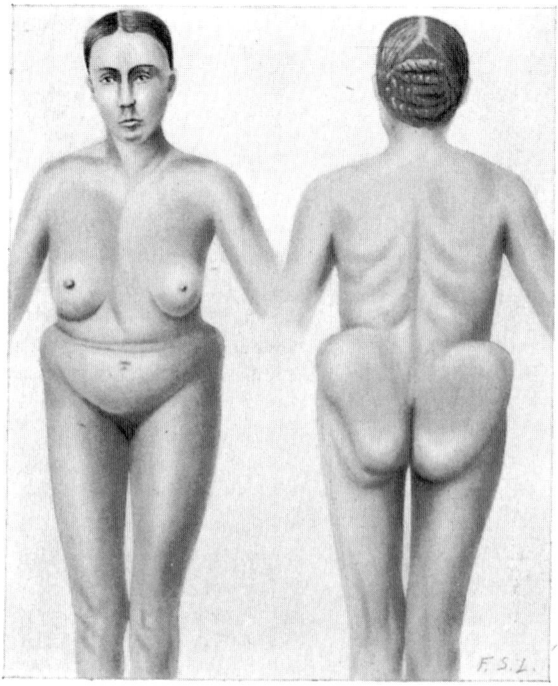

FIG. 582.—FRONT AND BACK VIEWS OF WOMAN WITH SPONDYLOLISTHESIS (Ahlfeld).

Effect upon Labour.—When the condition is but slightly marked its effect upon labour is similar to that of a flat pelvis, as the greatest contraction is in the conjugata vera, although it should be remembered that it is likewise associated with considerable contraction of the inferior strait. When the deformity is pronounced and the lower lumbar vertebræ overhang the superior strait, the degree of contraction, from an obstetrical point of view, is to be reckoned not by the distance between the symphysis pubis and the anterior portion of the last lumbar vertebra, but by the length of the pseudo-conjugate, whose posterior extremity may be at the fourth, third, or even second lumbar vertebra, and in many cases is so short as absolutely to preclude the possibility of the head entering the pelvis.

Diagnosis.—In typical cases, mere inspection of the patient should lead one to suspect the existence of this deformity, inasmuch as there is always marked lumbar lordosis and the entire trunk seems to have caved in, so that the ribs come almost in contact with the iliac crests. When viewed from the front, the abdominal walls appear redundant out of all proportion. Such patients have a peculiar duck-like walk or waddling gait, to which Neugebauer first directed attention. Since the posterior portion of the last lumbar vertebra retains its normal position while the rest of the vertebral column sinks forward, the spine of the last lumbar vertebra will sometimes form a marked prominence just above the sacrum. The condition, however, should not be mistaken for a deep-seated kyphosis.

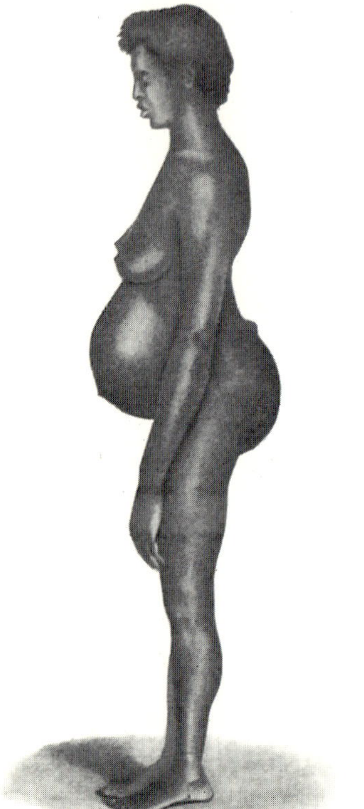

Fig. 583.—Side View of Woman with Spondylolisthesis, showing Projecting Spine of Last Lumbar Vertebra.

On internal examination the diagnosis, as a rule, is readily made, as the body of the last lumbar vertebra will be found lying in front of the anterior and upper portion of the sacrum and will be detected when one attempts to measure the diagonal conjugate. At the same time the ilio-pectineal line ends abruptly at the margins of the overhanging vertebral body instead of continuing uninterruptedly to the promontory of the sacrum.

Owing to the marked lordosis, which frequently accompanies the condition, the bodies of the lower lumbar vertebræ can readily be palpated and counted, and the bifurcation of the aorta, or at least the common iliac arteries, are not infrequently readily accessible to the examining finger.

Occasionally pronounced rhachitic changes in the sacrum may simulate spondylolisthesis, but a correct diagnosis can usually be arrived at. If such patients be anæsthetized, on careful palpation the ilio-pectineal lines will be found to terminate at the promontory of the sacrum instead of at the sides of the prolapsed body of the last lumbar vertebra.

A somewhat similar condition is presented in marked cases of lumbosacral kyphosis, particularly in the pelvis obtecta. Under such circumstances the promontory of the sacrum is destroyed, but a correct diagnosis can usually be made by carefully palpating the anterior surface of the sacrum and tracing the alæ to the body of the first sacral vertebra, which, of course, is impossible in spondylolisthesis.

Prognosis.—Generally speaking, spontaneous labour can occur only when the deformity is minimal, and accordingly, in pronounced cases, the outlook is uniformly bad for both mother and child unless radical operative measures be undertaken. Other things being equal, a spondylolisthetic pelvis offers a worse prognosis than a rhachitic one with the same antero-posterior measurements, for the reason that in the former the inferior strait is contracted, while in the latter it is usually enlarged.

In considering the probable outcome of labour, one should not only measure the distance between the symphysis pubis and the last lumbar vertebra, but should also estimate the pseudo-conjugate, inasmuch as the latter much more frequently than the antero-posterior diameter of the superior strait offers the greatest obstacle to labour. The fact that a patient with spondylolisthesis has had one or more spontaneous labours does not necessarily imply that the labour in question will be uneventful, for the reason that the degree of deformity not infrequently increases with age, as was clearly demonstrated in my own case.

Treatment.—With a pseudo-conjugate of 8 centimetres or over, the possibility of spontaneous labour, or delivery by forceps or version, should be borne in mind; but when it measures less than 8 centimetres Cæsarean section should be done at the onset of labour. Symphyseotomy does not seem applicable to the condition. It certainly proved ineffectual in Morisani's case as well as in my own, having been resorted to in the latter only after the patient had persistently declined to submit to Cæsarean section.

LITERATURE

Barbour. Spinal Deformity in Relation to Obstetrics. Edinburgh, 1883.

Boursier de Coudray, Louise. Abrégé de l'art des accouchements. Paris, 1759.

Breisky. Ueber den Einfluss der Kyphose auf die Beckengestalt. Zeitschr. der Gesellsch. der Aerzte in Wien, i, 1865.

Breus und Kolisko. Die path. Beckenformen. Bd. iii, I. Theil, 1900. Spondylolisthesis, 17–159. Kyphosen-Becken, 163–307. Skoliosen-Becken, 311–352. Kyphoskoliosen Becken, 355–359.

Champneys. The Obstetrics of the Kyphotic Pelvis. Trans. Lond. Obst. Soc., 1883, xxv, 166–194.

Chantreuil. Étude sur les déformations du bassin chez les cyphotiques. Thèse de Paris, 1869.

Chiari. Die Aetiologie und Genese der sogenannten Spondylolisthesis lumbo-sacralis. Zeitschr. f. Heilkunde, 1892.

Doktor. Ein Fall von conservativen Kaiserschnitt. Centralbl. f. Gyn., 1893, 630–633.

Fehling. Pelvis obtecta. Archiv f. Gyn., 1872, iv, 1–33.

Herrgott. Du spondylizème. Archives de Tocologie, 1877 (Fév.-Mars).

Kilian. De spondylolisthesi gravissimæ pelvangustiæ causa nuper detecta. Bonn, 1853.

Klien. Die Geburt beim kyphotischen Becken. Archiv f. Gyn., 1896, l, 1–128.

Königstein. Entstehungsweise spondylolisthetischer Becken. D. I., Marburg, 1871.

Lambl. Das Wesen und die Entstehung der Spondylolisthesis. Scanzoni's Beiträge, 1855, iii, 1–77.

LANE. Some of the Changes which are produced by Pressure in the Lower Part of the Spinal Column; Spondylolisthesis, etc. Trans. Lond. Path. Soc., 1885, xxxvi, 364–378.

LEOPOLD. Das skoliotische und kypho-skol. rachitische Becken. Leipzig, 1879.

Weitere Untersuchungen über das skoliotische und kypho-skol. rachitische Becken. Archiv f. Gyn., 1880, xvi, 1–23.

MORISANI. Ancora della Sinfisiotomia. Annali di Ost. e Gin., 1886, viii, 345–391.

NEUGEBAUER. Zur Entwickelungsgeschichte des spondylolisthetischen Beckens und seiner Diagnose. Halle u. Dorpat, 1882, 294.

Spondylolisthesis et spondylizème. Paris, 1892.

Die heutige Statistik der Geburten bei Beckenverengerung infolge von Rückgrätskyphose. Monatsschr. f. Geb. u. Gyn., 1895, l, 317–347.

ROBERT. Eine eigenthümliche angeborene Lordose, etc. Monatsschr. f. Geburtsk., 1855, v, 81–94.

ROKITANSKY. Anomalien der Gestalt des Rückgräts und seiner Theile. Lehrbuch der path. Anat., III. Aufl., 1856, ii, 162–172.

SCHROEDER-OLSHAUSEN-VEIT. Lehrbuch der Geb., XIII. Aufl., 1899, 649.

TREUB. Recherches sur le bassin cyphotique. Leyden, 1889.

WILLIAMS, J. WHITRIDGE. A Case of Spondylolisthesis, with Description of the Pelvis. Amer. Jour. Obst., 1899, xl, 145–171.

CHAPTER XXXVIII

PELVIC ANOMALIES RESULTING FROM THE ABNORMAL DIRECTION OF THE FORCE EXERTED BY THE FEMORA—ATYPICAL DEFORMITIES

Normally, in the case of an individual standing erect, the upward and inward force exerted by the femora is of equal intensity on either side, and is transmitted to the pelvis through the acetabula. In walking or running, the entire body weight is transmitted alternately first to one and then to the other leg. On the other hand, in a person suffering from disease affecting one leg, the other sound one has to bear more than its share of the body weight, and consequently the upward and inward force exerted by the femur is, as a rule, greater upon that side of the pelvis. To these mechanical factors are due the changes in shape which accompany certain forms of lameness, provided that the lesion, which gives rise to the latter, appears at an early period of life while the pelvic bones are still in a formative state.

The defect may be either unilateral or bilateral; in the former case it is usually due to coxalgia, luxation of the femur, infantile paralysis,

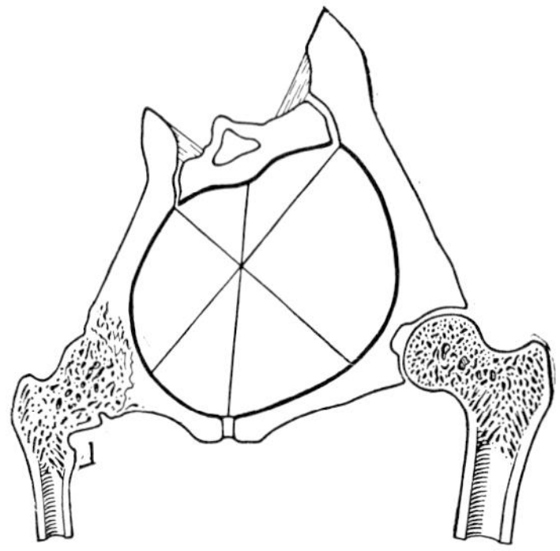

Fig. 584.—Diagram showing Coxalgic Pelvis before the Individual has Walked (Tarnier).

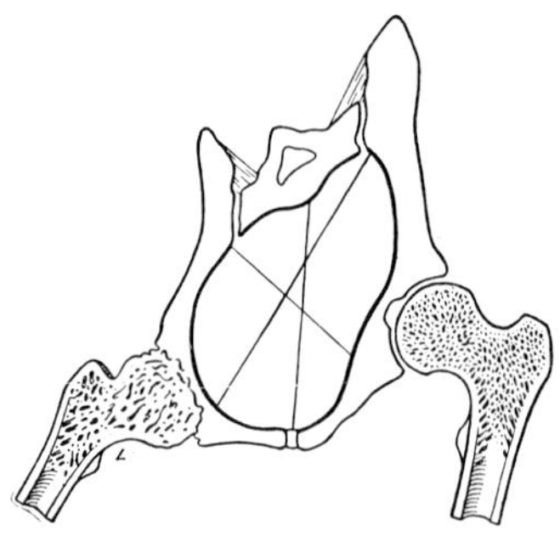

Fig. 585.—Diagram showing Coxalgic Pelvis after the Individual has Walked (Tarnier).

or shortening of one leg from various causes, while the most common causes of the latter are luxation of both femora and double club-foot. These conditions have been studied in detail by Prouvost, in whose article, as well as in the chapter of Tarnier and Budin upon the subject, full literature is to be found.

Pelvic Deformities Due to Unilateral Lameness.—*Coxalgia* occurring in early life nearly always gives rise to an obliquely contracted pelvis. If the disease makes its appearance before the patient learns to walk, or if the child is obliged to keep to its bed for a prolonged period, definite changes occur in the pelvis as a direct result of the disease. These are in great part

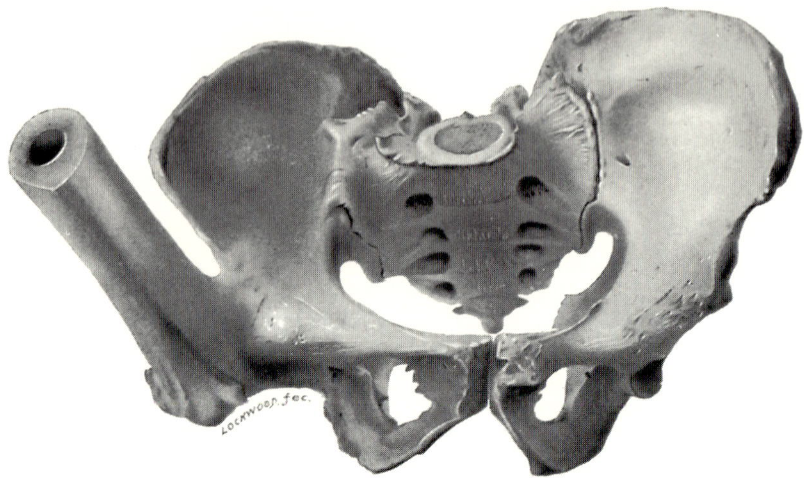

Fig. 586.

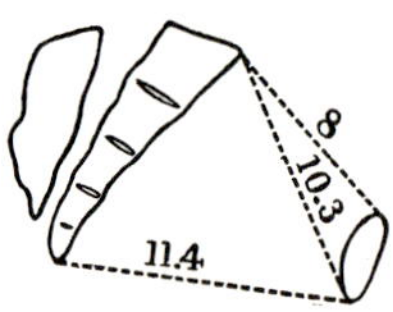

Fig. 587.

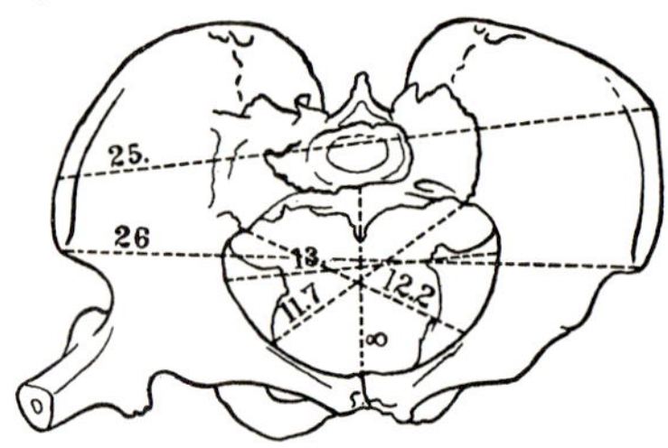

Fig. 588.

FIGS. 586–588.—COXALGIC PELVIS WITH ANKYLOSED FEMUR.

atrophic, and are manifested by imperfect development of the diseased side of the pelvis, the innominate bone being smaller than its fellow and the ilio-pectineal line represented by the arc of a circle having a smaller radius than upon the well side. At the same time, the sacral alæ are less developed upon the affected side, and the entire bone is somewhat rotated about its vertical axis, so that its anterior surface looks towards the well side (Figs. 584 and 585).

When the individual begins to stand, owing to the actual shortening of the diseased leg or to fear of placing it firmly upon the ground, the body weight is transmitted in great part to the well leg. As a result the pelvis becomes obliquely tilted, being higher on the well side, and a compensatory scoliosis appears. At the same time the upward and inward force exerted by the femur tends to push the well side of the pelvis upward, inward, and backward, whereby the ilio-pectineal line is markedly flattened and the asymmetry of the sacrum still further increased, thus giving rise to an obliquely contracted pelvis. The contraction is not limited to the superior strait, but involves the lower portion of the pelvis as well, the spine and tuberosity of the ischium being displaced towards the middle line.

Not uncommonly these changes are accompanied by irritative processes at the sacro-iliac articulations, which eventually lead to ankylosis. As a general rule, the oblique contraction is to be found on the well side of the pelvis, but, according to Tarnier, the reverse is the case when the affected leg is ankylosed in a position of adduction and internal rotation.

Similar though less marked changes take place in the pelvis when *unilateral luxation* of the femur occurs in early life. Under such circum-

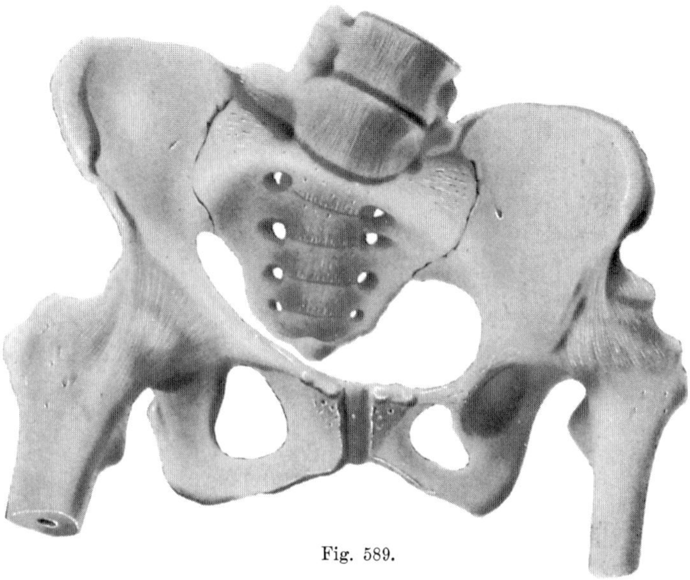

Fig. 589.

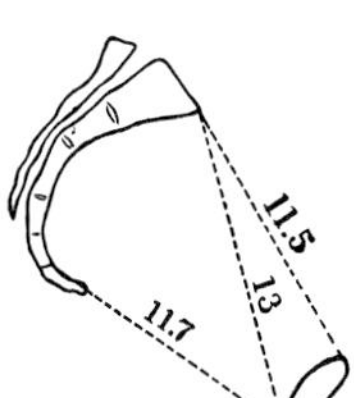

Fig. 590.

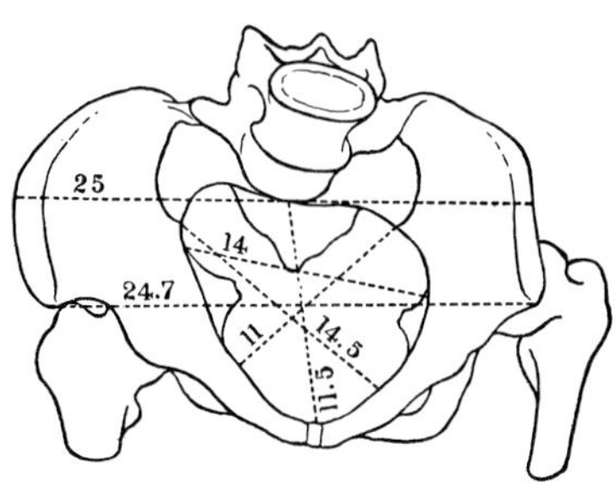

Fig. 591.

Figs. 589–591.—Obliquely Contracted Pelvis, Due to Unilateral Luxation of Femur.

stances the head of the bone is displaced backward and upward upon the outer surface of the ilium, where a new joint surface may occasionally be formed. The affected leg becomes considerably shortened, and accordingly an undue share of the body weight is transmitted through the well leg, which forces the corresponding side of the pelvis upward, inward, and backward, and leads to an oblique contraction, just as in coxalgia.

In unilateral *infantile paralysis,* and in those cases in which disease at the knee- or ankle-joint, or amputation has caused shortening of one leg, unless the patient has had the benefit of proper orthopædic treatment, similar changes occur in the pelvis, though it rarely assumes the extreme degree of obliquity which characterizes the coxalgic variety.

Diagnosis.—A limping gait at once suggests an obliquely contracted pelvis, and when, upon questioning the patient, it is found that the condition has been present since early childhood, the existence of pelvic deformity upon the side corresponding to the sound leg becomes highly probable.

More accurate information can be obtained by careful examination and noticing the relative position of the iliac crests and the presence or absence of compensatory scoliosis, and finally an absolute diagnosis can be arrived at by the employment of the measurements suggested by Naegele for the detection of the obliquely contracted pelvis due to imperfect development of the sacral alæ. An accurate conception concerning the degree of contraction, however, can be obtained only by careful exploration of the interior of the pelvis, preferably with the patient under the influence of an anæsthetic, although in many coxalgic patients this may be extremely difficult on account of the ankylosis of one leg.

Effect upon Labour.—The effect of this class of pelves upon labour varies with the extent and position of the deformity. If the affected side is so contracted as to prevent its being occupied by a portion of the presenting part, we have for all practical purposes a generally contracted pelvis, and engagement, if it can occur at all, will take place more readily when the biparietal diameter of the head is in relation with the long oblique diameter of the superior strait. But even after descent has occurred, all obstacles to labour have by no means been overcome, since in many cases the inward projection of the ischium may lead to abnormalities in rotation. Generally speaking, these pelves are not excessively contracted, Prouvost reporting that 40 out of the 50 cases of labour complicated by them ended spontaneously.

Treatment.—As the pelvic contraction is usually not very pronounced, Cæsarean section is rarely indicated, unless the fœtus is very large, or the history of previous labours has shown that the birth of a living child is out of the question. When the obstacle to the engagement of the head is not serious, version gives better results than forceps. This is especially true in coxalgic pelves when the ankylosed leg and the asymmetry of the pubic arch may make its proper application practically impossible.

Symphyseotomy is never a justifiable operation in these cases, particularly in those due to coxalgia, as we have no means of determining in advance whether the sacro-iliac synchondroses are synostosed; and if such be the case the operation cannot lead to an increase in the capacity of the pelvic canal.

Pelvic Deformity Due to Bilateral Lameness.—Occasionally children are born with *luxation of both femora*, the heads of the bones lying, as a rule, upon the outer surfaces of the iliac bones, above and posterior to their usual situation. In some cases the acetabula are entirely absent, but more frequently they are present in a rudimentary condition, new but imperfect substitutes being formed higher up. Strange to say, the condition does not usually seriously interfere with the individual in the matter of learning to walk at the usual age, though the gait is more or less wabbly.

The pelvic changes resulting from this condition have been studied particularly by Kleinwächter, Schauta, and Sassmann, the latter writer having collected 27 cases from the literature. Owing to the fact that the upward and inward force exerted by the femora is not applied in its usual direction through the acetabula, the pelvis becomes unduly wide, and more or less flattened antero-posteriorly. The transverse widening is particularly marked at the inferior strait, while the flattening, as a rule, is not very pronounced. Thus, the conjugata vera usually measures between 9 and 10 centimetres, and in only 2 of the cases collected by Sassmann was it as short as 7 centimetres. Hence, as might be expected, this pelvis rarely offers any serious obstacle to labour.

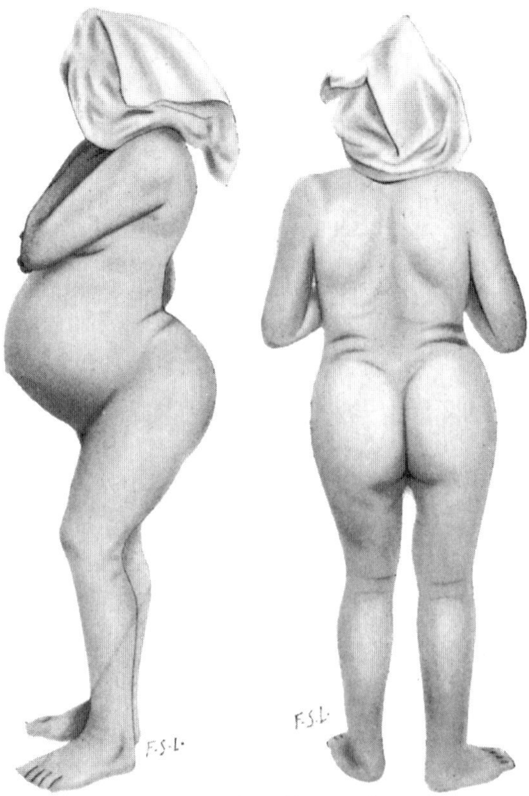

FIG. 592.—SIDE AND REAR VIEW OF PATIENT WITH BILATERAL LUXATION OF FEMORA.

The patient presents a characteristic appearance, which is suggestive of that observed in spondylolisthesis. Owing to the displacement of the femora the trochanters are more prominent than usual, and the width of the buttocks is increased. At the same time, owing to the increase in the pelvic inclination, there is marked lordosis, the back of the patient appearing considerably shortened and presenting a marked saddle-shaped depression just above the sacrum.

According to Schauta, Meyer described a pelvis obtained from an individual who had *double club-foot*, and found that it was markedly funnel-shaped. This condition he attributed to the absence of the usual spring at the foot and ankle-joints, and to the fact that the knees were held fixed during walking, accordingly, with each step a distinct shock was imparted to the acetabula, instead of the more gentle force which is exerted under ordinary circumstances.

Atypical Deformities of the Pelvis.—In rare instances the pelvis may be more or less deformed by the presence of bony outgrowths at various points, and less frequently by tumour formations. *Exostoses* are most frequently observed upon the posterior surface of the symphysis, in front of the sacro-iliac joints, or upon the anterior surface of the sacrum, though in occasional cases they may be formed along the course of the ilio-pectineal line.

Kilian, in 1854, directed attention to the fact that such structures may form sharp, more or less knife-like projections. He designated the condition as *acanthopelys* or *pelvis spinosa.* Such formations are rarely sufficiently large to offer any obstacle to labour, but owing to their peculiar structure may do considerable injury to the material soft parts. In fact, in several of the cases reported, they have cut through the lower portion of the uterus.

In rare instances *callus formation,* resulting from inflammatory processes within the pelvis, may attain such proportions as to lead to serious pelvic obstruction, as in a case reported by Ahlfeld.

Tumour formations of various kinds may spring from the walls of the true or false pelvis and so obstruct the pelvic cavity as to render labour impossible. Fibromata, osteomata, enchondromata, carcinomata, and osteosarcomata of the pelvis have been described, and sometimes assume very considerable proportions, and occasionally become cystic. Stadfeld was able to collect 49 such cases in 1879, and Goder 81 cases in 1895. Full literature is to be found in their articles and in the chapter of Schauta dealing with the subject.

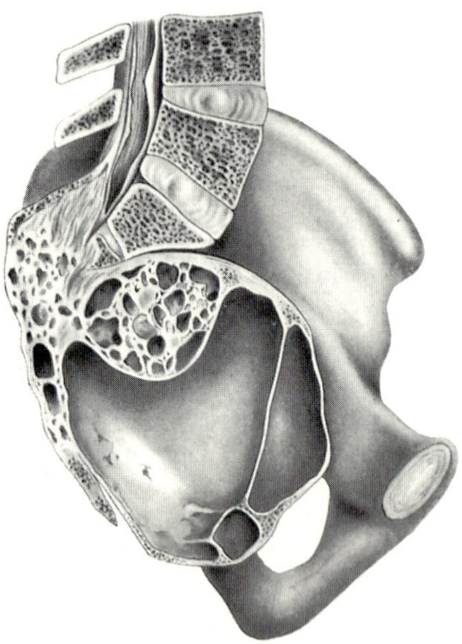

FIG. 593.—OBSTRUCTION OF PELVIC CANAL BY CYSTIC ENCHONDROMA (Zweifel).

The prognosis is very grave when the pelvis is obstructed by tumours from its walls, 50 per cent of the mothers and 89 per cent of the children having perished in the cases collected by Stadfeld, while in only 11 cases was labour terminated by spontaneous delivery, forceps, or version.

In rare instances, healed *fractures* of the pelvis may offer an insuperable obstacle to the birth of the child, owing either to an excessive formation of callus or to the projection of the broken ends of the bones into the pelvic cavity. This condition, however, is very rare, as it is stated that only 0.8 per cent of all fractures involve the pelvis, and in such cases the internal injuries are usually so severe as to lead to the death of the patient, so that only a small proportion of such women survive, and very few of them become pregnant.

The effect upon labour depends upon the location of the fracture and its manner of healing. Fig. 594 shows a pelvis described by Mars, and gives an

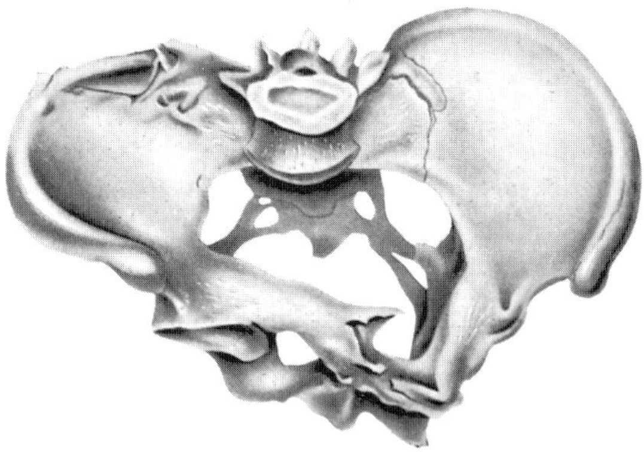

Fig. 594.—Fractured Pelvis (Mars).

idea of the extent of the changes which sometimes result. In a case reported by Neugebauer, in which there was a transverse fracture of the second sacral vertebra, the vertebral column prolapsed into the pelvic cavity and gave rise to a deformity suggestive of spondylolisthesis. For further details the reader is referred to the articles of Schauta and Tarnier.

LITERATURE

Ahlfeld. Das durch Knochenauswüchse verengte Becken. Lehrbuch der Geburtshülfe, II. Aufl., 1898, 336.

Goder. Von dem Becken ausgehende Tumoren als Geburtshinderniss. D. I., Halle, 1895.

Kilian. Das Stachelbecken (Akanthopelys); Schilderungen neuer Beckenformen, etc. Mannheim, 1854, 59–114.

Kleinwächter. Das Luxationsbecken, etc. Prager Vierteljahrsschr. f. Heilkunde, cxviii, cxix.

Mars. Schrägverengtes Becken infolge einer Fractur. Archiv f. Gyn., 1889, xxxvi, 289–300.

Prouvost. Étude sur les bassins viciés par boiterie. Thèse de Paris, 1891.

Sassmann. Das Becken bei angeborener doppelseitiger Hüftgelenksluxation. Archiv f. Gyn., 1873, v, 241–267.

Schauta. Müller's Handbuch d. Geb., 1889, ii.
Die Beckenformen bei doppelseitiger Luxation der Schenkelköpfe, 466–472.
Die Beckenform bei Klumpfuss, 472–473.

Stadfeld. Die Geburt bei Geschwülsten des Beckens. Centralbl. f. Gyn., 1880, 417–420.

Tarnier et Budin. Traité de l'art des accouchements. Paris, 1898, iii.
Malformations du bassin dans la claudication, 229–278.
Déformations atypiques du bassin, 338–352.

CHAPTER XXXIX

DYSTOCIA DUE TO ABNORMALITIES IN DEVELOPMENT OR PRESENTATION OF THE FŒTUS

Excessive Development.—As was stated in Chapter V, the child at birth rarely exceeds 12 pounds (5,600 grammes) in weight, though authentic accounts of much larger infants are to be found in the literature.

Provided the pelvis is not contracted, it is very exceptional for a normally formed child, weighing less than 10½ pounds (5,000 grammes), to give rise to dystocia by its mere size. In overdeveloped children the difficulty is generally due to the fact that the head tends to become not only larger but harder, and consequently less malleable with increasing weight; although it sometimes happens that after the head has passed through the pelvic canal without difficulty the dystocia may be due to the arrest of the unusually large shoulders either at the pelvic brim or outlet. On the other hand, when the pelvis is abnormal, great difficulty may be experienced in delivering even moderately sized children.

Excessive development of the fœtus can usually be traced to one of four causes: prolongation of pregnancy, large size of one or both parents, advancing age, or multiparity of the mother.

Cases in which three hundred days or more elapse between the last menstrual period and the onset of labour are not uncommon, but in the majority of these the prolongation of pregnancy is only apparent, and merely means that fertilization of the ovum took place just before the first period missed, instead of shortly after the last menstrual flow. On the other hand, actual prolongation is occasionally observed, and is liable to exert a serious influence upon the course of labour, inasmuch as the child increases steadily in size for every additional day it remains in the uterus. Accordingly, whenever it seems probable that gestation has gone on beyond the normal term, the patient should be carefully watched and examined at frequent intervals, so that labour may be induced as soon as there is any sign of disproportion between the size of the head and the pelvis.

More frequently the excessive size of the child is due to the fact that one or both of its parents are unusually large; moreover, it is a matter of common observation that the fœtal head in many instances resembles that of its father, large-headed men usually producing children with similar characteristics. The age of the mother has likewise an important influence upon the fœtal development. Thus, the children of elderly primiparæ often exceed the ordinary average, and in multiparæ the children are often larger with each successive pregnancy, provided they do not follow in too rapid succession.

As a rule, large-headed children have hard and well ossified heads. This is more particularly true for males, in whom the biparietal diameter is usually somewhat greater than in female children of the same size. In such cases the inability of the head to become moulded not only interferes with its engagement, but predisposes to certain injuries, such as spoon-shaped depressions of the skull, when artificial delivery becomes necessary.

Although in the case of a normal pelvis a moderate increase in the size of the child is usually without any practical significance, when any degree of contraction exists such a condition may make all the difference between an easy and a difficult labour. At the same time, it must be remembered that in multiparous women the dystocia is often due in great part to the loss of tone of the uterine musculature incident to repeated childbearing.

Inasmuch as we possess no perfectly satisfactory means of determining the size of the child, and particularly of its head, the diagnosis of excessive development is, as a rule, not established until after fruitless attempts at delivery have been made. Nevertheless, a careful routine examination will often enable the obstetrician to arrive at fairly accurate conclusions and prepare him to meet this complication.

Generally speaking, if the pelvis is normal, the failure of engagement in the last weeks of pregnancy in a primipara, or the existence of a face, brow, or transverse presentation should suggest the probability of an excessively large head. Accurate bimanual palpation frequently confirms such a suspicion, especially when Müller's method of impression fails to cause the head to enter the pelvis.

Treatment.—Owing to the difficulty of clinching the diagnosis, the treatment is usually very unsatisfactory. If the patient has gone several weeks beyond term, and examination shows that the head is probably excessively large, there should be no hesitancy in the immediate induction of labour, the operation being particularly indicated in multiparous women whose history shows that excessive fœtal development was the cause of the previous difficult labours. On the other hand, if the pregnancy is not prolonged, the condition is rarely suspected at the outset of labour, and the diagnosis is made only after Nature has shown that she is unable to effect delivery. In such cases it is often very difficult to determine upon the best method of dealing with the complication. If careful examination shows that the head is excessively large and well ossified, the advisability of Cæsarean section may be considered if the patient is intensely desirous of offspring; though it should be remembered that, owing to the manipulations which have usually preceded it, the prognosis is not so favourable as in frank cases, and accordingly the operation has only a limited field of usefulness. In most cases, however, when delivery appears imperative, better results are obtained by version than by the employment of forceps upon the freely movable head.

When the obstacle to delivery is due to excessive size of the shoulders rather than of the head, labour can often readily be terminated after diminishing the size of the shoulder girdle by cutting through the clavicles with a pair of heavy scissors—*cleidotomy.*

Malformations of the Fœtus.—*Double Monsters.*—For practical purposes 3 groups of double monsters may be distinguished: (1) Incomplete double formations at the upper or lower half of the body (diprosopus, dipagus); (2) twins which are united together at the upper or lower end of the body (craniopagus, ischiopagus, or pygopagus); (3) double monsters which are united by the trunk (thoracopagus and dicephalus).

The diagnosis of any one of these conditions is not made until the serious difficulty experienced in attempting delivery has led to careful exploration under anæsthesia with the entire hand, although in many cases the existence of a multiple pregnancy may have been suspected. As such monstrosities frequently present minor deformities as well, the detection of a clubfoot, hare-lip, etc., should always direct one's attention to the possible existence of some still more serious abnormality.

Fortunately the delivery of many monstrosities is much more readily accomplished than would appear possible at first sight. In the first place, such pregnancies rarely go on to full term, so that the monstrosity rarely exceeds a normal child in size. In the second place, the connection between the two halves is often of such a character as to permit of sufficient motility between the component parts as to make their successive delivery possible.

On the other hand, in the first group the large size of the doubled portion of the monster may lead to serious mechanical obstacles at the time of delivery. The fused head in a *diprosopus* is, as a rule, much more readily delivered when it forms the after-coming part than when it presents primarily. In the second group, a *craniopagus* presenting by the head usually causes only a moderate amount of difficulty; whereas, on the other hand, *ischiopagi* and *pygopagi,* as a rule, call for complicated and difficult manœuvres before delivery can be effected.

In the third group, the delivery of *dicephalic monsters* is facilitated when they present by the breech, as in many cases first one and then the other head can be extracted. On the other hand, in cephalic presentations the two heads may mutually interfere with one another and thus prevent engagement until one has been diminished in size by craniotomy. When engagement of one head occurs, delivery can be partially effected by forceps, but as a rule the head cannot be delivered beyond the pubic arch, for the reason that further descent is prevented by the arrest of the second head at the superior strait. Under such circumstances it is advisable to amputate the first head, after which delivery of the rest of the monster is, as a rule, best accomplished by version.

Thoracopagi usually offer a less serious obstacle to delivery, for the reason that they are frequently so loosely connected with one another that considerable motility is possible. Indeed, it is not unusual for the 2 children to present in a different manner. When possible, it is advisable to bring down all four feet at the same time, and to effect extraction in such a way that the posterior head is first delivered. In cephalic presentations, the head and body of the first child are expelled, and the second child is then born very much as in an ordinary twin pregnancy. If, however, the latter presents transversely, its delivery can be effected only by version and extraction.

Deformities of Fœtus.—In this place attention will be directed only to those abnormalities in fœtal development which may give rise to difficult labour. An *acardiacus* is a monster which is sometimes developed in single-ovum twin pregnancies as the result of inequalities in the communicating placental circulation. One twin is well developed and normal, while the other is imperfectly formed and lacks a heart. The way in which this is brought about was considered on page 329.

The most common variety of acardiac monster is the *acephalicus* or headless fœtus. Less common is the *amorphous* monster, which possesses neither a head nor extremities, but is round in shape and presents upon its surface a number of small nodules, which represent the rudimentary extremities. The umbilical cord may be attached to any portion of its surface. The interior of the monstrosity contains a rudimentary intestinal tract, cystic cavities, vertebræ, etc., but no trace of a heart. The rarest variety of acardiacus is the *acormus* or trunkless monster, which consists of an imperfectly developed head and a rudimentary body, the umbilical cord being attached to the cervical region.

As a rule such monsters do not attain any notable size, although exceptionally, as the result of obstruction in the umbilical vein, they may become œdematous and give rise to dystocia.

The *anencephalus* or *hemicephalus* is a monster possessing a trunk, but only an imperfectly developed head, from which a large part of the brain and skull is lacking. Ordinarily, such beings are of moderate size, but occasionally the shoulders may be so excessively developed as to give rise to serious dystocia.

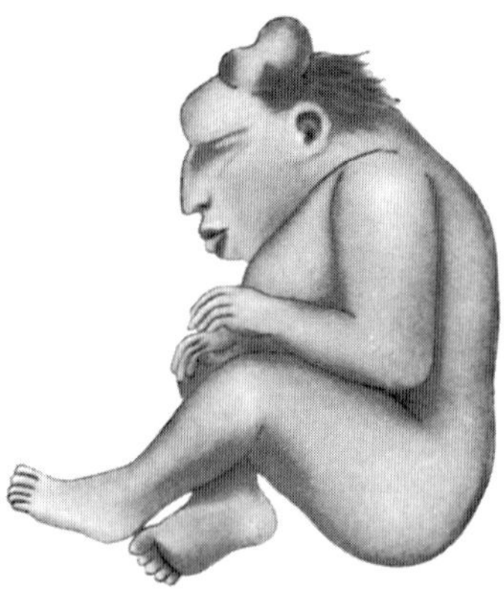

FIG. 595.—ANENCEPHALUS (Schroeder).

Owing to the absence of the cranial vault, the face is very prominent and somewhat extended, the eyes often protrude markedly from their sockets, and the tongue hangs from the mouth. The brain is in a rudimentary condition, and the base of the skull is accessible to the examining finger, so that the sella turcica can be distinguished. Owing to the exposed condition of the base of the brain and the upper part of the medulla, there is frequently a marked increase in the amount of amniotic fluid, its production being analogous to that noted in the picûre experiments of the physiologists.

In view of the abnormal shape of the head, face presentations are frequently observed, while those of the vertex are less common than with a normal fœtus. Transverse and foot presentations are likewise not unusual.

When the monstrosity presents by the face or head, a correct diagnosis is frequently made by vaginal touch, the characteristic bulging of the eyes being noted in the former, and the absence of the cranial vault and the presence of the sella turcica in the latter presentation.

Delivery, as a rule, occurs much more readily when the monster presents by the breech, for the reason that the imperfectly developed head is not an efficient dilating agent, though in many cases rapid and spontaneous delivery is observed. Even when the enlarged shoulders give rise to dystocia, delivery can usually be accomplished by means of version without any great difficulty.

Hydrocephalus.—In this not very rare condition, the cerebral ventricles are distended by an excessive amount of cerebro-spinal fluid (Fig. 596). As a result the skull becomes much increased in size, not infrequently attaining several times its normal dimensions, while the brain substance forms a layer only a few millimetres thick beneath it. At the same time the cranial bones are imperfectly developed, the sutures and fontanelles being much wider than usual.

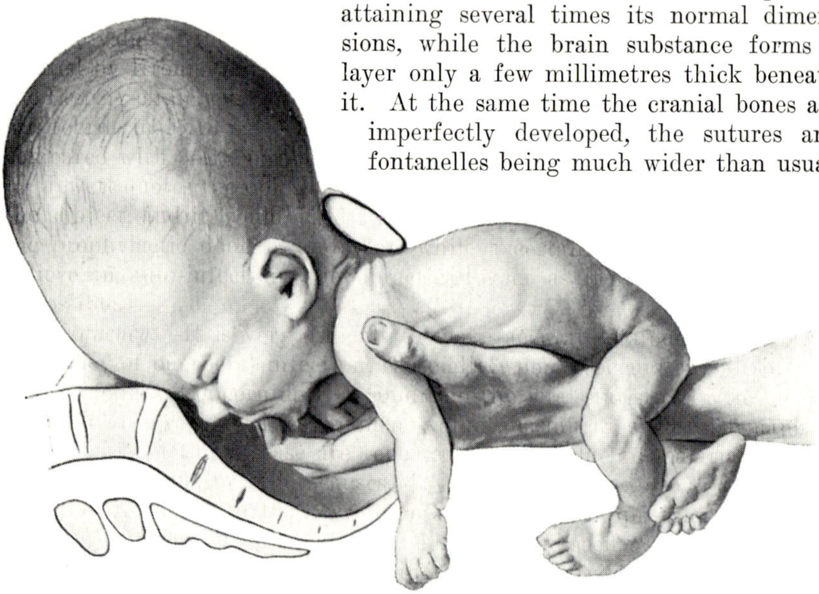

FIG. 596.—DYSTOCIA DUE TO HYDROCEPHALUS (Bumm).

If the enlarged head is not tensely filled with fluid, under the influence of the uterine contractions, it may undergo such changes in shape that its spontaneous expulsion becomes possible. This, however, is so rare a possibility that it should not be reckoned with in determining the treatment to be pursued in a given case. Still less frequently, owing to the pressure to which the head is subjected at the time of labour, the tissues forming a fontanelle or suture may give way, so that the cerebro-spinal fluid can escape, after which the head collapses and spontaneous delivery becomes possible. In the vast majority of cases, however, the condition gives rise to serious dystocia, which if not promptly relieved will lead to rupture of the uterus and the death of the patient from intra-abdominal hæmorrhage.

In hydrocephalic children, although cephalic presentations predominate, owing to the lack of accommodation between the head and the pelvic canal the breech is often substituted.

Diagnosis.—As a rule the condition is not recognised until several hours of fruitless second-stage pains have demonstrated the existence of an obstacle to delivery. On the other hand, careful examination should ordinarily lead to a correct diagnosis in the last weeks of pregnancy or soon after the onset of labour. In many cases the deformity can be detected by external palpation, the immensely large and movable head being isolated above the superior strait or in the fundus of the uterus. Furthermore, the examiner should always be on the lookout for the presence of fluctuation, while a peculiar crackling sensation can be elicited by pressure upon the skull. I have made a positive diagnosis in this manner upon several occasions without an internal examination.

As soon as the cervix is dilated, vaginal examination will reveal a large head with widely gaping sutures, through which fluctuation can be obtained by appropriate manœuvres. Of course this does not hold good in those cases in which the child presents by the breech, but here abdominal palpation will reveal the presence of the large fluctuant head in the fundus of the uterus, or just above the superior strait, in case attempts at extraction have been made.

Prognosis.—For the child the outlook is uniformly bad, for even if born alive it usually succumbs within a few days, and in the rare cases in which it survives, grows up a hopeless idiot. The maternal prognosis depends largely upon the obstetrician. If left to Nature, the usual termination of labour complicated by hydrocephalus is rupture of the uterus; whereas, if the condition be detected and proper treatment instituted, the results are almost universally favourable.

Treatment.—As soon as the cervix has become completely dilated, the head should be perforated, in order that the cerebro-spinal fluid can escape and the skull collapse, after which delivery can be effected by the unaided efforts of Nature, or may be accelerated by the employment of the cranioclast. On account of the nature of the disease and its effect upon the child, the operation may be undertaken without hesitancy, even by those who ordinarily do not consider craniotomy a justifiable procedure.

In evacuating the hydrocephalic head it should be borne in mind that, owing to the extreme thinness of the brain, mere perforation is not always synonymous with fœtal death. For this reason the perforator should be carried to the base of the skull and vigorously manipulated in order to destroy the medulla, as nothing could be more horrible than the extraction of a living child after such an operation.

Enlargement of the Abdomen of the Fœtus.—Enlargement of the abdomen sufficient to cause grave dystocia is usually the result of ascites, a very much distended bladder, or of tumours of the kidneys or liver.

Whenever the abdominal distention is marked, spontaneous labour is out of the question; but, unfortunately the condition usually escapes detection until fruitless attempts at delivery have demonstrated the existence of some obstruction and have led the obstetrician to introduce his entire hand into the uterus in the hope of discovering its nature.

Occasionally a fœtus affected with *general dropsy* may attain such immense proportions that spontaneous delivery is impossible. A number of such cases are recorded in Ballantyne's valuable monograph. In very rare instances the ascites associated with *fœtal peritonitis* may have a similar result, and exceptionally a fœtus suffering from *chondrodystrophia* or *fœtal rhachitis* may become so œdematous as to give rise to dystocia.

As the result of the dilatation of the superficial lymphatics associated with œdema of the subcutaneous tissues, the fœtus may assume immense proportions and take on a bizarre shape. This condition, which is designated as *elephantiasis congenita cystica*, has been studied in detail by Ballantyne, and is a very rare cause of difficult labour (Fig. 597).

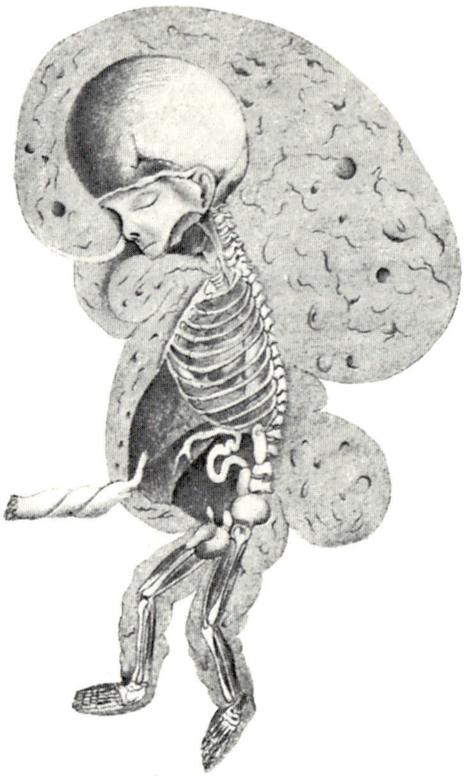

FIG. 597.—ELEPHANTIASIS CONGENITA CYSTICA (Ballantyne).

Defective development of the lower portion of the urinary tract may lead to the *retention of urine* accompanied by distention of the abdomen sufficient to render normal delivery impossible (Fig. 598). Examples of this condition have been reported by Walther, Schwyzer, and others, who also give details as to its ætiology.

A much more frequent cause of abdominal enlargement is the presence of *congenital cystic kidneys*. The growth, which is histologically an adenocystoma, may involve one or both organs, and give rise to tumours of immense size. The condition is frequently associated with dilatation of the ureters, and with dropsical effusions into the various body cavities. Fig. 599 gives an idea of the extent of the abdominal enlargement in a case which I delivered.

Mirabeau, Theilhaber, Hanau, Brouha, and many others have recently studied the condition in detail from an anatomical point of view, and have likewise considered its practical obstetrical bearings.

In rare cases the abdominal enlargement may be due to *tumours of the liver*, Porak and Couvelaire having reported a case of congenital cystic liver associated with a similar condition of the kidneys. Moreover, large tumours, arising from any of the abdominal organs, may give rise to dystocia. Thus, Rogers has described an immense *fibro-cystic testicle*, and Phaenomenow an aortic aneurysm so large as to interfere with delivery. In rare instances fœtal inclusions, such as the so-called *fœtus in fœtu*, may be responsible. Occasionally the invasion by Bacillus aerogenes capsulatus may be followed by such an extensive production of gas that the fœtus becomes more than double the normal size when spontaneous delivery is impossible.

In all of these conditions, if the dystocia is marked, delivery can be accomplished only after opening the body of the fœtus and allowing the fluid to escape, or removing a portion, at least, of the offending tumour formation. The latter operation is not always easy, for, owing to the constrained position of the hand *in utero* and the dense consistency of the growth in many cases, great difficulty is experienced in completing it.

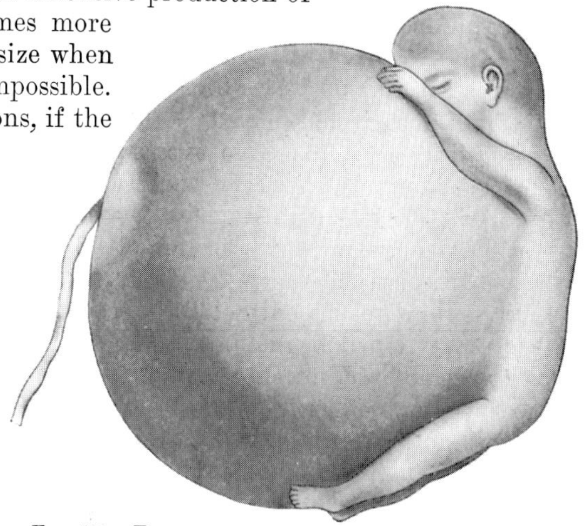

FIG. 598.—FŒTUS WITH IMMENSELY DISTENDED BLADDER (Hecker).

Tumours of the Body of the Fœtus.—In rare instances, abnormal growths arising from various portions of the body of the fœtus may seriously interfere with delivery. Cases are on record in which lipomata, carcinomata, angiomata, and various other tumours have given rise to such an enlargement that spontaneous delivery became out of the question. Exceptionally, dermoid cysts and teratomatous tumours about the perinæum and sacrum may offer a serious obstacle. Fig. 256 represents a fœtus in which an adenoma of the thyroid gland necessitated a destructive

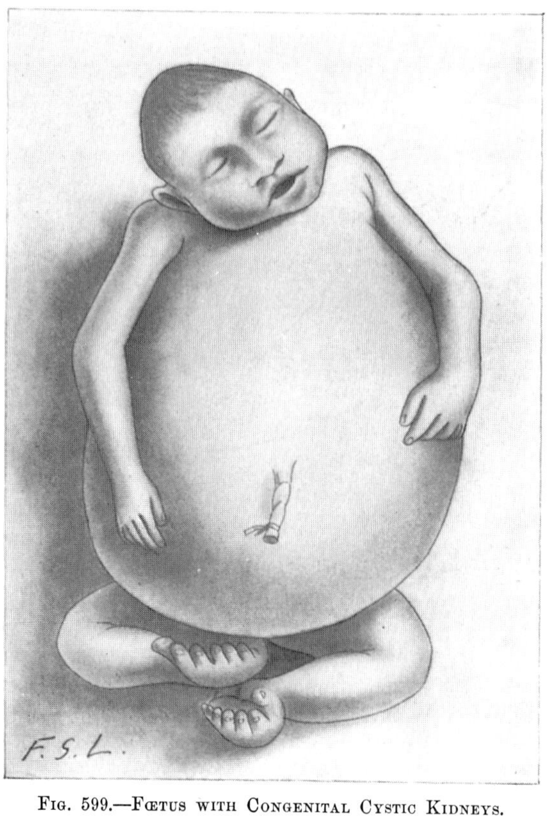

FIG. 599.—FŒTUS WITH CONGENITAL CYSTIC KIDNEYS.

operation. In rare instances parasitic fœtal tumours, a large umbilical hernia, a spina bifida, and other growths, give rise to difficult labour.

Dystocia Due to Abnormal Presentations of the Fœtus—*Transverse Presentations.*—In this condition the long axis of the fœtus crosses that of the mother at about a right angle. When it forms an acute angle we speak of an *oblique* presentation. The latter, however, is usually only transitory, becoming converted into a longitudinal presentation when labour supervenes.

In transverse presentations the shoulder usually occupies the superior strait, the head lying in one and the breech in the other iliac fossa (Figs. 600 and 601). Accordingly, such a condition is commonly spoken of as a *shoulder*, and less frequently as a *lateral plane presentation*. As the acromion process is one of the most characteristic features of the shoulder, these are usually designated as *acromio-iliac presentations*, the position being right or left according to the side of the mother towards which the shoulder is

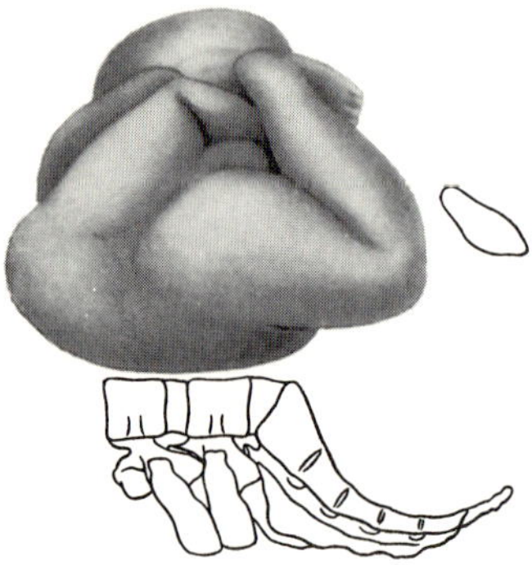

Fig. 600.—Diagram showing Left Acromio-iliac Dorso-posterior Presentation.

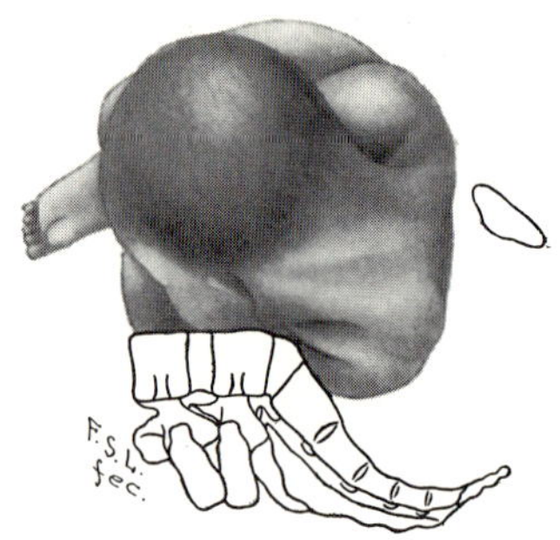

Fig. 601.—Diagram showing Right Acromio-iliac Dorso-anterior Presentation.

directed. Moreover, in either position, the back may be directed either anteriorly or posteriorly, and accordingly it is customary to distinguish between the *dorso-anterior* and *dorso-posterior* varieties. The recognition of the position of the back is of very considerable importance in connection with the proper performance of version—the treatment *par excellence* in this condition.

According to Schroeder, the shoulder is directed towards the left side of the mother 2.6 times more frequently than towards the right, while the back looks anteriorly 2.5 times more frequently than posteriorly.

Ætiology.—The existence of a transverse presentation in a primiparous woman is *prima facie* evidence of a lack of accommodation, usually the result of disproportion between the size of the head and the pelvis. In rare instances it may be due to hydramnios. In multiparæ, on the other hand, the most frequent ætiological factor is an abnormal relaxation of the abdominal and uterine walls, the result of repeated childbearing, which may be still further complicated by any of the causes already enumerated. Accordingly, transverse presentations are much more frequently observed in women who have borne a number of children, and in them, as a rule, the

PLATE XV.

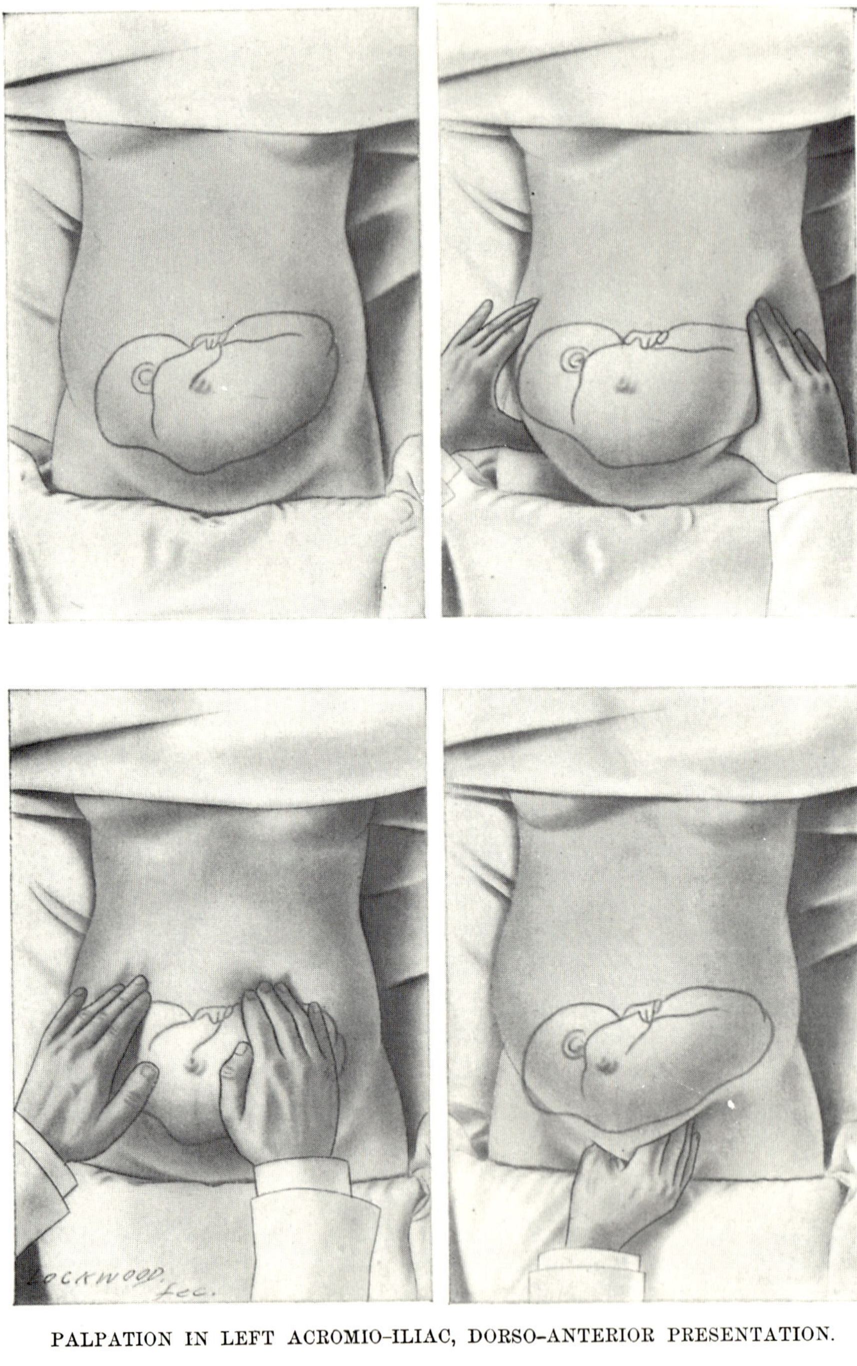

PALPATION IN LEFT ACROMIO-ILIAC, DORSO-ANTERIOR PRESENTATION.

condition is not so serious as in primiparæ, for the reason that in the former spontaneous reposition frequently ensues after the onset of labour pains, the child assuming a longitudinal presentation, whereas such an occurrence is exceptional in the latter.

This spontaneous conversion into a longitudinal presentation is rendered more difficult by premature rupture of the membranes, as well as by any condition which interferes with the descent or engagement of the head; for example, a contracted pelvis, placenta prævia, a pelvic tumour, or twin pregnancy. In rare instances longitudinal may become converted into secondary transverse presentations at the time of labour, although such an occurrence is exceptional, and is always indicative of disproportion between the size of the child and the pelvis.

Diagnosis.—The diagnosis of a transverse presentation is usually readily made, inspection alone frequently causing one to suspect its existence. The abdomen is seen to be unusually wide from side to side, while the fundus of the uterus frequently does not extend above the umbilicus.

On palpation the first manœuvre reveals the absence of the head or the breech from the fundus. On the second manœuvre a ballottable head will be found in one and the breech in the other iliac fossa, while the third and fourth manœuvres are negative, unless labour has been in progress for some time and the shoulder has become impacted in the pelvis. At the same time the position of the back is readily diagnosed. When it is situated anteriorly, a hard resistant plane will be felt extending across the front of the abdomen; when it lies posteriorly, irregular nodulations, representing the small parts, will be felt in the same location (Plate XV).

On vaginal touch in the early stages of labour, the side of the thorax, readily recognisable by the "gridiron" sensation afforded by the ribs, can be made out at the superior strait. When dilatation is further advanced, the scapula can be distinguished on one and the clavicle on the other side of the thorax, while the position of the axilla will indicate towards which side the shoulder is directed. Later in labour the shoulder becomes wedged down in the pelvic canal, and a hand and arm not infrequently prolapse into the vagina; whether it is the right or left can be readily determined by ascertaining to which one of the obstetrician's it corresponds, just as in shaking hands.

Course of Labour.—With very rare exceptions, spontaneous labour is impossible in persistent transverse presentations, since expulsion cannot be effected unless both the head and trunk of the child enter the pelvis at the same time, a manifestly impossible event when both are of normal proportions. Accordingly, both the fœtus and mother must inevitably perish if appropriate measures are not instituted.

After rupture of the membranes, if the patient is left to herself an arm usually prolapses and the shoulder becomes forced down into the pelvic cavity, but can descend for only a certain distance, being arrested by the head and trunk at the superior strait. The uterus then contracts vigorously in the attempt to overcome the obstacle, but in vain. After a certain time the contraction ring rises higher and higher, the lower uterine segment becomes more and more stretched and eventually gives way, when a part or the whole of the product of conception escapes into the abdominal cavity. Under such circumstances the patient usually succumbs within a short time to intraperitoneal hæmorrhage, while in other instances death occurs after a longer or shorter period from infection.

Possibly once in many thousand cases the uterus ceases to contract before rupture occurs, the child being retained within the uterus, may eventually become converted into a lithopædion, to be finally cast off by suppurative processes. So far as I know, such a condition has not been described in human beings, though it is well known to the veterinarians. Nevertheless, the experience of Resnikow, who removed the suppurating fragments of a fœtus from the uterus four years after the expected date of confinement, is very suggestive.

In transverse presentations, now and again, spontaneous delivery ensues. Bartholin, in the seventeenth century, pointed out that a child which has lain transversely during the later months of pregnancy may spontaneously assume a longitudinal presentation at the time of labour. This so-called *spontaneous version* is a not infrequent occurrence. Its mode of production has already been referred to.

A century later, Roederer pointed out that in very rare instances, if the child was small and the pelvis large, delivery might occasionally be accomplished in spite of the persistence of the abnormal presentation. This process he designated *spontaneous evolution*. The monograph of Payer is replete with historical allusions to the subject.

Spontaneous version occurs only in the early stages of labour, and its occurrence should not be looked for after the rupture of the membranes.

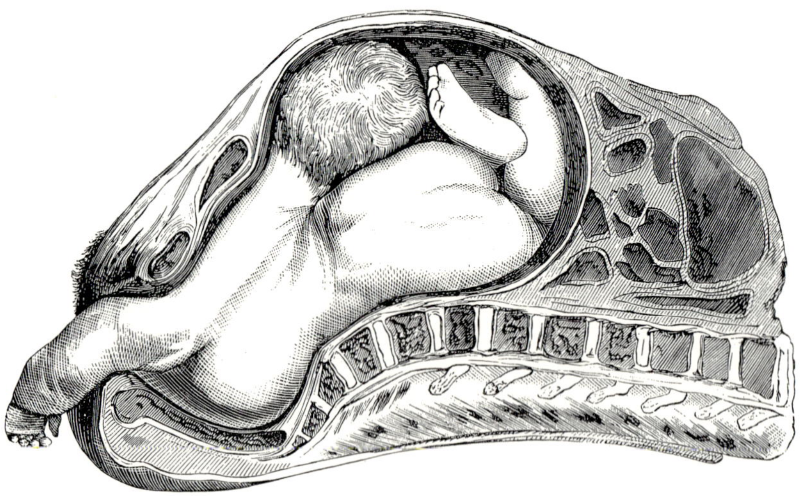

Fig. 602.—Frozen Section through Woman Dying in Labour with a Neglected Transverse Presentation (Chiara)

Spontaneous evolution, on the other hand, is possible only late in labour after the membranes have ruptured and the shoulder has become wedged down into the pelvic cavity. This, however, is met with so rarely, demands such peculiar conditions, and is attended by such risks to the mother, that its occurrence should never be counted upon in actual practice.

When, however, the pelvis is normal and the child undersized, and particularly if it is macerated, spontaneous evolution may be effected in one of two ways provided the pains are sufficiently strong. Thus, the impacted shoulder after being driven deeper and deeper into the pelvis may eventually rotate to the front and emerge from the vulva, its expulsion being followed by the rest of the thorax and then by the feet, while the head still remains above the superior strait (Fig. 603). Less frequently, particularly if the

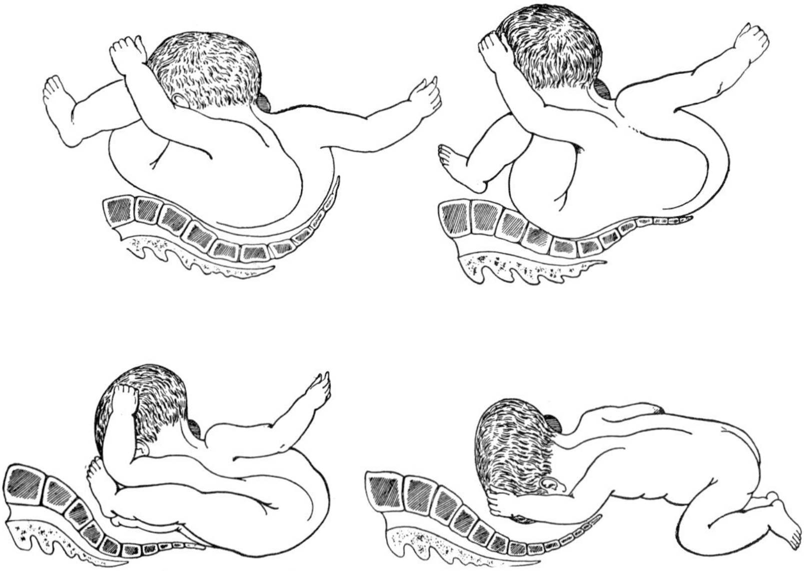

FIG. 603.—DIAGRAM ILLUSTRATING MECHANISM OF SPONTANEOUS EVOLUTION (Jungmann).

child is macerated, the shoulder may be forced down through the pelvis, while the body is so bent upon itself that the head and thorax come into close apposition and eventually enter the pelvis together. The birth of the shoulder is followed by that of the head and thorax, which emerge simultaneously from the vulva, and are followed by the breech and lower extremities. This mechanism is described as *partus conduplicato corpore* (Fig. 604).

In very rare instances spontaneous evolution may occur even when the child has attained considerable proportions. Thus, Payer has reported the case of a child weighing 2,650 grammes and measuring 50 centimetres in length, which was so born, and gives a list of 10 similar instances from the literature in which the children were of an equal or greater weight, one among them—Champion's case—being born alive.

Prognosis.—If spontaneous version does not occur within the first few hours after the onset of labour, and operative procedures are not instituted, the outcome for both mother and child is almost uniformly fatal, the child succumbing to asphyxia and the mother to hæmorrhage or infection, as a result of rupture of the uterus. On the other hand, if appropriate measures are instituted at the proper time, the prognosis for the child is fair, while for the mother it is excellent. In this class of cases prolapse of the cord is one of the most frequent causes of fœtal death.

Treatment.—If the diagnosis has been made in the last month of pregnancy and the pelvis is approximately normal, cephalic version should be effected by external manipulations, and the child held in its new position by means of a properly fitting bandage. On the other hand, if the pelvis is markedly contracted, such a procedure is not advisable, as Cæsarean section will probably be the operation of choice.

If the patient is not seen until after labour has set in, external cephalic version should likewise be attempted, provided the membranes have not

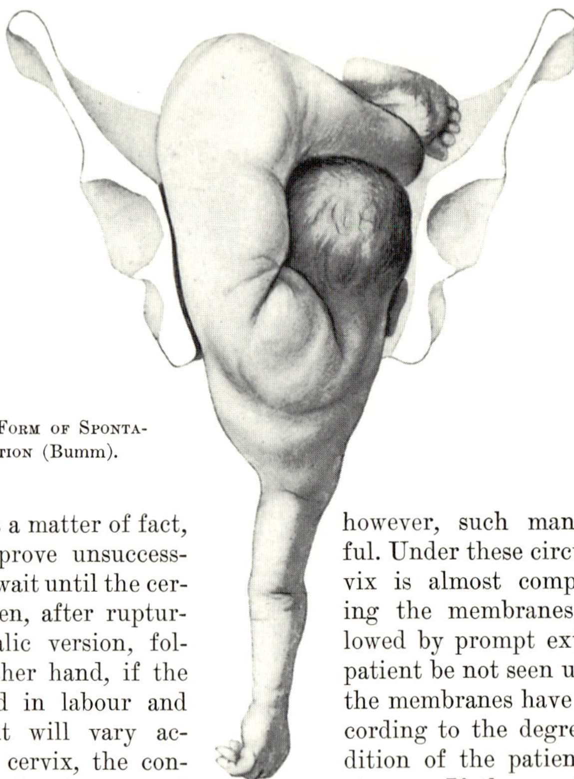

Fig. 604.—Rare Form of Spontaneous Evolution (Bumm).

ruptured. As a matter of fact, however, such manipulations will usually prove unsuccessful. Under these circumstances it is better to wait until the cervix is almost completely dilated, and then, after rupturing the membranes, perform internal podalic version, followed by prompt extraction.

On the other hand, if the patient be not seen until she is well advanced in labour and the membranes have ruptured, the treatment will vary according to the degree of dilatation of the cervix, the condition of the patient, as well as that of the fœtus and uterus. If the cervix is only partially dilated, while the child is alive and freely movable in the uterus, bipolar version may be attempted. After a foot has been brought down the cervix should be allowed to dilate still further before extraction is completed. On the other hand, if the condition is complicated by prolapse of the cord, the cervix should be dilated manually, and the child rapidly extracted after internal podalic version.

Whenever the cervix is fully dilated, internal podalic version should be performed at once, according to the rules already given, and followed by immediate extraction, provided the uterus is not so tightly contracted down over the child and the lower uterine segment so thinned out that such a procedure appears synonymous with rupture. In such cases, anæsthesia sometimes so relaxes the organ that version may be safely effected, even though at first glance it had appeared to be out of the question.

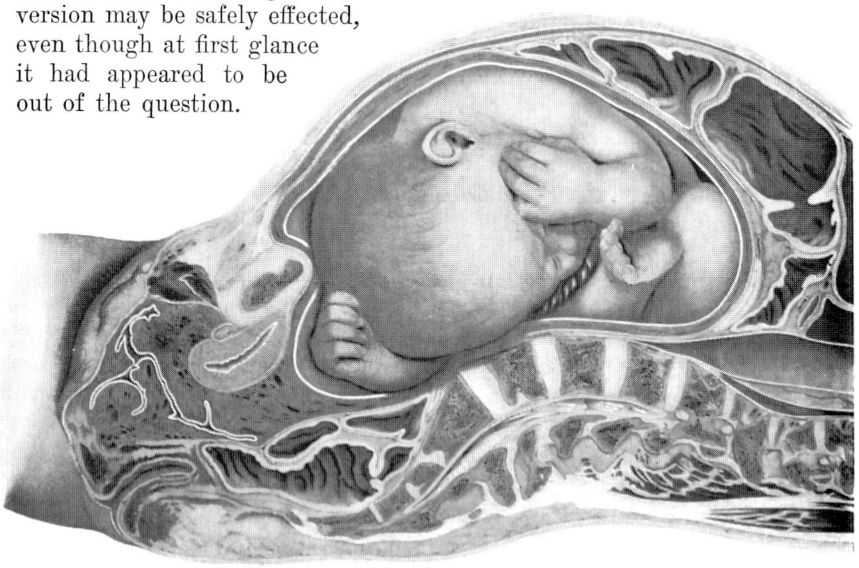

Fig. 605.—Frozen Section through Woman Dying at End of Pregnancy. Compound Presentation. (Braune.)

When version appears to be contra-indicated, *decapitation* becomes the operation of choice, even if the child is alive, although very exceptionally Cæsarean section might be thought of under the circumstances. It should not, however, be undertaken except at the express wish of the patient and her family, and then only after they have been made fully conversant with its inherent danger in the case of a patient who in all probability is already infected.

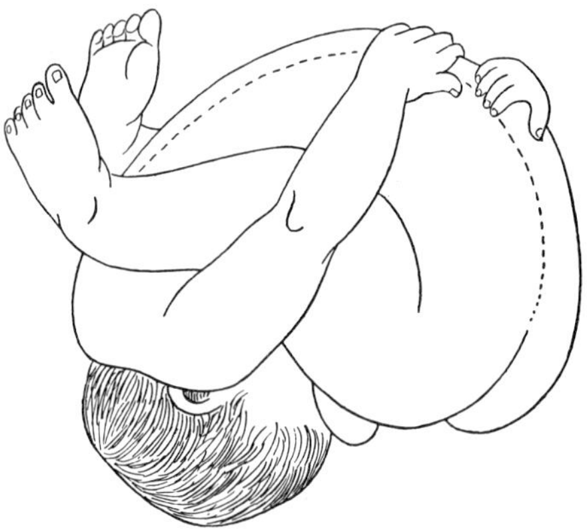

Fig. 606.—Compound Presentation (Hahl).

Compound Presentations. — By this term is understood the prolapse of an extremity alongside of the presenting part, both entering the pelvic canal simultaneously. It is not an infrequent occurrence, being observed about once in every 250 cases (Fig. 605).

As a rule, a hand or an arm comes down with the head; much less commonly both arms, or a hand and a foot, or both feet may present together. Hahl has reported a case in which the neck of the child was girdled by its legs, so that the scrotum and head were felt upon vaginal examination (Fig. 606).

Some idea of the relative frequency of the different combinations may be gained from the following table, taken from Pernice:

Head and hand	26 cases
Head and arm	8 "
Head, hand, and cord	5 "
Head and both hands	4 "
Head, one hand, and one foot	2 "
Head, two hands, one foot, and cord	1 case
Face, hand, and cord	1 "

Such a condition is frequently associated with a disproportion between the size of the head and the pelvis, owing to which early engagement has been interfered with, and as a result one or more of the extremities have prolapsed before the presenting part entered the pelvis.

Treatment.—Whenever, during the first stage of labour, a hand is distinguished alongside of the head, it should be pushed up if possible; but if it be firmly fixed between the head and the pelvic wall it should be left alone, since it will usually not interfere with labour. On the other hand, if the entire arm has prolapsed alongside of the head, an energetic effort should be made to replace it. If this is not possible, version should be performed, since if the arm retains its position it may give rise to serious dystocia, more especially if it extends around the child's neck, constituting the so-called *nuchal position.*

When, as happens only rarely, the foot prolapses, attempts should be made to replace it; if these fail, version should be resorted to.

LITERATURE

Ballantyne. General Fœtal Cystic Elephantiasis. The Diseases of the Fœtus, Edinburgh, 1892, i, 182–219.

Bartholin. Quoted by Payer.

Brouha. Du rein polykystique congénital. Revue de Gyn., 1901, v, 231.

Hanau. Ueber congenitale Cystennieren. D. I., Giessen, 1890.

Hahl. Strictur des os internum als Geburtshinderniss. Archiv f. Gyn., 1901, lxiii, 684–694.

Mirabeau. Beitrag zur Lehre von der fötalen Cystenniere. Monatsschr. f. Geb. u. Gyn., 1900, xi, 216–237.

Payer. Zur Lehre von der Selbstentwickelung. Volkmann's Sammlung klin. Vorträge, N. F., 1901, Nr. 314.

Pernice. Die Geburt mit Vorfall der Extremitäten neben dem Kopfe. Leipzig, 1858.

Phaenomenow. Beitrag zur Casuistik der durch die Frucht bedingten Geburtshindernisse. Archiv f. Gyn., 1881, xvii, 133–139.

Porak et Couvelaire. Foie polykystique cause de dystocie. Comptes rendus Soc. d'Obst., de Gyn. et de Pæd. de Paris, 1901, iii, 26–37.

Resnikow. Vierjährige Retention in utero eines Skeletes der im 7. Monate der Schwangerschaft abgestorbenen Frucht. Centralbl. f. Gyn., 1895, 244–247.

Roederer. Quoted by Payer.

Schroeder, Olshausen und Veit. Lehrbuch der Geburtshülfe, XIII. Aufl., 1899, 737.

Schwyzer. Ueber einen Fall von Geburtshinderniss, bedingt durch hochgradige Eierweiterung der fötalen Harnblase. Archiv f. Gyn., 1893, xliii, 333–346.

Theilhaber. Ein Fall von Cystenniere. Monatsschr. f. Geb. u. Gyn., 1899, ix, 496–504.

Walther. Dystokie infolge übermässiger Ausdehnung der fötalen Harnblase. Zeitschr. f. Geb. u. Gyn., 1893, xxvii, 333–347.

CHAPTER XL

ECLAMPSIA

ECLAMPSIA is an acute disease which may occur in the pregnant, parturient, or puerperal woman, and is characterized by clonic and tonic convulsions, during which there is loss of consciousness followed by more or less prolonged coma.

Frequency.—Statistical tables go to show that eclampsia occurs about once in every 500 labours, but it is almost impossible to determine its frequency with any degree of exactness, inasmuch as few practitioners see a sufficiently comprehensive series of cases in private practice to permit of trustworthy conclusions; while, on the other hand, hospital records by themselves give an exaggerated idea of its frequency, for the reason that many of the patients would have remained at home unless they had had convulsions. The following table would indicate that eclampsia occurs in about 0.75 per cent of the women entering lying-in hospitals—once in 133 cases:

Goldberg (Dresden, 1891)	in 10,717	labours,	81	cases	of eclampsia	(0.75%)
Cassamayor (Paris, 1892)	" 16,225	"	99	"	"	(0.61%)
Green (Boston, 1892)	" 3,500	"	36	"	"	(1%)
Knapp (Prag, 1900)	" 7,636	"	41	"	"	(0.53%)
Newell (Boston, 1900)	" 6,700	"	99	"	"	(1.17%)

The larger tabulations made by Löhlein in 1891, and by Veit in 1896, which are based upon statistics from the various clinics in Germany, afford almost the same conclusions. In the former there were 325 instances of eclampsia in 15,328 cases, and in the latter 905 in 149,366 cases—a percentage of 0.62 and 0.60 respectively—1 in 160 and 1 in 166. These statistics include all cases of eclampsia, but Löhlein differentiated between the total number of cases and those occurring in patients who were in the hospital at the onset of the disorder, and found that in the latter the ratio was only 0.3 per cent—one in 330.

Eclampsia varies markedly in frequency at different times, Cassamayor stating that in Tarnier's clinic in Paris it was observed many times more frequently in some years than in others. Thus, in 1872, there was 1 case to every 47 labours, as compared with 1 to 730 and 1 to 130 in the years 1882 and 1891 respectively.

Clinical History.—Zweifel has reported a case of eclampsia occurring in the third month, but as a rule it is not encountered before the second half of pregnancy, and becomes more frequent the nearer term is approached.

It is generally stated that 70 to 80 per cent of all cases occur in primiparous women, Knapp, Olshausen, Cassamayor, and Goldberg reporting a proportion of 71, 75, 77, and 86.4 per cent respectively. In all probability these figures are somewhat too high, inasmuch as they are based upon hospital practice. Nevertheless, be this as it may, it is certain that in the main primiparous women are much more liable to the disorder.

Twin pregnancy and hydramnios appear to act as predisposing factors, the former condition being noted by Olshausen and Cassamayor in 8 and 5.7 per cent of their cases of eclampsia respectively, whereas for all labours the usual ratio is 1.5 per cent. It is possible that heredity sometimes plays a part in its production, and Elliot, Olshausen, and Pinard have reported cases which apparently confirm this view.

An eclamptic convulsion sometimes occurs without warning, "like a bolt from a clear sky," in women who are apparently in perfect health. In the majority of cases, however, the outbreak is preceded for a longer or shorter period by premonitory symptoms indicative of the toxæmia of pregnancy, among the more common being œdema, headache, epigastric pain, and possibly disturbances of vision. At the same time the urine becomes decreased in quantity, while albumin and casts and a marked diminution in the amount of urea are demonstrable.

The attack may come on at any time, sometimes while the patient is sleeping. If she is awake, the first sign of the impending convulsion is a fixed expression of the eyes, which soon begin to roll from side to side. The pupils are usually dilated, less often contracted. The convulsive movements appear first about the mouth, which begins to twitch and is drawn to one side, the entire face becoming distorted. They extend rapidly to the arms, the body, and finally to the legs. They are usually clonic in character, though sometimes they take on a tonic form and the patient becomes rigid. The breathing is stertorous, the face congested and flushed, the patient foams at the mouth, and often bites her tongue. During the convulsion, which may last for a few seconds to two minutes, the woman is profoundly unconscious, and after the movements cease passes into a condition of coma which lasts for a longer or shorter period.

More particularly when the disorder appears in the latter part of labour or during the puerperium, a single convulsion only may be observed, an uninterrupted recovery ensuing after the patient emerges from the coma. Oftener, however, the first is the forerunner of other convulsions, which may vary in number from 1 to 2 in mild, to 100 or more in fatal cases, the intervals between them becoming shorter in inverse proportion to the number. In rare instances they follow one another so rapidly that the patient appears to be in a prolonged, almost continuous convulsion.

The duration of the coma is very variable. When the convulsions are infrequent, the patient usually recovers consciousness after each attack, while in severe cases the coma persists from one convulsion to another, and death may result without any awakening from it. In rare instances a single convulsion may be followed by profound coma, from which the patient never emerges, though, as a rule, death does not occur until after a frequent repetition of the convulsive attacks. The immediate cause of death is usually œdema of the lungs or apoplexy, though if the fatal issue is postponed for several days, it is usually attributable to an aspiration pneumonia or a puerperal infection.

In most cases during the seizure the arterial pressure is markedly increased, and the pulse is full and bounding. In severe cases, however, it is weaker and more rapid, becoming more compressible and filiform with each succeeding convulsion. In many cases the temperature rises to a very considerable height from the onset of the disease and gradually falls as the patient improves; sometimes, however, it remains normal. A temperature of 104 or 105 degrees is not unusual, and in fatal cases it may reach 107 or 108 degrees just before the end. As regards the cause of this elevation, there is much discrepancy of opinion. Olshausen believes that the poison which gives rise to the eclampsia also stimulates the thermal centres, while Zweifel holds that the fever is nearly always of infectious origin. The fact that the uterine lochia have been found to be perfectly sterile in a number of cases speaks against infection being the sole cause, but that it is often responsible, especially in those cases in which the fever persists for days after the cessation of the seizures, there can be but little doubt. Moreover, it would seem that women suffering from eclampsia are more susceptible to infection than usual.

According as the disorder first appears before or during labour or in the first hours of the puerperium, it is designated as ante-partum, intra-partum, or post-partum eclampsia. It is generally stated in the text-books that the last is the least common; but that the conclusions as to the relative incidence of the different varieties are by no means unanimous is shown by the following table:

	Ante-partum.	*Intra-partum.*	*Post-partum.*
Olshausen....	40%	46%	14%
Knapp.......	24.5%	60.9%	14.6%
Goldberg.....	26%	57%	17%
Green........	36%	22%	42%

Newell states that one third of his cases occurred after the birth of the child. Personally, I have observed the post-partum variety in only a few instances.

It would appear from the statistics of three of the authors just cited, that ante-partum eclampsia occurs less frequently than the intra-partum variety, but my own figures would be more nearly in accord with them than those of Green. Olshausen has reached a similar conclusion, and considers that the contrary statements of most authors are due to the fact that they have failed to remember that in the majority of cases uterine contractions set in with the first convulsion, so that if the patient is not seen before the seizure it is often very difficult to determine with which variety one has to deal.

Ante-partum eclampsia may terminate in several ways. As a rule, labour sets in and a premature child is born spontaneously, or the uterus is emptied by operative procedures. Sometimes the patient dies undelivered. In a small number of cases labour does not supervene, and if the woman survives the attack she may give birth to a dead or macerated fœtus some time afterward. In such cases it is believed that its death is the direct result of the eclampsia. Now and again the patient may recover from the attack and give birth to a living child at term, while in very exceptional cases, after being perfectly well for a longer or shorter period, she may have a recurrence of the seizure, which may terminate in any one of the ways mentioned above. Such cases have been described by Leudet, Olshausen, and Lafon.

If the attack occurs during labour, the pains usually increase in frequency and severity, so that the child will be born somewhat sooner than usual, after which the convulsions generally cease. On the other hand, in severe cases, or when there is some impediment causing dystocia, the patient may die undelivered, unless operative measures are undertaken.

In post-partum eclampsia the attack usually comes on soon after delivery, and recovery often occurs after a single convulsion. In other cases, however, the seizures follow one another in rapid succession, and occasionally cause death. The general belief that cases of this variety are comparatively benign is denied by Olshausen, who noted a mortality of 25 per cent.

A few instances have been reported in which the disorder did not appear until several weeks after the birth of the child. It is probable, as has been pointed out by Van der Velde, that the vast majority of such cases were not eclamptic at all, but that the seizures were due to other causes.

In rare instances the onset is preceded by a distinct aura (Olshausen), but this is usually lacking, the convulsion coming on either without warning or after the appearance of symptoms indicative of the toxæmia of pregnancy. As has been pointed out by Olshausen, severe epigastric pain is a frequent precursor of the seizure, and is a sign to which too much attention can hardly be paid.

The convulsions are always followed by unconsciousness, and, moreover, the patient may not only not remember the attack itself, but even have no recollection of occurrences which have taken place several hours previous to it. This is a not altogether uncommon observation, and may sometimes have an important bearing from a medico-legal point of view.

In 5 per cent of Löhlein's and in 13 per cent of Knapp's cases eclampsia was followed by marked mental derangement. My own observations lead me to believe that the experience of these authors was exceptional, although it must not be forgotten that mental derangement following eclamptic convulsions is one of the well-recognised varieties of puerperal insanity; but whether it is a direct result of the disease or is due indirectly to infection has not yet been demonstrated.

In rare instances, as the result of permanent cerebral lesions incident to eclampsia, a *hemianopsia* may develop during the puerperium. A case of this character, occurring in my practice, was reported in detail by Woods at the 1902 meeting of the American Ophthalmological Society.

More frequently the patient suffers from disturbed vision during the latter part of pregnancy, due to an albuminuric retinitis. As this is an accompaniment of an acute nephritis, eclampsia does not always develop.

The outcome in such cases is dependent upon the further course of the underlying disease. In other cases the visual disturbance is unattended by demonstrable changes in the retina or optic nerve, and is to be regarded merely as a manifestation of the general toxæmia, complete recovery usually following within a few days after the termination of pregnancy.

In a small number of cases the patient becomes markedly jaundiced, either during or just after the convulsive seizure. This sign is of grave prognostic significance, and indicates serious hepatic lesions.

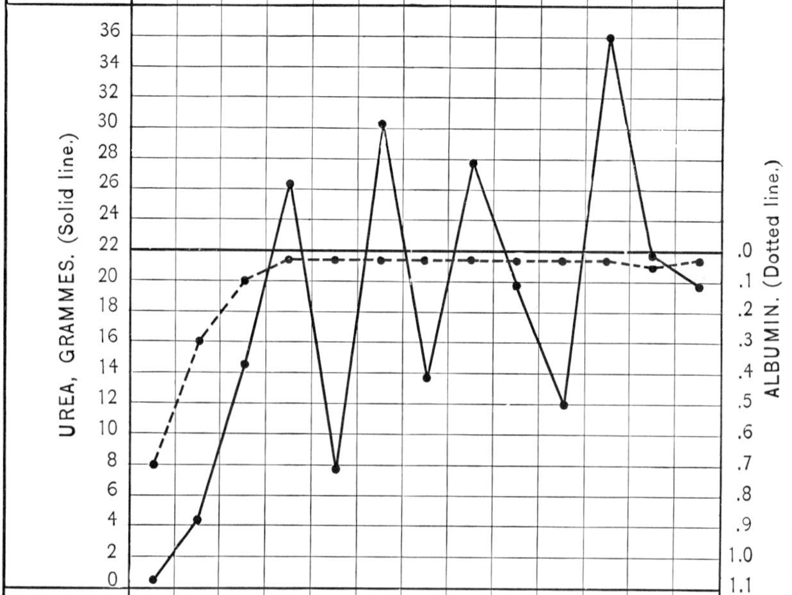

February	3	4	5	6	7	8	9	10	11	12	13	14	15
UREA, PER CC.	.002	.003	.005	.01	.006	.014	.01	.016	.01	.017	.015	.014	.016
UREA FOR 24 HOURS.	.42	4.1	15.5	26.5	7.8	30.6	13.8	28.	19.3	12.	36.	22.	19.8
AMOUNT OF URINE.	210	1520	3100	2650	1300	2190	1380	1750	1930	680	2400	1560	1200
STOOLS.	4	2	1	2	1	2	1	1	1	0	2	1	4
SWEATS.	3	0	0	0	0	0	0	0	0	0	0	0	0

Fig. 607.—Urea Chart.

Eclampsia followed by recovery. Chart shows marked quantity of albumin and almost total absence of urea at time of convulsions, with rapid disappearance of the former and immense increase in the amount of the latter in the following days.

Eclampsia may occur not only during the course of an ordinary gestation, but was observed by Maygrier in the false labour accompanying extra-uterine pregnancy.

During the eclamptic attack the urine is markedly diminished in amount, is loaded with tube casts and often contains a considerable quantity of blood, while occasionally the secretion is entirely suppressed. Chemical examination nearly always reveals the presence of an abundance of albumin and a notable diminution in the amount of urea. After the termination of the convulsions, in favourable cases, there is a rapid increase in the amount of urine and urea, together with a decrease in the amount of

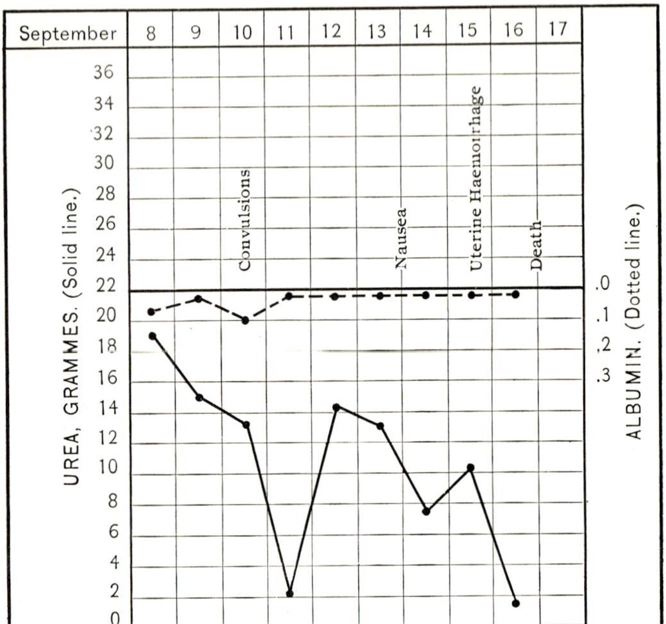

September	8	9	10	11	12	13	14	15	16	17
UREA, PER CC.	.017	.007	.006	.008	.006	.002	.003	.006	.003	.005
UREA FOR 24 HOURS.	19	15	13.7	2.	14.6	13	7.5	10.3	1.5	
AMOUNT OF URINE.	1120	2130	2100	160	2240	5160	2140	1710	460	
STOOLS.	4	4	2	3	7	11	12	6	5	
SWEATS.	0	0	0	4	4	4	4	4	3	

Fig. 608.—Urea Chart.

Eclampsia followed by death. Chart shows almost total disappearance of urea at time of convulsions, with rapid rise the following day, followed by a progressive fall as death approached.

albumin. In the majority of cases the urine rapidly becomes normal, and within a few weeks gives no evidence of the previous pathological condition. On the other hand, it sometimes contains albumin and casts for months after delivery—a finding that indicates the existence of a chronic renal lesion, which, as a rule, has been present before the eclamptic attack, although occasionally the nephritis appears to have been a direct result of the eclampsia. (See Figs. 607 and 608.)

Pathology.—After Rayer and Lever had demonstrated the presence of albumin in the urine of women suffering from this disorder, it was generally believed that the fundamental pathological lesion in eclampsia was a nephritis, and for a long time the condition was considered to be identical with uræmia.

This view, however, was gradually abandoned when it was found that only a small proportion of the women suffering from chronic nephritis had eclampsia; and still further modifications became necessary after it had been shown that the urine did not necessarily contain albumin at the time of the eclamptic attack, Schroeder, Ingerslev, and Charpentier having collected respectively 62, 112, and 143 such cases from the literature. Its absence, however, does not necessarily disprove the renal origin of the disease, since Van der Velde has reported two instances of eclampsia in which the kidneys were markedly diseased, notwithstanding the fact that albumin was not demonstrable in the urine.

For the most part, autopsy will reveal the presence of renal changes, which may be very marked in some and only slight in other cases. The lesions are usually those of an acute nephritis with marked necrosis of the renal epithelium. Ordinarily, this is the only lesion, though occasionally it may be engrafted upon a chronic process. Prutz found kidney changes in all but 7 out of 368 cases collected from the literature, in which the description was sufficiently accurate to be of value. Forms of acute or chronic nephritis were present in 46 and 11.6 per cent of his cases respectively, while degenerative changes were observed more frequently. His conclusions are stated as follows: "Notwithstanding the frequency of renal lesions, we are not justified, even in the majority of cases, in considering them as the anatomical substratum of eclampsia, for in many instances they are too insignificant; accordingly, it must remain a question whether they are not purely secondary in the greater proportion of the cases."

More or less similar results were obtained by Olshausen, Goldberg, Hughes and Carter, Lubarsch and Schmorl, all of whom stated that renal lesions were absent in a small proportion of their cases. Moreover, Bouffe de Saint Blaise, after studying the condition of the kidneys in 40 cases of eclampsia, states that these organs are often perfectly normal, and that the lesions when present should be considered as secondary. On the other hand, Pels Leusden, Winckler, and Knapp observed pronounced renal changes in all of their cases, and were inclined to consider them as the characteristic lesion of the disease.

Guénard and Potocki attempted to determine the permeability of the kidneys by administering methylene blue to 7 eclamptic patients. As the drug could always be demonstrated in the urine a short time after its administration, they concluded that the renal function was not markedly impaired, even though anatomical lesions might be present.

On the whole, the evidence at hand would seem to indicate that renal changes, while almost constantly present, are not, as a rule, sufficiently marked to justify one in considering them as the characteristic lesion of eclampsia, which must therefore be sought in some other organ.

Halbertsma, in 1876, pointed out that the ureters were often enlarged and dilated, and was inclined to attribute the production of the disease to this condition. Prutz noted a similar finding 37 times in his analysis of 500 autopsies.

In 1886, Jürgens and Klebs pointed out the existence of a *hæmorrhagic hepatitis* in certain cases of eclampsia. Their observations, however, created very little interest, and it remained for Pilliet, in 1888, to direct our attention to certain hæmorrhagic lesions in the eclamptic liver. His work was abundantly confirmed by Schmorl, who in a monograph published in 1893, and based upon the autopsies of 17 women dead of eclampsia, stated that he had found in every case lesions of the liver which he held to be more characteristic than those observed in the kidneys. These consist of irregularly shaped, reddish or whitish areas scattered through the entire organ, but more particularly in the neighbourhood of the smaller portal vessels. They are readily seen with the naked eye, and on section give the liver a mottled appearance. Under the microscope they are recognised as areas of necrosis, in which blood-cells may or may not be present. Schmorl attributed their formation to degenerative changes following thrombotic

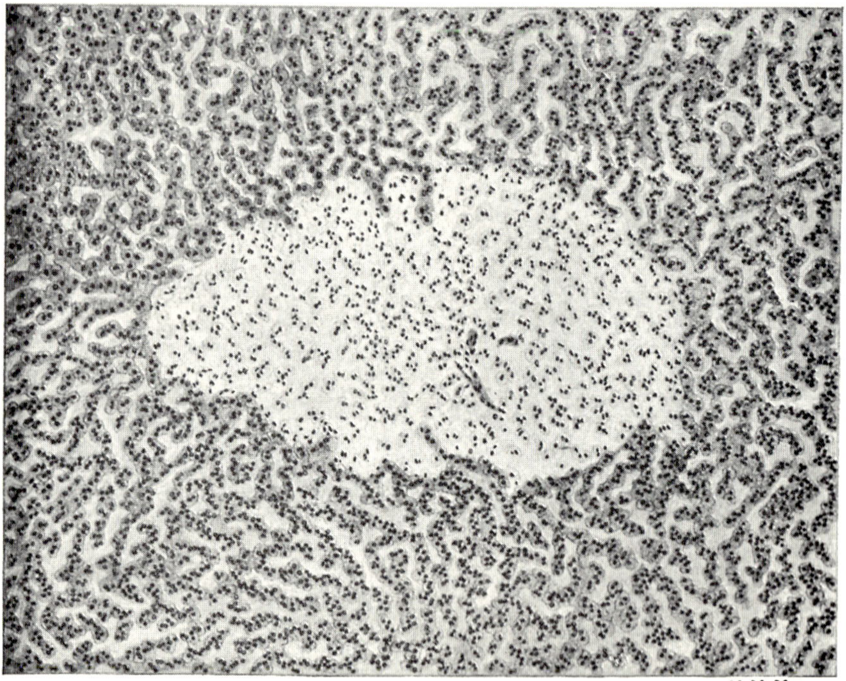

Fig. 609.—Area of Necrosis in Eclamptic Liver. × 90.

processes in the smaller portal vessels, and considered that their presence justified the diagnosis of eclampsia without further knowledge of the history of the case (Fig. 609).

These results were soon confirmed by Lubarsch, Prutz, Bar and Guyeisse, Bouffe de Saint Blaise, and many others, the last-named observer having demonstrated them in 42 consecutive cases, while Schmorl, in 1902, found them in 71 out of 73 autopsies. I have been able to demonstrate similar lesions in all the eclamptic livers which I have examined, although rarely so pronounced as described by Schmorl. Indeed, in several specimens they could be identified only with the aid of the microscope. At the same time they are extremely characteristic, and, as the researches of Schmorl

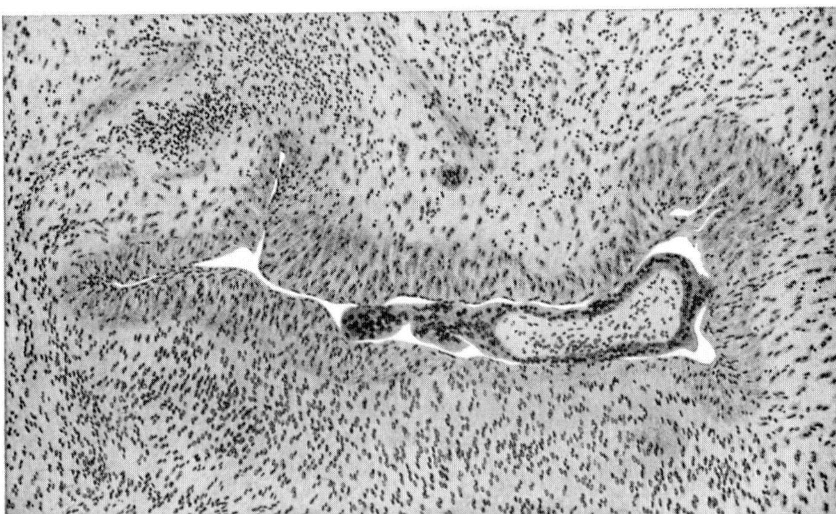

Fig. 610.—Placental Giant Cell and Chorionic Villus in Blood-vessel of Tube Wall Some Distance from Placental Site. × 80.

show that they do not occur with such regularity in any other disease, it must be admitted that they are intimately connected with eclampsia, although, as will be indicated later, they cannot be regarded as its primary cause.

The hepatic changes are so characteristic and constant that Bouffe de Saint Blaise and many French observers believe that they represent the primary lesion of the disease, and consider that the entire process is due to an impairment of the hepatic function—a *hepato-toxæmia.*

Several observers have described the presence of hæmatomata of varying size, just beneath the capsule of the liver, Prutz having recorded a fatal hæmorrhage from the rupture of such a structure into the peritoneal cavity.

Various statements have been made concerning the pathological findings in the brain—œdema, hyperæmia, thrombosis, and apoplexy being described as the main lesions. Prutz noted œdema in 42 per cent, hyperæmia in 35 per cent, and apoplexy in 13 per cent, while the brain was apparently normal in 10 per cent of his cases. Schmorl, in 58 out of 65 autopsies, in which the organ was examined, noted the presence of thrombi in the smaller cerebral vessels, and regarded them as the cause of the small areas of necrosis which are so often observed.

Marked degenerative changes are often noticed in the myocardium, which Schmorl regards as secondary lesions resulting from the prolonged use of chloroform in the treatment of the disease.

Most recent observers, notably Schmorl and Winckler, have demonstrated the presence of giant cells in the pulmonary capillaries which they have identified with the so-called giant cells of the placenta—namely, masses of syncytium. Schmorl formerly believed that their presence probably explained the origin of the thrombotic processes observed in various organs. But at present they are regarded as having no significance, as they are frequently found in pregnant women dead of other diseases. I have frequently seen similar giant cells and even portions of chorionic villi in the vessels of the uterus in cases of normal gestation, and in those of the tube in extra-uterine pregnancy (Fig. 610).

In patients who have died several days after the cessation of the convulsions, in addition to the lesions just described, broncho-pneumonia or various evidences of puerperal infection are frequently noted.

It is apparent, therefore, that the main lesions in eclampsia are found in the kidneys, liver, and brain; but in view of the marked discrepancy in the statements of the various authors concerning their relative frequency and importance, it would seem that the anatomical changes are not constant, although those in the liver are the most characteristic. Accordingly, we are forced to conclude either that under the term eclampsia are included a number of different disease entities, each with their own anatomical lesions; or, what is more probable, that the morbid process is caused by some as yet unknown poisonous substance circulating in the blood which may give rise to lesions of varying intensity in the several organs.

Ætiology.—So many hypotheses have been advanced concerning the ætiology of eclampsia that Zweifel has aptly designated it as "the disease of theories." Unfortunately, exact knowledge is still lacking.

From the earliest periods it was considered as a disorder of the nervous system peculiar to pregnancy. This conception is no longer entertained, though there is no doubt that the nervous system is in a condition of far less stable equilibrium during pregnancy than at other times. This fact has been conclusively demonstrated by Blumreich and Zuntz, who showed that convulsions could be produced by the application of far smaller quantities of powdered creatinin to the cerebral cortex in pregnant than in non-pregnant animals.

This theory was to a certain extent rehabilitated in 1892 by Herff, who held that, owing to a faulty development of the nervous system, a certain number of women are particularly prone to eclampsia, so that conditions which in healthy individuals are of but little significance would be sufficient to give rise to the disease.

As a result of the work of Lever, eclampsia was identified with uræmia, and this view was only slowly abandoned after it had been conclusively demonstrated that the two conditions had but little in common.

Spiegelberg, in 1870, advanced the theory that the circulation of ammonium carbonate in the blood was responsible for the seizures, but, chemical analysis having failed to substantiate this statement, the idea was soon abandoned.

The Traube-Rosenstein theory, which held that the convulsions were the result of anæmia and œdema of the brain, found widespread acceptance for many years, but was ultimately abandoned in view of the fact that such conditions could not be demonstrated at autopsy in the majority of cases.

Délore and Rodet, of Lyons, in 1884, suggested bacterial invasion as a possible ætiological factor, but adduced no evidence in support of such a view. The first investigations were made by Doléris in 1885. Following him a number of other observers, among whom may be mentioned Blanc, Combemale and Bué, Favre, Gley, Gerdes, Herrgott, Sourel, and Levinowitch, published work on similar lines. They cultivated various bacteria from the blood, urine, and tissues of eclamptic women, but their results were so contradictory as to be of but little value. On the other hand, Haegler, Döderlein, Schmorl, Lubarsch and Bar and Guyeisse, after finding that careful bacteriological examination of the fluids and tissues of women dead of eclampsia gave uniformly negative results, felt justified in asserting that the micro-organisms described by other observers could not be considered as ætiological factors.

My own investigations have been confirmatory of these latter observers, and up to the present time satisfactory proof has not been adduced in support of the bacterial nature of eclampsia, nor does it seem likely to be forthcoming.

A much more promising field of investigation was opened up by the work of Bouchard upon auto-intoxication. Rivière, in 1888, was the first to put forward the theory that eclampsia was an auto-intoxication resulting from the heaping up of some substance in the system during pregnancy, holding that its presence was indicated by an increase in the toxicity of the blood serum and a decrease in that of the urine.

This conception was placed upon an apparently solid foundation by the work of Chamberlent and Tarnier and their students, who showed that in a number of cases the urine of women suffering from eclampsia, or just about to be attacked by it, was far less toxic than usual, while the toxicity of the blood serum was markedly increased. They concluded, therefore, that some poisonous substance, which should have been excreted by the kidneys, was accumulating in the system and thereby increasing the toxicity of the blood serum, which in turn gave rise to the renal and hepatic lesions which still further accentuated the condition.

Their investigations were apparently confirmed by the work of Ludwig and Savor, who considered the offending product to be carbamic acid, which they believed was formed as the result of imperfect metabolic processes, especially in the liver. The most enthusiastic advocates of this theory are the students of Pinard. Thus, Bouffe de Saint Blaise considers that the main feature of the disease is an alteration in the function of the liver, which fails to render innocuous certain poisonous products of metabolism during their passage through it, and that these in turn give rise to an auto-intoxication which is designated as *hepato-toxæmia*. When the disturbance is slight, the patient merely suffers from nausea or headache; but when it is marked, secondary renal changes develop which in turn lead to a still further retention of the poison and the ultimate production of eclampsia.

The studies of Volhard in 1897 failed to substantiate this theory, as he was unable to show that the blood serum was more toxic in eclampsia than in other conditions. Moreover, the doctrine in general has received a severe blow from the work of Van der Bergh, Forchheimer, Stewart, and Schumacher, which showed the results obtained by the injection of blood serum and urine into animals to be so variable and dependent upon so many factors that they must be received with the greatest caution.

Their experiments proved that death depends in great part upon the rapidity with which the injection is made rather than upon the toxicity of the fluid injected. Moreover, Schumacher and Stewart have demonstrated that a large part of the urinary toxicity is due to bacterial products rather than to the presence of a definite organic poison in the urine, since they found that large quantities could be injected into animals with almost perfect impunity, provided the urine is thoroughly sterilized; whereas, if such precautions are not taken, small quantities of the same urine led to uniformly fatal results.

The present status of the question may therefore be summarized as follows: The clinical history and anatomical findings afford presumptive evidence that the disease is due to the circulation of some poisonous substance in the blood which gives rise to thrombosis in many of the smaller vessels, with consequent degenerative and necrotic changes in the various organs. But, at the same time, we are absolutely ignorant concerning the nature of the offending substance, and besides, the experimental evidence thus far adduced in favour of such an ætiological factor is not convincing.

Schmorl at one time believed that the thrombotic processes were made possible by the action of a fibrin ferment set free from placental cells which had escaped into the maternal circulation. His later investigations, however, tended to invalidate this assumption.

Bulius and Falk noted a marked proliferation of the syncytium in the placenta, and this they considered characteristic of the disease. Their results, however, have not been verified by other investigators, nor have I been able to confirm them in the eclamptic placentæ which I have examined.

Several observers believe that they have demonstrated the presence of other substances in the blood serum or urine which might explain the production of eclampsia. Thus, Massen described an increase in leucomaines, and Kollmann thought he demonstrated an unusual amount of globulin in the blood serum. Their researches have not yet been confirmed, and their conclusions must therefore be accepted with reserve.

During the past few years a number of authors, particularly Fehling and Dienst, have advanced the theory that the disease may be due to intoxication with products of the fœtal metabolism, the maternal organism being sometimes unable to accommodate itself to the increased work necessary for their elimination as well as that of its own excretory products. They argue, therefore, that under such circumstances certain poisonous materials could accumulate in the system and eventually give rise to organic lesions in the mother.

This view receives a certain amount of support from clinical experience, since, as is well known, the convulsions usually cease soon after delivery; while in rare cases the death of the fœtus during pregnancy is immediately followed by recovery. Moreover, Baron and Castaigne have lately demonstrated that the transmission to the mother of substances injected into the fœtus ceases almost immediately after its death.

The advocates of the fœtal origin of eclampsia also adduce as an argument the fact that convulsions sometimes appear in the child shortly after its birth. Cases of this character have been reported by Wilke, Woyer, Schmid, Dienst, and others, and in several instances characteristic lesions were observed in the organs of the fœtus. Furthermore, lesions identical with those in the liver and kidneys of the mothers have been observed in the corresponding organs of children which were born dead or died soon after delivery. Such observations have been made by Schmorl, Chamberlent, Bar and Guyeisse, Knapp, Dienst, and myself, and are considered critically in Dienst's monograph.

The observations of Krönig and Füth upon the osmotic pressure of the fœtal and maternal blood show that there is no fundamental objection to the acceptance of such a theory; but at the same time, I do not believe that the demonstration of lesions in the organs of the fœtus necessarily affords evidence of its correctness. To my mind such findings simply prove that they are the result of the circulation of some substance in the blood which leads to the formation of thrombi, with subsequent necrosis, although as yet the evidence is insufficient to indicate whether it is transmitted through the placenta from the fœtus to the mother, or in the opposite direction.

In summing up the ætiology of eclampsia, it appears that the evidence thus far adduced in support of the auto-intoxication theory, though not conclusive, is sufficiently suggestive to warrant its tentative acceptance, at least until some better explanation is forthcoming. I believe that it is probable that further studies of the metabolism in normal pregnancy as well as in eclampsia will eventually afford us definite information concerning its causation.

An interesting contribution to the subject has been made by Hélouin, who studied what he calls the "rapport azoturique"—the relation between the total nitrogen of the urine and the amount eliminated as urea—in the albuminuria of pregnancy and eclampsia. He found that in normal urine 80 to 90 per cent of the total nitrogen was eliminated in the form of urea, but only a much smaller proportion in diseased conditions.

Diagnosis.—The diagnosis of eclampsia usually offers no difficulty, especially when the patient has been under observation during the later months of pregnancy. When the woman is first seen in a seizure it becomes necessary to differentiate the condition from uræmia, epilepsy, and a hysterical convulsion.

Prognosis.—The prognosis is always serious, eclampsia being regarded as one of the most dangerous conditions with which the obstetrician has to deal. The maternal mortality varies from 20 to 25 per cent, and that of the fœtus from 33 to 50 per cent, although Porak and Stroganoff report series of 47 and 113 cases with a maternal mortality of 6.38 and 5.31 per cent respectively. Such favourable results, however, are very exceptional.

As a rule, the prognosis is more gloomy when the seizures come on before or during parturition, whereas post-partum eclampsia is considered less dangerous. Recent statistics, however, indicate that the last variety is more serious than is generally believed, Green, Zweifel, and Olshausen having lost 6.6, 9.5, and 25 per cent of their cases respectively.

There is considerable discrepancy of opinion concerning the relative prognosis in primiparous and multiparous women. Thus, Veit in 902 cases gives a corrected mortality of 14.3 per cent for the former and 19.5 per cent for the latter, and Goldberg states the disorder is twice as dangerous in the latter. Olshausen, on the other hand, believes that there is no difference in the two groups, and Zweifel states that the mortality among his patients was 3 times greater in primiparæ (16.6 to 5.5 per cent). In all probability the prognosis really depends much more upon the severity of the attack than upon the number of children that the woman has borne.

In individual cases it is often extremely difficult to predict the course of the disease, some patients dying in the first seizure while others recover after as many as 30. Winckel states that he has never observed recovery after more than 18 convulsions, but my own experience does not bear out this assertion. At the same time, there is no doubt that, other things being equal, the prognosis becomes more and more serious with each convulsion, although their absolute number is not of so much moment as the rapidity with which they follow one another and the duration of the coma after each attack.

Valuable prognostic data are also afforded by the condition of the pulse and temperature. When the former remains full and firm between the attacks, the outlook is usually good; whereas a weak, rapid, and thready pulse usually indicates a fatal issue, particularly if the temperature is high. Apoplexy, paralysis, and œdema of the lungs are most serious complications and usually end in death.

If the eclampsia comes on during pregnancy the prognosis is very favourably affected by the death of the fœtus, the convulsions usually ceasing soon afterward.

Treatment.—(*a*) *Prophylactic.*—The prophylactic treatment is most important, and is identical with that recommended for the toxæmia of pregnancy (p. 455). Indeed, the chief aim in treating the latter condition is to prevent the possible outbreak of eclampsia. Hence the necessity of regular and frequent examinations of the urine, and the immediate institution of appropriate treatment and diet as soon as any abnormality is detected or symptoms appear which indicate that the eliminative processes are at fault. By the employment of these precautionary measures, and by promptly inducing premature labour in those cases which do not improve or which become progressively worse under treatment, the frequency of eclampsia will be greatly diminished and many valuable lives saved. At present, however, despite all we can do, cases of eclampsia will still occur, and sometimes even in patients who apparently have responded most satisfactorily to prophylactic treatment. Thus, I could cite several instances in which, under appropriate measures, the subjective symptoms disappeared, the urine and urea increased in quantity and the albumin decreased, and yet, just as I was congratulating myself upon a most satisfactory result, a convulsion occurred. Moreover, one of my patients who was apparently perfectly well, and whose urine had shown no abnormality the day before labour, had an eclamptic seizure just after delivery.

Such experiences have convinced me that prophylactic treatment, while productive of untold good, is not invariably successful or always applicable, nor can I agree with Davis and Edgar that eclampsia is always a preventable affection. Such a satisfactory condition of affairs can hardly obtain until its ætiology is perfectly understood, and we are in possession of more accurate and reliable methods of foretelling the outcome in cases of toxæmia of pregnancy.

Experience goes to show that the cases accompanied by œdema are more readily amenable to treatment and less likely to eventuate in eclampsia than those in which it is absent. This point was emphasized many years ago by Stoltz.

(*b*) *Curative.*—In the presence of actual eclampsia, chloroform should be administered during the convulsive attacks in the hope of cutting them short, after which comparatively large doses of morphine should be given hypodermically, beginning with a quarter of a grain and repeating it, if necessary, until 3 doses have been administered.

Diuresis should be stimulated as much as possible, especially by the application of hot packs. The bowels should be moved by a strong cathartic, preferably 1 drop of croton-oil in a dram of olive-oil, placed on the back of the tongue if the patient is unconscious. At the same time a thick cork or folded towel placed between the teeth will prevent the patient from biting her tongue during the attacks. Food or medicine should not be administered by the mouth as long as the patient is unconscious, as in many instances particles find their way into the air-passages instead of being swallowed, and later give rise to an inspiration pneumonia.

When convulsions have once occurred, the pregnancy or labour, as the case may be, should be terminated as soon as is consistent with the safety of the patient. There is, however, considerable divergence of opinion upon this point. J. Veit and Charpentier advocate the administration of morphine in large doses, but not interfering until the cervix is completely dilated, and then employing forceps or version. Dührssen, Zweifel, and most American authorities, on the other hand, advocate emptying the uterus at an earlier period, provided it can be done without serious injury to the mother.

The question as to the advisability of early operative interference, in my opinion, can only be decided by determining the proportion of cases in which the convulsions cease after the birth of the child. Statistics bearing upon this point have been adduced by Dührssen, Olshausen, and Zweifel, who noted a cessation of the seizures either immediately or soon after delivery in 93.75 per cent, 85 per cent, and 66 per cent of their cases respectively. Zweifel reports a mortality of 28.5 per cent under expectant, and 11.25 per cent under active treatment. Judging from these figures it would appear that prompt delivery is indicated whenever it can be accomplished in a conservative manner.

In the majority of cases, even in ante-partum eclampsia, speedy delivery is facilitated by the fact that uterine contractions come on or increase in force soon after the onset of the disease, and labour usually pursues a more rapid course than usual. Thus, in many instances, after the first few convulsions the cervical canal is found to be already obliterated, the only resistance to the birth of the child being offered by the external os. When this is the case, delivery is readily accomplished by dilating the cervix by Harris's method, as described in Chapter XIX. In this way, provided that the external os will admit the tips of two fingers, complete dilatation can be readily and harmlessly accomplished in a surprisingly short space of time, often within eight or ten minutes. The child should then be delivered by forceps if the head is low down in the pelvis, or by version if it is only slightly engaged or movable above the pelvic brim.

If, however, labour has not set in and the cervical canal is intact, the question of rapid delivery becomes more complicated, and it becomes necessary to determine whether it is more advisable to adopt expectant treatment or to attempt to hasten delivery. In such cases, Dührssen advocates deep multiple incisions of the cervix followed by rapid extraction. I am not convinced as to the propriety of such a procedure, but prefer to bring about with steel dilators a degree of dilatation sufficient to permit the introduction of a Champetier de Ribes's balloon, which is then inflated with sterilized salt solution and allowed to overcome the resistance of the internal os, its action being hastened, if desired, by gentle traction upon the tube attached to the apparatus. In most cases the cervical canal yields promptly to the dilating bag, after which dilatation can be completed by Harris's method, or, if necessary, by multiple incisions. I do not advocate manual dilatation when the cervical canal is intact, as the operation is extremely tedious, sometimes requiring several hours, and nearly always results in deep tears of the cervix, which sometimes extend through the lower uterine segment.

In the rare instances in primiparous women in whom the external os and cervical canal are very resistant and almost cartilaginous in consistence, so that they cannot be dilated sufficiently to permit even the introduction of the bag, prompt delivery can be effected only by means of Dührssen's deep incisions or by Cæsarean section. In such cases, unless the obstetrician is a competent operator, I believe he will subserve the interests of the patient better by not attempting delivery, and placing his reliance upon medicinal treatment. On the other hand, if the case appears desperate, the child being viable and still alive, and the patient is in a well-conducted hospital, the advantages of Cæsarean section, as advocated by Halbertsma in 1889, should be carefully considered.

Certainly, in the class of cases under discussion, it will prove a more conservative procedure than forcible and brutal dilatation of a rigid cervix, but at the same time it should be resorted to only as a last expedient in a few very exceptional cases. Kettlitz, in 1897, collected 27 cases with a mortality of 47.3 per cent, while Hillmann, in 1900, reported a mortality of

52.5 per cent in 40 cases. It is true that these figures do not appear very encouraging, but it must be remembered that all the patients were in a desperate condition, and were operated upon as a last resort, so that in all probability even a greater number would have died under expectant treatment. Olshausen has performed the operation 3 times in his last 250 cases of eclampsia, saving 2 of the mothers and all of the children.

After the birth of the child no attempt should be made to hasten the third stage of labour, as a moderate loss of blood should be encouraged rather than checked.

After the delivery of the placenta one should continue to stimulate diuresis and diaphoresis, especially by means of hot packs, and a second dose of croton-oil should be administered if the first has been ineffectual. Diuresis is notably favoured by the subcutaneous injection of large amounts of salt solution. Thompson has lately demonstrated this fact for dogs, and showed that in some cases the flow of urine was increased by at least 300 per cent.

If the patient does not show marked signs of improvement shortly after delivery, from 300 to 500 cubic centimetres of blood should be withdrawn. If beneficial results follow, the procedure may be repeated if necessary. As the average woman possesses from $8\frac{1}{2}$ to 9 pounds of blood, 500 cubic centimetres would represent from $\frac{1}{8}$ to $\frac{1}{9}$ of its total bulk. Accordingly, if that amount of blood is drawn off and replaced by an infusion of an equal quantity of salt solution, the remainder of the blood is so diluted that, for practical purposes, $\frac{1}{4}$ or $\frac{1}{5}$ of the total poison has been removed, and this aid is often sufficient to tide the patient over sufficiently long to allow Nature to reassert herself.

It is generally stated that bleeding is indicated only when the pulse is full and bounding. Personally, I have bled with most excellent results a number of patients whose pulse was thin and weak. This experience would certainly seem to show that venesection is indicated in all cases in which delivery of the child is not followed by a cessation of the convulsions, no matter what the condition of the pulse.

Pilocarpine should never be used, on account of its tendency to produce œdema of the lungs, nor have I any experience with veratrum viride, which is so highly praised by many American writers.

In view of the marked liability of eclamptic women to infection, all operative procedures must be conducted in the most rigidly aseptic manner, particular care being taken to avoid the contamination of the vagina and the hands of the operator by fæcal material.

LITERATURE

Bar. Est-il démontré que l'éclampsie est une maladie microbienne? L'Obstétrique, iii, 1898, 481–505.

Bar et Guyeisse. Lésions du foie et des reins chez les éclamptiques et les fœtus issus des femmes éclamptiques. L'Obstétrique, 1897, ii, 263.

Baron et Castaigne. Contribution à l'étude de la pathogénie de l'éclampsie puerpérale, etc. Archives de méd. exp. et d'anat. path., 1898, x, 693–711.

Blanc. Pathogénie de l'éclampsie. Archives de Tocol., 1890, xvii, 747–754.

BLUMREICH und ZUNTZ. Exp. und kritische Beiträge zur Pathogenese der Eklampsie. Archiv f. Gyn., 1902, lxv, 736–785.

BOUCHARD. Leçons sur l'auto-intoxication. Paris, 1887.

BOUFFE DE SAINT BLAISE. Lésions anat. que l'on trouve dans l'éclampsie. Thèse de Paris, 1891.

Foie et éclampsie puerpérale. Annales de Gyn. et d'Obst., 1891, xxxv, 48.

Les auto-intoxications gravidiques. Annales de Gyn. et d'Obst., 1898, l, 342–373.

Quelques cas d'accès éclamptiques sans albuminurie. Annales de Gyn. et d'Obst., 1900, liv, 76–77.

BULIUS. Gutartige Wucherungen des Syncytiums. Centralbl. f. Gyn., 1897, 693–695.

CASSAMAYOR. Contribution à l'étude de l'éclampsie puerpérale d'après une statistique de la Clinique de 1872–1892. Thèse de Paris, 1892.

CHAMBERLENT. Toxicité de sérum maternal et fœtal dans un cas d'éclampsie puerpérale. Archives cliniques de Bordeaux, 1894, 271–284.

Recherches exp. et anat. path. sur les causes de la mort du fœtus dans l'éclampsie puerpérale. Nouv. Arch. d'Obst. et de Gyn., 1895, 175.

CHAMBERLENT et DEMONT. Recherches exp. sur la toxicité de l'urine dans les derniers mois de la grossesse. Comptes rendus Soc. de Biol., 1892, iv, 27–35.

CHARPENTIER. Éclampsie sans albuminurie. Traité pratique des accouchements. Paris, 1883, i, 699.

Traitement de l'éclampsie. Annales de Gyn., 1896, xliv, 488.

COMBEMALE et BUÉ. Faits à l'appui de la nature microbienne de l'éclampsie puerpérale. Comptes rendus Soc. de Biol., 1892, iv, 244–245.

DAVIS. The Prophylaxis and Treatment of Eclampsia. Therapeutic Gazette, July 15, 1895; also Trans. Amer. Gyn. Soc., 1895.

Eclampsia, Ante- and Post-partum. Amer. Jour. Obst., 1898, xxxvii, 467–480.

DÉLORE et RODET. Mémoire sur l'étiologie bactérienne de l'éclampsie. Résumé dans l'Arch. de Tocologie, 1884, ii, 921.

DIENST. Kritische Studien über die Pathogenese der Eklampsie, etc. Archiv f. Gyn., 1902, lxv, 369–464.

DÖDERLEIN. Zur Frage der "Eklampsie." Centralbl. f. Gyn., 1893, 1.

DÜHRSSEN. Ueber Eklampsie. Theil II, Archiv f. Gyn., 1893, xliii, 49–161.

EDGAR. The Treatment of Puerperal Eclampsia. N. Y. Med. Record, December 26, 1896, and January 2, 1897.

ELLIOT. Obstetrical Clinic, New York, 1873.

FALK. Partielle hydropische Degeneration der Placenta bei einer Eklamptischen. Centralbl. f. Gyn., 1897, 1073–1078.

FAVRE. Ueber eine Methode der Nephrectomie und über Schwangerschaftsniere und Eklampsie auf bakterial-physikalischen Basis. Virchow's Archiv, 1892, cxxix, 40–61.

FEHLING. Die Pathogenese und Behandlung der Eklampsie im Lichte der heutigen Anschauungen. Volkmann's Sammlung klin. Vorträge, N. F., 1899, Nr. 248.

Begriff und Pathogenese der Eklampsie. Verh. der deutschen Gesell. f. Gyn., 1901, 239–261.

FORCHHEIMER and STEWART. On the Toxicity of the Urine. Amer. Jour. Med. Sciences, September, 1899, 297–303.

GERDES. Zur Aetiologie der Puerperal-eklampsie. Centralbl. f. Gyn., 1892, 379–384.

GOLDBERG. Beitrag zur Eklampsie auf Grund von 81 Fällen. Archiv f. Gyn., 1891, xii, 295–329; and 1892, xiii, 87–102.

GREEN. Puerperal Eclampsia. Trans. Amer. Gyn. Soc., 1893, xviii, 141–174.

GUÉNARD. Étude de la perméabilité rénale chez les éclamptiques par le procédé du bleu de méthylène. Thèse de Paris, 1898.

HAEGLER. Zur Frage "Eklampsiebacillus" Gerdes. Centralbl. f. Gyn., 1892, 996–998.

HALBERTSMA. Ueber die Aetiologie der Eklampsia puerperalis. Volkmann's Sammlung klin. Vorträge, 1884, Nr. 212.

HALBERTSMA. Eklampsia gravidarum. Eine neue Indikationsstellung für die Sectio Caesarea. Ref. Centralbl. f. Gyn., 1889, 901.

HÉLOUIN. Contribution à l'étude du diagnostic de l'hepato-toxhémie gravidique. Thèse de Paris, 1899.

HERFF. Zur Theorie der Eklampsie. Centralbl. f. Gyn., 1892, 230–233.

HERRGOTT. Considération sur la pathogénie de l'éclampsie puerpérale. Annales de Gyn., 1893, xxxix, 1–8 ; 109–120.

HILLMANN. Ein Fall von Sectio Caesarea, ausgeführt wegen Eklampsie. Monatsschr. f. Geb. und Gyn., 1899, x, 193–207.

HUGHES and CARTER. A Clinical Experimental Study of Uræmia. Amer. Jour. Med. Sciences, 1894, cviii, 177–193 ; 265–295.

INGERSLEV. Beitrag zur Albuminurie während der Schwangerschaft, der Geburt und der Eklampsie. Zeitschr. f. Geb. u. Gyn., 1881, vi, 171–212.

JÜRGENS. Fettemboli und Metastase von Leberzellen bei Eklampsie, etc. Berliner klin. Wochenschr., 1886, 519.

KETTLITZ. Ueber Kaiserschnitt wegen Eklampsie. D. I., Halle, 1897.

KLEBS. Multipel Leberzellen-thrombose. Ziegler's Beiträge, 1888, iii, 1–30.

KNAPP. Klinische Beobachtungen über Eklampsie. Berlin, 1896.

Ueber puerperale Eklampsie und deren Behandlung. Berlin, 1900.

KOLLMANN. Zur Aetiologie und Therapie der Eklampsie. Centralbl. f. Gyn., 1897, 341–346.

KRÖNIG und FÜTH. Experimentelle Untersuchungen über Eklampsie. Verh. d. deutschen Gesell. f. Gyn., 1901, 313–332.

LAFON. Contribution à l'étude de quelques formes anormales d'éclampsie. Thèse de Paris, 1899.

LEVER. Cases of Puerperal Convulsions, with Remarks. Guy's Hospital Reports, 1843.

LEVINOWITCH. Bakteriologische Untersuchung des Blutes bei Eklampsie. (Vorläufige Mittheilung.) Centralbl. f. Gyn., 1899, 1385–1387.

LÖHLEIN. Zur Häufigkeit, Prognose und Therapie der Eklampsie. Verh. der deutschen Ges. f. Gyn., 1891, 177–179.

LUBARSCH. Die Puerperal-eklampsie. Ergebnisse der allg. Path. und path. Anat., 1896, i, 113–134.

LUDWIG und SAVOR. Experimentelle Studien zur Pathogenese der Eklampsie. Monatsschr. f. Geb. u. Gyn., 1895, 447–473.

MASSEN. Zwischenprodukte des Stoffwechsels als Ursache der Eklampsie. Ref. Centralbl. f. Gyn., 1896, 1208.

MAYGRIER. Quoted by Lafon.

NEWELL. Eclampsia in the Boston City Hospital for the Past Fifteen Years. Boston Med. and Surg. Jour., November 9, 1899.

OLSHAUSEN. Ueber Eklampsie. Volkmann's Sammlung klin. Vorträge, N. F., 1891, Nr. 39.

Sectio Caesarea wegen Eklampsie. Centralbl. f. Gyn., 1900, 63.

PELS LEUSDEN. Beiträge zur path. Anatomie der Puerperal-eklampsie. Virchow's Archiv, 1895, cxlii, 1–45.

PILLIET et LÉTIENNE. Lésions du foie dans l'éclampsie avec ictère. Nouv. Arch. d'Obst. et de Gyn., 1889, iv, 312–367.

PORAK. Traitement de l'éclampsie puerpérale. Annales de Gyn. et d'Obst., 1900, liv, 79–96.

PRUTZ. Ueber des anat. Verhalten der Nieren bei der Puerperal-eklampsie. Zeitschr. f. Geb. u. Gyn., xxiii, 1892, 1–52.

Ueber Eklampsie. Vereins-Beilage der deutsch. med. Wochenschr., 1897, 194.

RAYER. Traité des maladies des reins. Paris, 1839.

RIVIÈRE. Pathogénie et traitement de l'éclampsie. Paris, 1889.

ROSENSTEIN. Ueber Eklampsie. Monatsschr. f. Geburtsk. u. Gyn., 1864, xxiii, 413–430.

SCHMID. Eklampsie bei Mutter u. Kind. Centralbl. f. Gyn., 1897, 821–827.

SCHMORL. Path. anat. Untersuchungen über Puerperal-eklampsie. Leipzig, 1893.
Zur Lehre von der Eklampsie. Archiv f. Gyn., 1902, lxv, 504–529.

SCHROEDER. Quoted by Ingerslev.

SCHUMACHER. Exper. Beiträge zur Eklampsie-frage. Hegar's Beiträge zur Geb. u. Gyn., 1901, v, 257–309.

SOUREL. Contribution à l'étude des accès éclamptiques et plus particulière de leur pathogénie. Paris, 1894.

SPIEGELBERG. Ein Beitrag zur Lehre von der Eklampsie. Ammonia im Blute. Archiv f. Gyn., 1870, i, 383–391.

STEWART. Toxicity of the Urine in Pregnancy. Amer. Jour. Obst., 1901, xliv, 506–575.

STROGANOFF. Ueber die Behandlung der Eklampsie. Centralbl. f. Gyn., 1901, 1309-1312.

TARNIER et CHAMBERLENT. Note relative à la recherches de la toxicité du sérum sanguin dans deux cas d'éclampsie. Comptes rendus de la Soc. de Biol., 1892, iv, 179–182.

THOMPSON. The Influence of Sodium Chloride on the Secretion of Urine. British Med. Jour., April 1, 1899, 793.

VAN DER BERGH. Ueber die Giftigkeit des Harns. Zeitschr. f. klin. Medizin, 1898, xxxv, 52–79.

VAN DER VELDE. Eklampsia puerperalis tardiforma. Ref. Frommel's Jahresbericht, 1897, 752.

VEIT, J. Ueber die Behandlung der Eklampsie. Ruge's Festschrift, 1896, 101 120.

VOLHARD. Exp. und kritische Studien zur Pathogenese der Eklampsie. Monatsschr. f. Geb. u. Gyn., 1897, 411–437.

WILKE. Ein Fall von Encephalitis des Kindes bei Eklampsie der Mutter. Centralbl. f. Gyn., 1893, 385–392.

WINCKEL. Lehrbuch der Geburtshülfe, 1893, II. Aufl., 536–547.

WINCKLER. Beitrag zur Lehre von der Eklampsie. Virchow's Archiv, 1898, cliv, 187–233.

WOYER. Ein Fall von Eklampsie bei Mutter und Kind. Centralbl. f. Gyn., 1895, 329–334.

ZWEIFEL. Zur Behandlung der Eklampsie, Bericht über 129 hier beobachtete Fälle. Centralbl. f. Gyn., 1895, 1201–1218; 1238–1256; 1265–1277.

CHAPTER XLI

HÆMORRHAGE

PREMATURE SEPARATION OF THE NORMALLY IMPLANTED PLACENTA—PLACENTA PRÆVIA—POST-PARTUM HÆMORRHAGE—INVERSION OF THE UTERUS

A PROFUSE hæmorrhage occurring prior to or shortly after the birth of the child is always dangerous and not infrequently a fatal complication. Practically all classes of *ante-partum hæmorrhage*, with the exception of those originating from lacerations of the genital canal, are due to a partial or complete separation of the placenta from its attachment to the uterine wall. This accident is an inevitable accompaniment of labour when the placenta is implanted in the neighbourhood of the internal os—placenta prævia—but occasionally occurs when the organ occupies its normal site in the upper portion of the uterus.

Premature Separation of the Normally Implanted Placenta.—From the time of Hippocrates it had been customary to ascribe all cases of ante-partum hæmorrhage to this accident, but with the recognition of the nature of placenta prævia and the knowledge that its separation is unavoidably associated with hæmorrhage, the earlier view was abandoned and the former accident came to be regarded as of rare incidence.

Goodell, in 1869, collected 106 instances from the literature, while Holmes, in 1901, was able to find 200 additional cases. The latter writer, however, believes that these figures give a very inadequate idea of the frequency of the accident, and he himself considers that it occurs about once in every 500 labours. His contention is confirmed by Lyle's statistics, which show that 40 cases were observed in the Rotunda Hospital of Dublin during the ten years ending with 1899. Inasmuch as I have met with only 3 instances, my own experience leads me to believe that the condition is extremely rare.

Ætiology.—Unfortunately, the primary cause of the premature separation of the placenta is imperfectly understood, although a number of theories have been advanced concerning it. In 67 of Holmes's cases there was a history of a preceding traumatism which, according to Coe, is the most common ætiological factor. On the other hand, most German authorities attribute the accident to inflammatory changes in the decidua, which were present in every one of the 8 cases examined by Weiss, although in 2 of them the predominant lesion was a suppurative metritis.

Winter believes that a close relationship exists between nephritis and premature separation of the placenta, and many authors have subscribed to this opinion. Weiss, on the other hand, was able to demonstrate albuminuria in only 5 out of his 8 cases, and it would appear probable that in many instances, at least, such a combination is purely accidental; for, if renal lesions played anything like the prominent part assigned to them by Winter and his followers, premature separation of the placenta would be frequently observed, since nephritis complicating pregnancy is by no means uncommon.

Multiparity would appear to be a predisposing cause, only 19.2 per cent of the cases collected by Holmes having been noted in primiparæ. Moreover, the frequency of the accident increases directly with the number of pregnancies, and the advocates of the endometritis theory believe that these facts add to the force of their arguments.

Any of these conditions may come into play during pregnancy or at the time of labour. On the other hand, certain ætiological factors cannot

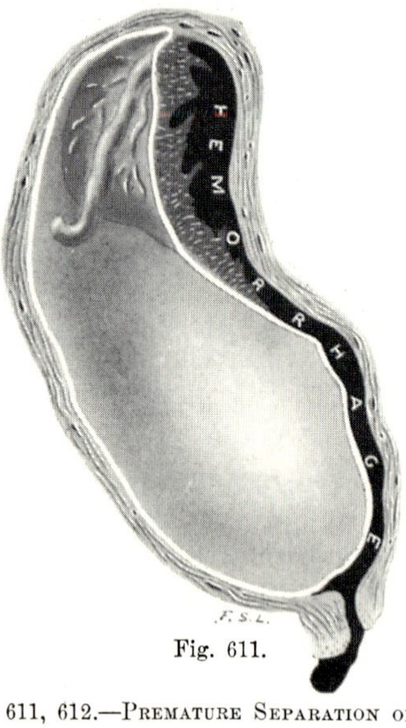

Fig. 611.

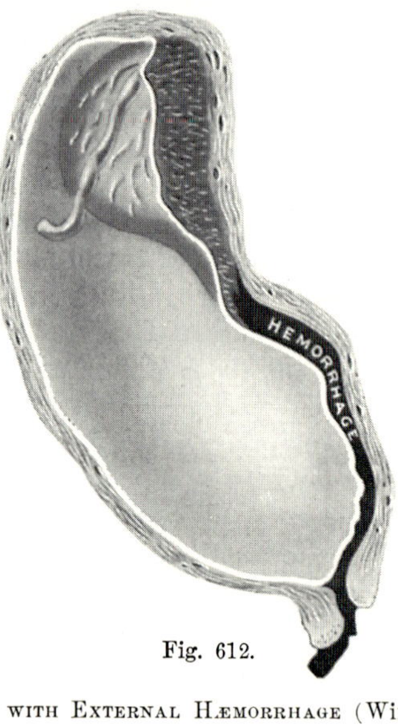

Fig. 612.

Figs. 611, 612.—Premature Separation of Placenta with External Hæmorrhage (Winter).

become operative until labour has set in. Among these may be mentioned traction exerted by an abnormally short umbilical cord, as well as a sudden diminution in the bulk of the uterine contents following the birth of the first child in a twin pregnancy or the too rapid expulsion of a large amount of amniotic fluid in hydramnios.

Pathology.—As the result of the separation of the placenta the vessels traversing the decidua serotina are torn through, and since the uterus, which is still distended by the product of conception, is unable to retract in the usual manner and compress them, hæmorrhage must inevitably result. The blood may make its way to the exterior or be retained within the uterus. According to Goodell, the latter condition, which constitutes what is termed *concealed hæmorrhage,* is liable to occur (1) when there is an effusion of blood behind the placenta, its margins still remaining adherent; (2) when the placenta is completely separated, while the membranes retain their attachment to the uterine wall; (3) when the blood gains access to the amniotic cavity after breaking through the membranes; and (4) when the head is so accurately applied to the lower uterine segment that the blood cannot make its way past it. In about two thirds of the cases, however, the membranes are dissected up and the blood eventually escapes from the cervix. Thus, in a series of 306 cases collected by Goodell and Holmes, the hæmorrhage was external in 193 and concealed in 113.

Rigby, in 1780, directed particular attention to this condition, and designated the hæmorrhage resulting from it as *accidental,* as contrasted with the *unavoidable* hæmorrhage following the partial separation of a placenta prævia. In many instances the prematurely separated organ may be seriously damaged by the hæmorrhage; and especially in the cases complicated by albuminuria, a large part of its bulk is often found occupied by fresh red infarcts or placental apoplexies. In other cases, however, the only anatomical indication of the condition visible in the placenta will be a few blood-clots upon its maternal surface or about one of its margins.

Clinical History.—Premature separation of the placenta may occur during the later months of pregnancy or at the time of labour. In the former case, the resulting external or concealed hæmorrhage is soon followed by the onset of uterine contractions. In either event, if the loss of blood is marked, the patient presents signs of acute anæmia, and passes into a condition of profound shock which may end fatally if delivery is not effected promptly.

In concealed hæmorrhage the uterus gradually becomes of a size considerably larger than would normally correspond to the duration of the pregnancy, and assumes an almost ligneous consistency, so that the results of palpation become very indefinite. At the same time the patient complains of intense pain. On the other hand, when the hæmorrhage is external, there is little or no enlargement of the uterus, and the pain is less severe. In the former case the pain and shock are often attributed to other conditions, and the patient is sometimes left to die undelivered.

When the premature separation of the placenta occurs at the time of labour as the result of traction upon an abnormally short cord, or of the sudden partial emptying of the uterine cavity in twin pregnancy or hydramnios, external hæmorrhage generally occurs, and in the former case the fœtal heart sounds become imperceptible.

In very exceptional instances the placenta may become separated from its attachment during the course of an otherwise normal labour, and be extruded in front of the child. No doubt most of the recorded cases were really instances of placenta prævia, although now and again, as in the case reported by Münchmeyer, such an accident may occur even when the placenta is inserted normally—*prolapse of the placenta.*

Diagnosis.—The appearance of acute anæmia, with manifestations of shock, in a patient in the later months of pregnancy should always suggest the possibility of concealed intra-uterine hæmorrhage, though similar symptoms may follow the rupture of an advanced extra-uterine pregnancy, or the very exceptional cases of spontaneous rupture of the uterus. In many instances the diagnosis is placed beyond doubt by the large size of the uterus and its ligneous consistence, though usually it is arrived at mainly by exclusion.

When, however, the hæmorrhage is external, the diagnosis is rendered practically positive by the failure to demonstrate the presence of a placenta prævia, though, of course, it is impossible to differentiate the rare cases of rupture of the circular sinus of the placenta to which Budin has directed our attention. When the accident occurs during labour and is attended by some loss of blood, the symptoms are suggestive of those following rupture of the uterus, though the latter accident rarely occurs except after a prolonged second stage, while premature separation may occur at any period of labour.

In the exceptional instances in which the hæmorrhage is entirely retroplacental, a localized elevation of the corresponding portion of the uterine wall can occasionally be detected on palpation.

Prognosis.—Accidental hæmorrhage, whether external or concealed, is one of the most serious complications of pregnancy and labour, practically all of the children and many of the mothers perishing. Thus, Goodell and Holmes report a maternal and fœtal mortality of 50.9 per cent and 94.4 per cent, and of 32.2 per cent and 85.8 per cent respectively.

Treatment.—In the more marked forms the life of the mother can be saved only by prompt evacuation of the uterus. On the other hand, when the separation is partial and the loss of blood but slight, the accident may be without serious significance. In the latter class of cases an expectant treatment should be pursued, and labour allowed to take its natural course, interference being indicated only when the symptoms become urgent. On the other hand, if the patient presents signs of acute hæmorrhage, whether of the concealed or external variety, the uterus should be emptied with the least possible delay, in order that it may retract and thus compress the bleeding vessels.

If labour has not yet set in, the cervix should be dilated instrumentally to a sufficient extent to permit the introduction of a Champetier de Ribes balloon, and as soon as the internal os has become obliterated further dilatation should be effected by Harris's method. On the other hand, if the condition of the cervix permits, manual dilatation should be employed from the outset and the child promptly delivered by version or forceps, as appears most advisable. In the rare cases in which the symptoms are urgent and the cervix so rigid that dilatation cannot be promptly accomplished, deep cervical incisions should be made without hesitation, and united by sutures after the extraction of the child.

Not uncommonly the tonicity of the uterus has been so impaired by the loss of blood and the distention to which it has been subjected that it fails to contract and retract during the third stage of labour, and as a result profuse post-partum hæmorrhage may follow. This possibility should always be borne in mind, and the operator should have in readiness the necessary materials for packing the uterus at a moment's notice.

Placenta Prævia.—The most common cause of ante-partum hæmorrhage is the partial separation of a placenta implanted in the neighbourhood of the internal os—placenta prævia.

Our knowledge concerning this abnormality may be said to date from the end of the seventeenth and the beginning of the eighteenth centuries, Portal, in 1685, and Schacher, in 1709, having accurately described the condition from a clinical and an anatomical point of view. Notwithstanding the fact that Smellie, William Hunter, and Rigby were well acquainted with placenta prævia and its dangers, very little advance was made in our knowledge concerning it until Barnes promulgated his views as to its mode of production and the methods of controlling the hæmorrhage arising from it. Since then many investigators have busied themselves in searching for its mode of origin and the most suitable treatment. An excellent historical *résumé* is contained in von Herff's monograph.

In this condition, the placenta, instead of being implanted high up upon the anterior or the posterior wall of the uterus, overlaps the internal os

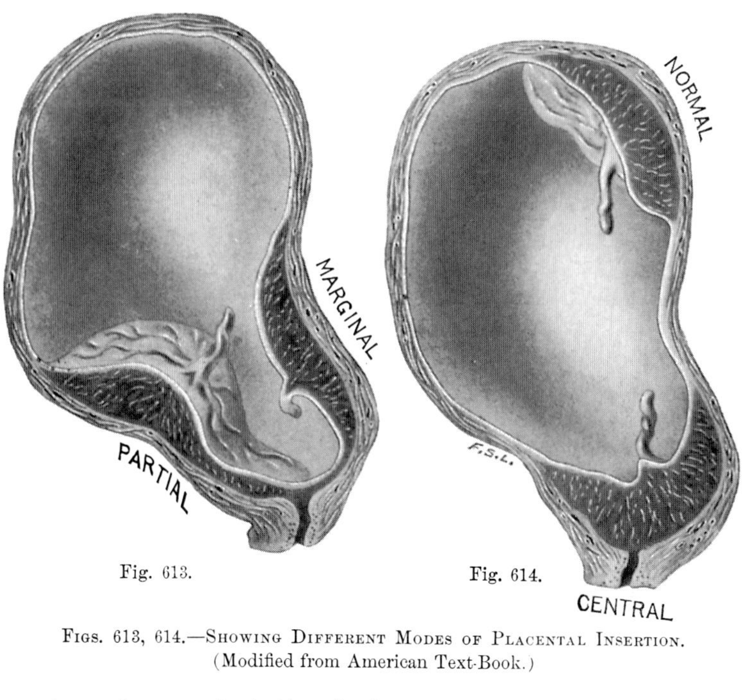

Fig. 613. Fig. 614.

Figs. 613, 614.—Showing Different Modes of Placental Insertion. (Modified from American Text-Book.)

to a greater or lesser extent, thereby becoming accessible to the examining finger. Ordinarily, three varieties are distinguished: *Placenta prævia centralis, lateralis* or *partialis*, and *marginalis*. In the first the internal os is completely covered by placental tissue, which is adherent to its margins; in the second the placenta encroaches more or less upon the internal os, but does not completely cover it; in the third the placenta is implanted higher up, its lower margin becoming palpable only after the cervix has undergone a certain degree of dilatation (Figs. 613 and 614).

Strictly speaking, only the central and partial varieties are entitled to be looked upon as true instances of placenta prævia, since in the third form the placental tissue does not overlap the internal os during pregnancy. Moreover, it is not always possible to differentiate between the first two before labour, for the reason that a partial placenta prævia, which may completely cover the internal os during pregnancy, will encroach upon only one margin of it when dilatation is complete. In both of these varieties partial separation of the placenta is an inevitable consequence of the formation of the lower uterine segment and the dilatation of the cervix. This is always associated with hæmorrhage, which was therefore designated by Rigby as *unavoidable.* In placenta prævia marginalis, on the other hand, hæmorrhage does not always occur, and as the placental tissue can be felt only after dilatation has proceeded to a certain extent, the existence of the condition is frequently unrecognised. Such cases are closely related to the so-called *vicious insertion* of the placenta described by Pinard and his pupils, which is of frequent occurrence.

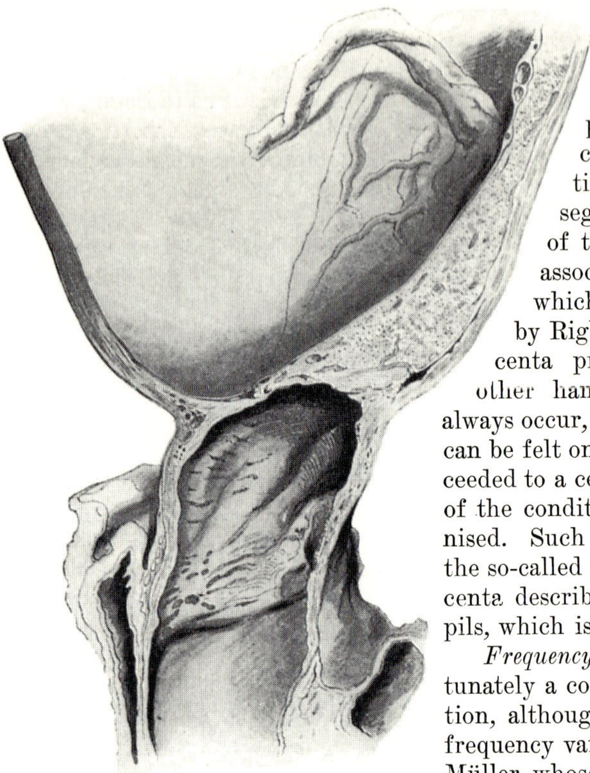

FIG. 615.—PLACENTA PRÆVIA, IN WHICH NO ATTEMPT AT DELIVERY HAD BEEN MADE (Ahlfeld).

Frequency.—Placenta prævia is fortunately a comparatively rare complication, although the statements as to its frequency vary considerably. Thus, W. Müller, whose statistics were based upon 876,432 labours, stated that it occurs once in 1,078 cases, while Lomer and Tarnier, on the other hand, estimated its incidence to be once in 723 and 207 cases respectively. In all probability it would be correct to say that it is met with about once in 1,000 cases in private, as compared with once in 250 cases in hospital practice.

Moreover, there is considerable variation in the statements as to the relative frequency of the several varieties, though it is generally admitted that the partial form is the one most frequently observed. Thus, Koblanck and Strassmann observed the central variety in 18.4 and 23.8 per cent, the lateral in 64.5 and 61.5 per cent, and the marginal in 17.1 and 15.2 per cent of their placenta prævia cases respectively. Pinard, on the other hand, states that he has never met with a placenta which was uniformly adherent to the margins of the internal os, and that the marginal is the most frequent variety. In favour of this view he adduces the fact that he had observed the so-called vicious insertion in 28.12 per cent of all normal labours. His conclusions must, however, be accepted with reserve, since they are based upon the measurement of the distance of the margin of the placenta from the point of rupture of the membranes, as determined from the examination of the after-birth, and it is clear that such a mode of investigation is not above reproach.

Ætiology.—Concerning the ætiology of placenta prævia comparatively little is known. Two factors, however, appear to favour its occurrence—endometritis and multiparity.

The abnormality occurs comparatively rarely in primiparæ, and increases in frequency with the number of children which the individual has borne. This point is strikingly illustrated by the following figures of Doranth, which are based upon 30,796 labours occurring in Chrobak's clinic. Placenta prævia was noted in 0.17, 0.48, 0.65, 1.37, 1.28, and 3.39 per cent of the patients, according as they had given birth to 1, 2, 3, 4, 5, or 6 children respectively; whereas, when the number of children varied between 7 and 10, the percentage was 5.51.

The occurrence of placenta prævia is not only favoured by the absolute number of children, but also by the rapidity with which the labours have followed one another, Strassmann finding that the average age of his patients was 32.9 years, and that the average number of labours was 6.38.

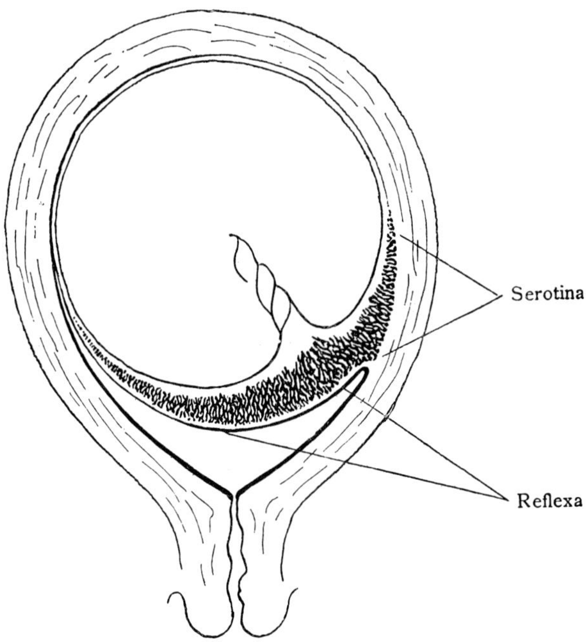

Fig. 616.—Diagram illustrating Hofmeier's Theory of the Formation of Placenta Prævia.

Mode of Formation.—The older authorities believed that placenta prævia was due to the primary implantation of the ovum in the lower portion of the uterus, or to the separation from its attachment of a normally implanted ovum, which, falling to the lower portion of the uterus, contracted new connections just before escaping through the cervix. Later it was urged that such a view failed to explain the production of the central variety, as it was inconceivable that the minute ovum could be prevented from escaping from the uterus sufficiently long to permit the formation of attachments between it and the margins of the internal os. At the same time, when one recalls the fact that with the uterus in its normal anteflexed position, the region of the internal os is frequently at a higher level than the fundus, such an occurrence is not so surprising as would appear at first sight.

Notwithstanding these objections, the former view was generally accepted until 1888, when Hofmeier and Kaltenbach advanced the theory that a part of the placenta developed from a portion of chorion in contact with the decidua reflexa. As pregnancy advanced, this so-called *reflexa placenta* gradually bridged over the internal os and eventually came in contact and fused with the decidua vera, after which vascular connections with the uterine wall became established (Fig. 616).

This view at once met with very favourable consideration, and at the 1897 meeting of the German Gynæcological Congress was again strongly advocated by Hofmeier. At the same time, while stating that he had examined numerous specimens which appeared to substantiate this mode of origin, he admitted that it was not the only manner in which a placenta prævia might originate; inasmuch as in certain instances the extension of the placental area might be rendered possible by a process of cleavage in the decidua vera, as the result of which the margin of the organ would extend beyond the serotina. Should such a process extend downward, it was readily conceivable that the placenta might grow on either side of the internal os, and, as the latter became obliterated, completely cover it. At that time Peters's ovum had not been described, so that Hofmeier was not aware that an analogous process probably occurs in every pregnancy at the normal placental site. Ahlfeld was not convinced by Hofmeier's arguments, and contended that the old theory of primary low implantation applied to the great majority of cases.

Strassmann, in 1901, pointed out that one of the most important factors in the development of placenta prævia was to be found in defective vascularization of the decidua, the result of inflammatory or atrophic changes, the latter being favoured by repeated and closely following pregnancies. Such conditions, he maintained, limit the amount of blood going to the placenta, so that in order to obtain its requisite supply of nutriment it becomes necessary for it to spread over a greater area of attachment, and in so doing its lower portion occasionally approaches the region of the internal os, completely or partially overlapping it as the case may be. Plausibility is lent to such a view by the fact that the placenta in this abnormality is spread over a greater area of the uterus than usual, while at the same time it is often considerably thinner.

In view, therefore, of Peters's work upon the normal implantation of the ovum and the development of the decidua reflexa, as well as Strassmann's theoretical deductions, it appears probable that in most cases placenta prævia results from the primary implantation of the ovum in the lower portion of the uterus, associated with extensive cleavage of the decidua vera, by which the extension of the placenta to the region of the internal os is facilitated. At the same time the possibility of its occasional development from a reflexa placenta must be admitted.

Very exceptionally, as reported by von Weiss, Keilmann, Ponfick, and others, a part of the placenta is developed upon the upper portion of the cervix. The possibility of such an occurrence must be admitted, and is sustained by the observation of Küstner, that in multiparous women the lining of the upper part of the cervical canal occasionally becomes indistinguishable from that of the lower portion of the uterus.

Symptoms.—The most characteristic symptom of placenta prævia is hæmorrhage, which usually does not appear until after the seventh month of pregnancy. At the same time it is probable that not a few cases of abortion are due to this condition, although the true state of affairs usually escapes observation. I have seen several abortions in the third month which were clearly due to this abnormality.

The hæmorrhage frequently comes on without warning in a pregnant woman who has previously considered herself in perfect health. Occasionally it makes its first appearance while the patient is asleep, so that on awakening and feeling the bedclothes moist, she is surprised to find that she is lying in a pool of blood. Ordinarily, the initial bleeding ceases spontaneously, to recur again when least expected, though in rare instances the first hæmorrhage may be so profuse as to prove fatal. In other cases the bleeding does not cease entirely, there being a continuous discharge of small quantities of a blood-stained fluid, which eventually so weakens the woman that a comparatively slight acute hæmorrhage may be sufficient to cause death. In a certain proportion of cases, particularly when the insertion is marginal, the bleeding does not appear until the time of labour, when it may vary from a slight, blood-stained discharge to a profuse or even fatal hæmorrhage. As a rule, it is less copious in this than in the other varieties.

The mode of production of the hæmorrhage is readily understood when one recalls the changes which take place in the lower uterine segment and in the cervix in the later weeks of pregnancy and at the time of labour. When the placenta is inserted centrally, it is evident that as dilatation of the internal os progresses the tissue connecting the placenta with its margins must inevitably be torn through, the rupture being necessarily followed by hæmorrhage from the intervillous spaces and from the vessels of the decidua. Moreover, as the lower uterine segment becomes developed, it is impossible for the ovum to follow its retraction, and consequently the connection between it and the placenta must of necessity be more or less completely severed and hæmorrhage result. At the same time, the bleeding is favoured by the fact that it is impossible for the stretched fibres of the lower uterine segment to compress the torn vessels, as is the case when the placenta becomes separated during the third stage of a normal labour.

As the placenta prævia occupies the lower portion of the uterus, it interferes with the accommodation between it and the fœtal head, and consequently abnormal presentations are unusually frequent, Müller having noted 272 transverse and 107 breech presentations in 1,148 cases.

In normal labour all danger is ordinarily past with the completion of the second stage; but in placenta prævia, as a result of abnormal adhesions or an excessively large area of attachment, the process of separation is sometimes interfered with. As a result, profuse hæmorrhage not infrequently occurs after the birth of the child, and exceptionally the manual removal of the placenta becomes necessary.

Diagnosis.—Placenta prævia should always be suspected in patients suffering from uterine hæmorrhage in the second half of pregnancy, and its possibility should be borne in mind until a careful examination has revealed some other satisfactory explanation for its origin. In the great majority of cases the cervix is softer and more succulent than usual, and its canal is more or less patulous, so that but little difficulty is experienced in carrying the finger through the internal os and feeling the characteristic sponge-like placental tissue, or at least making out a soggy, thick substance lying between the finger and the presenting part. When, however, the cervix is not patulous it should be dilated, under anæsthesia if necessary, sufficiently to permit the introduction of the finger, which is then passed through the internal os and swept around the adjacent portion of the lower uterine segment, when the presence or absence of the abnormality can be positively determined. It is true that such a procedure occasionally results in the induction of premature labour; but the risk is nevertheless quite justifiable, since we possess no other means of arriving at a definite diagnosis, which should be made at any cost on account of the very serious menace which the existence of the condition offers to the life of the patient.

Prognosis.—The prognosis is always serious. According to Müller, under expectant treatment the maternal mortality varied from 36 to 40 per cent, while for the children it was about 66 per cent, one half of those which are born alive perishing within the first ten days following delivery. The danger to the mother arises primarily from hæmorrhage, which is usually the direct result of the condition, though occasionally it may be due to deep cervical tears resulting from too hasty artificial dilatation or the extraction of the child through an imperfectly dilated cervix. Moreover, such patients are particularly prone to puerperal infection, which is favoured by the presence of the thrombosed sinuses in the lower uterine segment.

The fœtal mortality is due in great part to the fact that many of the children are born some weeks or months prematurely. In many instances they perish from asphyxiation, the result of placental hæmorrhage, while occasionally they succumb during attempts at extraction through an imperfectly dilated cervix.

Nowadays, the maternal mortality depends upon the variety of the placenta prævia, the method of delivery, and the condition of the patient when first seen. Thus, in 178 cases reported by Hofmeier, Behm, and Lomer, and treated by 11 different obstetricians by combined version by the Braxton Hicks manœuvre, the maternal mortality was 4.5 per cent, whereas 93 cases treated by the three operators mentioned showed a mortality of only 1 per cent. Koblanck reports a death-rate of 3.8 per cent in 467 cases treated in the Frauenklinik in Berlin, and Strassmann one of 5 per cent in 100 cases which he delivered personally. According to their figures, the prognosis is from 3 to 8 times more serious in central placenta prævia than in the other varieties. Moreover, the mortality depends upon the condition of the patient when first seen, it being evident that women who have suffered from profuse and repeated bleeding have far less chance of recovery than those who come under observation after the first slight hæmorrhage.

Unfortunately, the fœtal mortality has shown comparatively little decrease in recent years, Küstner and Strassmann giving percentages of 35 and 61.22 respectively. This difference is probably due to the fact that the former employed the rubber bag extensively, whereas the latter treated his cases by the Braxton Hicks method of version and gradual extraction. A very great improvement in this respect is hardly to be anticipated on account of the large number of premature children with which one has to deal.

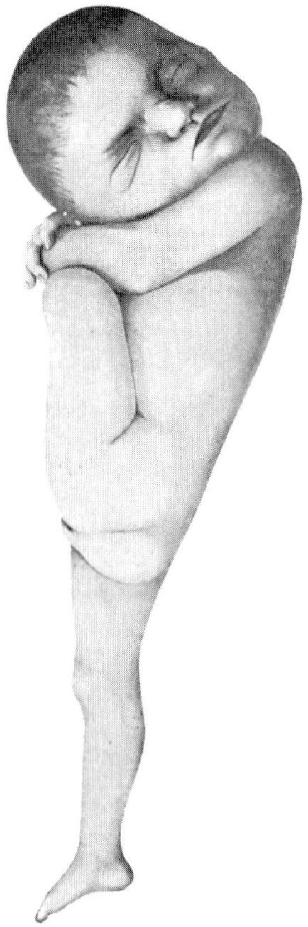

Fig. 617.—Fœtus partially extracted from a Patient Dying of Placenta Prævia, showing how it acts as a Tampon (Leopold).

Treatment.—On account of the danger of profuse and unexpected hæmorrhage, pregnancy or labour, as the case may be, should be terminated in the most conservative manner as soon as possible after a placenta prævia has been positively diagnosed. There is no single method of treatment applicable to all classes, and the obstetrician who understands how to differentiate his cases will obtain the best results.

If the diagnosis is made during pregnancy, the cervix should be dilated by means of the finger or by the Goodell or Hegar instrument sufficiently to permit the introduction of two fingers. This having been attained, further treatment will depend upon whether the child is viable or not. In the former case the best results are obtained by the introduction of a Champetier de Ribes balloon after rupture of the membranes or perforation of the placenta, according as one has to deal with a lateral or central insertion, dilatation being hastened by attaching a 2-pound weight to the end of the tube by a string and suspending it over the foot of the bed. On the other hand, if the child is not viable, equally good results are more readily obtained by bringing down a foot by Braxton Hicks's manœuvre and using the breech of the child as a tampon to control further bleeding. If the hæmorrhage ceases after the foot has been brought down, the expulsion of the child may be left to Nature; but if the oozing continues, gentle traction should be made upon the leg so as to compress the placenta with the child's buttocks. Whichever method is employed, extraction should not be attempted until the cervix is completely dilated, or at least sufficiently so as to permit the ready passage of the head. Too much haste is liable to cause deep cervical tears, giving rise to profuse hæmorrhage and requiring the application of sutures, while in other instances serious difficulty may be encountered in delivering the child.

Generally speaking, better results will be obtained in private practice by the employment of Braxton Hicks's bipolar version, no matter what may be the condition of the child, for the reason that the average practitioner will rarely be equipped with a suitable balloon and the necessary paraphernalia for its introduction. In hospital practice, however, its employment has undoubtedly aided materially in diminishing the fœtal mortality.

In very exceptional instances in primiparous women, the cervix may be so rigid that it is impossible to dilate it sufficiently to permit the employment of either of the above-mentioned procedures. Under such circumstances a tight cervical and vaginal pack of sterilized gauze bandage should be applied. This will check the hæmorrhage for the time being, and after remaining in place for a few hours will usually bring about sufficient dilatation to permit the employment of whatever manœuvres may be deemed necessary.

At the time of labour, the treatment depends upon the degree of dilatation and the condition of the patient. If the cervix is obliterated, immediate delivery by version or forceps is indicated. On the other hand, if the dilatation is only partial, the hæmorrhage slight, and the placenta inserted marginally, good results frequently follow rupture of the membranes, since the placenta is then able to follow the retracting uterine wall. In all other cases I prefer to complete the dilatation by Harris's method, provided the consistency of the cervix is such that it appears probable that the procedure can be readily and safely employed. The membranes are then ruptured or the placenta is torn through, according as one has to deal with a partial or complete placenta prævia, after which the child is turned and promptly extracted. I have obtained very satisfactory results by this method, as have also Harris, Didry, and many others.

If, however, it does not appear likely that the cervix can be readily dilated manually, or that such a procedure is liable to give rise to deep cervical tears, it is advisable to make use of a Champetier de Ribes balloon or to perform version by the bipolar method of Braxton Hicks, extracting the child only after satisfactory dilatation has been obtained.

If the patient is seen at the beginning of labour and before the cervix has undergone any great degree of dilatation, the same methods should be employed as during pregnancy.

Whenever the hæmorrhage has been profuse, and the patient presents the subjective symptoms of an acute anæmia, it becomes necessary to resort to the constitutional measures outlined under the treatment of post-partum hæmorrhage. Occasionally, when the patient is markedly exsanguinated when first seen, but is losing little or no blood at the time, it is better to devote one's attention to improving her general condition rather than to attempt immediate delivery.

In view of the danger to the mother, and particularly the marked fœtal mortality attending placenta prævia, as well as the fact that not a few children are sacrificed by Braxton Hicks's method of version, or by extraction through an imperfectly dilated cervix, Tait, Donoghue, Palmer Dudley, and others have recommended the performance of Cæsarean section, provided the child is viable and the patient in good condition.

As the results obtained by the methods of treatment outlined above are quite satisfactory so far as the mother is concerned, it seems doubtful whether Cæsarean section will come into very general use, particularly as the operation is applicable only to patients who are in a hospital, or the rich, who can be surrounded by every convenience and safeguard. If such a line of treatment were attempted among the poorer classes in their own homes, the death-rate, I am sure, would be much greater than that obtained by the usual methods. Moreover, as has been said, the fœtal mortality in any case is not susceptible of any material reduction, for the reason that the pregnancy is generally terminated before term, when the chances of extra-uterine life are relatively unfavourable. Ehrenfest, after carefully considering the subject, has arrived at the same conclusion.

At the same time, I am prepared to admit that Cæsarean section may be the operation of choice in a very small number of cases, as, for instance, when a primipara with a very rigid cervix and a living child is overtaken by profuse hæmorrhage. Such conditions, however, are so exceptional that it appears to me that the field of usefulness for the operation is very limited, and that its widespread employment would be productive of far more harm than good.

The mode of production and significance of slight ante-partum hæmorrhage, which sometimes follows intra-uterine *rupture of the cord* or the tearing of the vessels of the velamentously inserted umbilical cord, have already been considered in Chapter XXVIII.

Post-partum Hæmorrhage.—With the exception of the very rare cases incident to inversion of the uterus, a serious bleeding following the birth of the child is usually due to one of three causes. Of these the most common is retention of the partially separated placenta or of individual cotyledons; less often it is due to deep tears involving the tissues of the birth canal, and in very rare instances to defective functioning of the uterine musculature—atony.

Ætiology.—As long as the placenta remains firmly attached to the uterine wall the possibility of hæmorrhage is slight, but when it has become partially separated, the normal action of the uterine musculature is interfered with. As a result, the torn vessels at the partially denuded placental site are not constricted, and accordingly more or less profuse hæmorrhage occurs. Imperfect separation of the placenta can usually be attributed to improper management of the third stage of labour, particularly the too early and energetic employment of Credé's manœuvre. Exceptionally, it may result from an abnormally intimate attachment of the placenta, due to a decidual endometritis or some other morbid condition. The retention of isolated cotyledons or of a small succenturiate lobe interferes with the normal contraction and retention of the uterus in precisely the same manner as the partially separated placenta.

The part played by deep tears of the generative tract is perfectly obvious, and will be considered in detail in the following chapter.

In very rare instances serious hæmorrhage may result from rupture of large varicose veins, of an aneurysm of the uterine artery, or the disturbance of areas of thrombosis in the cervix.

Formerly, *atony* of the puerperal uterus was considered the most frequent cause of post-partum hæmorrhage, but more careful observation has shown that such a condition is seldom primary; for, with the exception of the rare instances in which it follows excessive distention of the uterus incident to twin pregnancy or hydramnios, serious abnormalities in the contractile function of the uterine musculature are usually associated with some mechanical cause, such as retention of portions of the placenta, the presence of myomata in the uterine walls, or in rare cases the existence of adhesions between the uterus and the surrounding organs. It is probable, however, that Veit goes too far in denying *in toto* the possibility of a primary atony, although the general tendency to overestimate its frequency must be admitted.

The rare cases of hæmorrhage following *paralysis at the placental site*, in which the rest of the organ remains firmly contracted, as in the cases reported by Chiari, Braun and Spaeth, Olshausen, and others, point to the possibility of a partial atony, while the occasional instances in which patients bleed profusely after each labour without demonstrable cause, likewise afford corroborative evidence. At the same time the possible existence of hæmophilia should always be borne in mind in such women, as in a case reported by Wehle.

Clinical History.—Hæmorrhage may occur either during or after the third stage of labour. In the first class of cases, as a rule, it is the result of tears or of partial separation of the placenta. Fortunately, hæmorrhage dependent upon the latter cause is usually not serious, for the reason that in the vast majority of such cases the condition is only transitory, complete separation occurring spontaneously as the result of uterine contraction, when satisfactory retraction checks the loss of blood. Exceptionally the bleeding may persist even after the placenta has become completely separated and lies free in the uterine cavity. In such cases, however, it is due either to tears or to imperfect functioning of the uterus.

Generally speaking, partial separation occurring during the course of placental expulsion by the Schultze mechanism is not accompanied by external hæmorrhage until the placenta escapes from the vulva, when the large amount of blood collected behind it is suddenly discharged. In Duncan's mechanism, on the other hand, the loss of blood continues throughout the entire placental period.

A hæmorrhage which persists after the extrusion of the placenta may be due to tears, retention of placental remnants, or to atony. In the first there is a steady flow of bright-red blood, which begins immediately after the delivery of the child. When the hæmorrhage is due to retention, the blood escapes in gushes, which are apt to be synchronous with the uterine contractions, and frequently in large clots; whereas in cases due to primary atony there is a continuous flow of blood, which may be so abundant as to cause death within a very few minutes.

In rare instances, even after the discharge of the placenta, the hæmorrhage may be *concealed*, several litres of blood sometimes accumulating in the uterine cavity.

The amount of blood lost during a post-partum hæmorrhage may vary from 500 to 3,000 cubic centimetres, the latter extreme, however, being usually incompatible with life. Generally speaking, the effect upon the patient depends more upon her general condition than upon the actual amount of blood lost. Thus, a woman who is already exhausted by a prolonged labour or weakened by antecedent disease, may succumb after a loss of from 1,000 to 1,500 cubic centimetres, which others suffer with impunity. As a rule, the loss of a small amount of blood is not attended by serious symptoms; but when the hæmorrhage is profuse the pulse becomes rapid and compressible, the face becomes pallid and assumes a drawn appearance, while at the same time the woman may complain of disturbed vision, chilliness, and shortness of breath. In extreme cases symptoms of air hunger appear, and the patient usually passes into unconsciousness before the fatal termination.

Diagnosis.—The diagnosis offers no difficulty, except in the rare instances in which the hæmorrhage has taken place into the uterine cavity and does not appear externally. It must, however, be distinctly stated that concealed hæmorrhage should never occur if the condition of the uterus is conscientiously watched, although, if routine precautions are neglected, the first indication of the condition is occasionally afforded by the pale and haggard appearance of the patient. On examination the pulse-rate will be found greatly accelerated, the uterus markedly increased in size, and presenting a doughy consistence instead of the characteristic firm, hard sensation offered by the normal puerperal organ. Pressure upon it is followed by a copious flow of blood from the vagina.

Although the source of the hæmorrhage is sometimes very hard to trace, yet inasmuch as the decision as to the proper treatment of the patient frequently depends upon its recognition, a differential diagnosis is of the utmost importance. Generally speaking, if the hæmorrhage commences immediately after the birth of the child, it is due either to tears of the genital tract or to partial separation of the placenta. In the latter case it usually ceases temporarily after energetic kneading of the uterus, but recurs as soon as it is allowed to relax. If manipulations of the uterus prove of no avail, it is probable that the hæmorrhage comes from a tear, although this is not a universal rule, since in a certain number of instances the loss of blood will continue until the placenta is expressed by Credé's method or is removed manually.

Again, a hæmorrhage persisting after the uterus has been emptied, while abdominal palpation shows that the organ itself is firmly contracted, suggests a serious tear of the birth canal, which should be sought for, and when found closed with sutures. In order to accomplish this, the patient having been brought to the edge of the bed, the external genitalia are carefully inspected. If the perinæum is intact, the cervix should be forced down towards the vulva by pressure upon the fundus, and if this fails to bring it into view, it should be examined by the fingers in the vagina. If a cervical lesion cannot be detected, the vaginal walls should be spread apart by means of a speculum and thoroughly inspected. A hæmorrhage which does not come on until ten or fifteen minutes after the birth of the child can hardly be due to a tear.

On the other hand, if the uterus does not contract and retract firmly after the expulsion of the placenta, or if it remains so only so long as kneading is kept up, the cause of the hæmorrhage must be sought for either in the retention of a placental cotyledon or in atony. Certainty with regard to the former point is usually obtained by careful inspection of the afterbirth, a large defect upon its maternal surface indicating the retention of a cotyledon, while a more or less circular defect in the membranes a short distance from the placental margin shows that a succenturiate lobe has been left behind. At the same time one should be careful not to confound mere fissures with defects due to loss of tissue. The diagnosis of primary atony should be made only in those cases in which every other explanation has been excluded.

Treatment.—With proper management, hæmorrhage during and immediately following the third stage of labour should be extremely rare. The most important prophylactic measures consist in watching the condition of the uterus after the birth of the child, and not resorting to Credé's manœuvre until the rising up of the fundus indicates that the placenta has become completely detached. Premature attempts at expression are a frequent cause of imperfect separation. Again, owing to the tendency towards relaxation following the birth of twins, as well as in hydramnios, concealed hæmorrhage, and placenta prævia, the condition of the uterus should be most carefully watched for the few minutes immediately following the birth of the child, and energetic kneading through the abdominal walls promptly resorted to upon the first sign of failing contraction.

The placenta should be carefully examined after its expulsion, for the purpose of ascertaining whether it is intact or not. If it shows any serious defect, immediate preparations should be made for the removal of the retained portion in case symptoms supervene.

In the presence of actual hæmorrhage, the treatment varies according as the placenta is still within the uterus or has already been expelled. In the former case the uterus should at once be grasped through the abdominal wall and firmly kneaded. If firm contractions come on, all is well, but if the hæmorrhage continues and the uterus relaxes as soon as the kneading is stopped, the placenta should be expressed by Credé's method; and if this cannot be accomplished and the patient's condition is alarming, manual removal may become necessary. This latter procedure, however, should be resorted to only in serious cases, and the directions given for its performance in Chapter XXIV should be most conscientiously followed.

If the hæmorrhage does not cease after the delivery of the placenta, the cause should be ascertained and suitable treatment instituted. Tears should be located and their edges brought together by sutures. On the other hand, if the hæmorrhage is the result of the retention of placental tissue, the carefully disinfected hand should be carried up into the uterus in order to seek for and remove the retained cotyledon. Under such circumstances the hand acts as a most efficient irritator, causing the uterus to contract energetically. After separating the retained portion of placenta the hand should not be withdrawn at once, but should be allowed to recede gradually as it is forced down by the contraction of the fundus.

If the hæmorrhage is due to atony, the uterus should be vigorously kneaded, and from 40 to 60 minims of ergot or of ergotol administered hypodermically. After careful disinfection of the skin, the needle should be plunged in at right angles to the surface, deep down into the tissues of the thigh, since in this way the chances of abscess formation are greatly diminished.

If these measures are not attended with the desired result, a very hot intra-uterine douche of several litres of sterile salt solution should be employed. In many cases this acts as a most efficient hæmostatic, effectively irritating the uterus and causing it to contract forcibly and permanently.

If the hæmorrhage persists in spite of the douche, our only hope of controlling it is by packing the uterus tightly with sterile gauze, which should be introduced according to the directions given in Chapter XXIV (see Fig. 419). Before resorting to the use of the pack it is always advisable to palpate the interior of the uterus, as occasionally a portion of the placenta may have been retained, even though immediately after expulsion the organ may have apparently been entire.

Formerly it was customary to recommend the introduction into the uterus of ice or solutions containing vinegar, the perchloride of iron, or other astringent substances. Their employment, however, is not advisable, since ice and ordinary vinegar are never sterile, while the iron solution accomplishes its purpose by the formation of dense coagula, which are later separated from the uterus by suppurative processes. Above all, none of them act as promptly or efficiently as the pack, the employment of which, although comparatively rarely indicated, in exceptional cases offers the only reliable means of coping with the condition. For this reason the obstetrician should always carry in his bag the materials necessary for it, as they cannot usually be obtained promptly in an emergency.

Too great stress cannot be laid upon the importance of observing the most rigorous aseptic technique in every intra-uterine manipulation undertaken for the purpose of checking post-partum hæmorrhage. The natural tendency of the physician is to forget all other risks in his attempts to check the bleeding at once. Such neglect, however, is frequently attended by most serious consequences, the patient being saved from death from hæmorrhage merely to perish of infection a few days later. For this reason, therefore, the obstetrician will usually best subserve the interests of his patient by taking the time necessary for carefully disinfecting his hands before beginning any manipulations. In fact, the only exception is offered by the very rare cases of atonic hæmorrhage in which it appears probable that a delay even of a few minutes means inevitable death.

After the actual hæmorrhage has been checked, attention must be directed to the general condition of the patient. When the shock is not profound and the pulse not particularly rapid, elevation of the foot of the bed and the application of hot bottles or bricks to the extremities will be all that is needed. In more severe cases, the administration of $\frac{1}{30}$ grain of strychnine hypodermically, 3 doses being given in prompt succession, if necessary, is attended by excellent results, which may be supplemented by hypodermic injections of whisky or ether. Hot rectal enemata of equal parts of black coffee and salt solution are also valuable.

When the patient is profoundly shocked, sterile normal salt solution in large quantities—500 cubic centimetres being injected under each breast, and repeated as soon as absorption has occurred—will prove the best restorative. When the condition is very serious and a suitable canula is available, even more striking results may be obtained by administering it intravenously. Occasionally, when the loss of blood has been very great, these measures may be supplemented by tightly bandaging the extremities or compressing the aorta, in the hope of retaining as large a quantity of blood as possible in the upper part of the body.

Inversion of the Uterus.—This condition is a very rare, but important cause of post-partum hæmorrhage. According to Beckmann, not a single case occurred in 250,000 labours in the St. Petersburg Lying-in Hospital,

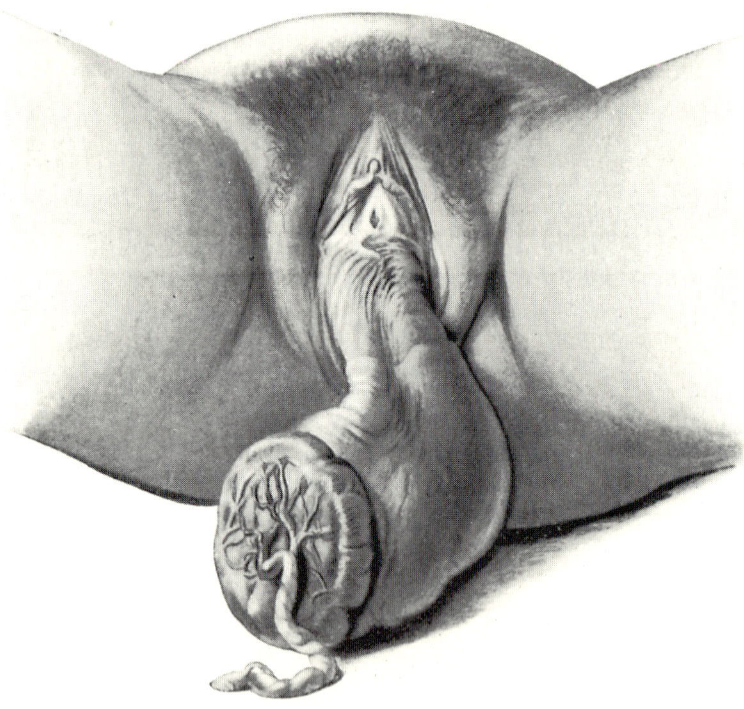

Fig. 618.—Complete Inversion of Uterus (Bumm).

while Madden noted it only once in 190,833 deliveries in Dublin. Many obstetricians in large practice have never seen a case, or have met with only a few examples of the condition. The historical and statistical aspects of the subject are fully dealt with in the articles of Beckmann, Browne, and Vogel.

Now and again the fundus of the uterus becomes inverted and comes into close contact with or may protrude through the external os; while in rare instances the entire organ appears outside of the vulva, the condition being respectively designated as *incomplete* and *complete inversion* and *prolapse of the inverted uterus* (Fig. 618). In not a few cases the placenta remains attached to the inverted organ.

Ætiology.—For the production of the accident two factors are necessary: marked laxity of the uterine walls, particularly at the placental site, and a patulous cervical canal. Inversion may occur spontaneously as the result of the intra-abdominal pressure or from the mere weight of the intestines, while in other cases it is attributable to violence resulting from the too vigorous employment of Credé's manœuvre or to traction upon the cord.

Beckmann, who has carefully analyzed 100 cases reported in the literature, believes that in the majority of instances the accident occurs spontaneously, while Vogel, in a similar review, holds that most cases are due to violence. His contention appears to be confirmed by Beckmann's statistics, as only 3 of the 100 cases occurred in hospital practice. Indeed, it is highly probable that the accident is excessively rare when labour is properly conducted, but that it occurs more frequently under the unfavourable conditions existing in private practice, particularly as conducted by midwives.

The complication usually follows a full-term labour, although a number of cases are recorded in which it was noted after abortion. It is also an interesting fact that more than 50 per cent of the cases recorded by both Beckmann and Vogel were in primiparous women.

Symptoms.—As a rule, inversion of the uterus is promptly followed by alarming symptoms, the patient presenting marked evidences of shock, with a rapid pulse and a tendency to syncope. In other cases convulsions occur and profuse hæmorrhage is not infrequently noted. On the other hand, the symptoms are sometimes very slight, and the condition may continue for several days without causing any serious annoyance to the patient.

In the rare instances the cervix may so retract about the completely inverted uterus that strangulation occurs, followed by gangrene. In other instances this does not take place, but the condition becomes chronic, necessitating operative procedures later.

Prognosis.—If the condition is detected promptly, and the uterus replaced immediately, the prognosis is fair, Beckmann reporting a mortality of 14 per cent. On the other hand, if strangulation or gangrene occur, the outlook is ominous.

Treatment.—In very recent cases reposition can usually be effected without difficulty by pressure exerted by several fingers in the vagina, it being important to remember that the force should be directed upward in the axis of the superior strait. Neglect of this precaution undoubtedly accounts for a certain number of failures. As the procedure is generally painful, anæsthesia should be employed.

If the placenta is still attached to the uterus, it is generally advisable to defer its separation until reposition has been effected, because the contractile function of the inverted uterus being in abeyance there is always the risk of profuse hæmorrhage. On the other hand, if the patient is not seen until well advanced in the puerperium, and when the cervix is so contracted that reposition cannot be accomplished so readily, operative procedures become necessary. Full particulars concerning these will be found in the current works on gynæcology.

LITERATURE

AHLFELD. Ueber Placenta prævia. Verh. d. deutschen Gesell. f. Gyn., 1897, 268–277.

BARNES. The Physiology and Treatment of Placenta Prævia. London, 1858.

Placenta Prævia. Lectures on Obstetric Operations, 4th ed. London, 1886, 398–422.

BECKMANN. Zur Aetiologie der Inversio uteri post partum. Zeitschr. f. Geb. u. Gyn., 1895, xxxi, 371–401.

BEHM. Die combinirte Wendung bei Placenta prævia. Zeitschr. f. Geb. u. Gyn., 1883, ix, 373–419.

BRAUN, CHIARI und SPAETH. Paralyse des Uterus. Klinik der Geb. u. Gyn., Erlangen, 1855, 202–204.

BROWNE. Inversion of the Uterus. Amer. Gyn. and Obst. Jour., 1899, xv, 115–129.

BUDIN. Hémorrhagies utérines et rupture du sinus circulaire. Femmes en couches et nouveau nés, 1897, 143–161.

COE. Accidental Hæmorrhage during the First Stage of Full-term Labour. Trans. Amer. Gyn. Soc., 1891, xvi, 35–50.

DIDRY. De la dilatation manuelle du col utérin dans les accouchements avec hémorrhagies placentaires graves. Thèse de Nancy, 1899.

DONOGHUE. Cæsarean Section for Placenta Prævia. Boston Med. and Surg. Jour., December 6, 1900, cxliii, 571.

DORANTH. Statisches über Placenta prævia. Chrobak's Berichte aus der 2ten geb. gyn. Klinik in Wien, 1897, i, 77–119.

DUDLEY. The Modern Cæsarean Section an Ideal Method of Treatment for Placenta Prævia. N. Y. Med. Jour., November 3, 1900.

EHRENFEST. The Impropriety of Cæsarean Section in Placenta Prævia, etc. Amer. Med., January 12, 1902, 64–68.

GOODELL. Concealed Accidental Hæmorrhage of the Gravid Uterus. Amer. Jour. Obst., 1870, ii, 281–346.

HARRIS. A Method of performing Rapid Manual Dilatation of the Os Uteri, and its Advantage in the Treatment of Placenta Prævia. Amer. Jour. Obst., 1894, xxix, 37–49.

HERFF. Zur Lehre von der Placenta prævia. Zeitschr. f. Geb. u. Gyn., 1896, xxxv, 325–372.

HOFMEIER. Zur Behandlung der Placenta prævia. Zeitschr. f. Geb. u. Gyn., 1882, viii, 89–101.

Ueber Placenta prævia. Verh. d. deutschen Gesell. f. Gyn., 1888, 159–163.

Zur Entstehung der Placenta prævia. Zeitschr. f. Geb. u. Gyn., 1894, xxxix, 1–17.

Ueber Placenta prævia. Verh. d. deutschen Gesell. f. Gyn., 1897, 204–225.

HOLMES. Ablatio Placentæ. Amer. Jour. Obst., 1901, xliv, 753–784.

HUNTER. Anatomical Description of the Human Gravid Uterus. Birmingham, 1774.

KALTENBACH. Zur Pathogenese der Placenta prævia. Zeitschr. f. Geb. u. Gyn., 1890, xviii, 1–7.

KEILMANN. Eine Cervixplacenta. Centralbl. f. Gyn., 1897, 857–858.

KOBLANCK. Placenta prævia. Sänger-Herff, Encyklopädie der Geb. u. Gyn., 1900, ii, 189–191.

KÜSTNER. Ueber Placenta prævia. Verh. d. deutschen Gesell. f. Gyn., 1897, 277–283.

LOMER. On Combined Turning in the Treatment of Placenta Prævia. Amer. Jour. Obst., 1884, xvii, 1233–1260.

LYLE. The Treatment of Accidental Hæmorrhage. The Physician and Surgeon, London, April 12, 1900.

MADDEN. Quoted by Browne.

MÜLLER, W. Placenta prævia. Stuttgart, 1877.

MÜNCHMEYER. Ueber den Vorfall der Nachgeburt bei regelmässigem Sitze derselben. Archiv f. Gyn., 1888, xxxiii, 486–497.

OLSHAUSEN. Paralyse der Placentar-insertionsstelle. Schroeder's Lehrbuch der Geb., XIII. Aufl., 1899, 775.

PETERS. Ueber die Einbettung des menschlichen Eies. Wien, 1899.

PINARD. De la rupture prématurée, dite spontanée, des membranes, etc. Annales d'Obst. et de Gyn., 1886, xxv, 171–179 ; 321–345.

PONFICK. Zur Anatomie der Placenta prævia. Archiv f. Gyn., 1900, lx, 147–173.

PORTAL. La pratique des accouchements, etc. Paris, 1685.

RIGBY. An Essay on the Uterine Hæmorrhage which Precedes the Delivery of the Full-grown Fœtus. London, 1776.

SCHACHER. De placentæ uterinæ morbis. Lipsiae, 1709.

SMELLIE. A Treatise on the Theory and Practice of Midwifery, 1752.

SPIEGELBERG. Die Inversion der Gebärmutter. Lehrbuch der Geb., 1891, III. Aufl., 599–607.

STRASSMANN. Ueber Placenta prævia. Zeitschr. f. Geb. u. Gyn., 1901, xliv, 529–546.
Placenta prævia. Archiv f. Gyn., 1902, xxvii, 112–275.

TAIT. On the Treatment of Unavoidable Hæmorrhage by Removal of the Uterus. Med. Rec., March 4, 1899, lv, No. 9.

TARNIER et BUDIN. Hémorrhagie par insertion vicieuse du placenta. Traité de l'art des accouchements, 1898, iii, 571–659.

VEIT. Ueber die Behandlung der Blutungen unmittelbar nach der Geburt. Zeitschr. f. Geb. u. Gyn., 1895, xxxi, 214–225.

VOGEL. Beitrag zur Lehre von der Inversio uteri. Zeitschr. f. Geb. u. Gyn., 1900, xlii, 490–525.

WEHLE. Ueber Hämophilie bei einer Gebärenden. Centralbl. f. Gyn., 1893, 672–675.

WEISS. Ueber vorzeitige Lösung der normal sitzenden Placenta. Archiv f. Gyn., 1897, xlvi, 256–291.
Zur Kasuistik der Placenta prævia centralis. Centralbl. f. Gyn., 1897, 641–649.

WINTER. Zur Lehre von der vorzeitigen Placentarlösung bei Nephritis. Zeitschr. f. Geb. u. Gyn., 1885, xi, 398–408.

CHAPTER XLII

INJURIES TO THE BIRTH CANAL

Injuries to the Vulval Outlet.—In the chapter upon the Conduct of Normal Labour reference was made to the frequency of perineal lacerations, and emphasis was laid upon the necessity for repairing them immediately after the birth of the child.

More rarely tears occur about the anterior portion of the vulva. In spontaneous labour these seldom amount to more than slight abrasions upon the inner surfaces of the labia minora, but in operative deliveries, especially when the handles of the forceps have been unduly elevated, serious lesions may be produced as a result of compression of the tissues between the pubic arch and the blades of the instrument. Now and again the labia minora are completely severed and torn loose from their connections, or deep tears occur on either side of the urethra implicating the vessels supplying the clitoris and giving rise to profuse hæmorrhage.

Injuries to the Vagina.—With the exception of the most superficial varieties, which are limited to the mucous membrane of the fourchette, all perineal lacerations are accompanied by more or less injury to the lower portion of the vagina. Such tears rarely occur in the median line, but extend a variable distance up one or both vaginal sulci, being almost always sufficiently deep to involve some fibres of the levator ani muscle. Bilateral lacerations of this variety are usually unequal in length and are separated from one another by a tongue-shaped portion of mucosa which represents the lower end of the posterior column of the vagina (Fig. 297).

These injuries should always be looked for, and their repair should form a part of every operation for the restoration of a lacerated perinæum. If this precaution is neglected and the external wound alone is attended to, the patient will eventually present symptoms due to *relaxation of the vaginal outlet*, even though the perinæum proper may be in perfect condition.

Isolated tears involving the middle third of the vagina, and unassociated with lacerations of the perinæum or cervix, are very rarely observed. They are usually longitudinal, and result from injuries sustained during a forceps operation, though now and again they follow spontaneous delivery. They frequently extend deeply into the underlying tissues, and may give rise to a copious hæmorrhage, which, however, is readily controlled by a few sutures. Their presence is usually overlooked, inasmuch as they can be recognised only after the vaginal walls are spread apart by means of a speculum.

More important are the *injuries to the levator ani muscle,* which are not associated with tears through the vaginal mucosa and therefore escape immediate detection. As the result of overdistention of the birth canal, there may occur a submucous separation of certain fibres of the muscle, or at least so great a diminution in its tonicity that it can no longer properly fulfil its function as the pelvic diaphragm. In these cases the patient sooner or later suffers just as severely from symptoms of relaxation as if a deeply lacerated perinæum had been left unrepaired. Although the accident can sometimes be avoided by an intelligent use of forceps when the second stage of labour is unduly prolonged, indications for prophylactic measures are not always at hand, since it not infrequently follows spontaneous and rapid delivery.

Lesions of the upper third of the vagina are extremely uncommon unless they represent the extension of deep cervical tears into the fornix. In very rare instances, however, the cervix may be entirely or partially torn loose from its vaginal attachment, rupture in other cases occurring in either the anterior, posterior, or lateral fornix. Hugenberger, in 1875, collected 40 cases of this accident from the literature, and designated it as *colpaporrhexis.* Schtschotkin, in 1891, published 40 additional instances, while Kaufmann, in 1901, estimated that something more than 100 cases have been recorded altogether.

The accident is somewhat analogous to rupture of the lower uterine segment, and follows energetic efforts on the part of the uterus to overcome some obstacle to the passage of the child. As a result of the retraction of Bandl's ring, so great a strain may be exerted upon the cervix that it is torn loose from its vaginal attachment. It is commonly taught that colpaporrhexis is possible only in those cases in which the lips of the cervix are not compressed between the presenting part and the pelvic wall, but are free to follow the retracting uterus. It sometimes occurs spontaneously, but more frequently follows ill-chosen operative procedures.

The *symptoms* are identical with those following rupture of the uterus, and will be considered under that heading. Immediately following the rupture, the child may escape into the peritoneal cavity, after which the intestines may protrude into the vaginal canal, as in a case reported by Ross.

The *diagnosis* is made solely by the sense of touch, as the clinical symptoms do not differ from those following rupture of the uterus. The prognosis is extremely unfavourable, 60 to 75 per cent of the cases reported in the literature having ended fatally.

Most authorities recommend treating the condition by means of a vaginal pack, a procedure which probably explains in part the high mortality. Everke recommends repairing the rupture through the vagina after extracting the child. I am inclined to agree with Schick that laparotomy offers the best chance for successfully coping with this emergency, since in this way one can obtain an accurate idea of the extent of the injury, when it may sometimes be possible to unite the torn surfaces by sutures, or, failing that, to remove the uterus.

Lesions of the Cervix.—Slight degrees of cervical laceration must be regarded as an inevitable accompaniment of childbirth. Such tears, however, heal rapidly and rarely give rise to symptoms. In healing they cause a material change in the shape of the external os, and thereby afford us a means of determining whether a woman has borne children or not.

In other cases the tears are deeper, not infrequently implicating one or both sides of the cervix and extending as far upward as the vaginal junction. In rarer instances the laceration may extend across the vaginal fornix or into the lower uterine segment, and occasionally open up the base of the broad ligament. Such extensive lesions usually involve vessels of considerable size, and are nearly always associated with profuse hæmorrhage.

Deep cervical tears occasionally occur during the course of spontaneous labour, and under such circumstances their genesis is not always readily explainable. More usually, however, they follow attempts at rapid manual or instrumental dilatation, especially in eclampsia, placenta prævia, and in women suffering from general œdema. Moreover, they are apt to result from attempts at delivery through an imperfectly dilated cervix, no matter whether forceps or version be employed.

Occasionally, even in spontaneous labours, the anterior lip of the cervix may be caught between the head and the symphysis pubis and compressed until it undergoes necrotic changes and separation occurs. In still rarer instances the entire vaginal portion may be torn loose from the rest of the cervix. According to Boudreau, this so-called *circular detachment of the cervix* usually occurs in elderly primiparæ when the pains are strong and a serious obstacle to delivery is offered by an imperfectly dilated os externum.

Symptoms.—In all lesions involving the cervix there is usually no escape of blood until after the birth of the child, when the hæmorrhage may be profuse. In many cases, however, the bleeding is so slight that the condition would pass unrecognised were it not detected upon an examination made for some other indication. When one lip of the entire vaginal portion of the cervix is torn off there is usually very little hæmorrhage, for the reason that the tissues have been so compressed before the occurrence of the accident that the vessels have undergone thrombosis; likewise, circular detachment of the cervix is often not followed by bleeding.

Most cervical tears heal spontaneously, provided the patient remains uninfected; but the deep wound affords to any pathogenic micro-organisms which may be present a ready port of entry into the lymphatics at the base of the broad ligament.

Diagnosis.—A deep cervical tear should always be suspected in cases of profuse hæmorrhage coming on during the third stage of labour, if the hand applied over the lower abdomen can feel that the uterus is firmly contracted. For a positive diagnosis, however, a vaginal examination is necessary, while the extent of the injury can be fully appreciated only after drawing the cervix down to the vulva and subjecting it to direct inspection.

Tears unaccompanied by hæmorrhage usually escape detection unless they are accidentally discovered during a vaginal examination made for some other reason. Annular detachment of the vaginal portion of the cervix should be diagnosed whenever an irregular mass of tissue having a circular opening is cast off before or after the birth of the child.

Treatment.—Deep cervical tears accompanied by hæmorrhage should be immediately repaired, the introduction of a few sutures readily checking the flow of blood. On the other hand, if the condition is not associated with hæmorrhage, it is advisable to leave the patient alone rather than subject her to the manipulations necessary for its repair, which inevitably expose her to additional risks of infection. Moreover, in the majority of such tears spontaneous healing ensues, and in the exceptional cases in which this does not occur, better results are usually obtained by a secondary operation performed in the latter part of the puerperium.

The treatment of cervical tears associated with hæmorrhage varies with the extent of the lesion. When the laceration is limited to the cervix, or

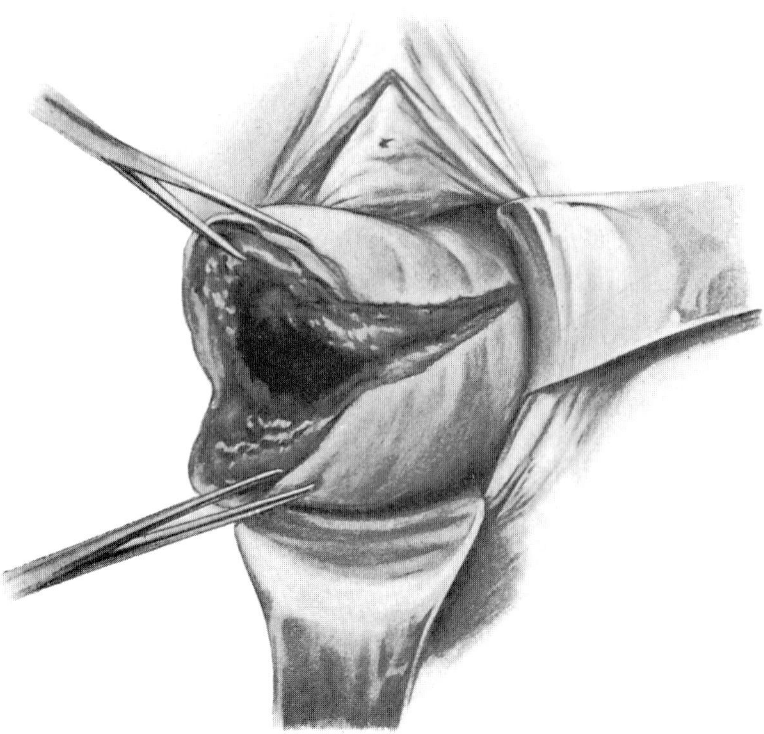

Fig. 619.—Lacerated Cervix drawn down to Vulva, Preparatory to Repair (Bumm).

even when it extends well into the vaginal fornix, most satisfactory results are obtained by the introduction of sutures after bringing the cervix into view at the vulva. This is effected by having an assistant make firm downward pressure upon the uterus, while at the same time the operator exerts strong traction by means of a bullet forceps inserted into either lip of the cervix, the vaginal walls, if necessary, being held apart by means of suitable retractors (Fig. 619). As the hæmorrhage usually comes from the upper angle of the wound, it is advisable to apply the first suture in this situation, since if the suturing is begun at the free end of the tear, a dead space is often left towards its upper end from which subsequent hæmorrhage may occur. Either silkworm or catgut sutures may be employed. The beginner is cautioned against too great a regard for appearances and attempting to give the cervix too normal a look, inasmuch as the retraction occurring within the next few days may lead to such constriction of its lumen as to cause retention of the lochial discharge.

Many authorities recommend a tight vaginal pack in this class of cases. This will usually check the hæmorrhage and may be employed in an emergency, but its employment does not compare in efficiency with repair by suture. In the rare cases in which the wound extends through the broad ligament into the peritoneal cavity, a tight pack may be introduced, provided there is no serious hæmorrhage; but in all other cases the only satisfactory method of dealing with the condition is by laparotomy.

The treatment of tears of the upper part of the cervix which involve the lower uterine segment will be considered when we take up the treatment of rupture of the uterus.

Rupture of the Uterus.—This accident, which is one of the most serious with which the obstetrician can be confronted, seldom occurs except in prolonged labours, although instances of spontaneous rupture during pregnancy are on record.

(*a*) *During Pregnancy.*—Reference has already been made to rupture which occurs during the course of gestation, in a rudimentary horn of a bicornuate uterus or in the interstitial portion of the Fallopian tube, as well as to the exceptional cases in which the uterine scar following Cæsarean section gives way in a subsequent pregnancy, and its mode of production is readily understood.

On the other hand, the ætiological factors concerned in spontaneous rupture of the apparently normal pregnant uterus are not so readily explained, many causes having been invoked, but none are of universal application. Thus, in some instances, the accident may be attributed to faulty hypertrophy of the uterine wall in the fundal region. Alexandroff, Jellinghaus, and others are inclined to attribute certain cases to inherent weakness of the uterine walls resulting from the excessive formation of connective tissue following the manual removal of an adherent placenta in previous pregnancies. Herzfeld holds that in one of his cases the accident was due to anatomical changes following curettage in a previous pregnancy. Poroschin considers that he was able to demonstrate in certain cases a faulty development or relative absence of the elastic-tissue fibres which are normally present in the uterine walls. All the possibilities which have been suggested in this connection have been considered in detail by Sänger, and while some of them are applicable to a certain number of cases, it is impossible to offer a satisfactory explanation for others. Blind, after the study of 22 cases reported in the literature, states that the rupture nearly always occurs in the upper part of the uterus, usually in the neighbourhood of the fundus.

The symptoms, diagnosis, prognosis, and treatment of this condition are identical with those following rupture of the uterus occurring at the time of labour. It should be noted, however, that in a number of the cases reported in the literature the hæmorrhage following the accident was so slight as not to give rise to symptoms, the condition escaping recognition until operative procedures became necessary for the removal of the fœtus lying free in the abdominal cavity.

In several instances, as in the cases reported by Leopold and Henrotin, the placenta remained in the uterus, while the fœtus, surrounded by its membranes, escaped into the peritoneal cavity, where it went on to further development—*utero-abdominal pregnancy.* Such an occurrence is very exceptional, as it is usually synonymous with fœtal death.

(*b*) *Rupture of the Uterus at the Time of Labour.*—This not very infrequent accident is one of the most serious complications of labour, as it nearly always leads to the death of the fœtus, and frequently to that of the mother as well.

Ætiology.—Practically we are indebted to Bandl for the first clear explanation as to the mode of its production, its ætiology being inseparably connected with the doctrine of the lower uterine segment and the formation of the contraction ring.

Normally, under the influence of labour pains the uterus becomes differentiated into two portions, separated by a circular ridge of tissue, to which the term *contraction ring* is usually applied. The upper, by its contractions, serves to expel the child, while the lower undergoes dilatation and merely forms part of the canal through which the contents of the uterus are forced. On the other hand, when a serious obstacle is opposed to the passage of the child, the active portion of the uterus is stimulated to more forcible efforts. As it contracts it likewise slowly becomes retracted, its lower margin—the contraction ring—eventually occupying a much higher level than usual. As a result, particularly if the lips of the cervix are caught between the presenting part and the superior strait, powerful upward traction is exerted upon the passive portion of the uterus, which becomes more and more stretched, and thinner and thinner. At the same time the contraction ring separating the two portions becomes thicker and more prominent, so that it can readily be distinguished as a transverse or oblique ridge extending across the abdomen just below or perhaps on a level with the umbilicus. The round ligaments, likewise, are subjected to an abnormal strain and remain tense even in the intervals between the uterine contractions.

As the process goes on the lower segment becomes extremely sensitive to pressure, the uterine contractions increase progressively in frequency and intensity, and cause the patient greater suffering. The pulse becomes more rapid, and the patient presents a worn and haggard appearance. Such a condition indicates that rupture is imminent and will occur unless delivery is promptly effected in a conservative manner.

Generally speaking, rupture is more apt to take place when one side of the lower uterine segment is subjected to greater stretching than the other. In transverse presentations this condition is most marked on the side of the uterus occupied by the head. A similar danger threatens the posterior wall when the child presents by the head and the patient has a markedly pendulous abdomen.

Excessive stretching of the lower uterine segment, and consequent danger of rupture, is favoured by any factor which interferes with the birth of the child, and more particularly with the entrance of the presenting part into the pelvis. Such conditions are most frequently afforded by contracted pelves, neglected transverse presentations, hydrocephalus, excessive size of the child, and, in fact, by any obstacle to labour. The following analysis by Merz shows the ætiological factors concerned in the production of 160 cases of rupture of the uterus:

Contracted pelvis	70
Neglected transverse presentation	26
Hydrocephalus	18
Large child or unfavourable presentation	10
Stenosis of birth canal	6
Trauma	5
Pelvic tumour	3
Ascites	1
Operative procedures	21

It is customary to distinguish between *spontaneous* and *violent rupture* of the uterus. In the former the accident occurs spontaneously, while in the latter it is usually the result of ill-judged manipulations on the part of the obstetrician in a uterus whose lower segment is so thinned out and distended that the slightest violence proves too much for its resistive powers.

Violent rupture occurs relatively frequently when version is attempted in neglected transverse presentations. The proper treatment of this class of cases requires the utmost nicety of judgment, as it is ofttimes extremely difficult to determine whether the lower uterine segment is so thinned out as to contra-indicate attempts at version, the operation having been readily accomplished under anæsthesia in some cases in which, at first sight, it had appeared impracticable; whereas in others, in which it seemed that the necessary manipulations would be without danger, rupture followed the mere introduction of the hand. Moreover, there is a marked difference in the rapidity with which overstretching of the lower uterine segment comes about, the condition supervening very rapidly in some cases, while in others many hours of strong, second-stage pains may be necessary for its production.

Certain women seem to possess a predisposition towards rupture of the uterus, this assumption being supported by the fact that not a few cases of repeated rupture appear in the literature. Thus, Mikhine found records of 13 patients, 6 of whom died as a result of a second rupture, and Peham has likewise reported similar instances. It is quite likely that under such circumstances the second rupture occurs in tissues already weakened by the previous accident.

Pathology.—Rupture of the uterus occurring at the time of labour is limited almost entirely to the lower uterine segment, the rent usually pursuing an oblique direction; although when it is in the immediate vicinity of the cervix it frequently extends transversely. On the other hand, it is usually longitudinal when it occurs in the portion of the uterus adjacent to the broad ligament.

It is customary to distinguish between *complete* and *incomplete rupture,* according as the laceration communicates directly with the peritoneal cavity or is separated from it by the perineal covering of the uterus or broad ligament. The former is apparently the more common, Merz having collected 118 complete as against 46 incomplete ruptures. Koblanck noted 58 and 24 respectively in 80 cases occurring in the Berlin Frauenklinik.

Incomplete ruptures not infrequently extend into the broad ligament; under such circumstances the hæmorrhage often occurs less rapidly than

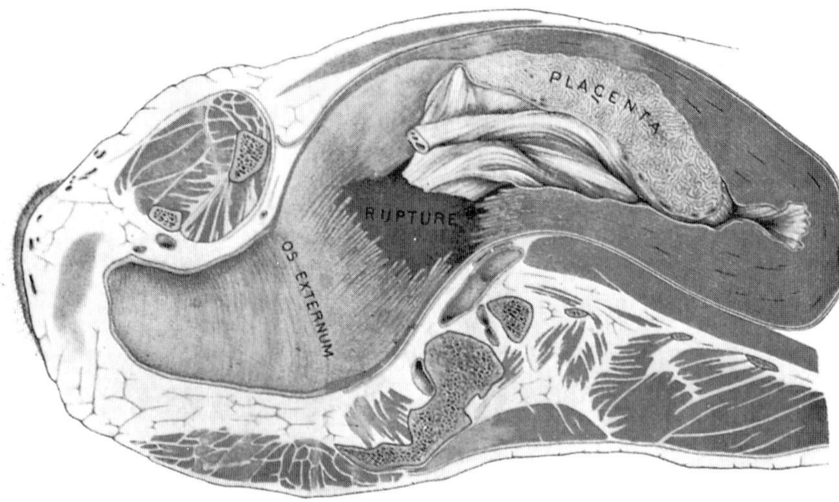

FIG. 620.—LONGITUDINAL SECTION THROUGH WOMAN DYING FROM RUPTURE OF THE UTERUS (Zweifel).

in the complete variety, the blood slowly accumulating between the leaflets and leading to the separation of the peritonæum from the surrounding viscera, with the consequent formation of a large *subperitoneal hæmatoma.* Occasionally, a hæmorrhage sufficiently copious to cause the death of the patient may remain inclosed between the structures. More frequently, however, the fatal issue does not occur until rupture of the hæmatoma into the peritoneal cavity relieves the pressure which had previously, to some extent, restrained the bleeding.

Although the rupture occurs primarily in the lower uterine segment, it is not unusual for the laceration to extend further upward into the body of the uterus or downward through the cervix into the vagina, primary lesions of the uterine body, as a rule, being observed only in the cases of spontaneous rupture occurring during pregnancy. The tear itself usually presents jagged, irregular margins which are stained with blood.

Following complete rupture, the uterine contents may escape into the peritoneal cavity, while in the incomplete variety they may come to lie beneath the serous covering of the uterus or between the leaflets of the broad ligament. In a certain number of cases of either variety, however, particularly when the presenting part is firmly engaged at the time of rupture, only a portion of the fœtus escapes, the rest remaining in the uterine cavity.

Symptoms.—The symptoms of actual rupture vary considerably. As a rule, the patient, after presenting for some time the premonitory signs of the accident, suddenly, at the height of an intense uterine contraction or during an intra-uterine manipulation, complains of a sharp, shooting pain in the lower abdomen, and frequently cries out that something has given way inside of her. At the same time the lower uterine segment becomes much more sensitive to pressure. Immediately following these symptoms there is an absolute cessation of the uterine contractions, and the patient, who has previously been in intense agony, suddenly experiences marked relief. At the same time there is usually more or less external hæmorrhage, though not uncommonly it is very slight in amount.

Palpation or vaginal examination shows that the presenting part has slipped away from the superior strait and has become movable, while a hard, round body, which represents the firmly contracted uterus, can be felt alongside of the fœtus. Naturally, if the uterine contents have escaped into the abdominal cavity, the presenting part cannot be felt on vaginal examination.

As a rule, shortly after the occurrence of complete rupture, the patient presents symptoms of collapse, the pulse increases markedly in rapidity, loses tone, and takes on a filiform character, the face becomes pallid, assumes a drawn appearance, and is often covered with beads of sweat. If the hæmorrhage has been copious, she may complain of chilliness, disturbances of vision, and air hunger, and eventually pass into an unconscious state.

Symptoms of collapse, however, do not always appear immediately, but are sometimes deferred for several hours after rupture, being less marked when the child remains partially within the uterus. After incomplete rupture, on the other hand, the immediate symptoms are sometimes very slight, but increase in severity as the subperitoneal hæmatoma becomes larger, while actual symptoms of collapse frequently do not appear until secondary rupture into the peritoneal cavity has taken place.

In a certain number of cases of incomplete rupture, emphysematous crackling can be elicited in the tissues of the anterior abdominal wall, 14 cases of this character having been collected by Dischler. It would appear probable that the condition is usually due to the invasion of the subperitoneal connective tissue by Bacillus aerogenes capsulatus. It is true that bacteriological proof has not been adduced in support of this statement, but the fact that the women had been in labour for many hours, and that many of the children were more or less putrefied, speaks strongly in favour of such a view.

Diagnosis.—The diagnosis is usually easy, especially in the cases in which the accident occurs while the patient is under supervision. If she is not seen until later, the characteristic history and the collapse are almost pathognomonic, the only other conditions in which the latter is noted before delivery being the cases of hæmorrhage following the rupture of an advanced extra-uterine pregnancy, or the premature separation of the normally implanted placenta.

If the child has escaped into the abdominal cavity, it is much more readily felt on palpation than usual, while on one side of it the hard, rounded body of the uterus can be detected. Moreover, vaginal examination frequently reveals the existence of a tear in the uterine wall through which the fingers can be passed into the abdominal cavity, where they come in contact with the intestines. Again, the fact that the presenting part cannot be felt is conclusive evidence that the fœtus has escaped from the uterus.

Prognosis.—The chances for the child are almost uniformly bad, since it frequently succumbs before the occurrence of the accident. On the other hand, if it has survived up to that time, its only chance of living is afforded by immediate extraction, asphyxia, the result of the separation of the placenta, being otherwise inevitable. If left to themselves, the vast majority of the mothers die from hæmorrhage or infection, although spontaneous recovery has been noted in exceptional cases.

Death from hæmorrhage usually occurs within the first few hours, though occasionally it may be deferred for forty-eight hours; in infection the fatal termination does not occur for some days.

Spontaneous recovery is least likely to occur when the child has escaped into the abdominal cavity, though isolated instances are on record in which the patient has survived even such an accident. Under such circumstances the child dies, and may then undergo any one of the several eventualities mentioned in the chapter on Extra-Uterine Pregnancy. So far as the women are concerned, even if they are properly treated, the mortality is very high, at least one third succumbing.

Treatment.—(*a*) *Prophylactic.*—Intelligent care of the lying-in woman should almost entirely do away with this accident. Whenever there is a possibility of the existence of an obstacle to the birth of the child, the obstetrician should always be on the alert for symptoms indicative of impending rupture. Transverse presentations should be promptly delivered by version as soon as the cervix is fully dilated; in head presentations failure of engagement after one hour of strong second-stage pains should be regarded with suspicion, and if the contraction ring rises up labour should be promptly terminated by the most conservative procedure. In neglected cases, decapitation in transverse and craniotomy in head presentations often promise the best results. Such procedures are the more justifiable under the circumstances, as the children are usually either already dead or exposed to such danger that their chances of being delivered alive are very slight.

(*b*) *Curative.*—If the child is still within the uterus, delivery should be promptly effected by the natural passages in the most conservative manner possible. On the other hand, if it has already escaped into the abdominal cavity, laparotomy should be performed, and followed, after removal of the child, by whatever operative procedures may be deemed necessary—suture of the tear, supravaginal amputation, or total removal of the uterus.

On the other hand, in the cases which are not seen until the child has already been delivered *per vaginam*, and in which the uterine rupture was not recognised until after its birth, various procedures have been suggested by different authorities.

Personally, I believe that the best results will follow laparotomy, no matter what the character of the tear or whether the patient is suffering from hæmorrhage or not, for the reason that it is ofttimes difficult to determine the extent of the laceration, and that it is absolutely impossible to foretell whether the hæmorrhage can be checked by simple procedures; and, even if these succeed, whether the result will be permanent. Fritsch is correct in stating that the only method by which we can assure ourselves against all further risk of hæmorrhage is by opening the abdomen. Varnier takes a similar view as the result of his experience in 23 cases, and holds that laparotomy should be resorted to whenever practicable.

On the other hand, certain authorities argue that, inasmuch as the danger to be apprehended in incomplete rupture is from hæmorrhage rather than sepsis, laparotomy should be performed only in those cases in which the loss of blood is profuse, and that in all others equally good if not better results may be obtained by draining or packing the rupture from the vagina. Such a procedure, however, would not appear rational, for not infrequently women, who are apparently in excellent condition shortly after the occurrence of the rupture, begin to bleed profusely some hours later, and are then in danger of dying before operative procedures can be carried out.

Schmit reports 83 cases treated by packing or drainage, and 32 by laparotomy, with a mortality of 48 and 75 per cent respectively; while Klien has collected a series of 125 and 149 cases, with a respective mortality of 39 and 44 per cent. The latter states that the mortality was only 17 per cent in the cases which were treated exclusively by drainage. He therefore concludes that laparotomy is justifiable only in those cases in which hæmorrhage is persistent and cannot be checked by other measures. Varnier, on the contrary, states that out of 11 cases in his experience which were treated by packing, 10 died; whereas 3 of the 6 patients operated upon recovered, 6 others dying before operative procedures could be instituted. The statistics thus far adduced can hardly be regarded as conclusive, inasmuch as it is probable that many of the cases were seen and operated upon only as a last resort.

Instrumental Perforation of the Uterus.—Reference has already been made to perforation of the uterus following attempts at criminal abortion or in the effort to remove placental tissue by means of the curette or polypus forceps, after an incomplete abortion. Similar accidents likewise occasionally occur as the result of want of skill on the part of the obstetrician in full-term labour. As has already been pointed out, not infrequently, in cases of this character, loops of intestine prolapse through the rupture. Under such circumstances laparotomy is the ideal treatment, though in the absence of prolapse of the intestines cases are recorded in which recovery occurred spontaneously under what were apparently most unfavourable circumstances.

Perforation of the Genital Tract following Necrosis.—In obstructed labour the tissues in various portions of the genital tract may be forcibly compressed between the head and the bony canal. If the pressure is transitory it is without significance; but if it is long continued, necrosis results, and after a few days the area implicated sloughs away so that perforation follows.

In most cases of this character the perforation occurs between the vagina and the bladder, giving rise to a *vesico-vaginal fistula*. Less frequently the anterior lip of the cervix is compressed against the symphysis pubis, and an abnormal communication is eventually established between the cervical canal and the bladder—*cervico-vesical fistula*.

If the patient is not infected, the fistulous tract frequently heals without further treatment. In other cases, however, it may persist, when a subsequent plastic operation becomes necessary for its cure.

Occasionally, the posterior wall of the uterus may be subjected to so much pressure against the promontory of the sacrum that necrosis results, and a connection is established with Douglas's *cul-de-sac*. If infection occurs, the accident is usually followed by septic peritonitis. Fortunately, recovery usually follows without further complications, inasmuch as a localized peritonitis leads to the formation of adhesions between the posterior wall of the uterus and the pelvic peritonæum, thereby doing away with the possibility of a general peritoneal infection. It should be remembered that similar lesions may occur in the rare cases in which exostoses or bony spicules protrude from the walls of the birth canal, as in *pelvis spinosa*.

LITERATURE

Alexandroff. Ein Fall von Uterusruptur während der Schwangerschaft. Monatsschr. f. Geb. u. Gyn., 1900, xii, 447–457.

Bandl. Ueber Ruptur des Uterus und ihre Mechanik. Wien, 1875.

Blind. Beitrag zur Aetiologie der Uterusruptur während der Schwangerschaft und unter der Geburt. D. I., Strassburg, 1892.

Boudreau. L'arrachement circulaire du col utérin pendant l'accouchement. Thèse de Toulouse, 1902.

Dischler. Ueber subperitoneales Emphysem nach Ruptura uteri. Archiv f. Gyn., 1898, lvi, 199–217.

Everke. Ueber Kolpaporrhexis in der Geburt. Monatsschr. f. Geb. u. Gyn, 1898, vii, 233–239.

Fritsch. Ueber die Behandlung der Uterusruptur. Verh. d. deutschen Gesell. f. Gyn., 1895, 1–19.

Henrotin. Utero-abdominal Gestation. The Practice of Obstetrics by American Authors, 1899, 386.

Herzfeld. Ruptur des schwangeren Uterus. Centralbl. f. Gyn., 1901, 1219–1227.

Hugenberger. Ueber Kolpaporrhexis in der Geburt. Petersburger med. Zeitschr., 1875, v, Heft 5, 26.

Jellinghaus. Ueber Uterusrupturen während der Schwangerschaft. Archiv f. Gyn., 1897, liv, 103–116.

Kaufmann. Ueber die Zerreissung des Scheidengewölbes während der Geburt. Monatsschr. f. Geb. u. Gyn., 1901, xiii, 464–470.

KLIEN. Die operative und nicht operative Behandlung der Uterusruptur. Archiv f. Gyn., 1900, lxii, Heft 2.

KOBLANCK. Beitrag zur Lehre von der Ruptura uteri. Stuttgart, 1895.

LEOPOLD. Ausgetragene secundäre Abdominalschwangerschaft nach Ruptura uteri traumatica, etc. Archiv f. Gyn., 1896, lii, 376–388.

MERZ. Zur Behandlung der Uterusruptur. Archiv f. Gyn., 1894, xlv, 181–271.

MIKHINE. Un cas de récidive de rupture utérine. Annales de Gyn. et d'Obst., 1902, lvii, 403–410.

PEHAM. Ueber Uterusrupturen in Narben. Centralbl. f. Gyn., 1902, 87–94.

POROSCHIN. Zur Aetiologie der spontanen Uterusruptur während Schwangerschaft und Geburt. Centralbl. f. Gyn., 1898, 183.

ROSS. Lacerated and Punctured Wounds of the Genital Tract. Amer. Jour. Obst., 1898, xxxvii, 449–469.

SÄNGER. Ruptura uteri. Verh. der deutschen Gesell. f. Gyn., 1895, 19–86.

SCHICK. Zerreissung des Scheidengewölbes während der Geburt. Prager med. Wochenschr., 1893, Nr. 29–30.

SCHMIT. Ein Beitrag zur Therapie der Uterusruptur. Monatsschr. f. Geb. u. Gyn., 1900, xii, 325–342.

SCHTSCHOTKIN. Quoted by Kaufmann.

VARNIER. Du traitement des ruptures de l'utérus. Annales de Gyn. et d'Obst., 1901, lvi, 249–279.

CHAPTER XLIII

PROLAPSE OF THE UMBILICAL CORD—ASPHYXIA NEONATORUM —SUDDEN DEATH DURING LABOUR

Prolapse of the Umbilical Cord.—It is customary to distinguish between *presentation* and *prolapse of the funis* or umbilical cord. In the former the cord can be palpated through the intact membranes, while in the latter a loop of it protrudes through the cervix into the vagina, and exceptionally emerges from the vulva.

Ætiology.—In general it may be said that any factor which interferes with the accurate adaptation of the presenting part to the lower uterine segment predisposes to prolapse of the cord. Accordingly, the accident occurs most commonly in transverse and foot, and less often in frank breech presentations. On the other hand, it is rarely observed when the child presents by the head, unless accommodation is interfered with as a result of a contracted pelvis, excessive development of the fœtus, hydramnios, or abnormal flaccidity of the lower uterine segment. For this reason it is much more common in multiparous than in primiparous women.

Symptoms.—Prolapse of the cord is without appreciable effect upon the course of labour so far as the mother is concerned. On the other hand, it is one of the most frequent causes of fœtal death, compression between the presenting part and the pelvic wall interfering with the circulation to such an extent that asphyxia and inevitable death often follow unless prompt delivery is effected. The danger is greater in vertex than in other presentations, for the reason that there is less likelihood that the cord will escape compression when the pelvic canal is filled out by the hard, rounded head than by the softer and more irregularly shaped part in other presentations.

Diagnosis.—Presentation of the funis is diagnosed when on palpation a soft, pulsating cord-like body can be felt through the membranes. In many instances, however, its recognition is only possible when the cord is in direct contact with the presenting part.

Prolapse of the cord, on the other hand, is readily recognised, since on vaginal examination the fingers come directly in contact with a loop, while exceptionally the structure may protrude from the vulva. Mistakes are hardly possible if the fœtus is alive, as distinct pulsations are felt, although in their absence the condition is sometimes overlooked on superficial examination.

The possibility of prolapse of the cord should be particularly borne in mind in multiparous women in whom the membranes rupture while the head is still freely movable above the superior strait. In such cases the sudden cessation of the fœtal heart-beat renders the diagnosis almost certain, even without vaginal examination.

Treatment.—The treatment to be pursued in any given case depends mainly upon the degree to which the cervix is dilated, and to a lesser extent upon the presentation. So long as the membranes remain intact there is no immediate danger of compression, and for this reason every precaution should be taken to avoid their premature rupture, vaginal examinations being made with the utmost gentleness. At the same time the obstetrician should hold himself in readiness to effect delivery as soon as the cervix is sufficiently dilated.

If the membranes have already ruptured, provided dilatation is complete and the child presents by the head, its life can often be saved by prompt delivery, which can usually be effected more rapidly by version than by forceps, unless the head is already deep down in the pelvic canal. In breech presentations, a foot should be brought down and followed immediately by extraction. In transverse presentations version is indicated.

On the other hand, when the cervix is only partially dilated, the chances of a favourable outcome for the child are markedly diminished. If the head is not deeply engaged the patient should be placed in the knee-chest position, the entire hand introduced into the vagina, and an attempt made to push the cord up into the uterus and, if possible, to carry it over some projecting portion of the child's body. If the cord remains in the uterus the patient should be made to lie upon the side towards which the child's back is directed in the hope of avoiding compression.

In the majority of cases, however, the prolapse recurs again as soon as the hand is removed. Under such circumstances an improvised repositor will sometimes serve us in good stead, although the results attending the use of such devices are often unsatisfactory. A piece of bobbin is firmly attached to the free end of a sterile bougie or catheter in such a manner as to leave a loop several inches long. This is then passed around the prolapsed cord and slipped over the tip of the bougie. By this means the cord can readily be carried up into the uterus, after which it may be freed from the repositor by bringing the loop in contact with a portion of the child and making traction upon it so as to cause it to slip off from the tip of the bougie. In the great majority of cases the condition recurs as soon as the repositor is removed; to insure against any risk of such an accident, the bougie may be left in the uterus.

Occasionally the tendency to prolapse may be overcome by placing the patient in the knee-chest position until engagement of the presenting part occurs, when the cord cannot get past it. In most cases, however, these manœuvres prove ineffectual, and the death of the child becomes almost inevitable in vertex, and only somewhat less so in breech and transverse presentations.

In exceptional cases, if the child is in good condition, excellent results may be obtained by manual dilatation of the cervix, followed by prompt version and extraction. On the other hand, if the pulsations in the cord are weak or have ceased altogether, such a procedure should never be adopted, inasmuch as the child has either already perished or will die before delivery can be effected. If, however, the cervix is fully dilated, such limitations do not hold good, as occasionally a child that is apparently hopelessly lost may be rescued.

Asphyxia.—Normally, the fœtus while it remains in the uterus is in a condition of apnœa, being satisfactorily supplied with oxygen by means of the placental circulation. As soon as delivery occurs, owing to the separation of the placenta or to a great diminution in its area of attachment, this source of oxygen is entirely cut off, or so greatly reduced that the necessity for active respiration arises. Generally speaking, imperfect oxygenation should be considered as the primary factor in the establishment of this function, although numerous accessory causes come into play during the act of delivery and just after birth.

Exceptionally, as the result of the death of the mother, compression of the prolapsed cord, premature separation of the placenta, or much less commonly of tetanic contraction of the uterus, the normal supply of properly aerated blood through the umbilical vessels may be cut off or interfered with while the child is still within the uterus. Occasionally, a similar condition may be brought about by compression against the symphysis of a cord which is wrapped around the neck of the child, while now and again asphyxia and even death may result when the head is on the perinæum, owing to excessive retraction of the active segment of the uterus, with a consequent diminution in the area of placental attachment.

As a result of the action of any of these factors, the child may take its first breath while still in the uterus or in the lower portion of the birth canal. In the former case it draws a certain quantity of amniotic fluid into its lungs, unless such an eventuality is rendered impossible by the fact that the mouth and nose are closely applied to the uterine wall or are covered by the fœtal membranes. When respiration begins while the head is in the vagina, a certain amount of mucus is liable to be aspirated. In either event the needed oxygen is not obtained, and the resulting air hunger leads to increased respiratory efforts, which are nevertheless of no avail. Gradually the accumulation of carbon dioxide and other excrementitious materials in the fœtal organism leads to such a pronounced decrease in the irritability of the medulla, that eventually the attempts at respiration cease, the intervals between the pulsations of the heart become longer and longer, and the child dies from asphyxia.

Again, pressure exerted upon the brain in difficult labours and operative procedures may lead to vagus irritation and consequent slowing of the heart. As a result of the interference with the fœtal circulation, the blood becomes poorer in oxygen and richer in excrementitious material; this goes on until at last the irritability of the medulla becomes so lowered that the usual stimuli fail to call forth the first respiratory movement and asphyxia results.

The most frequent causes of cerebral compression are attempts on the part of the uterus to force the head through a contracted superior strait, excessive pressure exerted by the blades of the forceps, and intra-cranial hæmorrhage. When limited to the cerebral hemispheres, a very considerable effusion of blood may occur without exerting a deleterious effect upon the fœtus; but if the base of the brain is implicated a much smaller amount may give rise to serious disturbances.

Diagnosis.—The importance of watching for manifestations pointing to threatened intra-uterine asphyxia cannot be overestimated, inasmuch as their recognition frequently affords the indication for operative delivery, without which the life of the child is inevitably lost.

The most characteristic symptom is afforded by changes in the fœtal pulse-rate. At first, as a result of momentary compression of the brain or interference with the placental circulation, it becomes slower with each uterine contraction, but regains its normal frequency in the intervals between the pains. As the condition becomes more serious the remissions fail to occur, and the pulse becomes slower and slower and eventually the heart ceases to beat. For practical purposes it is well to assume that a pulse-rate of 100 or less is incompatible with prolonged life for the fœtus, and under such circumstances rapid delivery is indicated, provided it can be accomplished without too great risk for the mother. Exceptionally, the first sign of asphyxia is a marked increase in the frequency of the fœtal pulse, which may vary from 160 to 200. The acceleration, however, is only transient, and, as a rule, soon gives place to a marked slowing, which becomes still more perceptible as the fatal termination is approached.

In vertex presentations another characteristic sign of impending asphyxia is the escape of meconium. This is due to relaxation of the sphincter ani muscle induced by faulty aeration of the blood. In breech presentations, of course, this symptom is without significance, and is to be regarded as a purely mechanical result of pressure applied to the abdomen of the fœtus. Accordingly, whenever the amniotic fluid in a vertex presentation presents a yellowish-green appearance and contains flakes of meconium, we may conclude that the child is in danger, and that the only hope for its safety lies in prompt delivery.

Especially in difficult breech extractions, when delay is experienced in delivering the head, signs of asphyxia may appear in a child which was apparently in excellent condition before the operation. Under such circumstances the finger in the child's mouth can readily appreciate the fact that vigorous inspiratory movements are being made. A similar phenomenon may occasionally be observed in vertex presentations, when the head is arrested on the pelvic floor, the movements of the mouth being felt or seen through the thinned-out perinæum.

Very exceptionally the child may not only make inspiratory efforts, but actually give utterance to sounds *in utero*—*vagitus uterinus.* For the production of this phenomenon it is essential that air gain access to the fœtus, its entrance into the uterus sometimes resulting from the introduction of the hand or instruments. A very characteristic example of this phenomenon has been recorded by Gummert, who has collated most of the recent literature bearing upon the subject.

After delivery, the asphyxiated child may present one of two appearances—*asphyxia pallida* or *asphyxia livida.* In both respiration is in abeyance or occurs only in gasps, while the heart beats slowly and feebly. In the former the surface of the body is pale and cold, the extremities hang limp, and the child fails to respond to the usual external stimuli. In the latter, on the other hand, it presents a congested or livid appearance, which is usually attributed to overdistention of the right heart and the inferior vena cava. This form of asphyxia is usually more amenable to treatment than the pallid variety.

Prognosis.—Asphyxia neonatorum is always serious. The prognosis is relatively favourable when the condition is due to mechanical interference with the placental circulation, but is far less so when it results from injuries to the brain, such as intra-cranial hæmorrhage, fractures, or depressions of the skull.

Treatment.—Normally, the child should make its first inspiratory movement a few moments after it emerges from the vulva. If this does not occur, the feet being grasped by the fingers of one hand and the child suspended with its head downward, its body should be slapped vigorously with the other. If this manœuvre does not prove immediately successful, and particularly if attempts at respiration are associated with a gurgling sound, a finger should be passed to the back of the pharynx for the purpose of removing any foreign material which may interfere with the free access of air to the laryngeal opening. Ordinarily, if the child is not deeply asphyxiated, these measures will bring about the desired results; but if they fail, artificial respiration should at once be instituted, the child's thorax being compressed 5 or 6 times to the minute.

In some instances, however, more radical measures will be found necessary. In such cases the cord should be ligated and cut through, and the child immersed in hot and cold water alternately, with only its head protruding, and rubbed vigorously. If there is any reason to believe that the bronchial tubes contain mucus or amniotic fluid, a small, soft-rubber catheter should be introduced into the larynx and the offending material removed by suction exerted by the obstetrician, or by the employment of a Ribemont-Dessaignes insufflator.

If these measures do not lead to the establishment of respiration, the child should be wrapped in a piece of blanket or flannel, to prevent too rapid cooling, and laid upon a table or chair, the head being allowed to hang over the edge. The tip of the tongue is then grasped by a small pair of artery forceps and drawn forward as far as possible and then allowed to recede, the manœuvre being repeated at regular intervals 10 or 15 times to the minute. After the first few tractions, an inspiratory movement usually follows, after which respiration goes on regularly. This procedure, known as *Laborde's method of resuscitation*, is based upon the principle that traction upon the tongue irritates the fibres of the superior laryngeal, glossopharyngeal and lingual nerves, which in turn give rise to a reflex stimulation of the phrenic nerves with consequent contraction of the diaphragm and the intercostal muscles. Generally speaking, it is the most effective measure at our disposal, and the prognosis becomes extremely gloomy if its employment is not attended by satisfactory results within a few minutes. Occasionally its efficiency may be heightened by practising it with the child immersed in a hot bath.

Before, however, despairing of saving the child's life, recourse may be had to *Schultze's method.* In this manœuvre, as shown in Figs. 621 and 622, the child is seized by both hands in such a manner that the index fingers of the operator lie under its axillæ, the thumbs over the thorax, while the palmar surfaces of the remaining fingers are applied to its back, the head at the same time being fixed by the balls of the thumbs. The obstetrician stands with his legs apart and at first allows the fœtus to hang down between them, he then slowly carries the child over his head in such a manner that the legs fall towards its face, so that the body becomes sharply flexed, after which he brings it back to its original position. The manœuvre is repeated 4 or 5 times a minute. The *rationale* of the method is readily appreciated: the thorax is markedly compressed when the child is elevated and expanded when it is lowered, the two positions favouring expiration and inspiration respectively.

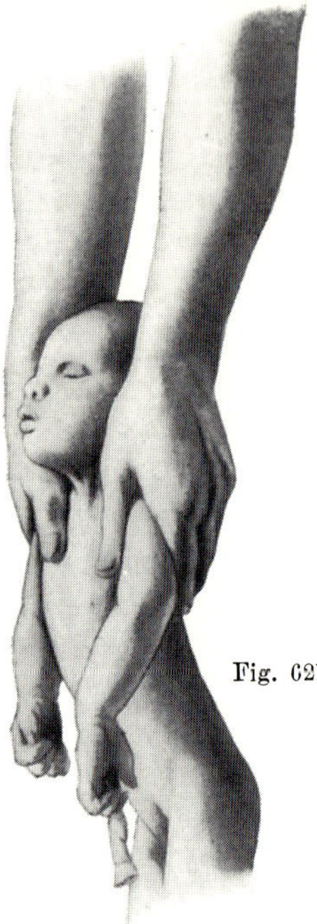

Fig. 621.

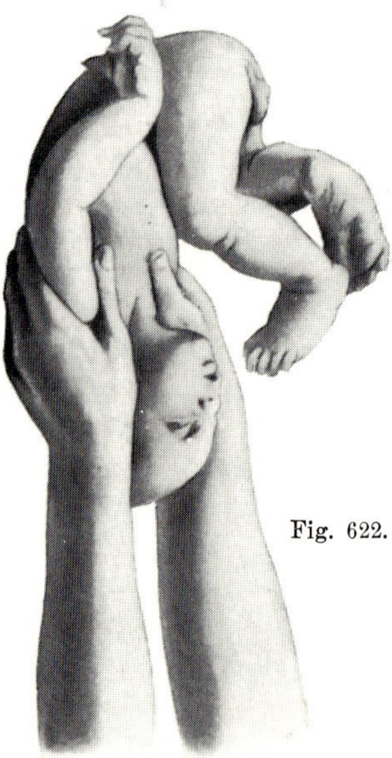

Fig. 622.

Figs. 621, 622.—Schultze's Method of Resuscitation.

Some idea of its efficiency may be gained by the fact that, when it is practised upon a dead child, air can be distinctly heard to enter and leave the lungs with each movement. The procedure, however, is not without peculiar disadvantages. In the first place, its employment sometimes gives rise to fracture of the clavicles or ribs, and occasionally to rupture of the liver or other serious lesions of the internal organs. Moreover, in view of the no small degree of violence associated with its use, the manœuvre is contra-indicated in those cases in which the clavicle or humerus have been fractured during a difficult extraction, inasmuch as the free ends of the bones are liable to cause serious injury to the soft parts.

Byrd, in 1874, suggested a convenient substitute for Schultze's method. He recommended that the back of the child be allowed to rest upon the palmar surface of both hands, the ulnar margins being almost in apposition, while the thumb of one hand is applied over the sternum and the other over the thighs. By approximating the radial margins of the hands, the operator can then bring the child's head and feet closely together, thereby compressing the thorax and causing expiration, while a movement in the opposite direction brings about extreme expansion and favours inspiration.

In obstinate cases, beneficial results sometimes follow the hypodermic injection of a few drops of whisky or ether.

When the asphyxia is the result of a depressed fracture of the skull it may be permissible to make a small perforation through which the blade of a pair of scissors or some other suitable instrument is introduced, and an effort made to replace the depressed portion and thus remove the source of compression. Such an operation, however, should be attempted only when other procedures have failed, and provided that the heart still continues to beat strongly, though slowly.

Efforts at resuscitation should be persevered in as long as the heart continues to beat, one method after another being given a trial. The necessity for persistence is shown by the fact that successful results are not unusual after trials lasting for thirty to sixty minutes, or even longer.

Sudden Death during or shortly after Labour.—Ordinarily, death occurring during labour, or in the first few hours immediately following it, is the result of some one of the abnormalities to which allusion has already been made, particularly acute œdema of the lungs or apoplexy complicating eclampsia, or acute anæmia the result of post-partum hæmorrhage, placenta prævia, premature separation of the normally implanted placenta, or rupture of the genital canal.

In rare instances, incomplete rupture of the uterus is unattended by symptoms at the time of its occurrence, the blood slowly accumulating between the folds of the broad ligament with a gradual development of symptoms of shock. A subperitoneal hæmatoma formed in this way is liable to rupture into the peritoneal cavity at any time within the first forty-eight hours after delivery and lead to sudden death.

Moreover, a woman in labour, or during the puerperium, may die suddenly from the effects of any condition which would give rise to a similar outcome under other circumstances. Thus, cases have been reported in which the fatal termination was due to rupture of an aortic or cardiac aneurysm, hæmorrhage from a gastric ulcer, or other accidents. Van der Velde has reported a case of a fatal retro-peritoneal hæmorrhage complicating an acute pancreatitis, while Node and Hines observed sudden death during labour following the rupture of an aneurysm of the splenic artery.

In the chapter dealing with the Pathology of Pregnancy reference was made to the consequences of labour in women suffering from valvular lesions of the heart, particularly stenosis of the mitral orifice. Less frequently, sudden death may be due to fatty degeneration or to changes in the myocardium. Such accidents are to be particularly dreaded in elderly and corpulent women.

Shock.—Formerly it was customary to attribute a certain number of deaths following labour to shock, which was supposed to occur in certain individuals after prolonged and very painful labours, the incidental loss of rest, imperfect nutrition, and mental excitement being looked upon as predisposing causes. In the present state of our knowledge, however, this explanation is hardly permissible, since in the majority of such cases a carefully performed autopsy will reveal the existence of some condition sufficiently serious to account for the unfavourable outcome, the most common being hæmorrhage following some severe injury to the genital tract.

Syncope.—Faintness is not an uncommon result of exhaustion following prolonged labour, and in neuropathic individuals may occur even after an easy and rapid delivery. In rare instances it may be due to cerebral anæmia resulting from lack of blood in the nervous centres following the sudden diminution in the intra-abdominal pressure incident to the rapid decrease in the size of the uterus.

The faintness usually passes off rapidly and does not lead to untoward results. On the other hand, it occasionally gives cause for serious alarm, the pulse becoming weaker and more rapid and the patient remaining in a condition of profound prostration. I have never seen a death from this cause, but can recall one patient who caused me the greatest possible anxiety, and who was in imminent danger for more than twelve hours.

Haig Ferguson reports 3 cases of serious exhaustion following labour in which he was inclined to attribute the condition to reflex irritation resulting from pressure upon the ovaries incident to the improper employment of Credé's method of expressing the placenta, the organ being grasped laterally instead of antero-posteriorly.

Profound Mental Depression.—In rare instances the only apparent explanation for death, or for a profound collapse which eventuates in recovery, is to be found in the mental condition of the patient, since the most careful examination, both at the bedside and at autopsy, may fail to reveal the slightest abnormality.

I recall a case in my own practice which apparently belongs in this category. The patient, who was unhappily married, had already passed through two very difficult labours. When I saw her, in the latter part of the first stage of her third labour, she was about the room. Just before going to bed at the beginning of the second stage she asked the nurse and myself to witness her will, as she said she felt sure she would not recover. The labour was rapid and uneventful, the placenta coming away spontaneously, and everything appearing to be most satisfactory. On approaching the bed to take leave of the patient half an hour later, I was struck with her haggard appearance. Fearing the possibility of hæmorrhage, I at once applied my hand over the uterus and found it tightly contracted, while the pulse was of excellent quality. Without any apparent reason, and in spite of energetic stimulation and the subcutaneous administration of salt solution, the patient grew slowly worse, the pulse becoming rapid and weak, the eyes sinking back in their sockets, and the face assuming a drawn and Hippocratic expression.

The most careful examination failed to reveal the slightest cause for the condition. The hand introduced into the uterus could find no trace of rupture. Eight hours after delivery I requested a colleague to see her in consultation, but he also was unable to offer any explanation. It then occurred to me that the condition might possibly be the result of her morbid forebodings, and acting upon this supposition I administered a large dose of morphine hypodermically, which was promptly followed by sound sleep, a marked improvement in the character of the pulse, and a rapid change for the better in the general appearance. Upon awaking a few hours later, the patient felt very comfortable and made an uninterrupted recovery.

Pulmonary Embolism.—This accident, usually noted only later in the puerperium, but occasionally occurring shortly after labour, is due to the detachment of a small particle of thrombus situated in a uterine or pelvic vein or elsewhere, which is carried to the right side of the heart and leads to more or less complete occlusion of the pulmonary artery. Under such circumstances the patient complains of intense and sudden precordial pain, becomes livid in appearance, and presents symptoms of profound dyspnœa and eventually of air hunger. These embolisms, however, are not always fatal, a small proportion of the patients recovering.

The treatment is purely palliative. The woman should be placed in the recumbent position, stimulants by the mouth and salt solution subcutaneously should be administered. Inhalations of oxygen, if obtainable, are also indicated.

Entrance of Air into the Uterine Sinuses.—Certain cases of death following intra-uterine manipulations in women suffering from placenta prævia or rupture of the uterus, are attributed by many authorities to the entrance of air into the uterine sinuses, whence it is carried to the heart. The exact cause of death is not understood, some holding that the air bubbles enter the coronary arteries, and others that the right heart, being unable to rid itself of them, becomes paralyzed as a result of its fruitless efforts.

The symptoms are analogous to those following pulmonary embolism. Cases of this character have been reported by Olshausen, Lesse, Perkins, Roger, and others.

That such a condition occasionally occurs is clear from the fact that several cases have been reported in which sudden death followed the injection of air into the pregnant uterus for the purpose of producing abortion. On the other hand, it is probable that its frequency has been much overestimated, and that not a few of the cases which have come to autopsy, and which were supposed to demonstrate such a possibility, are open to another and far more reasonable explanation. Thus, G. W. Dobbin, in my clinic, was able to demonstrate the presence of Bacillus aerogenes capsulatus in the tissues from one of Perkins's cases, in which the presence of air bubbles in the blood-vessels had been regarded as satisfactory evidence as to the cause of death. Wendeler had a similar experience, and it would therefore seem permissible to regard with scepticism all cases of supposed air embolism in which death did not occur almost instantaneously, or in which careful bacteriological investigation demonstrated the presence of gas bacilli.

Post-mortem Delivery.—In the literature, which has been carefully searched by Aveling and Reimann, a number of cases are recorded in which spontaneous birth of the child took place some hours or days after the death of the mother. Moreover, delivery sometimes occurs after burial, and when the body has been exhumed for some reason two individuals instead of one have been found in the coffin. These are instances of the so-called "coffin birth." The phenomenon is usually observed in multiparous women in whom the vaginal outlet is markedly relaxed, and is supposed to be due to a marked increase in the intra-abdominal pressure produced by putrefactive changes, though certain authorities are inclined to attribute isolated cases to rigor mortis of the uterine musculature.

LITERATURE

Aveling. On Post-mortem Parturition, with References to Forty-four Cases. Trans. London Obst. Soc., 1873, xiv, 240–258.

Byrd. A Speedy Method in Asphyxia. The Obst. Jour. of Great Britain and Ireland, 1874, i, 65–69, Amer. Supplement.

Dobbin. Bemerkungen zu den Arbeiten von Schnell, Wendeler und Goebel: Ueber einen Fall von Gasblasen im Blute einer nach Tympania uteri gestorbenen Puerpera. Monatsschr. f. Geb. u. Gyn., 1897, vi, 375–379.

Ferguson. On a Variety of Post-partum Shock, its Nature, Cause, and Prevention. Edinburgh Med. Jour., 1899, xxxv, 32–41.

Gummert. Ueber vagitus uterinus. Monatsschr. f. Geb. u. Gyn., 1899, ix, 492–496.

Laborde. Les tractions rhythmées de la langue, moyen rationnel et puissant de ranimer la fonction respiratoire et la vie. Paris, 1894.

Lesse. Ein weiterer Fall von Luftembolie bei Placenta prævia. Zeitschr. f. Geb. u. Gyn., 1896, xxxv, 184–191.

Nodes and Hines. Fatal Rupture of an Aneurysm of the Splenic Artery immediately after Labour. Trans. London Obst. Soc., 1900, xlii, 305–310.

Olshausen. Ueber Lufteintritt in die Uterusvenen. Monatsschr. f. Geburtsk., 1864, xxiv, 350–374.

Perkins. Air Embolism, etc. Boston Med. and Surg. Jour., 1897, February 18 and 29.

Reimann. Ueber Geburten nach dem Tode der Mutter. Archiv f. Gyn., 1877, xi, 215–255.

Roger. Étude clinique sur la phénomène de l'entrée de l'air par les sinus utérins dans l'étal puerpéral. Thèse de Paris, 1899.

Schultze. Ueber die beste Methode der Wiederbelebung scheintodt geborener Kinder. Jenaische Zeitschr. f. Med. u. Naturwissensch., 1866, iii, Heft 4.

Der Scheintod Neugeborener. Jena, 1871.

Van der Velde. Ein Fall von tödtlicher Pancreasblutung, etc. Ref. Frommel's Jahresbericht, 1898, 764.

Wendeler. Ueber einen Fall von Gasblasen im Blute einer nach Tympania uteri gestorbenen Puerpera. Monatsschr. f. Geb. u. Gyn., 1896, iv, 581–583.

PATHOLOGY OF THE PUERPERIUM

CHAPTER XLIV

PUERPERAL INFECTION

UNDER the general heading of "puerperal infection" are now included all the various morbid conditions which result from the entrance, during labour or the puerperium, of infective micro-organisms into the female generative tract. The older term, "puerperal fever," is at once too vague and misleading, and for many reasons should be discarded. In the first place, it suggests the old idea of the essentiality of the affection so strongly urged in this country by the late Fordyce Barker, and takes no account of the various ætiological factors which may be concerned. Moreover, it emphasizes the febrile phenomena of the affection, instead of laying stress upon its infectious nature and the consequent responsibility of the obstetrician and his assistants. Again, "puerperal septicæmia" and "puerperal sepsis," which are often used as synonymous terms, are hardly less satisfactory, inasmuch as in many instances the infection results in perfectly localized inflammatory processes, to which such terms cannot be applied without violating the established rules of diction.

It is probable that puerperal infection has occurred almost as long as children have been born, and passages in the works of Hippocrates, Galen, Avicenna, and many of the old writers, clearly have reference to it. As early as 1676, Willis wrote on the subject of *febris puerperarum*, but the English term "puerperal fever" probably was first employed by Strother in 1718.

The ancients regarded the affection as the result of retention of the lochia, and for centuries this explanation was universally accepted. In the early part of the seventeenth century Plater showed that it was essentially a metritis, and was followed in the next century by Puzos with his milk metastasis theory. From the time of Plater, until Semmelweiss proved its identity with wound infection, and Lister demonstrated the value of antiseptic methods, all sorts of theories were suggested concerning its origin and nature, which are comprehensively dealt with in the monographs of Eisenmann and Silberschmidt.

Organisms Causing Puerperal Infection.—In 1847, Semmelweiss, then an assistant in the Vienna Lying-in Hospital, began a careful inquiry into the causes of the frightful mortality attending labour in that institution, as compared with the small number of women succumbing to puerperal infection when delivered in their own homes. As a result of his observations, he concluded that the morbid process was essentially a wound infection, and was due to the introduction of septic material by the examining finger. Acting upon this idea he issued stringent orders that the physicians, students, and midwives should disinfect their hands with chlorine water before examining parturient women. In spite of almost immediate surprising results—the mortality falling from over 10 to about 1 per cent—his work was scoffed at by many of the most prominent men of his time, and his discovery remained unappreciated until the influence of Lister's teachings and the development of bacteriology had brought about a revolution in the treatment of wounds.

Among the principal organisms which have been proved to be causes of puerperal infection are the following:

(*a*) *Streptococcus.*—The Streptococcus pyogenes is the most frequent cause of the epidemic and fatal forms of puerperal infection. As early as 1865 this organism was observed in the tissues of women who had died during the puerperium, by Mayrhofer, whose findings were confirmed by Coze and Feltz, Recklinghausen, Waldeyer, Klebs, Orth, Heiberg, and Landau. Pasteur, in 1880, however, was the first to cultivate streptococci from cases of puerperal infection, and he called them " chapélets en grains." He was assisted in this work by Doléris, who carried it still further, and showed that the streptococcus was generally the infectious agent, but that staphylococci, and occasionally bacilli, were sometimes responsible for the infection. These researches were soon confirmed by Lomer, Bumm, Döderlein, Winter, Widal, and by all subsequent observers.

(*b*) *Staphylococcus.*—Further investigation gradually demonstrated the fact that the streptococcus is not necessarily the only organism which may be concerned, but that most of the pus producers, which give rise to wound infection in other parts of the body, may likewise at times be the exciting factors.

Brieger, in 1888, reported autopsies upon 7 women who had died after a febrile puerperium, in 5 of which he demonstrated Staphylococcus aureus. Doléris, in his thesis of 1880, stated that he had been able in similar cases to cultivate in pure culture cocci arranged in groups or bunches, but it was not until 1894 that he stated definitely that they were staphylococci.

The statement made by Fehling and Haegler that staphylococci usually give rise to mild forms of infection, has not been borne out by the observations of other investigators. Occasionally mixed infections with staphylococcus and streptococcus are observed, as reported by Döderlein and Bar and Tissier. It appears that Staphylococcus aureus is the variety observed in puerperal infection, the albus and citreus playing little or no part in its production.

(*c*) *Gonococcus.*—Although clinicians had long suspected that gonorrhœa not infrequently plays a part in the production of puerperal infection, Krönig was the first to adduce bacteriological proof of its action. In 1893 he reported 9 cases of mild infection, in all of which he was able to obtain pure cultures of gonococci from the uterine lochia. In a more recent communication he states that he was able to cultivate the same organism from the discharges of 50 out of 179 patients presenting febrile puerperia, thus showing that it plays an important part in the production of puerperal disease. None of these cases ended fatally, most of the patients recovering spontaneously.

Leopold has reported similar cases, and Maslowsky and Neumann state that they were able to demonstrate the gonococcus in the tissues of cases of endometritis deciduæ. As a rule, gonorrhœal infection in the puerperium pursues a favourable course, but occasionally fatal septicæmia may result, as in one of my cases reported by Harris and Dabney.

(*d*) *Bacillus Coli Communis.*—In the writer's article (1893) upon puerperal infection from a bacteriological point of view, it was stated that von Franqué had cultivated the colon bacillus from a case of puerperal infection, and the belief was expressed that it would be demonstrated more frequently in the future. Time has amply verified this prediction, and there are now on record a long series of cases due to this organism. *A priori*, this is what would be expected when one takes into consideration the proximity of the genital tract to the rectum, and the ease with which contamination can occur when the obstetrician fails to observe the strictest asepsis.

Some idea of the enormous numbers of colon bacilli present in the human body may be gained from the consideration of the figures of several French observers. Thus, Vignal states that 1 decigramme of fæces contains about 20,000,000, and Gilbert and Dominici estimate that from 12,000,000,-000 to 15,000,000,000 are daily excreted. It is therefore evident that the examining finger can hardly avoid contamination with these organisms if it comes in contact with a non-disinfected perinæum.

Gebhard demonstrated their presence in 7 cases of tympania uteri, either alone or in combination with other organisms, and Galtier states that it is the organism most frequently concerned in the production of this condition.

Not uncommonly it is associated with the streptococcus, as in cases reported by Marmorek, Charpentier, Bar and Tissier, and the writer. Some observers have thought that this combination augments the virulence of the streptococcus and gives rise to very intense infections.

(*e*) *Bacillus Diphtheriæ.*—Until very recently it was believed that the diphtheritic deposits upon the vagina and the interior of the puerperal uterus were due to the streptococcus alone, and were in no way connected with true diphtheria. That this is not always the case, however, has been shown by the recent observations of Nisot, Bumm, the writer, and others, who reported instances in which the Klebs-Loeffler bacillus was cultivated from the diphtheritic membrane in the vagina, the affection yielding promptly to the use of the anti-diphtheritic serum.

(*f*) *Bacillus Aerogenes Capsulatus* (Gas Bacillus).—The gas bacillus of Welch is occasionally concerned in puerperal infection. In 1896 the writer observed an instance of this kind, which was reported by Dobbin. Briefly stated, the case was as follows: An outdoor patient, a Bohemian woman, with a generally contracted pelvis, had been in labour for some three to four days under the care of a midwife. When she came into our hands the head of a macerated child was found firmly engaged in the superior strait, the uterus being in a state of tetanic contraction. A fœtid, dark-coloured discharge, which contained many gas bubbles, was escaping from the vagina with a crackling sound. Owing to the softened condition of the child's head delivery with forceps was out of the question, and was effected by means of Tarnier's basiotribe. The mother was profoundly infected at the time and died the next day. Within a few hours after death her body had nearly doubled its original size, as the result of the development of gas in the subcutaneous tissues. Similar changes were observed in the fœtus and in the placenta, and we were able to demonstrate the presence of the gas bacillus in the tissues of both, as well as in the uterine lochia. Unfortunately no autopsy was allowed upon the mother, and we were therefore unable to say to what extent the organisms had penetrated into her tissues.

Well-authenticated instances of infection with this organism have been reported by Stewart, Ernst, Norris, Wood, Halban, and others, and the entire literature upon the subject was exhaustively reviewed by Welch in 1900.

It is important to remember that the gas bubbles which are found in the blood-vessels of women supposed to have perished from the entrance of air into the uterine sinuses, are frequently the product of the bacillus in question. Attention was first directed to this point by Dobbin, and was still further insisted upon by Welch, so that at present the diagnosis of *air embolism* is not justifiable unless careful bacteriological examination has demonstrated the absence of the gas bacillus.

(*g*) *Bacillus Typhosus.*—In 1898, Dobbin and the writer isolated Bacillus typhosus, streptococcus, staphylococcus aureus, and an unidentified anaerobic gas-producing bacillus from the uterine lochia of a Bohemian woman who was admitted to the Johns Hopkins Hospital on the fifth day of the puerperium with high fever. Her blood gave the characteristic Widal reaction, but all the usual symptoms of typhoid fever were absent. The temperature fell to normal on the thirteenth day, and did not rise again. We were inclined to believe that the typhoid bacilli were introduced into her uterus by the midwife, along with other organisms, since she was delivered upon the same bed upon which her husband had died of typhoid fever a few days previously. A somewhat similar case has been reported by Blumer, in which the autopsy revealed an unsuspected typhoid fever.

(*h*) *Bacillary Infection.*—Isolated cases reported by Fraenkel, Doléris, Widal, Mixius, Goldscheider, and others, tend to show that certain cases of fatal infection may be due to bacilli with whose properties we are as yet unacquainted. But the bacteriological work upon which these statements are based is not of a character to enable us to identify the organisms in question, much less to classify them. At the same time, bacteriological examination of the uterine lochia in all cases of fever in the puerperium, as carried out by Krönig and the writer, clearly show that many bacteria with which we are as yet unfamiliar may take part in the process. I have recently seen a case of phlegmasia alba dolens in which the infectious agent was apparently a short, thick, anaerobic bacillus.

(*i*) *Sapræmia.*—Besides the cases in which the infection is due to the growth and extension of micro-organisms within the body, there is a large group in which the symptoms are due to the absorption of toxines produced within the uterus or elsewhere in the generative tract by organisms which do not invade the tissues deeply nor make their way into the blood current. To this form of infection Matthews Duncan some years ago applied the term "*sapræmia.*" It is usually thought to be due to the invasion of the uterus by putrefactive organisms with whose properties we are as yet almost totally unfamiliar.

No doubt the term has been greatly abused, and many cases have been included under it which were really due to infection with the ordinary pyogenic organisms. Nor are we justified in considering a case as sapræmic unless the lochia have been examined bacteriologically and found to be free from pyogenic organisms.

This statement is borne out by the observations of Bumm, who found streptococci in 8 out of 11 cases which were thought to present the clinical picture of sapræmia. Von Franqué also obtained somewhat similar results, and concluded that sapræmic fever in the puerperium is extremely rare, and should be diagnosed only after an accurate bacteriological examination of the uterine lochia has demonstrated the absence of pathogenic and the presence of saprophytic organisms.

The causative organisms in sapræmia are mostly of an anaerobic nature, and consequently do not grow on the usual culture media. Many of them are gas producers, and cause the frothy, ill-smelling secretion which is so characteristic of these cases. Many different varieties are undoubtedly concerned in its production, though only a few have as yet been isolated. Thus, Bumm cultivated from one case an anaerobic bacillus, which decomposed albumin and produced poisonous substances, while Döderlein isolated an anaerobic gas-producing coccus from a woman who presented a frothy, purulent vaginal discharge. Krönig, in 43 abnormal puerperia, found organisms which did not grow on the usual media, and in 32 of them obtained varieties which were pure anaerobes.

Besides the organisms already mentioned, it is not unlikely that further research will show still others which may play a part in the production of isolated cases of puerperal infection; but to summarize, it may be said that those most commonly concerned are the well-known pyogenic organisms (streptococcus, staphylococcus, bacillus coli, and gonococcus) and the various putrefactive varieties.

Some idea of the relative frequency with which the several organisms occur in puerperal infections may be gathered from the work of Krönig, who examined 179 cases of puerperal endometritis bacteriologically, and as a result of his observations divided them into 3 groups—pyogenic, gonorrhœal, and sapræmic. The pyogenic group comprised 79 cases, in 75 of which the infective agent was the streptococcus, and in 4 the staphylococcus. In 50 cases the gonococcus was isolated, while in 43 of the 50 sapræmic cases the organisms did not grow on the usual culture media, 32 of them being pure anaerobes.

Bacteriological examination of the uterine lochia in a series of 150 cases of my own, in which the temperature rose to 101° F., or higher, during the first ten days of the puerperium, gave the following results:

Streptococcus	31 cases
Streptococcus and bacillus coli	5 "
Streptococcus, staphylococcus, and bacilli	2 "
Streptococcus, bacillus coli, and gas bacillus	2 "
Streptococcus, staphylococcus, gas and typhoid bacillus	1 "
Streptococcus, staphylococcus, bacillus coli, and gas bacilli	1 "
Streptococcus and unidentified bacillus	2 "
Staphylococcus	4 "
Bacillus coli	11 "
Gonococcus	7 "
Gonococcus and bacillus coli	1 "
Unidentified aerobic bacteria	4 "
Unidentified anaerobic bacteria	8 "
Bacillus diphtheriæ	1 "
Bacillus typhosus	1 "
Bacteria seen in cover-slips, but which failed to grow on any of the more usual media	45 "
Absolutely sterile	25 "

Pathological Anatomy.—The lesions may vary widely even in cases clinically similar, and these variations afford a probable explanation for the failure of the older authors to appreciate the true nature of the affection. Thus, there may be an almost infinite series of gradations from a slight membrane covering a small perineal tear to an inflammatory process involving the entire generative tract, or extending beyond it to the parametrium or peritonæum, and sometimes resulting in a general pyæmic infection. In other cases the infectious elements pass through the port of entry with such rapidity that they do not excite local lesions, but produce a septicæmia which is rapidly fatal—the *sepsis foudroyante* of the French authors. In the majority of cases of puerperal infection, however, the endometrium is the portion affected, and the morbid process does not pass beyond it, the condition being termed a septic or putrid endometritis, according as it has resulted from the invasion of pyogenic or putrefactive organisms respectively.

In other cases the lesions may be situated in any part of the generative tract, more than one region being frequently implicated. Thus, at different times we have to deal with a puerperal vaginitis, endometritis, metritis, parametritis, metrolymphangitis, metrophlebitis, salpingitis, oophoritis, peritonitis, pyæmia, or phlegmasia alba dolens respectively.

Lesions of the Vulva and Vagina.—In former times the *puerperal ulcer* was of very common occurrence, but with the introduction of aseptic methods into midwifery its frequency has become markedly diminished, so that now it is only rarely encountered.

These ulcers appear on the surface of tears about the vulva and perinæum, soon take on a dirty, greenish-yellow appearance which is due to necrosis, and are bathed in a foul-smelling secretion. In some cases they are covered by a grayish-white membrane, and on this account were formerly designated as "diphtheritic ulcers." Careful bacteriological examination, however, has shown that, except for their external appearance, they have nothing in common with diphtheria. As a rule these give rise to very little systemic disturbance, and would frequently pass unnoticed were it not for ocular inspection.

Puerperal Vaginitis.—Of this there are two forms, the one being characterized by general inflammation, the mucosa becoming thickened, soft, reddened, and bathed with an abundant purulent secretion. In the other type, especially when torn surfaces are present, the vaginal walls may be the seat of a pseudo-diphtheritic membrane, which may vary in extent from a small patch covering a tear to a complete cast of the entire vaginal canal.

Until recently it was believed that none of the so-called cases of *diphtheria* of the vagina were due to the invasion of the Klebs-Loeffler bacillus; but the recent observations of Bumm, Nisot, myself, and others show that in a few cases that organism is undoubtedly the ætiological factor.

Endometritis.—The most common lesion in puerperal infection is an inflammation of the endometrium. When one recalls the condition of the uterus immediately after delivery, with its bleeding, raw surfaces and the large, gaping, thrombosed placental sinuses, it becomes apparent that any virulent material which has been introduced into the cavity during labour can easily find entry into its walls. Again, when one considers the mechanism by which the decidua is normally removed, one can readily see that an ideal culture medium is prepared by Nature for the reception and propagation of organisms introduced from without.

In puerperal endometritis the infection may be limited to the placental site, or may extend over the entire mucosa. When the former alone is implicated, the organisms are usually found growing into the thrombi and producing comparatively little local reaction. On the other hand, when the entire internal surface of the uterus is affected, the endometrium may become converted into a stinking, sloughing area made up of necrotic material and decidual *débris*, and bathed with a bloody, purulent discharge. The necrotic material soon takes on a dirty yellowish-green appearance, and in many instances ulcerated surfaces appear, coated with fibrin and presenting the clinical picture of diphtheria. This type was formerly designated as *diphtheritic endometritis*, but just as happens in the case of the vagina, the condition, as a rule, is not a true diphtheria, but simply represents a fibrinous exudation, the result of an intense necrosis following the invasion of the usual pyogenic organisms. Infections due to streptococcus or staphylococcus are usually associated with very little odour; whereas in those excited by bacillus coli or any of the various putrefactive organisms the interior of the uterus is bathed with a profuse foul-smelling discharge which frequently contains gas bubbles. The amount of necrotic material produced is often enormous, and may recur with great rapidity after curetting. Fig. 623 represents the uterus from a case of puerperal infection due to streptococcus and bacillus coli. The woman succumbed ten days after the birth of the child, having been curetted three or four days before death, the uterus at that time having been scraped perfectly clean. A glance at the drawing, however, shows that the entire cavity is filled with necrotic material, which in all probability had been reproduced in the interval elapsing between the curettage and the time of death.

Although the infection generally remains limited to the endometrium, in not a few cases it may progress beyond it, giving rise to a metritis, a

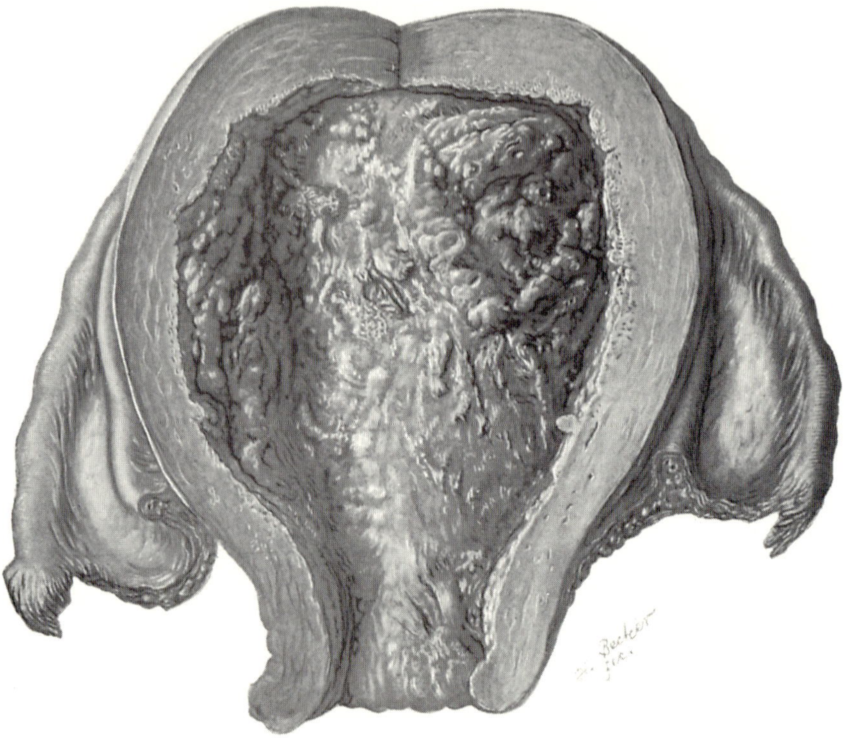

Fig. 623.—Uterus from Woman Dying Ten Days after Labour from a Mixed Infection, with Streptococcus and Bacillus Coli. × ⅜.

lymphangitis, or a phlebitis, as the case may be. This extension usually occurs through the lymphatics, and in such cases areas of inflammation can be traced along their course extending to the peritoneal surface of the uterus. At other times, especially when the infection has been limited to the placental site, the thrombi may be invaded by the micro-organisms, and there results a *phlebitis* which may remain limited to the uterine wall or may rapidly extend beyond it and give rise to the various thrombotic forms of puerperal infection.

The lesions produced in the endometrium vary considerably according to the micro-organisms concerned, and still more according to their virulence. In the cases in which one has to deal with a virulent streptococcus or staphylococcus infection, the local changes are comparatively slight, the process rapidly spreading through the lymphatics or veins past the uterus, and giving rise to a peritonitis or a general systemic infection. On the other hand, in the cases due to putrefactive organisms, to the colon bacillus, and to the ordinary pus-organisms of lesser virulence, the process remains more or less limited to the endometrium and causes marked local lesions. Fig. 624 represents the uterus from a woman dying of a virulent streptococcic infection. The walls of its cavity are seen to be almost perfectly smooth, and nothing is present which could have been removed by means of the curette. In this respect the case stands in marked contrast to the one represented in Fig. 623, in which the infectious agents were streptococcus and bacillus coli.

Moreover, when one studies the microscopical features of puerperal endometritis, one finds these differences still further accentuated. Most of our knowledge on this point we owe to the researches of Bumm and Döderlein, both of whom have shown that there are marked histological

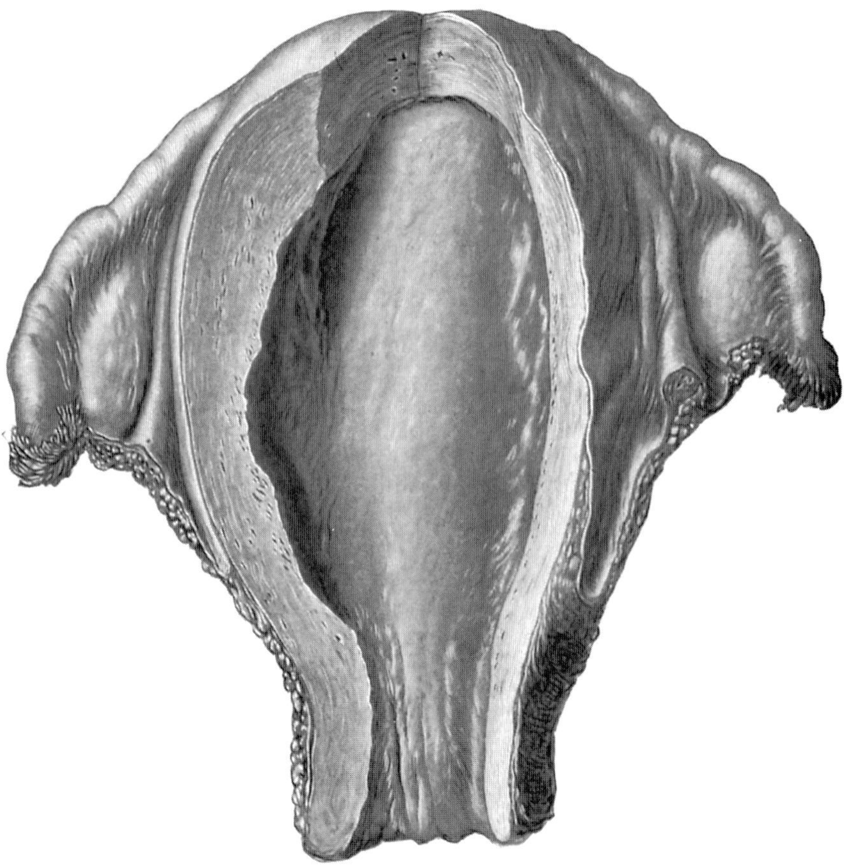

FIG. 624.—UTERUS FROM WOMAN DYING TEN DAYS AFTER LABOUR FROM STREPTOCOCCUS INFECTION. × ⅔.

differences between the putrid and septic forms. According to Bumm, in sections through the wall of a uterus the seat of a *putrid endometritis*, a thick layer of necrotic material is found lining the uterine cavity, embedded in which are large numbers of the offending micro-organisms. Beneath this is a thick layer of small-cell infiltration—the zone of reaction—and under this again, more or less normal tissue. Careful study of the sections shows that the micro-organisms are limited almost entirely to the superficial

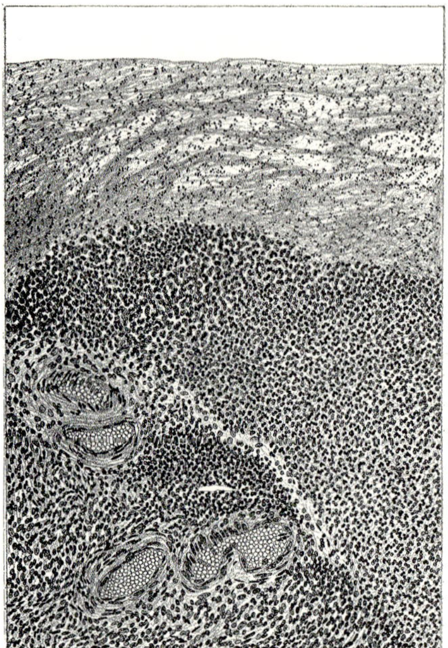

K. M. Montague, fec.

FIG. 625.—PUERPERAL ENDOMETRITIS DUE TO COLON INFECTION, SHOWING MARKED DEVELOPMENT OF LEUCOCYTIC WALL.

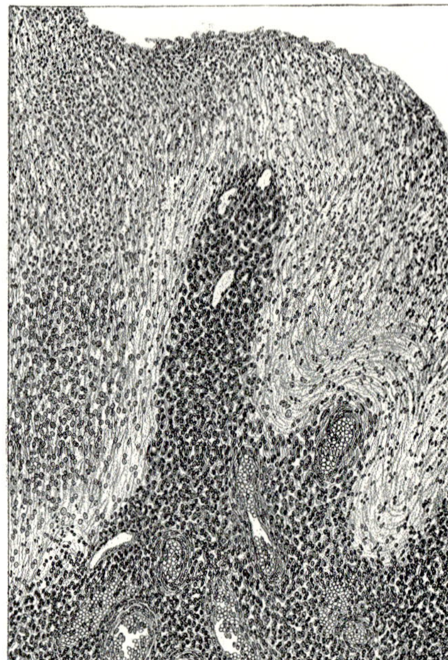

K. M. Montague, fec.

FIG. 626.—PUERPERAL ENDOMETRITIS DUE TO STREPTOCOCCUS INFECTION, SHOWING SLIGHT DEVELOPMENT OF LEUCOCYTIC WALL.

necrotic layer; and although a few may be present in the reaction zone, none can be made out in the tissues beneath it, thus showing Nature's mode of preventing the invasion of the body by the micro-organisms (Figs. 625 and 627).

These pictures are observed not only in the cases due to infection with the putrefactive bacteria, but also in those in which the pyogenic organisms possess only a slight degree of virulence. On the other hand, in cases of *septic endometritis*, and especially where the organisms are virulent, a totally different appearance is noted. Although here also a layer of necrotic material containing organisms is found adjoining the uterine cavity, it is usually thinner than in the preceding case. The zone of small-cell infiltration is either lacking or very imperfectly developed, and the micro-organisms can be observed making their way down through the decidua and along the lymphatics through the muscular wall of the uterus out towards its peritoneal surface (Figs. 626 and 628). I have been able to abundantly confirm the observations of Bumm, whose conclusions are amply justified (Plate XVI).

The effect produced by various micro-organisms was strikingly demon-

PLATE XVI.

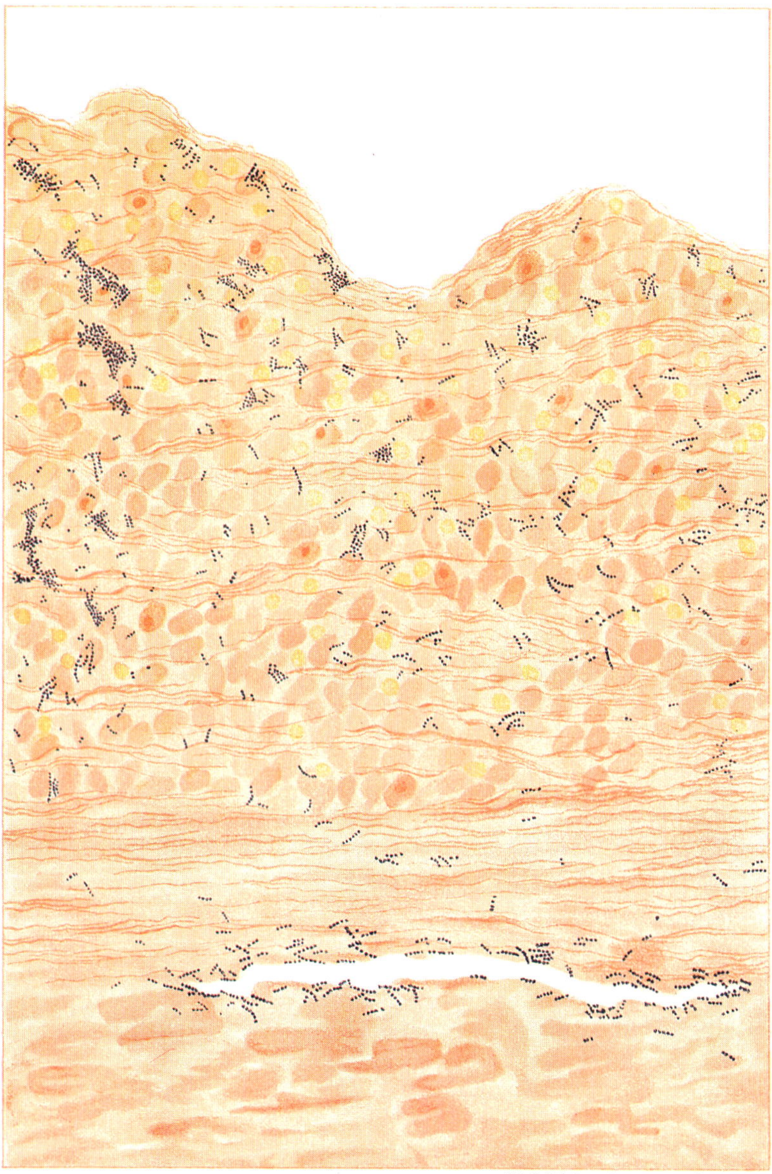

K.M.Montague, fec.

SECTION THROUGH ENDOMETRIUM IN STREPTOCOCCIC PUERPERAL INFECTION. × 1000.

strated in one of my own cases—a double infection with streptococcus and bacillus coli. On making sections through the uterine wall characteristic necrotic tissue was seen lining the cavity of the uterus, and in it appeared both forms of micro-organisms. Beneath this the zone of small-cell infiltration was fairly well developed, and in its upper part both forms of organisms were recognisable. In its lower portion, however, there were only streptococci, which had continued to pass through the uterine wall by way of the lymphatics, and on reaching the peripheral surface had given rise to a peritonitis.

It would appear, therefore, that Nature endeavours to confine the micro-organisms to the inner surface of the uterus by interposing between the necrotic layer and the deeper portions a barrier of small-cell infiltration, which acts as an efficient filter when the micro-organisms are attenuated, but fails to restrain them when they possess a marked degree of virulence.

Parametritis.—One of the more frequent complications of the uterine infection is parametritis, which is usually due to the transmission of the

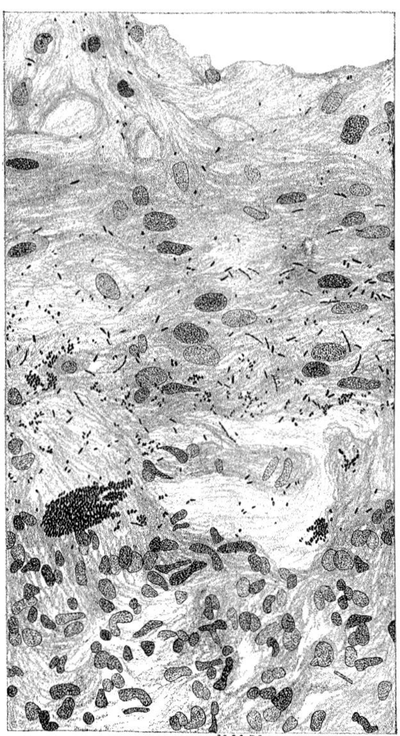

Fig. 627.—Colon Bacillus Endometritis. Leucocytic Wall not Invaded by Bacteria. × 800.

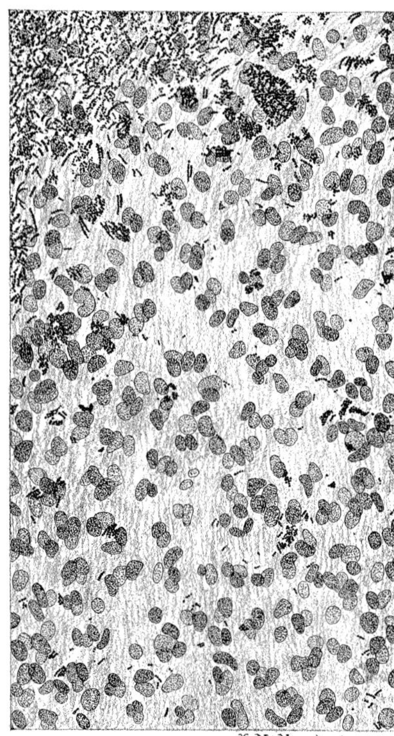

Fig. 628.—Streptococcic Endometritis, showing Invasion of Leucocytic Wall. × 800.

micro-organisms through the lymphatics to the peri-uterine connective tissue. The first effect of their invasion is a marked inflammatory œdema, with very little or no suppuration. In mild cases the process goes no further, but in the severer types it rapidly spreads to the surrounding connective tissue and eventuates in abscess formation. The infectious agents in severe cases follow the course of the lymphatics, and sometimes pass behind the peritonæum and give rise to *retroperitoneal phlegmons*, which may extend as high as the posterior mediastinum. On the other hand, when they are transmitted along those which go to the anterior portion of the pelvis, inflammatory phenomena occur about the inguinal canal. In still another class of cases they invade the connective tissue surrounding the greater vessels of the thigh, and give rise to a phlegmasia alba dolens.

Occasionally the parametritic implication originates from infected tears about the cervix, but as a rule it is secondary to infection from the uterine cavity.

As has already been pointed out, in a considerable number of cases the inflammatory process extends into the uterine wall, and there gives rise to divers lesions of *metritis*, which may vary from small areas of leucocytic infiltration to definite abscess formation. As a rule, however, multiple abscesses scattered through the uterine wall are due to implication of the lymphatics, and inasmuch as these channels are most numerous beneath its peritoneal covering, abscesses are most abundant in that situation.

Salpingitis.—In a small proportion of cases the process extends directly from the uterine cavity to the Fallopian tubes, and there gives rise to various inflammatory phenomena. Occasionally the salpingitis is due to infection through the lymphatics and not by continuity from the endometrium. Sometimes an *oophoritis* occurs, the ovaries being enlarged to several times their usual size and very œdematous. The process may stop here or go on to typical abscess formation. The ovarian infection in the majority of cases is due to lymphatic involvement, and is usually associated with affections of the parametrium. Much more rarely it results from direct infection of a ruptured follicle by means of the peritonitic fluid.

Peritonitis.—In the vast majority of cases the fatal termination in puerperal infection is due to a peritonitis. As was pointed out when considering the histological changes in puerperal endometritis, the streptococci or other infecting agents may rapidly make their way from the interior of the uterus to the peritoneal surface by means of the lymphatics, and there give rise to inflammatory changes. This is the usual mode of infection, but in rare instances it may be due to the escape of pus from the Fallopian tubes; though in none of the autopsies which the writer has witnessed upon women dead of puerperal fever has such a mode of origin been observed. In other cases, it may follow the rupture of a parametritic or ovarian abscess.

Pyæmia.—The pyæmic form usually results from the infection of thrombi at the placental site and the subsequent inflammatory changes occurring in the veins. The thrombosis may be limited to a comparatively small area and be entirely within the uterine wall, or it may extend beyond the uterus, so that occasionally all the pelvic vessels are thrombosed as far up as the junction of the renal veins with the inferior vena cava. By the breaking down of the thrombi small particles escape into the circulation and are carried by the blood current in various directions, giving rise to endocarditis and *metastatic abscesses*, from which no portion of the body appears to be exempt. In this form of puerperal infection such abscesses may be found in any of the internal organs, the synovial surfaces also being frequently implicated and giving rise to swellings about the joints, which, if not promptly treated, may lead to their complete destruction.

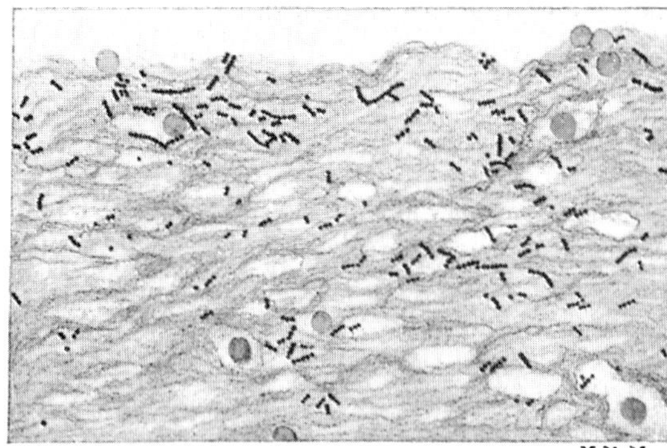

Fig. 629.—Section through Thrombosed Pelvic Vein, showing Streptococci. × 800.

In a number of other cases blebs or *bullæ*, due to the same cause, appear on various portions of the body, and in their contents the offending micro-organisms are readily demonstrable. Most cases of pyæmia present very little uterine involvement, and death, when it occurs, is due to general exhaustion following a prolonged suppurative process, rather than to peritonitis, which is the usual cause of death in the other forms of infection.

Phlegmasia Alba Dolens.—As was pointed out when the question of parametritis was considered, this affection is sometimes due to the extension through the lymphatics of a parametritis to the tissues surrounding the great vessels of the thigh. As a rule, however, it results from the extension of a thrombotic process from the pelvic veins, though sometimes it appears to be the only manifestation of the infection, and under such circumstances its mode of production is very difficult to explain. In a small percentage of cases it is possibly not of infectious origin.

Ætiology.—Careful investigation has demonstrated that the bacteria concerned in puerperal infection are identical with those with which we are familiar as causing wound infection. In fact, puerperal infection must be regarded as a wound infection caused by the introduction of pathogenic organisms into the generative tract either before, during, or immediately after labour. In other words, we have to deal with a direct infection from without, the offending bacteria being brought to the woman by the hands, instruments, or any other object which may come in contact with her generative organs.

Puerperal infection, then, is *contact infection*, this conception having been first definitely enunciated by Semmelweiss in the following words: "I consider puerperal fever, not a single case excepted, as a resorption fever, caused by the resorption of a decomposed animal-organic material. The first result of the absorption is a change in the blood, and the exudations are the result of this change. The decomposed animal-organic material, which when resorbed causes childbed fever, is brought to the individual from without in the great majority of cases, and this is infection from without. These are the cases which represent the epidemics of childbed fever. These are the cases which can be prevented."

In the latter part of the eighteenth century puerperal fever began to be considered as a contagious malady in England. This conception apparently originated with Thomas Kirkland, of Ashby, in 1774, but was first clearly enunciated in 1795 by Gordon, of Aberdeen, in his treatise "On the Epidemic of Puerperal Fever, as it prevailed in Aberdeen from December 1789 to March 1792," in which he gave a table of 77 cases which he had attended himself.

In this country we are mainly indebted to Oliver Wendell Holmes for introducing the conception of the infectious nature of the affection. In an article entitled Puerperal Fever as a Private Pestilence, first published in 1843, he clearly showed that it was a preventible affection, and owed its origin either to the accoucheur or midwife. His teachings, however, did not exert the influence which might have been expected, mainly because they were opposed by the leading obstetricians of the country, notably Meigs and Hodge, the former stating that he preferred to consider the disease as due to the workings of Providence, which he could understand, rather than to an unknown infection of which he could form no conception.

For many years the prevalent theory in Europe as to the causation of puerperal fever was that it was due to miasmatic, telluric, or atmospheric influences. This view held its ground until after the appearance of Semmelweiss's article in 1861; although in 1864, Hirsch, after studying the matter from an historical standpoint, came to the conclusion that the malady was of infectious rather than of miasmatic origin.

It was not, however, until Lister had introduced antiseptic methods into surgery, and Stadfeld, of Copenhagen, had recommended the use of bichloride of mercury in obstetrics, that the great mass of the profession began to understand that puerperal fever was due to contact infection, and could be prevented to a very great degree. The bacteriological work of Pasteur and his successors, and the almost constant presence of streptococci in fatal cases, decided the question, and at present no one doubts the infectious nature of the disease.

Modes of External Infection.—The most usual mode of infection is by the hands of the obstetrician or the midwife, and no one who has observed the way in which not a few medical men conduct labours can wonder that puerperal fever occasionally occurs. The employment of dirty instruments, as well as of dirty hands, also plays an important part.

Sources of infection, much rarer, it is true, but generally overlooked, are copulation during the later days of pregnancy, and, especially among the lower classes, self-inoculation by the patient fingering her genitalia or even making internal examinations. Contact with secretions from wounds of any kind also plays an important part in its production, and whether the purulent material be from an external wound or elsewhere within the body, the result will be the same. It is only necessary to recall in this connection the case of Dr. Rutter, of Philadelphia, who was followed wherever he went by an epidemic of puerperal fever, while his brother practitioners were practically free from it. It appeared later that the source of infection was an ozæna from which he was constantly contaminating his hands.

Wounds on the hands of the nurse, bone felons, and other affections of the fingers, and not infrequently a pustular eczema, are sometimes responsible.

For many years it has been known that puerperal fever often occurred when a woman in labour was cared for by a physician who at the same time was attending a case of erysipelas. As has already been said, one of the old ideas concerning the affection held it to be identical with the former disease, but it was not until bacteriology had proved that erysipelas and most of the serious cases of puerperal infection are due to the streptococcus that this relation was understood. At the present time the majority of observers believe that there is no essential difference between streptococcus erysipelatis of Fehleisen and the ordinary streptococcus pyogenes.

Puerperal fever has also been frequently observed to occur in the practice of those attending diphtheria, scarlet fever, and occasionally typhoid cases. Although no essential relationship between these affections has ever been proven, it is well known that in both diphtheria and scarlet fever complications due to the streptococcus are frequently met with, and these organisms may be conveyed to the woman in labour.

Air infection is supposed by some to play an important ætiological part, and many authors advise covering the external genitalia with an occlusive pad to prevent the entry of air into the vagina, and thus eliminate this source of infection. This, however, occurs very infrequently, if, indeed, it is ever the cause of the disease; nor are the statements of Garrigues convincing, in which he attributed an epidemic of puerperal fever in the New York Lying-in Hospital to the presence of a dead rat in the cellar, inasmuch as it is far more probable that the disease was due to imperfect hand disinfection on the part of his assistants, or to the introduction of pathogenic organisms within the vagina in some way or other by the patients themselves. Nevertheless, in England, and to a less extent in this country, *sewer gas* is believed to play a prominent part in the production of puerperal infection. But I believe that the danger of infection from such sources has been greatly exaggerated, and will be spoken of less and less frequently as medical men become better versed in the technique of rigorous hand disinfection.

To show how accurate a conception Semmelweiss possessed of the various modes of contact infection, it may be interesting to quote what he says concerning it: "The bearer of the decomposed animal-organic material is the examining finger, the operating hand, instruments, bedclothes, atmospheric air, sponges, the hands of midwives or nurses which come in contact with the excrement of women sick with puerperal fever, and after that handle pregnant or parturient women. In other words, the bearer of the decomposed animal-organic material is anything which is soiled by a decomposed animal-organic material and comes in contact with the genitalia of these patients."

Auto-infection.—Every one at the present time believes that the vast majority of cases of infection are the result of the introduction from without of pathogenic micro-organisms into the genital canal of the pregnant or parturient woman. Nevertheless, many authorities teach that in a certain number of cases the infection does not result in this manner, but owes its origin to micro-organisms which were already within the genital tract before the onset of labour. To infection arising in this way the term "*auto-infection*" is applied. The conception originated with Semmelweiss, who stated: "In rare cases the decomposed animal-organic material, which causes childbed fever when absorbed, is produced within the patient herself. These are the cases of auto-infection, and cannot be prevented."

With the enthusiasm which attended the introduction of antiseptic methods of midwifery, the possibility of auto-infection was lost sight of for a time, and it was only when the statistics of well-conducted lying-in establishments showed that a certain number of cases of infection still occurred, despite the rigorous application of antiseptic principles, that the idea was rehabilitated by Ahlfeld and Kaltenbach.

Of course, with the recognition of the fact that puerperal fever was a germ disease, the definition introduced by Semmelweiss fell to the ground, since the micro-organisms could not originate spontaneously within the body of the woman. Kaltenbach then advanced the view that pathogenic organisms are present in the vaginæ of a considerable number of healthy pregnant women, and that these might be introduced into the uterus by a finger which was perfectly sterile before being passed up the canal. Of course these would not be instances of auto-infection in the strict sense of the word, and much confusion might have been avoided had the term "indirect infection" been substituted for it, since the micro-organisms must have been introduced into the vagina at some period of life, and the question simply resolves itself into one of time. Many observers now hold that auto-infection, even in this modified sense, is not possible, and that all cases of puerperal infection are due to the introduction from without of pathogenic micro-organisms at the time of labour.

After all, the question can be finally decided only by the results of the bacteriological examination of the generative tract in the pregnant and non-pregnant conditions. If careful investigation shows that pathogenic micro-organisms are absent from the uterus and vagina of the pregnant woman, the doctrine of auto-infection must be abandoned. On the other hand, if they can be demonstrated in apparently healthy women during pregnancy, despite any preconceived opinion, we shall be forced to admit its possibility.

Practically all bacteriological investigators are united in claiming that the cavity of the normal uterus is free from micro-organisms both in the pregnant and non-pregnant conditions. This fact has been amply proved by the work of Gönner, Döderlein, and Winternitz; while Strauss and Sanchez-Toledo have demonstrated the same in the lower animals. On the contrary, Franz and Burckhardt state that bacteria can be isolated from the cavity of the uterus in the latter part of the puerperium in a large proportion of cases. Their results, however, are controverted by the recent work of Döderlein and Winternitz, and appear invalidated by the fact that the writer found the uterine lochia absolutely sterile in 25 out of 150 women who presented rises of temperature in the puerperium.

On the other hand, when we come to consider the bacterial contents of the cervical canal in the healthy woman, the conclusions are by no means so uniform. Some observers state that micro-organisms are present in most cases, whereas others consider that they are usually absent. These contradictory results were apparently satisfactorily reconciled by Walthard's work. He found that cultures taken from the lower portion of the cervical canal contained identically the same micro-organisms as the vagina, but that they became less plentiful as the internal os was approached, disappearing altogether about one third of the way up. It would appear, therefore, that the observers who found bacteria in the cervix had obtained the secretion from the lower portion of its canal, while those who reported negative results had examined material from higher up. Accordingly, we may conclude that both the uterus and upper portion of the cervix are practically, if not absolutely, sterile, and can therefore offer no possible chance for the occurrence of either auto- or indirect infection.

Ultimately the question narrows down to the demonstration of the presence or absence of pathogenic micro-organisms in the healthy vagina, and, according to the results of careful investigations on these lines, the doctrine of auto-infection must be generally accepted or absolutely abandoned. Ahlfeld, in all his articles upon the subject, assumes that "the vagina is swarming with various varieties of pathogenic organisms," and auto-infection can only be prevented by thoroughly disinfecting the vagina in every case by antiseptic douches.

Unfortunately, the bacteriological examination of the vaginal secretion of pregnant women until recently did not offer grounds for absolutely satisfactory conclusions. Thus, the work of Gönner, Thomen, Samschin, Krönig and Menge, Bensis, Bergholm, and the writer in 1898, appear to show that pyogenic micro-organisms, with the exception of the gonococcus, cannot be found in the vagina of pregnant women; while, on the other hand, numerous investigators have isolated the streptococcus in a varying proportion of their cases, as is shown by the following table:

Burckhardt..........	4%	Witte.............	12.5%
Steffeck.............	4%	Kottmann.........	13%
Döderlein............	4.1%	Winter............	15%
Burguburu..........	8.5%	Williams (1893)....	20%
Koblanck............	9.5%	Vahle..............	25%
Vahle...............	10%	Walthard.........	27%

Döderlein's studies on the vaginal secretion, published in 1892, promised for a time to reconcile the conflicting results. He pointed out that the vaginal secretion might occur in one of two forms, which he designated as normal and pathological. The former was a thick, dry, cheese-like material of a whitish colour and distinctly acid reaction. Microscopically it showed epithelial cells, a pure culture of tolerably long bacilli, and now and then a few yeast fungi. It did not contain pyogenic micro-organisms, and offered absolutely no support for the doctrine of auto-infection. The pathological secretion, on the other hand, was fluid, generally of a yellowish colour suggesting pus, and occasionally contained gas bubbles. In it were found large numbers of leucocytes, many micro-organisms of various kinds, and in a few cases streptococci. Its reaction was less acid than that of the normal secretion, occasionally neutral, and very rarely even alkaline.

Döderlein's work was based upon the examination of 190 pregnant women, 55.3 per cent of whom presented a normal and 44.6 per cent a pathological secretion, while in 10 per cent of the latter he was able to demonstrate the presence of streptococci by cultural methods. His investigations, accordingly, indicated that auto-infection was out of the question when the secretion was normal, whereas its occurrence was theoretically possible in 10 per cent of the pathological cases.

Döderlein supposed that the contradictory results of previous investigators could be reconciled by assuming that those obtaining negative results had worked with normal, whereas the positive results were obtained from the pathological secretion.

Krönig, in 1897, stated that he had examined the vaginal secretion in 167 pregnant women, and that in none of them was he able to demonstrate typical streptococci nor any other pyogenic micro-organisms, with the exception of the gonococcus. He therefore concluded that the vaginal secretion should be considered as practically sterile, and that it did not offer the slightest evidence in support of the doctrine of auto-infection. He surmised that the conflicting results of the various observers were due to differences in the methods of obtaining the specimens, and that whenever they were obtained by means of a speculum, pathogenic micro-organisms had probably been carried up along with the instrument from the vulva. To avoid this, he recommended the employment of a small tube, which could be introduced into the vagina under the guidance of the eye, without coming in contact with the labia minora or the margins of the hymen.

In 1898, I reported to the American Gynæcological Society the results of the examination of the vaginal secretion in 92 pregnant women, the specimens having been obtained by means of a small tube similar to that employed by Krönig and Menge. In none of these cases was Streptococcus pyogenes or Staphylococcus aureus demonstrated, but in 6 cases Staphylococcus epidermidis albus was present. Whether the latter really existed in the vagina, or whether its presence was due to contamination is open to doubt; but as this organism is never found in severe cases of puerperal infection, its presence in the vaginal secretion is a matter of indifference so far as the question in dispute is concerned. My researches, therefore, confirmed Krönig's observations as to the absence of pyogenic cocci from the vaginal secretion of pregnant women, and warranted the conclusion that auto-infection due to them was impossible, although it could not be absolutely denied that it might occasionally occur from other bacteria, especially in some of the cases of putrefactive endometritis.

These conclusions were absolutely contradictory to those at which I had arrived five years previously, when I confirmed Döderlein's original work, by finding streptococci in 20 per cent of the vaginal secretions which I examined. The only possible explanation for the different results obtained in the two series of investigations must be sought in the manner in which the specimens were obtained, as all the other conditions under which the work was carried out were identical. In the first series a sterile glass speculum was employed in obtaining the secretion, and in the second a Menge tube. It appeared highly probable that a number of bacteria were carried into the vagina by the speculum from the margins of the hymen and the inner surfaces of the labia minora with which it had come in contact; whereas, such contact having been avoided when the tube was employed, the secretion obtained was absolutely free from contamination.

The truth of this explanation was placed beyond doubt by the examination of 25 additional cases, 3 sets of cultures being made from each. The first was taken from the hymen and inner surfaces of the labia minora, the second from the vaginal secretion obtained by a Menge tube, and the third from the vaginal secretion obtained through a sterilized speculum. Pyogenic cocci or colon bacilli were demonstrated in 80 per cent of the first, in none of the second, and in 48 per cent of the third series of experiments, thereby showing conclusively that the vaginal secretion of healthy women is absolutely free from pyogenic cocci when obtained without contamination, but that bacteria are present upon the hymen and labia minora in most cases, and that it is impossible to introduce a speculum into the vagina without carrying them along with it in at least one half of such cases.

As a result, therefore, of the work of Krönig and Menge and myself, it has been fairly satisfactorily demonstrated that under normal conditions pyogenic cocci are never present in the vagina of pregnant women, and that therefore there is no possibility of auto-infection as far as these organisms are concerned, and whenever they are demonstrated in the uterine secretion of puerperal women they should be regarded as affording conclusive evidence of external infection. It is possible, however, that in rare cases auto-infection may occur from certain anaerobes contained in the vaginal secretion, but satisfactory evidence cannot be adduced in support of such an occurrence until methods have been devised which will enable us to isolate and grow satisfactorily in pure culture the organisms in question.

So far as is known, the gonococcus is the only pyogenic bacterium which can live and thrive in the vaginal secretion. But, although it is not infrequently the cause of an elevation of temperature during the puerperium, such cases should not be considered as supporting the doctrine of auto-infection, for the reason that the women had become infected before or during pregnancy, and the organisms had persisted in the crypts of the cervical canal, living there as parasites, and simply finding more suitable conditions for development in the first few days of the puerperium, when they make their way into the uterine cavity and manifest their presence by the production of fever and increased discharge.

An interesting fact in connection with the question of auto-infection is that those who believe most firmly in its possibility, and who are in the habit of employing prophylactic vaginal douches for the destruction of the organisms in the vagina, have thus far been able to present far less favourable statistics than their opponents. Thus, Ahlfeld finds that 38 per cent of his patients have a rise of temperature during the puerperium, even after the use of the prophylactic douche. Again, Kaltenbach, while chief of the Lying-in Clinic at Halle, always resorted to its routine employment, but the statistics show a very material improvement since his successor, Fehling, discontinued the practice. Furthermore, the results of Leopold and Mermann, who do not use the douche at all, show a constant improvement corresponding with the increasing precision with which objective asepsis is carried out.

The value of the prophylactic vaginal douche has recently been investigated by Krönig and Bretschneider. The latter followed 2,280 cases in the Leipzig clinic, every alternate woman being douched. The puerperium was febrile in 45.18 per cent of the cases in which the douche was used, as compared with 36.78 per cent of the cases in which it was omitted.

Jewett quotes the opinions of a number of American obstetricians upon the subject, and it would appear that the majority of them do not employ the prophylactic douche, and that, while a certain number theoretically believe in auto-infection, they practically act as if its occurrence were impossible.

Frequency.—It is very difficult to make accurate statements as to the frequency of puerperal infection, especially when it occurs outside of hospital practice. Concerning this condition the vital statistics of the health officers of the various cities are of no value, inasmuch as the vast majority of deaths from this disease are reported as being due to malaria, typhoid fever, pneumonia, or other causes.

Thus, Reynolds, in 1893, wrote an article upon the prevalence of puerperal fever in Boston. In that year he himself had seen 28 cases in hospital practice with 7 deaths; but, in looking over the statistics furnished by the health office, he found that, granting the reports of the department to be accurate, this number represented more than one fourth of all the cases of this character in Boston—a conclusion which would certainly appear incredible.

Since the introduction of antiseptic methods into midwifery, the mortality from puerperal infection has decreased very markedly in hospital practice. In the old Maternity of Paris, and in the Lying-in Hospital in Vienna, in some years the mortality from this affection varied from 10 to 15 per cent of all the women admitted, so that finally it attracted the attention of the public at large, and steps were being taken to abolish such institutions as a menace to public health. With the introduction of aseptic methods, however, all this was changed, so that at present in well-regulated lying-in hospitals the mortality from infection is usually only a small fraction of 1 per cent. Hence it happens that at the present time, in the discussions upon the subject, at least so far as hospitals are concerned, the question is not so much one of mortality, but mainly one of morbidity, and deals with the percentage of patients whose temperature rises above 38° C. or 100.4° F. during the puerperium.

On the other hand, in private practice it is doubtful whether the results are materially better to-day than they were before the introduction of antiseptic methods, for the reason that the doctrines of asepsis have not yet permeated the rank and file of medical men, much less of midwives, to whose care is committed a very large proportion of obstetrical cases. Though, at the same time, it must be admitted that we rarely hear of outbreaks of puerperal infection such as are mentioned in the historical work of Hirsch, who gives us the particulars of 216 epidemics occurring between the years 1652 and 1862.

Bacon, in an article based upon the records of the health department of Chicago for the forty years prior to 1896, shows that puerperal infection still plays a very prominent part in the death list, being the cause of death assigned in 12.75 per cent of the women dying between the ages of twenty and fifty years. In 1873, 20 per cent of all women dying in Chicago between these ages succumbed to puerperal sepsis. Happily, the mortality has gradually fallen, reaching 6 per cent in 1892, and being recorded as 7.3 per cent in 1895. These results are substantiated by those of Ingerslev, who states that, even at the present time in Denmark, with the single exception of tuberculosis, puerperal infection is the most frequent cause of death in women between the ages of twenty and fifty years.

The investigations of Boxall and Byers show a similar condition in England, where it may be said that outside of the lying-in hospitals this preventible scourge claims as many and perhaps more victims as it did twenty or even forty years ago.

Moreover, in trying to determine the frequency of puerperal infection, one cannot be guided altogether by the mortality statistics, inasmuch as the largest proportion of these cases do not end fatally. On the other hand, any one who deals mainly with gynæcological work cannot fail to be impressed with the very large proportion of patients whose troubles have originated from febrile affections during the puerperium, which in many cases were clearly due to the neglect of aseptic precautions on the part of the obstetrician or midwife.

Symptoms.—As was stated when considering the pathological anatomy of puerperal infection, the common lesion is an endometritis. This may be either of the septic or putrid variety, each type presenting a group of more or less characteristic symptoms.

In the cases of septic endometritis, after everything has gone smoothly for the first three or four days of the puerperium, the patient suddenly experiences some malaise, and may complain of headache and a feeling of chilliness, or she may have a well-defined chill, the temperature soon rising to 103° F. or higher. Generally, only one rigor occurs, after which the temperature remains constantly elevated. At the same time there is some tenderness in the lower part of the abdomen, the uterus is larger and more doughy in consistency than it should be, and is sensitive on pressure. The lochial discharge is sometimes increased in quantity, and is partly bloody, partly purulent in character, although in the purely septic forms it is practically devoid of odour. If the temperature is very high, the secretion is not infrequently diminished in amount, and occasionally disappears almost entirely.

The character of the uterine discharges in these cases often leads to a mistake in diagnosis, for the average practitioner associates puerperal infection with profuse and foul-smelling lochia; whereas, in reality in the most virulent cases, and especially in those due to a pure streptococcus infection, there is very little, if any, odour to be noticed, and its absence, therefore, is not necessarily a favourable indication, but rather the reverse.

Another point of importance is the faulty involution of the uterus. This must be looked upon as an important factor in the further spread of the disease, for, as has already been said, the micro-organisms make their way through the muscular walls of the uterus by means of the lymphatics, and when the organ is markedly relaxed these channels are more patent and offer far less resistance to the outward passage of the bacteria than when firm, normal contraction is present.

The further history of septic endometritis varies according as the process remains limited to the cavity of the uterus or extends beyond it. In the former case the temperature gradually falls, the secretion becomes less and less, and the patient is slowly restored to health. In the majority of cases, however, the mucosa is not restored to its normal condition at once, but for a long time remains the seat of a subacute or chronic inflammation. When the process has extended beyond the uterus, the symptoms will vary according to the organs involved, and those belonging to a parametritis, peritonitis, or pyæmia, as the case may be, are superadded.

The clinical picture presented by a putrid endometritis differs somewhat from that characterizing the septic form. Here we likewise have the initial chill and the high temperature, but the patient's condition does not usually appear so serious. The main difference, however, between the two varieties is to be noted in the character of the uterine discharge, which in the putrid cases is abundant, very foul-smelling, and frequently has a frothy appearance on account of the large number of gas bubbles contained in it. These cases usually eventuate in recovery, and only in rare instances terminate fatally.

Between these two well-marked classes of cases, however, there exist all gradations, and not uncommonly we have to deal with a mixed infection due to pyogenic as well as putrefactive organisms.

As has already been said, the chill and rise of temperature are occasionally associated with localized ulceration about the vulva or somewhere in the vagina. In the vast majority of cases, however, the puerperal ulcer or vaginitis does not occur alone, but is accompanied by an endometritis.

The extension of the process from the uterine cavity or from ulcers about the cervix to the parametrium produces an array of more or less characteristic manifestations. In many cases the initial rise of temperature lasts only for a short time, and we are congratulating ourselves that our patient has escaped so easily when suddenly another chill occurs, the fever rises again, to pursue a more or less irregular course, usually marked by evening exacerbations. This may continue for some time without any local manifestation; but, sooner or later, careful abdominal palpation will reveal the presence of a mass on one or both sides of the uterus, due to pus formation within the folds of the broad ligament. The abscess may be limited to the broad ligament itself, or may extend along the connective tissue upon the anterior portion of the pelvis up to the neighbourhood of Poupart's ligament; in other cases again, it extends backward towards the retroperitoneal region. The fever continues until the abscess ruptures spontaneously or has been opened, except in a few cases in which it undergoes gradual resorption, leaving a mass of cicatricial tissue to mark its former situation. If not operated upon, a parametritic abscess may burst spontaneously into the rectum or bladder, and occasionally through the abdominal wall in the region of the inguinal canal. Unless it ruptures into the peritoneal cavity the patient usually recovers.

In certain instances the infection extends from the uterine cavity to the Fallopian tubes, and there gives rise to a salpingitis with its accompanying symptoms. A large proportion of the cases of pyosalpinx, which come to operation months or years later, have originated in this manner, particularly after infection following abortions.

Unfortunately, it sometimes happens that the process does not remain limited to the uterus or to the parametrium, but the micro-organisms make their way through the lymphatics of the muscular wall of the uterus to the peritonæum, and there excite a peritonitis; though in exceptional instances it may result from an extension of the inflammation from the tubes, and occasionally from the rupture of a parametritic or ovarian abscess or of a pyosalpinx.

Somewhat rarely the peritoneal implication is limited to the portion lining the pelvic cavity—pelvic peritonitis. If the process does not spread, the chances are that the patient will recover, but if the peritonæum be invaded to any great extent death is almost inevitable. The characteristic symptoms of *peritonitis* may make their appearance at almost any time during the puerperium, but rarely come on before the third or fourth day, or later than the end of the first week, unless they are due to rupture of an abscess.

When the patient is infected with very virulent streptococci, the endometritic implication is usually very slight, and practically the first sign of infection appears from the side of the peritonæum. A marked rigor occurs, the temperature rises rapidly and remains constantly elevated, the pulse becomes rapid, and later on very weak and thready in character. The patient complains of intense pain, which is at first limited to the lower portion but gradually extends over the entire abdomen. At the same time there is marked tympanites, and the abdominal walls are rendered tense by the distended intestines. If a fatal issue ensues, death usually occurs within the first ten days of the puerperium, the patient gradually sinking, although she may remain conscious to the last. In rare cases the temperature is but little elevated and the pain slight, the serious character of the condition being indicated only by the rapid and compressible pulse.

In the cases of *pyœmia*, on the other hand, the clinical picture is very different. Here the initial chill does not occur so early, and the temperature does not remain constantly elevated, but instead we have a typical hectic fever, with the chill, high temperature, and remission recurring in succession. The symptoms of pyæmia vary very considerably, according as it is the result of the dislodgment of a single thrombus or of the constant entry into the blood of small infected particles. In the first instance we have a metastasis produced at some one point, the symptoms depending upon the organ involved. On the other hand, if thrombi are being constantly dislodged we may have symptoms referable to various organs.

One of the most constant manifestations of pyæmia is an infectious broncho-pneumonia, which contributes to the fatal termination. In other cases swellings occur at the various joints which frequently eventuate in suppuration and lead to total destruction of the tissues implicated. The course of pyæmia varies very materially according to the organs attacked and the resisting powers of the patient, but it is nothing like so uniformly fatal as the peritonitic form of infection.

In a certain number of cases the infection is so virulent that the organisms do not have a chance to become localized in any one organ, and both they and their toxines are found in abundance in the circulating blood, with very slight implication of the uterus. This happens in cases of so-called *septicæmia,* which represents the most rapidly fatal form of infection, the patients occasionally dying on the second or third day of the puerperium in a condition of shock, and without the development of local symptoms. A case of streptococcus septicæmia, observed recently in our out-patient department, ended fatally within eighteen hours after the initial rise of temperature.

In a small number of cases the thrombotic process involving the pelvic veins may extend to the femoral vein on one or both sides, giving rise to *phlegmasia alba dolens.* This accident, as a rule, does not make its appearance until some time in the second week of the puerperium, or even later, the first symptom being pain along the course of the femoral vessels, which in thin individuals may be felt as hard, sensitive cords. At the same time œdema appears in the feet and soon extends upward, though occasionally it may appear first in the thigh. This swelling is associated with severe pain, and usually lasts for a considerable time, months sometimes elapsing before the patient can walk with comfort. At the same time the condition is rarely fatal unless some complication occurs. At the onset of certain cases of phlegmasia the patients complain of severe pain about the chest. This symptom is attributed by Pinard and Wallich to the arrest of small thrombi in the pleural vessels which give rise to isolated areas of pleurisy.

In a certain number of cases infection may occur before the birth of the child. This is designated as *intra-partum infection,* and usually occurs in slow labours in which the membranes have ruptured at an early period. Under such circumstances the temperature may be markedly elevated and the patient present a profoundly septic appearance even before delivery. When the temperature during labour rises above 100.5° F., we should always think of this complication, and at once institute procedures to hasten the evacuation of the uterus.

Diagnosis.—The diagnosis of puerperal fever is usually made without difficulty, as the clinical history is very significant.

If a patient who has been doing well after delivery has a chill and a rise of temperature on the third or fourth day, we may be practically sure that we have to deal with an infection, unless we can account for the symptoms by some other satisfactory cause. In many cases the initial chill does not occur, and the first indication of the condition is a rise of temperature. In general, a temperature exceeding 100.4° F. (38° C.), and persisting for more than twenty-four hours, should be regarded as an *a priori* evidence of infection.

In the old times it was believed that the onset of the lacteal secretion was accompanied by fever, and the older observers were always ready to attribute a rise of temperature on the third or fourth day to this cause. At the present time, however, this so-called "*milk fever*" is no longer regarded as a morbid entity, as we know that the normal puerperium should be absolutely afebrile.

After the infection has become well established, either as an endometritis, peritonitis, or one of the other forms, the diagnosis is generally easy. In uncomplicated cases of puerperal endometritis usually very little pain is complained of, and it sometimes becomes a difficult matter to decide positively whether the temperature is due to a uterine infection or some other cause.

In a certain number of instances a febrile movement may occur on the third or fourth day which may justifiably be ascribed to *emotional causes*, such as excitement, fright, or grief. The temperature may rise suddenly, and after reaching a considerable height promptly fall to normal within a few hours. At first we should always suspect a beginning infection, and it is only after the rapid subsidence of the symptoms that such a diagnosis is permissible.

Now and again a post-partum rise of temperature is caused by *auto-intoxication from the intestinal tract.* Special attention has been devoted to this subject by Budin and Galtier, who state that in some instances such a condition may closely simulate puerperal infection. The diagnosis is readily arrived at, however, by the administration of a purgative, for after a copious movement of the bowels the temperature falls rapidly and remains normal.

Again, fever occurring in the early part of the puerperium is not uncommonly due to inflammatory troubles about the breasts, but the subsequent history of the case readily clears up the question of diagnosis.

In addition to the more usual causes of fever during the puerperium not due to infection, many intercurrent diseases may be accompanied by a chill and high temperature which for a short time may make one suspect a puerperal infection, although the subsequent history of the case may show that one's fears have been groundless. This is frequently so in angina and acute pulmonary affections which may occur at any time during the puerperium.

Occasionally, prolonged suppurative processes in the pelvis may be accompanied by symptoms which may readily be confounded with one or other of these diseases, but in the present state of our knowledge there is no reason why we should long remain in doubt as to the cause and origin of the fever in a given case.

There are two diseases, however—malaria and typhoid fever—that are frequently confounded with puerperal infection, and that are often made the scapegoat to shield the practitioner who has neglected aseptic precautions in the conduct of his case. While there is no doubt that either of these affections may occur during the puerperal period, in the vast majority of cases the diagnosis is open to question.

If the symptoms be due to malaria, one should be able to demonstrate the presence of the specific organisms; and in default of a positive examination of the blood one is not justified in regarding an elevated temperature and an occasional chill occurring during the puerperium as of malarial origin. Indeed, it would be far better to go still further and make it a rule that one is never justified in excluding a puerperal infection as a probable causative factor unless cultural methods have demonstrated that the uterine cavity is free from all pathogenic organisms; for it is possible that in a certain number of cases a puerperal infection may be associated with malarial poisoning, and without the bacteriological examination of the uterine lochia, after finding the specific plasmodia in the blood, one might be satisfied of the exclusive malarial origin of the symptoms, whereas, in reality they are partially due to infection. Judged by these criteria, a malarial fever complicating the puerperium will appear in health statistics far less frequently than at present.

At the same time, there is no doubt that occasionally a latent malarial infection may suddenly burst out again during the puerperium. Thus, in several of our cases the women had chills followed by fever, and we were able to demonstrate the presence of quartan malarial organisms in the blood, and at the same time to make sure of the absolute sterility of the uterine lochia.

The diagnosis of typhoid fever is very frequently made in prolonged cases of puerperal infection, being based by the average observer on the long-continued fever and the general prostration of the patient. No doubt typhoid fever may be an occasional complication, but every one, who will make a point of inquiring fully into the many instances of which he hears, will soon be convinced that only a small proportion of the cases so designated are really typhoid in origin, and that most of them depend upon an infection of the genital tract. In the present state of our knowledge, especially since Widal's discovery of the agglutinative action of the blood serum of typhoid patients upon cultures of typhoid bacilli, we are not justified in making a diagnosis of typhoid fever unless this specific action can be demonstrated.

On the other hand, typhoid fever complicating the puerperium may simulate very closely a puerperal infection, and Jung has recently described several cases in which this mistake was made, the true nature of the malady not being discovered until autopsy.

To sum up, it may be safely said that every rise of temperature observed in a puerperal woman should be regarded as due to infection until it has been clearly demonstrated that some other exciting cause is responsible. Hence it follows that in making a diagnosis of any affection complicating the puerperium, an accurate and complete physical examination of the patient is necessary, and at the same time all the aids which the recent advances in microscopy and bacteriology have placed at our command should be utilized.

Bacteriological Examination of the Lochia.—As the most common lesion in puerperal infection is an endometritis, it is a matter of some importance to decide whether one has to deal with the septic or putrid variety; but although in many cases the clinical symptoms will give tolerably definite indications, a positive conclusion can be arrived at only after a bacteriological examination of the uterine lochia, putrefactive organisms being obtained in the sapræmic and pyogenic organisms, more especially the streptococcus, in the septic types. In gonorrhœal infections the development of a purulent ophthalmia on the part of the child affords an almost positive diagnosis, but even in such cases one is not sure that other organisms may not be concerned.

Cultures may be taken from the interior of the uterus with comparatively little difficulty by means of a simple device first introduced by Döderlein. This consists of a glass tube 20 to 25 centimetres in length and 3 to 4 millimetres in diameter, with a slight bend at one end so as to conform to the anteflexed condition of the uterus. For practical purposes it is most conveniently sterilized by dry heat in a long tube of thick glass plugged with cotton, in which it can afterward be carried about ready for immediate use without fear of contamination. In an emergency, however, it may be sterilized by boiling.

When cultures are to be made from the uterus, the instruments and hands of the operator and the external genitalia of the patient having been thoroughly disinfected, the patient is placed in the Sims's or dorsal position and the posterior vaginal wall retracted by a suitable speculum. The cervix is then seized and brought into view with a volsellum forceps, and, its vaginal portion having been carefully cleansed with a bit of sterilized cotton, the lochial tube is removed from its container and introduced as far as possible into the uterus, care being taken to avoid touching the external genitalia with it during the manipulation. To the end of the lochial tube protruding from the vulva a large syringe is attached by means of a piece of rubber tubing. On making suction a certain amount of the uterine contents is drawn up into the tube, which is then removed from the uterus and its ends hermetically closed with sealing-wax. It is then replaced in its container and taken to the laboratory, where it is broken in its middle portion and cultures made from the contents (Fig. 630).

This method, although it may appear to be somewhat complicated, can be readily carried out by any practitioner who is conversant with the ordinary rules of surgical technique, and if the tube be sent to a competent bacteriologist for examination it can be determined within twenty-four hours whether the infection is due to pyogenic or putrefactive bacteria, and whether one has to deal with a dangerous or a comparatively harmless condition.

In my practice such a procedure forms a part of the routine examination in every case presenting a rise of temperature above 101° F. The satisfaction of knowing exactly with what form of infection we have to deal amply repays for the trouble taken, and at the same time the recognition of the infective agent gives important indications as to treatment.

After removing the specimens of lochia for bacteriological examination, provided the cervix is sufficiently patulous, it is well to introduce the sterile finger into the uterus and feel its interior, after which a douche of several litres of normal salt solution should be given. Palpation of the cavity of the uterus enables us in many cases to predict in advance the result of the bacteriological examination, and, what is of more practical value, gives us important information as to the line of treatment to be pursued. Thus, in putrid endometritis and infections due to the colon bacillus, we usually find the surface of the uterine cavity rough and covered with shreds of broken-down tissue; while in the septic forms its interior is often perfectly smooth.

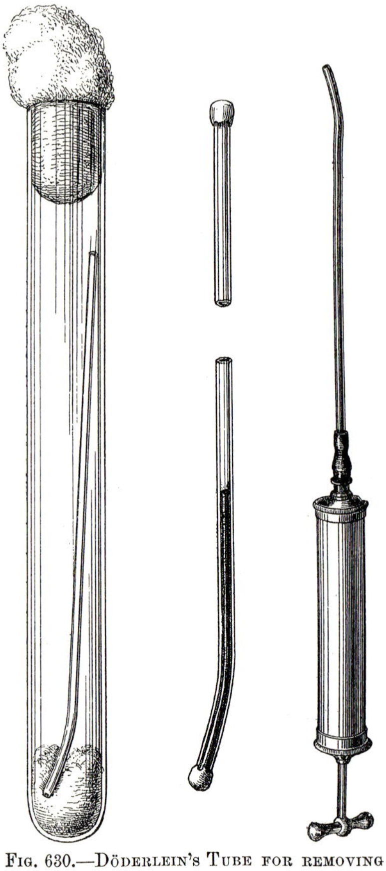

FIG. 630.—DÖDERLEIN'S TUBE FOR REMOVING UTERINE LOCHIA.

The macroscopic appearance of the lochia is also of considerable value, for in a putrid endometritis the discharge is frothy and frequently very offensive in odour, while in pure streptococcic infections it is very little changed from the normal. This distinction needs to be especially emphasized, since the first question which the practitioner usually asks the nurse in the presence of fever during the puerperium, is whether the lochia are foul-smelling or not, and if he receives a negative answer he is too apt to think that the fever is of other than uterine origin. As a matter of fact, the reverse is almost constantly true, and, as a rule, the foulness of the odour is in inverse proportion to the danger to which the patient is exposed.

When the process has extended beyond the uterus the diagnosis is much more readily made, and, provided that malarial or typhoid fever and acute miliary tuberculosis have been positively excluded, it is hardly possible to mistake the symptoms produced by a peritonitis or by a pyæmia. In the cases of parametritis and suppurative affections of the tubes and ovaries, bimanual examination will demonstrate the presence of a mass on one or other side of the uterus, if the tumour has not already made itself evident to abdominal palpation.

Prophylactic Treatment.—In considering the treatment of puerperal fever, prophylaxis should occupy the most important place. As has been repeatedly insisted, puerperal infection is wound-infection, and is due to the introduction of pathogenic micro-organisms by the hands or instruments of the doctor or nurse. Hence it naturally follows that the most scrupulous asepsis immediately before and during labour is the means upon which we have mainly to rely to limit its occurrence. Every physician who conducts a labour case cannot feel too strongly his personal responsibility in this connection, and he fails to do his full duty to his patient unless he regards the rules of asepsis as carefully as when performing a capital surgical operation. This question with all its various phases has been fully dealt with in the appropriate chapters.

All that has been said concerning the necessity of cleanliness and asepsis on the part of the physician applies equally well to the nurse, and in all her manipulations about the patient she should never forget her responsibility in this respect. Moreover, she should be strictly forbidden to make vaginal examinations or give douches except at the direct request of the physician in charge.

As long as vaginal examinations are made, no matter how carefully we may attempt to sterilize our hands, infection will occasionally occur. For this reason vaginal examinations should be dispensed with as far as possible, and with this end in view the *accoucheur* should never lose an opportunity of perfecting himself in the methods of external examination.

In view of what has already been said concerning the bacterial contents of the vagina, and the results of the experiments of Leopold and others, which have been confirmed by my own personal experience, I strongly advise against the employment of the *prophylactic douche* as a routine procedure, believing that it should be resorted to only when the vaginal secretion presents marked evidences of abnormality.

During the second stage of labour it is well to have the vulva covered with an aseptic pad in the form of a towel soaked in bichloride solution. This is done not so much for fear of infection from the air, as to prevent the possibility of contamination from the patient's hands.

The third stage of labour likewise offers many facilities for infection, and too much stress cannot be laid upon its proper conduct. Speaking broadly, the generative tract after the birth of the child should be regarded as a *noli me tangere*, unless an emergency, such as a hæmorrhage or an adherent placenta, necessitates the introduction of the hand.

The recommendation that a routine vaginal examination is called for at the conclusion of the third stage of labour in order to detect cervical tears with a view to their immediate repair, cannot be too strongly deprecated, and those who follow it will inevitably encounter a much larger percentage of abnormal puerperia than when vaginal examinations at the conclusion of the third stage of labour are reserved for exceptional and urgent cases.

Another point in the prophylaxis of puerperal infection is to close with sutures immediately after the conclusion of labour any perineal wound that extends beyond the mucosa, unless the procedure is contra-indicated by profound exhaustion on the part of the patient, or by a very œdematous condition of the tissues implicated. To save time, it is the writer's practice to introduce the sutures immediately after the birth of the child, and while waiting for the expulsion of the placenta.

To recapitulate, the liability to puerperal infection will be materially lessened by the strict observance of the following: (1) The maintenance of asepsis by the obstetrician and nurse before, during, and after delivery; (2) the restriction of vaginal examinations within the narrowest limits possible; (3) the omission of vaginal douches except in certain rare cases; (4) the immediate repair of perineal lacerations which might otherwise offer foci for infection; and (5) regarding the genital canal of the puerperal woman as a *noli me tangere,* into which neither finger nor instrument should be introduced except in emergencies.

Curative Treatment.—The curative treatment of puerperal infection is a question concerning which there is a great deal of dispute, and it is probable that what is said here may be directly opposed to the usual practice of many physicians.

If a puerperal ulcer is situated about the vulva or on the lower portion of the vagina, it should be occasionally touched with pure carbolic acid or tincture of iodine, and the parts kept as clean as possible. If the repaired perinæum breaks down and suppurates, the stitches should be removed in order that free drainage may be provided.

As has been said, puerperal endometritis is the form of infection most frequently encountered, and unfortunately the directions for its treatment differ widely and are often contradictory.

As soon as the patient's temperature reaches 102° F., unless a uterine infection can be excluded with a fair amount of certainty, the uterine lochia should be obtained in the manner described above, and submitted to a bacteriological examination. When feasible, immediately after having withdrawn the tube, the sterilized index finger should be introduced and the interior of the uterus carefully explored, after which, by means of careful bimanual examination, the condition of the appendages and the broad ligaments is determined. If the uterine cavity is perfectly smooth, a douche of several litres of boiled water or normal salt solution should be given, but curettage should not be thought of. On the other hand, if its interior is rough and jagged and contains more or less *débris,* it should be thoroughly cleaned out with the finger, after which an abundant saline douche should be employed.

Curettage as a routine measure in all cases of puerperal endometritis is by no means to be recommended, for the reason that in the most severe cases there usually is absolutely nothing in the uterine cavity which can be removed, and its employment can only do harm by breaking down the leucocytic wall which serves to prevent the invasion of the deeper layers of the uterus by the offending bacteria. On the other hand, when the uterus contains much *débris,* its removal is more readily effected by means of the finger than by the curette.

This teaching is directly contrary to that of many American and the majority of French writers, who enthusiastically recommend the use of the curette in all cases of puerperal infection. On the other hand, Fritsch, whose views represent the conservative German doctrines on the subject, would reserve its use for exceptional cases, and certainly the writer's experience has convinced him of the advisability of this restriction.

The routine use of *bichloride* or *carbolic intra-uterine douches* in the treatment of these cases is contra-indicated on several grounds. In cases due to virulent streptococci, a histological examination shows that the organisms have penetrated deep down into the tissues by the time the initial chill and rise of temperature occurs. Under these circumstances the employment of an antiseptic douche is not rational, inasmuch as the germicidal fluid cannot possibly penetrate the uterine wall sufficiently deep to reach the bacteria, which are giving rise to the symptoms and upon which the further spread of the disease is dependent.

Moreover, it has been shown experimentally by Bumm that bichloride injections penetrate the tissues only to a very slight extent. He took the liver of an animal dead of anthrax, and after soaking it for thirty minutes in a 1-to-1,000 bichloride solution placed it upon a freezing microtome and cut thick sections from it. After cutting off about $\frac{1}{10}$ of a millimetre, he inoculated the next section into another animal, which succumbed to anthrax, thus showing that the germicidal action of the bichloride had been exerted only upon the surface. If this be the case in the laboratory after the tissues have been immersed in the antiseptic solution, what effect can we expect upon organisms embedded in the muscular wall of the uterus from the transitory application to the surface of a few litres of a weak bichloride solution? Bumm likewise showed that the streptococci made their way through the uterus with great rapidity, travelling 2 centimetres or more in the space of six hours. What has been said concerning bichloride applies equally well to the other disinfectants.

On the other hand, their employment in cases of putrid endometritis is even less rational. In the vast majority of such cases simply cleaning out the uterus with the finger or curette, followed by a douche of sterile salt solution, will lead to a rapid fall of temperature and the amelioration of untoward symptoms. The object in giving a douche in these cases is simply to wash away the *dêbris* which has been left behind by the finger, and for this purpose sterile water or salt solution is far better than any antiseptic fluid.

In addition to these somewhat theoretical objections, there is this very practical one: that the employment of antiseptics may do an immense amount of harm. Not a few cases of sudden collapse following the use of carbolic-acid douches are on record, while in some instances intra-uterine injections of bichloride have been proved to have been the direct cause of death. Several years ago, at the autopsy upon a woman who was supposed to have died from puerperal sepsis, I found all the anatomical lesions of bichloride poisoning, so that, to say the least, it remained doubtful whether the infection or the treatment instituted for its relief was responsible for the fatal issue.

On reference to the literature at that time, I collected some 46 cases in which death had followed the employment of bichloride douches during the puerperium. In many instances, to be sure, excessive quantities had been employed, but in several a single injection of several litres of a 1-to-4,000 solution had resulted in fatal mercurial poisoning. When these facts are taken into consideration, along with the theoretical objections to the employment of antiseptics under these circumstances, it would appear that the benefit to be expected from their employment is at least very problematical, while the dangers are very real.

The results following the method of treatment just outlined are quite as good as those obtained with the various antiseptic douches, and this contention is sustained by the experience of Bumm and Krönig. By this means I have treated 52 cases of streptococcic endometritis, with 2 deaths attributable to the disease—a mortality of less than 4 per cent. In 30 cases I had to deal with a pure streptococcic infection, and all of the patients recovered; while of 12 cases in which it was associated with the colon bacillus or other organisms, 2 proved fatal. The latter figures apparently bear out the conclusions of Bar and Tissier, that combined infections with Streptococcus pyogenes and Bacillus coli are much more dangerous than infections due to either organism alone. At the same time it is not desired to give the impression that pure streptococcic infections are devoid of danger, as they are always serious and often fatal, and the writer feels sure that he must inevitably have deaths to report sooner or later. Nevertheless, the results in the cases just mentioned would appear to indicate that too energetic treatment may be harmful, and that an equally good or better outcome can be obtained by safer and more conservative measures.

To recapitulate, in dealing with a case of puerperal endometritis after having removed some of the uterine lochia for cultures, the cavity should be explored by the sterile finger and cleaned out or not according to its condition. The uterus should then be douched with several litres of boiled water or sterile salt solution. If the bacteriological examination shows the presence of streptococci, all local treatment should at once be omitted. If, on the other hand, one has to deal with a putrid endometritis, and the symptoms do not yield to the first injection, additional douches may be given. When the infection has extended beyond the uterus, local treatment should not be persisted in, as it will do more harm than good.

Bumm observed that in many instances involution had taken place very incompletely, and he therefore recommended the employment of ergot to secure better contraction, thereby occluding to a greater degree the lymphatics in the uterine wall. My own experience is in accord with this view, and in cases in which the uterus is larger than it should be at a given period of the puerperium the employment of the drug would certainly appear to be indicated.

In gonorrhœal endometritis active treatment is not required at the time, since in the vast majority of cases the slight rise of temperature associated with the onset of the disease soon falls to normal, and the patients recover spontaneously or are left with a chronic endometritis and diseases of the appendages, which can be treated much more advantageously at a later period.

In all severe cases, general tonic measures that will serve to keep up the strength of the patient and increase her resistance to the infective virus are most valuable. The most reliable drugs are strychnine and alcohol, and it is a matter of experience that these patients can bear much larger quantities of the latter than when in health. High fever should not be combated with antipyretics, the external application of cold, either in the form of spongings or cold baths, being far preferable. Hydrotherapeutic measures have been enthusiastically advocated by Macé, Runge, and Desternes, and in their hands have given very satisfactory results.

If the process has extended beyond the uterus, and we have to deal with a parametritis or a pelvic peritonitis, dry or moist heat to the lower portion of the abdomen in the form of poultices or other hot applications, is to be recommended.

Occasionally, surprisingly good results are obtained in profoundly septic conditions by repeated subcutaneous injections of sterile salt solution. Attention was first directed to this method of treatment by Bosc, and subsequent experience has in great part justified his predictions.

Of late a great deal has been written on the *operative treatment* of puerperal infection, nearly every prominent obstetrician and gynæcologist having made some contribution to the subject. Every one is agreed as to the advisability of opening parametritic abscesses as soon as fluctuation appears rather than allowing them to rupture spontaneously. Not uncommonly, in cases of parametritis, on palpation a semi-fluctuant sensation is conveyed to the examining finger which may lead one to suppose that one has to deal with pus, whereas upon opening the supposed abscess through the vagina or abdominal wall, as the case may be, the tumour turns out to be a mass of inflammatory exudate without pus formation, and only a small amount of serous fluid will escape when it is cut into. Fortunately, incision into these masses frequently gives as good results as if a considerable quantity of pus had been evacuated, just as happens in ordinary cases of cellulitis in other portions of the body.

When pus tubes or ovarian abscesses can be made out by bimanual palpation, their removal is urgently indicated, for as long as they remain the patient will continue in a septic condition. Whether these should be dealt with by laparotomy or by puncture through the vagina will depend upon the particular case. If they are freely movable, laparotomy should be performed; whereas if they are adherent and readily accessible from below, vaginal puncture with subsequent packing of the abscess cavity with gauze is to be preferred.

The chief point of discussion concerning the operative treatment of puerperal infection has been as to the advisability of removing the infected uterus at an early period. Here the various surgeons take quite opposite views, the more radical advocating its prompt removal, while the more conservative do not regard this step with favour.

For two reasons it would appear that *hysterectomy* is usually contraindicated in puerperal infection. In the first place, if one operates at a period sufficiently early to prevent the extension of the process to other organs, a large number of uteri will undoubtedly be removed unnecessarily; on the other hand, if one waits until a later period, when other organs have become implicated, the operation will also be useless. Nevertheless, there is a restricted field for hysterectomy in those cases in which the process has not extended materially beyond the uterus but has given rise to abscess formation within its walls. Again, in a putrid endometritis, when all other attempts to check the disease have proved futile, the operation would appear to be justifiable. Sippel has reported a case of this nature in which after total failure of all other methods of treatment hysterectomy was followed by complete recovery.

Lusk suggested that hysterectomy may sometimes be useful in the cases of pyæmia in which infected thrombi are carried from the uterus to various portions of the body, giving rise to a hectic condition. He declares that if the operation be done early enough—say after the second rise of temperature—it offers a very reasonable chance of success. No doubt in exceptional cases this may be true, but as a rule the thrombosis has extended far beyond the uterus by the time the pyæmic symptoms make their appearance, and the operation would have to be done through septic tissue. On the whole, the question of hysterectomy in this affection would seem to depend upon our ability to make a correct diagnosis and to foretell the course of the disease. This, however, is a most difficult matter, and until more accurate means of diagnosis and prognosis are at our disposal we do not believe that the operation will be very generally accepted. This question has been carefully considered by Bumm (1902), who arrived at practically the same conclusions.

The prospects of coping more successfully with puerperal infection were greatly brightened in 1895 by Marmorek's announcement of the discovery of an *antistreptococcic serum*. Unfortunately, up to the present time the results of serum therapy have not proved more satisfactory than other methods of treatment. In May, 1899, a committee of the American Gynæcological Society, of which the writer was chairman, made an exhaustive report upon this subject, giving the complete literature and collecting all the cases treated by serum reported up to that time. They found that 352 cases of puerperal infection had been so treated, with 73 deaths—a mortality of 20.74 per cent. In a large number of cases the lochia were not examined bacteriologically, and there was therefore considerable doubt as to whether the infections were due to the streptococcus; but in 101 cases in which its presence was demonstrated there were 33 deaths—a mortality of 32.69 per cent.

This is a very discouraging showing, especially when compared to the results obtained by Krönig and the writer without serum therapy, the former having treated 56 and the latter 52 cases of streptococcus endometritis, with a mortality of less than 4 per cent. The question therefore arises, Was the high mortality attending the use of the antistreptococcic serum due to its employment or to other causes? Our investigations having indicated that the serum was practically harmless, the poor results following its use can probably be explained in one of two ways: first, that only exceptionally severe cases were treated by it; and secondly, that a large number of the cases so treated had already been curetted—a procedure which is often followed by untoward results.

In view of these facts, the committee reported that there was no evidence in favour of the therapeutic value of antistreptococcic serum, although it apparently did not exert a deleterious effect upon the patient, and therefore might be employed if the physician so desired.

Although at first sight it would seem difficult to reconcile these conclusions with the enthusiastic reports of many observers, it is probable that the good results of individual practitioners must be attributed to the fact that they employed the serum only in a few cases, and seem to have forgotten that most cases undergo spontaneous cure if not interfered with.

It is always difficult to arrive at correct conclusions as to the value of any given therapeutic agent, unless large numbers of cases are used as a basis, and this is particularly true in the affection under consideration, for the reason that its clinical course is so very variable. Thus, it is not at all rare in cases of streptococcic infection to see the temperature rise rapidly to 103°–105° F., remain there for a day or so, and then fall as rapidly as it had risen. This may occur without the employment of any treatment, and had the specific serum been employed in such cases it is more than probable that the rapid amelioration of symptoms would have been attributed to its use.

That we as yet possess no satisfactory treatment for all cases of puerperal infection is indicated by the vast number of methods advocated from time to time. In this place only a few of the more recent need be mentioned.

Fochier advocates in pyæmic cases the production of what he calls *abscès de fixation*—that is, the production of abscesses on various portions of the body by the subcutaneous injection of turpentine. He thought he observed that the condition of the patient improved as soon as the abscesses made their appearance on the surface, and his method of treatment was intended to simulate Nature's process. Unfortunately, experience has failed to strengthen this view.

Kezmarsky, in 1894, reported 2 cases of severe venous sepsis in which he gave intravenous injections of 1 to 5 milligrammes of corrosive sublimate. He noted a marked effect following its exhibition, and both patients recovered. His work was enthusiastically taken up by Rissmann, who likewise reported several cures. In the hands of others, however, the method has not proved satisfactory.

Hofbauer, in 1896, reported 7 cases of puerperal sepsis in which he produced an artificial leucocytosis by the employment of nuclein. In some of his cases the temperature fell by a lysis and in others by crisis, and he believed that the artificial leucocytosis played a marked part in their cure. Thus far no one has substantiated Hofbauer's results, but Hirst states his belief that more is to be expected from this line of treatment than from serum therapy.

LITERATURE

AHLFELD. Beiträge zur Lehre vom Resorptionsfieber im Wochenbett und von der Selbstinfektion. Berichte und Arbeiten, 1883, 165.

Beitrag zur Lehre der Selbstinfektion. Centralbl. f. Gyn., 1887, 729.

Beiträge zur Lehre vom Resorptionsfieber in der Geburt und im Wochenbette und von der Selbstinfektion. Zeitschr. f. Geb. u. Gyn., 1893, xxvii, 466–519.

BACON. The Mortality from Puerperal Infection in Chicago. Amer. Gyn. and Obst. Jour., 1896, viii, 429–446.

BAR et TISSIER. La Semaine Méd., 1896, 155.

Sérothérapie dans l'infection puerpérale. L'Obstétrique, 1896, 97–128, 204–217.

BARKER. The Puerperal Diseases. 3d ed., 1874.

BENSIS. Recherches sur la flore vulvaire et vaginal chez femme enceinte. Thèse de Paris, 1900.

BERGHOLM. Ueber die Mikroorganismen des Vaginalsecretes Schwangerer. Archiv f. Gyn., 1902, xliv, 497–589.

BLUMER. A Case of Mixed Puerperal and Typhoid Infection, in which the Streptococcus and Typhoid Bacillus were isolated both from the Blood and Uterine Cavity. Amer. Jour. Obst., 1899, xxxix, 42–50.

BOSC. Injections de sérum artificiel dans les maladies infectieuses et les intoxications. Presse Méd., 1896, No. 49, 287–290.

BOXALL. The Mortality of Childbirth. Lancet, 1893, ii, 9–15.

BRETSCHNEIDER. Klinische Versuche über den Einfluss der Scheidenspülungen während der Geburt auf den Wochenbettsverlauf. Archiv f. Gyn., 1901, lxiii, 453–471.

BRIEGER. Ueber bakteriologische Untersuchungen bei einigen Fällen von Puerperalfieber. Charité-Annalen, 1888, xiii, 198.

BUDIN. La Semaine Méd., 1896, 155.

BUMM. Die puerperale Wundinfektion. Centralbl. f. Bakteriol., 1887, ii, 343.

Histologische Untersuchungen über die puerperale Endometritis. Archiv f. Gyn., 1891, xl, 398.

Ueber die verschiedenen Virulenzgrade der puerperalen Infektion und die lokale Behandlung bei Puerperalfieber. Centralbl. f. Gyn., 1893, 975.

Ueber Diphtherie und Kindbettfieber. Zeitschr. f. Geb. u. Gyn., 1895, xxxiii, 126–136.

Ueber die Aufgaben weiterer Forschungen auf dem Gebiete der puerperalen Wundinfektion. Archiv f. Gyn., 1899, xxxiv, 325.

Ueber die chirurgische Behandlung des Kindbettfiebers. Sammlung zwangloser Abhandlungen aus dem Gebiete der Frauenheilkunde und Geb., 1902, iv, Heft 4.

BURCKHARDT. Ueber den Einfluss der Scheidenbakterien auf den Verlauf des Wochenbettes. Archiv f. Gyn., 1893, xiv, 71–94.

Ueber den Keimgehalt der Uterushöhle bei normalen Wöchnerinnen. Centralbl. f. Gyn., 1898, 686–689.

BURGUBURU. Zur Bakteriologie des Vaginalsekretes Schwangerer. Archiv f. exper. Path. und Pharmak., 1892, xxx, November.

BYERS. Mortality from Puerperal Fever in England and Wales. Amer. Jour. Obst., 1901, xliv, 433–441.

CHARPENTIER. Sérothérapie anti-streptococcique appliquée au traitement de la fièvre puerpérale. La Semaine Gyn., 1896, No. 12, 89–92.

COZE et FELTZ. Gazette Méd. de Strasbourg, 1869, 30.

CZERNIEWSKI. Zur Frage von den puerperalen Erkrankungen. Eine bakteriologische Studie. Archiv f. Gyn., 1888, xxxiii, 73.

DESTERNES. Indications et rôle du bain froid dans le traitement de l'infection puerpérale. Thèse de Paris, 1895.

DOBBIN. Puerperal Sepsis Due to Infection with the Bacillus Aerogenes Capsulatus. Bull. Johns Hopkins Hosp., February, 1897.

A Case of Puerperal Infection in which the Bacillus Typhosus was found in the Uterus. Amer. Jour. Obst., 1898, xxxviii, 185–198.

DÖDERLEIN. Untersuchung über das Vorkommen von Spaltpilzen in den Lochien des Uterus und der Vagina gesunder und kranker Wöchnerinnen. Archiv f. Gyn., 1887, xxxi, 412.

Klinisches und Bakteriologisches über eine Puerperalfieberepidemie. Archiv f. Gyn., 1891, xi, 99.

Das Scheidensekret und seine Bedeutung für das Puerperalfieber. Leipzig, 1892.

Vorläufige Mittheilung über weitere bakteriologische Untersuchungen des Scheidensekretes. Centralbl. f. Gyn., 1894, 779.

Die Beziehungen der Endometritis zu den Fortpflanzungsvorgängen. Verh. d. deutschen Ges. f. Gyn., 1895, 224–242.

DÖDERLEIN und WINTERNITZ. Die Bakteriologie der puerperalen Sekrete. Hegar's Beiträge zur Geb. u. Gyn., 1900, iii, 161–174.

DOLÉRIS. Essai sur la pathogénie et la thérapeutique des accidents infectieux des suites de couches. Thèse de Paris, 1880.

Inflammation puerpérale. Nouv. Archives d'Obst. et de Gyn., 1894, ix, 97–122, 142–161.

EISENMANN. Wund- und Kindbettfieber. Erlangen, 1837.

ERNST. Ueber einen gasbildenden Anäroben im menschlichen Körper und seine Beziehung zur Schaumleber. Virchow's Archiv, cxxxiii, Heft 2.

FEHLING. Ueber Selbstinfektion. Verh. d. deutschen Gesellsch. f. Gyn., Freiburg, 1889.

Ueber die Erkrankungsziffern Entbindungshäuser. Deutsche med. Wochenschr., 1896, 426.

FOCHIER. Traitement de l'infection puerpérale par la provocation de phlegmons souscutanés. Annales de Gyn., 1892, xxvii, 356–362.

FRÄNKEL. Quoted by Lomer.

v. FRANQUÉ. Bakteriologische Untersuchungen bei normalem und fieberhaftem Wochenbett. Zeitschr. f. Geb. u. Gyn., 1893, xxv, 277.

FRANZ. Bakteriologische und klinische Untersuchungen über leichte Fiebersteigerungen im Wochenbette. Hegar's Beiträge zur Geb. u. Gyn., iii, 1900, 51–100.

FRITSCH. Ueber Auskratzung des Uterus nach reifen Geburten. Zeitschr. f. Geb. u. Gyn., 1891, xxi, 456.

GALTIER. De l'infection primitive du liquide amniotique après rupture prématurée des membranes de l'œuf humain. Thèse de Paris, 1895.

GARRIGUES. Puerperal Infection. Amer. Text-Book of Obstetrics, 1895, 683–734.

GEBHARD. Bacterium coli commune aus Fällen von Tympania uteri gezüchtet. Verh. d. deutschen Gesellsch. f. Gyn., 1893, 305.

GILBERT et DOMINCI. Recherches sur le nombre des microbes du tube digestif. Semaine Méd., 1894, 76.

GOLDSCHEIDER. Klinische und bakteriologische Mittheilungen über Sepsis puerperalis. Charité-Annalen, 1893, xviii, 164–242.

GÖNNER. Ueber Mikroorganismen im Sekrete der weiblichen Genitalien während der Schwangerschaft und bei puerperalen Erkrankungen. Centralbl. f. Gyn., 1887, 444.

HAEGLER. Quoted by Fehling. Physiologie und Path. des Wochenbetts. Stuttgart, 1890.

HALBAN. Uterusemphysem und Gassepsis. Monatsschr. f. Geb. u. Gyn., 1900, xi, 88–122.

HARRIS and DABNEY. Report of a Case of Gonorrhœal Endocarditis in a Patient Dying in the Puerperium. Bull. Johns Hopkins Hosp., 1901, xii, 68–76.

HEIBERG. Die puerperalen und pyämischen Processe, 1873.

HIRSCH. Historisch-pathologische Untersuchungen über Puerperalfieber. Erlangen, 1864.

HIRST. Modern Methods of Treatment of Puerperal Infection, and their Comparative Worth. Amer. Jour. Obst., 1896, xxxiv, 180-184.

HOFBAUER. Zur Verwerthung einer künstlichen Leukocytose bei der Behandlung septischer Puerperalprocesse. Centralbl. f. Gyn., 1896, 441-449.

HOLMES. Puerperal Fever as a Private Pestilence. Boston, 1865.

INGERSLEV. Die Sterblichkeit an Wochenbettfieber in Dänemark und die Bedeutung der Antiseptik für dasselbe. Zeitschr. f. Geb. u. Gyn., 1893, xxvi, 443.

JEWETT. The Question of Puerperal Self-Infection. Amer. Gyn. and Obst. Jour., 1896, viii, 417-429.

KALTENBACH. Zur Antisepsis in der Geburtshülfe. Volkmann's Sammlung klin. Vorträge, Nr. 295.

Ueber Selbstinfektion. Verh. d. deutschen Gesellsch. f. Gyn., Freiburg, 1889.

KEZMARSKY. Intravenöse Sublimatinjection bei venöser Sepsis im Wochenbette. Centralbl. f. Gyn., 1894, 906.

KIRKLAND. Treatise on Childbed Fever, 1774.

KOBLANCK. Zur puerperalen Infektion. Zeitschr. f. Geb. u. Gyn., 1899, xi, 85-92.

KOTTMANN. Beitrag zur Bakteriologie der Vagina. Archiv f. Gyn., 1898, lv, 615.

KRÖNIG. Klinische Versuche über den Einfluss der Scheidenspülungen während der Geburt auf den Wochenbettsverlauf. Münchener med. Wochenschr., 1900, Nr. 1.

Vorläufige Mittheilung über Gonorrhöe im Wochenbett. Centralbl. f. Gyn., 1893, 157.

Scheidensekretuntersuchungen bei ein Hundert Schwangeren. Aseptik in der Geburtshülfe. Centralbl. f. Gyn., 1894, 3-10.

Ueber Fieber intra-partum. Centralbl. f. Gyn., 1894, 749.

Discussion über Endometritis. Verh. d. deutschen Gesellsch. f. Gyn., 1895, 498-502.

KRÖNIG und MENGE. Bakteriologie des Genitalkanales der schwangeren, kreisenden und puerperalen Frau. Leipzig, 1897.

LANDAU. Ueber puerperale Erkrankungen. Archiv f. Gyn., 1874, vi, 147.

LEOPOLD. Ueber die Wochenbetten von nicht untersuchten und nicht ausgespülten Gebärenden. Verh. d. deutschen Gesellsch. f. Gyn., Freiburg, 1889.

Dritter Beitrag zur Verhütung des Kindbettfiebers. Archiv f. Gyn., 1889, xxxv, 149-162.

Ueber die Entbehrlichkeit der Scheidenausspülungen und Auswaschungen bei regelmässigen Geburten und über die grösstmögliche Verwerthung der äusseren Untersuchung in der Geburtshülfe. Archiv f. Gyn., 1891, xl, 349.

Ueber gonorrhöisches Fieber im Wochenbett bei einer innerlich nicht untersuchten Gebärenden. Centralbl. f. Gyn., 1893, 675.

Vergleichende Untersuchungen über die Entbehrlichkeit der Scheidenausspülungen bei ganz normalen Geburten und über die sogenannte Selbstinfektion. Archiv f. Gyn., 1894, xlvii, 580-635.

LEOPOLD und ORB. Die Leitung ganz normaler Geburten nur durch äussere Untersuchung. Archiv f. Gyn., 1895, xlviii, 304-323.

LEOPOLD und SPÖRLING. Die Leitung der regelmässigen Geburten nur durch äussere Untersuchungen. Archiv f. Gyn., xiv, 339-371.

LOMER. Ueber den heutigen Stand der Lehre von den Infektionsträgern bei Puerperalfieber. Zeitschr. f. Geb. u. Gyn., 1884, x, 366.

LUSK. Recent Bacteriological Investigations concerning the Nature of Puerperal Fever, Amer. Jour. Obst., 1896, xxxiii, 337-347.

MACÉ. Traitement de la septicémie puerpérale par la réfrigération et en particulier par les bains froids. Gaz. des Hôp., 1894, 1376, 1372.

MARMOREK. Sur le streptocoque. Comptes rendus de la Soc. de Biol., 1895, 10me série, ii, 122.

Le streptocoque et le sérum antistreptococcique. Annales de l'Institut Pasteur, 1895, ix, 593-620.

MASLOWSKY. Zur Aetiologie der vorzeitigen Ablösung der Placenta vom normalen Sitz. Monatsschr. f. Geb. u. Gyn., 1896, iv, 212–218.

MAYRHOFER. Zur Frage nach Aetiologie der Puerperalprocesse. Monatsschr. f. Geburtskunde, 1865, xxv, 112–134.

MEIGS. On Childbed Fever. Philadelphia, 1854.

MERMANN. Zur Antisepsis in der Geburtshülfe. Centralbl. f. Gyn., 1887, 439.

Die Entbehrlichkeit und Gefahren innerer Desinfektion bei normalen Geburten. Verh. d. deutschen Gesellsch. f. Gyn., Freiburg, 1889.

Fünfter Bericht über zwei Hundert Geburten ohne innere Desinfektion. Centralbl. f. Gyn., 1894, 786.

MIXIUS. Bakteriologische Untersuchungen einiger Fälle puerperaler Sepsis. D. I., Berlin, 1892.

NEUMANN. Ueber puerperale Uterusgonorrhöe. Monatsschr. f. Geb. u. Gyn., 1896, iv, 109–116.

NISOT. Diphthérie vagino-utérine puerpérale. Sérothérapie, guérison. Annales de Gyn. et d'Obst., 1896, xlv, 259.

NORRIS. A Report of Six Cases in which the Bacillus Aerogenes Capsulatus was isolated. Amer. Jour. Med. Sciences, February, 1899.

ORTH. Virchow's Archiv, lviii, 441.

PASTEUR. Septicémie puerpérale. Bull. de l'Acad. de Méd., 1879, 260–271.

PINARD et WALLICH. Traitement de l'infection puerpérale. Paris, 1896.

RECKLINGHAUSEN. Centralbl. f. med. Wissenschaften, 1871, 713.

REYNOLDS. The Frequency of Puerperal Infection in Massachusetts, etc. Boston Med. and Surg. Jour., cxxxi, 153–155.

RUNGE. Die Allgemeinbehandlung der puerperalen Sepsis. Archiv f. Gyn., 1888, xxxiii, 39–52.

SAMSCHIN. Ueber das Vorkommen von Eiterstaphylococcen in den Genitalien von gesunden Frauen. Deutsche med. Wochenschr., 1890, 232.

SEMMELWEISS. Die Aetiologie, der Begriff u. die Prophylaxis des Kindbettfiebers. Pest, Wien u. Leipzig, 1861.

SILBERSCHMIDT. Historisch-kritische Darstellung der Pathologie des Kindbettfiebers, Gekrönte Preisschrift. Erlangen, 1859.

SIPPEL. Supravaginale Amputation des septischen puerperalen Uterus. Centralbl. f. Gyn., 1894, 667–674.

STEFFECK. Bakteriologische Begründung der Selbstinfektion. Zeitschr. f. Geb. u. Gyn., 1890, xx, 339.

STEWART and BALDWIN. Bacillus Aerogenes Capsulatus. Columbus Med. Jour., Aug., 1893.

STRAUSS et SANCHEZ-TOLEDO. Septicémie puerpérale expérimentale. Nouv. Archive d'Obst. et de Gyn., 1889, cv, 277–295.

STROTHER. Critical Essay on Fevers. London, 1718.

THOMEN. Bakteriologische Untersuchungen normaler Lochien und der Vagina und Cervix Schwangerer. Archiv f. Gyn., 1889, xxxvi, 231.

VAHLE. Ueber das Vorkommen von Streptococcen in der Scheide Gebärender. Zeitschr. f. Geb. u. Gyn., 1896, xxxv, 192–215.

VIGNAL. Sur l'action des micro-organisms de la bouche et des matières fécales. Comptes rendus de la Soc. de Biol., août, 1887.

WALDEYER. Ueber das Vorkommen von Bakterien bei der diphtheritischen Form des Puerperalfiebers. Archiv f. Gyn., 1872, iii, 293.

WALTHARD. Bakteriologische Untersuchungen des weiblichen Genitalsekretes in der Gravidität und in Puerperium. Archiv f. Gyn., 1895, xlviii, 201–269.

WELCH. Morbid Conditions caused by Bacillus Aerogenes Capsulatus. Boston Med. and Surg. Jour., 1900, cxliii, 73–87.

WIDAL. Étude sur l'infection puerpérale. Thèse de Paris, 1889.

Infection puerperale et phlegmasia alba dolens. Gaz. des Hôp., 1889, 565.

WILLIAMS, J. W. Puerperal Infection considered from a Bacteriological Point of View, with Special Reference to the Question of Auto-Infection. Amer. Jour. Med. Sciences, July, 1893.

The Cause of the Conflicting Statements concerning the Bacterial Contents of the Vaginal Secretion of the Pregnant Woman. Amer. Jour. Obst., 1898, xxxviii, 807–817.

The Bacteria of the Vagina and their Practical Significance, based upon the Bacteriological Examination of the Vaginal Secretion in Ninety-two Pregnant Women. Amer. Jour. Obst., 1898, xxxviii, 449–483.

Diphtheria of the Vulva. Amer. Jour. Obst., 1898, xxxviii, 180–185.

Ein Fall von puerperaler Infektion, bei dem sich Typhusbacillen in den Lochien fanden. Centralbl. f. Gyn., 1898, Nr. 34.

Puerperal Diphtheria. Amer. Jour. Obst., August, 1898.

WILLIAMS, PRYOR, FRY, and REYNOLDS. The Value of Antistreptococcic Serum in the Treatment of Puerperal Infection. Trans. Amer. Gyn. Soc., 1899, xxiv, 80–126.

WINTER. Die Mikroorganismen im Genitalkanal der gesunden Frauen. Zeitschr. f. Geb. u. Gyn., 1888, xiv, 443.

WITTE. Bakteriologische Untersuchungsbefunde bei path. Zuständen im weibl. Genitalapparat, mit besonderer Berücksichtigung der Eitererreger. Zeitschr. f. Geb. u. Gyn., 1892, xxv, 1–30.

WOOD. Puerperal Infection caused by the Bacillus Aerogenes Capsulatus. Med. Rec., April 15, 1899. Ref. Centralbl. f. Gyn., 1900, 436, Nr. 16.

CHAPTER XLV

DISEASES AND ABNORMALITIES OF THE PUERPERIUM

We have already discussed in detail the more typical instances of puerperal infection. We shall now take up certain atypical varieties—tetanus, phlegmasia alba dolens, and cystitis—and shall then proceed to consider certain other diseases and abnormalities which may be encountered in the puerperium, but which are not due to the introduction of infective material into the genital tract. Thus, we shall find that fever associated with constitutional disturbances is not infrequently met with as the result of pathological conditions in the breasts, disorders of the intestinal tract, and in very rare instances of emotional causes. Moreover, it must be remembered that Nature has not rendered the puerperal woman exempt from the various disorders from which she might suffer at other times.

Tetanus.—The undoubted development of tetanus during the puerperium, although a very rare occurrence, has been fully established by the researches of Chantemesse and Widal, Heyse, Rubeska, and others, who have isolated the characteristic bacilli from the uterine lochia. The infection usually follows gross errors in antiseptic technique, especially during operative procedures. Thus, in several of the reported cases, it is recorded that the operator placed the forceps upon the dirty floor by the side of the bed, and afterward carried it directly to the genital tract of the patient. Occasionally, however, such an explanation cannot be adduced, as in the recent epidemic in the Prague Lying-in Hospital, the disease, in one instance, at least, occurred in a woman who had not even been examined internally.

The disease follows abortion more frequently than full-term labour, and as a rule gives rise to untoward manifestations between the sixth and tenth days of the puerperium, and sometimes later, though in rare instances the first symptom has been known to appear before the completion of labour. The prognosis is very grave. All of the 20 patients mentioned by Rubeska succumbed, while Vinay reports a similar result in 94 out of the 106 cases included in his statistics.

Beyond affording means for temporarily controlling the symptoms, therapeutic measures are valueless, and thus far the results obtained from the employment of anti-tetanus serum have not been encouraging, although its prophylactic employment has been attended by excellent results. In view of the hopelessness of other lines of treatment, Pawlik and Rubeska removed the uterus in several of their cases, but without avail.

Thrombosis of the Vessels of the Lower Extremities.—Thrombosis occurring in the crural, popliteal, or saphenous veins—*phlegmasia alba dolens*—is usually a manifestation of infection, and follows the direct extension of a thrombotic process from the pelvic veins, although occasionally it results from a localized phlebitis or periphlebitis. The lumina of the large veins rarely undergo complete obliteration, so that the circulation, while markedly interfered with, is not completely shut off.

Symptoms of phlegmasia do not usually make their appearance until the latter part of the second week of the puerperium or even later. In most cases the first manifestation is pain in one leg extending along the course of one of the larger veins; this is soon followed by œdema, which usually begins in the foot and extends upward, although occasionally it appears first in the neighbourhood of the groin. The leg soon becomes much swollen, the skin being tightly stretched and presenting a glazed appearance, and at first pitting can be elicited only after prolonged pressure with the finger-tip. If the crural vein is implicated, a cord-like structure, which is very sensitive to pressure, can often be palpated just beneath Poupart's ligament and for a certain distance down the thigh.

The inflammatory changes are usually attended by some elevation of temperature, the pulse being more or less accelerated. High fever and a very rapid action of the heart usually indicate that a similar process is taking place in other portions of the body, and that the patient is suffering from a general infection or pyæmia. The pain, swelling, and temperature continue for several weeks, and then gradually subside, though occasionally months elapse before the patient regains the full use of the leg.

Ordinarily, the process is limited to one side, more rarely both extremities are affected, an interval of a week or ten days elapsing before the second leg becomes implicated. If properly treated, most cases undergo spontaneous cure, the condition being dangerous only when it forms part of a generalized infection, or when the thrombus undergoes suppuration and softening, so that infected particles are carried to other parts, giving rise to metastatic abscesses and occasionally to sudden death from pulmonary embolism.

Treatment.—Perfect rest is absolutely essential. The lower part of the leg should be elevated, and the entire member encased in absorbent cotton and protected from the weight of the bedclothes by a suitable contrivance. If the pain is severe morphine may be required, though ordinarily the application along the course of the thrombosed vein of cloths soaked in lead water and opium is followed by marked relief. Excellent results have been reported from painting the leg with a 15- or 20-per-cent solution of ichthyol.

On account of the danger of detaching portions of the thrombus, the leg should never be rubbed. The patient should be kept in a horizontal position for at least a week after the pain has disappeared and the temperature subsided, and after being allowed to get up she should be cautioned against making sudden movements.

Small varicose veins of the lower extremities sometimes undergo thrombosis during pregnancy, but more often during the first weeks of the puerperium. In pregnancy this occurrence is favoured by the interference with the circulation due to the pressure exerted by the uterus upon the vessels returning from the extremities. During the puerperium its development is occasionally favoured by pressure exerted upon the intrapelvic veins by inflammatory exudates. In small veins the thrombosis is usually unattended by symptoms, although now and again the development of a localized phlebitis or periphlebitis may cause pain, and exceptionally eventuate in the formation of a small localized abscess.

Gangrene of the Lower Extremities.—In very rare instances, as the result of extensive thrombosis of the venous channels or of embolism of the crural artery, the circulation in the foot and ankle may become so impaired that gangrene results. One or both feet may be affected in this way. This accident, first described by Churchill and studied more particularly by Wormser and Burckhard, is one of the most serious complications of the puerperium, and usually ends fatally. Thus, 62 per cent of the 34 patients mentioned in Lafond's thesis died, in spite of the fact that in several instances amputation was resorted to in order to check the further development of the process.

Diseases of the Urinary Tract.—A *cystitis* occurring during the puerperium is usually the result of infection following catheterization, during which the rules of asepsis have not been scrupulously followed. The occurrence of the condition is favoured by the presence of slight lesions of the vesical mucosa which frequently accompany easy and spontaneous labours, and are almost universally associated with difficult deliveries.

In view of the impossibility of thoroughly disinfecting the vulva and urethral orifice, cystitis will occasionally occur, despite the most rigid precautions. For this reason catheterization should be restricted to the greatest possible extent, and employed only in those cases in which the patient is unable to evacuate her bladder after being placed in a sitting position. In rare instances, the affection results from the direct extension of areas of inflammation about the urethral orifice and vulva.

As the process demands a certain period of incubation, symptoms do not usually appear for several days. The patient first experiences a frequent desire to micturate, but passes only a small quantity of urine at one time, the act being accompanied by a burning sensation in the urethra and a tendency to tenesmus after each evacuation. At the same time, the bladder and the urethra become sensitive on pressure. The urine is usually cloudy, and upon microscopic examination is found to be loaded with mucus, leucocytes, epithelial cells, and bacteria. Occasionally it contains a large proportion of blood. The acid reaction is usually retained, although, more especially when the process is prolonged, the secretion may become alkaline, and very offensive in odour.

Now and again cases are encountered in which the infection is so severe that larger or smaller portions of the mucosa become exfoliated and are cast off with the urine, their expulsion being associated with cramp-like pains.

In these virulent types, and also in the milder but obstinate processes, the disease tends to extend up the ureters and to involve the pelvis of the kidney, giving rise to a *pyelo-nephrosis* or even a *pyelo-nephritis*, though several weeks are usually required for the development of these latter conditions. Thus, in some cases the patient who has previously had a cystitis, but has recovered satisfactorily from the puerperium, may suddenly experience intense pain in one renal region, associated with the development of a temperature characterized by marked remissions and the passage of large quantities of urine laden with pus. The condition not infrequently apparently passes off, to recur again when least expected.

In mild cases of cystitis the *treatment* consists in the ingestion of large quantities of fluids, particularly milk and the carbonated and alkaline waters. The vesical irritability is often satisfactorily allayed by the administration of the various balsams, such as copaiba or sandalwood, 3 to 5 drops in capsules or upon a lump of sugar 4 times a day, or by the exhibition of 5-grain capsules of salol or urotropin repeated every four to six hours. Ordinarily, simple treatment leads to recovery in a comparatively short time, but if the process drags on, daily irrigation of the bladder with a 2-per-cent solution of boric acid or a 1-to-20,000 or 30,000 solution of bichloride should be practised.

Most cases of pyelo-nephrosis recover spontaneously after rest in bed and the administration of large quantities of fluids and the usual renal antiseptics; but whenever a pyelo-nephritis develops and is accompanied by prolonged febrile manifestations, drainage and occasionally extirpation of the organ becomes necessary.

Retention of Urine.—In Chapter XVI, upon the care of the patient during the puerperium, reference was made to the retention of urine, which frequently causes annoyance during the first few days of that period.

Incontinence of Urine.—In multiparous women, for the first few days of the puerperium, coughing, sneezing, or other factors leading to a sudden increase in the intra-abdominal pressure, often produce an involuntary discharge of a small quantity of urine.

More marked incontinence at this time is usually the result of lesions about the neck of the bladder following operative delivery, though when the condition does not manifest itself until the end of the first week it is usually the first sign of the development of a *vesico-vaginal fistula.* In the majority of such cases scrupulous attention to cleanliness will be followed by spontaneous recovery; but when the fistulous opening is extensive, a cure can be effected only by operative procedures at a later period.

Hæmorrhages during the Puerperium.—Ordinarily, if there has been no serious loss of blood during the first hour or hour and a half following delivery, it may be assumed that the danger of post-partum hæmorrhage has practically passed, and that the only loss of blood for the next few days will be represented by the lochial discharge.

Occasionally, however, in the latter part of the first week, and more often still later in the puerperium, more or less severe uterine hæmorrhages are encountered. They are nearly always due to the retention of portions of a placental cotyledon or of a succenturiate lobule which may not have been discovered at the time of labour in spite of the most rigid precautions; although the presence of large portions of placenta can hardly be overlooked unless the obstetrician is grossly negligent. If the retained tissue is not cast off spontaneously or removed, it undergoes gradual necrosis, while at the same time fibrin becomes deposited about its periphery, giving rise to a polypoid growth of varying size—*placental polyp*—a certain amount of hæmorrhage, although not enough to cause alarm, continuing as long as it remains in the uterus.

Large portions of the fœtal membranes retained in the uterine cavity rarely give rise to serious hæmorrhage, as the tissues gradually disintegrate and are cast off with the lochial discharge. The presence of a remnant of decidua of any considerable size which has failed to undergo the usual regressive changes, may act as an irritant upon the regenerating endometrium, giving rise to a hyperplasia which is usually associated with more or less hæmorrhage. This condition is designated as *endometritis post-partum* or *post-abortion*, according as it follows full-term labour or abortion.

The diagnosis of the retention of a placental remnant or the existence of a polyp can only be verified by the sense of touch. Therefore, whenever a patient suffers from an acute loss of blood during the puerperium, the interior of the uterus should be carefully palpated, and any abnormal substance found in it should be promptly removed by means of the finger or curette.

The treatment of the slight hæmorrhage following retroflexion and subinvolution of the uterus will be referred to under those headings. The loss of blood associated with an endometritis post-partum also demands curettage. If the patient does not begin to bleed until late in the puerperium, and more particularly after the expulsion of an hydatidiform mole, the possibility of the existence of a deciduoma malignum should always be considered. Whenever possible, the tissues obtained by curetting should be submitted to microscopical examination, since in this way one receives timely warning of the existence of any serious process.

Puerperal Hæmatoma.—A tumefaction resulting from the escape of blood into the connective tissue beneath the vaginal mucosa or the skin covering the external genitalia is known as a *vaginal* or *vulval hæmatoma.* This condition, first studied in detail by Deneux, in 1830, is a rare complication of labour and the puerperium, occurring about once in 1,500 or 2,000 cases. It occasionally originates during pregnancy, but more often follows injury to a blood-vessel during the act of labour without laceration of the superficial tissues. Now and again it does not occur until later, and is then attributable to the sloughing of a vessel which has become necrotic as the result of prolonged pressure.

The site at which the hæmatoma develops varies according as the torn vessel lies beneath or above the pelvic fascia. In the former case the tumefaction involves the vulva and perineal region, while in the latter it protrudes into the vaginal canal, and as it increases in size separates the peritonæum from the underlying tissues, so that at times the hæmatoma gradually extends up into the false pelvis.

If the tumour is large, it not only causes discomfort by its mere size, but gives rise to great suffering, which becomes more intense the more rapidly it is formed, as the result of the tearing and stretching of the tissues. In rare instances, such large quantities of blood may be contained in the hæmatoma that the patient suffers from an acute anæmia, and should the mass rupture into the peritoneal cavity or through the external covering, a profuse external hæmorrhage may occur which sometimes proves fatal. On the other hand, a hæmatoma of a moderate size is usually absorbed spontaneously. In other cases the tissues covering the tumour may undergo pressure necrosis and give way, profuse hæmorrhage resulting, or the contents may be discharged in the form of large clots. In either event the interior of the hæmatoma is very prone to become infected, the condition sometimes ending fatally.

A vulval hæmatoma is readily diagnosed by the sudden appearance at the vulva of a tense, elastic, fluctuating, and sensitive tumour of varying size, covered by the discoloured skin. When the mass develops in the vagina it may escape detection for a time, but pressure symptoms soon ensue, and on a vaginal examination one discovers a round, fluctuant tumour which encroaches upon the lumen. On the other hand, when a hæmatoma extends upward between the folds of the broad ligament, it is liable to escape detection, unless symptoms of anæmia or infection appear. In such cases careful palpation reveals the presence of a rounded tumour mass to one side of the uterus; although if the patient is not seen until after infection has occurred, the differential diagnosis between such a condition and a pelvic inflammatory mass becomes difficult.

The prognosis is usually favourable, though very large hæmatomata occasionally lead to death from hæmorrhage, whereas in rare cases the fatal termination is the result of infection.

Treatment.—Small hæmatomata should be left alone, as spontaneous resorption usually takes place, provided the parts be kept clean and infection avoided. On the other hand, since a steady increase in the size of the swelling indicates a continuance of hæmorrhage, the tumour in such cases should be laid widely open and packed with gauze, which usually effectually controls the loss of blood. The strictest antiseptic precautions are imperative, inasmuch as infection is a frequent complication.

Diseases and Abnormalities of the Uterus.—*Subinvolution.*—This term is used to describe an arrest or retardation of the process of involution, by which the puerperal uterus should be gradually restored to its original proportions.

Normal involution is to be attributed to atrophy of the individual muscle cells rather than to fatty degeneration, as was formerly supposed. Its proximate cause is to be sought in the sudden and marked diminution of the blood supply to the uterus; and, as this can be brought about only by satisfactory contraction and retraction of the organ, it is apparent that any interference with the process may be followed by subinvolution.

Among the most frequent ætiological factors in its production are imperfect exfoliation of the decidua, retention of portions of the afterbirth, inflammatory lesions of the endometrium, the presence of myomatous nodules in the uterine wall, abnormalities of circulation which frequently accompany displacements of the uterus, the existence of pelvic inflammatory lesions, and insufficient rest during the puerperium. In other words, subinvolution is practically always the result of local conditions and not of constitutional disorders, and accordingly careful investigation will nearly always reveal the underlying cause, and appropriate treatment, if undertaken sufficiently early, will lead to its cure.

The existence of subinvolution is manifested by a prolongation of the lochial discharge beyond the usual period, its cessation being followed by a persistent leucorrhœa and pains in the back, a general feeling of dragginess, and a delayed return to perfect health. Similar symptoms accompany uterine displacements, but in all probability are in great part due to the coincident subinvolution.

The diagnosis is established by bimanual examination, the uterus being found to be larger, softer, and more succulent than it should be at a given time following delivery. Normally the fundus should have descended to the level of the upper margin of the symphysis by the tenth day of the puerperium, although the organ does not regain its original size for six weeks or more after delivery.

Inasmuch as subinvolution is dependent mainly upon local conditions, very little can be expected from medicinal treatment, although the administration of 20 drops of the fluid extract of ergot every three or four hours for several days is sometimes followed by improvement. Local measures afford much better results. If the uterus is displaced it should be put in proper position by bimanual manipulation and held in position by a suitably fitting pessary. When disease of the endometrium or retention of portions of the after-birth are responsible, prompt curettage offers the most efficient method of treatment. On the other hand, procrastination may lead to serious results, as the subinvolution may become permanent, and prove a constant source of irritation.

Lactation Atrophy of the Uterus.—Occasionally, in women who suckle their children, the uterus may undergo excessive involution, becoming smaller than in the virginal state. This condition, which usually becomes most marked during the third or fourth month after delivery, is attributed to reflex irritation emanating from the breasts and incident to lactation and nursing. It usually disappears spontaneously after weaning, though when the child is nursed for a longer period than usual the uterus may begin to increase in size before the end of a year, even though lactation be continued. It is probable that the cessation of menstruation, which is usually observed during lactation, should be attributed to this form of atrophy.

The condition was first definitely described by Jacquet, in 1871, and since the publication of his paper has been carefully studied by numerous investigators, particularly Thorn, Gottschalk, Döderlein, and Vineberg.

In rare instances the atrophy may persist after weaning and become permanent, the uterine cavity sometimes measuring only a few centimetres in length. This abnormality, first described by Chiari, Braun, and Spaeth, in 1855, was later designated by Simpson as *superinvolution.* It is probable that it may occasionally be the causative factor in the unusually early appearance of the menopause.

Displacements of the Uterus.—Immediately following the birth of the child, the lower uterine segment and cervix are represented by a flabby, collapsed structure which is freely movable upon the rest of the organ (see Fig. 304). Under these circumstances a comparatively trivial cause, such as a slight increase in the intra-abdominal pressure or distention of the rectum, may lead to a bending over of the upper part—*anteflexion of the uterus.* The condition is usually without significance, but occasionally the angle formed between the upper and lower portions of the organ may be so acute as to occlude the cervical canal and lead to the retention of the lochial discharge—*lochiometra.* As a rule, the retention, when it occurs, is only transitory, but if it be prolonged the lochia may undergo putrefactive changes which are accompanied by the formation of toxines, the absorption of which may give rise to constitutional symptoms. The complication is readily overcome by allowing the retained discharge to drain away through a douche-tube, after which the uterine cavity should be irrigated with sterile salt solution.

So long as the body of the uterus lies above the promontory of the sacrum, retrodisplacement cannot occur, as the falling backward of the enlarged fundus is prevented by the convex surface offered by the lumbar vertebræ. But as soon as the organ has descended into the pelvic cavity a *retroflexion* or *retroversion* immediately becomes possible. Their development is occasionally favoured by the use of an abdominal binder which may cause the abdominal contents to exert pressure upon the fundus of the uterus, forcing it downward and backward. More often the retroflexion merely represents a recurrence of a similar condition existing prior to pregnancy, while in other cases it may be the result of extreme distention of the bladder. Not uncommonly its mode of production is difficult to understand.

Backward displacements of the uterus rarely give rise to symptoms so long as the patient remains in bed, but as soon as she begins to move about their presence is apt to cause more or less inconvenience. The earliest and most characteristic manifestation is a marked increase in the amount of lochial discharge or the reappearance of the flow if it has already ceased. Sometimes the patient suffers from pain in the back and lower abdomen, although in other cases she may only be conscious that she is not regaining her strength as rapidly as she had expected.

The presence of these symptoms should always suggest the existence of a retroflexion, although they are sometimes due to subinvolution produced by other causes. A positive diagnosis can always be made upon vaginal examination.

The restoration of the uterus to its normal position by bimanual manipulations, and the introduction of a properly fitting pessary, as a rule will afford prompt relief, and on removal of the pessary some months later it will usually be found that a permanent cure has resulted. On the other hand, if its employment is postponed too long much less favourable results are obtained. This fact serves again to emphasize the necessity for making a final examination before discharging the puerperal patient. When the patient has suffered from retroflexion before pregnancy, an examination made at the end of the second week of the puerperium will usually show that the uterus has returned to its abnormal position. In such cases it should be replaced and a pessary at once introduced.

Relaxation of the Vaginal Outlet and Prolapse of the Uterus.—Reference has already been made to the frequent occurrence of perineal lacerations at the time of labour and the consequent relaxation of the vaginal outlet which follows neglect to repair them.

Moreover, the changes following childbearing predispose to the occurrence of *prolapse of the uterus,* and an exacerbation should be expected during the puerperium in women who have presented moderate degrees of descensus uteri before labour. In order to obtain the best results, and to prevent serious disability, an early operation is imperative, since the difficulty of rectifying the condition depends largely upon the extent of the prolapse and the length of time that it has been allowed to exist.

Obstetrical Paralysis.—Paralytic conditions may develop in either mother or child during the puerperium. That branches of the sacral plexus sometimes suffer from pressure during labour is demonstrated by the fact that many patients complain of intense neuralgia or of cramp-like pains extending down one or both legs as soon as the head begins to descend into the pelvic canal. As a rule, of course, the compression is rarely severe enough to give rise to grave lesions. In some instances, however, the pain continues after delivery, and is accompanied by the development of paralysis in the muscles supplied by the external popliteal nerve—the flexors of the ankles and the extensors of the toes—the gluteal muscles occasionally becoming affected to a lesser extent.

The subject has been carefully studied by Hünermann and H. M. Thomas. The investigations of the former supplied a very satisfactory explanation of the common localization of the paralysis by showing that the external popliteal nerve receives fibres from the fourth and fifth lumbar roots, and that these on their way downward to join the sacral plexus pass over the brim of the pelvis, where they are exposed to danger from compression, whereas the lower roots which lie upon the pyriformis muscle are more protected.

Hünermann considers that the chances of injurious pressure are greatest where the pelvis is generally contracted, and less so in the rhachitic varieties, inasmuch as the projecting promontory in the latter tends to prevent the head from coming in contact with the nerve. In the majority of cases the injury is the result of direct pressure exerted by the child's head, and only exceptionally is caused by the forceps.

In view of the fact that only one oblique diameter of the superior strait is occupied by the greatest diameter of the head, it is readily understood why the paralysis is usually limited to one leg, Thomas's case being the only instance on record in which both legs were affected. The paralytic symptoms usually appear immediately after delivery, and may become permanent unless suitable therapeutic measures, more particularly the use of electricity, are promptly instituted.

In other cases paralytic symptoms accompanied by intense neuralgic pains following the course of the sciatic nerve, follow pelvic inflammatory troubles. The condition is sometimes due to the development of a neuritis affecting certain branches of the sacral plexus, while in other cases pressure exerted by an inflammatory exudate is responsible. I have seen a case of the latter character which persisted for years in spite of continuous treatment, and which disappeared as if by magic after laparotomy and the separation of the adherent appendages from the posterior and lateral portions of the pelvic wall.

Winscheid has directed particular attention to the rare cases of *neuritis* which follow delivery. The inflammation may be general or localized. In the latter, only one or two nerves are affected—the median, ulnar, or crural —and atrophic symptoms soon make their appearance. In the former, since a number of nerves are implicated simultaneously, sometimes even those of the face not escaping, the symptoms may be manifold and the condition become most serious. In either event we are ignorant concerning the mode of production of the nerve lesions, though they are supposed to be due to toxic influences. The prognosis is fair for the localized but poor for the generalized variety.

It is also important to bear in mind that separation of the symphysis pubis, or of one or other sacro-iliac synchondrosis during labour, may be followed by pain and so marked an interference with locomotion as at first sight to suggest the existence of paralysis. Moreover, the disturbances in the function of the psoas muscles and the adductors of the thigh, which so frequently accompany the early stages of osteomalacia, might readily lead to a similar error.

As a result of a difficult labour, and exceptionally after an easy one, the child is sometimes born presenting an affection of the arm which is commonly known as *Duchenne's paralysis.* In this form, paralysis of the deltoid, infraspinatus, and the flexor muscles of the forearm causes the entire arm to fall close to the side of the body, and at the same time to rotate inward, while the forearm becomes extended upon the arm. The motility of the fingers is usually retained.

Erb pointed out that such a paralysis could be due only to a lesion involving the fifth and sixth roots of the brachial plexus, and showed that electrical stimulation at a point from 2 to 3 centimetres above the clavicle and in front of the transverse process of the sixth cervical vertebra —now known as Erb's point—produces contractions of the muscles involved. He considered that the paralysis frequently follows compression of the plexus by the clavicle in the Prague method of extraction, more particularly when the arms have become extended over the head. In other cases its production is attributed to traction with the fingers in the axilla of the child, and occasionally to the use of forceps.

That compression may be exerted during the employment of either of the first two of these manœuvres is at once evident from a consideration of the anatomical relations. On the other hand, the experiments of Stolper show that the plexus cannot possibly be compressed by the tips of the forceps so long as the child presents by the vertex, although it may occur in face or brow presentations.

Carter, in 1893, was the first to direct attention to the fact that the condition is due to stretching of the upper roots of the brachial plexus more frequently than to abnormal pressure. His results were confirmed by the experimental work of Fieux, Schoemaker, and Stolper, all of whom demonstrated that the plexus was readily subjected to extreme tension as a result of pulling obliquely upon the head, thus sharply flexing it towards one or other shoulder. As traction in this direction is frequently employed in order to effect delivery of the shoulders in vertex presentations, it is readily seen that Duchenne's paralysis might follow comparatively simple or even spontaneous labours. In view of these considerations, therefore, in extracting the shoulders care should be taken not to bring about too great lateral flexion of the neck. Moreover, in breech extractions the Prague manœuvre should be employed only when absolutely necessary, and particular attention should be devoted to preventing the extension of the arms over the head, as it not only materially complicates delivery, but adds considerably to the danger of infantile paralysis.

The *prognosis* is usually fair, the majority of the children recovering. Occasionally, however, a case may resist all treatment and the child may remain hopelessly paralyzed. All of the five instances which I have personally observed ended in recovery, but in some of them prolonged treatment was necessary. In this form of paralysis the children should be promptly put under the care of a competent neurologist, as the intelligent use of the electrical current is frequently the only means by which degenerative changes in the nerves and muscles can be obviated, and neglect in this regard may result in the condition becoming permanent.

Abnormalities and Diseases of the Breasts.—Complete *absence of both breasts* is one of the rarest anomalies of development, while the absence of one and the normal development of the other breast has been noted in a few isolated cases.

Hypertrophy of the breasts is more frequently observed, but is nevertheless an infrequent occurrence. In a large proportion of the recorded cases the condition developed rapidly in young unmarried women, both breasts being implicated and occasionally attaining such immense proportions that amputation became necessary. Cases have been reported in which a single breast weighed more than 50 pounds. The hypertrophy sometimes recedes during lactation, so that the abnormality does not always afford an absolute contra-indication to suckling the child. Overdevelopment of the mammæ is sometimes observed in men, a number of cases having been collected by Laurent.

Supernumerary Breasts.—Probably one in every few hundred women has one or more accessory breasts—*polymastia.* Reference to 262 such cases are to be found in Goldberger's article.

The supernumerary breasts rarely attain any considerable size, and occasionally are so minute as to be mistaken for small pigmented moles. They are usually provided with distinct nipples. They are most commonly situated upon the anterior thoracic or abdominal walls, usually near the mammary line; less frequently they are found in the axillæ, and occasionally upon other portions of the body—the shoulder, flank, or groin, and in rare instances the thigh. They vary greatly in number, Neugebauer having described a patient with 10 breasts.

The condition is usually regarded as an atavistic reversion, though it is not associated with an increased tendency towards multiple pregnancy. In not a few instances an apparent hereditary influence can be traced. Not all observers, however, accept this view, Ahlfeld holding that the distribution of the mammary tissue is to be attributed to the transference at an early period of development of some of the cells, which ordinarily go to form the breasts, to other portions of the body by means of the amnion. The condition has no obstetrical significance, though occasionally the enlargement of supernumerary breasts occupying the axillæ may result in considerable discomfort to the patient.

Abnormalities of the Nipples.—The typical nipple is cylindrical in shape and projects well beyond the general surface of the breast, its exterior being slightly nodular but free from fissures. Variations from the normal, however, are not uncommon, some of them being so pronounced as to interfere seriously with the act of suckling.

In some women the lactiferous ducts open directly into an area which forms a depression at the centre of the areola. In pronounced instances of this so-called *depressed nipple*, nursing is out of the question, although when the depression is not very deep the breast may occasionally be made available by the employment of a nipple-shield.

More frequently, although not depressed, the nipple is so stunted that it hardly projects above the surface of the breast, and in consequence can be seized by the child's mouth only with the greatest difficulty. In the presence of this anomaly daily attempts should be made during the last few months of pregnancy to draw the nipple out by traction with the fingers, and a wooden nipple-shield should be constantly worn in the hope that by exerting pressure upon the periphery of the areola the nipple itself may be gradually made to protrude through the opening of the shield (see Fig. 173).

Again, it sometimes happens that nipples which are normal in shape and size may present so fissured or nodular a surface as to be especially susceptible to injury from the child's mouth during the act of nursing. In such cases small cracks or *fissures* almost inevitably appear, and render nursing so painful that the mother dreads the approach of the child, and the mental distress so induced often has a deleterious influence upon the secretory function. Moreover, such injuries are still more serious in that they offer a convenient portal of entry for pyogenic bacteria which are liable to invade the breast and give rise to a mastitis.

Abnormalities in the Mammary Secretion.—Marked individual variations exist in the amount of milk secreted, many of which are dependent not upon the general health and appearance of the individual, but upon the degree of development of the glandular portions of the breasts. Thus we often find that a woman who possesses large, well-formed breasts, and who apparently should be an excellent milk-producer, secretes only a small quantity; while, on the other hand, one is often surprised at the abundant supply produced by another whose mammæ are small and flat. It is a matter of common observation that stout women with well-formed but redundant breasts usually have a very deficient secretion, the bulk of the organ being made up of fatty tissue while the glandular elements are poorly developed. Deficient secretion is likewise frequently noted in very young women and in elderly primiparæ. In the former, the defect is to be attributed to imperfect development; in the latter, to regressive and atrophic changes in the breasts.

In very rare instances there is an absolute lack of mammary secretion—*agalacia*. As a rule, however, the defect is not absolute, as it is nearly always possible to cause at least a small amount to exude from the nipple on the third or fourth day of the puerperium. On the other hand, relative deficiency is frequently observed, a large number of women secreting an amount of milk quite insufficient for the nutrition of the child. In Chapter XVII reference was made to the variations in the quantity of the milk as well as the various factors which may be concerned in their production.

Occasionally the mammary secretion is excessive—*polygalacia*—and may even be so abundant that milk is constantly escaping from the nipples. This latter condition, which is known as *galactorrhœa*, sometimes continues for years after the birth of the child, and is extremely intractable to treatment. Nothing is known as to its cause. Although in rare instances the health of the woman may remain unimpaired, as a rule she soon begins to show evidences of the continuous drain upon her system, becoming irritable, querulous, and eventually developing symptoms of cachexia.

Galactorrhœa is best treated by the application of tight bandages and the internal administration of fairly large doses of potassium iodide. Good effects are also said to have been obtained from the use of chloral. In a certain number of cases the condition is combined with atrophy of the uterus, and several observers have reported improvement following procedures which tend to bring about an increase in size of the uterus, such as the use of the vaginal douche, local applications to the cervix, or the employment of electricity.

Diseases of the Nipples.—The mode of production and treatment of fissures of the nipples has already been considered in detail in Chapter XVII.

Engorgement of the Breasts.—For the first twenty-four or forty-eight hours following the development of the lacteal secretion, it is not unusual for the breasts to become immensely distended, and to offer on palpation a firm, nodular resistance. This condition, which is commonly known as "*caked breast*," often gives rise to a considerable degree of pain, and is frequently accompanied by a slight elevation of temperature. Within a day or so the engorgement usually passes off spontaneously or as the result of appropriate treatment, though in some cases it persists in spite of all that can be done, and may be a forerunner of the development of a mammary abscess. It is probable that the excessive distention of the glandular portion of the breast leads to slight tissue changes, thereby offering a locus minoris resistentiæ for invasion by bacteria, which are usually present in the lactiferous ducts.

Whenever the breast becomes markedly engorged, immediate steps should be taken to relieve the condition. This is most readily accomplished by evacuating a portion of its contents. When the child is unable to draw off a sufficient quantity, an English breast-pump should be employed to remove the excess. In many cases, however, when this procedure proves ineffectual, proper massage often gives immediate relief. The nurse having anointed the palmar surfaces of her hands with olive-oil, mixed with equal parts of laudanum if the breasts are very sensitive, makes stroking movements, beginning at the periphery of the breast and gradually approaching the nipple. At first the manipulations should be made very gently, but as the patient becomes accustomed to them more force may be employed, which will soon cause the milk to exude from the nipple. After the breast has been emptied, it should be thickly covered with cotton batting and firmly compressed against the thoracic wall by means of a tightly applied bandage, which not only relieves pain by preventing the overloaded organ from sagging downward, but at the same time serves to diminish the amount of secretion by diminishing the blood supply.

Occasionally the engorgement persists in spite of all that can be done. In such cases, if several days of persistent effort prove unavailing, the interests of the patient will be best subserved by drying up the breasts, as a continuance of the condition is almost sure to eventuate in abscess formation.

Inflammation of the Breasts—Mastitis.—Parenchymatous inflammation of the mammary glands is a not infrequent complication of the puerperium. The symptoms hardly ever appear before the end of the first week, and as a rule not until considerably later. Marked engorgement usually precedes the inflammatory trouble, the first sign of which is afforded by chilly sensations or an actual rigor, which is soon followed by a considerable rise in temperature and an increase in the rate of the pulse. The breast becomes hard, its surface is reddened, and the patient complains of acute pain. In many instances, by the end of twenty-four hours the condition disappears spontaneously without treatment, being often favourably influenced by the application of a tightly fitting bandage. But if the symptoms persist for longer than forty-eight hours, suppuration is to be expected. The process may remain limited to a single lobe if the first abscess is opened promptly; but if left to itself the breast is liable to become undermined in all directions, and as a result the destruction of tissue is extensive, and the external surface may be left riddled with numerous fistulous tracts.

In some cases the constitutional symptoms attending a mammary abscess are very marked, whereas the local manifestations may be so slight as to escape observation. Such cases are usually mistaken for puerperal infection, and give rise to no little anxiety until the examination of cultures from the uterine cavity has demonstrated the absence of bacteria. On the other hand, a certain number of cases pursue a subacute or almost chronic course, the breast being somewhat harder than usual and more or less painful, but constitutional symptoms are either lacking or very slight. Under such circumstances the first indication of the true state of affairs is often afforded by the detection of fluctuation.

Ætiology.—Mastitis is always the result of infection, pathogenic bacteria from outside gaining access to the breast through fissured nipples by way of the lymphatics; or else some of those already present in the lactiferous ducts meet with conditions which enable them to invade the tissues. The researches of Bumm, Hönigmann, Koestlin, and others, have demonstrated that Staphylococcus albus is present in 80 to 94 per cent of all breasts. Ordinarily, this micro-organism lives in the milk as a harmless parasite, but when the tissues are seriously altered as the result of engorgement, it is possible for it to become pathogenic. That this occurs, however, in only a small proportion of cases has been shown by the researches of Rubeska, who reported the following bacteriological findings in 16 cases of mammary abscess:

Staphylococcus aureus	9 cases
Staphylococcus aureus and albus	3 "
Staphylococcus albus	3 "
Streptococcus	1 case

Exceptionally, other bacteria are causative agents, Sarfert having demonstrated the gonococcus in one instance.

When the infection occurs through fissured nipples, the inflammation is usually phlegmonous in character. In some cases it involves only the connective tissue beneath the breast, a large collection of pus being formed between it and the thoracic wall—retromammary abscess. Again, the infection may be limited to the areola, beneath which small abscesses, rarely exceeding 1.5 centimetre in diameter, may develop—*subareolar mastitis.*

According to Winckel, 67.6 per cent of all cases of mastitis occur in primiparæ, but its actual incidence varies according to the care given the patients during pregnancy and the puerperium. Thus, the statistics of Rubeska show a frequency of 0.54 to 4.1 per cent in the various German clinics. Generally speaking, it may be said that the occurrence of mastitis in more than 1 per cent of a large series of cases is indicative of neglect on the part of the physician or nurse.

Treatment.—The occurrence of mastitis can be prevented in great part by suitable prophylactic measures, which mainly consist in preventing the development of fissured nipples or treating them properly after they have appeared.

The most suitable measures for hardening the nipples during pregnancy so as to enable them to better withstand the strain of nursing, have already been mentioned in Chapter XVII. When lactation becomes established the strictest cleanliness should be observed and the nipples watched most carefully. As soon as a fissure begins to develop a nipple-shield should be employed, the child not being allowed to apply the mouth directly to the nipple until healing has taken place. In the intervals between the feedings the sore nipple should be covered with a clean cloth or a piece of absorbent cotton soaked in a saturated solution of boric acid. The various applications which are usually recommended, however good in themselves, will prove practically valueless unless the nipple can be placed at comparative rest, which is best afforded by the use of a suitable nipple-shield. If the condition becomes worse after some days' trial of this treatment, it is advisable to wean the child rather than take the risk of infection which is so prone to follow if the deeply fissured nipple be used for any length of time. Finally, it may be said that too great stress cannot be laid upon prompt attention to engorgement of the breasts, as its prolonged persistence is nearly always followed by abscess formation.

On the first symptom of mammary infection, the breast should be put at rest as far as possible by not allowing the child to nurse it, and withdrawing the milk, if necessary, by means of a breast-pump. After being emptied the breast should be thickly covered with cotton, and by means of a tightly fitting bandage subjected to the greatest possible pressure consistent with the comfort of the patient. In many cases such treatment apparently cuts short the process, the symptoms disappearing within twenty-four hours, after which the patient is able to resume suckling her child. Usually, however, the process sooner or later eventuates in abscess formation. In such cases the breasts should be carefully watched and incised as soon as the slightest evidence of fluctuation can be obtained. Procrastination is not permissible, delay being synonymous with extension of the process, which frequently leads to such extensive destruction of tissue as to permanently destroy the physiological function of the organ.

The incisions should be made radially, extending from near the areolar margin towards the periphery of the gland, in order to avoid injury to the lactiferous ducts. In early cases, a single incision over the most dependent portion of the area of fluctuation is usually sufficient, but when multiple abscesses are present several incisions may be required. The operation should always be done under anæsthesia, and the obstetrician should not consider that it has been completed until he has introduced a finger through the incision and carefully explored the interior of the breast, breaking down the partition walls between the various pockets of pus, so that only a single abscess cavity is left to be dealt with. This should then be loosely packed with gauze, which is removed at the end of twenty-four hours and the cavity washed out with sterile salt solution or a 2-per-cent boric-acid solution, after which another pack is inserted. If the pus has been thoroughly evacuated the abscess cavity becomes obliterated with a rapidity which is sometimes surprising.

Galactocele.—Very exceptionally, as the result of clogging of a milk duct by inspissated secretion, an accumulation of milk may take place in one or more lobes of the breast. Ordinarily, this is limited in amount, but may become excessive and form a fluctuant tumour which may give rise to pressure symptoms. In many instances, massage and the application of a tight bandage will cause it to disappear, while in others the structure may attain such a size that puncture becomes imperative.

Puerperal Psychoses.—Reference has already been made to the alterations in the mental condition which may accompany pregnancy. These vary from slight changes in disposition to actual insanity, though fortunately the latter is of relatively rare occurrence.

The insanity of pregnancy is usually a manifestation of autointoxication, and may be accompanied by melancholic or maniacal symptoms. It usually persists throughout the remainder of gestation, but disappears shortly after labour, unless the patient has an hereditary tendency to mental derangement.

Puerperal insanity, on the other hand, is much more common, and according to the statistics compiled by Berkley is noted once in every 616 labours, though my experience would lead me to believe it less frequent. In former times it was a comparatively common complication of the puerperium, and it would seem that the introduction of aseptic methods into midwifery is responsible for a reduction by one half in its incidence.

The affection usually makes its appearance within the first two weeks following delivery. When it occurs at a later period it is designated as *lactational insanity.*

Puerperal psychoses may be due to one of three causes: infection, auto-intoxication, or direct lability of the nervous system. Of these, infection is by far the most important. This fact has long been recognised, but it is only of late that the bacteria concerned have been identified, and then only in a small proportion of the cases. In 2 of the 3 instances which have come under my observation, the infection was due to the streptococcus, and in the third to the streptococcus and colon bacillus. Berkley likewise reports a case due to the organism first mentioned.

Auto-intoxication is also a frequent ætiological factor, and it is probable that the vast majority of mental derangements following eclampsia are due to this condition. Ordinarily, insanity is regarded as a rare complication of eclampsia, though Olshausen observed it in 6 per cent of his 515 cases. According to Hansen, infection and auto-intoxication are responsible for more than 80 per cent of all cases, while the remainder are to be attributed to other causes, occurring particularly in women afflicted with hereditary tendencies, the exciting cause of the insanity being shock, extreme mental depression, or the rapid loss of a large quantity of blood.

The puerperal psychoses are usually characterized by great excitement during the first few days, associated with all sorts of hallucinations. Later the maniacal symptoms disappear, and the patient passes into a condition of depression, and frequently exhibits suicidal tendencies.

The prognosis is most favourable in the cases following eclampsia, the majority of these patients recovering. On the other hand, those following infection are very tedious, and 20 to 40 per cent of the women fail to regain their mental equilibrium. It is not unusual for the mental derangement to last for from three to six months, although the prospect for recovery is poor if the latter period is exceeded. It is generally stated that from 5 to 10 per cent of the patients afflicted with puerperal insanity die, this high mortality rate being due, of course, to the underlying infection and not to the mental derangement itself.

In cases following infection, the treatment should first be directed to the underlying condition, and the directions described in Chapter XLIV rigorously followed. The acute maniacal symptoms should be met by the administration of sedatives, and the patient should be watched most carefully throughout her entire illness, more particularly during the periods of depression, during which she should never be left alone for fear that she may do an injury to herself. If prompt improvement does not follow the disappearance of the symptoms ascribable to infection, the patient should be placed in charge of a competent psychiatrist.

Typhoid Fever.—This is not an infrequent complication of the puerperium. Its course, however, varies but little from that observed under other conditions, although the prognosis is necessarily somewhat influenced by the fact that the patient is already debilitated by the strain incident to labour. The diagnosis should never be made unless a definite Widal reaction can be demonstrated, inasmuch as all the other symptoms of the disease may be associated with a prolonged puerperal sepsis, especially when the endocardium is involved. Furthermore, the so-called typhoid condition is often encountered in various forms of pyæmia.

Malarial Fever.—In certain districts the puerperium is not infrequently complicated by malarial infection. Although the course of the disease is not materially influenced by the fact that the patient has recently given birth to a child, it is interesting to note that labour, no less than surgical procedures, seems to predispose to a recrudescence of the disorder in women who have already suffered from it, the typical phenomena often appearing during the first few days of the puerperium.

Too many sins of omission and commission on the part of the obstetrician have undoubtedly been cloaked under the diagnosis of "malaria." At the present day, whenever a patient presents a temperature characterized by marked remissions and possibly by chills, puerperal infection should be suspected, and the existence of malarial fever should never be seriously entertained unless all other possibilities have been practically eliminated and the characteristic parasites have been found in the blood.

As soon as a positive diagnosis has been made, quinine should be given in sufficiently large doses to break up the attack, as it exerts no appreciable influence upon the mammary secretion or the well-being of the child.

Pneumonia.—Croupous pneumonia is a rare complication of the puerperal state, unless the disease has existed before the onset of labour. The outlook is always serious.

The lobular variety, or broncho-pneumonia, is often a terminal process, and is one of the most common causes of death in patients who succumb within a few days following an eclamptic attack. The treatment does not differ essentially from that employed at other times.

Scarlet Fever.—Although scarlet fever is rarely encountered during the puerperium, its occurrence has given rise to a great deal of discussion and a very considerable literature. The interest manifested in the disease is largely to be accounted for by the fact that a scarlatiniform rash is occasionally observed during the course of a puerperal infection, so that in many cases a differential diagnosis becomes very difficult.

Epidemics of scarlet fever in the puerperium have been reported by Boxall, Meyer, Ahlfeld, and others. Nevertheless, it would appear that the puerperal woman is to a certain extent immune from the disease, inasmuch as statistics go to show that only a small proportion of those exposed to the contagion become infected. Thus, Meyer found the rate of morbidity to be about 1 per cent among his patients.

It is generally stated that infection may occur in the usual manner as well as by the entrance of the specific poison through wounds about the genitalia. The belief in the possibility of the latter eventuality is based upon the fact that the rash occasionally appears first in the neighbourhood of the vulva, and thence spreads to other portions of the body. Moreover, the frequent association of pelvic inflammatory troubles, and the occasional localization of diphtheritic patches in the vulva or vagina, instead of in the throat, are advanced in support of the view. Modern bacteriological investigation, however, has destroyed the force of this last argument, since it has shown that the so-called diphtheritic deposits occurring in the throat in scarlet fever are due to a coincident streptococcic infection. Moreover, since such conditions about the genitalia usually have a similar origin, it would appear difficult to differentiate between those complicating scarlet fever and the varieties occurring during the course of puerperal infection. It is also urged that the appearance of the disease on the third or fourth day of the puerperium speaks in favour of transmission of contagion through the genitalia.

In frank cases, the diagnosis is readily made from the existence of a characteristic rash, which is later followed by desquamation. Moreover, the strawberry tongue, the development of pseudo-diphtheritic patches in the pharynx, the appearance of albumin in the urine, together with a history of exposure to possible contagion, usually remove all doubt. On the other hand, in the absence of characteristic manifestations, the diagnosis cannot be made, it being often impossible to differentiate between scarlet fever and puerperal infection, even when a distinct history of exposure to contagion can be elicited.

The prognosis is largely the same as under other circumstances, mild forms, as a rule, ending in recovery, whereas patients affected with the hæmorrhagic variety usually die. The puerperium appears to exert little effect upon the course of the disease, the death-rate not being higher than under ordinary conditions. The child may or may not be infected.

Measles and *small-pox* occasionally occur during the puerperium, but their course does not differ materially from that observed in women who have not recently given birth to children.

Diphtheria.—True diphtheritic patches, in which the Klebs-Loeffler bacillus can be demonstrated, occasionally occur upon denuded portions of the vulva and vagina. They may be due to a primary genital infection, or be merely part of a process primarily localized in the throat. Inasmuch as pseudo-diphtheritic patches in the genital tract during the course of puerperal infection are not of rare occurrence, the presence of a fibrinous exudate about the vagina or vulva should lead to a diagnosis of diphtheria only in those cases in which the characteristic bacilli can be demonstrated. If the process is limited to the genital tract, the constitutional symptoms are not severe, and the disease usually pursues a benign course, readily yielding to the employment of the anti-diphtheritic serum.

LITERATURE

AHLFELD. Spaltung der Anlage der Brustdrüse, Polymastie. Die Missbildung des Menschen. Leipzig, 1880, 110–113.

Ueber Exantheme im Wochenbette, etc. Zeitschr. f. Geb. u. Gyn., 1893, xxv, 31–44.

BERKLEY. The Insanities of the Puerperal Period. A Treatise on Mental Diseases, 1900, 307–328.

BOXALL. Scarlatina during Pregnancy and in the Puerperal State. Trans. Lond. Obst. Soc., 1889, xxx, 11–77; 126–154.

BUMM. Zur Aetiologie der puerperalen Mastitis. Archiv f. Gyn., 1886, xxvii, 460–484.

BURCKHARD. Gangrän der unteren Extremitäten im Wochenbette. Centralbl. f. Gyn., 1900, 1381–1384.

CARTER. Obstetrical Paralysis, etc. Boston Med. and Surg. Jour., May 4, 1893.

CHANTEMESSE et WIDAL. Recherches sur l'étiologie du tétanus. Le Bull. Méd., 1889, No. 74.

CHIARI, BRAUN und SPAETH. Acquirirte Volumsabnahme des Uteruskörpers. Klinik der Geb., 1854, 371–372.

DENEUX. Mémoire sur les tumeurs sanguines de la vulve et du vagin. Paris, 1830.

DÖDERLEIN. Die Atrophia uteri. Veit's Handbuch der Gyn., 1897, ii, 391–402.

DUCHENNE. Paralysies obstétricales infantiles du membre supérieur. De l'électrisation localisée. Paris, 1872, 3me éd., 357.

FIEUX. De la pathogénie des paralysies brachiales chez le nouveau-né. Annales de Gyn. et d'Obst., 1897, xlvii, 52–64.

GOLDBERGER. Ein seltener Fall von Polymastie. Archiv f. Gyn., 1895, xlix, 272–277.

GOTTSCHALK. Beitrag zur Lehre von der Atrophia uteri. Volkmann's Sammlung klin. Vorträge, N. F., Nr. 49.

HANSEN. Ueber das Verhältniss zwischen der puerperalen Geisteskrankheit u. der puerperalen Infection. Zeitschr. f. Geb. u. Gyn., 1888, xv, 60–127.

HEYSE. Ueber Tetanus puerperalis. Deutsche med. Wochenschr., 1893, Nr. 14, 318.

HÖNIGMANN. Bakteriologische Untersuchungen über Frauenmilch. D. I., Breslau, 1893.

HÜNERMANN. Ueber Nervenlähmung im Gebiete des Nervus ischiadicus infolge von Entbindungen. Archiv f. Gyn., 1900, xlii, 489–512.

JACQUET. Ueber Atrophia uteri. Berliner Beiträge zur Geb. u. Gyn., 1873, ii, 1–11.

KENTMANN. Tetanus puerperalis. Monatsschr. f. Geb. u. Gyn., 1900, xi, 527–539.

KÖSTLIN. Beiträge zur Frage des Keimgehaltes der Frauenmilch u. zur Aetiologie der Mastitis. Archiv f. Gyn., 1897, liii, 201–277.

LAFOND. De la gangrène des membres inférieurs dans les suites de couches. Thèse de Bordeaux, 1901.

LAURENT. Gynäkomastie, etc. Bibliothek für Socialwissenschaft. Leipzig, 1896, vi.

MEYER. Ueber Scharlach bei Wöchnerinnen. Zeitschr. f. Geb. u. Gyn., 1888, xiv, 289–351.

NEUGEBAUER. Eine bisher einzig dastehende Beobachtung von Polymastie mit 10 Brustwarzen. Centralbl. f. Gyn., 1886, 729–736.

OLSHAUSEN. Beitrag zu den puerperalen Psychosen, speciell den nach Eklampsie auftretenden. Zeitschr. f. Geb. u. Gyn., 1891, xxi, 371–385.

RUBESKA. Beiträge zum Tetanus puerperalis. Archiv f. Gyn., 1897, liv, 1–12.

Zur Behandlung von wunden Warzen und Mastitiden im Wochenbett. Archiv f. Gyn., 1899, lviii, 177–184.

SARFERT. Diplokokken im Eiter bei Mastitis. Deutsche med. Wochenschr., 1894, Nr. 8.

SCHOEMAKER. Ueber die Aetiologie der Entbindungslähmungen, etc. Zeitschr. f. Geb. u. Gyn., 1899, xli, 33–53.

STOLPER. Ueber Entbindungslähmungen. Monatsschr. f. Geb. u. Gyn., 1901, xiv, 49–65.

THOMAS. Obstetrical Paralysis, Infantile and Maternal. The Johns Hopkins Hospital Bulletin, 1900, xi, 279.

THORN. Beitrag zur Lehre von der Atrophia uteri. Zeitschr. f. Geb. u. Gyn., 1889, xvi, 57–105.

VINAY. Du tétanus puerpéral. Archives de Tocologie, 1892, xix, 179.

VINEBERG. A Further Contribution to the Study and Practical Significance of Lactation Atrophy of the Uterus. Amer. Gyn., 1902, i, No. 2.

WINCKEL. Entzündung des Brustdrüsenparenchyms, etc. Die Pathologie u. Therapie des Wochenbetts. III. Aufl., 1878, 428–439.

WINSCHEID. Neuritis gravidarum und Neuritis puerperalis. Graefe's Sammlung zwangloser Abhandlungen auf dem Gebiete der Frauenheilkunde und Geb., 1898, iii, Heft 8.

WORMSER. Nochmals zur puerperalen Gangrän der unteren Extremitäten. Centralbl. f. Gyn., 1901, 110–112.

INDEX

(1)

THE END